# PRACTICAL PAEDIATRICS

EDITED BY

**Professor Mike South** MBBS DCH MD MRCP FRACP FJFICM FCICM
Paediatrician & Intensivist,
Director, Department of General Medicine
Royal Children's Hospital;
Fellow, Murdoch Children's Research Institute,
Professor of Paediatric Medicine, Department of Paediatrics,
University of Melbourne
Australia

**Professor David Isaacs** MBBCHIR MD(Cantab) FRACP FRCPCH
Senior Staff Specialist
Department of Infectious Diseases & Microbiology
Clinical Professor in Paediatric Infectious Diseases,
University of Sydney
Australia

SEVENTH EDITION

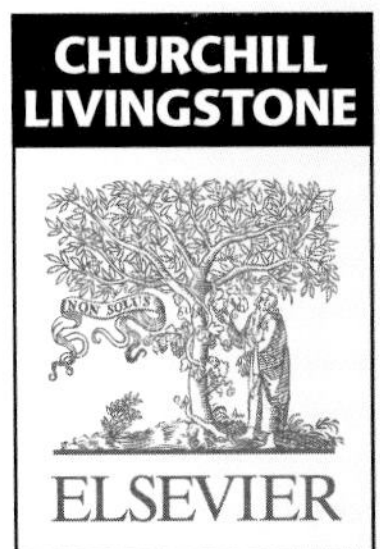


Edinburgh London New York Oxford Philadelphia St Louis Sydney Toronto 2012

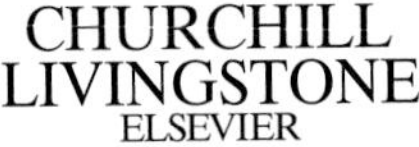



First edition 1986
Second edition 1990
Third edition 1994
Fourth Edition 1998
Fifth Edition 2003
Sixth Edition 2007

ISBN 9780702042928

**British Library Cataloguing in Publication Data**
A catalogue record for this book is available from the British Library

**Library of Congress Cataloging in Publication Data**
A catalog record for this book is available from the Library of Congress

**Notices**
Knowledge and best practice in this field are constantly changing. As new research and experience broaden our understanding, changes in research methods, professional practices, or medical treatment may become necessary.

Practitioners and researchers must always rely on their own experience and knowledge in evaluating and using any information, methods, compounds, or experiments described herein. In using such information or methods they should be mindful of their own safety and the safety of others, including parties for whom they have a professional responsibility.

With respect to any drug or pharmaceutical products identified, readers are advised to check the most current information provided (i) on procedures featured or (ii) by the manufacturer of each product to be administered, to verify the recommended dose or formula, the method and duration of administration, and contraindications. It is the responsibility of practitioners, relying on their own experience and knowledge of their patients, to make diagnoses, to determine dosages and the best treatment for each individual patient, and to take all appropriate safety precautions.

To the fullest extent of the law, neither the Publisher nor the authors, contributors, or editors, assume any liability for any injury and/or damage to persons or property as a matter of products liability, negligence or otherwise, or from any use or operation of any methods, products, instructions, or ideas contained in the material herein.



Printed in China

The Publisher's policy is to use **paper manufactured from sustainable forests**

# Preface

Welcome to the 7th edition of Practical Paediatrics.

Practical Paediatrics is used by medical students, doctors training in paediatrics and other specialty areas of medicine, primary care practitioners, nurses and allied health trainees and practitioners, and many other health professional groups.

Practical Paediatrics is intended to bridge the gap between some of the highly summarized handbooks of paediatrics and the bigger textbooks. It gives more than the bare dot-points of paediatric learning without going into highly advanced detail. It covers all of the common and important childhood conditions seen in the more resource-rich countries, and also covers many aspects of normal child development, family influences, and topics such as Indigenous child health.

Practical Paediatrics was first published in 1986. The concept was to provide a paediatric text for medical students that would be user-friendly, practical in its approach, relevant to curricula in Australia and New Zealand, the Asia–Pacific region and internationally, be up to date in its information, and available at a reasonable price. Practical Paediatrics has more than met all of these objectives. There has been a new edition approximately every 4 years and we are pleased that it remains so popular that we now to have the opportunity to publish the 7th edition.

Max Robinson founded the book and was an editor of all editions up to and including the 5th edition. Don Roberton joined Max for the 3rd edition and continued until the 6th. The 6th edition was co-edited by Mike South, and he has been joined for the 7th edition by David Isaacs.

In this edition, all content has been revised, often extensively. There are now 78 chapters with a total of 120 authors (51 of them new for this edition). They are all highly acknowledged experts in their field and prominent teachers in paediatrics in Australia and New Zealand.

Reading lists and up-to-date websites that give useful academic and parent and family information have been included as in the last two editions. These, along with a comprehensive set of Self Assessment Questions, are now available on a website which is accessible to purchasers of the textbook. This allows easy searching of the reading lists, linkages to the websites, and also linkages to online sections of the textbook itself. There are many new Self Assessment Questions, which have been a popular feature, providing a practical assessment of learning by testing problem-solving skills. The answers to each question are accompanied by a rationale explaining the reasons for the answers.

Many new Clinical Examples have been incorporated to assist the reader in placing information in context and to aid the learning process. Highlighted Practical Points in each section serve to emphasize key issues, and also function as an aid to revision.

We are grateful to all the contributing authors, and to staff from Elsevier including Veronika Watkins, Clive Hewat and Vinod Kumar, who have made much of our task easy and pain-free.

We hope that you will find this edition of Practical Paediatrics useful, and that it assists in developing an understanding and interest in the health needs of children, their families and their communities.

Mike South
David Isaacs

# Contributors

**Frances Abbott** BScN MRCNA
Clinical Nurse Consultant – Culture,
Royal Darwin Hospital,
Darwin, Australia
*Indigenous culture and health*

**Navid Adib** MBBS FRACP PhD
Paediatric Rheumatologist,
Queensland Paediatric Rheumatology Services,
Brisbane, Queensland, Australia
*Arthritis and connective tissue disorders*

**George Alex** MBBS MMed, MRCP FRACP PhD
Consultant
Gastroenterologist/Hepatologist,
Royal Children's Hospital,
Melbourne, Victoria, Australia
*Diarrhoea*

**Jane Alsweiler** MBChB FRACP PhD
Senior Lecturer in Paediatrics,
University of Auckland,
Auckland, New Zealand
*Low birth weight, prematurity and jaundice in infancy*

**Antoinette Anazodo** MBBS MSC
Diploma Adolescent Cancer FRACP
Director of Youth Cancer Services,
Sydney Children's Hospital and Prince of Wales Hospital,
Sydney, New South Wales, Australia
*Cancers*

**Chris Barnes** MBBS(Hons) FRACP FRCPA
Haematologist, Royal Children's Hospital,
Melbourne, Victoria, Australia
*Abnormal bleeding and clotting*

**Christopher Barnett** MBBS FRACP FCCMG
Consultant Clinical Geneticist,
SA Clinical Genetics Service,
Women's and Children's Hospital,
North Adelaide, South Australia,
Australia
*The dysmorphic child*

**Paul Bauert** OAM FAMA BSc MBBS FRACP
Director of Paediatrics, Royal Darwin Hospital,
Darwin, Australia
*Indigenous culture and health*

**Louise A Baur** AM MBBS(Hons) BSc(Med) PhD FRACP
Professor, Discipline of Paediatrics & Child Health,
Sydney Medical School,
The Children's Hospital at Westmead,
Sydney, New South Wales, Australia
*Obesity*

**Spencer Beasley** MBChB(Otago) MS(Melbourne) FRACS
Clinical Director, Department of Paediatric Surgery,
Christchurch Hospital,
Christchurch, New Zealand
*Abdominal pain and vomiting*
*Surgical conditions in the newborn*
*Surgical conditions in older children*

**Sean Beggs** MBBS MPH FRACP
Staff Specialist, Department of Paediatrics
Royal Hobart Hospital,
Hobart, Australia
*The clinical consultation*

**Julie Bines** MBBS MD FRACP
Victor and Loti Smorgon Professor of Paediatrics,
University of Melbourne, Melbourne, Victoria;
Department of Gastroenterology and Clinical Nutrition, Royal Children's Hospital,
Melbourne, Victoria;
Murdoch Childrens Research Institute,
Melbourne, Australia
*Nutrition*

**Helen L M Bird** MBChB, FRANZCR
Consultant Paediatric Radiologist,
Royal Children's Hospital,
Melbourne, Victoria, Australia
*Imaging*

**Robert Booy** MBBS(Hons) MSc MD FRACP FRCPCH
Head, Clinical Research, National Centre for Immunisation Research & Surveillance,
Discipline of Paediatrics and Child Health and School of Public Health, The University of Sydney,
Sydney, Australia
*Meningitis and encephalitis*

**David Brewster** BA(Hons) MD MPH FRACP PhD AM(Honorary)
Professor of Paediatrics, University of Botswana,
Gaborone, Botswana, South Africa
*Infections in tropical and developing countries*

**Justin Brown** MA MBBChir MRCP MRCPCH FRACP
Paediatric Endocrinologist,
Monash Children's Hospital,
Monash Medical Centre, Melbourne;
Senior Lecturer, Monash University,
Melbourne, Victoria, Australia
*Thyroid disorders*

**Leo Buchanan** MBChB FRACP
Taranaki and TeAtiawa
Senior Clinical Lecturer Paediatrics,
University of Otago, Wellington, New Zealand
*Indigenous culture and health*

**Mariam Buksh** MBBS Dip. Paediatrics FRACP(Paediatrics)
Neonatal Paediatrician,
Auckland City Hospital,
Auckland, New Zealand
*Low birth weight, prematurity and jaundice*

**David Burgner** BSc(Hons) MBChB MRCP MRCPCH DTM&H FRACP PhD
Principal Research Fellow and Consultant in Paediatric Infectious Diseases,
Murdoch Children's Research Institute,
Royal Children's Hospital and Monash Children's Hospital,
Melbourne, Victoria, Australia
*Infectious disease*
*Refugee health*

**Fergus Cameron** BMedSci MBBS DipRACOG FRACP MD
Professor and Head, Diabetes Services and Deputy Director,
Department of Endocrinology and Diabetes, and Centre for Hormone Research,
Royal Children's Hospital and Murdoch Children's Research Institute,
Melbourne, Victoria, Australia
*Thyroid disorders*

**Jonathan Rhys Carapetis,** MBBS FRACP FAFPHM PhD
Professor and Director, Menzies School of Health Research,
Darwin, Northern Territory, Australia
*Bone and joint infections*

**Susan M Carden** MBBS FRANZCO FRACS PhD
Senior Lecturer, University of Melbourne;
Senior Ophthalmologist, Royal Children's Hospital,
Melbourne, Victoria, Australia
*Eye disorders*

**Daniel Cass** MBBS FRACS FRCS PhD
William Dunlop Professor of Paediatric Surgery,
Department of Surgery, Children's Hospital at Westmead,
Sydney, Australia
*Trauma*

**Anne B Chang** MBBS MPHTM FRACP PhD
Professor, Child Health Division, Menzies School of Health Research,
Charles Darwin University, Darwin, North Territory;
Queensland Children's Respiratory Centre, Queensland Medical Research Institute, Royal Children's Hospital,
Brisbane, Queensland, Australia
*An approach to chronic cough and cystic fibrosis*

**Michael Cheung** BSc MBChB MD MRCP (UK) FRACP
Director of Cardiology,
Royal Children's Hospital,
Melbourne, Victoria, Australia
*Heart disease*
*Suspected heart disease: assessment*

**Kevin J Collins** MBBS FRACP GDipArts(French)
Paediatric Neurologist, Departments of Neurology and Developmental Medicine,
Royal Children's Hospital,
Melbourne, Victoria, Australia
*Cerebral palsy and neurodegenerative disorders*

**David Coman** MBBS MPhil FRACP
Staff Specialist, Department of Metabolic Medicine,
University of Queensland,
Brisbane, Australia
*Inborn errors of metabolism*

**Carolyn Cottier** MBBS BA FRACP
Staff Specialist, Sydney Children's Hospital, Randwick and Campbelltown Hospital,
Campbelltown, Sydney, Australia
*Developmental surveillance and assessment*

**Jennifer Couper** MBChB MD FRACP
Head, Deptartment of Diabetes and Endocrinology,
Women's and Children's Hospital Network,
Discipline of Paediatrics, University of Adelaide,
Adelaide, South Australia, Australia
*Diabetes*

**Peter Cundy** MBBS FRACS
Head of Orthopaedic Surgery,
Women's & Children's Hospital,
Adelaide, South Australia, Australia
*Orthopaedic problems*

**Brian A Darlow** MA MBBChir MD FRCP FRACP FRCPCH
CureKids Professor of Paediatric Research, University of Otago,
Christchurch, New Zealand
*Newborn infant: stabilization and examination*

**Geoffrey Davidson** MBBS MD FRACP
Senior Gasroenterologist,
Women's & Children's Hospital,
Adelaide, South Australia, Australia
*Gastro-oesophageal reflux and Helicobacter pylori infection*

**Mark William Davies** MBBS DCH PhD FRACP
Eminent Senior Staff Specialist in Neonatology (Consultant Neonatologist),
Royal Brisbane & Women's Hospital;
Associate Professor of Neonatology,
University of Queensland,
Brisbane, Queensland, Australia
*Breathing problems in the newborn*

**Andrew Day** MBChB MD FRACP AGAF
Associated Professor and Head of Department, Paediatrics,
University of Otago,
Christchurch, New Zealand
*Abdominal pain and vomiting*

**Martin Delatycki** MBBS FRACP PhD
Professor and Director,
Clinical Genetics, Austin Health Heidelberg,
Victoria, Australia
*Genetic counselling*

**Terence Donald** MBBS FRACP
Senior Consultant, Child Protection Unit,
Women's and Children's Hospital,
Adelaide, South Australia, Australia
*Child abuse*

**Trevor Duke,** MD FRACP FCICM
Director, Centre for International Child HealthUniversity,
Department of Paediatrics,
Royal Children's Hospital,
Melbourne, Victoria, Australia
*Child health in a global context*
*Fluid replacement therapy*

**Shoma Dutt** BMedSci MBBS PhD FRACP
Staff Specialist, Department of Gastroenterology,
The Children's Hospital at Westmead;
Lecturer, Discipline of Paediatrics & Child Health,
Sydney Medical School, University of Sydney,
Sydney, Australia
*Chronic diarrhoea and malabsorption*

**Daryl Efron** MBBS FRACP MD
Consultant Paediatrician,
Royal Children's Hospital,
Melbourne, Victoria, Australia
*Failure to thrive*

**Dawn Elder** MBChB DCH FRACP PhD
Associate Professor,
Department of Paediatrics and Child Health,
University of Otago,
Wellington, New Zealand
*Sudden unexpected death in infancy*

**James E Elder** MBBS FRANZCO FRACS
Consultant Ophthalmologist, Department of Ophthalmology,
Royal Children's Hospital, Melbourne;
Department of Paediatrics, University of Melbourne;
Melbourne, Australia
*Eye disorders*

**Jan Fairchild** MBBS FRACP
Senior Staff Specialist, Department of Endocrinology and Diabetes,
Women's and Children's Hospital, Adelaide, South Australia, Australia
*The child of uncertain sex*

**Peter Flett** MBBS FRACP FACRM FAFRM(RACP)
Associate Professor and Paediatric Rehabilitation Specialist,
State-wide Director, Paediatric Rehabilitation,
Royal Hobart Hospital,
Tasmania, Australia
*Neural tube defects, large heads and hydrocephalus*

**Jeremy L Freeman** MBBS FRACP
Staff Specialist, The Royal Children's Hospital,
Melbourne, Victoria, Australia
*Seizures and epilepsies*

**Michael Gold,** MBBChB DCH MD FCP FRACP
Senior Staff Specialist and Associate Professor,
Department of Allergy and Immunology & Discipline of Paediatrics,
University of Adelaide,
Adelaide, South Australia, Australia
*Atopy*

**Brian Graetz** PhD MPsych(Clin)
Program Director,
beyondblue: The National Depression Initiative,
Melbourne, Victoria, Australia
*Common mental health problems*

**Stephen M Graham** MBBS DTCH FRACP PhD
Associate Professor of International Child Health,
University of Melbourne Department of Paediatrics,
The Royal Children's Hospital, Melbourne, Australia;
Consultant in Child Lung Health,
International Union Against Tuberculosis and Lung Disease,
Paris, France
*Infections in tropical and developing countries*

**Sonia Grover** MBBS FRANZCOG MD
Head of Department, Paediatric and Adolescent Gynaecology, Royal Children's Hospital;
Honorary Principal fellow, Department of Paediatric, Melbourne University. (Consultant gynaecologist Mercy Hospital for Women; consultant gynaecologist Austin Health.)
Deptartment of Paediatric and Adolescent Gynaecology, Royal Children's Hospital, Melbourne, Australia
*Gynaecology*

**Wolfram Haller** MD MRCPCH (UK)
Fellow Paediatric Gastroenterology,
Royal Children's Hospital, Melbourne,
Parkville, Victoria, Australia
*Liver diseases*

**Kerrod B Hallett** MDSc MPH FRACDS FICD
Director, Department of Dentistry,
Royal Children's Hospital,
Melbourne, Australia
*Teeth and oral cavity disorders*

**Paul Hammond** MBBS FRACP
Senior Staff Specialist, Gastroenterology Unit, Women's and Children's Hospital,
Adelaide, Australia
*Gastro-oesophageal reflux and Helicobacter pylori infection*

**Winita Hardikar** MBBS FRACP PhD
Associate Professor and Head of Liver and Intestinal Transplantation,
Department of Gastroenterology,
Royal Children's Hospital,
Melbourne, Victoria, Australia
*Liver diseases*

**Jane Harding** MBChB Dphil FRACP
Professor of Neonatology, Liggins Institute, University of Auckland,
Auckland, New Zealand
*Low birth weight, prematurity and jaundice in infancy*

**A Simon Harvey** MD FRACP
Neurologist and Epileptologist,
Department of Neurology,
The Royal Children's Hospital,
Melbourne, Victoria, Australia
*Seizures and epilepsies*

**Helen S. Heussler** MBBS FRACP MRCPCH PGCAP DM
Associate Professor and Senior Staff Specialist,
Developmental Paediatrics and Sleep Medicine,
Mater Children's Hospital,
Brisbane, Queensland, Australia
*Sleep problems*

**Harriet Hiscock** MD FRACP Grad Dip Epi
Associate Professor and General Paediatrician,
Centre for Community Child Health;
NHMRC Post-doctoral Research Fellow,
Murdoch Children's Research Institute,
The Royal Children's Hospital, Melbourne;
Principal Fellow, Department of Paediatrics,
University of Melbourne,
Melbourne, Victoria, Australia
*Life events of normal children*

**Neil Hotham** BPharm
Senior Specialist Drug Information Pharmacist,
Women's and Children's Hospital,
North Adelaide, South Australia, Australia
*Birth defects, prenatal diagnosis and teratogens*

**David Isaacs,** MBBChir MD(Cantab) FRACP FRCPCH
Senior Staff Specialist,
Department of Infectious Diseases & Microbiology,
The Children's Hospital at Westmead;
Clinical Professor in Paediatric Infectious Diseases,
University of Sydney,
Sydney, New South Wales, Australia
*Infectious disease*

**Adam Jaffé** BSc(Hons) MBBS MD FRCP FRCPCH FRACP
Consultant in Respiratory Medicine;
Head of Respiratory Department,
Sydney Children's Hospital;
Conjoint Professor, School of Women's and Children's Health,
University of New South Wales,
Sydney, New South Wales, Australia
*Asthma*

**Luke Anthony Jardine** MBBS FRACP MClinEpid
Neonatologist, Mater Mother's Hospital, South Brisbane;
Honorary Researcher, Mater Medical Research Institute;
Senior Lecturer, University of Queensland,
Queensland, Australia
*Breathing problems in the newborn*

**Cheryl Jones** MBBS (Hons) Phd FRACP
Clinical academic, Paediatric infectious diseases specialist,
Deptartment of Infectious Diseases & Microbiology,
University of Sydney,
Sydney, Australia
*Meningitis and encephalitis*

**Colin Jones** MBBS FRACP PhD
Professor and Director, Department of Nephrology,
Royal Children's Hospital,
Parkville, Victoria, Australia
*Urinary tract infections and malformations*
*Bone mineral disorders*

**Timothy W Jones** MD DCH FRACP
Head of Department, Department of Endocrinology,
Princess Margaret Hospital for Children and Telethon Institute for Child Health Research,
Perth, Australia
*Diabetes*

**Nitin Kapur** MBBS MD PhD
Associate Lecturer, School of Medicine,
University of Queensland,
Brisbane, Australia
*An approach to chronic cough and cystic fibrosis*

**Joshua Y Kausman** MBBS FRACP
Paediatric Nephrologist,
Royal Children's Hospital,
Melbourne, Victoria, Australia
*Urinary tract infections and malformations*
*Bone mineral disorders*

**Andrew Kennedy** MBBS, FRACP
General Paediatrician and Adolescent Physician,
Princess Margaret Hospital,
Perth, Western Australia, Australia
*Care of the adolescent*

**Nicky Kilpatrick** BDS PhD
Professor, Paediatric Dentistry,
University of Bristol,
Bristol, UK
*Teeth and oral cavity disorders*

**Sebastian King,** BSc(Med) MBBS PhD
Paediatric Surgical Registrar,
Christchurch Hospital,
Christchurch, New Zealand
*Surgical conditions in the newborn*
*Surgical conditions in older children*

**Andrew J Kornberg** MBBS(Hons) FRACP
Associate Professor and Director of Neurology,
Royal Children's Hospital,
Parkville, Victoria, Australia
*Neuromuscular disorders*

**Peter Le Souëf** MBBS MD FRACP
Professor of Paediatrics, School of Paediatrics and Child Health,
University of West Australia,
Perth, Western Australia, Australia
*Lower respiratory tract infections and abnormalities*

**Jan Liebelt** MBBS(Hons) FRACP(Clin Genet), MSc
Clinical Geneticist,
South Australian Clinical Genetics Service,
Adelaide, South Australia, Australia
*Birth defects, prenatal diagnosis and teratogens*

**Zoe McCallum** MBBS FRACP
Department of Gastroenterology and Clinical Nutrition,
Royal Children's Hospital,
Melbourne, Australia
*Nutrition*

**Brett McDermott,** MBBS MD FRANZCP CertChildPsych
Executive Director, Child and Youth Mental Health Service,
Mater Children's Hospital,
Brisbane, Australia
*Major psychiatric disorders*

**James McGill,** MBBS(Hons) FRACP FRCPA HGSA Certified Clinical Geneticist
Director, Department of Metabolic Medicine,
Royal Children's Hospital,
Brisbane, Australia
*Inborn errors of metabolism*

**Sarah Kate McMahon** MBBS(Hons) PhD FRACP
Staff Specialist, Department of Endocrinology and Diabetes,
Royal Children's Hospital,
Brisbane, Queensland, Australia
*Growth and variations of growth*

**Sarah McNab** MBBS FRACP
General Paediatrician,
Royal Children's Hospital,
Melbourne, Victoria, Australia.
*Fluid replacement therapy*

**Steven McTaggart** MBBS FRACP PhD
Associate Professor and Director, Child & Adolescent Renal Service,
Royal Children's and Mater Children's Hospitals,
Brisbane, Queensland, Australia
*Glomerulonephritis, renal failure and hypertension*

**Craig Mellis,** MBBS MPH MD FRACP
Associate Dean and Head, Central Clinical School,
University of Sydney,
Sydney, New South Wales, Australia
*Acute upper respiratory infections*

**Paul Monagle** MBBS MSc MD FRACP FRCPA FCCP
Stevenson chair, Head of Department,
Department of Paediatrics, University of Melbourne,
Melbourne, Victoria, Australia
*Anaemia*

**Kevin J Murray** MBBS FRACP
Head of Department, Department of Rheumatology,
Princess Margaret Hospital for Children,
Perth, Western Australia, Australia
*Arthritis and connective tissue disorders*

**Ed Oakley** MBBS FACEM
Director, Paediatric Emergency Medicine
Monash Children's, Southern Health,
Melbourne, Victoria, Australia
*Poisoning and envenomation*
*Resuscitation*

**Tracey O'Brien** FRACP MBChB MHL BSc DCH
Head, Cord & Marrow Transplant Program, Senior Staff Specialist,
Centre for Children's Cancer & Blood Disorders,
Sydney Children's Hospital,
Sydney, Australia
*Cancers*

**Michael O'Callaghan** MBBS MSc FRACP
Director, Child Development and Rehabilitation,
Mater Children's Hospital,
Brisbane, Queensland, Australia
*Developmental disability*

**Edward V O'Loughlin** MD(Syd) FRACP
Senior Staff Specialist,
Department of Gastroenterology,
The Children's Hospital at Westmead,
Sydney, New South Wales, Australia
*Chronic diarrhoea and malabsorption*

**Georgia Paxton** MBBS(hons) BMedSci MPH FRACP
Paediatrician, Medical Coordinator, Immigrant Health Department of General Medicine,
Royal Children's Hospital,
Parkville, Victoria, Australia
*Refugee health*

**Roderic J Phillips** BSc MBBS FRACP PhD
Paediatric Skin Specialist,
Royal Children's Hospital,
Melbourne, Australia
*Skin disorders*

**Nicola K Poplawski** MBChB DipPaed FRACP MD
Clinical Geneticist,
Women's and Children's Hospital, North Adelaide;
SA Pathology, University of Adelaide, Adelaide,
South Australia, Australia
*Modern genetics*

**Jeremy Raftos** MBBS(Hon) FRACP
Senior Staff Specialist, Paediatric Emergency Department,
Women's & Children's Hospital,
North Adelaide, South Australia, Australia
*Emergencies: causes and assessment*

**Dinah Reddihough** MD BSc FRACP FAFRM
Paediatrician, Developmental Medicine,
Royal Children's Hospital;
Clinical Professor, Department of Paediatrics,
University of Melbourne;
Group Leader, Developmental Disability and Rehabilitation Research, Murdoch Childrens Research Institute,
Melbourne, Australia
*Cerebral palsy and neurodegenerative disorders*

**Peter Richmond** MBBS MRCP(UK) FRACP
University of Western Australia School of Paediatrics and Child Health;
Director, Vaccine Trials Group, Telethon Institute for Child Health Research;
Consultant Paediatric Immunologist and Paediatrician,
Princess Margaret Hospital for Children;
Director, Child Health Research Network, Children and Adolescent Health Service,
Perth, Western Australia, Australia
*Imumunization*

**Gehan Roberts** MPH PhD FRACP
Developmental-Behavioural Paediatrician,
Centre for Community Child Health;
NHMRC Post-doctoral research fellow,
Murdoch Children's Research Institute,
The Royal Children's Hospital,
Melbourne, Victoria, Australia
*Life events of normal children*

**Maureen Rogers** MBBS FACD
Emeritus Consultant Dermatologist,
Deptartment of Dermatology, The Children's Hospital at Westmead,
Westmead, New South Wales, Australia
*Skin disorders*

**Elizabeth Rose** MBBS FRACS
Consultant Otolaryngologist,
Royal Children's Hospital and Royal Victorian Eye and Ear Hospital,
Melbourne, Australia
*Ear, nose and throat disorders*

**Jeremy Rosenbaum,** MBBS(Hons) FRACP
Department of Gastroenterology, Hepatology and Nutrition,
Royal Children's Hospital,
Melbourne, Victoria, Australia
*Diarrhoea*

**Remo (Ray) N Russo** PhD MBBS FRACP FAFRM (RACP)
Director, Paediatric Rehabilitation Department,
Women's and Children's Health Network,
Women's & Children's Hospital Campus,
Adelaide, South Australia, Australia
*Neural tube defects, large heads and hydrocephalus*

**Monique Ryan** M Med BS, FRACP
Senior Staff Specialist, Children's Neurosciences Centre,
Royal Children's Hospital, Melbourne, Australia
*Neuromuscular disorders*

**Michael G Sawyer** MBBS, PhD, Dip Child Psych FRANZCP FRCPC
Head, Research and Evaluation Unit,
Women's and Children's Hospital,
Adelaide;
Professor, Discipline of Paediatrics, University of Adelaide,
Adelaide, South Australia, Australia
*Common mental health problems*

**Susan M Sawyer** MBBS MD FRACP FSAHM
Director, Centre for Adolescent,
Royal Children's Hospital,
Department of Paediatrics,
University of Melbourne;
Murdoch Children's Research Institute
Melbourne, Victoria, Australia
*Care of the adolescent*
*An approach to chronic cough and cystic fibrosis*

**Ben Saxon** MBBS FRACP FRCPA
Haematologist, Children, Youth and Women's Health Service,
North Adelaide, South Australia, Australia
*Abnormal bleeding and clotting*

**Hiran Selvadurai,** MBBS FRACP PhD
Associate Professor and Paediatric Respiratory Physician;
Staff Specialist,
The Children's Hospital at Westmead,
Sydney, New South Wales, Australia
*Wheezing disorders other than asthma*

**Jill Sewell** MBBS FRACP RACP RCPCH(Hon)
Deputy Director centre for Community Child Health
The Royal Children's Hospital,
Melbourne, Australia
*Hyperactivity and inattention*

**Peter D Sly** MBBS MD FRACP DSc
Professor and Deputy Director, Queensland Children's Medical Research Institute,
University of Queensland,
Brisbane, Queensland, Australia
*Stridor*

**Mike South,** MBBS DCH MRCP(UK) FRACP FJFICM FCICM MD
Professor and Director, Department of General Medicine,
Royal Children's Hospital,
Melbourne, Victoria, Australia
*Resuscitation*
*The clinical consultation*

**Zornitza Stark** MA(Oxon) BM BCh FRACP
Clinical Geneticist, Genetic Health Services,
Melbourne, Victoria, Australia
*Genetic counselling*

**Mike Starr,** MBBS FRACP
Paediatrician; Infectious Diseases Physician; Consultant in Emergency Medicine;
Director of Paediatric Physician Training, Royal Children's Hospital,
Melbourne, Victoria, Australia
*Congenital and perinatal infections*

**David Starte** MBBS MRCPCH FAFPHM FRACP
Senior Staff Specialist,
Child Development Service,
Royal North Shore Hospital,
Sydney, New South Wales, Australia
*Developmental surveillance and assessment*

**Andrew Steer** MBBS
Clinical and Public Health Research Fellow,
Medical Coordinator, Fiji, Suva, Fiji Islands
*Bone and joint infections*

**Gopinath Musuwadi Subramanian** MD DNB(Paed) DM DNB(Neurology) FRACP
Staff Specialist in Paediatric Neurology,
John Hunter Children's Hospital,
Newcastle, New South Wales, Australia
*Headache*

**Sadasivam Suresh** MBBS, MRCPCH, FRACP
Staff Specialist, Paediatric Respiratory & Sleep Medicine,
Mater Children's Hospital,
Brisbane, Queensland, Australia
*Stridor*
*Sleep problems*

**Barry Taylor** MBChB FRACP
Head of the Department of Women's and Children's Health, Dunedin School of Medicine and Consultant Paediatrician, Southern DHB, NZ,
University of Otago,
Dunedin, New Zealand
*Sudden unexpected death in infancy*

**Rita L. Teele** MD RANZCR
Consultant Paediatric Radiologist and Honorary Professor of Radiology with Anatomy,
Department of Radiology, Starship Children's Hospital and Auckland School of Medicine,
Auckland, New Zealand
*Imaging*

**Elizabeth Mary Thompson** MBBS MD FRACP
SA Pathology at the Women's and Children's Hospital,
Adelaide, South Australia, Australia
*The dysmorphic child*

**James Tibballs** BMedSc(Hons) MBBS MEd MBA MD MHlth&MedLaw DALF PGDipArts(Fr) FANZCA FCICM FACLM
Associate Professor and Deputy Director; Paediatric Intensive Care Unit & Resuscitation Officer,
Royal Children's Hospital,
Melbourne;
Principal Fellow, Departments of Paediatrics and Pharmacology (Australian Venom Research Unit),
University of Melbourne,
Melbourne, Victoria, Australia
*Poisoning and envenomation*

**Graham Vimpani** AM MBBS PhD FRACP FAFPHM
Clinical Chair, Kaleidoscope Greater Newcastle,
Newcastle, Australia
*Child health and disease*

**Neil Wigg** MBBS FRACP MPolAdmin
Associate Professor and Director, Community Child Health Services,
Fortitude Valley, Queensland, Australia
*The child and the family*

**Ian Wilkinson** MBBS (University of Queensland) FRACP
Staff Paediatric Neurologist,
John Hunter Children's Hospital,
Newcastle, New South Wales, Australia
*Headache*

**Ken Winkel** MBBS BMedSci PhD FACTM
Director, Australian Venom Research Unit,
Department of Pharmacology,
University of Melbourne,
Melbourne, Australia
*Poisoning and envenomation*

**Li-Chuen Wong** MBBS(Hons) MM DCH FACD
Visiting Medical Officer (VMO), The Children's Hospital at Westmead,
Sydney, New South Wales, Australia
*Skin disorders*

**Melanie Wong** MBBS(Hons) PhD FRACP FRCPA
Senior Staff Specialist,
Department of Allergy and Immunology,
The Children's Hospital at Westmead
Sydney, New South Wales, Australia
*Immunodeficiency and its investigation*

**Karen Zwi** MBBCh MSc MMed MRCP FRACP
Community Paediatrician and Head of Department of Community Child Health;
Senior Lecturer, University of New South Wales,
Sydney Children's Hospitals Network,
Sydney, New South Wales, Australia
*Child health and disease*

# Contents

## Part 5
## Paediatric emergencies



## Part 6
## Fluid replacement



## Part 7
## Principles of imaging



## Part 8
## Common orthopaedic problems and fractures



## Part 9
## Common paediatric surgical problems



## Part 10
## Inherited and metabolic problems



## Part 11
## Neonatal problems



## Part 12
## Infections



## Part 13
## Allergy, immunity and inflammation

## Part 14
## Respiratory disorders



## Part 15
## Cardiac disorders



## Part 16
## Haematological disorders and malignancies



## Part 17
## Seizure disorders and disorders of the nervous system



## Part 18
## Urinary tract disorders and hypertension



## Part 19
## Endocrine disorders



## Part 20
## Gastrointestinal tract and hepatic disorders

## Part 21
## Skin disorders



## Part 22
## ENT, eye and dental disorders

PART 1

# CURRENT PAEDIATRICS

# 1.1 Child health and disease

Karen Zwi, Graham Vimpani

## Setting the scene

Globally deaths in children under the age of 5 years are at their lowest level ever. They fell by over three million to 10 million deaths annually in the 15 years prior to 2006. Australian children are amongst the healthiest children in the world, generally have access to high-quality health care, and infant and child mortality rates halved between 1986 and 2006, which compares favourably with other high-income countries. However, there are significant groups of children in Australia that have relatively poor health and access to care. These include Aboriginal and Torres Strait Islander children, refugee children, children living in out-of-home care (foster or kinship care), children with disabilities, children from socioeconomically disadvantaged backgrounds, and children living in rural and remote Australia. There are also new emerging morbidities, such as the rising rates of childhood obesity, diabetes, dental decay and emotional–behavioural disorders. In addition, many of our childhood deaths are still preventable, especially those due to injuries such as motor vehicle incidents and drowning. Fortunately children are living for longer with chronic diseases and as long-term survivors of cancer. Therefore, the role of the health system in offering high-quality, child-centred care close to home is becoming increasingly important. This chapter discusses the key child health issues facing Australian children today and ways to improve the health of our children.

## What do we know about children and young people in Australia today?

Children and young people (up to the age of 24 years) comprise approximately one-third of the 22.5 million population of Australia, but, as in most other developed countries, this proportion is falling.

- 19.4% of the Australian population is now aged 0–14 years (4.1 million children), compared with over 28% in 1971, although children in the Northern Territory comprise about 25% of the population.
- 4.8% of Australian children are Indigenous and 38% of the Indigenous population is aged less than 14 years. This reflects the higher birth rate amongst Indigenous women (2.1 births per 1000 compared with 1.8 per 1000 in the total population) and the younger age structure of the Indigenous population due to shorter life expectancy.
- 5.9% of Australian children were born overseas in 2009 and 33% have at least one overseas-born parent. Sudan-born had the highest proportion (21%) of residents aged 0–14 years, followed by the USA (16%), Afghanistan (14%), South Africa, Singapore, Pakistan and Zimbabwe (12–13% each). Most migrants enjoy health that is equal to or better than that of the Australian-born population, often with lower rates of death, mental illness and disease risk factors.

Almost 1% of all Australian children are refugees, nearly a quarter of them from Sudan. These children have higher health needs on arrival than the local population due to their adverse environmental circumstances and restricted access to health care in their countries of origin.

The number of children in out-of-home care has more than doubled since 1997, from 11 600 to 26 700 in 2008, with the rate increasing from 3.0 placements per 1000 children in 1997 to 6.5 per 1000 in 2008. Children enter statutory care most often because of child abuse and neglect. Some of the risk factors include low family income, parental substance abuse, mental health issues, and community and family violence. Across the country, Indigenous children are nine times more likely to be placed in out-of-home care (foster care, kinship care, residential care) than non-Indigenous children. Australian surveys have shown that the majority of these children have chronic physical, developmental or mental health conditions arising from their earlier neglect and trauma.

## Where do Australian children live and why is this important?

The majority (86%) of Australian children aged 0–14 years in 2007 live in the south-eastern mainland states: almost one-third in New South Wales, a quarter in Victoria and one-fifth in Queensland.

Two-thirds of Australian children aged 0–14 years live in major cities. Three per cent of children live in remote and very remote areas. Indigenous children are eight times more likely to live in remote and very remote areas, accounting for 38% of all children in these areas, despite accounting for less than 5% of all children. Children comprise a larger proportion of the total population living in rural and remote areas. Access to high-quality health care is poorer in these areas and children experience higher death rates, higher rates of neural tube defects and lower rates of cancer survival than those in major cities.

## What are the circumstances of Australian households?

### Family composition

The type of family in which children live has changed minimally in the decade to 2007. Some 83% live in couple families (including 10% in blended and step families) and around 17% in one-parent families, 87% with their mother.

### Family income and work

Poverty is well known to affect the health of children. Australia is ranked behind many developed countries, with 10 of 24 Organisation for Economic Co-operation and Development (OECD) countries having a lower proportion of children living in relative income poverty than Australia.

- In 1999, 12% of Australian children aged 0–17 years lived in households with equivalent income of less than 50% of the median household income (*relative poverty*).
- In 2005–2006, low-income households (those in the second and third income deciles) with children aged 0–12 years accounted for 421 300 households Australia-wide and received on average $347 a week ($218 a week less than median-income households with children aged 0–12 years).
- Jobless families are disproportionately likely to be reliant on welfare, to have low incomes and to experience financial stress. In 2006, 15% of Australian children aged 0–14 years lived in jobless families, a decline from 19% in 1996.
- Nearly half (42%) of Indigenous children aged 0–14 years live in jobless families, three times the proportion of all children. The higher proportion of Indigenous children living in one-parent families contributes to this higher rate, as 45% of Indigenous children live in one-parent families compared with 20% of all children. 68% of Indigenous children living in one-parent families do not live with an employed parent.
- Australia had the second highest proportion of working-age, jobless families with children aged 0–17 years of 24 OECD countries in 2000, largely due to the relatively high rate of one-parent households in Australia and the high rate of joblessness (51%) among this group.

### Why does this matter?

Members of jobless households report worse physical and mental health and lower life satisfaction than members of households where someone is employed. There are causal relationships between parental joblessness and family conflict, family breakdown and child abuse. Secure employment provides financial stability, self-confidence and social contact for parents, with positive effects flowing on to children.

## Childcare and early childhood education

### Why are early childhood education and care important for health and wellbeing?

Most Australian children participate in child care or early education prior to school entry. Early experiences in a child's life strongly influence the biological pathways that affect cognition, behaviour, language development, capacity to learn, memory, stress response, and physical and mental health and wellbeing throughout life. Early childhood education is important for successful transition to formal schooling. It is also associated with a lower incidence of personal and social problems in later life, such as school dropout, welfare dependency, unemployment and criminal behaviour. Preschool programmes may be especially positive in the lives of children from disadvantaged backgrounds, where children may not be receiving the stimulation they require from the home environment. An English study of over 3000 preschool children found that the increased risk of antisocial or worried behaviour among disadvantaged children at school entry can be reduced by high-quality preschool care at 3 and 4 years of age.

### Australian children's experiences of child care and early education

In 2008, 50.2% of Australian under 2-year-olds were in formal or informal child care, compared with 41% in care in 2002. Around half (47%) of children in child care spent less than 10 hours per week in care. A further 37% were in care for 10–29 hours, and 16% of children spent more than 30 hours per week in child care. It is within this latter group where British and American studies have raised concerns about the increased prevalence of disruptive behaviour in later childhood.

Overall, the most commonly used type of child care was informal care, used by 29% of all children aged 0–12 years. Care provided by grandparents was the most common type of informal care and was used by 19% of children.

Social Trends 2010 reported that the use of child care was highest (78%) for children in one-parent families where the parent was in full-time employment. Around two-thirds (64%) of children attended care if their parent was employed part-time, whereas the proportion of children attending care dropped to 40% if the parent was not employed.

The story was similar for couple families. When both parents were in full-time employment, 60% of children usually attended child care. This fell to 51% for children in families where one parent was employed full-time and the other part-time. The proportion of children in child care was lower when both parents were employed part-time (41%) or if only one parent was employed full-time (25%) or part-time (26%). The proportion of children in child care was only 17% for couple families where neither parent was employed.

It is difficult to estimate the number of children who participate in formal early childhood education programmes in the years before the first year of primary schooling owing to the varied nature of children's services throughout Australia and differences in data collection between states and territories. According to the Australian Bureau of Statistics (ABS) 2005 Child Care Survey, 68% of children aged 3–4 years attended preschool or a long day-care centre. Nearly half (48%) of long day-care services offered a preschool (or structured educational) programme.

In terms of children's participation in pre-primary education, Australia is one of the worst performers in the OECD, despite growing evidence that preschool education has major long-term benefits for the child's educational and social trajectory.

## Why is the proportion of children in the population declining and what does that mean for children of the future?

Since the last century there has been a general decline in fertility in Australia to the current level of 1.77 children per woman. In addition there has been a significant increase in life expectancy leading to ageing of the population. Consequently, the projected child population proportion (aged 0–14 years) will drop from almost 20% in 2010 to 12–15% in the year 2051. Whilst it can be argued that expenditure on quality, evidence-based services for children and young people is a cost-beneficial investment likely to promote better health and wellbeing in the population generally, the ageing population is likely to create pressure on the allocation of resources for children's services in the future.

## Child health

### What affects child health?

The health of a child reflects a complex interaction between biological susceptibility and the child's experience of the environment. The child's environment affects health in both immediate and long-term ways, with physical factors such as pollution or hunger due to neglect having a short-term impact as well as possibly affecting the child's wellbeing and health in the long term. Many factors previously thought to be short-term problems (such as low birth weight) are now known to produce adverse health effects well into adult life.

The context in which a child grows up plays a major role in that child's lifetime health. A child's health can be deeply affected by the family circumstances, the community in which the child is raised, and the cultural and social factors operating in society. Factors such as the protection of children's rights in society, community support to new parents, how a society deals with poverty or discrimination, the availability of maternity leave or welfare grants to unemployed parents all affect the health of that society's children.

There is convincing evidence that home visiting to high-risk, disadvantaged parents before and after the birth of their child and good-quality early childhood education can significantly affect the life trajectory of those children, affecting their cognitive development and successful transition to formal schooling. These interventions are associated with lower incidence of personal and social problems later in life, such as school dropout, welfare dependency, unemployment and criminal behaviour. These effects are more marked in children from disadvantaged backgrounds and therefore may be particularly effective in closing the gap between advantaged and disadvantaged children.

Greater understanding of the role of gene–environment interactions on child health outcomes (epigenetics) has demonstrated the combined impact of biological susceptibility and adverse environmental factors. For example, a Canadian study has shown that adults who have committed suicide and were abused as children have reduced *NR3C1* gene expression (through methylation) and reduced total glucocorticoid expression in the hippocampus compared with those who committed suicide with no history of childhood maltreatment. This combination leads to reduced feedback inhibition and thus to higher cortisol levels in response to stress, enhancing its effects in adulthood, vulnerability to mood disorders and increasing suicide risk.

## How do we describe child health?

We use rates of mortality and morbidity to evaluate the health status of a community. Mortality is a very crude index of health and is of limited value in assessing the health status and health needs of a community. Morbidity is a measure of the presence or absence of medical diseases or conditions. A widely accepted view is that to describe health adequately involves also measuring a broad range of social and economic risk and protective factors. In 1946, the World Health Organization (WHO) defined health holistically as 'a state of complete physical, mental, and social wellbeing and not merely the absence of disease or infirmity'. A child's physical, mental and social wellbeing is inextricably linked to the environment and social values surrounding that child. Furthermore, children and adolescents are growing and developing rapidly, and may be more susceptible than adults to adverse environmental influences (Fig. 1.1.1).

## Individual and social determinants of health

Levels of health and wellbeing depend on two broad forces: determinants (factors that influence health) and interventions (interventions to improve health). There are many determinants and they interact in complex ways. They range from individual behaviours (such as smoking or drink-driving) to much broader factors such as socioeconomic background. All of these interact with our genetic makeup to produce health outcomes, such as reduced life expectancy, and increased illness or disability. Interventions can range from personal services to treat the sick to broad preventive campaigns such as encouraging breastfeeding.

Protective factors promote positive health and development and include factors such as infant breastfeeding, physical activity and sound nutrition. Factors that increase the risk of ill-health in children include overweight and obesity, exposure to tobacco smoke or alcohol use in pregnancy. From a practical point of view, complete paediatric clinical assessment requires a consideration of all aspects of the child's life, such as the home circumstances, the access to health care, the physical and mental health of the parents, and the quality of community support available. This applies equally to every child whether they present with leukaemia, cystic fibrosis, acute bacterial meningitis, developmental delay, child maltreatment, behaviour problems or even a well-child review (Fig. 1.1.2).

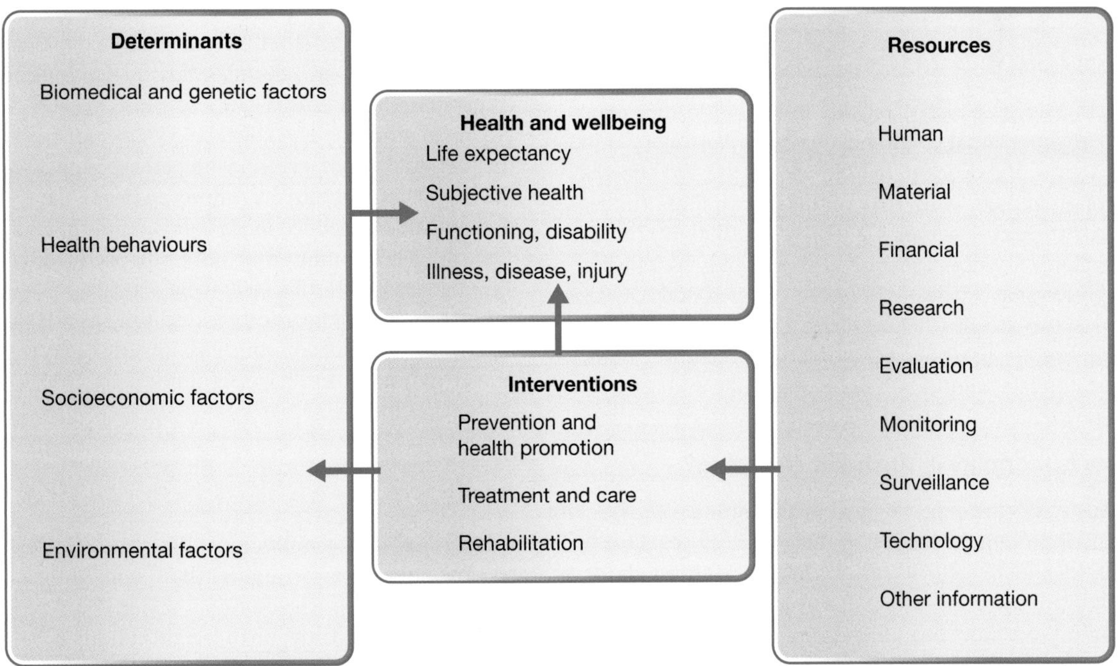


Fig. 1.1.1 A conceptual framework for Australia's health. (From Australian Institute of Health and Welfare 2010 Australia's health 2010: the twelfth biennial health report of the Australian Institute of Health and Welfare. AIHW, Canberra, p 4, with permission.)

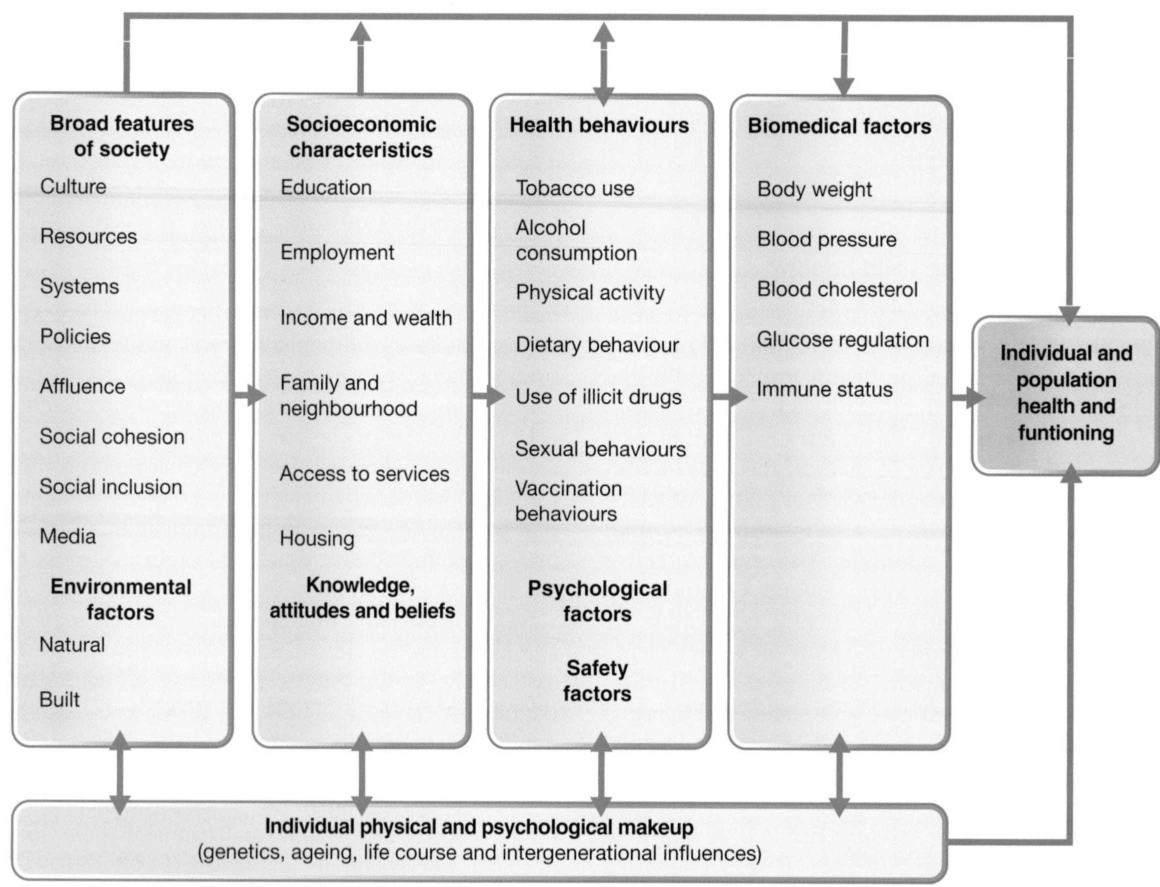


Fig. 1.1.2 A conceptual framework for determinants of health. (From Australian Institute of Health and Welfare 2010 Australia's health 2010: the twelfth biennial health report of the Australian Institute of Health and Welfare. AIHW, Canberra, p 65, with permission.)

## Mortality

Death rates in children provide insights into the social and environmental conditions in which Australia's children grow and develop. In 2007 there were 1709 deaths among children, with 70% of these in infants (under 1 year of age), a rate of 4.2 deaths per 1000 live births. The number of deaths among 1–14-year-olds was considerably lower at 506 deaths (a rate of 13 per 100000). Over the last two decades there has been a steady decline in the death rate for those aged 1–14 years. In contrast, infant mortality rates almost halved between 1986 and 2006.

### How is mortality in Australia changing?

- Australia's life expectancy at birth continues to rise and is among the highest in the world (79 years for males and almost 84 years for females), although for Indigenous people it remains about 20 years less.
- Infant mortality has fallen from a rate of approximately 100 per 1000 live births at the turn of the 20th century to the 2007 rate of 4.2 per 1000 live births. Figure 1.1.3 shows the decline over the last two decades.
- Death rates among children and young people have halved in the last two decades, largely due to fewer transport-related deaths.
- Neonatal mortality has fallen below 3 per 1000 for the first time, in association with better perinatal care.
- Post-neonatal mortality has improved due to the declining rate of sudden unexplained deaths in infancy.
- The Indigenous infant mortality rate declined by 47% between 1991 and 2006 (Fig. 1.1.3).
- Infectious disease mortality is declining as a result of improved socioeconomic circumstances and universal immunization programmes.

## Spotlight on Indigenous children

In Australia, Indigenous mortality and morbidity rates are substantially higher than non-Indigenous rates at all ages.

- The proportion of low birth weight infants is 5.9% overall, but 12.5% for Indigenous births.
- The proportion of preterm infants is 7.9% overall, but 13.7% for Indigenous births.

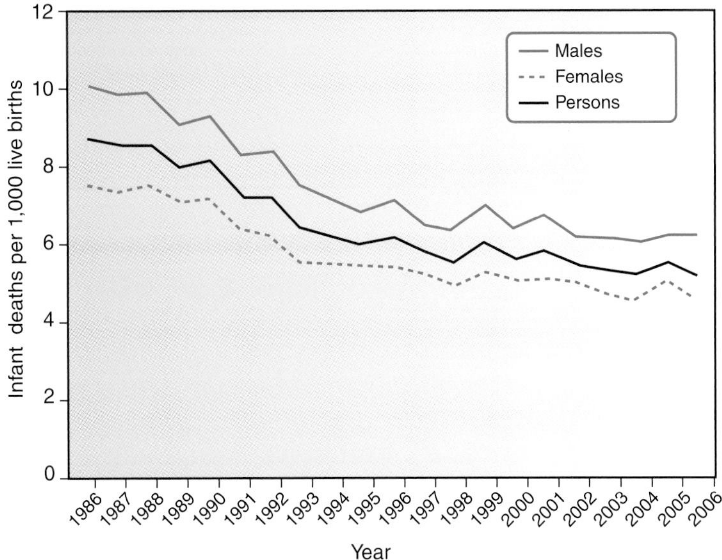


Fig. 1.1.3 Infant mortality rate, 1986–2006. (From Australian Institute of Health and Welfare 2010 A picture of Australia's children 2009. AIHW, Canberra, with permission.)

- The Indigenous perinatal mortality rate is two times higher than the non-Indigenous rate (20 per 1000 versus 10 per 1000).
- The Indigenous infant mortality rate is three times higher than the non-Indigenous rate (13 per 1000 versus 4.2 per 1000), although the gap is closing.
- The Indigenous 1–14 years mortality rate is three times higher than that of non-Indigenous Australians (39 per 100000 compared with 13 per 100000).
- Some 70% of the 'excess' deaths in rural and remote areas (observed deaths in rural and remote areas compared with what would be expected if city death rates had applied) occur in Indigenous children.
- Injury (which is largely preventable) was the leading cause of death for Indigenous children, accounting for almost half of all deaths (46%).
- Indigenous Australians have the highest recorded rates of acute rheumatic fever and rheumatic heart disease in the world, almost exclusively restricted to the Northern Territory and Central Australia, and extremely rare in other Australians.
- The teenage birth rate is five times higher in Indigenous women (80 births per 1000 compared with 15 per 1000), and increases the risk of adverse health outcomes. The rate increases with increasing remoteness.

### How can we explain the health of Indigenous children?

The health inequality of Indigenous Australians compared with the rest of the population reflects disadvantage across a range of socioeconomic factors that affect health and wellbeing. The low socioeconomic status arises from lower levels of education, employment and income, and results in greater exposure to factors such as smoking, poor nutrition, alcohol misuse, overcrowded living conditions and violence. However, not all the health inequalities are explained by socioeconomic differences and there are complex historical, cultural, access and political factors impacting on Indigenous health. On the positive side, Indigenous children are just as likely to be fully immunized at 2 years of age as non-Indigenous children, and Indigenous households with children aged 0–14 years are just as able to get support during a time of crisis (reflecting extended family and community support structures – 'social capital') as non-Indigenous households. The Council of Australian Governments has committed to halving the mortality gap for Indigenous children aged under 5 years within a decade. Improvements in Indigenous child mortality (Fig.1.1.4) require better access to antenatal care, teenage reproductive and sexual health services, child and maternal health services, and integrated child and family services.

## Infant mortality

Infant mortality rates are important indicators of child health, and refer to infant deaths within 1 year of birth. The leading causes of death in this age group in 2007 were:

- Perinatal conditions (48%)
- Congenital anomalies (26%)
- Ill-defined conditions, mostly sudden infant death syndrome (SIDS) (12%).

Part of infant mortality is neonatal mortality, which is death within 28 days (ABS definition) of birth. Neonatal

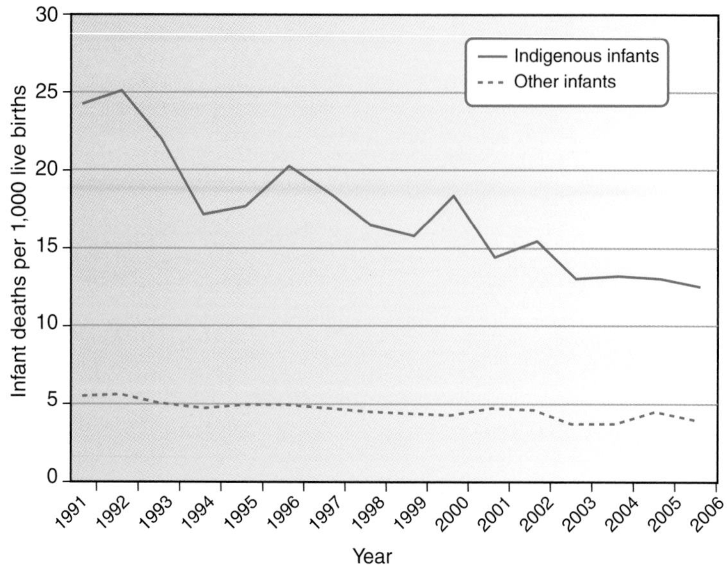


Fig. 1.1.4 Infant mortality by Indigenous status, 1991–2006. Deaths are based on year of registration and state of usual residence (Western Australia, South Australia or Northern Territory). The average of births over 1993–1995 in Western Australia was used as the denominator for infant mortality rates for 1991 and 1992 to correct for errors in births recorded for 1991 and 1992. (From Australian Institute of Health and Welfare 2010 A picture of Australia's children 2009. AIHW, Canberra, with permission.)

mortality has reduced substantially since the 1920s in Australia. Some 60% of neonatal deaths occur on the day of birth, with most being due to extreme prematurity, poor fetal growth, congenital malformations or pregnancy complications. With the advent of neonatal intensive care in the late 1960s, the neonatal mortality rate declined even further. Other important factors contributing to the decline have been the use of periconceptional folate to prevent neural tube defects (anencephaly, spina bifida and encephalocele) and improved understanding of the determinants of premature labour, intrauterine growth restriction, and some developmental anomalies. Figure 1.1.5 shows Australia's Infant Mortality Rate as compared to other selected OECD countries.

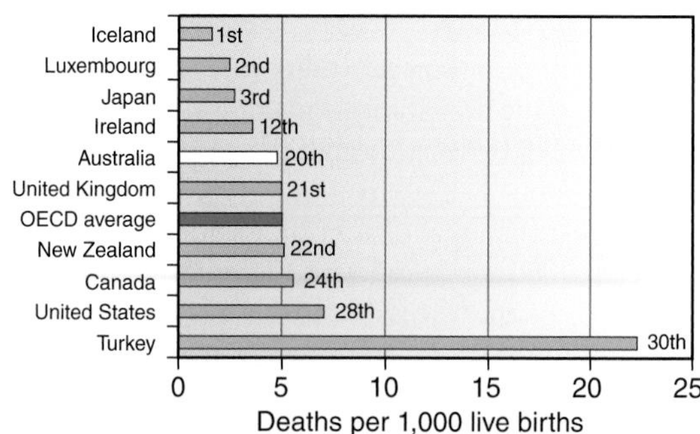


Fig. 1.1.5 Infant mortality rates among selected OECD countries, 2006. Data for Canada and the USA are for 2005. Based on data from 30 OECD countries, using the most recent year of available data. (From Australian Institute of Health and Welfare 2010 A picture of Australia's children 2009. AIHW, Canberra, with permission.)

## Sudden infant death syndrome

A major contributor to the recent decline in post-neonatal mortality (children aged over 1 month and under 1 year) has been the decline in deaths from SIDS. SIDS is the commonest cause of sudden unexplained death in infancy (SUDi), for which strict diagnostic criteria must be satisfied. Between 1982 and 2002, the SIDS death rate fell from 180 to 46 deaths per 100000 live births. Public education campaigns during the 1990s, emphasizing that babies should be placed on their back when placed to sleep, contributed to the decline. Apart from sleeping position, other risk factors have also been identified consistently from epidemiological studies. These include maternal cigarette smoking, lack of breastfeeding, overheating of the baby and a parental history of illicit drug use. Unfortunately, the rate of SIDS in Indigenous infants remains higher than in non-Indigenous infants, probably because of a higher prevalence of the risk factors.

## Causes of death between 1 and 14 years

More than 98% of children survive from birth to 15 years of age (Fig. 1.1.6). The mortality rate for children aged 1–14 years declined by 52% between 1983 and 2003.

The three main causes of death in 2007 were:

- injury (37%)
- cancer (17%)
- diseases of the nervous system (10%). (Figure 1.1.7)

The leading causes of injury death in this age group are road transport incidents (involving occupants,

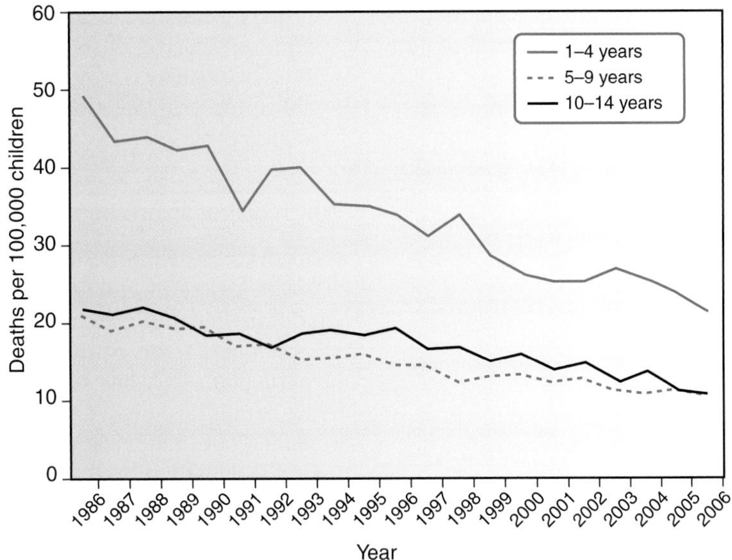


Fig. 1.1.6 Death rates for children aged 1–14 years, 1986–2006. (From Australian Institute of Health and Welfare 2010 A picture of Australia's children 2009. AIHW, Canberra, with permission.)

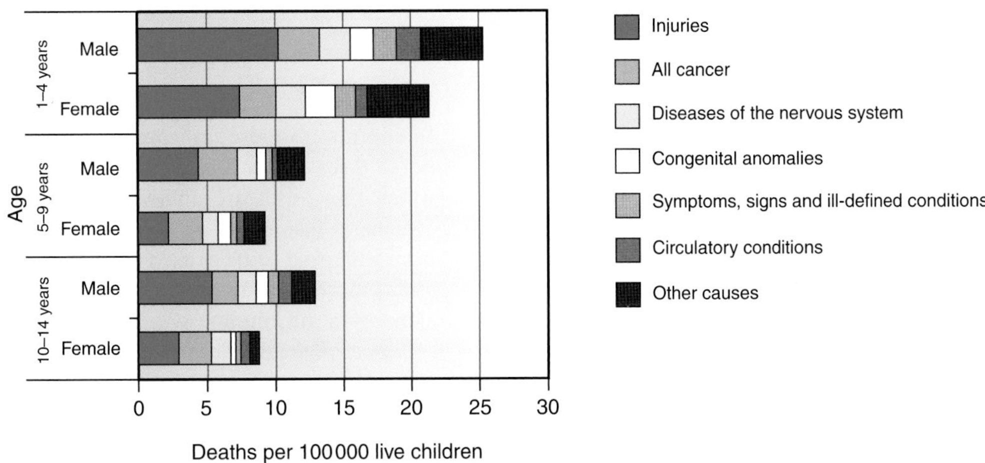


Fig. 1.1.7 Leading causes of death among children aged 1–14 years, 2004–2006. 'Other causes' accounted for 17% of child deaths among 1–14-year-olds in 2004–2006. (From Australian Institute of Health and Welfare 2010 A picture of Australia's children 2009. AIHW, Canberra, with permission.)

pedestrians and cyclists) and drowning (domestic swimming pools, bathtubs, dams and drains, rivers and sea, and domestic buckets). Swimming pool drowning accounts for about half of all drownings in those aged under 5 years, a proportion that has shown no significant change since the 1990s.

The decline in injury mortality has been due to a number of preventive actions, including:

- child-resistant packaging of medication
- traffic control measures (such as infant and child seat-restraint legislation, improved vehicle design, traffic control through speed cameras, random breath-testing, school speed zones and young driver regulations)
- domestic pool isolation fencing.

Another important cause of preventable mortality in children is bacterial meningitis. Introduction of universal immunization for *Haemophilus influenzae* type b (Hib), meningococcus C and pneumococcal infections has resulted in a significant decrease in invasive disease due to these organisms.

## Causes of death between 15 and 19 years

Mortality rates in this age group are about five times higher than in children aged 5–14 years, although substantially lower than in the 0–4-year group. The principal causes of death in adolescents are injury (50%), suicide (20%) and cancer (10%). Traffic-related causes are the most important contributor and alcohol use is the key risk factor. The mortality rate for males is twice that of females in this age group. The disturbing increase in adolescent male suicide that occurred between 1979 and 1998, with the rate increasing by 40%, has begun to fall for reasons that are unclear; in 2002 rates were at their lowest since 1984. The male rate is currently four times higher than the female rate.

## Morbidity

### Changes in disease patterns

#### How is children's health changing?

- The prevalence of asthma in children and young people rose during the 1980s and 1990s (from 12.3% to 19.2%), but there has been no further increase since then. Currently, 12% of children report asthma as a long-term condition, one of the highest rates in the world. Around 40% of children with asthma live with a person who smokes; higher exposure rates occur among socioeconomically disadvantaged children.
- There has been increasing concern about problems of developmental health and wellbeing, with 35% of new paediatric consultations for behaviour problems and 13% for learning problems. Around one in seven (14%) of Australian children aged 4–14 years had mental health problems in the latest National Survey of Health and Wellbeing (1998).
- One in four children (25%) aged 5–17 years are overweight or obese.
- The prevalence of disability has increased from 5.3% in 1981 to 8.3% in 2003. Almost half of these children had severe or profound core activity limitations, so that they needed assistance with one or more of the core activities of daily living (self-care, mobility or communication tasks). Some 75% of 5–19-year-olds with a disability also experienced schooling restrictions that resulted in them needing special assistance, arrangements or equipment at school, attending special classes or a special school, needing frequent time off school or having difficulty with aspects of school work or the school environment. A quarter of those with a disability had asthma and others had autism, disruptive behaviour and intellectual impairment. More than 90% of children with autism had severe or profound core activity limitations, and all had schooling restrictions.
- There has been a rising incidence of cerebral palsy in births under 1500 g (from 10 to 70 per 1000 live births) during the last 25 years, largely due to the improved survival of these children.
- Rates of sexually transmitted infections (chlamydia and gonococcal infections) are increasing amongst young people aged 15–24 years.

#### Which diseases are declining and why?

Paediatrics has changed dramatically during the past 50 years, as the mortality rate for all life-threatening conditions has declined. The most dramatic change has been as a result of declines in infectious diseases in particular. This has been the result of improved living conditions, higher levels of education, and the availability of immunization and antibiotics.

Of particular importance is the greatly reduced incidence of tuberculosis; chronic suppurative diseases of the chest, bone and ear; rheumatic fever and rheumatic heart disease; and streptococcal infections. It should be noted that the incidence of all infections was falling well before the advent of antibiotic and chemotherapeutic drugs, which are often credited incorrectly for control of infection.

#### Which diseases are increasing?

In contrast to these improvements, some other childhood diseases have shown a rising prevalence, for which the causes are unclear. The incidence of type 1 diabetes has increased since 2000. The increase has been too rapid to be caused entirely by genetic factors and is more likely to be environmental factors causing changes in the immune system that trigger the disease.

New challenges have also been posed by the emergence of problems of developmental health and wellbeing that are related to extensive changes in social and family life during the past 30 years. Examples are child maltreatment, behaviour and learning problems, youth suicide, obesity and other eating disorders, substance misuse and early onset of criminal behaviour.

### Burden of disease and long-term health conditions

Chronic and long-term conditions account for a large proportion of the burden of disease among children, and can affect growth and physical, social and emotional development. In 2003, almost a quarter of the burden of disease in children was due to mental disorders such as anxiety and depression, attention-deficit disorder and autism spectrum disorders. A further 18% was due to chronic respiratory conditions (mainly asthma) and 16% to neonatal conditions (Table 1.1.1).

Conditions such as cancer and diabetes are uncommon in childhood but a considerable number of children are affected by them each year. Type 1

**Table 1.1.1 Burden of disease and mortality in 0–14-year-olds in Australia**

| Parent-reported prevalence (2007–2008) | | Hospitalizations (2007–2008) | | Infant mortality (2007) | | Child (1–14 years) mortality (2007) | | Burden of disease and injury (DALYs)* (2003) | |
|---|---|---|---|---|---|---|---|---|---|
| Condition | % of children | Condition | % of all child hospitalizations | Condition | % of all infant deaths | Condition | % of all child deaths | Condition | % of all child DALYs |
| Respiratory diseases | 17.4 | Respiratory conditions | 18.6 | Perinatal conditions | 47.7 | Injury and poisoning | 36.8 | Mental disorders | 22.6 |
| Eye and adnexa disorders | 10.1 | Injury and poisoning | 12.1 | Congenital anomalies | 25.8 | Cancer | 17.0 | Chronic respiratory conditions | 18.1 |
| Ill-defined conditions† | 6.7 | Perinatal conditions | 10.3 | Ill-defined conditions† | 12.1 | Diseases of the nervous system | 9.9 | Neonatal conditions | 15.6 |
| Mental and behavioural problems | 5.3 | Digestive conditions | 10.2 | Injury and poisoning | 3.0 | Circulatory conditions | 6.3 | Congenital conditions | 11.6 |
| Ear and mastoid disorders‡ | 3.2 | Ill-defined conditions† | 6.9 | Diseases of the nervous system | 2.3 | Ill-defined conditions† | 6.3 | Injuries | 7.4 |

*Disability-adjusted life-years.

†Parent-reported prevalence, hospitalizations and deaths from ill-defined conditions include those for which a more specific diagnosis could not be made or where signs or symptoms could not be determined.

‡Diseases of skin and subcutaneous tissue were in equal fifth position with ear and mastoid disorders.

Note: The conditions listed above are based on the International Classification of Diseases, tenth revision (ICD-10), chapter level headings, except for the burden of disease data, where conditions are grouped using a different methodology.

Source: Australian Institute of Health and Welfare 2010 Australia's health 2010: the twelfth biennial health report of the Australian Institute of Health and Welfare. AIHW, Canberra, p 299.

diabetes most often appears during childhood or adolescence and requires ongoing management to control and reduce the risk of complications. The rate of new cases in 2007 (24 per 100 000 children) has increased significantly since 2000 (19 per 100 000 children). For cancer, the rate of 14 per 100 000 children in the 5-year period from 2002 to 2006 has not increased since 1996–2000. The most common cancer types are lymphoid leukaemia, cancer of the brain and myeloid leukaemia. Overall survival from cancer and leukaemia in particular continues to improve. The 5-year survival rate for children with leukaemia increased from 64% to 83% between 1982–1986 and 1998–2004.

### Is birth weight important?

A key indicator of infant health is the proportion of infants with low birth weight. 'Low birth weight' is defined as less than 2500 g at birth; 'very low birth weight' is under 1500 g and 'extremely low birth weight' is under 1000 g. There has been little change in the incidence of low birth weight in recent generations. Indeed, there has been a slight rise in its incidence in the last decade (from 6.3% to 6.8%), which is explained partly by a higher proportion of older mothers giving birth. In 1998, the birth rate in women over 35 years of age exceeded that in those less than 19 years for the first time. Low birth weight babies have a greater risk of poor health and dying, require longer periods of hospitalization after birth and are more likely to develop significant disabilities.

Low birth weight has been found to have enduring effects on health and is associated in adulthood with type 2 diabetes, high blood pressure, metabolic and cardiovascular disease, and possibly obesity. Many of the risk factors for low birth weight are modifiable by providing good antenatal care to pregnant women, reducing smoking, and optimizing general health and nutrition before and during pregnancy.

## Australian health services

- Health expenditure in 2007–2008 exceeded $100 billion for the first time and equalled 9.1% of gross domestic product (GDP).
- In 2007–2008, just over 2% of total health expenditure was for preventive services or health promotion.

In addition to the risk and protective factors discussed above, the capacity of the system to deliver a high-quality service plays a major role in improving the health and wellbeing of children. Care should be accessible, responsive to the population it serves and cost-effective. Some key performance indicators are used to reflect how well the system is performing in delivering quality health care to Australian children. These include the coverage of screening programmes such as the neonatal hearing screening programme, and preventive interventions such as childhood immunization. In general, preventive activity is more cost-effective than interventions designed to treat health problems that have already occurred. Nonetheless our health-care expenditure is heavily weighted towards treatment rather than preventive services. Health-care costs are rising steadily in Australia and redirecting more funding towards prevention of disease may help to reduce this escalation.

## Why are children taken to a health service?

### Hospitalizations

Around 10% of hospital admissions in Australia are for children under 15 years. Respiratory conditions were the most common reason for hospitalization in 2007–2008, followed by injury and poisoning. Boys were 1.6 times more likely to be hospitalized for injury as girls, with falls accounting for 39% and land transport incidents for 13%.

### Children and adolescents presenting to general practitioners

From an ongoing national survey of general practice statistics, it is known that 15.8% of total general practice encounters in Australia are for children aged 0–14 years, with a further 9.8% for young persons aged 15–24 years. The top reasons for consulting a doctor, including but not limited to general practitioners (GPs), in children aged under 15 years were respiratory conditions (upper respiratory infection, including tonsillitis, asthma and acute bronchitis) and immunization. Rates of presentation to GPs for asthma fell by almost one-third in 0–4-year-olds between 1998–1999 and 2001–2002.

### Children and adolescents presenting to specialized paediatric services

In the Australian health-care system, children may be referred to a consultant or specialist paediatrician by a general (or primary care) practitioner for consultation on difficult problems, or for management of rare or difficult-to-treat chronic illnesses. Paediatricians work in the community and/or in general hospitals with paediatric facilities (secondary paediatric services) or children's hospitals with extensive subspecialty services (tertiary hospitals). In addition, public and some private hospitals provide accident and emergency services for children. The pattern of injuries and acute and chronic illnesses seen in these settings varies according to the mix of private and public paediatric hospitals serving urban and rural communities. The case mix (pattern of clinical problems) differs for outpatient clinic attendances, emergency department presentations and hospital admissions.

A 12-month survey of the practice profile of paediatricians in the Barwon region of Victoria in 1996–1997 found that 10% of the childhood population had consulted a paediatrician practising in the community during this period: 68.9% of consultations concerned medical problems, with central nervous system/disability and the respiratory system each accounting for 16%, and gastrointestinal problems a further 14%. Nearly 35% of children seen had behavioural problems, with 76% of these relating to attention-deficit/hyperactivity disorder (ADHD), which was the most common diagnosis overall. A further 14.5% of consultations concerned children with epilepsy or disability, 13% were for children with learning problems and 10% were for asthma. Just over 4% of all consultations involved children with significant social problems. At least 50% of these paediatric medical consultations involved children with a chronic illness.

Attendances at an emergency department provide a further component of the picture of child injury and acute illness. Gastroenteritis, asthma and injuries dominate the mix of clinical conditions treated in this setting. Children aged 0–4 years with asthma attend emergency departments relatively more often than people of other ages who have asthma.

## Health behaviours

The health status of children and young people is changing as evidenced by health behaviour changes:

- Increased immunization uptake has followed the establishment of the Australian Childhood Immunisation Register (ACIR): 90.5% fully immunized at 1 year in 2002, 87.8% at 2 years and 80.6% at 6 years.
- There has been a plateau in rates of adolescent smoking but with persisting higher rates among girls (32% versus 28% for boys).
- Rates of obesity and overweight are rising: 25% of 7–18-year-olds in Sydney and Melbourne are overweight.

A number of factors that rely on public participation have a profound impact on child health, and on future good health as an adult. In traditional societies, parenting was a responsibility of the clan, not just the biological parents. The quality of parenting provided in developed countries is now arguably one of the major determinants of public health, being implicated in the high prevalence of academic failure, disruptive behaviour and other mental health problems, intentional and unintentional injuries, substance misuse and juvenile crime.

Other health behaviours may also have benefits or adverse effects; for example, high rates of breastfeeding and immunization, use of child restraints in motor vehicles, sun exposure protection using clothing and sun-screen creams, healthy nutrition, active lifestyles, pool fences and swimming competence, and bicycle helmets all have a beneficial impact on disease and injury prevention.

### Smoking and sun exposure

The massive increase in the incidence of lung cancer in men over the age of 50 years preceding the 1980s and, in more recent years, the rise in women, along with the increase in melanoma in both sexes, stands in stark contrast to the relatively stable incidence of most other cancers. What have these outcomes to do with paediatrics? The answer is that the behaviours associated with an increased risk of these diseases commence in childhood and adolescence.

#### Smoking-related disorders

The current patterns of lung cancer incidence and mortality in men (a 2% per year decline) and women (a 1.6% per year increase) probably reflect smoking behaviour patterns 20 years ago. Most smokers commence smoking in adolescence and this behaviour, once established, may be difficult to change. In addition, the number of pack-years of smoke exposure is directly related to the risk of smoking-related cancers, cardiovascular disease and numerous other health problems. The relationship between media exposure to cigarette promotion and the likelihood of young people becoming smokers is strong and well established. With increasing awareness of the profound and irrefutable causal relationship between cigarette smoking and disease, and with new laws restricting the way in which cigarettes may be advertised, the prevalence of adolescent smokers in Australia has finally started to decline during the past 15 years, although daily smoking rates are higher in 16–17-year-old girls (14.5%) compared with boys (7.95%).

Furthermore, the recent widespread recognition of the harmful effects of both prenatal and postnatal passive smoke exposure in children (low birth weight and prematurity, and all of their consequences, respiratory infections, asthma, otitis media, impaired lung growth) has led to rapid changes in public policy, laws and community practices aimed at reducing environmental tobacco smoke exposure, especially for children. The clinician's role is to assist in the education of young parents, to provide access to professional quit programmes and to encourage smokers in the meantime to smoke only outside the family home and wear protective clothing while doing so, and never in the family vehicle or in the company of children.

### Melanoma

In the case of melanoma, the incidence rates have increased markedly since 1983, especially for males. Australian melanoma rates are among the highest in the world, with a 10-fold difference in incidence between Australia and England and Wales. Melanoma risk is related to ultraviolet radiation exposure and the incidence is higher in individuals with many moles, those with fair, sun-sensitive skin, and those who have intermittent high recreational exposure. It is thought that exposure in childhood may be particularly important. It is therefore disconcerting to note that surveys have found that between 9% and 12% of children and young people in all age groups who have been exposed to the sun have not used sun protection.

### Obesity and physical fitness

There has been growing concern about the increasing levels of obesity and lack of physical fitness in children and young people in Australia. In 1985, 4% of boys and 6% of girls were classified, according to their body mass index (BMI – a measure of weight for height) as being overweight. More recent studies found that about 25% of children aged 7–18 years in Sydney and Melbourne were overweight, had sedentary lifestyles, and consumed a diet high in fat and low in the intake of fruit and vegetables. It is of some concern that around one-third of children under 12 years of age do not eat any fruit or fruit products, and more than 1 in 5 do not eat any vegetables or vegetable products. Childhood obesity is now being tackled as part of a national strategy developed by the National Obesity Taskforce.

## Future directions

There is widespread recognition that social, environmental, family and technological changes during the past half century have contributed to the changing pattern of childhood mortality and morbidity. There is also increasing awareness that exposures and behaviours occurring in fetal life and childhood have lifelong implications for physical, developmental and mental. The benefits of investing in children flow through to the entire population, with outcomes as diverse as greater productivity, lower burden of disease, stronger families, and safer and more connected communities. The health and wellbeing experience of children is thus increasingly being seen as having wide ramifications for the competence, coping and adaptability of human populations undergoing massive social changes associated with their transformation from industrial to globalized, information-based economies. Child health, as it was at the turn of the 20th century but for very different reasons, is once more at centre stage in the grand vision of improving the health and wellbeing of human populations.

**What are our ongoing challenges?**

- The health of Indigenous children remains significantly poorer on a range of indicators compared with the health of all Australian children.
- Some 40% of deaths in 1–14-year-olds are due to unintentional injury, a preventable cause of death.
- Rates of severe disability and diabetes are rising in children.
- An 'excess' of deaths of young children (100 per year) occurs in rural and remote areas.
- The teenage birth rate in Australia is higher than the OECD average, at 18 births per 1000 15–19-year-olds, 42% of whom smoke during pregnancy.

# Child health in a global context 1.2

Trevor Duke

## Introduction

In the 20th century there were dramatic reductions in child mortality and general improvements in child health in Western countries. These resulted from economic development, public health interventions, urbanization, better nutrition, maternal health and education, immunization and advances in health technology and curative care. Child mortality rates have fallen from over 100 per 1000 live births in the UK, North America, Australia, New Zealand, Japan, Scandinavian countries and western Europe at the end of the 19th century, to around 4–5 per 1000 live births at the beginning of the 21st century. The vast majority of the world's people who live in developing countries have not shared in this prosperity and progress. Although progress is being made in most countries, gross inequity exists, with sub-Saharan African and South Asian countries carrying the greatest burden of child deaths and morbidity.

The World Health Organization (WHO) estimated in 2000 that 10.7 million children under the age of 5 years die annually and 99% of these deaths occur in developing countries. By 2008, the estimated number of deaths had fallen to 8.8 million. Figure 1.2.1 shows the distribution of child mortality globally, the majority of under-5 deaths being concentrated in sub-Saharan Africa and South Asia. In 2010, it is estimated that 26 countries had child mortality rates greater than 100 per 1000 live births, all in sub-Saharan Africa except two, Afghanistan and Haiti. A further 30 countries had under-5 mortality rates above 50 per 1000 live births.

## Child health inequity

Inequity is unfair distribution, and child health has many layers of inequity. Inequity between regions and countries is brought into sharp focus in the 21st century because of globalization and freedom to travel. Countries that are half a day's flying time away from capital cities in Australia, for example, have child mortality rates 10 times higher than that of non-Indigenous children in Sydney or Melbourne.

Inequity exists also within countries. For example, in Papua New Guinea in 1999 the median child mortality rate was 89 per 1000 live births, but some provinces had under-5 mortality rates as low as 49 and others as high as 164 per 1000 live births. Similarly in Cambodia, the child mortality rates in various provinces ranged from 50 to 229 per 1000 live births. Urban child mortality is generally lower than rural mortality, for example: 43 versus 71 per 1000 live births respectively in South Africa. The neonatal mortality rate in remote mountainous areas of Vietnam is three times higher than in urban areas. In general, the rapid trend towards urbanization has contributed to lower child mortality, but some city slums in developing countries have rates of child disease and death that are higher than their nation's average.

Income is a major determinant of child mortality risk. In 2003, the average under-5 mortality rate was 123 deaths per 1000 in low-income countries, 39 in lower-middle-income countries and 22 in upper-middle-income countries. In high-income countries the rate was less than 7 per 1000. Within-country income inequity also has a great effect on child mortality risk. Among the poorest quintiles (the poorest 20%) of the populations of Cambodia and Vietnam, child mortality rates are two to three times higher than in the richest quintiles. Equity of income distribution is also an important determinant: countries with low gross domestic product (GDP) but a more even income distribution have much lower rates of mortality than other countries with higher GDP but inequitable income distribution. Maternal education and access to health services are also closely related to child mortality risk.

Disparities exist in the financial, technical and human resources available for child health, globally and within countries, and this is closely related to mortality risk. In 1973, Professor David Morley said of Nigeria: 'Three quarters of our population are rural, yet three quarters of our medical resources are spent in the towns where three quarters of our doctors live; three quarters of the people die from diseases which could be prevented at low cost, and yet three quarters of medical budgets are spent on curative services.' Unfortunately, the same is still true today of many developing countries. The doctor: population ratios

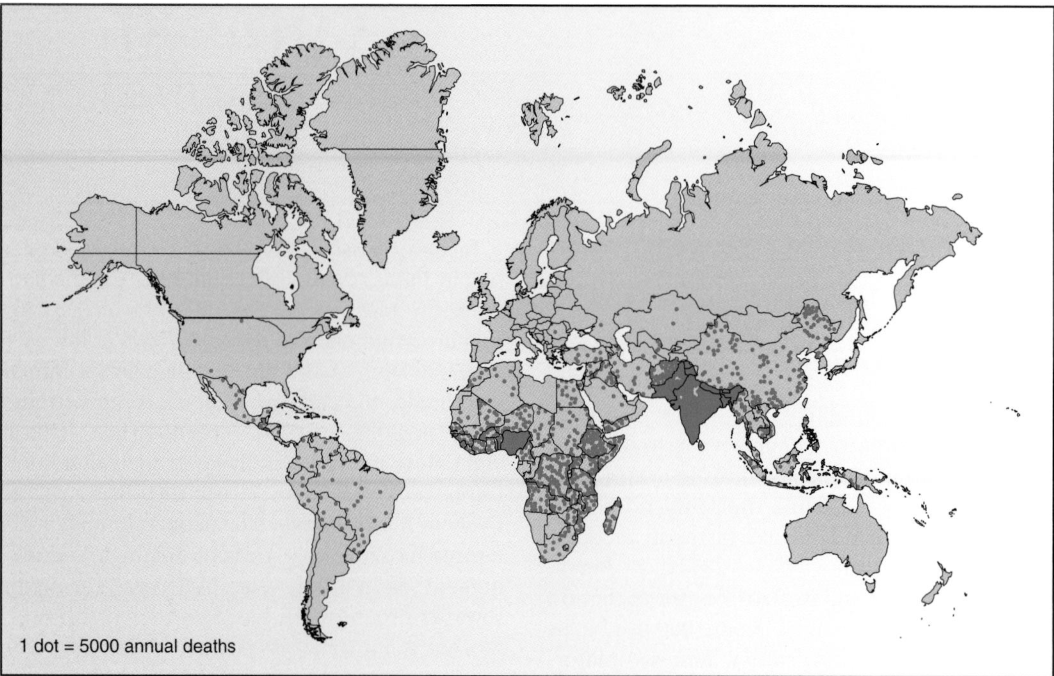


Fig. 1.2.1 The distribution of global child mortality. 1 dot = 5000 annual deaths. (Source: Black RE, Morris SS, Bryce J 2003 Where and why are 10 million children dying each year? Lancet 361: 2226–2234.)

of many countries are 20 times higher in cities than in rural areas. Differences in health service access between rural and urban populations manifest in disparities of functional outcomes as well as mortality risk. For example, compared to urban children with epilepsy, children with epilepsy in rural Zimbabwe are less likely to receive treatment (63% rural versus 95% urban), have a greater seizure burden (2.3 versus 1 per month) and are more likely to have problems that impair social and educational attainment.

Human resources in low-income countries are being further eroded by the drain of doctors and nurses migrating to richer countries. Human immunodeficiency virus/acquired immune deficiency syndrome (HIV/AIDS) has exacerbated this human resources crisis; to implement effective antiretroviral treatment programmes requires increased numbers of trained health workers. However, the cruel irony is that HIV/AIDS is claiming a major proportion of the young population of doctors and nurses in countries, particularly in Africa, that most need effective prevention and treatment programmes.

Research in child health is also disproportionate to the burden of diseases and inequitably distributed. While $73 is spent on health research per disability-adjusted life-year lost (DALY: an index that combines both mortality and disability) for diseases overall and $8.40 is spent on research into HIV, malaria and tuberculosis, only $0.51 per DALY is spent on research into acute respiratory infection and $0.30 per DALY on diarrhoea. Some 86% of scientific publications and 97% of patents are held by 16% of the world (the advanced economies), while the remaining 84% publish a mere 14% of the world's scientific papers and hold 3% of the world's patents. Therefore, between countries and for all major diseases, capacities to deal with child health problems are inversely proportional to the magnitude of the problems.

## Causes of global child mortality

The major causes of death in children aged under 5 years globally are listed in Table 1.2.1. The percentages vary widely across regions, with skewed distribution in the Africa region. For example, 94% and 89% of the world's malaria and HIV/AIDS deaths occur in Africa.

More than one-third of children who die in developing countries have moderate or severe malnutrition, and malnutrition is implicated in deaths from diarrhoea (61%), malaria (57%), pneumonia (52%) and measles (45%). However, malnutrition is often under-reported in national statistics and under-recognized

**Table 1.2.1 Major causes of death in children under 5 years of age globally, with estimates for 2000–2003 and 2008**

| | No. of deaths, in thousands | |
|---|---|---|
| | 2000–2003 | 2008 |
| **Deaths in children aged 1 month to 5 years** | 6685 (63%) | 5220 (59%) |
| Acute respiratory infections | 2027 (19%) | 1189 (14%)* |
| Diarrhoeal diseases | 1762 (17%) | 1257 (14%) |
| Malaria | 853 (8%) | 732 (8%) |
| Measles | 395 (4%) | 118 (1%) |
| HIV/AIDS | 321 (3%) | 201 (2%) |
| Injuries | 305 (3%) | 279 (3%) |
| Meningitis | | 164 (2%) |
| Pertussis | | 195 (2%) |
| Congenital anomalies | | 104 (1%) |
| Other | 1022 (10%) | 981 (11%) |
| **Neonatal deaths** | 3910 (37%) | 3573 (41%) |
| Pre-term birth | 1083 (10%) | 1033 (12%) |
| Severe infection | 1016 (10%) | |
| Sepsis | | 521 (6%) |
| Pneumonia | | 386 (4%) |
| Birth asphyxia | 894 (8%) | 814 (9%) |
| Congenital anomalies | 294 (3%) | 272 (3%) |
| Neonatal tetanus | 257 (2%) | 59 (1%) |
| Diarrhoeal diseases | 108 (1%) | 79 (1%) |
| Other | 258 (2%) | 409 (5%) |
| **Total deaths in children under 5 years** | 10 595 (100%) | 8793 (100%) |

Values in parentheses are percentages of total annual global deaths.

*The apparent dramatic reduction in pneumonia deaths in 2008 compared with 2000–2003 was highly dependent on data from China, the validity of which is uncertain. Note also that deaths from pertussis and meningitis were reported separately in 2008, and neonatal pneumonia was not specifically reported in 2000–2003 data.

Data from: World Health Organization 2005 The World Health Report 2005 – make every mother and child count. WHO, Geneva, p 190 (http://www.who.int/whr/2005/en/) and Black RE, Cousens S, Johnson HL et al. 2010 Global, regional, and national causes of child mortality in 2008: a systematic analysis. Lancet 375:1969–1987.

in clinical settings where childhood malnutrition is so common as almost to be the norm. The situation is even more complex than Table 1.2.1 suggests: although children often present with a single condition (e.g. acute respiratory infection), those who are most likely to die will often have experienced several other infections in recent months, have more than one infection concurrently (e.g. pneumonia and diarrhoea, or pneumonia and malaria) and have malnutrition with micronutrient (such as iron, zinc or vitamin A) deficiency.

## Progress in child mortality globally

Since 1990 there have been substantial reductions in deaths in children under 5 years of age. The child mortality rate was 11.9 million in 1990, 10.6 million in 2000, and one modelled projection for 2010 was 7.7 million, a 35% reduction over 20 years. Now no country has a rate of under-5 mortality more than 200 per 1000 live births, whereas in 2000 there were 10 such affected countries. The causes of this progress are many, but include better coverage of health interventions including immunization, vitamin A, insecticide-treated nets, prevention of parent-to-child transmission of HIV, the beneficial effects of urbanization and improved education for girls. In several low-income countries in sub-Saharan Africa there has been an accelerated decline in child mortality since 2000. One factor behind this is resolution of civil wars, allowing health services to re-establish and enabling basic health, education and community interventions to be more widely accessible. Understanding the broader determinants of child survival is crucial to understanding the potential impact of any intervention and the obstacles to reducing child mortality. A recent analysis of data from 152 countries found that gross national income (GNI) per capita, female illiteracy and income equality predicted 92% of the variance in child mortality. A recent study from the Gambia showed that community and social networks, personal support for caregivers in the home, and financial autonomy were more important determinants of child mortality than access to health services. Several large prospective studies have shown that access to community mothers' groups which support skills and care-seeking results in fewer neonatal deaths.

## Child disability and development

Like mortality, the capacity of countries to prevent and treat child disability is inversely proportional to the burden of the problems. Child disability and developmental problems occur at high rates in poor countries because of the frequency of neurological disease (including perinatal asphyxia, bacterial and tuberculous meningitis, cerebral malaria, viral encephalitis and neurocysticercosis), the contribution of undernutrition to developmental retardation (maternal malnutrition, low birth weight, iron and iodine deficiency), high rates of trauma and injury, *in utero* exposure to drugs and alcohol, congenital syphilis and rubella syndromes, and exposure to environmental toxins. Institutionalization of orphans and disabled children in some countries also contributes to severe developmental delay, because of emotional neglect and malnutrition. The lack of primary prevention, screening and rehabilitation services that might mitigate the effect of disabilities on function also worsens the impact of these conditions on individuals and the community.

In some countries, community rehabilitation services have improved the lives of many disabled children, iodine and other micronutrient supplementation and fortification programmes are under way, programmes for the primary prevention of injuries are starting, and increasingly developing countries are gaining access to vaccines that will prevent meningitis. However, more work in these areas is urgently needed.

## Neonatal health

More than one-third of all under-5 deaths occur in the first month of life (see Table 1.2.1) and the majority of neonatal deaths occur in the first few days after birth, making the neonatal period the most hazardous time of life. The majority of the 3.5 million annual neonatal deaths occur in socioeconomic deprivation in developing countries. Programmes to improve neonatal survival are focusing on supervised clean deliveries, essential care of the newborn (early breastfeeding, skin-to-skin warmth), steroids for preterm labour, antibiotics for premature rupture of membranes, maternal tetanus toxoid to prevent neonatal tetanus, prevention of parent-to-child transmission of HIV and identification of sick neonates requiring referral to hospital. Improving obstetric services is essential to addressing neonatal mortality, especially that due to birth asphyxia. WHO has produced guidelines for the management of seriously ill neonates in hospitals in developing countries. Improving neonatal health, particularly the reduction in low birth weight through improved maternal health, may reduce the risk of adult diseases such as hypertension, coronary artery disease and non-insulin-dependent diabetes, which form a large and increasing burden of non-communicable diseases in developing countries. As neonatal mortality falls, resources need to be available to deal with the increased morbidity that will occur in survivors. Such morbidities include malnutrition, chronic lung disease and neurological disease among survivors of prematurity. Mechanisms to follow up very low birth weight babies in low income countries are needed to optimize outcomes.

## Adolescent health

The health of young people (defined by WHO as aged 10–24 years) in developing countries has relatively recently been recognized as a high priority. Four out of five people between 10 and 24 years of age live in developing countries. Although mortality rates for adolescents in developing countries are much lower than for children under 5 years, the proportion of deaths occurring in adolescents is several times higher in developing countries than in industrialized countries. However, it is the future costs of current morbidity and the adoption of unhealthy behaviours by young people that pose the greatest risk and provide the greatest opportunities for prevention. As countries pass through economic transition, as the HIV/AIDS pandemic has developed and with increasing urbanization, the health problems of young people are increasingly on the global agenda. WHO estimates that half of all HIV infections have occurred in people less than 25 years old. There is high potential for prevention of many of the major diseases in adults by interventions targeted at adolescents. Indeed, improving the health of young people may be a major key to improving health at all ages: improving adolescent education, delaying reproductive age, improving nutrition and exercise, reducing smoking and drug and alcohol consumption, and preventing sexually transmitted infections will have beneficial effects on the young people themselves now and in decades to come, and reduce the burden of disease among newborns and children in future generations.

## Children in complex emergencies

Complex emergencies are identified as acute situations in which there is excess mortality (more than 1 death per 10 000 population per day). They may be due to natural (e.g. flood, tsunami or earthquake) or unnatural (war, famine) disasters, or both. With climate change and population growth placing increasing demands on the environment, conflict over basic resources is likely to increase. Complex emergencies are dynamic, with variable durations of emergency, recovery, resettlement, rehabilitation and development phases. After the initial disaster, high mortality rates are usually due to diarrhoeal disease, cholera and dysentery, measles, malaria, meningococcal disease, tuberculosis, neonatal causes, trauma, malnutrition and micronutrient deficiency. High rates of mental health problems, including post-traumatic stress disorder, depression and anxiety, have been reported in many studies of children living in refugee camps or exposed to violence or armed conflict. At the end of 2009, there were 10.4 million refugees under the mandate of the United Nations High Commission for Refugees (UNHCR), 4.6 million of whom came from Afghanistan and Iraq. In addition, there were 27 million conflict-generated, internally displaced persons, mostly in these two countries and in Somalia.

Many factors impede the delivery of health care in such situations, including lack of human resources and referral services, security constraints, poor supervision and coordination, and failure of integration with local health services or transition to a sustainable health system. In addition, lack of comprehensive guidelines and approaches, especially for the management of neonatal problems, HIV infection, mental health problems, and child and sexual abuse, limit the impact of health care in these situations.

## Climate change and child health

Like poverty, climate change has a disproportionate effect on the health of children, and is a major threat to progress in child survival. There is increasing evidence that many of the main killers of children (malaria, diarrhoea and malnutrition) are highly sensitive to climatic conditions. The regions of the world affected by malaria and dengue are expected to extend. In many Asian countries cholera is no longer a seasonal disease but occurs year round, likely because of increases in sea temperatures. Mass displacement because of rising sea levels in low-lying Pacific island nations and food shortages in other countries because of reduced arable land have their greatest effects on children in the poorest communities.

## The effect of poor child health on communities

Childhood disease has major effects on the economy and lives of families, communities and developing nations (see Clinical example). Poor health among children or a family member is a common reason for families sliding into poverty. For affected families, the cycle of poverty, poor nutrition, chronic ill-health and low educational attainment is common.

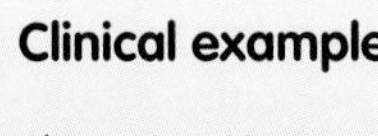

**Clinical example**

Chinua is a 10-year-old Nigerian boy who has sickle cell disease (HbSS). He has had repeated episodes of severe acute vaso-occlusive crises, and recently had a stroke, which left him with a mild left hemiparesis. Previously he had *Salmonella* osteomyelitis of the right femoral head. He walks with a crutch made by his father. He must take penicillin and folic acid daily. A doctor suggested that he could also take hydroxycarbamide (hydroxyurea) to reduce the frequency of crises, but Chinua's family cannot afford this. His mother, a weaver, can no longer trade because of Chinua's frequent need for hospitalization and care at home, and his father has used all the spare cash they had for transportation to the district hospital, clinical care and medicines.

## International conventions and child health

There have been several United Nations (UN) conventions designed to improve global child health in the last 30 years. The Declaration of Alma Ata in 1978 was one of the first to identify primary health as being crucial to child survival, and stressed that improvements in food security, clean water, sanitation, appropriate housing and education were crucial to progress. In 1990, the UN Convention on the Rights of the Child stated that all children have the right to the highest attainable standard of health, and access to care and medicines when they are sick, and held governments responsible for providing comprehensive health services. The mantra of the Declaration of Alma Ata was 'Health for all by the year 2000'. Sadly, for many reasons – the emergence of the HIV/AIDS pandemic, lack of political commitment, inadequate financing, a drastic human resources shortage and inadequate attention to non-health-sector elements – this ambitious aim did not come close to being realized. In 2000, the UN developed the Millennium Development Goals (MDGs) plan, which was signed by all UN member states and set specific goals in eight areas (Box 1.2.1). The fourth MDG calls for a reduction in child mortality. Specifically, MDG-4 states that countries should aim to reduce child mortality by two-thirds of what it was in 1990, by 2015. Some national governments have signed up to a modified target for MDG-4 to reflect what is feasible and realistic. Other MDGs are crucial to child health and development including: to halve the proportion of the population living on less than US$1 per day; to ensure universal primary education; to eliminate gender disparity in all levels of education; to reduce by three-quarters the maternal mortality ratio; to reverse the rising incidence of HIV, malaria and other diseases; to halve the proportion of people without sustainable access to safe drinking water and sanitation; and targets in development aid, market access, debt relief, employment and information access. Each of these goals has specific targets and indicators that can be used as benchmarks.

## Evidence for effective interventions in reducing child mortality

In 2003, *The Lancet* published a series on child survival, outlining the evidence for effectiveness of interventions in reducing child mortality. Twenty-three interventions (15 preventive and 8 curative) aimed at the commonest causes of child mortality had

**Box 1.2.1 The eight Millennium Development Goals and key indicators**

**1 Eradicate extreme poverty and hunger**
- Population below $1 a day (%)
- Percentage share of income or consumption held by poorest 20%
- Prevalence of child malnutrition (% of children under 5)
- Population below minimum level of dietary energy consumption (%)

**2 Achieve universal primary education**
- Net primary enrolment ratio (% of relevant age group)
- Percentage of cohort reaching grade 5 (%)
- Youth literacy rate (% ages 15–24)

**3 Promote gender equality**
- Ratio of girls to boys in primary and secondary education (%)
- Ratio of young literate females to males (% ages 15–24)
- Share of women employed in the non-agricultural sector (%)
- Proportion of seats held by women in national parliament (%)

**4 Reduce child mortality**
- Under-5 mortality rate (per 1000)
- Infant mortality rate (per 1000 live births)
- Immunization, measles (% of children under 12 months)

**5 Improve maternal health**
- Maternal mortality ratio (modelled estimate, per 100 000 live births)
- Births attended by skilled health staff (% of total)

**6 Combat HIV/AIDS, malaria and other diseases**
- Prevalence of HIV, female (% ages 15–24)
- Contraceptive prevalence rate (% of women ages 15–49)
- Number of children orphaned by HIV/AIDS
- Incidence of tuberculosis (per 100 000 people)

**7 Ensure environmental sustainability**
- Forest area (% of total land area)
- Nationally protected areas (% of total land area)
- GDP per unit of energy use (PPP $ per kg oil equivalent)
- Carbon dioxide emissions (metric tons per capita)
- Access to an improved water source (% of population)
- Access to improved sanitation (% of population)

**8 Develop a Global Partnership for Development**
- Youth unemployment rate (% of total labour force aged 15–24)
- Fixed line and mobile telephones (per 1000 people)
- Personal computers (per 1000 people)

high-grade evidence for effectiveness (i.e. large randomized controlled trials and/or systematic reviews). These interventions were selected for being low cost and having potential for implementation at near-universal scale in low-income countries. Some interventions protect against deaths from many causes. For example, breastfeeding protects against deaths from diarrhoea, pneumonia and neonatal sepsis, whereas insecticide-treated materials (bed-nets, sheets, etc.) protect against deaths from malaria and also reduce deaths from preterm delivery. However, with the exception of breastfeeding (estimated global coverage of 90%), global coverage of known effective interventions for reducing child deaths from common conditions is low.

To promote a comprehensive model of care for the sick child, in 1995 WHO developed the Integrated Management of Childhood Illness (IMCI). IMCI is a case management and training strategy that focuses on primary health workers managing the most important causes of childhood illness, including identification and treatment of children with multiple pathologies. Evaluation of IMCI in Bangladesh and Tanzania showed improvements in the quality of case management, and increased health-service utilization, increased rates of breastfeeding and nutrition practices, and lower prevalence of stunting. Now, more than 90 countries have adopted the strategy, albeit often in pilot projects with moderate coverage.

In recognizing that primary health care will have an optimal impact on child mortality only if there are effective referral services, WHO has produced complementary guidelines on paediatric care for district or provincial hospitals. These guidelines emphasize that diagnosis and drug treatment are not sufficient for optimal care of the seriously ill child, and that triage, supportive care (including fluids, oxygen, nutrition), monitoring, discharge planning and follow-up are also essential. These processes of care were found to be deficient in audits of practice in many developing and transitional countries, and there is now good evidence that mortality rates can fall substantially when these issues are addressed.

To move closer to MDG-4 in all countries by 2015, the focus will need to be on achieving universal access to health services and on improving equity. Limited resources may need to target interventions towards marginalized populations within low- and middle-income countries. These populations include the poor, refugees and internally displaced persons, families living in remote rural areas and urban slums, disaster areas and war zones, ethnic minorities, Indigenous populations, new immigrants, AIDS orphans, child workers, child soldiers and abandoned children. There is also a need for an 'enabling environment' for child health and survival: political commitment, adequate funding, human resources, community awareness and support, improvements in water, sanitation and the environment, and improvements in education and gender equality. The quality of care provided in health facilities and the nature of interactions between health systems, families and communities have major consequences for child health, human rights, poverty alleviation and development.

## How can child health professionals in developed countries contribute to global child health?

There are many pathways to meaningful contributions to global child health. However, they all require experience, technical expertise, perspective and cultural understanding. These prerequisites can best be gained by an extended time living and working in a developing country. This early experience, and the eventual expression of this work, can be immensely varied: working as a medical officer, nurse, teacher or researcher in a government hospital, university, public health service, mission hospital, research institute, non-governmental organization working with children, UN organization or collaborative institute for child health. A contribution can be made from virtually any specialty, but clinicians familiar with Western models of curative health care need to appreciate the central importance of public health. Skills in teaching, epidemiology, research and infectious diseases are especially valuable. In the forthcoming decades, increasing numbers of doctors and other health professionals from developed countries will make substantial, ongoing and career-long contributions to global child health, as part of their core work. For others, financial contributions to child health programmes in developing countries may be a preferred option. Whatever the pathways, there are several principles of international health collaboration that should be followed (Box 1.2.2).

**Box 1.2.2 Principles of global child health**

1. Focus on children who have least access to services
2. Support simple, low-cost interventions that can achieve high coverage
3. Improvement in nutrition is vital
4. Support national and local services and institutions, and deliver services where possible through existing local structures
5. Seek out, respect and support local human capacity; it is often greater than you think
6. Local ownership of ideas and strategies is essential for sustainability
7. Support multidisciplinary and multisector collaboration
8. Use a framework that incorporates human rights and equity
9. Critical evaluation of programmes is crucial to the efficient and ethical use of resources
10. Be patient – progress that incorporates these principles may not be fast, but it may be longlasting

The highest priorities for paediatrics in the 21st century are located firmly in the poorest areas of the developing world. Solutions will be largely local, although regional and global support for local initiatives and priorities is essential. Increasingly this is being recognized by individual health professionals, education and research institutions, medical journals and professional societies in developed countries.

PART 2

# CLINICAL ASSESSMENT

# 2.1 The clinical consultation

Mike South, Sean A. Beggs

The clinical consultation is the central act of medicine, with its primary aim being to arrive at a diagnosis and management plan that will assist the patient. For children, as with adults, there are three main pillars for arriving at a diagnosis, namely history, examination and investigations. In most presentations, the majority of the information required for a diagnosis comes from the history, with a smaller amount coming from the physical examination. In many cases, no investigations are required. A common paediatric scenario is one in which a difficult diagnosis is able to be made by an experienced clinician who simply takes a thorough history.

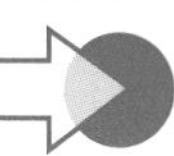

**Practical points**

- Skills in history-taking and examination cannot be acquired adequately by reading a textbook. Ensure you have lots of practice with children of all ages and in different clinical settings.
- Learn to appreciate what constitutes normal growth, development and physical findings on examination. Take every opportunity you can to observe normal children (who might be visiting the hospital or community health centre, in the cafeteria, or even travelling on public transport). Try to guess their ages from your observations (based on size, development and behaviour) and then ask how old they really are.
- Adapt the content and techniques of history-taking and examination to fit the age of the child and the urgency of the medical problem.
- Learn to be flexible in your approach – some patients will need to be examined on the floor, while in a play area, or from a distance.

## Planning your approach

To ensure you gain as much information as possible it is important to have given consideration to how you will approach the consultation. The basic structure of the clinical consultation is to take an accurate history and elicit all the relevant clinical signs in order to generate a differential diagnosis list and management plan. The use of a framework such as the SOAP note (below) is of great assistance when planning your initial approach to a consultation. This framework is also of great use when it comes to recording your notes. It facilitates recording them in a clear and concise manner that is easily understood by others involved in the care of the patient.

S – subjective: the history as given by the carers and child
O – objective: physical examination and results of investigations
A – assessment: primary diagnosis and differential diagnosis
P – plan: immediate and long-term plan to manage the patient.

When planning your approach to a paediatric consultation it is important to understand how children differ from adults. Consideration needs to be given to the age and developmental stage of the child, the setting and acuity of the presentation and how to best establish rapport with the child and family.

### Age and developmental stage of the child

The approach to clinical history-taking and physical examination of children differs from that used for adults; it also differs with the age and developmental stage of the child. These differences relate to the fact that children are growing and are acquiring new developing skills. There is also generally a third party (parent or caregiver) present, providing a significant component of the history. Therefore the description of symptoms may be modified by the parent's perceptions or interpretations, and by factors such as anxiety. These factors vary with age also. You will need to modify your approach to establishing rapport with the patient and how the examination is conducted according to the age and developmental stage of the patient. There are differences in the techniques of physical examination and in expected findings at different ages. Different aspects of the history will require emphasis at different ages. For example, details of the pregnancy and birth are relevant in infancy, whereas immunizations, growth and developmental milestones are important in preschool-aged children, and behaviour and schooling need to be explored in older children.

### Acuity of the presentation

The urgency of the presenting problem will impact significantly on how the consultation is conducted. In an emergency presentation, urgent treatment will obviously take priority over obtaining a complete history. It is, however, usually appropriate to return to aspects of the history at another time. For example, a complete past history and developmental assessment would not be necessary in a 4-year-old presenting with acute diarrhoea and vomiting, prior to commencing rehydration. However, it would be essential if the presentation was because of parental concern over the child's speech. In other cases it may be appropriate to *split the consultation into more than one session*. This is often appropriate for the assessment of more complex problems. Young children often become bored, tired, hungry or irritable if a consultation lasts more than about 30 minutes. This can limit their ability to concentrate or cooperate with the assessment.

**Clinical example**

Louise, a 4-month-old girl, was the first baby in her family. She was taken to the general practitioner by her mother, Mary, who was very anxious because she felt that her baby was constipated, with a bowel action only once every 3 days. Mary was worried that this was because she was not producing enough breast milk to meet Louise's needs. Mary had been advised by a relative to give Louise laxative drops and to switch to bottle-feeding.

Careful history-taking revealed that Louise was feeding well and was passing a partly formed stool every third day without difficulty. There were no abnormalities on examination. Her growth chart showed that she was gaining weight well and was tracking just above the 50th centile for her age. Mary was shown the chart to reassure her that her baby was thriving. It was explained that Louise's stool frequency was within the normal range for breastfed babies. Mary was encouraged to continue breastfeeding.

## Establishing rapport with the child and family

Your success in obtaining valuable information from the history and physical examination will depend on establishing a good relationship with the child and family. The parents need to know who you are, and to understand the purpose and likely outcome of the consultation. The child needs to feel comfortable in the environment and with you, particularly as you move on to the physical examination. Stranger anxiety, especially in children from about 8 months to 5 years of age, can be a significant obstacle. Experience and understanding help to overcome this.

Introduce yourself to the parents and, for almost all ages, to the child. Explain who you are and your role in the child's care. A common concern from parents of recently hospitalized children or children attending clinics is that they met many doctors and other health professionals, not really knowing who they were or who was 'in charge'.

Ask what name the child likes to be called by. How much you should talk directly to the child at this stage will vary with the age of the child and with your assessment of how relaxed the child is. Some children respond well to questions and comments about their favourite sports team, school or a toy they have brought with them, whereas others are shy and anxious if you address them directly. Learn to read children's responses and adapt accordingly. Young children may initially be very shy and cautious, and become much more confident and interactive later in the consultation.

Children's behaviour will often reflect how their parents are feeling. It is common for parents to be anxious when attending a medical consultation. If you can form a good relationship with the parents, they will feel more at ease during the consultation and you will also have a better relationship with the child.

Sometimes it is appropriate to reassure the child at the start that nothing unpleasant is going to happen during the consultation (e.g. no blood tests or 'needles'). The child may associate visits to the doctor with memories of past uncomfortable experiences. Never hesitate to explain why you are asking a certain question or why you are performing a particular part of the examination.

## The setting

The physical environment makes a big difference to how children feel. An adult may tolerate undressing in a cold room to be examined, but a 2-year-old will probably cry. A bright, colourful room with pictures on the wall and toys on the floor is much more conducive than a 'sterile' clinical environment. A good range of toys, drawing materials, puzzles and other activities for all ages will be helpful.

## Observation

It is important to remember that you can gain a significant amount of information regarding a child's state of health and development, prior to launching into the formal history and examination, simply by observation. It is important when planning your consultation to allow time to sit back and observe the child's interaction with their parent/carer and the environment. You should be able to assess whether the child looks well or unwell, is appropriately grown and developmentally appropriate for age. Your ability to do this will increase with experience.

## Referral information

You will often have referral information from another doctor in the form of either a referral letter from a general practitioner or the notes from the emergency department doctor. You need to take this information into consideration, but not trust it implicitly.

It is vital that you assess the child yourself and determine what you believe is the cause of the problem. Parents/patients often dislike having to repeat themselves several times, so it is important to explain clearly why you are asking them to repeat the story again.

## Taking the history

As mentioned above, the history is the most important component of the clinical consultation, as this is where the majority of information for making a diagnosis comes from. The basic outline or structure of paediatric history is the same as in adult medicine, but with the need for some variation in the areas that are focused on. This structure includes the following areas, which are described in more detail below:

- Presenting problem
- Past history
- Systems review
- Family history
- Social history
- Developmental history
- Behaviour
- Sleep
- Immunizations
- Medications
- Reviewing your understanding of the history.

It is worth remembering that a number of factors may impact on the taking of a paediatric history, such as how distressed the child is, the level of parental anxiety and sleep deprivation, which is common when looking after sick children. There will also be cases where the family do not speak English and it is vital to use an interpreter.

### The presenting problem

Start by asking the parent (and/or child) about the current problem or problems. It is important to find out what they perceive to be wrong and why they have chosen to seek medical attention at this time, and to get this information in their own words. It is also useful to ask what they believe the cause of the problem may be. Remember to use open-ended questions such as: 'Why have you come to see me today?' Allow the parent/child to provide the whole story before interrupting to clarify symptoms as this will disrupt their flow and may result in the omission of key information. Understanding the sequence and evolution of symptoms can be just as important as otherwise listing the symptoms themselves. Ensure you get the story from the beginning. Questions such as: 'When was she last completely well?' can be very helpful. The pattern of evolution will often reveal the diagnosis (e.g. central abdominal pain, later moving to the right iliac fossa in appendicitis). Parents know their children best and are generally good judges of when something is wrong. Their concerns should be taken seriously.

You then need to explore the symptoms in more detail; for example, if the presenting symptom is cough, you will want to learn its character, whether it is repetitive, whether it occurs under certain circumstances and whether it is moist or dry. When seeking extra detail or clarification, ensure your questions are open (e.g. 'Can you tell me about his bowel actions?') rather than closed (e.g. 'So he has not had any diarrhoea?'). It is important to gain information from the child as well as the carer. How you go about this will depend on the age of the child. For an infant it will be by observation alone, whereas an adolescent may well be the primary provider of the history.

Be sure that the parent understands the terminology you use and always avoid medical jargon. It is also important that you ensure you and the parents have the same understanding of terms that are used in everyday language but are also medical. For example, when a parent uses the term diarrhoea they may mean loose, but not frequent, stools. Or when they say, 'He vomited bile', are they referring to yellow gastric juices, which is often the case, or do they mean true bright green bile? You will want to enquire about appropriate epidemiological features such as whether anyone else in the family or other contacts has had similar symptoms, or whether anyone at home is a smoker.

Summarize your understanding of the symptoms and discuss this with the child and their parents once you feel you have a complete picture of the presenting problems and symptoms, to ensure that you have understood the information correctly and also to allow further information to be added if needed.

#### Clinical example

William, a 5-year-old boy, was brought by his parents for assessment because they noticed that he was tired each day in the late afternoon. He would lie on the sofa for up to an hour and be uninterested in playing during that time. Following this, he would seem to be his normal self.

This had been going on for nearly a year, since he started school. The rest of the history and examination were unremarkable. The parents' concerns seemed out of proportion to what is fairly common behaviour in early school-age children. When asked why they had chosen to seek a medical opinion now, they revealed that a child of one of the mother's work colleagues had recently been diagnosed with leukaemia, and tiredness had been one of the features of her illness. The parents' major concern was that William might have the same diagnosis.

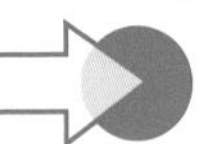

**Practical points**

- To obtain the trust of a child, you also need to gain the trust of the parent/s.
- Do not use abbreviations or medical jargon during discussion with the family (say 'blue' rather than 'cyanosed' and 'breathing difficulty' rather than 'dyspnoea').
- When the family use descriptions such as 'wheezing' or 'croupy', make sure that these words mean the same to them as they do to you.

## Past history

The initial enquiry about the past history seeks to gain information relevant to the current problem and age of the child. It is important to ask whether the current problem has ever occurred in the past and about past illness that might relate to the current presentation (e.g. a past history of meningitis will be very relevant for a 2-year-old who now presents with a seizure disorder). Then move on to the child's general state of health. Are they usually active and healthy? Have they had any other significant illness, operations or hospital admissions in the past?

For infants, it is important to obtain a history of the mother's pregnancy (her health, nutrition, use of medications, alcohol intake and smoking during the pregnancy, etc.), details of the birth (gestation, problems during labour, breech delivery, use of forceps or caesarean section) and the condition of the infant at birth (including the Apgar score, if known, and the need for any medical interventions such as oxygen therapy). What were the birth weight and other measurements? Ask about the infant's course in the first few weeks, including any illness and details of feeding and weight gain. Parents may have the child's health record, which will provide many of these details. Simple questions such as, 'Was the mother allowed to hold her baby immediately after birth?' and 'How soon was the baby discharged from hospital after birth?' can probe for problems. In young children, the early feeding history is also important.

Details of the pregnancy, birth and early course of postnatal life are usually of less significance for an older child presenting with an acute illness. They will be important, however, for an older child if the presenting problem is neurological or there is a concern about developmental progress.

## Systems review

A brief check for other symptoms should be undertaken, using the usual organ systems approach. Questions should be relevant to the current problem and the age of the child, rather than a long list of routine items. Ask about recent travel or potential environmental exposures if they are relevant to the presenting problem.

## Family and social history

These are in fact separate but closely aligned, and therefore are often enquired about at the same time. The young child's world is the family and it is important to obtain an understanding of the family and social contexts of the child's illness and management. Ask about the age and health of the child's parents and siblings. Who else lives in the same household, and who provides most of the child's care? Does the child live in more than one household, as is often the case when parents are separated? Does the child attend day care, kindergarten or school? Is there a family history relevant to the child's presenting problems?

Find out about the family's housing and economic situation. Are the parents employed? Do they receive any financial allowances or community services? Look for factors that might adversely affect the child's health (e.g. smoking by household members), or that may influence management decisions (e.g. if the family lives a long way from hospital and has no car).

It is usually useful to draw a brief family tree (Fig. 2.1.1).

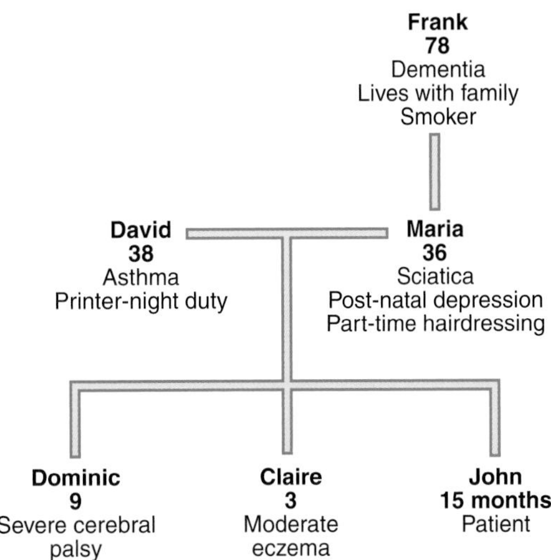


Fig. 2.1.1 This brief family tree reveals a lot about the genetic and environmental factors that affect John, who now presents with recurrent cough and wheeze.

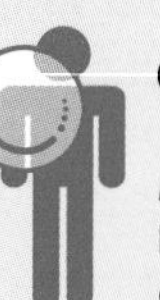

**Clinical example**

Mrs Baker brought her 10-year-old daughter, Ruth, for assessment. Ruth had previously been an outgoing and active girl but recently had seemed tired and listless, had lost her appetite and would often miss days of school because of headaches and abdominal pain. Mrs Baker was concerned that Ruth had an underlying illness such as glandular fever. Mrs Baker had had glandular fever herself when she was in her teenage years.

As part of the history-taking, enquiry was made about the family's current circumstances. Ruth's parents had recently separated, and Ruth, who had been close to her father, saw him only occasionally. Unfortunately, her parents were no longer on speaking terms. On examination, Ruth appeared well although she was rather withdrawn. Blood tests did not suggest any evidence of glandular fever. Ruth's symptoms were due to the changes in her parents' relationship and she was assisted by counselling and support from a child psychologist.

## Growth and development

One of the aspects of childhood that clearly differentiates it from adult life is that children are growing physically and acquiring new developmental skills. The achievement of a child's full growth and developmental potential is a central component of childhood and it follows that progress in this area requires careful assessment during the clinical consultation. During the history you should assess this via questions regarding the parents' perception and later confirm during the examination phase.

In infancy, growth is assessed mainly by checking for adequate weight gain, whereas in older children linear growth and appropriate body weight are both assessed. Where possible, birth measurements and any other previous growth measurement should be plotted on appropriate length/height, weight and head circumference centile charts (see Chapter 19.1). This provides two types of information: an estimate of growth achievement in comparison with that expected for the 'normal' population, and also growth progression with time in relation to expected genetic potential by observing 'tracking' along centile channels. Measurements are recorded most commonly in the parent-held child health record. An appropriate nutritional intake is an obvious and important prerequisite for normal growth: you should find out the usual daily pattern of food intake (breastfeeding in early childhood, type of formula feeds and intake pattern in later childhood) (see Chapter 3.3).

You should also ask questions to ascertain whether developmental progress is within normal expectations. This can be done for young children by asking specific 'screening' questions that determine developmental progress at hallmark ages for each of the four major areas of development: gross motor, fine motor/adaptive, language and special senses, and personal–social. This assessment has its greatest importance in the early years of life to enable early detection of developmental difficulties (e.g. hearing impairment, motor difficulties due to cerebral palsy) and allow early intervention.

For older children, ask about progress at kindergarten or school, including parents' assessment as to motor skills and cognitive abilities in comparison with siblings and peers. For school-aged children, enquire about special abilities that their child exhibits both in learning and in skills in sports or other activities. Ask children what they enjoy most in their learning activities ('What things are really fun to do?') and in what activities they see themselves as having special abilities ('What are you really good at?').

If this screening raises concerns, a more detailed developmental assessment is required (see Chapter 2.2).

## Behaviour

A brief history of the child's general behaviour is appropriate. Sometimes a perceived behavioural difficulty is the presenting problem and a more detailed history is necessary (see Chapters 4.1–4.3).

## Sleep

Sleep issues can often be a major concern for parents of young children. Poor sleep has been shown to have significant impact on a child's behaviour and development. It is important always to ask some screening questions regarding sleep; if these raise any concern, a more detailed history should be taken.

## Medications

Enquire about current and past medications, including any adverse reactions and suspected drug allergies. Ask specifically about prescription medications and over-the-counter items. Complementary or alternative therapies are now frequently used in children, but parents often forget or are reluctant to mention their use.

## Immunization status

Full details of past immunizations should always be obtained. Don't just ask: 'Is she up to date with immunizations?' or 'Has he had all his needles?' The answer you get will often be 'yes' and may be incorrect. Take time to go through what has been administered and compare this with the recommended schedule. Again, the child health record will be useful if available. Remember that, unless there is a specific contraindication, every clinical consultation should be seen as an opportunity to check immunization status and to offer immunizations that are due or have been missed (see Chapter 3.5).

### Closing questions

Complete the history-taking by providing the parent and child with the opportunity to add extra information that may have been left out and to air their own concerns about causes of the presenting problem. The following closing questions will sometimes bring out very important information:

- Is there anything else that is worrying you?
- Is there anything else I should know or anything I have forgotten to ask you?
- Do you have any ideas of your own about what may be causing your child's symptoms?

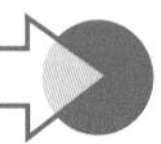

**Practical points**

- Always undertake a brief but accurate assessment of growth and development at any consultation.
- Remember to ask about all types of therapy used. Specifically enquire about complementary or alternative medications and other therapies.
- Always take the opportunity to check that the child has received all his/her immunizations at the appropriate ages.
- The closing questions will often be the ones to bring out the parents' deepest concerns regarding their child's problem. Don't omit this important opportunity, and leave yourself enough time to ask.
- Be observant of the child's physical activities and the child–parent interactions during the history-taking. These unstructured observations are an important part of the information-gathering process.

## The physical examination

### Introduction

The purpose of the physical examination is to provide additional information to aid in the diagnosis, assessment of the response to therapy, clues to co-morbidities, and important screening data on growth and development. By the time you are ready to move to the examination you need to ensure you have gained as much information as possible from observation. This is a very important technique with young children as they will not understand why they are being approached and touched by a stranger. Shyness and stranger anxiety may limit their cooperation and some will simply refuse any physical contact. This is particularly the case for children between approximately 9 months and 3 years of age. Obtaining cooperation and a successful examination requires skill, understanding and practice. Don't be surprised or concerned if you are unsuccessful sometimes: this also happens to experienced paediatricians. Try coming back to the examination at a different time or with a different approach.

Privacy during physical examination is just as important to children as to adults. You need to be friendly and relaxed, with a quiet and calm voice, and use gentle, unhurried physical movements. In young children you will often have to be opportunistic in your examination and be prepared to vary the sequence of the examination according to what the child is doing, examining them where they are most comfortable. For example, if a 2-year-old is asleep on his father's shoulder, take the opportunity to auscultate while they are quiet. In young children, ask yourself what are the most important items that you need to examine and do these first rather than adopting the more traditional sequence of examination used in adults and older children. Leave any potentially distressing components until last (e.g. examination of ears and throat). You may not be able to undertake all aspects of the examination at one time because it is tiring or frightening for the child. Do not push the child; be prepared to come back at a later stage to continue. Undressing a young child completely will often upset him or her, and you should consider what it is necessary to expose according to the clinical situation.

Hand hygiene is also very important. It is vital that you wash your hands, or use an alcohol-based hand rub, before and after every patient contact. This is the single most important measure to prevent hospital-acquired infections.

**Clinical example**

Ravi, an 18-month-old boy, presented to hospital with a history of cough and noisy breathing. His elder sibling had recently had a cold. Ravi was obviously frightened and upset when placed on the couch for the physical examination. He cried and clung to his mother's blouse when the emergency department resident tried to undress him.

David, the paediatric registrar, suggested that Ravi be placed on his mother's lap while he observed him from a short distance. The nurse handed Ravi a brightly coloured toy. He stopped crying and started to examine the toy. David was able to note that Ravi was well grown, did not look seriously unwell and was alert. He was pink in room air, there was a clear nasal discharge, and he had an obvious barking cough and mild stridor when resting. David asked that Ravi's mother lift his upper clothing to expose most of his chest. Ravi looked apprehensive but did not cry. David was able to observe good symmetrical chest movements with a respiratory rate of 22 per minute, and there was minimal indrawing of the intercostal soft tissues. David approached with his stethoscope but again Ravi looked as if he was about to cry. David knew that auscultation of the chest would not add much additional useful diagnostic information in this setting and so he desisted.

Ravi was diagnosed as having viral croup of mild to moderate severity.

Most paediatricians develop their own techniques or 'tricks' for obtaining a child's cooperation with aspects of the examination. Some techniques rely on distraction (e.g. producing a previously unseen toy just prior to auscultation of the precordium). Some may use an incremental approach to obtaining the child's confidence. For example, in an anxious child, one might commence auscultation of the lungs by placing the stethoscope on a less threatening area than the chest, such as the child's thigh, then moving it on to the chest once the child has learned that it is not uncomfortable. Alternatively one might auscultate the father's arm or back first so the child can see that nothing unpleasant is involved. With practice you need to learn methods that suit your own style of interacting with children of various ages. These skills cannot be learnt simply from a book but must be gained from experience of working with children of various ages.

It is important to emphasize that successful physical examination of children is not only about ticking boxes in a checklist. Knowing exactly what to examine in any given situation, how to perform the examination techniques in children of differing ages and how to interpret the results are much more important, and come only from experience in caring for children. Box 2.1.1 includes a list of the items that are commonly included during the physical examination as a guide only – don't use it as a checklist for every child.

## General observation and behaviour

What are your first impressions of the child? Does she look well or unwell, is she happy and relaxed, or does she seem tense and uncomfortable? Is she in pain? Is she of normal appearance or different from what you expect? Is she normally grown or small/large/obese/malnourished? Does she respond normally and in an age-appropriate way to her parents and siblings? How does she respond to you and to the surroundings? Is her understanding and language or other communication age-appropriate? Does she appear to hear and see normally? Is there anything obvious such as noisy breathing, increased work of breathing, jaundice, cyanosis, bruising, an abnormality of limb movement, skin rash or abnormal pigmentation? Does she move/crawl/walk/run/climb normally? Are her fine motor movements while playing, drawing or getting undressed and dressed normal?

These initial impressions can be of great importance and provide useful clues for your overall assessment of the nature of the child's health problems and their impact.

**Box 2.1.1 Items commonly included in the physical examination**

- Height*
- Weight*
- Head circumference
- Pulse rate*
- Respiratory rate*
- Blood pressure*

**General appearance**
- Looks well/unwell/sick/very sick*
- Alertness*
- Distressed/cooperative
- General body build
- Overall development including speech
- Facial appearance/dysmorphism*
- Posture, movement
- Interaction with parents*

**Skin**
- Colour/pigmentation/jaundice/cyanosis/pallor*
- Bruising/petechiae/rashes/scars
- Turgor
- Visible blood vessels
- Subcutaneous fat

**Nails/hair**
- Cyanosis/pallor/clubbing
- Haemorrhages
- Distribution and colour of hair

**Lymph nodes**
- Size/mobility/tenderness of nodes in each group (cervical, occipital, axillary, inguinal, etc.)

**Head**
- Size/shape/posture
- Fontanelles: presence/shape/tension
- Bruit/percussion

**Eyes**
- Appearance/blinking/ptosis/nystagmus
- Visual acuity/fields
- Ocular movements/squint
- Lids/discharge
- Fundoscopic appearance
- Light and corneal reflex

**Ears**
- Position/shape
- Discharge
- Hearing*
- Appearance of tympanic membranes

**Nose**
- Shape/flaring with respiration/discharge/bleeding
- Patency of airway/mucosal appearance/polyps

**Mouth/lips/teeth/gums/palate/pharynx**
- Colour of lips, tongue and buccal mucosa
- Presence of exudates/coating/ulcers
- Lip swelling or scaling/fissuring

*Continued*

- Number of teeth and presence of caries
- Breath odour/salivation
- Petechiae/bleeding
- Colour of pharyngeal mucosa
- Size, colour and presence of exudate on tonsils

**Chest/lungs**
- Shape/symmetry/deformities (including Harrison's sulcus, rickety rosary)
- Expansion of chest and pattern of breathing
- Soft tissue indrawing with respiration
- Pattern and rate of breathing
- Cough/stridor/wheezing
- Percussion note
- Breath sounds/added sounds

**Breasts**
- Development (Tanner stage)

**Heart**
- Appearance of precordium: deformity/activity
- Pulse: rate/rhythm/strength/nature
- Blood pressure
- Apex beat/cardiac impulse/thrills
- Percussion of cardiac dullness
- Heart sounds/added sounds
- Features of cardiac failure

**Abdomen**
- Shape/distension/visible mass/movement with respiration
- Visible veins/peristalsis
- Percussion/ascites
- Tenderness on palpation
- Enlarged organs/palpable mass
- Anus/rectum (avoid examination in children unless specifically indicated)

**Genitalia**
- Development (Tanner stage)
- Presence of testis in scrotum
- Scrotal swellings/hernia
- Urethral/vaginal discharge
- Evidence of injury

**Spine**
- Posture/deformity/hair/dimples/tenderness

**Limbs**
- Deformity/contractures
- Muscle development
- Hip dislocation (see Chapter 8.1)
- Joints: tenderness/swelling/range of movement
- Temperature/colour

**Nervous system**
- Alertness/responsiveness/general ability
- Abnormal movements/gait/posture
- Tone/power/coordination/symmetry of movement
- Reflexes/primitive reflexes
- Special sensory examination
- Sensation
- Cranial nerves

**Developmental assessment**
- See Chapter 2.2

Items marked with an asterisk (*) are usually included, whereas others will be noted in selected situations only.

## Measurements

Except in emergencies, measurement of weight and height (or length) and plotting these variables on centile charts should be a routine part of the examination for *all* children. Children are ideally weighed in only light undergarments, and in babies the nappy should be removed. In children under 2 years of age linear growth is assessed by measuring a lying length (Fig. 2.1.2), and the head circumference should also be measured and plotted. Length is best measured using a horizontal stadiometer. Head circumference should be measured using a tape measure that will not stretch. The aim is to measure the child's largest head circumference to the nearest millimetre. As a guide, place the tape measure above the ears, midway between the eyebrows and the hairline at the front and on the occiput at the back, then adjust to obtain the maximal measurement. Repeat this once or twice and record the largest measurement. After 2 years of age, linear growth is assessed by vertical height, and is best done using a stadiometer. In adolescents, it is important to assess the pubertal stage. This is obviously a delicate and potentially embarrassing examination for a teenager, and the required information can often be gathered from history and self-report rather than direct inspection (see Chapters 3.11 and 19.1).

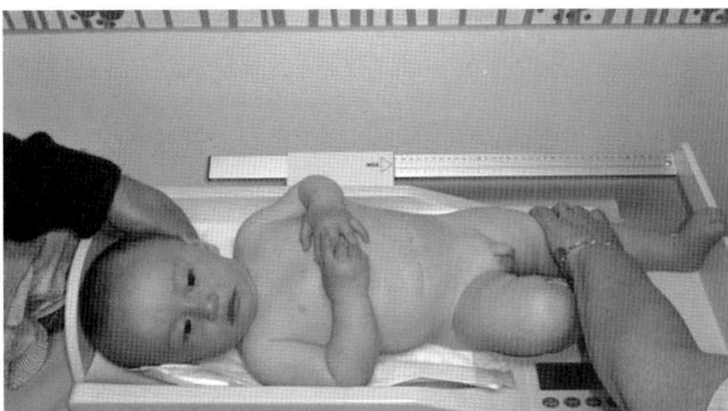

Fig. 2.1.2 Measuring the length of a young infant.

## Specific examination

It is assumed that the reader already has a good understanding of normal examination technique and expected findings for adult patients. There are many differences in the techniques and expected findings in children; these are emphasized below.

## Vital signs

Normal ranges for heart rate, respiratory rate and blood pressure vary with age. Table 2.1.1 gives approximate values for children at rest. Note that upper normal values for blood pressure can be different in boys and girls. If hypertension is suspected, consult age- and sex-specific graphs for blood pressure. Selection of an appropriately sized cuff for the age and size of the child is important for accurate measurement of blood pressure. The measuring of blood pressure can be quite upsetting so it is often best left until late in the examination.

## Respiratory system

Respiratory presentations are very common in children, so it is important to have a good understanding of how to examine the respiratory system in children. Initial inspection should look for any signs of increased work of breathing, such as nasal flaring, use of accessory muscles, head bobbing in infants, intercostal and subcostal recessions. The pattern of respiration in young infants often has a large abdominal component. The chest wall is compliant, so conditions that cause reduced lung compliance or airway obstruction will more readily be manifest by indrawing of the soft tissues of the chest wall, and in more serious disease the rib cage itself may be drawn in during inspiration. You should also inspect the shape of the chest wall and look for any asymmetry of chest wall movement. Listen for any added respiratory sounds such as an expiratory grunt or inspiratory stridor. As mentioned above, it is important to be opportunistic, so if the child is settled you may want to start with auscultation prior to moving on to other aspects of the respiratory examination. The breath sounds in infants are more readily heard because of the thin chest wall, and they often sound harsher on auscultation than in older children and adults. These normal differences in auscultation findings are even more pronounced in the upper parts of the right lung, sometimes leading inexperienced examiners to suspect pathology in this area in young children when in fact the breath sounds are normal for this age. Part 14 outlines the findings you would expect with various respiratory illnesses.

## Cardiovascular system

Cardiac disease affects approximately 1 in 100 children in developed countries, with the majority of these being congenital heart disease (CHD). Thus the focus of the cardiac examination in children is to detect signs of CHD, including potential secondary heart failure. Again, if the child is quiet, take the opportunity to start with auscultation before moving on to the other components of the cardiac examination. Listen to the heart rate: is it regular? Pay attention to the heart sounds: What is the quality and intensity, particularly of the second heart sound? Is there abnormal splitting or an added heart sound? Are there any murmurs? If so, are they systolic or diastolic? What is the quality and location of the murmur? Does it radiate? Then, if the child remains cooperative, you can go on to complete a full cardiovascular examination if indicated. A thorough description of examination of the child with suspected heart disease is provided in Chapter 15.1.

## Abdomen

Compared with older children, the abdomen of a young infant appears protuberant, and the umbilicus may be everted as a normal finding. The liver is normally palpable up to 2 cm below the right costal margin, and it is sometimes possible to feel the tip of a normal spleen and the lower pole of the right kidney.

When examining the abdomen it is important to consider the reason for the examination and thus what you are expecting to find or exclude. Is it simply part of a routine physical examination and you want to

**Table 2.1.1 Some normal ranges for vital signs at different ages in childhood**

| Age | Respiratory rate (breaths/min) | Heart rate (beats/min) | Systolic blood pressure (mmHg) |
|---|---|---|---|
| Newborn | 40–60 | 100–160 | 50–75 |
| 1 week to 3 months | 30–50 | 80–160 | 50–85 |
| 3 months to 2 years | 20–40 | 80–140 | 60–100 |
| 2 years to 10 years | 14–24 | 60–100 | 70–110 |
| >10 years | 12–20 | 50–100 | 85–120 |

exclude any asymptomatic masses or hernias, are you doing it for recurrent abdominal pain or a possible acute surgical abdomen? The indication will determine how you approach it. If there is pain, remember to start away from the pain; while palpating, always look at the child's face for indications of discomfort that would otherwise be missed.

When palpating the abdomen, the ideal position of the patient is lying flat on an examination couch, with relaxed abdominal muscles. This will often not be possible in young children as they will become distressed and cry, thus tensing their abdominal muscles. For young children it is often possible to examine them lying on their parent's lap, or a combination of the parent's and examiner's laps. If this is not successful, you may need to resort to palpating the abdomen with the patient sitting or standing.

Rectal examination should not be performed routinely. If indicated by the presenting problem, it should be undertaken only once and by the person who will be making management decisions based on the findings (e.g. a surgeon).

### Genitalia

In infant boys, assessment of the penis and scrotum should be considered part of the normal routine examination, as unsuspected inguinal herniae, undescended testes and urethral abnormalities may be detected. It is normal for the prepuce to be non-retractile and adherent to the glans up to around 4 years of age.

In girls, examination of the genitalia is usually undertaken only when indicated because of a specific problem. In instances where a genital examination beyond simple external observation is required in a girl, this should be done by an appropriate specialist.

### Central nervous system

Formal examination of the nervous system is time-consuming and many aspects require cooperation from the patient. In young children, observation of movement and behaviour can provide most of the necessary information, with specific neurological examination being reserved for children where the primary concern is the nervous system. Routine sensory examination is necessary only rarely.

### Skin

Examination of the skin is important not only in dermatological problems: congenital skin lesions may give diagnostic clues to other conditions. For example, the characteristic pale patches of tuberous sclerosis may provide the diagnosis in a child who is being assessed for developmental delay and seizures (see Chapter 21.1).

### Musculoskeletal system

As with the neurological system, a great deal of information regarding the musculoskeletal system can be obtained by observation, and a full formal examination is required only when it involves the primary problem. An important exception to this is that examination for developmental dysplasia of the hips should be routine in young infants (see Chapter 8.1).

### Special senses

From the history and general observation, you should be able to assess that the child can see and hear adequately. Screening examination for hearing and vision must be age-appropriate (see Chapters 22.1 and 22.2), and formal assessment by an audiologist or optometrist should be organized if there are concerns.

### Development

A brief screen of developmental achievements and progress should be undertaken; a significant amount of information regarding development will again be gained from observing the child. Can she walk? How well does she manipulate the toys? Is she using appropriate language for her age? Detailed assessment is not routine unless indicated by the clinical problem, or concerns are raised during the consultation (see Chapter 2.2).

### Head and neck

In babies it is important to examine the head shape, to palpate the fontanelles and the sutures, and to plot the head circumference as outlined above. The posterior fontanelle is often closed by 2 months of age, and the anterior fontanelle usually closes between 8 and 24 months of age. However, there is a wide range of normal with some closing by 3 months. The more important factor to consider, however, is head growth; it is reassuring if this is tracking along the centiles.

Examine the teeth, if present, for their number, pattern of eruption, and the presence of caries or abnormalities (see Chapter 22.3). Take this opportunity to remind parents of the importance of good dental care and of regular attendance at a dentist.

Examination of the mouth, throat and ears requires good cooperation or appropriate positioning of the child. It also has the potential to upset the child, so is usually best left until last. For examination of the ears, the recommended positioning is to have the child sitting on their parent's lap facing sideways; the parent then cuddles the child's head into the chest with one hand and places the other over the child's arms (Fig. 2.1.3), and if necessary has the child's legs

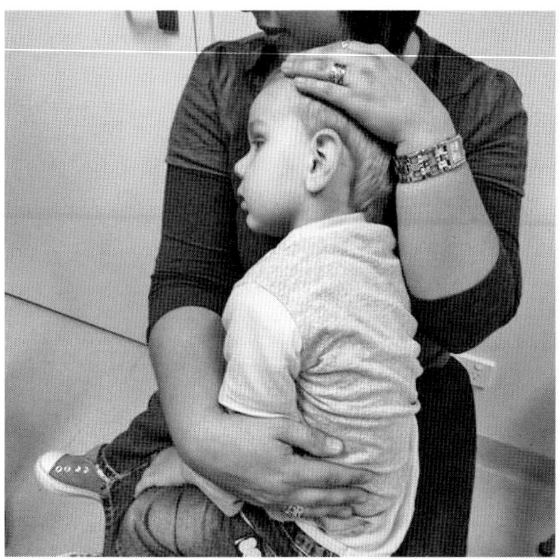

Fig. 2.1.3 Holding a child ready for ear examination. Note the position of the mother's hands.

between theirs, while the ear is examined. The child is then turned to face the opposite direction and the procedure is repeated to examine the other ear. To examine the mouth and throat, the child is then turned to face forwards; the parent then cuddles the child's head into their chest again with one hand and the other cuddles their arms (Fig. 2.1.4). The doctor can then examine with or without the aid of a tongue depressor. Observation of experienced practitioners will assist with learning these techniques.

### Concluding the examination

As for taking the history, it can be helpful to ask the parent or child whether there is anything else they would like you to check at this point. Your examination may also have revealed findings that prompt you to return and take further details in the history.

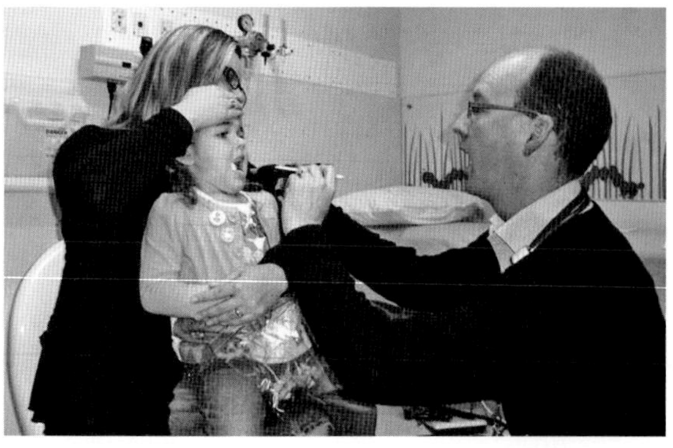

Fig. 2.1.4 Examining the throat. Note the mother's hands restraining the child's head and arms.

### Examinations at specific ages

There are several specific ages that differ sufficiently from your general paediatric examination that they deserve individual mention. They include the examination of the newborn, the 6-week review and the approach to an adolescent.

#### Newborn

It is recommended that all newborn infants have a full and detailed physical examination within the first 48 hours of life. The findings of this examination should be recorded in the child health record and conveyed to parents. The purpose of this examination is to check that the infant is healthy, check for significant abnormalities, and establish a baseline including weight, height and head circumference for future assessments. A detailed outline of the newborn examination is provided in Chapter 11.1.

#### 6-week review

This is generally the first medical review and examination of a baby after leaving hospital. It provides an opportunity for health promotion advice, and for the parents to express any concerns. The main purpose of the examination at this age is to detect congenital heart disease, developmental dysplasia of the hip, congenital cataracts and undescended testis.

#### Adolescence

This is often a time of increasing self-awareness and self-consciousness regarding body and appearance. This can mean that the idea of a physical examination is quite confronting. It is important that this is handled in a sensitive manner. This is covered in detail in Chapter 3.11.

## Note-taking

It is important that you produce an accurate and clear record of the history and examination findings. This will be needed to help you later and as a record for future staff involved in the child's care. A few items will need to be jotted down briefly as you go along, but the rest of the record should be written after the consultation is completed. You will not develop a good rapport with the family if you are constantly gazing at your papers and writing notes.

In younger children, you will have adapted the order of the physical examination to fit the clinical problem and their tolerance of the examination process.

Whatever the sequence in which you obtain your information, it is still important to record your findings in a logical and structured format. It is also vital that you record what your assessment is, including a differential diagnosis and what your short- and long-term management plan is. The use of the SOAP note format may facilitate this.

## The consultation as part of the therapy

Doctors often think of the management of a clinical problem as a chronological sequence commencing with history-taking and examination, followed by formulation of a differential diagnosis, appropriate investigations, final diagnosis, treatment, assessment of response and outcome. Most families who have an ill child will not arrive at the consultation with you with that same perspective. They will have come because they perceive that their child has a problem and they will often be anxious that it might turn out to be serious. They will be in a foreign environment and one that may have frightening associations for them. They may not know who exactly you are nor whether you are the best person to help them with their child's problem.

You will be in a position to help ease at least some of the family's anxieties long before you have even arrived at a diagnosis. You can achieve this by being friendly, by explaining who you are, and by conveying that you are genuinely interested in their concerns and that you value their time and opinions as much as your own. Use language they understand, give them time and opportunities to express their concerns fully, be gentle and caring during your examination, and give a clear explanation of what you think the problem might be and the nature and purpose of any investigations or treatment that you recommend. In this way, you will help to obtain the family's confidence and trust, which in turn will improve their willingness to cooperate with the plan of investigation and treatment that is required.

You will not acquire all of these skills overnight but learning them is rewarding and fun, and you will be a much more effective doctor for children and their families at the end of the process.

# 2.2 Developmental surveillance and assessment

David Starte, Carolyn Cottier

## Introduction

### Development as part of life

We continue to develop new skills throughout life, but it is during childhood, particularly the first 5 years of life, that the majority of basic skills are acquired.

Doctors learning about child development often wish to memorize lists of milestones, but fail to appreciate the diversity of normal variation. We do not expect an even distribution of talents among adults, yet we often assume children all develop similarly. It is the variability in normal patterns of development that makes the area fascinating and creates complex challenges in screening and diagnosis.

### Parents know their own children best

Child development starts with a good history. Parents are often remarkably accurate at recalling recent developmental achievements and changes, but more distant events may require prior notice so that sources such as relatives and baby books can be reviewed. A simple questionnaire filled in before the interview can allow parents to consider these details in the waiting room or at home. Parents should be asked open-ended questions about their child's progress, such as 'Tell me how she is getting around', as they are more likely to elicit revealing answers than 'Is she walking now?'. This process is time-consuming and parents need to feel relaxed and unhurried if they are to give their best information. Some of the information may well be sensitive, especially when there are problems, and a private setting without interruptions is important. Developmental interactions are best scheduled for a well-child visit or review to avoid confusing illness behaviour with developmental delay.

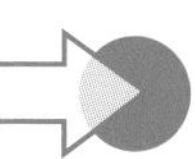

**Practical points**

- Always take any parental concerns or history of regression in skills very seriously (worried parents are usually right!).
- Surveillance and screening take place to ensure there are no warning signs of potential problems – if in doubt refer for therapy/intervention and then review.
- False reassurance must be avoided. Do not reassure unless you are certain of normality.
- All developmental diagnosis is dimensional across different areas of development and behaviour. It's not black and white, but which shades of which colours blend to make up the rainbow.
- Discussion of diagnosis/prognosis requires time, privacy, empathy, honesty, cultural sensitivity and both parents whenever possible. Details of what is said may be forgotten, so written reports are essential.
- Each assessment must produce a practical written action plan that is given to the family and others involved. Otherwise, it is at risk of being ineffective.

**Clinical example**

Sinclair, a 3-year-old child of English-speaking parents, had a vocabulary of only 20 words. His medical history was normal. The parents were reassured by his normal hearing assessment, as well as by the father's own history of initial poor speech development as a child. However, the preschool staff became concerned about the degree of his language difficulty and whether it was part of a global developmental delay. The words he knew were used singly, were clearly articulated and were used in their appropriate context, but, to indicate his needs, he resorted to leading an adult by the hand. No phrases or small sentences were heard. He understood two-step commands and used facial expressions, hand gesturing and eye-to-eye contact appropriately. At preschool, he was interested in the other children, but they often excluded him in play when he couldn't talk properly. He showed examples of imaginative, constructive and cooperative motor play. There were no behavioural concerns and he was an affectionate child.

Assessment with the Griffiths Mental Developmental Scales showed that his abilities tested within the average range for his age, other than a mild delay in speech and language skills. During the assessment, he was cooperative and persevered with the tasks at hand. Sinclair therefore had an isolated expressive language disorder of presumed familial origin, and was referred to a speech pathologist for assessment, therapy and liaison with the preschool teacher to modify his preschool curriculum.

### History is everything

A good developmental history starts with the pregnancy and delivery, and progresses through the neonatal, infancy, toddler and preschool years; it should be a routine part of all paediatric interactions. The doctor requires a working knowledge of normal development

**Table 2.2.1 Areas of development**

| Area | Description |
|---|---|
| Gross motor | Large muscle movements – walking, running, jumping, climbing and riding |
| Fine motor | Small muscle movements – grasp, release, drawing, speech clarity |
| Language | Receptive – understanding others<br>Expressive – own thoughts output<br>Pragmatic – social use, conversation |
| Social and daily living skills | Adult and child interaction<br>Feeding, dressing, washing, toileting |

and needs to be aware of the significance of variations that may indicate a developmental disorder. Child development progresses in many areas simultaneously (Table 2.2.1). It is as necessary to know the various developmental systems as it is to know the physical systems. Each will have its component parts, and the rate of progress in all of these components may be similar (when all are delayed, this is described as global delay) or discrepant (described as a specific delay in one area).

## Checking the normal (surveillance)

### What are the normal ranges?

The key is to look for areas of development delayed beyond the normal range and not to compare the child with 'normal milestones', which are merely the average age of achievement. By definition, half of the population will not meet median milestones, and their use can worry parents unnecessarily ('milestones are millstones'). It is preferable to use the normal ranges in Table 2.2.2. Many developmental patterns are familial, but so are many developmental disorders, so it is unwise to accept delay as a normal variation. Just because an uncle did not talk until he was 4 years old does not mean he did not also have a developmental language disorder or deafness. Other 'causes' such as being a twin, bilingualism or tongue-tie can produce minor variations, but not significant delays needing more formal diagnostic assessment. Assuming that the child's delay is caused by these minor variations is a common source of late diagnosis and delayed effective intervention. The most important conclusion that needs to be drawn from this surveillance is that there are no warning signs of a potential problem (Table 2.2.3). Should doubt exist, it is always better to seek a second opinion and to arrange some therapy or intervention than to provide false reassurance. It may make you feel better to reassure, but families who waste months finding help for their child will often feel let down.

### Any interaction is an opportunity to examine

As each area is reviewed through the different stages of childhood, any apparent delays or unusual features can be clarified with the family. This allows the developmental examination to be targeted. Although many children are shy and perhaps fearful, a quiet and patient approach will often bring out the show-off in children, especially for tasks about which they are

**Table 2.2.2 Normal ranges for children's developmental progress (approximately 25th to 90th percentile)**

| Age | Gross motor control | Vision and fine motor | Language and hearing | Social and daily living skills |
|---|---|---|---|---|
| 2–4 months | Head steady in sitting | Follows object through 180° | Squeals with pleasure | Smiles |
| 5–8 months | Sits without support | Passes cube from hand to hand | Turns to soft voice<br>Baba/Gaga babble (to 10 months) | Feeds self biscuit |
| 9–14 months | Stands with support | Neat pincer grasp of raisin | Mama or Dada specifically | Indicates needs by gesture |
| 12–16 months | Walks well alone | Stacks two cubes (to 21 months) | Three words (to 21 months) | Drinks from a cup |
| 15–24 months | Walks up steps | Scribbles spontaneously | Points to one body part | Removes garment |
| 21–36 months | Jumps on the spot | Draws vertical line in imitation | Uses plurals and phrases | Puts on clothing<br>Plays tag with other children |
| 3–4½ years | Balances on one foot for 5 seconds | Copies a ladder<br>Draws a face | Understands cold, tired and hungry<br>Asks 'Wh' questions | Separates from mother |

**Table 2.2.3 Warning signs to worry about; be concerned if the child is *not* doing this (but items marked with an asterisk (*) are a worry if they *are* present)**

| Age (months) | Gross motor control | Vision and fine motor | Language and hearing | Social and daily living skills |
|---|---|---|---|---|
| 3 | Complete head lag* | Following with eyes | Searching for sounds with eyes | Smiling |
| 6 | Persistent Moro reflex* | Preference for one hand*<br>Squint* | Head turn to soft voice | Interest in people |
| 9 | Sitting with support | Persistent hand regard* | Ba-ba-ba babble | Awareness of strangers |
| 12 | Pulling to stand<br>Standing with support | Pincer grasp | Trying one or two words | Constant mouthing* |
| 18 | Walking alone | Constructive play with blocks<br>Casting toys* | Six words<br>Constant dribbling* | Pointing at items<br>Finger-feeding |
| 24 | Running | Turning book pages | Fifty single words | Interested in other children<br>Helps with dressing |
| 36 | Kicking a ball | Drawing lines<br>Preference for one hand | 2–3-word phrases<br>Echolalia* | Interactive play with peers |
| 48 | Pedalling and hopping | Drawing a face | Sentences and 'Wh' questions | Imaginative role play<br>Toilet-trained by day |

confident. For this reason it is best to start looking at non-verbal areas (blocks, puzzles, drawing, etc.) and having appropriate furniture at the child's height will enable you to get down to the child's eye level. Simple equipment (Table 2.2.4) can be used to elicit a range of skills and the session should remain a play activity. Remember that too much direct eye contact, especially from above, can be threatening, and a relaxed tangential approach across the child may be more successful. Refusal to cooperate is a regular occurrence and it is better to reschedule than to persist and teach the child the sessions are going to be unpleasant.

The aim of the medical examination (see Chapter 2.1) is to detect any condition that might be causing the developmental delay, or indeed any general medical problem that may be exacerbating it. You should note the child's growth parameters, especially head circumference, and any signs of dysmorphism or neurocutaneous disorders.

**Table 2.2.4 Developmental equipment**

| Area | Equipment | Activity |
|---|---|---|
| Gross motor | Steps<br>Tennis ball<br>Tricycle | Crawling and walking up and down<br>Throwing, kicking and catching<br>Riding and pedalling |
| Fine motor | Raisins<br>Small blocks<br>Inset puzzles<br>Crayon<br>Paper (with child scissors) | Pincer grasp and feeding<br>Building, colour matching and counting<br>Matching and sorting shapes<br>Scribbling, drawing lines and shapes<br>For above plus cutting and folding |
| Language | Doll<br>Simple picture book<br>Toy telephone or dictaphone | Identifying and naming body parts<br>Pointing to items and describing the action<br>Encouraging speech samples |
| Social and daily living skills | Mirror<br>Toy cup, plate and cutlery | Watching baby's response to self<br>Feeding the doll and pretend tea party |

Although a thorough physical examination is desirable, particular attention needs to be paid to the neurological system, looking for signs of cerebral palsy and other neuromotor disorders (see Chapter 17.2). Some ingenuity may be needed after a long developmental session to re-engage the child in play.

Vision and hearing are vital for children's learning. For intervention to be as effective as possible, these senses need to be sharp. It may therefore be of more service to the child to arrange an opinion from a vision or hearing professional than to perform a rough screening test, which can miss minor problems that are easily remediable. Again, avoid false reassurance at all costs.

## Looking for problems (screening)

Screening is the process of detecting presymptomatic disorders in order to intervene and change their natural history. Screening uses tests of known accuracy in healthy or at-risk populations to uncover those with the target problem before symptoms arise. Further diagnostic testing can then be performed, before appropriate intervention is carried out. In the developmental context, tests are sometimes used to formalize the screening process. Examples are:

- Parent's Evaluation of Developmental Status (PEDS) – 10 simple questions about parental concerns (www.pedstest.com)
- Denver II – American observation schedule of four areas of development (www.denverii.com)
- Australian Developmental Screening Test (ADST) – Australian observation schedule (www.pearsonpsychcorp.com.au)
- Ages and Stages Questionnaires (ASQ) – structured parent questions for different ages (www.brookespublishing.com).

As developmental delays produce detectable symptoms, regular review of the various developmental areas at all doctor visits may well be a more effective method of detection than formal screening procedures at specified intervals. This surveillance is enhanced when combined with parent education about child development.

## Diagnosing disability (assessment)

Whilst this process is broadly a more detailed version of simple surveillance, it is common for doctors with particular experience in the area to be involved in teams with other professionals with specific expertise. These professionals may be:

- social workers or community nurses, who are skilled in family support/interactions
- psychologists, skilled in intelligence testing and behavioural interventions
- physiotherapists, with skills in movement and coordination
- speech pathologists, with language and oromotor assessment skills
- occupational therapists (OTs), with daily living skills, seating and manual dexterity expertise.

### Team benefits

In good teams, all members learn from one another and considerable role release can occur. Some specialized teams will need specific expertise from orthoptists, audiologists or orthotists, as well as technical support personnel to help with specific equipment. Clinics specializing in developmental assessment may be located in major hospitals with paediatric services or in community-based health centres.

It is important to be clear about the family's expectations of the assessment, so that their agenda is covered fully. It may be helpful to arrange a home visit by one of the team initially to break the ice with the family and see the child in more natural surroundings. Most families are understandably anxious about a formal developmental assessment, as it may lead to bad news. Anything done to reduce the family's apprehension will also be likely to reduce the child's fears and improve the reliability of the assessment as a sample of the child's development. To this end, the venue for the assessment should not be overly clinical and the staff should be understanding and welcoming.

### Clinical example

Max was a 3-year-old boy with an unremarkable past medical or family history. However, from the age of 2 years there had been concerns about his development, in particular his language and gross motor skills. A previous speech pathology assessment revealed a mild receptive and expressive language delay. Despite progress with speech therapy, a review of his general development was requested because of concerns that he was also stumbling when running. Compared with his sister, he was slightly later in sitting (8 months) and walking (15 months), and he initially had difficulties in climbing frames, but he still could jump or kick a ball well, and walked up and down stairs one step at a time. Max was examined using the Griffiths Mental Developmental Scales, which showed age-appropriate puzzle skills, low-average range for fine motor and language skills, and slightly more delayed gross motor skills. On examination, he had a lordotic posture, a waddling gait, only slightly overdeveloped calf muscles, and mild difficulty getting up from a sitting position on the ground. A proximal myopathy was suspected in association with his very mild developmental delay. The initial creatine kinase level was 33 000 units/litre and a dystrophin gene analysis was arranged. Max went on to have a muscle biopsy, which showed the typical changes of Duchenne muscular dystrophy.

Important aspects of the developmental assessment process are:

- multidisciplinary team approach
- colleagues working as equals
- good information gathering before the assessment
- standardized tests of development and intelligence
- standardized behavioural questionnaires
- specific therapist reviews as clinically indicated (physiotherapist, OT, speech therapist)
- ample time and privacy to discuss the findings with the family
- written reports to the family with a plan of action
- follow-up on any recommendations made.

### Test batteries

Most teams attempt some form of formal test of developmental status, often carried out by the psychologist or doctor, to assess the degree and distribution of any developmental delay or disability. This is not just to gain a score, but to provide a structured way of reviewing all aspects of cognitive development in an age-appropriate framework. In young children, this may be a developmental test such as the Griffiths or Bayley scales. In older children a standard intelligence test is often used such as the Weschler tests (WPPSI or WISC), or the Stanford–Binet scales.

A developmental quotient (DQ or GQ) derived from the former tests includes aspects of self-care and motor development, and is a broader concept than intelligence quotient (IQ), which relates more specifically to cognitive capacity. It is usual to talk about a delay in development when the child is young (say under 3 years of age) and the prognosis uncertain. When it seems that the child has a permanent developmental disorder, it is better to call it a disability, as many parents assume that any delay will eventually resolve. In addition, specific behavioural questionnaires may be used to assess the severity of symptoms suggestive of autism, attention deficit/hyperactivity disorder (ADHD), or other behavioural disorders such as oppositional defiant disorder or anxiety disorders.

### Medical investigations

Investigations that may be useful and should be considered in situations of possible developmental delay are:

- formal hearing and vision testing
- low average to borderline delay alone: consider degree of variation from family norms to judge need for investigation
- mild/moderate/severe/profound delay with language delay: chromosomes or comparative genomic hybridization (CGH) array, DNA for fragile X, thyroid function, creatinine kinase
- severe intellectual deficit: as above, plus lactate/pyruvate, amino and organic acids
- large head, central nervous system or skin signs: computed tomography (CT)/magnetic resonance imaging (MRI); consider neurologist opinion
- small head: TORCH titres; mild maternal phenylketonuria; MRI, consider neurologist opinion
- loss of speech skills: sleeping electroencephalography (EEG); neuro-metabolic tests
- old houses, renovations, pica: blood lead
- syndromic or dysmorphic features: genetics opinion before specific DNA studies.

#### Clinical example

When Jesse was 2 years 1 month old, he was referred for assessment of his development because of speech and language delays. On the developmental assessment he displayed a mild developmental delay overall, with an age equivalent level of 1 year 5 months. His weaknesses were in the areas of personal–social, language and fine motor skills, which were moderately delayed (1 year age equivalent level). His strength was in gross motor skills, which were normal (2 years 4 months age equivalent level). Speech therapy and occupational therapy were arranged and when he started preschool an individualized educational programme was established for him. Jesse was reviewed again at the age of 3 years 11 months and still showed an overall mild delay (2 years 7 months). Gross motor skills remained his personal strength, being within normal limits, and his puzzle-solving skills had improved to a borderline level. However, his weakest areas continued to be language and fine motor skills, which were still moderately delayed.

Speech therapy and occupational therapy programmes continued, and a special needs teacher was arranged to provide further educational support at preschool. At the age of 5 years 2 months a reassessment was arranged to plan for school placement based on his general learning progress and support needs. He was assessed using the Differential Ability Scales (an IQ test), which demonstrated a general conceptual ability around the first percentile (IQ = 63), in the mild deficit range. When considered together with parental, teacher and therapist reports, and his two previous developmental assessments, it was clear that Jesse had a long-term intellectual disability of mild degree. Mainstream kindergarten placement with integration support was arranged, with possible progression to an appropriate smaller support class at primary school age. Gross motor skills are not a good guide to intellectual development.

It should be remembered that investigations in these situations should be explained and offered rather than being just ordered: not all families are as focused on aetiology as medical staff. (See http://www.genetics.edu.au/factsheet for patient-friendly information about inheritance and genetic conditions.) Many parents' decisions about investigations will be influenced by whether they are planning to have further children.

Many children referred to developmental teams will already have a diagnosis such as Down syndrome or cerebral palsy, but some conditions are less obvious and need particular vigilance, for instance velocardiofacial syndrome, fragile X syndrome (see Chapter 10.3), thyroid deficiency or lead excess and, in boys, muscular dystrophy. Investigations or further opinions should be recommended to families as needed, to help exclude any conditions that appear possible. Modern genetic arrays looking for known deletions and rearrangements have the highest positive yield in most developmental presentations. Imaging and EEG testing are less rewarding unless specific signs or symptoms of neurological disorder are present.

## Practical outcomes

A feedback session after team members have discussed their opinions can be scheduled on the same day or later. It is always helpful if both parents are present and any close family supports they request, such as grandparents. Once the team's view has been clearly stated, it is normal to ask for the family's reaction and to discuss this. This will hopefully lead to discussions covering investigation, aetiology, prognosis, genetic advice and a plan of action. Recommendations can be formulated with the family as to what needs to be done by whom, where and when. This all needs to be recorded carefully and copies given to the family on the day, as much of what is said may be forgotten, especially when the news is shocking. However, the manner in which it is imparted is likely to be remembered for all time, and care taken with the time available, privacy and, if necessary, the use of interpreter services will help to optimize a potentially traumatic session.

All parents need copies of all the reports generated; further copies can be sent to professionals involved with the child if the family agrees. Follow-up can be arranged to review any investigations or to help establish intervention services. Many parents feel a sense of grief if the child has a serious developmental problem, and it may be necessary to provide written material and counselling to help them understand that this is a normal reaction. Failure to resolve the grief reaction can lead to ongoing anger, depression or marital conflict, and may delay important remedial action for the child.

### Clinical example

At 4 years 3 months, Adrian had only three recognizable words. He avoided eye-to-eye contact, and paid little attention to what was asked of him, preferring to play alone. He made sounds as he wandered around a room, laughing and giggling for no apparent reason, looking at himself in the mirror and often flapping his fingers close to his face. He was quiet, becoming upset only with the sound of a vacuum cleaner or a passing police car siren. He appeared distant, not giving or accepting affection spontaneously. He was toilet trained and could undress completely, but needed assistance to get dressed. He could not pedal a tricycle, and had poor ball-playing skills and an immature pencil grip with only circular scribbling. At preschool he needed constant direction and encouragement by the staff, and he had not developed any friendships.

Assessment with the Griffiths Mental Developmental Scales indicated a moderate developmental disability with non-verbal skills at around 2–2.5 years, but his verbal skills were found to be further delayed at 12–18 months. His behaviour was consistent with a diagnosis of autistic disorder, as he had a specific impairment in forming social relationships, in communicating and in playing imaginatively, in addition to his developmental disability. Adrian had high support needs and required intensive educational programming and behaviour modification to develop to his optimum potential. It was suggested that he be enrolled in a special school for children with disabilities.

PART 3

# SOCIAL AND PREVENTATIVE PAEDIATRICS

# 3.1 The child and the family

Neil Wigg

## Introduction

The ecological model of the determinants of children's health, development and wellbeing places the child at the centre of expanding spheres of influence. Surrounding the child is the family, the family's community and the wider society. A child's family exerts direct influences on the growing child and mediates the potential influences, both positive and negative, of the community, society and culture of origin.

The vast majority of the developmental health needs of children are met within the context of their family. A healthy child is one who is physically well, whose emotional needs are met and who is socially adjusted. Each of these needs has several parameters, which are discussed below.

### The physical needs of the child

- Care and protection from violence
- An adequate diet to provide for nutritional needs
- Protection against heat and cold in early life, and protection against physical dangers, such as fire, electricity, water, poisons and motor vehicles
- Prevention of illness through good living standards, education, health surveillance, immunization and other public health measures. A home environment that is free of tobacco smoke, lead and other toxins.

Children grow and thrive in the context of close and dependable relationships that provide love and nurture, security, responsive interaction and encouragement of exploration. Without at least one such relationship, development is disrupted and the consequences can be severe and longlasting.

### The emotional and social needs of the child

- The opportunity to grow up in a family context with close and dependable relationships with one or more adults (parents)
- Consistent, positive caregiving
- Reasonable limits to be set on the child's behaviour
- Feelings of being worthwhile and concern for the wellbeing of others
- The development of self-help skills and a sense of achievement
- Opportunities for play, recreation and companionship
- Opportunities to learn and explore
- Sensitive responses to emotional needs during illness, particularly in chronic illness
- Recognition of each child's individuality
- Recognition of the basic rights of every child, as outlined by the United Nations Declaration of the Rights of the Child.

To meet the physical, social and emotional needs of their children, parents and others in a caring role must fulfil their own needs. Caregiver needs include:

- adequate housing and transport
- freedom from unnecessary economic stress
- freedom from community and domestic violence
- easy access to family support and early childhood services, such as child care, health and education services
- knowledge of how to access community supports and services
- social networks and extended family supports, community and cultural connections
- an understanding of child development and behaviour.

The growth and development of a child in the family and community context are determined by the interplay of genetic, physical, social and emotional factors, and experience. The balance of risk and resilience factors influences a child's developmental pathway.

*Risk* factors preventing optimal progress might include:

- family conflict and disintegration
- economic disadvantage (low household income)
- parental mental health disorders
- individual child factors, such as low intellectual ability or difficult temperament
- external factors, such as unsafe neighbourhoods, environmental threats, war, etc.

Balanced against these are *resilience* factors, which are protective and promote wellbeing:

- safe, nurturing home environment
- consistent, supportive caregiving
- individual factors, e.g. normal intellectual ability
- sense/experience of success, self-determination and achievement.

### The building blocks for intellectual development

There are many components of the family and societal environment that are important in the intellectual development of the child. Some of these are:

- a loving and nurturing caregiving/family environment
- child-rearing beliefs and practices that are designed to promote healthy adaptation
- the opportunity to play, learn, explore and communicate
- the growth of self-regulation of physiological systems, emotions, behaviours and social interactions
- positive and consistent human relationships
- access to developmentally appropriate educational settings: children are active participants in their own development and learning
- good physical health.

As a child grows from a newborn infant to an independent young adult, his or her social environment expands and diversifies. A young infant has all its needs met within the immediate family. Contact with other young children is important for the social and emotional development of the preschooler. A young teenager may spend more time with peers than with her or his family. The structure of the family, the style of parenting and the capacity to support the growing child's progressive independence are all important determinants of the health and wellbeing of children.

## The family

'Families are big, small, extended, nuclear, multigenerational, with one parent, two parents, and grandparents. We live under one roof or many. A family can be as temporary as a few weeks, as permanent as forever. We become part of a family by birth, adoption, marriage or from a desire for mutual support. As family members, we nurture, protect, and influence each other. Families are dynamic and are cultures unto themselves, with different values and unique ways of realizing dreams. Together, our families become the source of our rich cultural heritage and spiritual diversity. Each family has strengths and qualities that flow from individual members and from the family as a unit. Our families create neighbourhoods, communities, states and nations.'

(Developed and adopted by the New Mexico Legislative Young Children's Continuum and New Mexico Coalition for Children, June 1990.)

## The Australian family

Australian society is multicultural, with pluralistic values and child-rearing practices. Child- and family-centred health care of children and young people should be carried out within the cultural and values framework relevant to the child.

**Clinical example**

Leanne was the 4-year-old daughter of professional parents who had migrated from another country in Asia. Her behaviour was demanding, overly active and often aggressive. Her communication skills were delayed. Both parents stated that in their families of origin children were not disciplined until school age and were cared for by the extended family.

Behavioural intervention needed to include these views of parenting.

Traditionally, Australian families have been made up of mother (usually at home), father, and two or more children. However, this picture of the 'nuclear' family no longer represents the Australian family. Families may be comprised of:

- couples with or without co-resident children of any age (85% of Australian families in 2006–2007)
- lone parents with co-resident children of any age (14% in 2006–2007)
- other families of related adults, where no couple or parent–child relationship exists (1%).

The proportion of Australian couple families with children has been decreasing over the last 10 years (down to 45% of couple families in 2006–2007). The proportion of one-parent families with children of any age declined slightly in 2006–2007 compared with previous years (14% in 2006–2007, down from 15% in both 2003 and 1997).

Many families in Australia do not contain dependent children. The Australian Bureau of Statistics (ABS) reports that, in 2006–2007, for families with dependent children aged 0–17 years:

- 80% of children lived in couple families (73% with both natural parents, 4% in step families and 3% in blended families)
- 20% of children lived in one-parent families
- of children living in one-parent families, 85% lived with the mother and 15% with the father (17% and 3% of all families with children, respectively)
- in 2006–2007, there were also 7000 foster families where there was one or more co-resident foster child.

Three demographic trends have altered the structure of Australian families with children:

- the rate of parental separation and divorce
- the age of having the first child
- the decision of women/couples not to have children.

During the past 20 years, marriage rates have fallen, and the age at first marriage and age of first birth have increased. The median age of first birth is now over 28 years. Consequently, family size is smaller.

- In 2006–2007, 15% of all adults reported that while they were children (under 18 years of age) their parents or guardians had either divorced or separated.
- There has been an increase in *de facto* relationships, which have become more socially acceptable in the last 20 years, including those in which children are involved. Marriage rates are not a measure of family formation.
- Family size and fertility rate are falling for all Australian women, both Indigenous and non-Indigenous, although these remain higher for Indigenous women.

### Families at work

Workforce participation rates for family members have increased in many developed countries in recent years. However, unemployment is also common, particularly in single-parent families. These changes have the potential for significant effects for children.

- In 2003, in couple families where the youngest child was under the age of 15 years, at least one parent was in employment in 94% of families. Both parents worked in 59% of these couple families.
- In lone-mother families where the youngest child was under 15 years of age, nearly 55% of mothers were not employed.
- In lone-mother families where the youngest child was aged 0–2 years, only 28% of mothers were employed.
- Couple families with children under 15 years of age had an average income 2.8 times that of lone-parent families.
- The proportion of all children under 15 years living in families without a parent employed fell from 19% in June 1994 to 17% in June 2004.

In 2006–2007:

- Both parents were employed in 63% of couple families with co-resident dependent children.
- There were 508 000 dependent children (10%) living in a household where no-one was employed.
- For lone mothers with dependent children, 34% of those whose youngest child was 0–4 years were employed, mostly on a part-time basis.

For many Australian families with children it is essential financially for both parents to have paid employment. 'Mum at home and Dad at work' is not the reality for most children. Accessible and affordable childcare, family day care, after-school care or other informal childcaring/minding arrangements are needed.

Coincident with these changes in families and communities, the incidence of child abuse (physical, emotional and sexual) is thought to have risen over the past three decades; however, data about the rates of abuse are incomplete and much goes unrecorded.

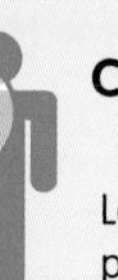

**Clinical example**

Lone parent Sharon, aged 24, and her three preschool-aged children live in an outer metropolitan suburb in a shared house. Jack, her second child, has delayed speech development and difficult behaviour. Jack was diagnosed by the local general practitioner as having chronic middle ear disease, but the waiting list for ear surgery at the children's hospital in town is almost 2 years. Sharon cannot afford private health insurance (and faster access to surgical care) or the long-term medication required for Jack.

## Children of families in distress

### Economic disadvantage/poverty

Poor people are more likely to have poor health. There is a gradient of socioeconomic effects on health: the more affluent you are, the more likely you are to experience good health; the poorer you are, the worse your health is likely to be. There is no particular cut-off point for economic advantage above which health is protected.

Low household income is associated with lower purchasing power, material deprivation and reduced ability to participate in everyday community activities.

Low-income households tend to occur in neighbourhoods that have fewer communal resources and where the social and physical environments are hazardous. Being poor is often also associated with much greater stress, feelings of lowered self-worth, powerlessness and helplessness. Mental and physical health problems follow.

International standards define poverty as a household income of less than 50% of the median income for that nation or state. In 2005, 12.8% (1 in 8) of Australian children lived in poverty.

Single-parent families are much more likely to live in poverty. The resulting inadequate diet, lack of opportunities and emotional stress may be coupled with the emotional turmoil that children and parents experience in separation and divorce. In general terms, children in one-parent families have poorer mental and physical health than their peers in two-parent families. However, much of this difference can be explained by lower household income and the stress of financial hardship. Fortunately, the majority of children in one-parent families still experience good health.

Low family income may affect the health of the children in many ways, such as:

- lower birth weight
- lower rates of breastfeeding
- poor vaccination rates
- poor growth
- higher rates of infectious disease.

A recent study by the Benevolent Society (2010) of unemployment and the well-being of children aged 5–10 years demonstrated a marked increase in conduct problems, peer relationship problems, emotional problems and hyperactivity problems of children from 'unemployed families' compared with those from families where an adult was employed.

### Indigenous families

Indigenous Australians (Aboriginal and Torres Strait Islander peoples) have poorer health than other Australians. Indigenous children have poorer nutrition and growth, higher rates of infectious disease, higher injury rates, and high rates of infant and child mortality (see Chapter 3.2).

The reasons for the persistence of the relatively poor health of Indigenous children are complex. Certainly living conditions, fewer educational opportunities, and poor access to goods and services all contribute. So do cultural disruption, high levels of poverty, lack of access to culturally acceptable health care, and racism.

The meaning and structure of family varies with culture. Aboriginal and Torres Strait Islander peoples have diverse and enduring cultures that endow families with special responsibilities for the care of children, the social life of communities, and the continuance of culture and customs. Family takes on more than biological and parenting relationships to include communal, customary and spiritual relationships. In many parts of Australia, Indigenous cultures are under major threat.

#### Clinical example

Taliah is the third child of a 21-year-old Aboriginal mother. The family lives in a small town in the Northern Territory. Taliah is 6 months old, growing and developing well, is breastfed and is free of illness. Her older brother and sister have much poorer health. Before her birth, Taliah's mother had joined the local 'strong women, strong babies, strong communities' programme.

Approximately half of all Aboriginal and Torres Strait Islander Australians now live in major metropolitan areas. Family structures and supports and communities are increasingly diverse and non-traditional. The health care of each individual Aboriginal and Torres Strait Islander child and family needs to take these changes into consideration, and provide care with respect given to family, community and cultural expectations.

### Immigrant families

Multicultural Australia includes many immigrant groups whose children are at greater health risk. Many families come to Australia to escape persecution and civil disruption in their own countries, and they bring with them the legacy of trauma and loss.

The major problems experienced by ethnic minority groups include lack of employment opportunities (and associated low household income), social isolation, unfamiliarity with health care and other social services, and barriers due to communication problems and cultural differences.

Culturally sensitive health-care services that include bilingual workers and interpreter services are essential. Doctors and other child health workers should recognize the vast range of child-rearing and health-care practices of ethnic groups in Australia.

### Families affected by mental health problems and drug abuse

Children's early development and health depends on the health and wellbeing of their parents. Postnatal depression is relatively common, affecting about 15% of mothers. Severe postnatal depression impacts on the establishment of infant–mother relationships (known as attachment). Disorders of attachment result in infant health problems, such as sleep problems, failure to thrive, disturbed behaviour such as excessive crying, and subsequent emotional and behavioural problems.

Children who grow up in families where one or both parents have a mental health problem frequently experience inconsistent parenting and disturbed relationships within the family. The scene is set for such children to develop behavioural, emotional and mental health problems.

The Western Australian Child Health Survey in 1995 identified that 20% of 12–16-year-olds had a significant mental health problem. Thus 1 in 5 teenage schoolchildren will have a mental health problem and most will not seek or receive treatment (see Chapter 4.2).

Alcohol is by far the most widely used and abused drug in our society. Drinking alcohol is not only accepted but is expected behaviour in Australia. Approximately two of three men and one in two women drink alcohol at least once a week. Of those who drink, about 10% of men and 6% of women are in the medium- to high-risk groups. The abuse of alcohol by one or both parents has a profound effect on the family.

**Clinical example**

Six-year-old twins Jonas and Jonno are now in long-term foster care, after lengthy periods of intermittent parental and temporary out-of-home care arrangements. Jonas is overactive, aggressive toward other children and his caretakers, and attention-seeking. Jonno is failing at school and is encopretic. Formal developmental assessment of both boys indicates 'normal potential'. The boys' mother has a history of substance abuse, postnatal depression and ongoing mental health issues. Alcohol abuse and violence perpetrated by their father led to parental separation 2 years ago.

Children of alcohol-dependent parents suffer anxiety and unhappiness, and may be exposed to violence and argument. In many cases this leads to the child becoming antisocial, engaging in alcohol/drug use, and developing mental health problems such as depression. Alcohol and drug (e.g. heroin) addiction frequently leads to financial stress in a family, together with deterioration in family relationships and parental separation. The consequences on children are severe.

### Family violence

Some 16% of Australian couples experience violence in the relationship. For 4% of couples the level of physical violence is such that physical harm is a likely outcome.

Our society tolerates high levels of violence in the media, in sport and in the community generally. However, violence in the family context has a profound effect on children. Violence between parents is frequently associated with violence towards their children.

Children who witness violence as a 'problem-solving' technique at home may adopt similar patterns of behaviour, particularly when they themselves become parents.

## Family-centred care

The hallmarks of family centred care are:

- Respect and dignity. Health-care practitioners listen to and honour patient and family perspectives and choices.
- Information sharing. Health-care practitioners communicate and share complete unbiased information with patients/families: patients/families receive timely, complete and accurate information in order to participate effectively in care and decision-making.
- Participation. Patients and families are encouraged and supported in care and decision-making at the level they choose.
- Collaboration. Patients/families are also included in service policy and development, facility design and professional education.

## Services for the child and family

General or primary care practitioners (family doctors) provide the mainstay of health services for children and families. These primary health-care services are complemented by a range of government-funded community health and social services, and non-governmental services. The following are given as examples and constitute a 'system of services' that promotes the developmental health of children and support families in the care of children.

For families with young infants:

- well-child care in child health centres
- home visiting programmes for families with additional needs, e.g. Family Care Program, Good Beginnings
- residential services
- parent help lines, child health lines (24-hour, 7-day telephone advice lines)
- printed and online information services.

For families with preschoolers:

- health surveillance, including immunization and health promotion
- injury prevention and safety promotion
- health service component to childcare and preschool services
- telephone and other information services
- health screening prior to school entry – provided by child health nurses, general practitioners (Healthy Kids Check)
- developmental assessment clinics and early intervention services.

For families with school-aged children:

- support services provided by education departments, e.g. guidance officers, counsellors
- assessments of children by child health nurses
- health education
- community mental health services
- school oral health (dental) services.

The Federal government in Australia provides a number of pensions or benefits administered by Centre Link and the Department of Family and Community

Services. These include the family allowance, childcare supplements, supporting parents and carer benefits.

State governments and non-governmental agencies (often church-affiliated) provide many family and community support services.

Similar government-funded services are provided for families in many other countries.

The field of family support services is complex and accessing 'the right service at the right time' is frequently a major problem for families experiencing distress. Family doctors and other child health workers need to know about the child and family services available in their area, and about government benefits for families.

# 3.2 Indigenous culture and health

The word Indigenous, meaning native, is used to describe the ancient or native population of a country. Indigenous populations have almost always been affected by colonization and migration of other populations and are almost always in a position of social disadvantage relative to the rest of the country's population. This social disadvantage is reflected in major inequalities of health.

There are Indigenous populations in countries throughout the Asia–Pacific region, as well as elsewhere in the world. For this chapter, the editors asked Paul Bauert and Francis Abbott to write about Aboriginal and Torres Strait Islander children in Australia, and Leo Buchanan to write about the Maori and Pacific island populations in New Zealand.

## PART 1 ABORIGINAL AND TORRES STRAIT ISLANDERS

Paul Bauert, Francis Abbott

### A definition of Aboriginal and Torres Strait Islander people

In Australia, the word Indigenous is used to refer to the Aboriginal and Torres Strait Islander peoples of Australia and is used by the Australian Bureau of Statistics (Indigenous Statistics for Schools), which also outlines the most widely adopted definition of Aboriginal or Torres Strait Islander (the 'Commonwealth working definition'):

> 'An Aboriginal or Torres Strait Islander is
> - a person of Aboriginal or Torres Strait Islander descent,
> - who identifies as being of Aboriginal or Torres Strait Islander origin and
> - who is accepted as such by the community with which the person associates.'

Australian Indigenous peoples are many diverse groups, with varying cultural ways, languages, traditions and names for themselves. The health-care professional should use a formal, accepted and respected name that people in the local community use to refer to themselves, some examples of which are:

- New South Wales – Koori
- Victoria – Koorie
- Queensland/North New South Wales – Murri
- South Australia – Nungah
- Western Australia (south-west) – Noongar
- Tasmania – Palawa
- North-east Arnhem Land, Northern Territory – Yolngu
- Tiwi Islands, Northern Territory – Tunuwi
- Jabiru region, Northern Territory – Binjing.

### Health care and cultural safety

Expressions such as 'cultural awareness', 'cultural safety', 'cultural security' and 'cultural competence' are often used and discussed in the literature in relation to organizations, health services and health care, and to individual service providers' abilities to interact appropriately and effectively with people of other cultures. Individual cultural competence has been described by the Northern Territory Government as having four components:

- Awareness of one's own cultural world view
- Attitude towards cultural differences
- Knowledge of different cultural practices and world views
- Cross-cultural skills.

Many jurisdictions and organizations, both governmental and non-governmental, have developed organizational policies, frameworks, resources and training around this cultural competence continuum. The National Health and Medical Research Council produced a guide to cultural competency, and a number of regions have developed various frameworks and resources based on this guide.

None of our diverse cultures, including Australian Indigenous culture, can be adequately described in one short chapter. However, this information can be a starting point in the progression from cultural awareness to cultural competence. Online generic courses concerning Indigenous culture are also available, including both free and accredited courses. Cultures, including Australian Indigenous culture, are never static but constantly changing with time, and there is much diversity within cultures.

Generic information and courses need to be built on by accessing any available face-to-face courses, resources and local Indigenous 'cultural brokers', in order to learn location-specific and role-specific cultural information, historical information, cultural contexts and protocols concerning the community being served. 'Cultural brokers' may be people such as: community elders, community workers, Aboriginal Health Workers, people working in Aboriginal Liaison roles, community/local councils, local Boards, and Aboriginal Controlled Services.

### Implications for a health-care professional's practice

- For an individual to be 'culturally competent' requires a willingness to change, to be empathic, adaptable and 'other centred', and to develop along a continuum that starts with a level of awareness, to being able to practice in a culturally competent manner.
- All health-care professionals working with Indigenous people should endeavour to access cultural competency training and resources relevant to Australian Indigenous culture in order to achieve this.
- Research any cultural competency guides, frameworks and resources that may have been developed for the local region and health services.
- Organizations' and individuals' cultural competence affects Indigenous people's ability and willingness to be able to access and use services.
- Find out who are the appropriate local cultural brokers to learn from.

## Population

Accurate figures for the number of Indigenous people living in Australia at the time of white settlement are not known. Anthropologists and others have suggested various numbers ranging from 300000 to 1000000. Archaeological research has suggested that the land could have supported 750000 people before white settlement.

Whatever the numbers were before 1788, they 'declined dramatically under the impact of new diseases, repressive and often brutal treatment, dispossession, and social and cultural disruption and disintegration' (*Year Book Australia, 1994* – Australian Bureau of Statistics). 'The decline of the Indigenous population continued well into the twentieth century', according to *Australia's Health 2010*, the 12th biennial health report of the Australian Institute of Health and Welfare.

By 2009, the estimated Indigenous population had increased to about 550000, comprising 2.5% of Australia's population (Australian Bureau of Statistics). These figures include 6% who identified as being of Torres Strait Islander origin and 4% as being of both Aboriginal and Torres Strait Islander. These increases are 'in excess of those which can be attributed to natural increase in the Indigenous population'. 'Changing social attitudes, political developments, improved statistical coverage, and a broader definition of Indigenous origin have all contributed to the increased likelihood of people identifying as being of Aboriginal or Torres Strait Islander origin' (*Australia's Health 2010*). Some 32% live in major cities, 43% in regional areas, and 25% in remote or very remote areas. Approximately 30% of the Northern Territory population are Indigenous people, the highest proportion in Australia. In comparison, Victoria has the lowest proportion, at 0.7%.

The Aboriginal and Torres Strait Islander population of Australia is very different from the rest of the population in age range as a result of higher birth rates and earlier age at death. In 2006, the median age was 21 years for Indigenous people and 37 years for the non-Indigenous population.

### Implications for a health-care professional's practice

- Find out whether the population in the area your health service covers includes Indigenous people.
- Consider whether the service is accessible and culturally appropriate for those people.
- Consult with the community as to what measures, if any, the people would like to see introduced to assist with this.
- Are there local Indigenous people employed in the service, or training and employment opportunities to help increase the numbers of Indigenous people in the organization?
- Are there health programmes that cater for the needs of the Indigenous community's age demographics?

## Mortality

The Australian Institute of Health and Welfare (AIHW) considers data from New South Wales, Queensland, Western Australia, South Australia and the Northern Territory as the most complete. The combined data from 2003–2007 demonstrate that mortality rates for all age groups of Indigenous males and females were approximately twice as high as for non-Indigenous people, except for those aged 75 years and over, where the ratio was only 1.2.

Life expectancy at birth is approximately 67 years for Indigenous males and 73 for females (compared with 78 and 83 years respectively for non-Indigenous males and females).

The AIHW considers that the mortality rate for children aged under 5 years is a key indicator of the general health and wellbeing of a population. In the period 2003–2007, the 692 deaths of Aboriginal and Torres Strait Islander children aged 0–4 years was around twice the rate for non-Indigenous children during this period. 'For injury and poisoning, and respiratory diseases, which were common causes of death among children of this age group, Indigenous children died at 3 and 4 times the rate of non-Indigenous children respectively' (*Australia's Health 2010*).

### Implications for a health-care professional's practice

- Indigenous people accessing care away from home may need assistance with planning for early return home as they may be culturally obliged to return for funeral ceremonies and 'sorry business' and/or may want the company of family while grieving.
- Unresolved or ongoing grief is highly likely to be impacting on the mental health and social and emotional wellbeing of people who have relatively frequent losses of close relatives.
- There may be reluctance to attend a health service where a relative has died. There may be a need to have a ceremony to 'cleanse' such an area. Seek guidance from local Indigenous people as to their wishes regarding this.
- People will be likely to want (and have a right to) a thorough and meaningful explanation of the cause of death of a family member. Keep in mind and respect the fact that people may also have their own cultural explanations for the cause of death.
- A dying person will usually want to return to 'country' (the land they are connected to) and family for particular processes and ceremonies associated with dying and to pass away there. The health-care professional may need to put processes in place to help facilitate this as soon as possible.
- Many Indigenous people do not use the name of a deceased person for a long time, if at all, after someone has died. A health-care professional talking with a family about someone who has passed away should use a relationship term instead, such as 'your aunty', 'grandfather', etc., or the local term specifically used for this situation.

## Health and illness beliefs

A definition of health as perceived by Aboriginal peoples was developed by the National Aboriginal Health Strategy in 1989:

> "Aboriginal health" means not just the physical wellbeing of an individual but refers to the social, emotional and cultural wellbeing of the whole community in which each individual is able to achieve their full potential as a human being thereby bringing about the total wellbeing of their community. It is a whole of life view and includes the cyclical concept of life – death – life.

For many Indigenous people, the spiritual or supernatural side of life remains an unquestioned reality. Many still retain a strong traditional belief in the causes of illness different to that of the western biomedical model, even if that is well explained, understood and accepted. The cause can be attributed to 'sorcery' or as a consequence of having transgressed some traditional law. The person may have to put this right to bring about a complete cure; they may want to continue 'western' medical treatment but may also need to return home to carry out correct traditional practices to restore health. Many people still access their own traditional healer, traditional medicines and healing practices.

*Men's business/Women's business:* This term refers to health and treatment matters of a personal nature concerning the bowels, bladder, genital areas, sexual matters, childbirth, etc. It is usually very difficult and 'shameful' for a male or female Indigenous person to discuss these or be treated in this area by someone of the opposite sex. However, Indigenous people, like others, are of course practical and, with adequate and respectful explanation, appreciate that sometimes a same-sex staff member is not available, although it is really preferable not to cross these boundaries.

### Implications for a health-care professional's practice

- When providing a service, keep in mind the holistic definition of health as defined above and work within this.
- Be guided by any available community cultural brokers as to people's concept of health and any traditional resources they access.
- If the community wishes, collaborate in incorporating these in the service.

- If the person is far from their community accessing health care, it may be necessary to help facilitate ongoing care and return to the community so that the person can also attend to cultural matters surrounding their illness beliefs.
- Endeavour to have sufficient numbers of both male and female staff, including Indigenous staff, employed in the service.
- If possible and appropriate, when no professional of the same sex as the client is available, have a 'chaperone' of the same sex as the person to accompany and support the professional and client while treating or discussing 'men's/women's business' matters.

## History, disadvantage and health

For a discussion on Australian Indigenous history since 1788, and its devastating impact on past and current health and welfare, the reader is encouraged to examine the Australian Indigenous Health*InfoNet.* Dispossession, introduction of new diseases, epidemics causing depopulation and consequent disruption in family systems and culture, loss of autonomy, destruction of traditional food and economic systems and ceremonial life and culture, separation of families and family members (including policies and practices that led to the Stolen Generations), and loss of control over much of daily life, are among the many contributing factors discussed. The 'clear relationship between the social inequalities experienced by Indigenous people and their current health status' is described. Loss of control over daily life is increasingly acknowledged as a significant cause of chronic stress, a contributor to chronic disease.

In their regular reporting of key indicators of Indigenous disadvantage, the Productivity Commission describes six 'headline indicators': post-secondary education; disability and chronic disease; household and individual income; substantiated child abuse and neglect; imprisonment and juvenile detention; family and community violence. In all of these indicators, Australian Indigenous people suffer substantial disadvantage compared with the rest of the population, despite some minor gains in some indicators over recent years:

- Australian Indigenous people endure an overall burden of ill-health that is 2.5 times that of the total Australian population.
- The leading causes of morbidity and mortality for Australian Indigenous people include: cardiovascular disease (including rheumatic fever and rheumatic heart disease); mental health problems and social and emotional wellbeing issues ('7 out of 10 Indigenous children were living in families that had experienced three or more major life stress events such as death in the family, serious illness, family breakdown, financial problems or arrest … and 22% had experienced seven or more of such events'); respiratory diseases; type 2 diabetes; chronic kidney disease; and injury.
- Co-morbidity of cardiovascular disease, diabetes and chronic kidney disease often occurs in the general population. However, this particular co-morbidity is even more common among Indigenous Australians.
- Cancer rates are lower for Indigenous people, but cancer death rates are approximately 1.5 times higher for Indigenous males and females than for non-Indigenous people. The main causes of Indigenous cancer deaths include cancers of the digestive organs and lung cancer. Among Indigenous people, smoking-related cancers are more common than among non-Indigenous people.
- Ear disease and hearing loss is higher than for the general Australian population, predominantly among children and young adults.

Other determinants and risk factors impacting on the health and welfare of many Indigenous Australians include: lower socioeconomic status; lower employment and educational levels; overcrowded housing conditions; remoteness (which includes lack of access to health services and adequate food supplies); food; poor nutrition; physical inactivity; overweight or obesity; higher rates of smoking (Indigenous people are more than twice as likely to be daily smokers than other Australians); alcohol consumption (although Indigenous people are considerably less likely to drink alcohol than other Australians, many of those who do drink, tend to drink at risky or high-risk levels). Low birth weight, ear infections (leading to hearing loss) and gastrointestinal infections also impact negatively on child health.

### Implications for a health-care professional's practice

- Find out the historical and social history of the community and build relationships and collaborations with any Indigenous-controlled organizations to help increase access to the health service by the local community.
- People may experience a feeling of powerlessness in the face of large organizations such as hospitals and health services.
- People are likely to be reluctant/uncomfortable accessing health services where there are no Indigenous people employed or that do not have culturally safe systems in place.

- They may take a while to develop rapport, preferring to take time to see whether the health-care professional is caring, friendly and respectful.
- They may have been separated from family and supportive kinship systems.
- Many are likely to have a loss of control over many aspects of their life; this has implications for following health-care advice and treatments.
- What are the common physical health problems among the local community's Indigenous people, and are there treatment resources available?
- Are there culturally appropriate mental health and social and emotional wellbeing services available?
- It may be appropriate to advocate for, or support the people's efforts to advocate for, socioeconomic and community development – particularly Indigenous community-controlled services and primary health care.
- Issues such as a lack of financial resources, transport, homelessness and food security may impact on a person's ability to follow lifestyle advice, attend for appointments and treatment, and purchase prescription and over-the-counter medicines.

## Family and kinship

Most Aboriginal people are members of an extensive, close kinship system and are very relationship focused. Relationship underpins most interaction, activities and responsibilities of daily life and communication. Some people may have lost connection to kinship systems but often still retain some relationship practices passed on, which originated in these kinship systems.

Kinship relationship has a bearing on roles, responsibilities, obligations to each other in caring and sharing, giving physical and emotional support, marriage, child-raising and teaching of culture. Old people (elders) are highly regarded and respected. The 'rules' and the way the kinship system works varies across different areas.

In many regions of Australia, the family related by 'blood' and marriage follows the pattern outlined in Figure 3.2.1. For a person in this system: your mother's sisters are also your mothers and, therefore, their children are your brothers and sisters. The opposite applies on the father's side: your father's brothers are also your fathers and their children are also your brothers and sisters. Accordingly, for an adult, you also have obligations and responsibilities towards the children of your sisters or brothers as they are also your children. Various fathers, mothers, aunts and uncles in this system have varying levels of significance and are afforded particular respect, especially in relation to providing cultural knowledge and learning.

People not necessarily related by blood or marriage may be 'adopted' into a kinship system, or given a kinship title (e.g. aunty, uncle, etc.) as acceptance or as a means of the family knowing how to relate to that person. Aboriginal people, who may or may not be related by blood or marriage, are often also related to one another by a relationship system loosely termed 'Skin Groups'. This has nothing to do with skin colour, but with relationships, and is also often connected to moieties. 'Skin' groupings and names vary across areas in number and 'rules'. Aboriginal people from near or far, known or unknown, from various related or unrelated language groups, can find a relationship from within this 'Skin Group' relationship system.

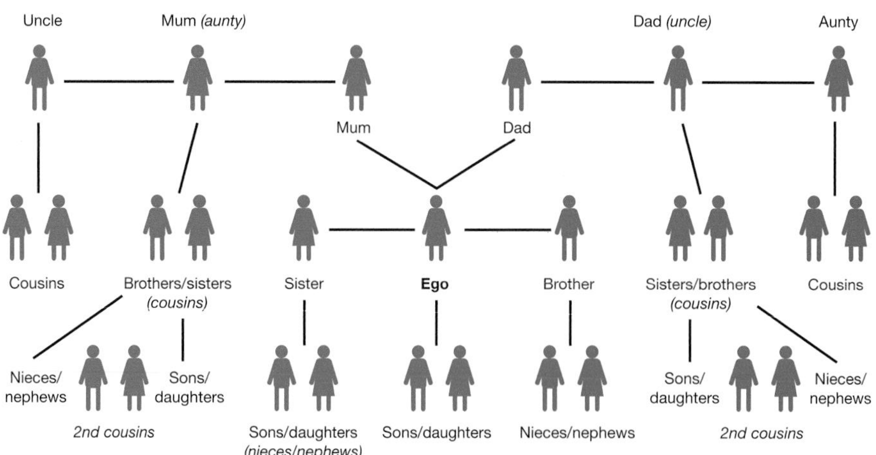


Fig. 3.2.1 The basic kinship family. Terms in italics denote the Caucasian Australian equivalent.

Within the kinship system avoidance relationships exist (sometimes referred to as 'poison cousins'), which is a reverence/respect relationship and involves various levels of avoidance. This varies from area to area, but some examples are: a man may not be able to speak to his mother-in-law; he may not be able to touch his brother or say his sister's name or be alone with her.

Thus, an Aboriginal person is most likely to have many people to whom they are closely related, are probably in frequent contact with, and/or who live in their area or community. When having to leave home to access health services many, many kilometres away, separation from family members and familiar surroundings is usually very stressful for Indigenous people and they often feel isolated, alone and scared. They are often also worrying about the welfare of their children and family back at home.

These kinship systems are usually collectivist based and have a consensus decision-making process which therefore differs from the 'mainstream' individualist-based culture of much of Australia and Australian health-care systems.

### Implications for a health-care professional's practice

- Be aware of the family relationship system of the person/family you are working with.
- Find out whether they wish to involve other family members and help facilitate this if necessary.
- In some cases there may be a family spokesperson who will speak for the patient.
- Often an Indigenous person culturally cannot really give consent to treatment by themselves but should involve various family members in care-planning whenever possible. Some relations can discuss relatively minor medical issues, but when the issue is complex or serious often only certain persons in the kinship system can be involved. Check with the client and/or those involved before these discussions.
- More than one person may be 'next of kin', depending on the particular situation.
- Usually, family relationships and obligations are more important than individual autonomy.
- An adult presenting with a child for treatment may not necessarily be the child's birth parent but another relative who also has responsibility for the child and who may also have more say in that child's welfare than the birth parent.
- A person accessing care may need extra support from family members if available and/or Indigenous staff such as Indigenous Health Workers or Indigenous Liaison/Social Support staff.

## Language and communication styles

Although many Australian Indigenous people speak English as their first language, others speak it as their second, third or more language, speaking Indigenous languages on a daily basis. There are varying levels of English proficiency among Indigenous language speakers, from very proficient to those who rarely speak it. Indigenous people may also regularly use Kriol or 'Aboriginal English'.

Communication styles often differ a lot from Caucasian Australian styles. Indigenous people often take time to 'size people up'. Most are good at observing body language and can see when there is a genuine, caring approach and the speaker wants to communicate properly. Communication usually requires a gentle and respectful approach with lowered tones.

Obvious attention to them can make an Indigenous person feel very uncomfortable, as most do not like to be made to 'stand out in the crowd' and describe this as a feeling of 'shame'. An abrupt, 'bossy' or loud assertive manner is, of course, most inappropriate and cuts off all hope of good communication.

Many Indigenous people do not always answer a question immediately as it is generally considered rude to do so because, out of respect for the questioner, the question deserves to be considered before it is answered. Where English is not the first language, there is also much mental exercise going on listening across languages and interpreting the question and answer before answering. A lot of direct questioning can be intimidating and may cause the person to 'clam up' or to say what they think you want to hear, because they wish to please, or in the hope that further in to the conversation they will gain more understanding.

Prolonged eye contact during conversation can make some Indigenous people feel uncomfortable. It is generally not a polite thing to do in their communication with each other. They may not be looking at the speaker, but may have eyes downcast or looking in another direction. This can vary, as some are more used to using direct eye contact with people than others.

Unnecessary, unfamiliar body contact – sitting too close and close touching – may offend unless you have established a good rapport with the patient. Many will use handshakes, both among themselves and with non-Indigenous people. However, if this is not done it should not be taken as an offence.

A lot of medical and general health information given to patients may be new information. Many Indigenous people have a world view and explanations for body and organ function that may not correlate with much of the biomedical world view. They have a right to this information and a right to consider it at length, discuss it with family and revisit it with staff. Research has shown that Indigenous people want to have the full story about their condition and treatments and that in many instances, for many years, this has not been provided in their interactions with health services. Many people who speak Indigenous languages do not use abstract thinking and concepts and, if used, the abstract is still grounded in the reality of the issue being discussed. For a good discussion on this and the resulting miss-communication that can occur when non-Indigenous people use abstract concepts in communication with Indigenous language speakers, the reader is encouraged to read: *White Men Are Liars – Another Look at Aboriginal–Western Interactions* (by M Bain, published by AuSIL, Alice Springs, 2005).

Indigenous staff, interpreters and family members can help with good communication, especially when the person appears quiet and withdrawn. Some areas such as the Kimberley region of Western Australia and the Northern Territory have formal interpreter services.

### Implications for a health-care professional's practice

- When working with or without an interpreter, when English is not the person's first language, speak clearly, use plain standard English, slow it down (not too slow) and break it up.
- Avoid using jargon and colloquialisms.
- 'Aboriginal English' and Kriol are languages with their own distinct structures. Do not attempt to speak these by using your own version of 'broken English' as it will probably not make sense (and may sound insulting).
- Use pictures/diagrams where possible to assist understanding.
- Do not assume understanding or a lack of understanding – find out what the person knows and build from the known to the unknown.
- It is necessary to be a good listener and not interrupt 'pause intervals'. When an Indigenous person can see someone knows how to listen, they will often volunteer more information than expected.
- Try to reduce some 'routine' questioning by getting information from a person's file, if available and appropriate.
- Avoid asking two questions at once as this can be confusing and difficult when listening across languages.
- Ask open-ended questions rather than questions that need just a 'yes' or 'no' answer.
- If English is not the first language, try to learn some of the language used, such as commonly used words and phrases. As well as helping communication, this helps build rapport and mutual respect.
- Check frequently that your message has been understood. Asking 'Do you understand?' is not a valid way to assess comprehension. Ask the person to tell you what they think you have said in their own words and summarize/check your understanding of what they have said.
- If direct eye contact is not being used, take cues from the person. You can be beside them so both are looking to the front.
- Find out whether there are Interpreter services in the area and if so, how to access these.

## PART 2 MAORI VIEW OF CHILD HEALTH AND ILLNESS

Leo Buchanan

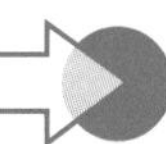

### Practical points

**Key cultural concepts**

- A child can never be seen in isolation from the family.
- Full health involves the integration of spiritual, emotional and physical matters along with family health.
- The child is seen as a gift.

**Clinical problems in Maori children**

- Some clinical problems are a reflection of persisting socioeconomic disadvantage for many Maori.
- Some clinical problems are uncommon but important conditions of genetic origin.
- Physical abuse of children is distressingly common amongst Maori.

**Some potential key ways forward**

- For many Maori to regain familiarity with what it is to be truly Maori.
- For the skilled sensitive promotion of significant breastfeeding consistent with World Health Organization recommendations.
- For more doctors of good will to become familiar with and responsive to Maori cultural values.

## Maori children in New Zealand

Maori children are an interesting, colourful and at times challenging part of the New Zealand landscape. They accounted for 22% of New Zealand's 64 120 births in 2009. They are, therefore, highly visible in both urban and rural New Zealand. They also have a significant presence throughout Australia as part of what is whimsically described as the 120 000-strong Ngati Skippy Maori immigrants. The broad ethnic breakdown of New Zealand's children under the age of 15 years in the 2006 census was as follows:

| | |
|---|---|
| European | 56% |
| Maori | 22% |
| Pacific Island | 11% |
| Asian | 10% |

## Who is Maori?

Until the 1980s, the official census definition was based on a child having 'half or more' Maori origin. Now, however, census data and common usage define Maori as a person of Maori ancestry who chooses to identify as Maori. It is important to be aware that the unifying term Maori really dates from the time of European occupation of New Zealand. Historically, tribal divisions were quite marked. Informed observers as recently as the 1930s referred to Aotearoa (New Zealand) as a series of islands joined by narrow strips of land.

## What are the particular features defining health for Maori?

Sir Mason Durie brilliantly summarized the wholeness or wellness of Maori as being thought of as the four walls of a house – each needing to stand to support the others. The four walls were listed as:

- *Taha wairua* (recognizing the intrinsic spiritual nature of humans)
- *Taha hinengaro* (concerned with thoughts and feelings)
- *Taha tinana* (the physical side of body functioning)
- *Taha whanau* (the role of the extended family).

Measuring all these aspects of health is not easy, with the spiritual side perhaps being the most challenging. Yet some would see *Taha wairua* as the most important aspect – the need to acknowledge or have a faith in a 'life force' – a God outside of yourself.

This turning outwards is consistent with the importance for Maori of being at one with the environment. Indeed, the special relationship between the person and the created environment is reflected in the shared meaning of some key words: *whanau* means birth, but is also the word for the child's more immediate family; *whenua* is the word for the placenta, but is also the word for land. Again the meaning of words illustrates the difficulty of seeing areas of health as being containable in isolated compartments. The word for intense anger is *pukuriri* – literally 'fighting within the stomach'. Likewise, the word for depression is *manawapouri* – 'blackness within the heart'.

In essence, the concept of health and wellness is therefore seen as always involving an interplay between spiritual matters, thoughts and feelings, the physical functions of the body, the family and the environment. In *te ao Maori* (the Maori World), all manner of possible explanatory links between events occurring around the same time or on a certain day would be considered as potentially contributing to an illness. There is empathy within Maoridom with the kind of Hippocratic notion that medicine is primarily an art that uses science for its own purposes on occasions. Maori would struggle with the idea that the only proper approach in medicine should hinge around randomized controlled trials or other manifestations of evidence-based medicine. A Maori doctor's practice would look to both science and art for guidance. This approach would be seen as no different from that of a brilliant scientist such as Pascal believing firmly in the basic Christian concept that God could become human.

## The significance of the child within Maori culture

The fourth concept of the four walls of health helps place the child – *Taha whanau*. The health of the child cannot be considered without regard to the family as a whole. The child is seen as a *taonga* (a special gift) to the *whanau* (family). The child brings a continuation of the inheritance lines (*whakapapa*). The child is seen as the hope for the future. The care and upbringing of the child would be seen as not belonging just to the parents but to the extended family, with grandparents playing a special role. Maori has been described as a culture that puts others before self, so that a young child would be expected to receive considerable *arohatanga* (warmth and love) and *awhinatanga* (help and assistance).

## Historical issues of significance to Maori health

### The Treaty of Waitangi

The document serving as a partnership for the English Crown with Maori and thus forming the basis for the modern New Zealand nation was the Treaty of Waitangi.

Maori far outnumbered Europeans in the New Zealand of the 1840 Treaty signing. The Treaty was constructed in both Maori and English with debate continuing to this day over important nuances in the differing meanings of key words in the English and Maori versions. In the discussions over what the Treaty might have guaranteed for the health of Maori, importance is placed on the second article promising protection to Maori of their *taonga* (treasures). Health is seen as one of these. Likewise attention has been frequently drawn to the third article promising to Maori the same rights (taken to include health rights) as their new English brothers and sisters. Other commentators have drawn attention to the importance of the so-called fourth clause of the Treaty in recognizing the spiritual component of health for Maori. This was read only at the important first signings at Waitangi itself. It read: 'The Governor says the several faiths of England, of the Wesleyans, of Rome and also the Maori custom, shall alike be protected by him.'

### The New Zealand wars

Overlapping with the implications for Maori health arising from breaches of the Treaty of Waitangi are the New Zealand land wars. These were strung out over about 40 years from the late 1840s and led to huge confiscations of Maori Land by the Crown as 'Reparation' for the armed conflicts that arose especially in the Waikato and Taranaki areas. The land confiscations suited the Government's purposes admirably to give it an income and to meet the land demands of rapidly escalating numbers of British immigrants. The land confiscations were quite disproportional to the numbers of soldiers killed or costs incurred. In Taranaki, for instance, nearly two million acres of land were taken. These conflicts led to the loss of life of key Maori leaders; the loss of land on which Maori could stand tall as well as land from which to generate an income; and for some a sense of shame and identity confusion that persists to this day. In recent years the government has attempted to readdress these land confiscations and Treaty of Waitangi breaches, with combinations of apologies and very modest monetary compensations.

## Cultural competency in working with Maori families

Cultural competency has come more to the fore in New Zealand since a legislative change initiated by the Medical Council of New Zealand that any medical practitioner must be culturally competent as well as clinically competent. My own view has always been that it is not possible to be clinically competent without being culturally competent. A working diagnosis of cultural competency could be the capacity to recognize and interact respectfully with any individual's particular culture.

In all situations, the approach to the family has to be one of courtesy and respect. Welcoming or acknowledging every member of the supporting family is a good start. Some general enquiries about what is happening in the family and where they are from are advisable in the non-emergency situation before plunging into defining the particular concerns about the child. This comment illustrates the importance of hastening slowly in working with Maori families. Polynesians as a whole prefer not to be rushed in exchanges as important as those concerning health. Ward rounds need to be a bit longer if the real face-to-face and heart-to-heart encounters that Maori seek in these matters are to be achieved.

A doctor, especially if young, should tend towards formality in dress code when working with Maori. In one sense the doctor may be partly seen as having a similarity within Maoridom to a *tohunga* – a person with special training and responsibilities to guard things that are special and sacred. In outpatient clinic settings, some distance and space between the doctors and the *whanau* should be organized, as this initial encounter can then mimic the rituals of engagement when Maori first meet in the very special area within Maori reserves called *marae*. Consultants on teaching ward rounds or in multidisciplinary clinic sessions might like to introduce or refer to others present with them as their supporting *whanau*.

## The organization of health services for Maori

In the 2006 census, only 3% of New Zealand medical practitioners identified themselves as Maori, whereas the total Maori population was 15%. Even among doctors identifying as Maori, a wide variation exists in their knowledge of *Taha Maori* (Maori things). Currently, fewer than 10 of New Zealand's 292 vocationally registered paediatricians have any Maori affiliation, so in the short to medium term it is difficult to deliver health services by Maori for Maori – which is the preferred option for many Maori. Rather, non-Maori medical practitioners of good will – sensitive to Maori nuances – need to support Maori children and their families. Doctors working with children should become familiar with specific local Maori health initiatives that relate to children. Most public hospitals have a definitive Maori liaison service, and community-based Maori health facilities are becoming more common.

## Socioeconomic and cultural contact issues

Maori continue to be significantly over-represented in less favourable socioeconomic clustering within New Zealand. Socioeconomic disadvantage includes lower income levels, higher unemployment rates, greater use of temporary or rental accommodation, and lower levels of education achievement. The higher hospitalization rates of Maori infants (in 2009, Maori infants comprised 35% of all public hospitalizations compared with 22% of births) and high rates of respiratory illness, rheumatic fever and skin sepsis are all seen as examples of the price of socioeconomic disadvantage as conventionally defined. One frustration for Maori, though, is that the measurements of 'Internal Forces' that may shape health or wellbeing are more problematic. How does one measure the presence or absence of shame at having too much or too little Maori, at losing contact with one's own tribal roots, being cut off from extended family, or just losing the notion of what it is to be Maori? The 2006 census showed that 84% of Maori now live in urban areas. Contact with *Taha Maori* (Maori things) is likely to be more of a challenge in urban areas. It is true that some measurable socioeconomic markers have improved for Maori over the last 10 years. Maori unemployment rates, for instance, may be dropping, but what if this is at the price of family-unfriendly work hours or is associated with the increased frequency of Maori infants and toddlers spending substantial amounts of time in day-care arrangements away from their family?

**Clinical example**

Rangi is a 6-year-old boy who presented to the emergency department (ED) with a history of intermittent fevers for some days and then, on the day of referral, a complaint of back pain on walking and some abdominal pain. He was admitted under the general surgeons who noted a C-reactive protein (CRP) level of 122 mg/L and haemoglobin level of 85 g/L, and felt that appendicitis was possible. A normal appendix was removed and the child's symptoms seemed to settle before discharge home. Rangi re-presented to the ED 2 weeks later with a history of limping on the left leg and intermittent fevers over a week. There was evidence of swelling over the left ankle and tenderness of the left big toe. His CRP level was 174 mg/L and there was a persisting normochronic anaemia and mild neutrophilia. He was admitted under the orthopaedic service with a suspected diagnosis of osteomyelitis or septic arthritis.

The left ankle was aspirated, with 56 000 white cells found in a murky aspirate. Treatment for osteomyelitis was commenced, but 1 week later there was again evidence of arthritis of the left ankle and no growth from the aspirate. A general paediatrician was consulted for the first time and heard a pansystolic murmur at the apex. An urgent echocardiogram showed moderate mitral valve incompetence. Antistreptococcal antibody titres were markedly raised. Rangi was diagnosed as having acute rheumatic fever. Rheumatic fever should be strongly considered in the differential diagnosis of any Maori child presenting with persistent fevers and joint pains or arthritis.

## Genetics and environment in clinical situations

There is a tendency to look towards adverse environmental conditions as major contributors to those clinical conditions seen more commonly in Maori children than in children of European ethnicity. These are certainly significant factors in the markedly increased incidence of rheumatic fever, skin sepsis, respiratory tract infections and glue ear. However, other conditions such as $\alpha$-thalassaemia trait (10% incidence), a particular type of congenital nephrotic syndrome, and the rare but fatal non-ketotic hyperglycinaemia are entirely genetic in origin. It is likely that the increased incidence of biliary atresia in Maori is also genetic in origin. Yet other conditions, such as the common entity of attention-deficit disorder, would appear to reflect both genetic and environmental factors.

In infancy, gastro-oesophageal reflux, infantile colic and food allergies, although all occurring amongst Maori, are much less often presented to paediatricians as a perceived problem by Maori families. Whereas obesity may be over-represented amongst Maori, anorexia nervosa appears to be very uncommon – partly one suspects in both situations a result of cultural perceptions of desirable body size.

In the development and behavioural areas, practitioners need to be careful not to attribute the various behavioural manifestations associated with either attention-deficit/hyperactivity disorder (ADHD) or autism to the Maori child living in a dysfunctional family. The family dysfunction may well result from the fact that the same conditions are present to varying degrees in one or both parents.

It is always important to consider what special significance a child's diagnosis may have to the *whanau* (extended family). The word tuberculosis may trigger

**Clinical example**

Rawinia is an 18-month-old toddler referred to paediatric outpatients because of anaemia, unresponsive to iron. A blood count aged 15 months, performed by her GP because of recurrent upper respiratory tract infections, showed a haemoglobin level of 95 g/L and a mean corpuscular volume (MCV) of 60 fL. Microcytosis and hypochromia were noted on the film smear. A repeat blood count after 6 weeks of oral iron showed no improvement. The paediatrician was confident that the iron had been given and, noting the Maori ethnicity of the child, established that iron and ferritin levels were normal after finding no clinical abnormality on examination. He suspected the harmless entity of $\alpha$-thalassaemia trait, which needs no treatment, and in due course confirmed this suspicion with appropriate DNA studies.

recall of the ravages this malady caused to family members in earlier generations. Likewise, a diagnosis of asthma or epilepsy will have added meaning if any family members have died from these conditions.

Finally, in assessing various diagnostic possibilities, it is worth remembering that some conditions such as cystic fibrosis or coeliac disease are much less likely amongst children with a major Maori ethnic component.

## The physical abuse problem

Notwithstanding the shadows over morbidity and even mortality data arising from the infections amongst Maori children, the longest blackest shadow in my view is that of physical abuse. Compared with non-Maori children, Maori are two to three times more likely to be hospitalized for injuries sustained as a result of deliberately inflicted physical harm than any other ethnic group. The death rates and permanent serious neurological handicap rates in Maori from the shaken baby syndrome are amongst the highest recorded internationally for any ethnic group.

It may be a matter of opinion as to whether any link can be construed between these facts and the high rate of induced abortions evident amongst Maori women in more recent years. What is undeniable is that Maori birth rates have plummeted dramatically since the 1970s to be now only a little higher than non-Maori rates, except amongst adolescents.

A number of one-off solutions to the Maori physical abuse scourge have been suggested. They have included lowering the relatively high teenage pregnancy rate; targeting alcohol and drug abuse; recognizing and reducing family violence; promoting positive parenting programmes or offering intervention services quickly to families dealing with a powder-keg crisis such as a persistently screaming baby. Regrettably, the truth is that none of these interventions seems to have had a major impact on lowering the incidence of physical abuse.

## A way forward

Could the key in reality to this challenge be the need to work toward an attitudinal change within Maoridom towards children – to recapture the idea that children are a gift? One of the oldest words in Maori for defining a woman is *Ukaipo* – literally the breastfeeder in the night. Yet the breastfeeding rate amongst Maori now is lower at 17% at the 6-month mark than for any other ethnic group in New Zealand. It does not seem unreasonable to suggest that a vigorous but sensitively promoted plan of supporting the World Health Organization's recommendations that women should significantly breastfeed to at least 12 months of age might, through its bonding powers, reduce physical abuse in the young as well as reduce early respiratory tract infections and glue ear. Such a programme, however, would have to be part of a wider undertaking to promote to all Maori a clearer appreciation of what it is to be truly Maori. In this way Te Rangi Hiroa's 1930 claim that Maori is a culture that puts other before self might have a more robust ring to it. One starting point for such an undertaking could be an emphasis on Sir Mason Durie's notion that four walls of the house need to be in order if true full health is to become realized. It is a case of back to the future.

*Kia Kaha! Kia Manawanui! Tihei Mauriora!*

# Nutrition 3.3

Zoe McCallum, Julie Bines

Adequate and appropriate nutrition is vital for a child's optimal growth and development. Many diseases in adult life have their antecedents in childhood nutrition, including, hypertension, type 2 diabetes, obesity, hyperlipidaemia and some cancers. In the hospitalized child, nutritional requirements may be increased as a result of inadequate intake, malabsorption or due to disease-related increased requirement for specific nutrients. In some situations oral feeding may be inadequate to support weight gain and growth. Options for nutritional support and nutritional therapy including specialized enteral formulas and supplements or parenteral (intravenous) nutrition may be required.

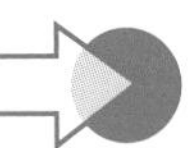

**Practical points**

- Nutrition in childhood, starting from *in utero*, is a key determinant of a child's growth and development, and future adult health status.
- Nutritional assessment requires a dietary history, physical examination and sometimes blood tests.
- Breastfeeding has many benefits over infant formula for both mother and infant.
- A range of infant formulas are available with differing protein sources and indications.
- Solids may be introduced after 6 months.
- 'Fussy' toddler eating is a normal developmental phenomenon; threats, scolding, bribery and use of food as a reward are likely to create rather than resolve problems.
- Water is the best non-milk drink for children (not juice or other sugar-sweetened drinks).
- Low-fat milk is appropriate for children over the age of 2 years.

## Nutritional requirements

### Nutrients and dietary guidelines

Nutrients are food components that are required for optimal growth, development and body function. Macronutrients (protein, fat and carbohydrate) are the basic building blocks for energy, lipid and nitrogen components of the body, and are essential for cellular homeostasis. Micronutrients (vitamins, minerals and trace elements) are required in much smaller amounts. Individual nutrient requirements vary with age, size, growth and health status.

In 2003, the Australian National Health and Medical Research Council (NHMRC) released a document that includes '*Dietary Guidelines for Children and Adolescents in Australia*' (available at: http://www.nhmrc.gov.au/_files_nhmrc/file/publications/synopses/n31.pdf). These guidelines provide complete nutritional advice for healthy children from birth to 18 years of age. They have been updated and will be available from 2011 on the website www.nhmrc.gov.au.

#### Dietary Guidelines for Children and Adolescents in Australia (National Health and Medical Research Council 2003)

Encourage and support breastfeeding

Children and adolescents need sufficient nutritious foods to grow and develop normally

- Growth should be checked regularly for young children
- Physical activity is important for all children and adolescents

Enjoy a wide range of nutritious foods

- Children and adolescents should be encouraged to:
  - Eat plenty of legumes and fruits
  - Eat plenty of cereals (including breads, rice, pasta and noodles), preferably wholegrain
  - Include lean meat, fish and poultry and/or alternatives
  - Include milks, yoghurts, cheese and/or alternatives
  - Reduced fat milks are not suitable for young children under 2 years, because of the high energy needs of young children, but reduced fat varieties should be encouraged for older children and adolescents
  - Alcohol is not recommended for children
- And care should be taken to:
  - Limit saturated fat intake and moderate total fat intake. Low-fat diets are not suitable for infants
  - Choose foods low in salt
  - Consume only moderate amounts of sugars and foods containing sugars

Care for your child's food: prepare and store it safely

### Energy

Food is metabolized and provides energy required by the body for growth and synthesis of new tissue, for metabolic processes, and for physiological functions and activity.

Fat, carbohydrate and protein provide energy, which is measured in kilojoules (kJ) or kilocalories (1 kcal provides 4.182 kJ). Fat provides a concentrated source of energy, contributing 37 kJ/g, approximately twice that provided by an equivalent amount of protein or carbohydrate. Fat contributes 50% of the total energy in breast milk or standard infant formula. The average diet of older children provides 30–40% of total energy from fat, 45–55% from carbohydrate and about 15% from protein. Most of the energy intake in children is used for growth and development. Recommendations for energy intake are difficult to determine, even for individuals of similar age, sex and size, because requirements vary. The NHMRC recommends that for children aged 5–14 years approximately 30% of energy intake should be fat, with no more than 10% coming from saturated fat.

## Nutritional assessment

Nutritional assessment is the process by which the individual is evaluated for normal growth and health, for risk factors contributing to disease, and for early detection of nutritional deficiencies and excesses.

Comprehensive nutritional assessment includes:

- dietary assessment
- physical examination, including anthropometry
- laboratory studies.

### Dietary assessment

The primary care giver(s) should be asked what the child usually eats in a typical day, in all settings that the child is in (i.e. home, child care, outings). Children derive up to 30% of their energy from snacks, so it is important to include these in the assessment of all food and fluids consumed.

Qualitative methods include a dietary history and food frequency questionnaire. These do not allow for the precise calculation of energy or nutrient intakes but rather determine the pattern, style and types of foods eaten.

Quantitative methods calculate precise energy and nutrient intakes and include a 24-hour food record and a 3-day food record.

If the initial dietary assessment raises concerns, referral should be made to a dietitian.

### Physical examination and anthropometry

Physical examination gives a general impression of nutritional status, including signs of anaemia, jaundice, wasting, oedema, lethargy, muscle weakness and fat stores.

Examination may reveal evidence of specific micronutrient deficiency, including pallor, bruising or bleeding, skin, hair and gum abnormalities, and neurological or ophthalmological disorders. In adolescents, the stage of puberty should be documented.

Anthropometry refers to the measurement of physical dimensions and body composition. Measurement of height/length and weight gives the most useful assessment of overall nutritional status, although normal growth can still occur in marginally malnourished children. Serial measurements of growth add valuable information about the impact and chronicity of nutritional compromise. The following routine measurements are used:

- recumbent length before 2 years of age, or height after 2 years of age
- weight for age
- weight for length/height
- head circumference (used until 36 months of age)
- growth velocity
- skinfold thickness (triceps and other sites as indicated)
- mid-arm circumference.

Growth charts for height or length, weight and head circumference are used to monitor growth at different chronological ages (see Chapter 19.1). Specific ethnocultural and syndrome-specific (Down, Turner) growth charts exist. Intrauterine growth curves have been developed for gestational ages 26–42 weeks using birth weight and length data for infants born at successive weeks of gestation. Premature infants should have the weight corrected until the child is 24 months of age, length until the child is 36 months of age, and head circumference until the child is 18 months of age.

Patients requiring long-term monitoring of nutritional status should have serial measurements of mid-arm circumference and triceps skinfold thickness to assess fat and muscle stores.

### Body mass index

Serial body mass index (BMI) is used as a representative measure of body fatness in children (see Chapter 3.4). It cannot, however, distinguish between excess weight produced by adiposity, muscularity or oedema. In children with nutritional deficiency, and in the setting of overweight and obesity, it is a useful measure of adiposity. It is calculated from the formula BMI = weight [kg]/height [m]$^2$. A BMI greater than the 85th percentile is defined as overweight and a BMI greater than the 95th percentile as obesity.

**Table 3.3.1 Laboratory parameters for assessing nutritional status**

| Status | Parameters |
|---|---|
| Protein | Albumin, total protein, pre-albumin, urea, 24-hour urinary nitrogen, carnitine |
| Fluid and electrolyte, and acid–base | Serum electrolytes, acid–base, urinalysis |
| Glucose tolerance | Serum glucose, HbA1c, insulin |
| Iron | Serum iron, serum ferritin, full blood examination |
| Minerals | Calcium, magnesium, phosphorus, alkaline phosphatase, bone age, bone density |
| Vitamins | Vitamins A, D, E/lipid ratio, C, $B_{12}$, folate, PT/PTT |
| Trace elements | Zinc, selenium, copper, chromium, manganese |
| Lipids | Serum cholesterol, HDL cholesterol, triglycerides, free fatty acids |

HbA1c, haemoglobin A1c; HDL, high-density lipoprotein; PT, prothrombin time; PTT, partial thromboplastin time.

### Laboratory assessment

Laboratory assessment is used to detect subclinical deficiency states or to confirm a clinical diagnosis. It provides an objective means of assessing nutritional status. Laboratory assessment is summarized in Table 3.3.1.

## Nutrition *in utero*

Research into the fetal origins of adult health has identified fetal nutrition as being of critical importance. Maternal nutrition is a powerful epigenetic determinant of not only birth size and subsequent growth, but also the future risk of metabolic syndrome (hyperlipidaemia, hypertension, coronary artery disease, type 2 diabetes) in adult life. The 'Barker' hypothesis states that adaptations undergone by the starved fetus *in utero* to become 'thrifty', that is to make maximum use of scarce nutrients, may in the setting of adequate, or even abundant, nutrition become counterproductive.

Most *in utero* malnutrition in Western societies, however, results from placental insufficiency. Periconceptual and antenatal folate supplements markedly reduce the risk of neural tube defects and are advised.

## Breastfeeding

Breastfeeding is the best form of nutrition for the growing infant. Australian hospitals are encouraged to adopt the '10 steps to successful breastfeeding' listed in Box 3.3.1.

The weight percentiles and body composition of breastfed infants differ from those who are formula-fed. In general, breastfed infants tend to grow rapidly in the first few months and then grow at a slower rate than current percentiles. This may result in their weight appearing inadequate when plotted on current growth charts, even when they are healthy. Current NHMRC recommendations for weight gain in infancy are 150–200 g/week at age 0–3 months, 100–150 g/week at age 3–6 months, and 70–90 g/week at age 6–12 months. Preterm breastfed infants require iron supplements from 4–8 weeks of age. Those born at a gestation of less than 32 weeks usually require fortification of breast milk with protein and calories in the preterm period to prevent growth failure. All breastfed infants should receive vitamin K on the first day of life.

Breastfeeding has many benefits for both the infant and the mother. Breast milk is tailored to the infant's needs and contains many factors protective against infection (see Infant formulas, below) and growth factors.

**Box 3.3.1 Ten steps to successful breastfeeding**

Every facility providing maternity services and care for newborn infants should:

1. Have a written breastfeeding policy that is communicated routinely to all health-care staff
2. Train all health-care staff in skills necessary to implement this policy
3. Inform all pregnant women about the benefits and management of breastfeeding
4. Help mothers initiate breastfeeding within half an hour of birth
5. Show mothers how to breastfeed, and how to maintain lactation even if they are separated from their infant
6. Give newborn infants no food or drink other than breast milk, unless indicated medically
7. Practise rooming-in (allow mothers and infants to remain together), 24 hours a day
8. Encourage breastfeeding on demand
9. Give no artificial teats or pacifiers (also called dummies or soothers) to breastfeeding infants
10. Foster the establishment of breastfeeding support groups and refer mothers to them on discharge from hospital or clinic

Source: World Health Organization 1989 Protecting, promoting and supporting breastfeeding: the special role of maternity services, a joint WHO/UNICEF statement. WHO, Geneva. Available at: http://www.unicef.org/newsline/tenstps.htm

Breastfed infants, in comparison with formula-fed infants, have improved neurodevelopment and a lower incidence of infection, diabetes, necrotizing enterocolitis and gastro-oesophageal reflux. Although there is some evidence that breastfeeding may protect against allergic disease in atopic families, the evidence for a population-wide protective effect is inconclusive. Breastfeeding may partially protect women against premenopausal breast cancer, ovarian cancer and osteoporosis. Lactational amenorrhoea may act as a contraceptive adjunct, especially in the developing world.

### Breastfeeding initiation

Information about the advantages and management of breastfeeding, including where to obtain advice and support, if needed, should be made available to all new mothers. Reasons given by mothers for stopping breastfeeding include pain and discomfort (e.g. sore nipples, mastitis, thrush), anxiety regarding the adequacy of milk supply, and a return to work.

### Common problems with breastfeeding

Problems may exist with both maternal breastfeeding technique and anatomy, as well as with the infant's suck and oropharyngeal anatomy. In addition, insufficient milk supply is often perceived to be a major problem, which may lead to unnecessary cessation of breastfeeding. Most women are physiologically able to produce sufficient milk. Appropriate education, encouragement and support may be all that is needed.

> **Clinical example**
>
> Isabella was born at term following an uneventful pregnancy and delivery. Her mother was very keen to feed her first baby but experienced considerable pain from sore, cracked nipples soon after discharge from hospital. She returned to the hospital to seek advice from a lactation consultant, who noted that Isabella was incorrectly positioned and attached.
>
> Correct positioning and attachment, which is vital for successful breastfeeding, resolved the problem of sore nipples, enabling Isabella's mother to continue to breastfeed without discomfort.
>
> Isabella breastfed on demand, approximately 3-hourly. At 4 weeks of age she started sleeping longer between feeds and suckled less vigorously. Her mother became very anxious and was concerned that her milk supply was inadequate, particularly as it became apparent that Isabella had not gained weight when weighed at a clinic visit. It was evident that the feeding difficulty was the result of infrequent feeding and maternal anxiety. She was encouraged to feed her baby more frequently, including during the night, and to ensure that Isabella drained the first side before offering the second. Her husband was encouraged to bring Isabella to her for feeding during the night. As a result, the milk supply increased and Isabella gained weight appropriately. Timely advice, and encouragement and support prevented this mother from ceasing breastfeeding unnecessarily.

## Infant formulas and other milks

When breast milk is not available, an infant formula is required. All infant formulas used in Australia are required to be manufactured in accordance with the *Australia New Zealand Food Standard Code*, which specifies the requirements for composition, quality and labelling for infant formulas.

Although the nutritional composition of infant formulas resembles that of human milk, it is not possible to incorporate the many immunological factors that have been identified in human milk. These include specific immune factors such as immunoglobulin A, maternal lymphocytes and macrophages, and other non-specific protective factors such as lactoferrin and lysozyme.

### Feeding requirements of infants

The infant's appetite determines the volume and number of feeds required. Demand feeding for bottle-fed infants is appropriate. Term infants require approximately 120–160 mL per kg per day to meet their fluid and nutrient needs during the first 4–6 months of life when milk feeds provide the sole source of nutrition. The number of feeds per day changes as the infant grows, and the number of feeds per day decreases with increased feed volumes. Infants under 6 weeks of age usually feed every 3 hours and rarely sleep through the night before 8 weeks. Infants experience an appetite spurt at 2 weeks, 6 weeks and 3 months.

Establishment of a feeding pattern is often easier for mothers of breastfed infants, as they respond to the infant's demands and do not focus on the volume consumed at each feed. The actual number and volume of feeds taken by bottle-fed infants causes considerable anxiety for some parents. Reassurance should be provided that the infant's appetite is the best guide, and as long as the infant gains weight consistently, but not excessively, and is thriving and active, intake is satisfactory.

### Composition of standard infant formulas

Standard infant formulas are recommended for healthy term infants who are not breastfed. The nutrient compositions of these standard formulas are very similar, with minor variations in the protein, fat and carbohydrate content (Table 3.3.2).

**Table 3.3.2 Breast milk and artificial formula compositions**

| | Energy (kJ (kcal)/100 mL) | Protein source | Fat source | Carbohydrate source | Indication | Concerns |
|---|---|---|---|---|---|---|
| Breast milk | 289 (69) | Protein source is whole protein | Short-, medium- and long-chain fats | Lactose | The preferred infant feed | HIV infection in mother |
| Breast milk fortified with FM85 (5%) and Poly-Joule (4.2%) | 432 (103) | Protein source is whole protein | Short-, medium- and long-chain fats | Lactose | Preterm infant | |
| Preterm formula (e.g. S26-LBW LCPs) | 340 (81) | Whey : casein: 60 : 40 | Coconut, oleic, palm, soy. LCPs, MCT (12.5%) | Lactose | Preterm infant | Does not contain immunoglobulins, and other non-specific protective and growth factors |
| Term formula – cow's milk based (e.g. S26, Nan1) | 273 (65) | Whey : casein: 60 : 40 | Oleo, coconut, soy, oleic, palm, canola, corn | Lactose | If breast milk not available | Does not contain immunoglobulins, and other non-specific protective and growth factors |
| Soy formula (e.g. Infasoy) | 274 (65) | Soy isolate | Oleo, coconut, soy, oleic | Corn syrup solids, sucrose | Soy formulas should be used in galactosaemic infants, and for infants of vegetarian families reluctant to use cow's milk | The presence of phytates in soy formulas may inhibit absorption of minerals, particularly calcium. Up to 50% of children with cow's milk protein intolerance will also be allergic to soy protein; it is preferable for these children to be given a formula with hydrolysed protein |

*Continued*

**Table 3.3.2 Breast milk and artificial formula compositions—cont'd**

| | Energy (kJ (kcal)/100 mL) | Protein source | Fat source | Carbohydrate source | Indication | Concerns |
|---|---|---|---|---|---|---|
| Lactose modified formulas (e.g. De-Lact) | 286 (69) | Casein dominant | Vegetable oil | Maltodextrin, glucose, galactose | Low-lactose or lactose-free formulas are the feeds of choice for formula-fed infants with true lactose intolerance | In older children with lactose intolerance, enzymatic drops containing lactase may be used with cow's milk |
| Hydrolysed formulas (peptide) (e.g. Pepti-Junior, Alfare) | 280 (67) | Whey hydrolysate, The protein in these formulas is partially hydrolysed to peptides and free amino acids | Vegetable oil, MCT (50%) | Corn syrup solids | Semi-elemental formulas are designed to meet the needs of infants who are intolerant of intact protein, who maldigest protein and fat, or who have problems with severe diarrhoea, food intolerance or allergy | These formulas are expensive and should be used only with medical guidance |
| Extensively hydrolysed (amino acid) formulas (e.g. Neocate, EleCare) | 298 (71) | Amino acids (elemental) | Safflower, soy, coconut | Dried glucose syrup | Infants with multiple food allergies or abnormal gut may require elemental formula in which the protein has been totally hydrolysed to amino acids | These formulas are expensive and should only be used with medical guidance. Taste bitter |

HIV, human immunodeficiency virus; LCP, long-chain poly-unsaturated fatty acids; MCT, medium-chain triglycerides.

- *Protein*. All standard infant formulas have cow's milk protein as a basis, which is modified in order to produce a protein composition more like that of human milk. The cow's milk protein is modified through heat treatment processes, with the addition of whey in order to modify the casein : whey ratio so that it is similar to that of human milk. Despite this, the amino acid profiles of infant formulas remain different from those of human milk.
- *Fat*. The fat sources in standard infant formulas are a mixture of vegetable oils with or without butterfat. It is possible to achieve ratios of saturated to unsaturated fatty acids that are similar but not identical to those of human milk. Although the degree of saturation may be similar, the structure of the fats is not the same, resulting in differences in digestion and absorption. The fatty acid composition of human milk also varies with the maternal diet, and can be modified favourably by substituting some of the saturated fats in the diet with appropriate mono- and poly-unsaturated fatty acids. Some manufacturers now add long-chain poly-unsaturated fatty acids to formulas, as there is evidence that these play an important role in infant development, with advanced visual pathway maturation and a postulated benefit for intelligence. The fat composition in formulas may also promote the formation of soaps in stools, contributing to constipation in some infants.
- *Carbohydrate*. The carbohydrate source in standard infant formulas is lactose.

All formulas are supplemented with vitamins and minerals. These standard infant formulas are suitable for the first 12 months of life. The practice of changing from one formula to another because an infant is irritable or unsettled should be strongly discouraged. This usually does not help settle the infant and has the potential to lead to mistakes in reconstitution, as scoop size and methods of preparation can vary between formula brands.

Soy formulas are sometimes recommended for use in infants with suspected cow's milk protein intolerance, colic, and in an attempt to prevent allergies. However, up to 50% of children with cow's milk protein intolerance will also be allergic to soy protein; a hydrolysed formula may be more appropriate.

## Preparation of formula

Having selected an appropriate formula, it is essential that it is prepared correctly and hygienically, using safe water and sterilized utensils and equipment. Formulas should be prepared according to the manufacturer's directions, using the scoop provided to measure the powder carefully. Studies have highlighted significant inaccuracies in measuring the amount of powder for formula reconstitution, and other mistakes in preparation of formula. Both diluting and concentrating formula can lead to serious electrolyte disturbance in the infant and should be avoided.

Breastfed babies do not require other fluids, even in hot weather, if they are fed frequently. Formula-fed infants may be offered small amounts of cooled, boiled water between feeds during very hot weather.

## Other milks

Cow's milk is appropriate to be introduced to infants over 12 months. The fat in milk is an important source of energy, fat-soluble vitamins and fatty acids for young children.

Cow's milk has lower iron content and higher levels of protein, sodium, potassium, phosphorus and calcium than human milk or formula. It also has a higher renal solute load and lacks vitamin C and essential fatty acids. Low-fat (2%) cow's milk can be given to children over 2 years of age. Skim milk (no fat) is not recommended unless there is a specific medical condition, such as hypercholesterolaemia. Soy milk should not be used for children under 2 years of age. Calcium-supplemented brands should be chosen if used for older children.

Goat's milk is not recommended for infant feeding. It has a similar macronutrient composition to cow's milk but there are micronutrient deficiencies. If parents insist on using goat's milk, a goat's milk infant formula fully supplemented with vitamins and minerals should be used, because goat's milk is markedly deficient in folate and other vitamins. If fresh goat's milk is used, it must be pasteurized or boiled and supplemented with folic acid and vitamins $B_{12}$, $B_6$, A and C. Infants with cow's milk protein intolerance are usually also intolerant to goat's milk protein.

### Clinical example

Thao brought her 13-month-old child, Madison, to the doctor for review of her cold. She reported that Madison constantly had a cold and was always tired, but she had attributed this to the fact that Madison was still little and had recently started child care. Madison's height and weight were both on the 50th centile. The GP noticed that she was pale, however, and asked about her diet. Thao replied that Madison was a 'fussy eater' but loved her milk. On further questioning the GP discovered that she had commenced cow's milk at 9 months of age and was currently consuming 800 mL per day. Iron studies and a blood count revealed iron-deficiency anaemia. Thao was advised to reduce Madison's milk intake to less than 500 mL daily and to offer a diet rich in meat and leafy green vegetables. It was explained that the cow's milk was 'filling Madison up' but was not providing her with iron and the other vitamins essential for her growth. Madison was commenced on an iron supplement. Thao was advised to delay the introduction of cow's milk until after 12 months of age in future children.

## Nutrition in the well child in the community

### Timing of introduction of solids

Breast milk or an appropriate formula is sufficient to meet the needs of the healthy, growing infant until 4–6 months of age. At this time solid foods can be introduced safely, supplementing the milk intake, which remains the major source of nutrition until about 12 months of age.

By 4–6 months of age infants have lost the tongue thrust or extrusion reflex, have head control, and are able to sit without support, allowing them to manipulate solid foods. Most infants at this age are showing an interest in the world around them and are receptive to trying new foods. Healthy full-term infants are born with iron stores that are sufficient for the first 4–6 months of life, after which these become depleted and milk feeds need to be supplemented with other dietary sources of iron, particularly haem-derived iron.

Introduction of solids before 4 months of age can displace breast milk or formula, but the solids do not necessarily supply sufficient energy and nutrients for the rapidly growing infant. Solids can also result in decreased breast milk supply, as a result of reduced frequency and intensity of sucking. Delaying the introduction of solids until later during the second 6 months of life may compromise growth and nutritional status, as breast milk alone is insufficient after 6 months to supply energy and micronutrient needs.

### The first foods

The introduction of a variety of foods is often referred to as the 'educational diet' as it begins the child's lifetime experience of food. The first foods to be introduced should be soft and smooth, although the infant quickly learns to manage foods of different textures, with the 'chewing reflex' using the gums developing around 7–9 months. Iron-fortified infant cereals are usually introduced first, as these can be mixed to the desired consistency with breast milk or formula. Fruit and vegetables are introduced gradually. Sources of haem iron such as meat and poultry are recommended at about 7 months of age. Custard, yoghurt and cheese can also be introduced. Most infants will be eating a variety of modified family meals by 12 months of age.

### Feeding the toddler

Between 1 and 3 years of age, growth and appetite slow markedly. The child displays independent thought and action. Young children have limited control over their food choices and rely on caregivers to provide a variety of foods. Often a child's natural satiety and refusal to finish all food provided is interpreted as 'fussy eating'. Unrealistic expectations may create feeding problems. Parental education regarding appropriate portion sizes for children and the concept of offering a new food on many (on average eight!) separate occasions is required. Threats, scolding, bribery and use of food as a reward are likely to create rather than resolve problems.

If a very limited diet is consumed, a dietitian should be consulted in order to assess the adequacy of energy and nutrient intake. Speech pathologists can assist with oral stimulation and the introduction of different tastes and textures.

Bottle-feeding should be avoided beyond 18 months of age. Excessive milk intake may result in iron deficiency. Infants should not be settled in bed with a bottle, as this can cause nursing-bottle caries (see Chapter 22.3).

Excessive intake of milk or fruit juice may reduce appetite and, as a result, may limit the variety of food intake. Excessive fruit juice consumption, particularly apple and pear juice, can result in toddler diarrhoea due to saturation of the facilitated diffusion of fructose. Fruit juice is high in sugar and does not contain the vitamins and fibre that are found in fresh fruit. It should not replace the consumption of water as the best drink for children.

### Daily food needs of preschoolers

Many parents are surprised at how little children of this age need.

- Milk group: 2 servings
  1 serving = 250 mL milk, 200 mg yoghurt or 35 g cheese
  Full-cream products recommended up to 2 years; from 2 years, reduced fat products.
- Bread and cereal group: 4–5 servings
  1 serving = 1 slice of bread, ½ cup pasta or 2 cereal wheat biscuits.
- Fruit and vegetable group: 4 or more servings
  1 serving = 1 piece of fruit or 2 tablespoons of vegetables; focus on variety rather than quantity.
- Meat or protein group: 2 servings
  1 serving = 30 g lean meat, fish or chicken, ½ cup beans or 1 egg.

### Specific nutritional concerns during childhood

#### Vegetarian diets

The lower energy and higher fibre content of vegetarian diets can limit children's total energy intake, as they may not consume sufficient volume to meet their needs.

Children on well planned semi-vegetarian, lacto or lacto ovo vegetarian diets are adequately nourished if appropriate attention is given to selection of suitable iron sources, and sufficient vitamin C is consumed to maximize iron absorption. Vegan diets place children at risk of iron deficiency anaemia. Children on vegan diets require calcium-fortified soy milk to ensure adequate calcium intake. The risks of vegetarian diets for adolescents, particularly vegans, are significant, because of the rapid growth that occurs during puberty. Sufficient energy and an adequate intake of iron, calcium, zinc and, if vegan, vitamin $B_{12}$ must be ensured.

Providing that the mother is consuming an adequate vegetarian diet, infants can be successfully breastfed. Strictly vegan mothers who are not receiving vitamin $B_{12}$ place their child at considerable risk of profound neurological impairment. Vegetarian mothers who formula-feed prefer not to use formulas based on cow's milk. An appropriately fortified infant soy formula may be used. Solid introduction should commence in the usual way, between 4 and 6 months of age, but particular attention needs to be given to iron, if haem iron-containing foods are being avoided. Infants placed on vegan diets are most at risk of nutritional deficiencies. Children who develop iron deficiency anaemia may be at risk of persistent minor neurocognitive impairment, even with iron repletion. Breastfed infants whose mothers get little direct sunlight (including cultures where women are veiled), require vitamin D supplements to prevent rickets.

#### Hypoallergenic diets

There is a role for elimination diets in children with documented multiple food allergy. However, food restriction in children places them at risk of macronutrient and micronutrient deficiency. This highlights the importance of communication with the treating doctor and/or dietitian to ensure that the diet is nutritionally sound.

### Nutrition issues in adolescence

Common features of teenage eating include skipping meals, consumption of a limited variety of foods, frequent consumption of high-fat, high-sugar, low-nutrient foods, a lack of fibre and fad dieting. Fast-food consumption may contribute to the increasing prevalence of adult obesity in Western society, particularly when combined with a sedentary lifestyle (see Chapter 3.4). Poor and sometimes inappropriate body image may account for the fad diets that are quite common among teenage girls and boys. Girls, in particular, often modify their diets to avoid foods that they see as being high in fat and energy, such as meat or milk; this may result in an entire food group being omitted from their diet. The avoidance of milk and milk products during the time of peak accumulation of bone mass and calcium accretion may play a role in osteoporosis later in life. Limiting sources of iron, such as red meat, can lead to iron deficiency. Appropriate nutrition education and role modelling needs to be provided both at home and in the school setting.

## Overnutrition

The dramatic rise in the prevalence of obesity amongst Australian children over the last three decades indicates that the aetiology is not purely genetic. Clearly there are complex genetic and environmental factors at play. These are discussed fully in Chapter 3.4. Importantly, overweight children may still be at risk of micronutrient malnutrition, such as iron, vitamin D and calcium deficiency. A poor-quality diet rich in excess calories may lack adequate micronutrients.

## Undernutrition

### Malnutrition

Malnutrition is the leading cause of childhood morbidity and mortality worldwide. Currently ample food is produced to feed the world's population but social and political forces, such as war, lack of transport infrastructure and degradation of arable land, conspire to keep food from the most needy.

A malnourished child has a weight-for-length (or height) of less than 70% or less than −3 standard deviations (SD) of the normalized reference figure (2009 World Health Organization Child Growth Standards and the Identification of Severe Acute Malnutrition in Infants and Children; available at http://www.who.int/child_adolescent_health/documents/malnutrition/en/index.html/). Children below 60% of weight-for-age may be stunted, and not severely wasted.

The reduction of all food intake or starvation leads to protein-energy malnutrition, resulting in marasmus (from the Greek 'to waste away'). Children who have a proportionately greater deprivation of protein than energy may develop kwashiorkor (from the Ghanaian 'deprived child'). These children are malnourished and oedematous. Children with kwashiorkor have a typical appearance consisting of a protuberant belly, muscle wasting, dependent oedema, flaking skin with depigmentation ('flaky paint' dermatitis), glossitis and angular cheilitis. Children suffering from severe protein-energy malnutrition may also have vitamin deficiencies, especially deficiencies of B vitamins such as thiamine, leading to beriberi, and niacin, leading to pellagra. Vitamin A deficiency can result in blindness and may significantly worsen mortality from diarrhoea and measles. Long-term consequences include insulin-dependent diabetes mellitus secondary to tropical pancreatitis, and also a significant reduction in IQ and school performance.

If malnutrition has occurred relatively acutely, height and weight discrepancies may result. If malnutrition has been severe and protracted, stunting may occur and often future growth is compromised, even after adequate energy provision.

### Malnutrition in the developing world

Malnutrition and kwashiorkor frequently date from the interruption of breastfeeding due to maternal ill-health, work requirements or the arrival of a new infant. In some parts of the developing world, high-quality protein, particularly meat, poultry and fish, is in short supply. Breast milk has many immune factors that provide passive protection as well as promoting the infant's own immune system; therefore, it is not surprising that cessation of breastfeeding predisposes the child to respiratory and diarrhoeal disease. The increased metabolic demands of infection may result in further nutritional 'stress'. Infection with human immunodeficiency virus (HIV) is a major contributor to malnutrition in the infected mother and her child, particularly in Africa. These factors all combine to contribute to the synergistic spiral of malnutrition and disease.

### Malnutrition in the developed world

Poverty plays a role in malnutrition in the developed world. However, other factors such as ignorance, food faddism and psychopathology also contribute.

In Australia, marasmus rarely develops in a malnourished child, usually because of intervention from social agencies or because medical intervention occurs. Kwashiorkor is virtually never seen, even in the Indigenous population, where protein-energy malnutrition often occurs. Both food intake and increased metabolic demands secondary to infectious disease burden contribute to protein-energy malnutrition.

Malnourished children may also have specific vitamin and trace element deficiencies. These should be assessed and corrected. By far the most common deficiencies in developed societies are in iron and folate and vitamin D. Low vitamin D levels have been increasingly recognized as a health problem in children over recent years.

## Nutrition in the hospitalized child

Acute and chronic protein-energy malnutrition is not uncommon in children in a tertiary hospital (Fig. 3.3.1). Malnutrition in hospitalized patients is associated with increased infectious and non-infectious complications, mortality, costs and length of stay.

Nutritional assessment of patients at admission and during the period of hospitalization provides the basis for the identification and treatment of nutrition deficits. Indicators for early nutritional intervention include:

- height-for-age and weight-for-age percentages or z scores more than 2SD below the mean for age
- height-for-age <95% expected

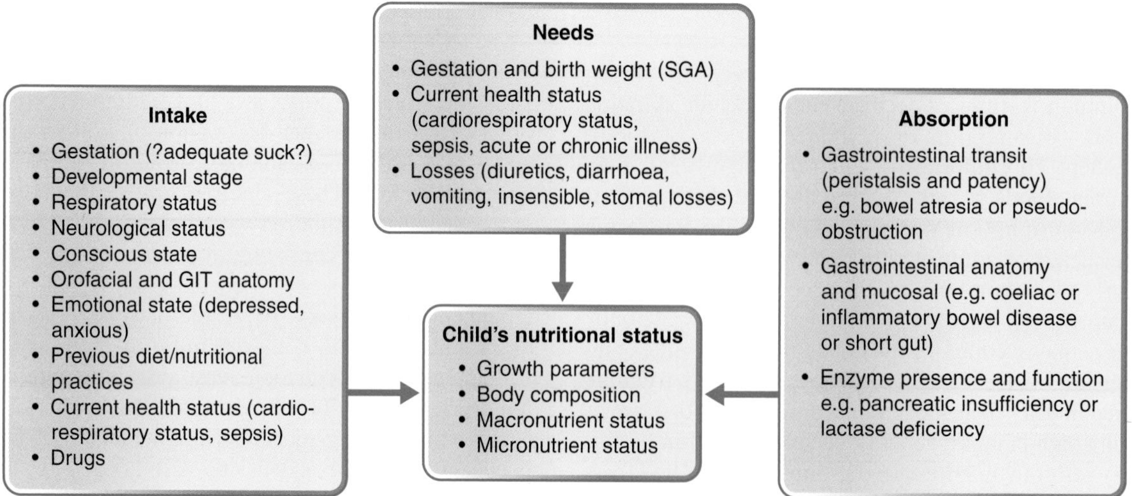


Fig. 3.3.1 Factors affecting a hospitalized child's nutritional status. GIT, gastrointestinal tract; SGA, small for gestational age.

- weight-for-height <90% expected or >120% expected
- height velocities <5 cm/year after 2 years of age.

In contrast to prolonged fasting, which responds to simple protein-energy repletion, the nutritional management of a patient with metabolic stress due to critical illness requires consideration of glucose metabolism, and specific micronutrient and energy requirements. Energy requirements during critical illness are usually reduced but will increase during the rehabilitation phase. The total energy expenditure (TEE) is the sum of:

$$\text{TEE} = \text{BMR} + E_{activity} + E_{growth} + E_{losses} + \text{Thermic effect of feeding } (\sim 10\%).$$

Basal metabolic rate (BMR) is the largest component of TEE and can be estimated in children using predictive equations (e.g. Schofield equation). BMR is increased by clinical conditions including fever, major surgery, cardiac failure, sepsis and burns. See Table 3.3.3.

## Feeds for infants

- Breast milk feeding should be the primary aim for very sick babies. If too premature or ill to suckle at the breast, expressed breast milk (EBM) can be fed via a nasogastric or orogastric tube until the baby is well enough to be placed on the breast.
- Breast milk fortifiers are available to add to EBM to increase its content of protein, energy and other nutrients in very low birth weight (VLBW – birth weight lies below the 10th centile for gestational age) babies. Fortifier should be added only once feeds are fully established (i.e. 150–200 mL per kg per day) unless the baby has a condition requiring fluid restriction (e.g. congestive cardiac failure or chronic lung disease). In addition, VLBW babies may require folate, iron, sodium and vitamins C, D and E. Iron should not be started until 12 weeks of age and VLBW babies who receive multiple blood transfusions may not need supplemental iron.
- If breast milk is not available, an infant formula is required. Low birth weight (LBW) formulas are designed for very premature (<32 weeks) babies. These formulas contain more energy, protein, calcium, phosphorus, trace elements and certain vitamins than standard formulas. They include long-chain poly-unsaturated fatty acids as part of their fat content, based on evidence that this improves neurodevelopmental outcomes. LBW formulas are used until a weight of 2.5 kg is achieved.
- Standard infant formulas provide approximately 280 kJ/100 mL (20 kcal/30 mL) and 1.5 g protein/100 mL. Fortification (to 350 kJ/100 mL or 420 kJ/100 mL) should be implemented only under the supervision of a paediatrician or dietitian.
- Infants and young children who develop an intercurrent gastroenteritis should have all fortification ceased until vomiting and diarrhoea resolve, to avoid the potential complication of hypernatraemic dehydration.

**Table 3.3.3 Reference values for energy and protein enteral requirements**

| Age | Energy (kcal per kg per day) | Protein (g per kg per day) |
|---|---|---|
| 0–6 months | 115 | 2.2 |
| 6–12 months | 95 | 2.0 |
| 1–3 years | 95 | 1.8 |
| 4–6 years | 90 | 1.5 |
| 7–10 years | 75 | 1.2 |
| 11–14 years (male/female) | 65/55 | 1.0 |
| 15–18 years (male/female) | 60/40 | 0.8 |

## Feeds for children

In some cases additional energy needs to be added to oral feeds, via:

- energy supplements, such as glucose polymers or fat emulsions added to oral foods and fluids
- complete supplements (e.g. PediaSure, Fortisip or Sustagen drinks), which can increase energy, protein and nutrient intake.

## Routes of feeding

Acute illnesses such as gastroenteritis and respiratory infections can result in inadequate oral intake to meet increased metabolic needs. This usually results in transient weight loss. Children may require supplemental hydration, receiving fluids by either nasogastric tube or the intravenous route. Children with chronic illness, however, may require long-term assistance to meet nutritional requirements. This may be in the form of supplemental feeding through either a nasogastric tube or a gastrostomy tube. The latter form of feeding is especially useful in chronic illness or neurological compromise, such as cystic fibrosis or cerebral palsy, and in children with chronic illness for whom re-establishment of oral feeding has not been possible (Table 3.3.4).

**Table 3.3.4 Diseases that increase micronutrient requirements**

| Disease | Increased requirement |
|---|---|
| Burns | Vitamins C, B complex, folate, zinc |
| HIV/AIDS | Zinc, selenium, iron |
| Renal failure/dialysis | Vitamins C, B complex, folate (reduce or omit copper, chromium, molybdenum) |
| Haemofiltration | Vitamins C, B complex, trace elements |
| Protein-energy malnutrition | Zinc, selenium, iron |
| Refeeding syndrome | Phosphate, magnesium, potassium |
| Short bowel syndrome, chronic malabsorption states | Vitamins A, $B_{12}$, D, E, K, folate, zinc, magnesium, selenium |
| Liver disease | Vitamins A, $B_{12}$, D, E, K, zinc, iron (reduce or omit manganese, copper) |
| High fistula output, chronic diarrhoea | Zinc, magnesium, selenium, folate, B complex, $B_{12}$ |
| Pancreatic insufficiency | Vitamins A, D, E, K |
| Inflammatory bowel disease | Folate, $B_{12}$, zinc, iron |

HIV/AIDS, human immunodeficiency virus/acquired immune deficiency syndrome.
Source: Thomson K, Tey D, Marks M (eds) 2009 Paediatric handbook, 8th edn. Wiley, Chichester.

Some children are unable to feed enterally and require parenteral (intravenous) nutrition. These include extremely premature or ill neonates, children recovering from intestinal surgery and children with intestinal failure.

## Prematurity

Premature infants have increased nutritional metabolic demands due to a rapid growth phase, tissue development, stress of illness, poor temperature control and the increased demands of small for gestational age (SGA) infants. These factors, combined with immature organ function, poor nutrient stores and altered feeding patterns, mean that the majority of premature infants require a combination of parenteral and/or specialized enteral nutrition. The former provides the recommended fluid and electrolyte requirements until the latter is tolerated at sufficient volumes for growth and development.

## Chronic illness

Monitoring of nutritional status should be an integral component of the routine care of children with chronic illness. Malnutrition and growth failure is common in children with cerebral palsy due to abnormalities in feeding skills, oromotor incoordination, gastro-oesophageal reflux, constipation and behavioural problems. Nutritional deficits place these patients at increased risk of pressure sores, skeletal abnormalities and infection. Enteral nutrition provided by a nasogastric or gastrostomy tube has been associated with improvement in energy levels, behaviour and mobility. Patients with renal disease, liver disease and cystic fibrosis are at risk of developing specific micronutrient abnormalities in addition to protein-energy malnutrition.

## Short bowel syndrome

Short bowel syndrome (SBS) is the clinical syndrome of severe malabsorption and maldigestion that occurs after a major surgical resection or a congenital shortening of the intestine. In a full-term neonate the small intestine is about 250±40 cm at birth. SBS occurs when the small bowel remnant is less than 30% of normal length, equivalent to less than 75 cm. Some patients with SBS require long-term parenteral nutrition to provide the nutrition, fluid and electrolytes necessary to sustain life (Fig. 3.3.2). Failure to wean from parenteral nutrition in children with SBS is associated with less than 30 cm jejunoileum, lack of enterocolic continuity, residual disease of the intestine and lack of early feeding tolerance.

## Parenteral nutrition

Infants and children who are unable to feed enterally require intravenous nutrition using a combination of nutrient and lipid solution (Fig. 3.3.3). These are delivered either by a peripheral intravenous line (maximum dextrose concentration of 10%) or via a central venous line (maximum dextrose concentration of 30%). The nutrient solution is comprised of amino acids (both essential and non-essential), glucose, electrolytes, minerals, vitamins, trace elements and water, and may contain heparin. The main source of non-protein calories is D-glucose (dextrose). The lipid emulsion is a concentrated source of calories with low osmolarity. Patients receiving parenteral nutrition require daily weighing and fluid balance. Baseline and frequent subsequent blood tests are required to monitor for electrolyte imbalance, glucose metabolism and to tailor the parenteral nutrition accordingly.

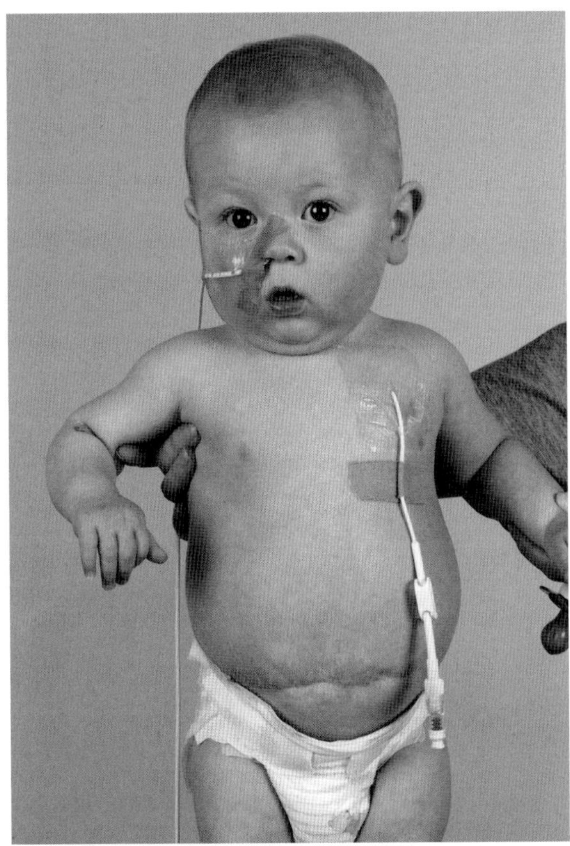

Fig. 3.3.2 Twelve-month-old boy born with gastroschisis, complicated by bowel resection resulting in short bowel syndrome. Treatment involved a nasogastric tube for enteral feeds and a central venous catheter for parenteral nutrition.

Parenteral nutrition can be complicated by life-threatening electrolyte imbalance, hypoglycaemia, hyperglycaemia, line sepsis, thrombosis and extravasation of the nutrient into the tissues, resulting in a parenteral nutrition 'burn'. Most infants and children are on parenteral nutrition for short periods of time during acute illness or recovery from surgery. However, children with intestinal failure may require lifelong total parenteral nutrition (TPN). In addition to the acute complications, these children are at risk of vitamin and micronutrient deficiency, growth failure, parenteral nutrition liver disease and vascular access complications.

## Refeeding syndrome

Refeeding syndrome is the term used for the metabolic complications that may occur when aggressive nutritional therapy is used to treat the severely malnourished patient. In particular, the delivery of intravenous or enteral carbohydrate loads may precipitate these potentially fatal electrolyte disturbances. The potential metabolic disturbances that may occur include hypokalaemia, hypophosphataemia, hypomagnesaemia and hyponatraemia. Potential side-effects of these electrolyte and mineral disturbances include: cardiac failure, respiratory compromise, seizures, myocardial infarction and arrhythmias.

Under most circumstances of prolonged starvation or significant weight loss, renourishment should commence slowly with small increases in nutrition delivered once electrolyte and mineral disturbances have been corrected. For example, commence feeding at basal energy requirements, increasing to full requirements over 7–10 days. Patients most at risk during refeeding include those with anorexia nervosa and those with weight loss more than 10–20% body weight, prolonged fasting or a minimal intake of longer than 7–10 days.

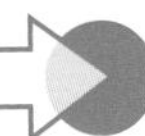

### Practical points

- Malnutrition is the leading cause of childhood morbidity and mortality worldwide.
- Malnutrition continues in Australia's own Indigenous population, with up to 20% of hospitalized Aboriginal children in Australia's Northern Territory estimated to be malnourished.
- The most common micronutrient deficiencies in developed societies are of iron and folate and vitamin D.
- Hospitalized children are at particular risk of malnutrition and require careful nutritional assessment of needs, losses, intake and absorption.
- Nutrition is safer when given enterally. Parenteral nutrition should be used only when enteral nutrition is contraindicated or unsuccessful.
- Refeeding syndrome describes the metabolic complications that occur when aggressive nutritional therapy is used to treat the severely malnourished patient in which the delivery of intravenous or enteral carbohydrate loads may precipitate potentially fatal electrolyte disturbances.

Monitoring of refeeding is essential and includes daily/regular monitoring of glucose, electrolytes, urea, creatinine, phosphate, magnesium and fluid balance until stable. Enteral or parenteral feeds may need to be ceased until electrolytes have been corrected. Supplementation of potassium, phosphate and magnesium may be required during the initial feeding period, guided by blood levels.

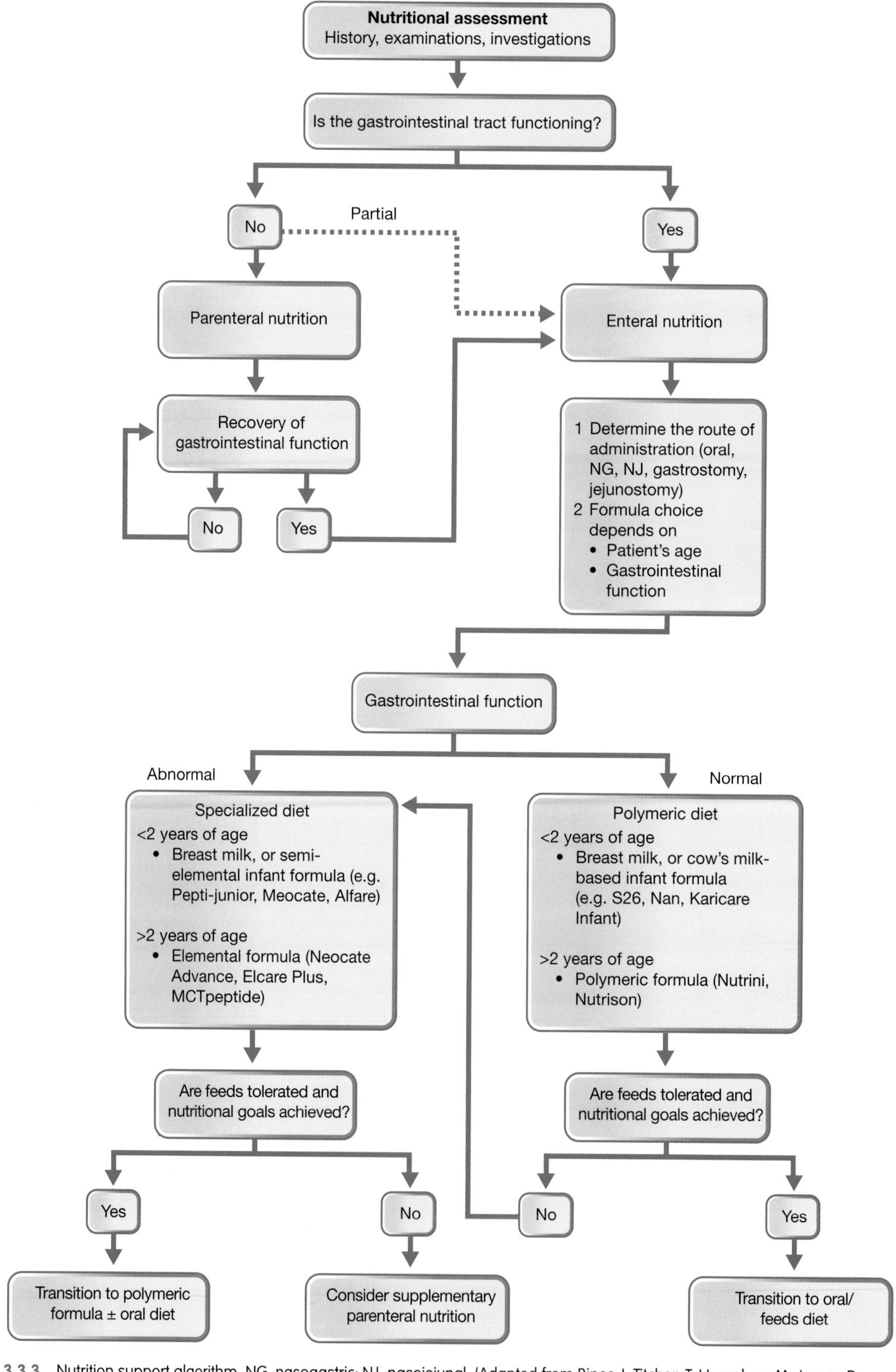


Fig. 3.3.3 Nutrition support algorithm. NG, nasogastric; NJ, nasojejunal. (Adapted from Bines J, Titchen T, Humphrey M, Jessen D 1997 A practical guide to paediatric nutrition support. Department of Gastroenterology and Clinical Nutrition, Royal Children's Hospital, Melbourne.)

# Obesity 3.4

Louise A. Baur

## Introduction

Paediatric obesity is a major public health problem in both developed and developing countries. Obese children and adolescents may suffer from a host of co-morbidities, some of which are immediately apparent, whereas others act as warning signs of future disease. Obesity can be a serious, chronic, relapsing disease. It is a disorder of energy imbalance that arises as a consequence of a complex interaction between genetic, social, behavioural and environmental factors. Although investment in primary prevention is vital in curbing the epidemic, effective treatment of those children and adolescents who are currently obese is also needed to improve both their immediate and long-term health outcomes.

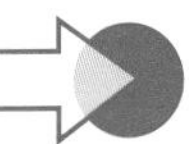

**Practical points**

- Obesity is a chronic disorder of energy imbalance – focus upon both sides of the energy balance equation: energy in and energy out.
- Measure body mass index (BMI) and plot on a BMI-for-age chart. Measure and record waist circumference, and calculate waist : height ratio.
- In pre-pubertal children, weight maintenance or reduction in the rate of weight gain, may be appropriate goals of therapy. Weight loss is often necessary for moderately obese younger children, and for adolescents.
- For younger children, focus upon the parents as agents of change. Adolescents will require a different, developmentally sensitive, approach.
- Long-term behavioural change is required, involving an increase in incidental physical activity, a reduction in sedentary behaviour and a sustainable change to a lower energy intake.
- There is a role for drug therapy in adolescents who have moderately severe obesity, or those with clinical insulin resistance.
- Prevention of obesity requires a whole-of-system approach in which many aspects of the broader food and physical activity environment are targeted.

## How is paediatric overweight and obesity defined?

### Body mass index – a measure of total body fatness

Body mass index (BMI; weight/height$^2$; kg/m$^2$) is a simple measure of body fatness. BMI varies dramatically with age and sex during childhood and adolescence: it increases in the first year, falls during preschool years, and then rises once more into adolescence. The point at which BMI starts to increase again, between 4 and 7 years of age, is termed the point of 'adiposity rebound' (Figs 3.4.1–3.4.4).

Several countries have their own BMI-for-age growth charts that can be used clinically to chart an individual's BMI and monitor changes over time. The World Health Organization has also developed BMI-for-age charts for international use for children aged 0–5 and 5–19 years (see Figs 3.4.1–3.4.4). Until further research helps establish the relation between BMI-for-age cut-points and health outcomes in childhood and adolescence, the decision as to which specific centile lines denote overweight and obesity in clinical settings ultimately remains arbitrary.

### Waist circumference and waist : height ratio – measures of fat distribution

In children and young people, just as in adults, waist circumference is correlated with abdominal fat, as well as with cardiovascular risk factors. Although waist circumference charts are available for some individual countries, there are no internationally accepted criteria for high- or low-risk waist circumference in this age group. Nationally developed waist circumference-for-age charts can be used to monitor clinical progress of an individual patient.

Waist-to-height ratio (waist/height) is an additional measure of fat distribution that is easy to calculate and reasonably independent of age and sex for individuals aged above 6 years. Waist-to-height ratios greater than 0.5 are associated with increased cardiometabolic risk factors. The clinical message is: 'Keep your waist to less than half your height'.

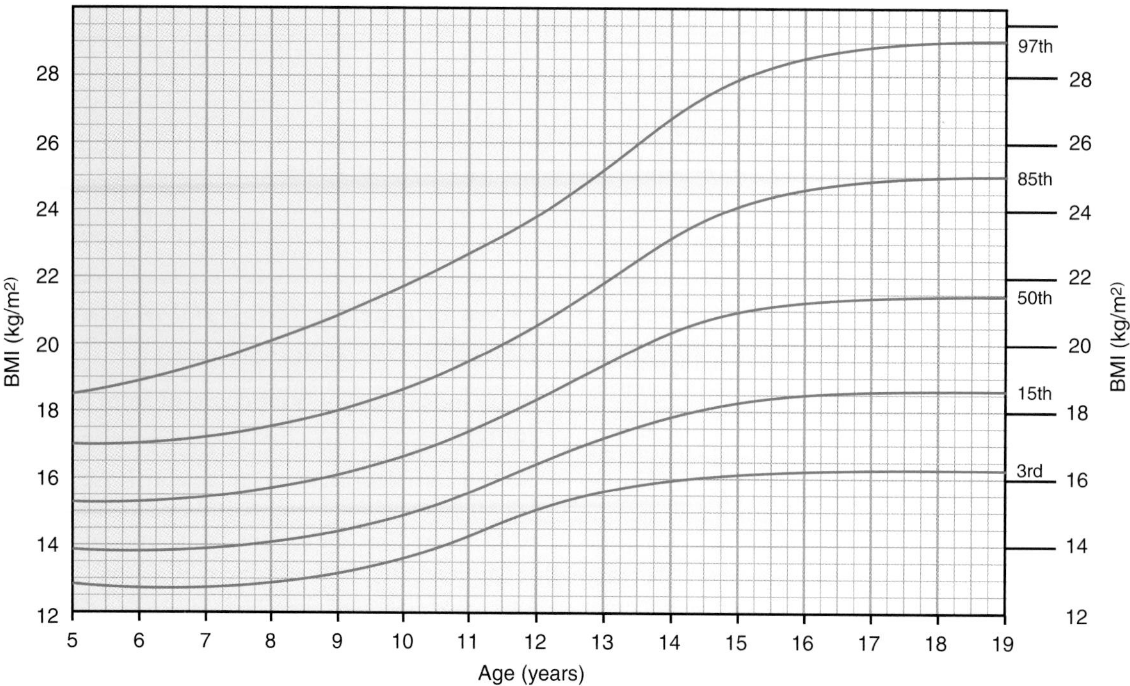


Fig. 3.4.1 Body mass index-for-age chart for girls aged 5–19 years. Source: 2007 World Health Organization Reference. Available at: http://www.who.int/growthref/cht_bmifa_girls_perc_5_19years.pdf

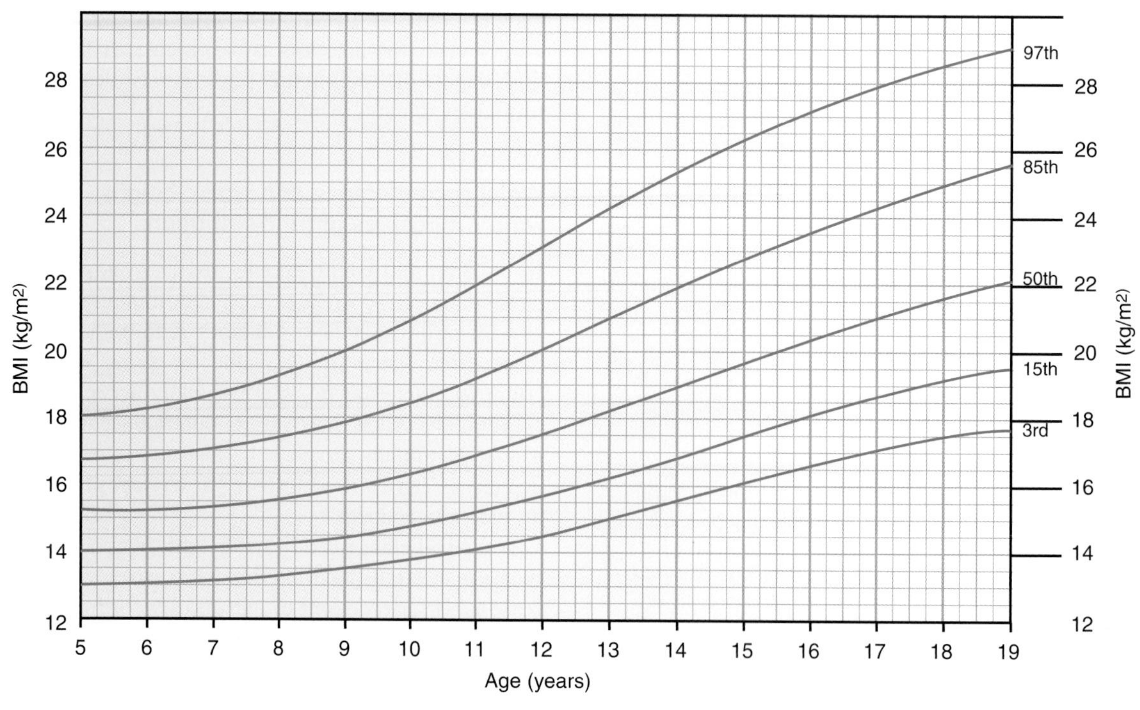


Fig. 3.4.2 Body mass index-for-age chart for boys aged 5–19 years. Source: 2007 World Health Organization Reference. Available at: http://www.who.int/growthref/cht_bmifa_boys_perc_5_19years.pdf

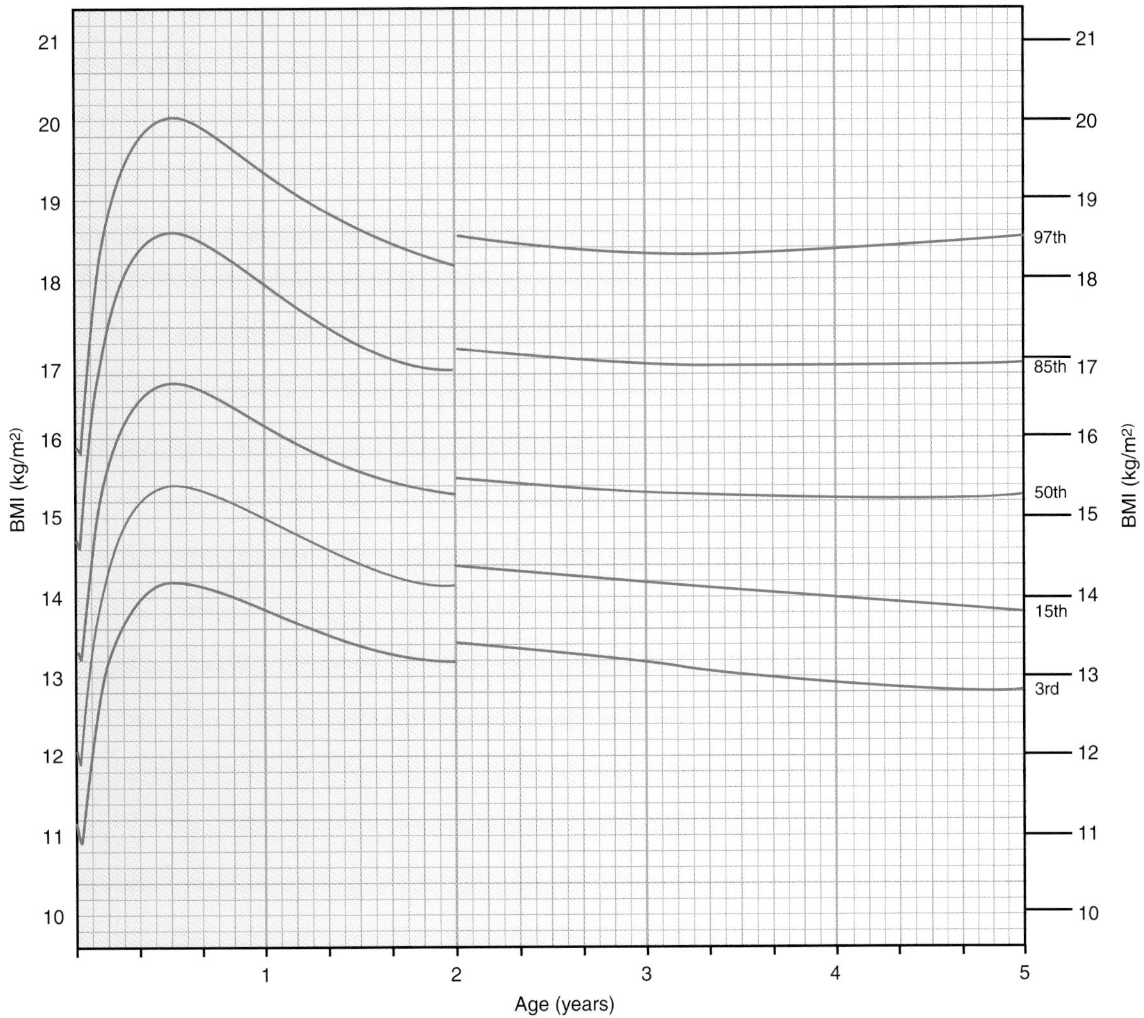


Fig. 3.4.3 Body mass index-for-age chart for girls aged 0–5 years. Source: World Health Organization Child Growth Standards. Available at: http://www.who.int/childgrowth/standards/cht_bfa_girls_p_0_5.pdf

### Racial and ethnic variations in definition

There are racial and ethnic variations in the biological response to excess adiposity. Among adults, Asians generally have a higher percentage body fat for a given BMI and an associated increased health risk at lower BMI values compared with Europeans, whereas Pacific populations generally have a lower percentage body fat and a decreased health risk at the same BMI levels. These differences are also likely within the child and adolescent age group, and ultimately require the development of ethnic- or race-specific definitions or criteria for obesity.

## What is the prevalence of paediatric overweight and obesity?

### International prevalence rates and secular trends

Worldwide, approximately 10% of school-aged children and adolescents are overweight, with 2–3% being obese. Prevalence rates vary across regions, with higher rates in children from the Americas, Europe and the Pacific than in those from sub-Saharan Africa or Asia.

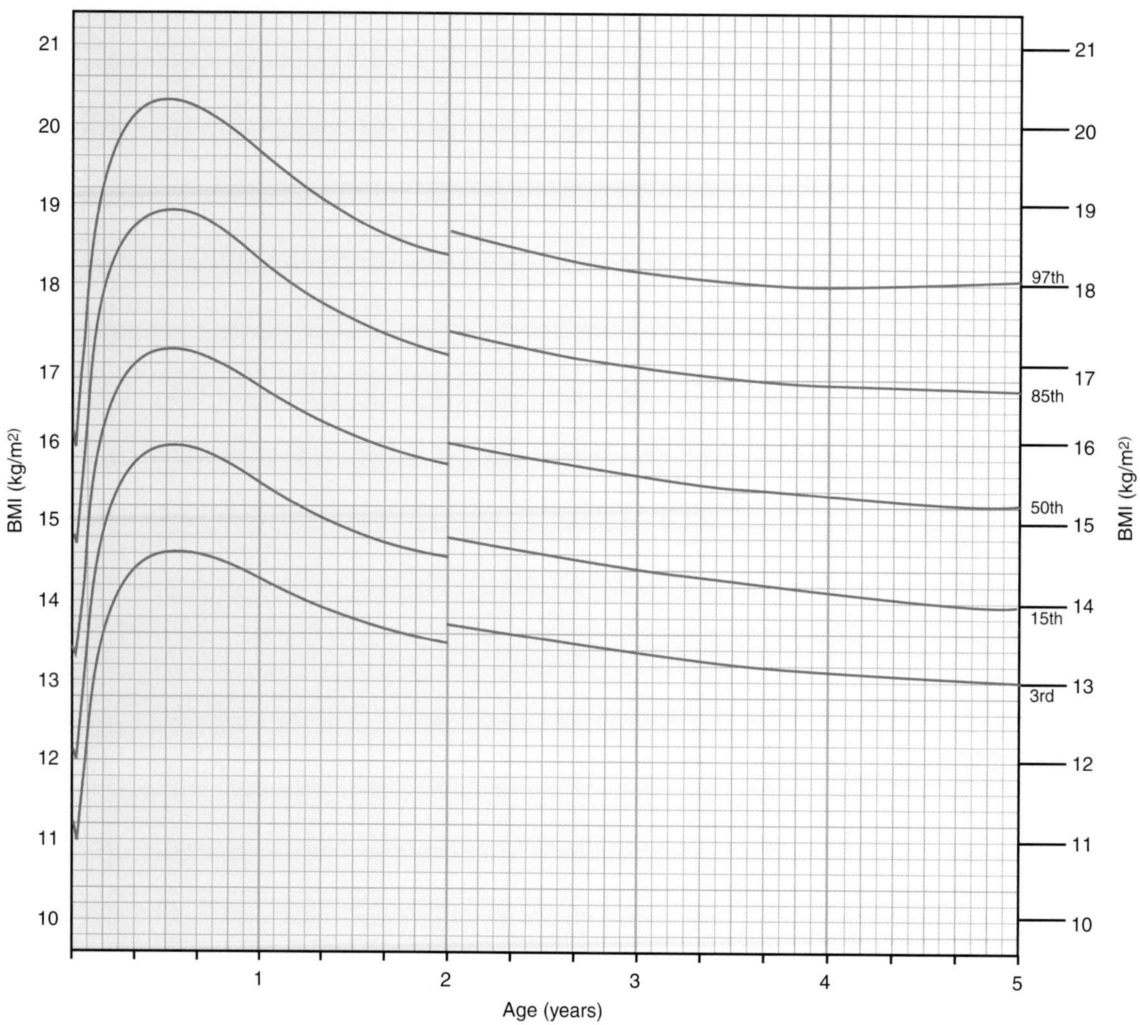


Fig. 3.4.4 Body mass index-for-age chart for boys aged 0–5 years. Source: World Health Organization Child Growth Standards. Available at: http://www.who.int/childgrowth/standards/cht_bfa_boys_p_0_5.pdf

In 2007 in Australia, approximately 1 in 4 children and adolescents were overweight or obese. In 2006–2007 in New Zealand, 29% of children and adolescents were overweight or obese, with higher rates being found in Pacific and Maori children.

Of most concern are the rapid changes in obesity prevalence in many countries in several continents. Several Asian countries that are experiencing rapid changes in urbanization and nutrition have seen increasing rates of obesity in paediatric populations in recent years. For example, urban Chinese and Vietnamese younger children now have similar obesity rates to those of children in Australia. In addition, overweight children are heavier than in the past. Such findings have very significant implications for future population health strategies.

## What are the complications of paediatric obesity?

The complications of obesity among children and adolescents may be immediate or may not manifest until the medium- to long-term. They affect many body systems, as outlined in Table 3.4.1.

### Complications during childhood and adolescence

#### Psychosocial complications

The most common consequences of obesity in childhood and adolescence are those related to psychosocial dysfunction and social isolation. In pre-adolescent children, physical appearance and athletic competence self-esteem are lower than in their normal weight peers, although global self-esteem appears to be preserved. In adolescent girls, excess weight is significantly related to body dissatisfaction, drive for thinness and bulimia. Cross-sectional studies of teenagers show an inverse relationship between weight and both global self-esteem and body-esteem. The pervasive, negative social messages associated with obesity in many communities may have a particular impact during adolescence.

There are differences in health-related quality of life between obese and non-obese children. In randomly sampled populations, the physical and social domains of health-related quality of life for obese children are lower than for non-overweight children. Severely obese patients have significantly reduced health-related quality of life compared with healthy children, having similar quality of life scores to children diagnosed with cancer.

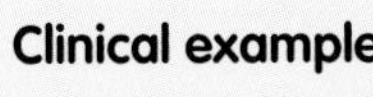

### Clinical example

**Trudy, a 13-year-old girl with obesity**

Trudy presented to her general practitioner (GP) with a respiratory tract infection. Her mother commented incidentally that Trudy was concerned about her weight and was being teased at school. Indeed, she had left her previous school because of bullying and now it appeared to be starting afresh in the new school.

Trudy is an only child, with a good relationship with her parents and some peers. She is in good general health, apart from the weight gain. Several family members are obese (mother and three grandparents), her paternal grandfather has type 2 diabetes, and her maternal grandfather has hypercholesterolaemia and ischaemic heart disease. Trudy leads a sedentary lifestyle: she enjoys playing music, sewing, reading and talking on the phone. Trudy is driven to and from school each day and watches 3 hours of television per day. Her dietary intake includes skipping breakfast, full-cream milk, 'something nice' for morning and afternoon tea, buying food at the milk-bar in the afternoon, a daily intake of 500 mL of soft drink and free access to biscuits at home.

On examination, Trudy's height was 161.5 cm (<75th centile), weight 74.3 kg (>97th centile), BMI 28.4 kg/m$^2$ (>95th centile for age; adult overweight range), waist circumference 89 cm (adult female 'at significant risk of metabolic complications' range) and waist : height ratio 0.55 (>0.5, indicative of cardiometabolic risk). She was in mid-puberty, and had abdominal and upper thigh striae. Blood pressure was 120/80 mmHg. A fasting blood test showed a normal glucose (4.6 mmol/L; normal range 3.5–5.5), mild hyperinsulinaemia (115 pmol/L) and a lipid profile characteristic of central obesity: total cholesterol 5.3 mmol/L (normal range 2.6–5.5), high-density lipoprotein (HDL) cholesterol 0.8 mmol/L (normal >0.9), triglycerides 1.9 mmol/L (normal range 0.6–1.7).

**Management**

The GP arranged to see Trudy and her mother, separately and together, initially every 3 weeks, and then less frequently. Two visits to a local dietitian were also arranged; more frequent follow-up could not be organized. Trudy was encouraged to set her own goals for food and activity changes; these goals were re-visited at the consultations. She was helped to look at ways in which eating cues could be recognized and modified. The family was supported to make changes to their eating patterns and the use of the television in the home.

**Progress**

In time, Trudy's mother lost some weight as a result of altered cooking practices and being more active. Water was offered at the evening meal instead of soft drink, less healthy snacks were no longer stored in the cupboards, and the family started eating more vegetables and had smaller meat and rice/potato portions at the evening meal. Trudy ate something for breakfast each morning and started walking to and from school. She started tennis lessons and found an interest in tap dancing.

Ten months later, Trudy's weight was 69.3 kg, height 163.0 cm, BMI 26.1 kg/m$^2$, waist circumference 81 cm and waist : height ratio 0.50. She reported being fitter and said she was greatly enjoying school and was no longer being bullied. A repeat fasting blood test showed an improved lipid profile (total cholesterol 4.8 mmol/L, HDL cholesterol 1.0 mmol/L, triglycerides 1.4 mmol/L) and a decreased insulin concentration (85 pmol/L), consistent with a reduction in central obesity.

## Orthopaedic complications

Slipped capital femoral epiphyses occur much more commonly in obese young people and much earlier than in non-obese patients. Blount disease (tibia vara) is a deformity of the medial portion of the proximal tibial metaphysis that arises as a result of increased weight-bearing on cartilaginous bone with subsequent compensatory overgrowth and bowing of the tibia. Obese young people also have low bone area and bone mass relative to their body weight, making them more prone to fractures than lean individuals.

Minor orthopaedic obesity-associated complications include knock knee (genu valgum), a decreased recovery from soft tissue ankle injuries, and flat, wide feet with increased static and dynamic plantar pressures. These conditions may seem relatively trivial in health terms, but could have a significant impact on a child's ability to participate fully in activities.

## Hepatobiliary complications

Obese children and adolescents may experience a range of gastrointestinal and hepatobiliary disorders, the most significant being non-alcoholic fatty liver disease (NAFLD). NAFLD is an umbrella term that includes steatosis as well as steatohepatitis. It typically

**Table 3.4.1 Potential obesity-associated complications in children and adolescents**

| System | Health problems |
|---|---|
| Psychosocial | Social isolation and discrimination, decreased self-esteem, learning difficulties, body image disorder, bulimia<br>*Medium and long term:* poorer social and economic 'success', bulimia |
| Respiratory | Obstructive sleep apnoea, asthma, poor exercise tolerance |
| Orthopaedic | Back pain, slipped femoral capital epiphyses, tibia vara, ankle sprains, flat feet |
| Hepatobiliary | Non-alcoholic fatty liver disease, gallstones |
| Reproductive | Polycystic ovary syndrome, menstrual abnormalities |
| Cardiovascular | Hypertension, adverse lipid profile (low HDL cholesterol, high triglycerides, high LDL cholesterol)<br>*Medium and long term:* increased risk of hypertension and adverse lipid profile in adulthood, increased risk of coronary artery disease in adulthood, left ventricular hypertrophy |
| Endocrine | Hyperinsulinaemia, insulin resistance, impaired glucose tolerance, impaired fasting glucose, type 2 diabetes mellitus<br>*Medium and long term:* increased risk of type 2 diabetes mellitus and metabolic syndrome in adulthood |
| Neurological | Benign intracranial hypertension |
| Skin | Acanthosis nigricans, striae, intertrigo |

HDL, high-density lipoprotein; LDL, low-density lipoprotein.

presents as an asymptomatic increase in the level of aminotransferases. The degree of steatosis is associated with the severity of obesity, a central fat distribution, hypertriglyceridaemia, insulin resistance and the presence of raised aminotransferases, with an increased level of alanine aminotransferase being most specific for steatosis. Liver fibrosis and even evolving cirrhosis have been identified in liver biopsy findings of paediatric patients with NAFLD.

Several clinical audits from paediatric surgical units have demonstrated an association between cholesterol cholelithiasis and obesity in children and adolescents. Gastro-oesophageal reflux is more prevalent in obese individuals, possibly secondary to increased intra-abdominal pressure.

### Neurological complications

Idiopathic raised intracranial pressure (pseudotumour cerebri) is a rare but potentially very serious complication of obesity. The role played by obesity in the pathogenesis of the disorder is unknown.

### Asthma and sleep-disordered breathing

Respiratory outcomes can be poor in obese children. Asthma is more prevalent in obese than non-obese children. Compared with lean children with asthma, overweight and obese children use more antiasthma medications, have more wheezing episodes and experience more unscheduled visits to hospital. Obese children also have a lower exercise tolerance than their lean peers, presumably compounding their obesity.

Potentially more serious is the complication of obstructive sleep apnoea. Between 1 in 10 and 1 in 4 obese children have obstructive sleep apnoea. Obstructive sleep apnoea is associated with severity of obesity, insulin resistance and dyslipidaemia. Profound hypoventilation and even sudden death have been reported in severe cases of obesity-associated sleep apnoea.

### Risk factors for cardiovascular disease

Risk factors for cardiovascular disease are one of the most common problems facing the obese young person. In the famed Bogalusa Heart Study from the USA, 60% of overweight 5–10-year-olds had one cardiovascular risk factor, such as hypertension, high low-density lipoprotein (LDL) cholesterol or high triglycerides, and over 20% had two or more risk factors. Overall, when compared with their lean peers, overweight children were 2.4 times as likely to have raised total cholesterol and diastolic blood pressure, and 4.5 times as likely to have increased systolic blood pressure. A central fat distribution is particularly associated with clustering of cardiovascular risk factors.

### Endocrine complications

Overweight children are much more likely to have raised fasting insulin concentrations (indicative of insulin resistance), impaired fasting glucose or glucose intolerance than their lean peers. Although still rare among children and adolescents, the incidence of type 2 diabetes mellitus is increasing and is inextricably linked to the prevalence of obesity among young people. Type 2 diabetes is more common in adolescents and those who are obese, have acanthosis nigricans (thickened pigmented skin at the base of the neck and in flexures, characteristic of insulin resistance; Fig. 3.4.5), have a family history of type 2 diabetes or are female.

The metabolic syndrome, a term describing a cluster of highly prevalent disorders in Western countries that are linked to insulin resistance and central obesity, was initially identified among adults. Among adolescents in the USA, the overall prevalence of the metabolic syndrome is approximately 10%, but the syndrome affects almost one-third of overweight adolescents.

### Reproductive system complications

Menstrual abnormalities occur more frequently in obese girls, including the early onset of puberty and menarche, as well as menstrual irregularities and polycystic ovary disease. There is a strong association between abdominal fat, increased levels of androgenic hormones, hirsutism, insulin resistance and polycystic ovaries, which grouped together is termed polycystic ovary syndrome.

### Skin complications

Obese children suffer from overheating as their fat tissue acts as insulation, resulting in profuse sweating with any physical activity. Thrush occurs more commonly in obese subjects, especially in such moist, overheated areas as skin-folds or the groin. Striae can also occur, particularly on the abdomen and thighs.

Acanthosis nigricans can occur in insulin-resistant states, such as obesity. It is characterized by thickened areas of hyperpigmentation, with later development of hypertrophy and sometimes papillomatosis (see Fig. 3.4.5). The skin lesions typically occur in intertriginous regions such as the base of the neck, axillae, groin, antecubital and popliteal fossae, and umbilicus. The condition occurs more frequently in dark-skinned ethnic groups.

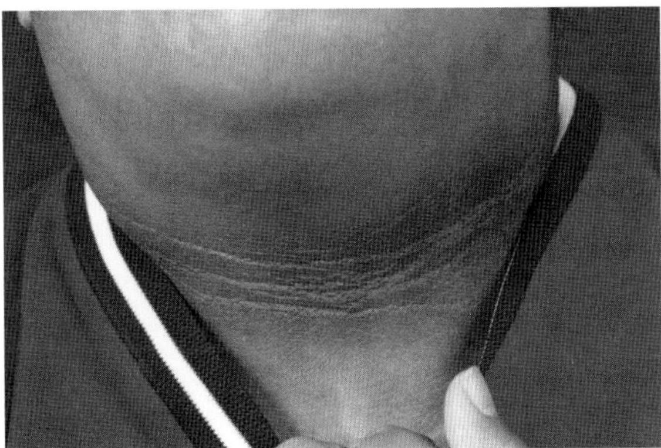

Fig. 3.4.5 Acanthosis nigricans, seen at the base of the neck of an adolescent male with obesity and hyperinsulinaemia.

## Adult complications arising from child and adolescent obesity

### Obesity in adulthood

The most significant health risk faced by obese young people is that they are at risk of becoming obese adults, who are at increased risk of cardiovascular disease, diabetes and some cancers. Tracking of obesity from childhood and adolescence through to adulthood is more likely with a family history of parental obesity, the presence of obesity in late childhood or adolescence, or with increased severity of obesity.

### Long-term cardiovascular complications

Obesity in childhood and adolescence is associated with an increased risk of cardiovascular disease risk factors, and an increased carotid intima–media thickness in young adults. Long-term (>50 years) follow-up of cohorts in the USA and the UK show that both all-cause and cardiovascular mortality is associated with higher adolescent BMI: study participants who, as young people, were heavier than the 75th centile for BMI were twice as likely to die from ischaemic heart disease than those who had a BMI between the 25th and 75th centile.

### Long-term endocrine and metabolic complications

Childhood BMI predicts the development of diabetes in adulthood. Results from the Bogalusa Heart Study show that childhood obesity is the strongest predictor of the development, in adulthood, of the cluster of risk factors that characterize the metabolic syndrome: children in the top quartile of BMI were 11 times more likely to develop the metabolic syndrome as adults than their lean peers.

### Long-term psychosocial complications

Overweight in adolescence may also be associated with later social and economic problems. Obese adolescent females and young women are more likely, as adults, to have lower family incomes, higher rates of poverty and lower rates of marriage than women with other forms of chronic physical disability but who are not overweight, a finding suggesting that discrimination plays a role in adverse outcomes. However, obesity limited to childhood does not appear to be associated with adverse socioeconomic, educational, social, and psychological outcomes in adulthood.

## What causes obesity?

Obesity is a complex condition, with interactions between genetic, metabolic, behavioural and environmental factors all contributing to its development (Fig. 3.4.6).

### Physiological basis of obesity

Obesity is a chronic disorder affecting the balance between energy intake and energy expenditure. This balance is influenced by a complex set of physiological pathways, of which the hypothalamus acts as the central regulator of energy homeostasis and energy intake. The resultant energy regulation system is very protective against weight loss, which has been the dominant physiological threat to the individual until the past couple of decades in most westernized societies. However, the system is not protective against weight gain.

### Genetic associations of obesity

#### The heritability of obesity

There is a strong familial association with obesity, with numerous studies indicating that a major part of this association is via a shared genetic predisposition.

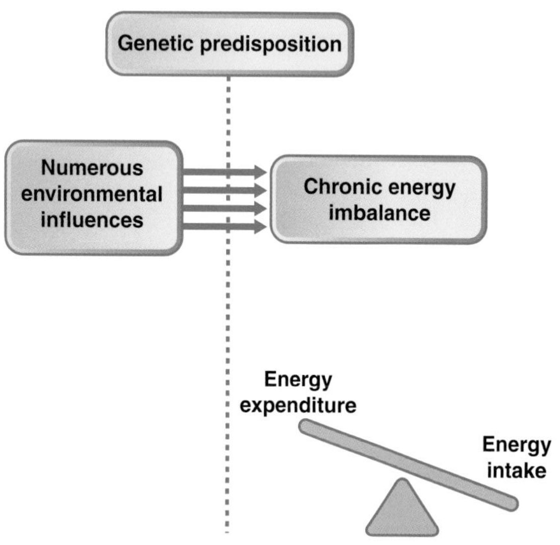


Fig. 3.4.6 Obesity is a disorder of chronic energy imbalance. Many environmental factors influence energy balance, through the filter of genetic predisposition.

Twin, family and adoption studies suggest an overall heritability of BMI and body composition of 25–50%.

#### Genes associated with common obesity

More than 200 different candidate genes have been associated with obesity-related phenotypes. The range of actions, or presumed actions, of the many gene products of candidate genes is extremely varied, reflecting the numerous physiological pathways influencing total body energy balance and fat distribution. Thus, genes influencing appetite and satiety signals, fat-cell differentiation, fat-cell signalling, adrenal action, resting metabolic rate, diet-induced thermogenesis, nutrient partitioning, peripheral insulin action, deposition of visceral fat and obesity-related co-morbidities are all the subject of intense investigation.

#### Monogenic forms of obesity

Mutations in several genes that encode proteins with probable roles in central appetite regulation have been described but are rare. Most of the mutations are associated with severe early-onset obesity and have a recessive form of inheritance, with the exception of mutations in the melanocortin-4 receptor gene, which has an autosomal dominant mode of inheritance.

#### Syndromic forms of obesity

Many rare syndromes that are caused by discrete genetic defects or chromosomal abnormalities have obesity as one of a constellation of physical and development abnormalities. The most frequent of these syndromes is Prader–Willi syndrome, characterized by diminished fetal activity, obesity, muscular hypotonia, mental retardation, short stature, hypogonadotropic hypogonadism, and small hands and feet, as well as a number of other features.

### Environmental and behavioural associations of obesity

The increased prevalence of obesity in recent decades in genetically stable populations highlights the central role of recent important environmental trends in the development of the obesity epidemic.

#### Television viewing

The association between television viewing and obesity in childhood and adolescence has been demonstrated in both cross-sectional and longitudinal studies, although as yet there are no clear data linking obesity with the viewing of interactive video games, computers or other 'small screen' recreation. Several possible mechanisms for the association between television viewing and obesity include:

- increased exposure to food marketing
- increased snacking of energy-dense foods and drinks while watching television
- displacement of time spent in more physical activities
- reinforcement of sedentary behaviour
- reduction in basal metabolic rate while watching television
- television viewing is a proxy for a generally obesity-conducive lifestyle, reflecting parenting style and limit-setting around food choices and recreational choices.

### Physical activity and sedentary behaviour

Lower physical activity levels and sedentary behaviours are associated, cross-sectionally, with a higher prevalence of obesity in children. Prospective studies suggest that physical activity has a protective effect on the development of excess weight gain in childhood. Major changes in urban and transport planning and the broader physical activity environment have contributed to a reduction in physical activity and an associated increase in obesity through the following:

- loss of public recreation space
- increased high-rise housing
- increased motorized transport
- decreased access to public transport
- increased use of passive forms of entertainment (e.g. television, computers)
- perceptions of lack of safety in local neighbourhoods.

### Dietary intake and eating patterns

The increased prevalence of obesity in recent decades has resulted, in part, from changes in dietary intake. Factors that are likely to have contributed to this include:

- an increased consumption of energy-dense, nutrient-poor foods
- a high intake of sugar-sweetened drinks
- heavy marketing of energy-dense foods and fast-food outlets
- increased dining at fast-food restaurants
- early feeding style – parental feeding restriction is associated with increased child eating and weight status.

Breastfeeding has a small but protective effect against obesity. Additional protective factors include high dietary fibre, low glycaemic index foods, and school environments that support healthy food choices for children. The relative contributions of dietary fat (versus energy) intake, portion sizes and specific eating patterns to the development of obesity remain unclear, although all may play an important role.

### Socioeconomic conditions

Overweight is high among the poorer children in developed countries and the richer children in developing countries. Potential contributors to obesity in urbanized developing countries include increased availability of cheap energy-dense foods and widespread access to television which would favour a more sedentary, indoor lifestyle.

## Medical conditions associated with obesity

Obesity may occur secondary to a range of medical conditions, some of which are outlined in Table 3.4.2.

## Other factors associated with obesity

- Growth patterns associated with an increased risk of subsequent obesity include an earlier adiposity rebound and rapid catch-up growth in the first 2 years.
- Parental obesity more than doubles the risk of adult obesity among both obese and non-obese children aged less than 10 years, and having two obese parents increases the risk of mid-childhood obesity by a factor of more than 10 when compared with children where neither parent is obese.
- Parental (especially maternal) dietary disinhibition is associated with development of excess weight gain in the child.

**Table 3.4.2 Medical conditions associated with obesity**

| System/effect | Conditions |
|---|---|
| Endocrine | Hypothyroidism, hypercortisolism, growth hormone deficiency or resistance |
| Central nervous system damage | Hypothalamic–pituitary damage due to surgery, trauma or cranial irradiation |
| Postmalignancy | Acute lymphoblastic leukaemia |
| Side-effects of drug therapy | Glucocorticoids, some antiepileptics (e.g. sodium valproate), some antipsychotics (e.g. risperidone, olanzapine), insulin |

## How is child and adolescent obesity managed?

### Clinical assessment

#### Clinical history

The clinical history should be conducted sensitively. The features that should be covered in a clinical history are outlined in Table 3.4.3.

#### Anthropometry

BMI, waist circumference and waist: height ratio are most useful when measured serially and used to monitor change over time:

- BMI is calculated as weight/height$^2$ and then plotted on a BMI-for-age chart (see Fig. 3.4.1).
- Waist circumference is measured at the midpoint between the lower edge of the ribs and the iliac crest, approximately at the level of the umbilicus, although in severely obese patients with a fatty apron this measurement can be difficult to ascertain.
- Waist: height ratio greater than 0.5 in people aged above 6 years is associated with increased cardiometabolic risk factors.

#### Physical examination

Features to be sought on physical examination include:

- hypertension (ensure that cuff width is adequate)
- skin findings (e.g. acanthosis nigricans, striae, intertrigo, skin chafing, hirsutism)
- adenotonsillar hypertrophy
- clinical signs of asthma
- hepatomegaly (fatty liver; note – may be difficult to palpate), right upper-quadrant tenderness (gallstones)
- an abnormal gait due to joint or other musculoskeletal problems; clinical signs of hip, knee or ankle problems; bowing of the tibia.

Findings on physical examination that may indicate other causes for obesity (e.g. hypothyroidism, hypercortisolism or Prader–Willi syndrome) and which call for further assessment include:

- short stature
- dysmorphic features
- violaceous striae
- intellectual disability
- visual or neurological defects indicative of a central nervous system lesion.

**Table 3.4.3 History to be sought as part of the clinical assessment of the obese patient**

| History | Details |
|---|---|
| General | Pregnancy details, including maternal gestational diabetes<br>Early medical history<br>Ethnicity |
| Weight | History of obesity including onset and duration of obesity<br>Pubertal history (including menstrual history if relevant)<br>Impact of obesity on the life of the patient and their family<br>Reasons for seeking clinical help |
| Complications | Psychological effects of obesity, including teasing and bullying<br>Presence of sleep apnoea/disturbed sleep<br>Asthma<br>Specific symptoms such as knee/hip pain<br>Menstrual history (girls)<br>Exercise tolerance |
| Family history of obesity and disorders associated with insulin resistance | Relative weights or BMIs of family members<br>Family history of obesity, type 2 diabetes, cardiovascular and cerebrovascular disease, fatty liver disease and obstructive sleep apnoea |
| Lifestyle | Physical activity, including transport to/from school, participation in organized sports or other activities, access to recreation space or equipment for games, availability of friends or family for games or play<br>Sedentary activities including television, video games, computer use, other passive entertainment time, mobile phone use<br>Dietary history including meal patterns, fast-food intake and snacks, soft-drink intake |

BMI, body mass index.

### Laboratory investigations

For overweight and mildly obese children, laboratory investigations are generally not necessary. However, if a child or adolescent is very obese (especially if centrally obese), has a family history of disorders associated with insulin resistance, or history and examination suggest the presence of complications of obesity or other risk factors, the following biochemical screening for dyslipidaemia, insulin resistance, glucose intolerance and liver abnormalities is recommended:

- Fasting lipid profile (total cholesterol, LDL cholesterol, HDL cholesterol, triglycerides)
- Fasting glucose
- Liver function tests (specifically alanine aminotransferase)
- Consider fasting insulin
- Consider oral glucose tolerance test.

Further assessment of liver function (e.g. liver ultrasonography, exclusion of other causes of liver dysfunction) may be required. More detailed endocrinological assessment may be needed if there is short stature, hirsutism or menstrual irregularities. If obstructive sleep apnoea is suspected then referral for polysomnography is warranted.

## Defining treatment outcomes

The goals of therapy should be clarified initially with the parents or young person, as appropriate. Markers of a successful outcome of therapy may include:

- changes in weight status: weight loss, and, in prepubertal children, slowing of weight gain or weight maintenance
- a decrease in waist circumference or waist : height ratio ('waist loss') is a useful indicator of reduction in abdominal obesity
- resolution of medical complications
- improvement in self-esteem and psychosocial functioning
- an increase in level of fitness or aerobic capacity
- improvement in family functioning.

Education of the family and, where appropriate, the young person about the nature of obesity, including the realization that it is a chronic disorder of energy balance, is also important, as the need for long-term changes in behaviour will then be more readily apparent. Helping the family or young person identify small, achievable goals is important; examples may include aiming initially for two extra walks per week, or reducing television viewing by 1 hour per day every few weeks.

## Broad principles of management

The broad principles of management include:

- clarification of treatment outcomes
- family involvement
- a developmentally appropriate approach
- long-term behaviour change
- long-term dietary change
- increased physical activity
- decreased sedentary behaviour.

## Conventional treatment approaches

### Family focus

Long-term maintenance of weight loss (i.e. from 2 to 10 years) is achieved when the intervention is family based. Families influence food and activity habits, and thus it is not surprising that effective therapy of obesity must take this into account. Altered food patterns within the whole family, as well as support of the child and parental reinforcement of a healthy lifestyle, are important factors in successful outcomes.

### A developmentally appropriate approach – pre-adolescent children

Treatment of pre-adolescent obesity with the parents as the exclusive agents of lifestyle change is superior, in terms of long-term weight and psychosocial outcomes, to a child-centred approach. Thus, when dealing with the obese pre-adolescent child, sessions involving the parent or parents alone, without the child being present, are likely to be the most effective.

### Adolescent-focused interventions

With adolescents, consider separate sessions for the young person and parents. Short-term weight management success is associated with a range of interventions, all involving intense support for behavioural change, such as increased physical activity, phone- and mail-based behavioural interventions initiated in primary care settings, pharmacological therapy and a low glycaemic load diet.

### Behaviour modification

There is a range of potential behavioural modification strategies that can be used in the management of childhood obesity, including:

- monitoring behaviour (e.g. weighing weekly, keeping a television-time chart)
- setting goals
- rewarding successful changes in behaviour through praise
- controlling the food and physical activity environment.

The nature of each of these strategies will vary depending upon the age and developmental status of the patient.

### Dietary management

Involvement of the entire family in making the change to a sustainable and healthy food intake is vital. The focus should be on behaviour change, healthier food choices, and a reduction in the consumption of energy-dense, micronutrient-poor foods and high-sugar drinks. Avoidance of severe dietary restriction may be important both in helping the development of the child's capacity to self-regulate dietary intake and in avoiding the subsequent development of disordered eating.

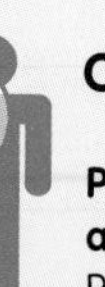

**Clinical example**

**Peter, a 15-year-old boy with central obesity and metabolic syndrome**

Peter, an Australian boy of Lebanese ethnic origin, with a strong family history of central obesity, type 2 diabetes, premature heart disease and hypertension, had significant central obesity (weight 102.8 kg, BMI 39.3 kg/m$^2$, waist circumference 115 cm and waist : height ratio 0.71). He had a very sedentary lifestyle and a large intake of soft drink and 'fast food' meals. Peter was aware that he was 'not able to keep up with my mates', but was otherwise unconcerned about his large size. He had a wide circle of friends. Findings on physical examination included hypertension (blood pressure 130/85 mmHg with a wide cuff; >95th centile for age, sex and height) and marked acanthosis nigricans at the base of his neck and in his axillae and groin flexures, indicative of insulin resistance.

Fasting blood tests showed normoglycaemia (4.8 mmol/L), hyperinsulinaemia (280 pmol/L), low HDL cholesterol (0.8 mmol/L), hypertriglyceridaemia (2.2 mmol/L) and a mildly raised alanine aminotransferase level (60 U/L; normal range 10–50). An oral glucose tolerance test excluded glucose intolerance and diabetes. Liver ultrasound findings were consistent with diffuse fatty infiltration (in keeping with NAFLD). Thus, Peter had several features of the metabolic syndrome: hyperinsulinaemia, dyslipidaemia, central obesity, hypertension, acanthosis nigricans and fatty liver disease.

Peter was encouraged to limit his television viewing and he also took out gym membership, although he found it difficult to attend regularly. A dietitian counselled about dietary change and provided initial frequent review, but again Peter was unable to sustain the lifestyle change, largely because of lack of motivation for change. Weight gain continued. Orlistat was prescribed, but Peter found the side-effects (bloating, steatorrhoea, abdominal pain) unacceptable and discontinued therapy. After review by a paediatric endocrinologist, Peter was commenced on the insulin-sensitizing agent, metformin. There was some initial weight loss on this therapy (2 kg in the first month of therapy), but Peter was relatively non-adherent to therapy after the first couple of months.

Dietary interventions should follow national nutrition guidelines and have an emphasis on the items listed in Box 3.4.1.

### Physical activity and sedentary behaviour

Participation of obese children in a lifestyle programme (e.g. walking, running, cycling or swimming, based on the family's preference) leads to greater long-term reductions in overweight when compared with a programme of isocaloric programmed aerobic exercise. Targeting decreased sedentary behaviour may be as effective as targeting increased physical activity in terms of medium-term weight and fitness outcomes.

**Box 3.4.1 Interventions for changes in dietary intake, physical activity, sedentary behaviour and weight**

**Dietary interventions**

- Modified eating patterns (e.g. regular meals, eating breakfast, eating together as a family, avoiding eating while watching the television)
- Parents modelling healthy food choices
- Food choices that are lower in energy and fat, and that have a lower glycaemic index
- Increased vegetable and fruit intake
- Healthier snack-food options
- Decreased portion sizes
- Reduction in soft-drink ('soda'), cordial, other sweetened drinks and fruit juice intake
- Water as the main beverage

**Physical activity and sedentary behaviour**

- Focus on increasing incidental activity (e.g. playing with friends or family, walking to the local shops, helping with housework)
- Look at active transport options (e.g. walking, cycling, using public transport)
- Choose organized activities that the child enjoys
- Improve access to recreation spaces and play equipment (e.g. balls, frisbees, skipping ropes)
- Limit time spent watching television, or using the computer, playstations or other such 'small screens', to less than 2 hours per day
- Consider alternatives to motorized transport

**Other behaviour modification strategies to promote healthy behaviours and monitor outcomes**

- Monitor behaviours (e.g. television viewing, time on Facebook and other recreational computer pursuits), having breakfast
- Monitor weight during weight loss phase (e.g. weekly, keep a record)
- Role-modelling of healthy lifestyle behaviours by family members
- Stimulus control (e.g. avoid having biscuits, soft drinks and unhealthy snack choices in the household, or on display in the home)

Recommendations regarding physical activity and sedentary behaviour are also listed in Box 3.4.1.

### Settings for treatment

Time-efficient interventions such as group sessions, holiday camps or mail- and phone-based behavioural interventions may do at least as well as individual sessions in the management of child and adolescent obesity.

### Non-conventional approaches to therapy

In adolescents, orlistat (a gastrointestinal lipase inhibitor) may play a role in management of moderately severe obesity. Metformin should be considered in obese adolescents with evidence of clinical insulin resistance. Both forms of drug therapy should be used only when the benefits of therapy have been weighed over the risk of adverse events. There is as yet little information to guide the use of Very Low Calorie Diets in adolescents. Any such therapies should occur in the context of a behavioural weight management programme and be restricted to specialist centres with expertise in managing severe obesity.

There is one randomized controlled trial of bariatric surgery (laparoscopic banding surgery) versus lifestyle intervention in adolescents with moderately severe obesity. The study showed improved weight outcomes at 2 years in those who underwent surgery. There are very few nationally relevant position statements on bariatric surgery in adolescents.

#### Clinical example

**Anna, a 2-year-old girl with excess weight gain**

At a consultation for an intercurrent illness, Anna, aged 2 years 2 months, had her height and weight assessed by her GP. Her height was 92 cm (97th centile for age) and she was noted to be obese, with weight of 19.8 kg (>97th centile for age) and BMI 23.4 kg/m$^2$ (>95th centile for age).

Anna's birth weight was 3.7 kg. Review of her growth records showed that her weight had tracked along the 90th centile for the first 6 months, and that from 12 months of age her weight had steadily veered above the 97th centile. In the past 14 months, Anna had been eating the same foods as her parents and two older siblings. This included two or three 'fast food' meals per week, several 'treat' snacks per day (e.g. biscuits or a packet of crisps) and a regular soft drink intake. When outside, Anna tended to sit and play in the sandpit rather than play actively. There were three televisions in the household and Anna was estimated to watch 3–4 hours of television per day. Both of Anna's parents were mildly obese and her siblings were also overweight.

The GP sensitively raised the issue of Anna's excess weight gain with Anna's mother and encouraged a whole-family approach to lifestyle change. Support for change was given by the GP, and the mother also attended a children's healthy nutrition group programme offered in the local community health centre. Changes that occurred over the next 6 months included offering the children water instead of soft drink, reducing portion sizes at the evening meal and providing healthy snack choices. The parents instituted some rules about television viewing, limiting it to less than 90 minutes per day. The children, including Anna, were encouraged to play outside more often. The sandpit was covered and Anna spent more time in active play.

Six months later, Anna's weight remained unchanged and her height was now 97 cm (97th centile for age). The resultant BMI was 21.0 kg/m$^2$, which was still above the 95th centile, but there was a marked 2.4-unit decrease over the time period.

## Primary prevention of child and adolescent obesity

Because child and adolescent obesity is so common in many countries and has such pervasive consequences, it is important that not just the overweight and obese are targeted with treatment interventions, but that effective primary prevention strategies are also identified and put into place. Interventions simply focusing on educating individuals and communities about behaviour change have had limited or no success in modifying obesity prevalence. This is because the broader environment in many communities does not readily support healthy food choices for physically active lifestyles.

Many upstream factors (physical, economic and sociocultural) contribute to obesity in individuals and can operate at both a microenvironmental level (the settings where individuals live, eat, play or go to school) as well as at a macroenvironmental level (the broader sectors that ultimately influence dietary intake and physical activity and that are beyond the ability of an individual to influence). Microenvironments relevant to obesity include homes, schools, community groups (e.g. clubs, churches), food retailers (e.g. supermarkets), food service outlets, recreation facilities and local neighbourhoods (e.g. cycle paths, street safety). Macroenvironments relevant to obesity include food production and importing, food manufacturing and importing, food marketing (e.g. fast-food advertising), the sports and leisure industry (e.g. instructor training programmes), urban and rural development (e.g. town planning, local government) and the transport system (e.g. public transport systems).

Considering this, a range of opportunities exists for prevention strategies in a given community or country. These might include:

- Reshaping the food supply and encouraging physical activity:
  - Review taxation systems to enable access to healthier foods and active recreation (e.g. tax breaks for fitness products and providing healthy foods in schools and workplaces; tax energy-dense foods and sugary drinks)
  - Regulate the amount of fats, trans-fats, sugar and salt in foods
  - Subsidize transport of fresh foods to rural and remote areas.
- Curbing inappropriate marketing of unhealthy foods and beverages.
- Improving public education and information:
  - Effective long-term marketing to improve eating and physical activity
  - Develop national systems of simple, comprehensible food labelling to support healthier food choices.
- Reshaping urban environments towards healthy options:
  - School communities that support healthy eating and physical activity
  - Comprehensive community-based interventions
  - Employers that support healthy eating and physical activity
  - Town planning and building design that encourage physical activity (e.g. public transport, cycle paths, footpaths, protect open spaces)
  - Incentive schemes that encourage healthy behaviours (e.g. gym memberships, active travel included in expense policies).
- Primary healthcare and public health workforce to support people in making healthier choices.
- Encouraging and supporting breastfeeding.
- Closing the gap for disadvantaged communities.
- Monitoring the prevalence of obesity and obesity-conducive behaviours, and evaluating the effectiveness of interventions.
- Implementing national food strategies that harmonize policies related to sustainability of the food supply, agriculture, food production, food distribution and health.

Such interventions will require intersectoral and inter-governmental cooperation, supported by adequate resourcing and significant community ownership.

# Immunization 3.5

Peter Richmond

Immunization provides protection against specific infectious diseases and is one of the greatest achievements of medical science and public health. It is the right of every child to be protected against vaccine-preventable diseases: parents, caregivers and health professionals need to ensure that immunization is available to all children.

Protection against subsequent infection after surviving the initial challenge has been recognized for many centuries for some infections. The use of material from smallpox lesions for vaccination was practised in early dynasties in China. Edward Jenner recognized that vaccination with cowpox virus could protect against challenge with smallpox. Smallpox was declared eradicated worldwide in 1979.

Diphtheria immunization began in the 1920s, and immunization campaigns against pertussis (whooping cough) were initiated in the 1940s. In the 1950s, triple antigen vaccine (DTP: diphtheria, tetanus and pertussis) was introduced and polio immunization campaigns began, leading to its elimination in the developed world. It is likely that poliomyelitis will be the second vaccine-preventable disease to be eradicated worldwide. Measles immunization has been available for more than 40 years, and the last decade has seen the introduction of many new vaccines with rapid impact on rates of serious infections such as meningococcal and pneumococcal disease.

Immunization remains one of the most important public health priorities in developed and developing countries. In the developing world, many millions of childhood deaths occur each year from vaccine-preventable diseases such as tetanus, pneumonia, diarrhoea and measles because of lack of access to vaccines and vaccine provider services. Thus, immunization and its promotion remains one of the major activities of the World Health Organization, with the aim of achieving universal immunization for children.

## Principles of immunization

Immunization may be passive or active.

### Passive immunity

Passive immunity refers to the acquisition of preformed antibody. The fetus receives maternal immunoglobulin (Ig) G antibodies during the later weeks of pregnancy, and breastfeeding supplies IgA antibody at the mucosal surfaces of the gastrointestinal tract.

Passive immunization as a means of disease prevention is used in the form of:

- normal human immunoglobulin for protection against measles and hepatitis A, and in children with immunodeficiency
- specific high-titre preparations against cytomegalovirus (CMV), varicella, tetanus, rabies, hepatitis B and diphtheria (for use as post-exposure prophylaxis in high-risk situations or in immunocompromised children), and as
- humanized monoclonal antibody against respiratory syncytial virus (RSV) infection (may be used as primary prophylaxis in children with chronic cardiac and lung disease).

Passively acquired immunoglobulin has a relatively short half-life and does not lead to active immunity or long-term protection.

### Active immunization

Active immunization involves administering a vaccine antigen so that a protective immune response develops that is similar to that occurring after naturally acquired infection. This immune response should be one that entails the development of persistent immunological memory, and long-term protection from the infectious disease.

Active immunization to prevent infection or the effects of infection may be performed using:

- whole organisms (live attenuated or killed)
- purified components of organisms (subunit vaccines, polysaccharide vaccines)
- modified products of the infecting organisms (toxoid vaccines)
- manufactured components of organisms (recombinant vaccines).

### Requirements of vaccines

Ideally, a vaccine should:

- give complete protection from the disease caused by the infection
- give lifelong protection
- cause minimal transient adverse effects
- need to be given once only

- be able to be given in combination with other vaccines
- be able to be administered easily and without discomfort
- be stable under a wide range of storage conditions
- have a long storage life
- be easy and cheap to manufacture.

## Principles of vaccine selection

Common infectious diseases and the vaccine types used for prevention of these diseases are listed in Table 3.5.1. The immunization strategies used for these diseases have been developed to take account of the following factors:

- *The nature of the disease process.* For example, toxoid vaccines are used to prevent diseases in which exotoxins are responsible for the disease such as diphtheria and tetanus.
- *The route of infection.* For example, oral rotavirus vaccines have been developed to provide protective mucosal immune responses to rotaviruses, which are a major cause of severe gastrointestinal tract infections in infants.
- *Variability of the organisms causing disease.* For example, influenza vaccines need annual modification to provide protection from prevalent circulating strains; polio vaccines (oral and inactivated) contain the three strains of the poliovirus that cause disease, and pneumococcal vaccines contains polysaccharide from 7 to 23 of the most common strains that cause disease out of more than 90 strains of pneumococci.
- *The nature of the immune response at different ages.* For example, *Haemophilus influenzae* type b (Hib) vaccines, meningococcal C vaccine and pneumococcal vaccines are much more effective in infants when given as polysaccharide–protein conjugate vaccines rather than purified polysaccharide vaccines because of the poor immune response to polysaccharides at this age.
- *The effects of maternal antibodies on vaccine responses in infants.* Measles immunization is not undertaken until the age of 9–12 months in most countries because passively acquired maternal antibody remains in sufficiently high concentration to neutralize the administered live attenuated vaccine virus strain in the infant prior to this age.
- *The age at which children are most susceptible to infection.* Meningococcal C conjugate vaccines are given as a single dose at 12 months of age in Australia as meningococcal C disease was rare before that age, whereas in the UK it is given to infants at 2, 4 and 12 months of age as the peak incidence was between 6 and 12 months of age.
- *The ability to reduce transmission in the community and induce herd immunity.* For example, rubella immunization is given to all children to provide longlasting immunity for girls before their childbearing years, and to decrease the circulation of rubella in the community, and therefore the

**Table 3.5.1 Vaccine types for schedule vaccines and other commonly available vaccines**

| Disease | Vaccine type |
|---|---|
| **Schedule vaccines** | |
| Hepatitis B | Recombinant subunit vaccine |
| Diphtheria | Toxoid (formaldehyde-treated toxin) |
| Tetanus | Toxoid (formaldehyde-treated toxin) |
| Pertussis | Acellular vaccine containing 2–5 protein antigens from *Bordetella pertussis* |
| *Haemophilus influenzae* type b (Hib) | Polysaccharide protein conjugates (PRP-OMP, PRP-T) |
| Poliomyelitis | IPV: inactivated poliovirus vaccine (types 1, 2 and 3) |
| Measles, mumps and rubella | Attenuated live viruses (freeze-dried) |
| Varicella | Attenuated live virus (freeze-dried) |
| Pneumococcal infections | Conjugate vaccine containing 7, 10 or 13 pneumococcal serotypes |
| Meningococcal C disease | Meningococcal C conjugate vaccine |
| **Other commonly used vaccines** | |
| Influenza | Subunit vaccine derived from inactivated virus |
| Hepatitis A | Inactivated hepatitis A strain |
| BCG | Live attenuated bacteria |
| Pneumococcal infections | Polysaccharide vaccine containing 23 pneumococcal serotypes (not conjugated) |
| Meningococcal infections | Quadrivalent vaccine containing A, C, W135 and Y polysaccharides (both conjugated and unconjugated available) |

BCG, bacille Calmette–Guérin.

risk of exposure of pregnant women to rubella. These strategies have resulted in a dramatic decrease in fetal rubella infection and the associated malformations that occur in early pregnancy (congenital rubella embryopathy).
- *The ability to optimize immunization coverage for the high-risk population.* A targeted strategy of hepatitis B vaccination in newborns of mothers who are hepatitis B carriers to prevent perinatal transmission was ineffective in immunizing the at-risk infants so universal newborn hepatitis B immunization has been implemented in Australia.

## Immunization schedule for routine childhood immunization

The national immunization schedule in countries is generally recommended by an expert committee and is then funded by the government at a later stage. The current Australian schedule is presented in Table 3.5.2. There are differences in the schedule in individual countries and sometimes within countries because of variations in the epidemiology of some diseases, the registration and prices for supply of different types of vaccine, and national priorities and public demand. The immunization schedule has changed significantly in recent years with the availability of new vaccines and is likely to change frequently in the future, so it is important to keep up to date.

Vaccines are provided to registered immunization providers and generally are free of charge for children. Immunization providers are general practitioners, local authority immunization services, some hospital services (particularly in children's hospitals), and some maternal and child health agencies. All immunization providers must be familiar with:
- the immunization schedule
- vaccine storage and handling requirements
- requirements for informed consent for vaccine administration
- adverse effects of immunization
- potential contraindications to immunization.

Information regarding schedules, vaccines and procedures needs to be updated regularly; in Australia this is provided at regular intervals by the National Health and Medical Research Council (NHMRC) Immunization Technical Advisory Group as *The Australian Immunisation Handbook*, which is made available to all immunization providers and to other health-care providers who have a role in immunization services, and is also available as an up-to-date electronic version on the internet (http://www.health.gov.au/internet/immunise/publishing.nsf/content/handbook-home). Similar immunization handbooks exist in electronic and hard copy format in the UK (http://www.dh.gov.uk/en/Publicationsandstatistics/Publications/PublicationsPolicyAndGuidance/DH_079917) and New Zealand (http://www.moh.govt.nz/moh.nsf/indexmh/immunisation-handbook-2011).

**Table 3.5.2 National Health and Medical Research Council National Immunization Programme for Australian children**

| Age | Vaccine | Route |
|---|---|---|
| Birth | HBV | IM |
| 2, 4 and 6 months | DTPa* | IM |
| | Hib* | IM |
| | IPV* | IM |
| | HBV* | IM |
| | PCV | IM |
| | RV | Oral |
| 12 months | MMR | SC |
| | Hib† | IM |
| | MenCC† | IM |
| 18 months | Varicella | SC |
| 4 years | DTPa-IPV | IM |
| | OPV | Oral |
| | MMR | SC |
| 12–15 years | dTpa | IM |
| | Varicella‡ | SC |
| | HBV§ | IM |
| | HPV¶ | IM |

*These antigens are currently given as a single injection as part of a hexavalent vaccine in infants in Australia and New Zealand, whereas HBV is not routinely used in the UK.

†May be given as a combined Hib–MenC conjugate vaccine (also used in the UK as a 2–4–12-month schedule).

‡Varicella vaccine is given only where children have not previously received varicella vaccine and have no history of chickenpox.

§This course of HBV (2 doses of adult formulation) is only for children not previously vaccinated against hepatitis B in infancy.

¶Currently, HPV vaccine is only given to girls as a 3-dose schedule, but is also licensed for boys.

HBV, recombinant hepatitis B vaccine; DTPa, infant formulation of acellular diphtheria, tetanus and pertussis vaccine; Hib, *Haemophilus influenzae* type b conjugate vaccine; IPV, inactivated poliovirus vaccine; OPV, oral poliovirus vaccine; PCV, pneumococcal conjugate vaccine (3 licensed formulations containing 7, 10 or 13 serotypes); RV, rotavirus vaccine (2 licensed formulations given as either 2- or 3-dose schedule); MMR, measles, mumps and rubella vaccine (a combined formulation with varicella vaccine (MMRV) is also licensed); MenCC, meningococcal C conjugate vaccine; dTpa, reduced antigen formulation of diphtheria–tetanus–acellular pertussis vaccine for adolescents and adults; HPV, human papillomavirus vaccine (both bivalent and quadrivalent HPV vaccines are licensed); IM, intramuscular; SC, subcutaneous.

## Administration of vaccines

### Storage of vaccines

Most vaccines need to be stored in a temperature range between 2° and 8°C. Maintenance of the cold chain is required from the time of manufacture until the time of administration. Vaccine storage temperature conditions must be monitored continuously, using thermometers capable of recording maximum and minimum temperatures, preferably in a purpose-built vaccine refrigerator. Generally, freezing of vaccines is more deleterious to vaccine efficacy than short periods of time above the recommended temperature range.

**Clinical example**

Holly was brought in by her mother to her general practitioner (GP) at 18 months of age to discuss her varicella immunization. Her parents were confused as they had heard she was better off getting chickenpox as an infection because it gave longer-lasting immunity and giving the vaccine at this age would put her at risk of more severe disease as an adult. Also they were concerned that, if she had the vaccine, she would be at risk of giving the disease to her brother Tom (4 years of age) who was undergoing chemotherapy for acute lymphoblastic leukaemia and had not had chickenpox or been vaccinated.

The GP advised Holly's parents that varicella vaccine provided good long-term protection against varicella infections and any breakthrough infections (1–2% per year) were mild. In contrast, although chickenpox infection is generally self-limiting, there are risks of severe varicella infection or secondary bacterial infection, which results in 1 in 200 children being hospitalized. The GP also advised that vaccinating Holly was the best way of protecting her brother, as vaccinated healthy children do not pass on the infection and this will decrease the risk of her brother being exposed to a potentially dangerous infection.

### Consent for immunization

Parents or guardians must be given adequate information that will allow them to make an informed decision about immunization for their child. The information given should include:

- the benefits and risks of immunization
- the common side-effects of the various vaccines.

This information preferably should be available in written form, and is provided in a form suitable for parents and guardians in *The Australian Immunisation Handbook*. Valid consent is necessary prior to each immunization episode.

### Pre-immunization questionnaire

In some circumstances, the risk of adverse reactions to immunization is increased in the presence of some conditions. A standardized questionnaire should be used routinely prior to each immunization episode. The questionnaire should enquire whether the child:

- has had any previous severe reactions to any vaccine
- has any condition that may lower immunity (for example, treatment with systemic steroids or chemotherapy, pre-existing immune deficiency disorder or disease affecting immunity, such as leukaemia) or lives with someone with lowered immunity
- might be pregnant (for girls of childbearing age)
- has had a vaccine containing live viruses within the last month
- has any severe allergies (although this is not a contraindication to scheduled immunizations)
- has received a blood transfusion or immunoglobulin preparation in the last 3 months
- identifies as being Aboriginal or Torres Strait Islander person (to ensure that they receive any additional immunizations required).

Children should be assessed to ensure that they are well enough to have vaccine administered: immunization should be deferred only rarely, but may be delayed temporarily if there is a temperature over 38.5°C, if the child has diarrhoea or vomiting (for oral vaccines only), or if he or she is obviously unwell for other reasons.

### Sites of vaccine administration

Intramuscular vaccine administration in infants under the age of 1 year should be at the junction of the upper and middle one thirds of the anterolateral thigh. If three separate intramuscular vaccines are being given, two vaccines are given in one thigh at least 2.5 cm apart and the other vaccine in the other thigh. In children over the age of 1 year, intramuscular vaccines are given into the mid-deltoid region of the upper arm. Vaccines should *not* be given in the buttocks because of possible suboptimal immune response or sciatic nerve damage.

### Adverse effects of immunization

Immunization promotes a protective immune response. As part of this, there is often some evidence of minor inflammation in association with parenterally administered vaccines which may result in local redness and swelling at the injection site or mild transient systemic symptoms including crying, irritability and fever. These were more common with whole-cell pertussis vaccines and are now much less frequent with the acellular pertussis combination vaccines and conjugate vaccines. Large local reactions may occur, especially in older children. Measles immunization may be followed by a mild and transient measles-like illness, with fever and a brief rash, about 7–10 days after immunization. All of these side-effects are generally transient, require no specific treatment and do not preclude further vaccination.

Rarely, there may be major events in association with immunization procedures. Anaphylaxis is very rare (less than 1 in 100 000 immunizations), but every immunization provider must have the appropriate equipment and training for dealing with anaphylaxis. The most important components of management of anaphylaxis are maintenance of the airway and the administration of adrenaline (epinephrine).

Convulsions sometimes are seen in association with immunization procedures. Simple febrile convulsions may occur in conjunction with febrile responses to any vaccine in children predisposed to febrile convulsions; however, these are not contraindications to further immunization. Immunization is not associated with sudden or unexpected infant death syndrome (SIDS). Several studies, including a recent well controlled study in New Zealand, have shown that the relative risk for SIDS is decreased in immunized children.

### Disorders that are not contraindications to immunization

Immunization is not contraindicated in children:

- with minor upper respiratory tract illness (colds, cough, sore throat) or low-grade fever at the time immunization is due
- using inhaled steroid medications for control of asthma, or topical steroids for dermatitis
- with allergies
- receiving antibiotics
- with controlled epilepsy, a history of febrile convulsions, a family history of epilepsy or stable neurological disorders
- who have been premature or who are growing poorly.

Children who have documented egg allergy can be safely immunized, as egg proteins are not found in vaccines in the routine childhood immunization schedule, including measles–mumps–rubella (MMR) vaccine. However, advice should be given about immunization with influenza and yellow fever vaccines, which are not recommended for children with anaphylaxis to egg due to the trace amounts of egg protein in these vaccines.

## Specific immunization considerations

### Prematurity

Premature infants should receive their immunizations at the appropriate age after birth, regardless of their gestational age. For example, an infant born 8 weeks prematurely should commence the immunization schedule at the age of 2 months, even though the gestational age would only be at 'term' if not born prematurely. Premature infants are generally at greater risk of infectious diseases and generally achieve similar protection following vaccination as term infants. For some vaccines such as hepatitis B and Hib, extremely premature infants (<29 weeks' gestation) may require additional doses to ensure protection.

#### Clinical example

Jake was born at 26 weeks' gestation after his mother unexpectedly went into premature labour. He had significant respiratory distress in the first 3 weeks after birth, requiring surfactant, and he was ventilated for 2 weeks. He then needed supplementary oxygen for 4 weeks. He needed parenteral nutrition for the first 4 weeks of life, then nasogastric tube feeding for 4 weeks, before he was able to suck and be fed expressed milk from a bottle.

The day he was born, Jake received his first dose of hepatitis B vaccine as part of the routine schedule of vaccines. At 8 weeks after birth, when he was still equivalent to 34 weeks' gestation, he received pneumococcal conjugate vaccine (PCV), DTPa vaccine, Hib and inactivated polio vaccine, and his second dose of hepatitis B vaccine as part of the routine immunization schedule. The DTPa , IPV, hepatitis B and Hib vaccine were given as a single combination vaccine, DTPa–HBV–IPV/Hib, into his lateral thigh, and the PCV vaccine was given at the same time into the other thigh. His equivalent gestation when he was discharged was 38 weeks. At the time of discharge, arrangements were made for Jake to have his 4-month schedule immunizations, DTPa–HBV–IPV/Hib and PCV, 4 weeks after discharge, when he was 4 months old and again at 6 months of age. This was followed by meningococcal C, MMR and Hib on his first birthday.

### Missed or delayed immunizations

If a child has not received immunization at the appropriate ages, 'catch up' immunization schedules are used. The immunization schedule does not have to be recommenced and additional doses of vaccine are not needed. Schedules for catch-up immunization for DTPa combination, hepatitis B virus (HBV), pneumococcal and Hib vaccines are outlined in the immunization handbook. Many opportunities for catch-up immunization are missed when children present to their general practitioner or hospital for unrelated problems and an accurate immunization history is not taken or checked in the parental hand-held record or immunization register.

### Live virus vaccines

Live virus vaccines such as MMR and varicella can be given on the same day if necessary, for example for catch-up immunization; however, if different live virus vaccines cannot be given on the same day, they should be given at least 4 weeks apart.

## Comparison of effects of diseases and vaccines

The benefits of immunization greatly outweigh the risks of any adverse events associated with administration of vaccines used in the childhood immunization schedule. Table 3.5.3 lists some comparisons for vaccine-preventable diseases and adverse effects, which may be associated with the corresponding vaccines. A more complete listing of adverse events is available in immunization handbooks and vaccine product information sheets.

## Recording of immunization administration

Accurate recording of vaccine administration is essential. This must include:

- the vaccine administered
- the vaccine batch number and any other appropriate identifying information
- identification of the immunization service provider
- the date at which the next immunization is due.

This information should be recorded in a parent-held Child Health Record, and in the records of the immunization service provider. It should also be entered in nationwide immunization databases. The Australian Childhood Immunization Register (ACIR) was commenced in 1996 for this purpose, and similar registers are used in New Zealand and the UK. The register is used for providing a reminder system to inform parents and caregivers when the next immunization is due for their child, as well as for monitoring vaccine coverage. Uptake of immunization may be encouraged by using financial incentives for both parents and immunization providers.

## Other vaccines

Other vaccines are available that are not part of the routine childhood immunization schedule.

**Table 3.5.3 Benefits and side-effects of childhood immunizations**

| Infection | Effects of infection | Side-effects of immunization |
|---|---|---|
| Hepatitis B | Persistent carrier state common after infection<br>Long-term risk of chronic hepatitis and primary liver cancer | Minor fever in 2–3%; local inflammation in 5–15% |
| Diphtheria | Toxin causes nerve and heart damage<br>Mortality rate 1 in 15 | DTPa may cause minor local reactions such as swelling, redness and discomfort in approximately 15% of recipients |
| Tetanus | Toxin causes nerve and muscle changes resulting in paralysis, convulsions<br>Mortality rate 1 in 10 | As for diphtheria |
| Pertussis | Whooping cough. Mortality and morbidity rate highest in infants. Mortality 1 in 200 if infected in first 6 months of life | As for diphtheria |
| Poliomyelitis | Febrile illness, followed by paralysis in many<br>Mortality rate 1 in 20 hospitalized patients<br>Permanent paralysis in many | Paralysis related to vaccine strain virus in 1 in 2.5–5 million recipients or close contacts |
| *Haemophilus influenzae* b | Systemic infections such as meningitis, epiglottitis, bone and joint infections<br>Meningitis mortality rate 1 in 20; longlasting morbidity 1 in 4 | Discomfort or local inflammation in 5%; fever in 2% |
| Measles, mumps and rubella | Measles encephalitis in 1 in 1000–2000; mumps encephalitis in 1 in 200<br>Congenital rubella syndrome if infected in first trimester of pregnancy | Minor fever, local inflammation in up to 10%<br>1 in 1 million may develop measles vaccine strain encephalitis; 1 in 3 million may develop mumps vaccine strain encephalitis |

Source: Modified from The Australian Immunisation Handbook, 9th edn, National Health and Medical Research Council, 2008.

### Influenza vaccine

The H1N1 influenza pandemic in 2009 highlighted the at-risk groups for hospitalization with influenza and its complications, as well as confirming the burden of influenza in young children.

Annual immunization with influenza vaccine is recommended for:

- children receiving immunosuppressive therapy, for example chronic steroid use and with malignancy, and those with human immunodeficiency virus (HIV) infection
- children over 6 months with chronic heart conditions, including cyanotic congenital heart disease
- children with chronic suppurative lung diseases, including cystic fibrosis
- children over 6 months of age with chronic illnesses requiring regular medical follow-up (diabetes mellitus, chronic renal failure, chronic metabolic disorders, haemoglobinopathies)
- contacts of high-risk patients, particularly household members.

### Bacillus Calmette–Guérin (BCG)

Immunization with BCG is no longer provided for all children in most developed countries where the overall prevalence of tuberculosis is low. However, it may be recommended for:

- neonates in Aboriginal and Torres Strait Islander communities in regions of high incidence
- neonates or young children in households containing immigrants from countries of high incidence
- children who are going to live in countries with a high tuberculosis prevalence.

### Hepatitis A vaccine

Hepatitis A vaccine normally is given as a two-dose schedule for travellers to endemic areas, and is recommended for Aboriginal and Torres Strait Islander children at 18 months of age in northern parts of Australia, owing to the incidence of hepatitis A with significant morbidity in that population, and in children with chronic liver disease.

### Pneumococcal vaccines

In addition to infants, pneumococcal immunization also is important in older children at high risk of pneumococcal disease, such as those with nephrotic syndrome, asplenia, sickle cell disease, immune deficiency, immunosuppressive therapy, renal failure, cardiac disease, cancer or chronic lung disease. These children may require additional boosters of pneumococcal conjugate vaccine or polysaccharide vaccine.

### Meningococcal quadrivalent $ACW_{135}Y$ polysaccharide vaccine

This is used for the control of outbreaks of meningococcal disease, in those with complement deficiency disorders, in those with asplenia or splenic dysfunction, and is required for pilgrims attending the Hajj as well as being recommended for travellers to sub-Saharan Africa, and other countries where these strains are common. Protection following the polysaccharide vaccine is short term so the quadrivalent $ACW_{135}Y$ conjugate vaccines are likely to become the preferred vaccine for these conditions.

> **Clinical example**
>
> Joshua, aged 6 months, was brought to the community health centre by his 18-year-old mother to see a doctor for advice about a rash on his cheeks, behind his ears and over his upper trunk. The rash was due to infantile eczema. On questioning, it was found that he had not yet received any of his childhood immunizations. His mother said that this was because he always seemed to have a runny nose when due for immunization, and she had been concerned that immunization might make his rash worse.
>
> She was reassured that immunization was not contraindicated in the presence of rhinitis or eczema and that immunization was important in infancy. Advice on the management of eczema was given. Joshua received his first DTPa, Hib, hepatitis B, IPV (poliovirus vaccine) and pneumococcal immunizations that day from the health centre's immunization clinic. The immunizations were recorded in his health record and in the Childhood Immunization Register, and appointments were made for further DTPa, Hib, hepatitis B, IPV and pneumococcal immunizations at ages 8 and 10 months. He achieved his second immunization 'milestone' by receiving MMR, meningococcal C vaccine and HBV on his first birthday.

## Immunization in special circumstances

### Travel

Advice for specific vaccines to protect against infection while travelling in other countries depends on the nature of endemic infections in those countries. Information can be obtained in Australia from the Commonwealth Department of Health and Aging, the National Travel Health Network and Centre in the UK, the World Health Organization, or from the US Centers for Disease Control and Prevention. It is important for all children travelling to be up to date for all their routine childhood immunizations as these infections are prevalent in many countries, and for parents to be aware of simple hygiene and protective measures for preventing infection.

### HIV infection

Infected or potentially infected infants and children should receive the standard immunization schedule including MMR vaccine, and it is recommended that inactivated poliovirus vaccine (IPV) be given in place of OPV if still used. Pneumococcal conjugate vaccine booster is recommended for HIV-infected infants, and pneumococcal polysaccharide vaccine for older children. Varicella vaccine can be given to HIV-infected children who are asymptomatic or mildly affected with a normal CD4 count. Annual influenza vaccination is also recommended. BCG should not be given to children with HIV infection because of the risk of disseminated disease.

### Bone marrow transplantation

Following allogeneic and autologous stem cell transplantation, pre-existing immunity to vaccine-preventable diseases is completely or partially lost and re-immunization is necessary. All routine childhood immunizations should be included, although the timing and number of doses required will vary between units and the degree of the patient's immune reconstitution, and expert advice should be sought.

### Asplenia

Children with asplenia (congenital; after splenectomy, for example for hereditary spherocytosis or trauma) or splenic dysfunction (for example in sickle cell disease) should receive pneumococcal vaccine (conjugate vaccine if less than 5 years of age and polysaccharide vaccine for older children) and meningococcal C conjugate vaccine followed by quadrivalent meningococcal polysaccharide vaccine. Hib vaccine should be given if it has not been received in infancy.

### Primary immunodeficiency disorders

Live viral vaccines and BCG should not be used in children with primary immunodeficiency disorders.

## Future vaccines and vaccine development

Potential changes to immunization strategies for children in the near future in Australia and many other countries include:

- new combination vaccines such as MMR–varicella
- meningococcal B vaccines for infants (a strain-specific vaccine has already been used in New Zealand with great success).

Other developments in immunization during the next 5–10 years are likely to lead to the availability of serotype-independent pneumococcal vaccines, live-attenuated nasal vaccines for RSV, parainfluenza virus and genetically modified chimeric dengue virus vaccine. There is a great need for vaccines against malaria and other parasitic diseases causing widespread morbidity globally, and for vaccines with greater efficacy against tuberculosis. Public health strategies will have as their primary focus procedures and community campaigns to ensure the highest possible uptake, in both developing and developed countries, of the highly effective vaccines already available.

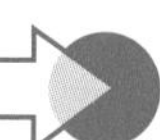

### Practical points

- Immunization is one of the most effective medical interventions for children to maintain their health.
- Immunization coverage needs to be maintained to prevent recurrence of infectious disease epidemics.
- There are few contraindications to immunization, and opportunistic immunization needs to be considered by all health providers.
- Informed consent needs to be taken from parents with an outline of potential benefits and adverse events prior to immunization.
- The effectiveness of immunization has led to the frequent introduction of new vaccines into the routine schedule, so immunization providers need to keep up to date.

# Trauma 3.6

Danny Cass

## Introduction

Children have never been safer. The rates of death and serious injury in developed countries have never been lower. In many OECD countries the decrease over the last 25 years has been in the order of 300%. Nevertheless, it is a testament to the size of the problem of paediatric trauma that, despite this significant decrease, trauma is still the largest single cause of death and severe disability in children. A lot has been done but there is still significant room for further improvement.

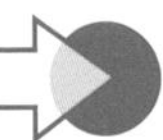

**Practical points**

- Injury is the leading cause of death in children over 1 year in developed countries.
- Injuries are not 'accidents' but predictable, preventable events.
- Cognitive and physical factors contribute to the developmental vulnerability of the child to injury.
- Environmental modification is more effective at preventing injury than education and supervision.
- Falls are the leading cause of injury in children of all ages.
- In toddlers, drowning is the leading cause of death and poisoning the most common cause of admission to hospital.
- Bicycles are the most common consumer product associated with injury in children.
- Suicide is the leading cause of death in children aged 10–14 years.

In developing counties the epidemic of trauma is increasing or at a peak. It is sad to see that rapid economic development in these developing countries has not included measures to prevent the errors developed countries had made during their phases of rapid urbanization after World War II. With the lessons learnt, many of the injuries could have been avoided. The priorities of children have again been overlooked and the same struggles for childhood safety have to be repeated. It behoves clinicians in developed counties to assist childhood advocates in developing countries to accelerate improvements and where possible avoid the unnecessary loss of life as a result of injury.

This chapter will firstly cover the sequence of care of the individual paediatric trauma patient, secondly describe specific injuries and their management, and finally discuss prevention strategies.

## Paediatric trauma care

Skill, knowledge and the ability to make decisions with incomplete information are essential. There is nothing potentially more terrifying to a clinician to be standing next to an injured child with no clear idea as to what body systems may be injured or how severely. Will this be a simple fracture or could there be a potentially fatal haemorrhage or a lurking extradural haematoma? However, with a systematic approach, the care of the injured child is straightforward and should not be daunting.

### Preparation

The care of such an injured child starts well before the arrival at your clinic or hospital. At medical school, ensure that you have done a first-aid course. After graduation, enrol in a trauma course suitable to your level of experience and vocation. Each of these skills courses teaches a systematic approach that deals logically with the sequence of potentially life-threatening injuries, work in teams, and how to communicate with the broader trauma system.

When starting any new job, ensure that you know the local trauma system. Is there a trauma team? What is your role? Are you likely to be the only clinician at some time during the night or weekend? Where is the equipment? How do you contact more senior clinicians?

### Initial care

Remember that most (97%) paediatric trauma is simple and involves a single system of the body. These injuries are easily dealt with calmly with a careful, well documented history, a detailed documented examination, appropriate investigations and, if necessary, referral to the appropriate surgical registrar. There can be tricky penetrating injuries such as a fall on to knitting needles with an entry point on the flank resulting in a spinal cord injury, but these are usually identified with the routine medical process described above. In the case just noted, it was the lack of passing urine and a percussible bladder that alerted the clinician to a potential spinal cord injury. The most common error in these injuries is lack of history-taking, a cursory examination, with poor and illegible documentation and poor handover.

About 3% of paediatric trauma cases are potentially more serious and involve multisystem injuries. These patients need a different structure of care. The essential ingredients are to transport such a patient quickly to a facility that can provide definitive care of the injuries. If such a patient is brought by parents to your surgery or small hospital, then management of the airway, pressure on points of obvious bleeding and arranging of transfer is all that is possible.

Ideally, such patients have an emergency call that brings emergency services to the scene, and with modern communication there is often forewarning that the child is coming to your hospital.

Upon arrival in the emergency department (ED) there is a structured and pertinent handover from the prehospital team. The first examination (*primary survey*) identifies and corrects immediate life-threatening injuries. Then focused tests (such as a chest or spinal X-ray) can be done and quick adjuncts to care instituted (e.g. inserting a urinary catheter or nasogastric tube) followed by a comprehensive *secondary survey*, which is a head to toe examination in association with a detailed history. In children, the same process is followed as in adults, but with refinements that take into account paediatric anatomy, physiology and psychology. In the moment of immediate care, if in doubt, do not hesitate because the patient is an injured child: do the same as you would for an adult. If the conscious state is such that you would intubate in an adult, then do not try to get by with a bag and mask in a child because of uncertainty: intubate. If the child is screaming and agitated, do not become so anxious that you are feeling you must intubate. Be guided by the objective signs and symptoms, as you would in an adult.

However, in your training take every opportunity to understand the refinements of paediatric trauma care. In this way you will provide optimal care for the injured child. The fluids must be calculated on a milligram per kilogram (mL/kg) basis. The endotracheal tubes have to be the correct size.

It is increasingly realized that trauma patients do not need aggressive fluid resuscitation in many instances. In fact, this can be counterproductive. The aim is to support cellular function, not to return all physiological parameters to normal. It is best to insert an intravenous line and be poised to give fluids. If there is a palpable radial pulse and the child is speaking or crying appropriately, then the heart and brain are getting sufficient oxygen, and fluids can be given judiciously. The respiratory rate is a good indicator of cellular hypoxia and metabolic acidosis (see Chapter 5.2 for age-associated normal values). Brain function is an exquisite indicator of cellular function. Even when the child is pale and has tachycardia, if he or she can have a coherent conversation then hold off excessive fluids as this can restart bleeding. Where there is continuing severe blood loss the patient is confused and breathing rapidly, often leading to confusion that the patient has a head or chest injury. It is these patients who need rapid and aggressive fluid resuscitation.

In this early phase, making decisions is more important than defining the precise diagnosis. The child should go directly to theatre if there is uncontrolled bleeding. However, this is a rare event. With faster computed tomography (CT), especially if located in the ED, a head and chest and/or abdominal scan can be performed. In children we are reluctant to perform whole-body scans routinely because of the radiation doses. Every test should be done looking for an injury that may need early treatment. CT is especially indicated for neurosurgical injuries where the precise location and extent of the injuries assists surgery.

Handover in the acute trauma situation is paramount. There needs to be clear and concise communication, both spoken and written. For this reason, the trauma team leader should be the most senior person who can also offer continuity of care. A consultant may be able to offer more expert care for a few minutes of care but then have to hand over. Frequent handover in the acute, fast-moving situation will often fail to hand over small but potentially critical pieces of information. A registrar who can be with the patient for some hours is often a better team leader, because continuity of care up to the point of deciding on the need for definitive surgical care outweighs the transient expertise of a consultant. A key contribution to care is clear, legible notes.

## Ongoing care

The next day it is important to review the whole situation (*tertiary survey*). This includes a complete history as many aspects at the scene and in the first few hours can be confused or misinterpreted. Therefore, it is important to start afresh and not merely to transcribe the ambulance or ED notes. A tertiary history is a precise description of the injury events including diagrams, documentation of safety issues such as seat belts or helmets, previous injuries and social circumstances that may verge on child neglect. A complete physical examination looks for any injuries that may have been overlooked initially, for example forearm fractures close to a drip site or a fractured jaw in an initially intubated patient.

A comprehensive discharge summary that ensures the local doctor is fully informed and an outpatient follow-up for all multisystem-injured patients contributes to optimal care. Often, problems with sleeping, fatigue, behaviour and school performance will be identified in outpatients. Sometimes a new aspect of the history comes to light.

## Specific organ injuries

### Spleen

The spleen is one of the most commonly injured organs. Over the last 25 years surgeons have gradually learned that most splenic injuries can be treated non-operatively. The key observation is to treat the patient clinically and not be overly influenced by radiological appearances. Most splenic injuries result in a brisk bleed, which quickly settles. Treatment is required only when there is significant continuing bleeding. Only about 50% of the most serious splenic injuries (grade 5) require surgical or radiological intervention.

### Liver

A similar strategy has evolved for paediatric liver injuries. Most lacerations and haematomas resolve without surgical intervention. However, at the severe end of the spectrum liver/caval injuries result in persistent blood loss and require early aggressive surgery aimed at damage control, which consists of compressive packing of the liver.

### Kidney

Renal injuries almost never need acute surgical intervention. The bleed is usually contained by fascia and, although it can be considerable on CT, there is usually no clinical deterioration. Surgery is reserved for significant urinary leaks with fever, and then usually consists of insertion of a double J stent.

### Small bowel perforation

This can be difficult to diagnose and can be fatal if missed, especially in the very young where the resultant peritonitis can be fulminant over a 24-hour period. There is usually a history of focused force to the abdomen, such as a handlebar of a bicycle or a pole or rock. CT may not show free gas, but there are often subtle features such as small bubbles of air, a thickened bowel wall or unexplained free fluid. Repeated examination, preferably by the same clinician, is the best way to pick up the evolving clinical deterioration and operate before serious complications result.

### Head injuries

The greatest concern is of an extradural or large subdural injury, where early recognition and removal of the compressive blood clot can transform a potentially fatal injury into a full recovery. History of a lucid interval, and localizing signs are the classical features. The more frequent use of CT has assisted.

In general, CT is recommended if consciousness is lost for more than 5 minutes. The practical problem is clearly documenting the period of any loss of consciousness.

From a practical point of view, the attending clinician should take and document a complete history and examination. After this, if there are no clear indications for CT, it is reasonable to observe for a 4–6-hour period and be prepared to perform CT if there is clinical change.

### Cervical spine

A frequently controversial area is when and how to clear for the potential of a cervical spine injury. In an awake cooperative patient, lack of any midline tenderness and active movement is sufficient. The problem is the intubated unconscious patient who was ejected from a car and needs to go to surgery the next day for a complex facial flap, as this will require repeated repositioning of the patient's neck and head. In this instance, CT and magnetic resonance imaging are thought by some clinicians still to be inadequate.

### Limb fractures

Limb fractures are the most common injuries requiring hospitalization and surgical treatment. Most are straightforward single-system injuries. However, the clinician must be alert to a 'limb at risk', as indicated by an absent or weak pulse, or a white cold limb. Such rare cases can be a problem as many children's hospitals may not have the vascular surgery expertise on staff and arrangements may have to be made with adult institutions or plastic surgery to provide this service.

## Prevention

Although there is evidence that a fully functioning trauma service can reduce the mortality rate by 20%, most reductions in childhood mortality have been achieved by prevention. Analysis of injuries reveals interventions that can prevent the incidence or minimize the resultant harm. By a combination of education of the public, engineering of the environment and enforcement of laws, many injuries can and have been prevented. The concepts are often simple but strong advocacy, constant education and a public that accepts the benefits of changes in behaviour are required to achieve tangible results.

### Road trauma

Road trauma is the single biggest cause of death and serious injury (40–50%) in almost all countries. In developed countries a concerted effort over 40 years has resulted in a significant improvement. Most of the reduction in paediatric trauma deaths has been the result of road trauma initiatives. The restraint of passengers, including age-appropriate child restraints, random alcohol testing and an acceptance by the public that drink driving is a serious crime, safer vehicles, bicycle helmets, and school and school-bus speed restrictions have all contributed to a reduction in road trauma.

Problems such as low-speed rollover injuries continue to recur, and engineering of vehicle cameras and education to 'spot the tot' is required to achieve further reductions. Newer hobbies such as off-road vehicles need analysis to determine patterns of injury and to balance these against the benefits to children's development.

In developing countries road trauma is increasing and there needs to be advocacy by clinicians to try to stem the epidemic.

### Drowning

Prevention is almost the only strategy for reducing this important cause of childhood death. Immediate resuscitation can help, but the main messages are direct arm's length supervision backed up by fencing and pool gate barriers. There has been a reduction in deaths over the last 25 years, especially in relation to the number of private swimming pools. However, with a new generation of parents of toddlers every few years, campaigns need to be continuous and relentless.

Until recently it was not appreciated how large a problem childhood drowning was in developing countries. Most deaths never came to the attention of hospitals or health authorities. More detailed community analysis has shown drowning to be a significant problem and advocacy has started.

### Burns and scalds

The incidence of burns and scalds has decreased significantly in European countries but still remains a problem in many communities. Almost all burns and hot water scalds could be prevented by public campaigns that separate children from flames and boiling water.

### Falls

As developed countries respond to increasing urbanized populations by encouraging high-density living, more children will live in high-rise accommodation. Any window opening or balcony above 2 metres is a serious potential health risk to children. Falls from windows have increased in most developed countries. It is a fundamental lack of the concern for infants and young children (often in their own bedrooms) that has allowed building codes that do not make window openings safe. The simple solution is to be able to restrict lower openings to 10 cm. This should be engineered at the time of building, but existing dwellings could be modified for as little as $10 and 10 minutes' work.

Childhood injury prevention requires effort by the whole community, with all clinicians (medical students, doctors, nurses, ambulance, allied health professionals and administrators) in important leadership roles. Clinicians have to look after paediatric trauma patients and therefore know the details of the injuries intimately, are motivated and have community credibility. They are therefore ideally placed to be at the forefront of ongoing prevention efforts. Meticulous tertiary trauma histories during the admission (often taken by medical students and interns) help to develop prevention data and guide likely solutions. Injury prevention information in doctors' surgeries and EDs helps to educate the community.

Most injury prevention campaigns are assumed to be based on careful data collection with this information then resulting in engineering and legislative change. However, this is rarely the case, with vehicle manufacturers, building industries and bureaucracies often resisting change. It often requires strong persistent advocacy by clinicians, parents and concerned citizens for change to occur. Some important injury prevention changes have occurred as the result of a single person being aware of a problem, devising a solution and advocating until change has occurred.

## Summary

Paediatric trauma is an important health issue as it is still the greatest cause of death and serious disability in most countries.

Medical students can prepare by doing first-aid courses, and being involved in detailed history-taking during their clinical rotations.

Interns and residents can improve their skills by attending trauma training courses, and being meticulous in their history-taking and physical examination.

Registrars and consultants can attend more advanced skills courses in trauma team training, advanced surgical techniques and trauma conferences, and participate in websites on trauma topics, multicentre studies (i.e. spinal cord injuries) and consensus statements.

Trauma care is mostly simple, but occasionally very challenging. Clinicians can contribute most by being prepared, sticking to basics in history-taking and examination, writing clear, legible notes regarding their decision-making, and using the skills that they feel comfortable with. When the situation is progressing beyond your skills level, discuss the issues with a more senior clinician.

Trauma prevention is everyone's responsibility.

# 3.7 Failure to thrive

Daryl Efron

Satisfactory growth is a key marker of good health in infancy and early childhood, and so the failure of a child to grow as expected is naturally a cause for concern for parents and health professionals. Failure to thrive (FTT) can result from a broad range of organic and environmental factors, with a combination of influences usually operating. The family often feel confused, worried and guilty, so evaluation needs to be conducted sensitively.

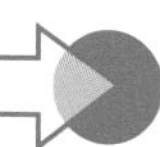

**Practical points**

- Failure to thrive is commonly due to a combination of factors, with psychosocial issues often prominent.
- Chronic illness in any system can result in failure to thrive.
- Investigations are unlikely to reveal a cause that was not apparent from a thorough history and examination.
- A multidisciplinary approach is necessary, with input from paediatricians, maternal and child health nurses, dietitians, speech pathologists and sometimes mental health professionals.
- Admission to hospital is required in severe malnutrition, unwell infants, or where there are concerns about the child's care at home.
- Infants who have had a period of failure to thrive are at risk of long-term problems with growth and development.

## Definition

FTT can be defined using various criteria. The term is generally applied to infants, although on occasion it is used in children up to 2–3 years of age. Concern is often raised when an infant's weight is below the third centile, that is, more than approximately two standard deviations below the population mean. However, this occurs normally in 3% of infants, most of whom are healthy but who are genetically destined to be small. Of more interest are the weight:length ratio, and particularly the growth trajectory with time. The criterion of weight crossing two major centile lines with time is more meaningful clinically, and a useful standard by which to decide when to describe an infant as having FTT, and to evaluate accordingly.

## Growth patterns

When a child is failing to thrive, weight gain is affected first, but if the problem persists, length also may be affected. If length is affected disproportionately, the possibility of a skeletal dysplasia syndrome or endocrinopathy should be considered. Head circumference is affected only when failure to thrive is severe.

Irrespective of birth weight, full-term infants tend to assume their genetically determined growth pattern some time in mid to late infancy. This often results in babies who were born large 'crossing down' to reach their predestined track on the growth chart. Measures should be plotted against age corrected for prematurity until 2 years of age.

It is often possible to identify a critical point or period at which a child's growth began to falter. This may enable recognition of an important factor that has adversely influenced growth, such as the introduction of a food to which the child is intolerant, intercurrent infection or change in environmental circumstances causing family stress.

## Causes

In developed countries, failing to thrive usually relates to inadequate caloric intake in the context of psychosocial difficulties. Poverty, parental mental illness, substance abuse, social isolation, family violence or intellectual disability may result in limited parental capacity or other priorities competing with adequate care of the child. The relationship between mother and infant is often disturbed. Maternal depression is very common in these situations, often present from the postnatal period or developing as a consequence of feeding difficulties and associated FTT.

Prematurity, intrauterine growth retardation and embryopathic intrauterine exposures increase the risk of FTT. Chronic or recurrent illness in any system can result in impaired growth (Table 3.7.1).

Mechanisms of growth failure include reduced intake (most common), inadequate nutrient absorption and, in some cases, increased energy utilization. Malnourished infants are vulnerable to infection, which may further compromise their nutritional state.

In some cases, parents hold alternative belief systems that influence their care of their child. These

| Table 3.7.1 Organic causes of failure to thrive | |
|---|---|
| System | Examples |
| Craniofacial | Cleft palate<br>Pierre Robin syndrome |
| Neurological | Cerebral palsy with pseudobulbar palsy<br>Raised intracranial pressure (vomiting)<br>Embryopathy (e.g. *in utero* infection, fetal alcohol syndrome) |
| Genetic | Chromosomal abnormality (e.g. trisomy 18)<br>Dysmorphic syndrome (e.g. Smith–Lemli–Opitz syndrome) |
| Gastrointestinal | Gastro-oesophageal reflux disease<br>Malabsorption (e.g. coeliac disease, lactose intolerance)<br>Chronic liver disease |
| Renal | Recurrent/persistent urinary tract infection<br>Chronic renal failure<br>Renal tubular acidosis |
| Respiratory | Chronic lung disease (e.g. bronchopulmonary dysplasia, cystic fibrosis)<br>Chronic upper airway obstruction |
| Metabolic | Inborn errors of metabolism (e.g. amino acidopathies, mitochondrial disorders) |
| Cardiac | Chronic congestive cardiac failure |
| Endocrine | Thyroid disease<br>Adrenal insufficiency |
| Immunological | Severe atopic disease<br>Food protein allergy<br>Severe combined immune deficiency |
| Infectious | Human immunodeficiency virus<br>Tuberculosis |

may include unconventional diets and feeding practices, opposition to immunization and mistrust of mainstream health-care providers. These cases can be extremely challenging and great skill is required to maintain a therapeutic relationship with the family.

There are often multiple contributing causes for failing to thrive. For example, an infant may have an underlying syndromic diagnosis that is associated with growth restriction but also results in recurrent infections, gastro-oesophageal reflux and irritability with poor feeding behaviour. Psychosocial problems may also be present in the family of a child with organic illness.

## Assessment

### Growth pattern

The initial step in the evaluation of a child who is failing to thrive is to chart the growth pattern to determine whether it is a cause for concern. Birth measures should be plotted against gestation, and then serial weight, length and head circumference should be plotted on percentile charts through to the present time. Where available, it is preferable to use a chart constructed from a population of the child's particular ethnic group or syndrome (e.g. Down syndrome). Mid-parental height gives an indication of the child's genetic growth potential. The point at which growth began to falter may provide a clue as to the cause, for instance after the introduction of wheat products in coeliac disease.

### History

A careful evaluation of dietary intake is necessary in the assessment of a child with FTT. A detailed history of feeding patterns is required, including frequency, duration and quality of breastfeeds, or total daily volume of formula. If the infant is breastfed, the mother's milk supply should be assessed. If formula-fed, check that the feeds are being prepared correctly. It is important to know both the range and quantity of solids being consumed, and how well the child can manage foods of different textures. A 3-day feed diary can be helpful in quantifying the nutritional intake. This history can be difficult to obtain reliably when there is psychosocial disadvantage or neglect.

A detailed systems review is necessary to identify any organic illness that might be contributing to the growth failure, either as the primary cause or as an exacerbating factor. Particular enquiry needs to be made about vomiting, diarrhoea, respiratory symptoms, lethargy and irritability.

Failing to thrive is commonly associated with developmental delay. Infants with FTT often fall behind in their gross motor development. Poor muscle bulk and tone results in immature truncal and neck posture, and generalized weakness. Commonly the infant's emotional development is also delayed. Malnourished and deprived infants may demonstrate apathy, anxiety, irritability and poorly regulated behavioural states. Some underfed infants become depressed and withdraw from social contact with primary caregivers. Important signs include gaze aversion, lack of a responsive smile, and lack of interest in social overture or reciprocal play activities. On the other hand, poor feeding may result from neurodevelopmental impairment, with irritability, oromotor dysfunction and an abnormal swallowing mechanism.

A good social history is critical. The family's social circumstances may be a central factor in the cause of the growth failure, and may also influence therapeutic effectiveness.

### Examination

A thorough physical examination is required in infants with FTT. The child's general appearance is important. Note whether the child appears small but well (i.e. good colour, alert, active) or malnourished and unwell (i.e. pale, miserable, lethargic).

A poor state of hygiene such as unclean skin and clothes, as well as a marked flattening of the occiput with hair loss, raise the possibility of neglect. The quality of the child's interaction with the mother should be noted. Is there good eye contact and reciprocal warm engagement? Temperamental characteristics should be noted. Irritability, withdrawn behaviour or an anxious, hypervigilant appearance are important signs.

Gross indicators of nutritional state include fat stores, particularly around the buttocks and thighs, and muscle bulk. The severely malnourished infant has prominent ribs, thin limbs, sparse hair and a bony face. Signs of micronutrient deficiency include pallor, rashes and sparse hair. Dysmorphic features raise the possibility of a genetic syndrome. Each system

**Clinical example**

James, aged 9 months, was referred by his maternal and child health nurse with concerns about his weight crossing the major centiles. He was born at 38 weeks' gestation with a birth weight of 3.6 kg (90th centile) and his current weight was 7.9 kg, which was just above the 10th centile. He had generally been a healthy infant, apart from some upper respiratory tract infections (URTIs) and had had a nocturnal cough for 3 weeks since his most recent URTI. He was still breastfed. Solids were introduced at 6 months and he was taking small amounts of rice cereal, vegetables and fruits, as well as some meat and chicken. Examination was normal. He was an alert, interactive infant and responded well to his mother.

His mother's height was 154 cm (3–10th centile) and his father's was 170 cm (10th centile).

James' parents were reassured that he appeared to be a healthy infant and seemed to have settled into his genetically determined growth pattern. Arrangements were made to see James again in 2–3 weeks to ensure that the cough had settled, or, if not, for a chest X-ray to be performed. He would have ongoing review to ensure that he continued to gain weight along the 10th centile as expected.

needs to be examined carefully for signs of malformation or disease. Candidiasis raises the possibility of an immune deficiency, although this is more likely to be secondary to malnutrition than the primary cause.

A developmental assessment should be completed as part of the examination. Direct observation of the child's feeding is important to enable better understanding of the feeding behaviour, for instance the intensity of demanding/interest in food, parent's feeding technique, coordination and vigour of suck and swallow, acceptance or rejection of bottle/spoon, duration of the feed (e.g. rushed or prolonged), distractibility and fatigue. Videotape recordings (taken by the parents at home) can be valuable in outpatient settings. Observe how the parents respond to the child's distress or signs of hunger (such as the rooting reflex, or biting his or her own fist in hunger), and how they hold, comfort and care for the child. Does the parent appear to enjoy caring for the child, or appear disengaged or coercive?

## Investigation

If there are no specific signs or symptoms, a diagnosis of organic disease is uncommon. Investigations undertaken to identify a hidden cause for FTT have a low yield. It is appropriate, however, to check electrolytes, serum creatinine, full blood examination, ferritin, and urine microscopy and culture. Other investigations may be indicated if there are specific findings on history or examination. These might include inflammatory markers, thyroid function tests, sweat test, karyotype, immune function tests, stool microscopy, coeliac disease serology, urine organic acid profile and brain imaging. If severe malnutrition is present, additional laboratory investigations are indicated, including liver function tests, alkaline phosphatase, calcium, phosphate, vitamin D, zinc, vitamin $B_{12}$ and folate.

## Management

The management of FTT depends on the severity, whether the child appears healthy or unwell, and psychosocial factors. Establishment and maintenance of rapport and trust with the family is an essential element of successful treatment. Clearly, any identified organic causes need specific therapy.

Mild FTT in an otherwise well child can be managed initially with dietary advice and close monitoring. Catch-up growth requires increased caloric intake. If the infant is breastfed, supplementation after breastfeeds, with either expressed breast milk or formula by bottle, may be necessary. For formula-fed infants, an increased caloric intake can be achieved by increasing the concentration of formula by 25%, or by adding a spoonful of glucose polymer powder to bottles. Depending on the age of the infant, the introduction of solids or adding extra calories to solids (using formula milk, butter, cream or margarine) may be indicated.

Admission to hospital may be necessary for children with severe FTT, those who are unwell, where the parents are very anxious, or where there is concern about the quality of care of the child. A thorough evaluation of the feeding behaviour and routines, mother–infant interaction, and the emotional status of both mother and infant can be achieved over several days. A multidisciplinary team approach is optimal in the assessment and management of these children. This includes a dietitian to assess nutritional intake, a speech pathologist to assess feeding, and a social worker to assess psychosocial stressors and the family's support system.

In some cases a mental health assessment of mother and/or infant is required. Contact should be made, with parental permission, with professionals in the community who have been involved with the family. This may include a lactation consultant, maternal and child health nurse, general practitioner and/or psychiatrist. Child protection services may need to be involved if there are concerns regarding the child's care. Strengths in the family should be identified and promoted.

Satisfactory growth with feeding in hospital (or out-of-home care) suggests that the FTT is psychosocial. In some cases, refeeding may be required using a nasogastric tube. This must be done carefully to avoid complications such as vomiting, diarrhoea, and electrolyte disturbances such as hypophosphataemia, hypomagnesaemia and hypokalaemia (see Chapter 3.3).

The desired feeding pattern for care at home needs to be established first in hospital. On discharge a clear, written feeding plan is essential. Professional supports in the community need to be engaged to continue monitoring and support. Frequent medical review is necessary initially. Children who have suffered severe FTT in infancy or early childhood are at risk of long-term growth, developmental and behavioural problems, and so should be followed up by a paediatrician into the school years.

### Clinical example

Taylah, aged 11 months, was brought for assessment by her mother, who was concerned that she 'wouldn't eat'. Her mother also said that Taylah would not sleep during the day, whinged too much and was often 'so worked up she made herself vomit'. Taylah's mother said that she was finding it extremely difficult to look after Taylah on her own. She reported that Taylah had diarrhoea at times, as well as a constantly runny nose. She was bottlefed but lately had not been enjoying her milk. She had little interest in solids.

Taylah's birth weight was 2.3 kg at 36 weeks (10th centile). Her mother did not have the Child Health Record and reported that she did not like the local maternal and child health nurse. Her mother did not interact with Taylah, who was sitting in the pram during the consultation. At one point, when Taylah cried, her mother said: 'See! This is what she's like all the time!' Taylah's mother appeared pale, thin and anxious. She appeared defensive and angry when asked some questions about her support system.

On examination, Taylah appeared thin, pale and miserable. Her clothes were soiled. She had an extensive nappy rash, as well as facial and scalp dermatitis. Her hair was sparse, particularly over the occiput, which was flat. Her weight was 6 kg (below the third centile, corrected for prematurity). Her length was 68 cm (10th centile) and her head circumference was 43 cm (2–50th centile). Physical examination was otherwise negative. She was unsteady when placed in a sitting position. It was not possible to elicit a smile from her. Her urine was negative on a dipstick test.

Taylah was referred to a paediatrician, who admitted her to the regional hospital. Taylah spent a week in hospital, where she fed well and gained 300 g within a few days. The hospital arranged a mental health assessment for Taylah's mother. Her mother was diagnosed with chronic depression and anxiety, and a follow-up appointment was arranged for soon after Taylah's discharge. The enhanced home visiting maternal and child health service was engaged for home-based support, along with close paediatric follow-up.

# 3.8 Developmental disability

Michael O'Callaghan

## Definition

Disability describes lack of skill in important areas of development that affect age-appropriate functions and participation of the child in the activities of daily life. The World Health Organization International Classification of Function (ICF) for disability and health describes not only how a condition affects body structures and function but also its influence on how a person may perform their personal, family and social roles, together with personal and environmental factors that affect this. Legislative frameworks, recognition of rights, opportunities for education and work, access and community attitudes all influence participation and ultimate quality of life. The biopsychosocial approach, with emphasis on the child as a person and on their overall function and wellbeing, together with a strong developmental and family perspective, provides a necessary framework for care of children with developmental disability.

A developmental disability may arise from genetic causes, during pregnancy, perinatally, or during childhood. Approximately 3–5% of children have a moderate to severe disability and up to 20% have a mild disability. Many of these disorders are more common in males. The disability may affect movement, cognitive, speech and sensory functions or behaviour, and it may vary in severity. A child may have multiple disabilities.

Commonly included low and higher prevalence disorders are shown in Box 3.8.1; because they affect brain function, they are also called neurodevelopmental disorders. Although the lower prevalence disorders are usually more severe, all of these conditions may have a substantial effect on the quality of life for the child and family. A number of low-prevalence severe disabilities affecting the brain, including hearing and visual impairment, cerebral palsy, spina bifida and autism, are covered in other sections of this book. The focus of this section includes general issues of management for all children with a developmental disability; the child with intellectual impairment and selected syndromes associated with this; and children with high prevalence but less severe disorders occurring singly or in combination.

## General issues of management

Developmental disabilities are chronic disorders, and this perspective is also required for management, in addition to the interventions that are specific for individual disorders. Four important general aspects of management are:

- *Family-centred care.* This includes an ongoing partnership with families, advocacy, the provision of information regarding the disorder, support groups, access to treatment and respite services, and to sources of financial support. When initially discussing the diagnosis with families, the consultation should include the presence, if possible, of both parents, sufficient uninterrupted time, a realistic and balanced acknowledgement of potential problems and strengths, and the opportunity for follow-up discussion. Long-term care of the person with severe developmental disability is likely to be stressful to parents, siblings and marriages, with major transitions such as commencing or finishing school and adolescence and transition to adult services often being challenging periods.
- *An individual child.* The focus is not only on the management of the medical disorder or disability but also the child's longer-term growth, health, development, emotional wellbeing, independence and adult function. Associated behavioural difficulties may be of equal or greater concern to the family than medical aspects of the disability, and also influence successful function in the school and community.
- *Prevention.* Knowledge of the genetic implications, natural history of a disorder, and common management issues may allow prevention of some problems and early identification of others (see, for example, Table 3.8.2).
- *A team and a plan.* As interventions are frequently multidisciplinary and may involve more than one professional or service, they should be coordinated, have an outcome focus and should involve families in considering realistic short- and long-term goals. Interventions should begin early and be focused on the needs of the child and family with programmes that occur, where possible, in the child's own home or community.

**Box 3.8.1 Developmental disabilities**

**Low prevalence**
- Cerebral palsy
- Moderate–severe intellectual impairment
- Autism
- Spina bifida
- Severe sensory impairment

**Higher prevalence**
- Developmental delay
- Mild intellectual impairment
- Speech and language
- Developmental coordination disorder
- Learning difficulty
- Attention-deficit/hyperactivity disorder
- Mild autistic spectrum disorder

The medical role in the management of a developmental disability includes initial diagnosis, advocacy, accessing services, and meeting normal and specialist health and developmental needs of the child. Trials of medication to modify genetic expression are occurring in a number of syndromes, including fragile X, and specific therapeutic medical interventions may emerge in future. Management is facilitated by seeking to understand the 'predicament' of the child and family – how they may feel, think and experience the situation. There is a need also for an evidence-based approach in discussing traditional and alternative interventions. The role requires acceptance of cultural and ethnic differences, realistic hope, advocacy and helping families to maintain their overall wellbeing. The needs of a child and family, however, can be met only by a range of professionals.

**Clinical example**

Angie was aged 6 years and had a mild intellectual impairment of unknown aetiology. Her behaviour had always been difficult and had recently become more difficult. She also had a diagnosis of attention-deficit/hyperactivity disorder in association with aggression that was only partially responsive to stimulant medication. Reviewing the situation using a biopsychosocial approach, her doctor realized that her behaviour had become worse when her father started working away from home, as a result of which Angie's mother, who always assumed the majority of Angie's care, had to cease her studies. Her mother described feeling socially isolated and depressed. Angie was in an integrated classroom with a modified programme, although she was acutely sensitive to her lack of academic success compared with her peers. Medication was still required and the dose adjusted, although this further understanding allowed additional interventions that markedly improved Angie's aggressive outbursts and adjustment.

## Intellectual impairment

### Terminology

Medical terms such as mental retardation (Diagnostic and Statistical Manual of Mental Disorders, edition IV; DSM-IV), intellectual impairment and general learning difficulty are often used synonymously. Although these terms all focus on important deficits in the child, they may be offensive to families, and do not describe competencies of individual children.

### Definition

Mental retardation, the term used in DSM-IV, is defined as significantly sub-average intellectual functioning accompanied by limited adaptive function, with onset before 18 years. Adaptive function describes activities of daily living and social competence. Tests of general intellectual function, such as the Stanford–Binet and Weschler Intelligence Scales, have a distribution that is approximately normal, with a mean intellectual quotient (IQ score) of 100 and a standard deviation of 15. The individual's score is, however, an estimate, as performance is affected by a range of child, tester and environmental factors.

Mild intellectual impairment is diagnosed in children with an IQ score between 70 and 55–50 who also have impaired adaptive function. Although the normal curve distribution suggests that 2–3% of children will be in this category, studies generally report a lower prevalence and an association with social disadvantage or family history of similar difficulties. The children may present with speech or behavioural difficulty, or may be identified with developmental concerns in early childhood education centres or with learning difficulty in the early school years. Physical and neurological examinations are usually normal.

Moderate intellectual impairment is defined as an IQ of 35–50, with more severely or profoundly affected children having an IQ score below this. Only approximately 0.3% of children have an IQ score lower than 50. These children often have a dysmorphic appearance, a recognized syndrome or other known aetiology for their intellectual disability. Presentation may be by recognition at birth or with global developmental delay during early childhood. Inexperienced parents may present with concerns regarding specific speech and gross motor delays. More severely affected children may also have other physical and sensory disorders, with many having multiple disabilities.

### Medical assessment

A standard medical and family history and physical and neurological examination are important, as is understanding the family's concerns, their belief regarding this, and the outcome they hope for from the consultation. Development is assessed from maternal concerns, milestones, current abilities on history and testing as required. Milestones are helpful if delay or regression has occurred, whereas developmental testing also allows the opportunity to interact with the child and informally assess social engagement, attention and quality of performance. The aetiology is not always identified, especially for children with less severe disorders, but is more likely if there are:

- minor physical anomalies present (e.g. simian crease or low-set ears)
- disturbances of growth (e.g. microcephaly or macrocephaly, extremes of stature or weight)
- abnormal skin lesions (e.g. multiple depigmented or pigmented naevi)
- malformations or abnormal findings in several organ systems
- behaviour characteristics of specific disorders (i.e. behavioural phenotype)
- family history of a similar disorder.

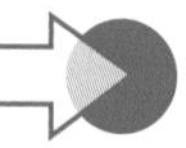

**Practical points**

**Examination of the child with suspected developmental disability**

*Informal observation*

- Appearance
- Behaviour (eye contact, social engagement, attention, activity level and anxiety)
- Play (symbolic, imaginative or repetitive)
- Movement (skills, symmetry and quality)

*Formal observation*

- Developmental assessment (strengths and weaknesses)
- Minor physical anomalies
- Vision and hearing
- Physical and central nervous system examinations
- Growth (plot percentiles)

## Differential diagnosis

The differential diagnosis of intellectual impairment includes children:

- who have been severely deprived or abused
- with a progressive neurodegenerative disorder or unrecognized epilepsy
- with severe sensory or specific developmental disorders
- where the child's apparent lack of skills is due to cultural differences, mental health disorders, ill health or refusal to participate
- infants with severe movement difficulties.

There are many prenatal, perinatal and postnatal aetiologies for intellectual impairment and multiple associated syndromes. A child with intellectual impairment may have other associated specific developmental delays, behaviour problems and health difficulties. This section describes a limited number of causes of intellectual impairment as examples. Although an approximate stereotype of disorders is described, the expression of the disorder varies and each child requires individual assessment.

## Investigations

Investigations and their indications are shown in Table 3.8.1. Genetic testing is evolving rapidly and may require consultations with the geneticist or laboratory.

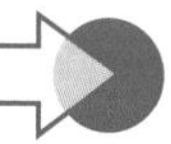

**Practical points**

**Assessment goals for the child with developmental disability**

- Developmental diagnosis
- Aetiological diagnosis
- Presence of associated disorders (co-morbidity)
- The psychosocial context (predicament)

## Fragile X syndrome

X-linked intellectual impairment may explain the male predominance among children with intellectual impairment. It exists in overlapping syndromic and non-syndromic forms (see Chapter 10.3).

Fragile X syndrome is the commonest form of X-linked intellectual impairment and is the most common inherited cause, with population estimates in males of approximately 1 in 3600. The condition arises because of an expanded CGG triplicate repeat sequence at Xq27.3 that interferes with the production of fragile X mental retardation protein (FMRP). A repeat sequence of less than 55 is considered normal, and a sequence of more than 200 copies results in loss of function of the gene affecting biochemical pathways. Individuals with 55–200 repeats, a premutation, are usually normal, although they may have learning, behavioural, mild cognitive difficulties or, later, early ovarian failure or develop an ataxic–tremor syndrome. Clinical testing should include DNA studies for the trinucleotide repeats.

The condition predominantly affects males as they have a single X chromosome. Girls are less commonly affected and the expression of the disorder is less marked. Genetic counselling is complex as expansion of the repeat sequence occurs only in female carriers in pregnancy, though the extent of this is not predictable. Males with this disorder will have normal sons and all of their daughters will be carriers.

Affected individuals may look normal, especially when younger. Typical physical characteristics and co-morbidities are shown in Box 3.8.2. Recurrent otitis media, strabismus or refractive errors in vision, and seizures may also occur. The intellectual impairment is usually of a moderate degree. DNA testing for fragile X syndrome should be considered in all children with intellectual impairment, and especially in males,

**Table 3.8.1 Investigations and indications for mental retardation**

| Test | Indication |
|---|---|
| Chromosome microarray (CMA) | Identifies submicrosopic deletions and duplications<br>Different types of arrays available. Because of normal copy number variation between individuals, interpretation may be difficult and require geneticist |
| Chromosomes (G banded karyotype) | Recognized chromosomal syndrome, a family history of chromosomal rearrangement (balanced translocation) |
| Fragile X | Consider in all children with intellectual impairment, especially male children, those with a family history of X-linked intellectual impairment or children with other clinical features of the syndrome |
| Fluorescent in situ hybridization (FISH) | Quicker than CMA and may be useful for specific clinically identified syndromes e.g. Williams |
| Thyroid function | Short stature, constipation, dry skin or hair, goitre or no neonatal screen |
| (CPK) | If muscle weakness or prominent calves are present. Duchenne dystrophy is associated with developmental disorders |
| Metabolic screen | Hypoglycaemia, acidosis, altered consciousness level, unusual odour or multiple body systems affected. Low yield if neonatal screening program |
| Ca, $PO_4$ | Short fourth metacarpal, short stature in pseudohypoparathyroidism |
| Electroencephalography (EEG) | If clinical seizures or history of sleep-related seizures |
| Magnetic resonance imaging (MRI) or computed tomography | If abnormal neurological signs, possible regression or moderate-severe intellectual impairment of unknown cause. MRI also for developmental disorders of brain |
| Lead | Exposure history, at-risk environment |
| Ferritin | Iron deficiency anaemia associated with delayed development |
| Other tests | For specific rare clinical indications |

where there is an X-linked family history of intellectual impairment, or the child's appearance or behaviour is characteristic of fragile X syndrome.

**Box 3.8.2 Clinical features of fragile X syndrome**

**Appearance**
- Prominent jaw
- Long, narrow face
- Large ears
- Joint hypermobility
- Testicular enlargement in adolescence

**Development**
- Moderate mental retardation
- Reduced coordination
- Risk of epilepsy

**Behaviour**
- Attention-deficit/hyperactivity disorder
- Social shyness
- Autistic spectrum disorder features

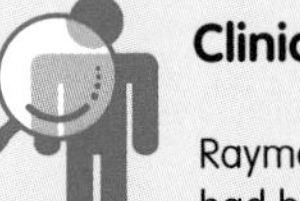

**Clinical example**

Raymond was 4 years old, and his mother had become concerned that his development was mildly delayed for his age and that he was active and impulsive. On questioning, her particular concern was that Raymond might be intellectually impaired, as were her own brother and maternal uncle. Physical and neurological examinations were normal. Genetic testing indicated that Raymond had fragile X and that his mother was a carrier for this disorder. Genetic counselling and formal assessment were provided.

## Down syndrome

Down syndrome or trisomy 21 (see Chapter 10.3) is the commonest genetic cause for moderate intellectual impairment, with an overall incidence of approximately 1 in 800 births. Risk varies, however, increasing especially with maternal age. Screening programmes in pregnancy vary though may involve combinations of first- and second-trimester serum markers such as low α-fetoprotein levels and pregnancy associated plasma protein A, high human chorionic gonadotrophin levels, low blood oestriol levels and ultrasound findings including nuchal thickening or characteristic malformations (see Chapter 10.1). Chromosomal studies indicate a full trisomy 21 secondary to non-disjunction in 95% of affected children, with translocation or more rarely mosaicism in the remainder.

At birth, the diagnosis is usually made from the overall dysmorphic appearance of the infant and clinical findings (Table 3.8.2). Confirmation by genetic testing is always necessary. Children with Down syndrome have an increased risk of malformations; 30–50% have congenital heart disease. A spectrum of cardiac lesions may be found, although abnormalities of the atrioventricular canal or ventricular septal defect are most common. Gastrointestinal malformations that may be found include duodenal atresia, imperforate anus and Hirschsprung disease.

Intellectual impairment is generally moderate, with a high risk of Alzheimer disease from 40 years of age onwards. The majority of children do not exhibit marked behavioural difficulty, although there is an increased prevalence of oppositional and autistic disorders. Health surveillance recommendations are shown in Table 3.8.2.

**Table 3.8.2 Down syndrome: clinical features and surveillance**

| Issue | Comment |
|---|---|
| Neonatal clinical features | Hypotonia<br>Brachycephaly<br>Eyes slanted, epicanthic folds, Brushfield spots<br>Tongue appears large<br>Ears poorly formed and small<br>Hands broad, simian crease<br>Gap between first and second toes |
| **Health surveillance** | |
| Growth | Use Down syndrome growth charts<br>Initial feeding difficulties common<br>Avoid obesity |
| Thyroid | Yearly thyroid tests |
| Coeliac disease | Consider testing if symptoms, or screen at 3–4 years |
| Neck | X-ray atlantoaxial joint if symptoms of neck pain or central nervous system signs in legs |
| Leukaemia | No routine screen, although increased risk of leukaemia or neonatal leukaemoid reaction |
| Hearing | Initial screen and repeat as indicated for chronic otitis media |
| Sleep | Risk of obstructive sleep apnoea |
| Vision | Cataracts, refractive errors, strabismus |
| Development | Early intervention/educational plan<br>Specific therapy if needed<br>Behaviour/adjustment/autism |
| Family | Genetic counselling, knowledge of condition, support, groups, respite, financial benefits |

## Prader–Willi syndrome

This is a rare disorder (1 in 25 000 live births per annum) due to loss of paternal expressed genes at 15q11–13. In 75% of cases, a paternal deletion is present, whereas in 20% of children two maternal copies of the gene are present. A small number of children with Prader–Willi syndrome have other rare genetic causes involving this region. Prader–Willi syndrome illustrates the complex nature of developmental disabilities, the burden on families especially when behaviour difficulty is marked, and the need for multidisciplinary services.

Children with Prader–Willi syndrome have a characteristic appearance and clinical expression involving health, growth, development, learning and behaviour, with the last often being the greatest burden for families. Initial severe neonatal hypotonia, often with a need for nasogastric feeds, is followed by the development of excessive appetite, lack of satiety and risk of obesity from 3 to 5 years. During this period, marked behavioural difficulties emerge, including food-seeking, oppositional and obsessive compulsive behaviour, difficulties with concentration and often mild features of autistic spectrum disorder. Skin picking may be a particular problem. The risk of psychosis as an adult is increased. Gross motor skills and speech are initially most markedly delayed in association with hypotonia. Affected children are usually mildly intellectually impaired and experience learning difficulties. Endocrine problems secondary to hypothalamic dysfunction affect growth, and the risk of type 2 diabetes is increased. Sleep disorders with central and obstructive apnoea are common and need to be monitored if growth hormone is given. The risk of scoliosis is increased.

*Angelman syndrome* is a similarly complex, although different, neurodevelopmental disorder arising from loss of maternal expressed genes in the same chromosomal region. The children are generally happy, ataxic, lack speech, and have severe intellectual impairment and a characteristic appearance.

## Microdeletion syndromes

*Velocardiofacial syndrome* arises from a chromosomal microdeletion at 22q11.2. There is a wide spectrum of clinical findings including cardiac anomalies, commonly involving the conotruncal region, thymus-associated immune deficiencies, developmental problems of speech, often in association with nasal escape from a cleft of the soft palate, intellectual and learning difficulties, behavioural difficulties and risk of later psychosis.

*Smith–Magenis syndrome* arises from a chromosomal deletion at 17p11.2. It has a wide spectrum of findings, and is associated with severe behavioural difficulty, particularly involving sleep and aggression to self or others.

### Environmental causes

Teratogens in pregnancy include intrauterine infection and significant alcohol intake. Fetal alcohol syndrome is an important cause of developmental delay and, in more severely affected children, is associated with microcephaly, growth retardation, characteristic facies and later intellectual, learning and behaviour problems. Brain damage from causes such as infection or trauma and severe emotional deprivation and neglect can all lead to intellectual impairment. Severe neonatal encephalopathy leads only rarely to isolated intellectual impairment and is usually associated with the presence of other disabilities, especially cerebral palsy. The interaction of both nature and nurture are important in influencing the development and health of children.

## High-prevalence disorders

### Developmental delay

Children show a broad range of skills at any age. Separating normal variation from mild delays is difficult and depends on the degree of delay or disorder, although it is also influenced by the extent of parental concern, the past medical and developmental history of the child, and family history, including the development of siblings and parents. A developmental disability results in a clinically meaningful degree of functional impairment. The pace of development may vary in individual children and predictors from early childhood have limited accuracy unless development is substantially delayed or disordered, or is associated with a condition of known poor prognosis. Delays may affect all or most areas of development, or may be restricted to specific domains such as speech or coordination. Because ill-health, motor or sensory impairment, and family adversity may all affect performance in young children, the term 'global developmental delay' is often used initially, even if intellectual impairment is suspected. The term may also be applied where two or more aspects of development are affected. Parents need, however, to understand that 'global developmental delay' does not imply either that their child will necessarily 'catch up' or that the extent of the delay in months is fixed. The ratio between developmental and chronological age, sometimes termed the developmental quotient, is more stable and a better guide to longer-term prognosis, whereas the actual gap in months may increase with age.

**Clinical example**

At age 2 years, John's parents were concerned that he was not speaking. He was able to jump and run, and responded to his name and 'no', although he knew no body parts and had just begun to attempt to stack blocks and use a pencil. From the Denver Test, his skills, apart from age-appropriate gross motor skills, were approximately those of a 12-month-old child. Referral for further assessments and investigation confirmed that John had a global developmental delay and possible intellectual impairment. When John was seen at age 4 years, his skills developmentally were at approximately a 2-year level. He had continued to gain skills in accordance with his developmental quotient of approximately 50, although his delay in development has increased from 12 to 24 months.

### Speech and language impairment

Disorders of communication may affect voice, fluency, articulation of words, grammar, comprehension, the pragmatics of language and non-verbal communication. The term 'pragmatics' describes the social use and understanding of communication. Because of the number of areas of speech and language that are potentially affected and the continuous nature of the distribution of these skills, defining what constitutes a meaningful delay to parents or child health professionals may be imprecise unless delays are moderate or development disordered. The doctor has a responsibility to consider the differential diagnosis of speech and language delays (Box 3.8.3). For any child with speech or language impairment

**Box 3.8.3 Differential diagnosis of speech and language disorders**

- Hearing impairment
- Intellectual impairment
- Autism
- Environmental deprivation
- Anatomical (e.g. palate abnormality)
- Bulbar or pseudobulbar palsy
- Seizures (Landau–Kleffner syndrome)
- Developmental speech and language disorder

a formal hearing test is mandatory. Children with global developmental delay or intellectual impairment will present not only with problems of speech and comprehension but also with impaired nonverbal abilities with block construction, puzzles or drawing, and deficits in self-care and social skills. Children with associated autism will manifest the behavioural features of that disorder.

### Clinical example

Mary presented at age 3 years with speech delay. She recited jingles but did not use words to communicate. The doctor assessing her was unable to gain her attention or make eye contact with her. Her parents stated that they experienced similar difficulties with Mary and that she spent her time in isolated repetitive play, lining up toys, rather than in imaginative play. She was not interested in other children and became distressed if they attempted to join her play. A diagnosis of autism was later confirmed.

Where other causes of speech and language delay are excluded and development is otherwise normal, the term 'developmental or specific speech and language disorder' is used. Twin studies indicate a strong genetic role in aetiology. Co-morbid disorders, especially difficulties with attention and coordination, are common. More moderate or severe delays may be followed by learning, cognitive and social difficulties as adults.

Interventions include not only assistance provided by a speech pathologist but also recognition of the importance of playgroups, educational programmes and management of co-morbidities.

## Developmental coordination disorder

Other terms used to describe the lack of motor skills in these children include dyspraxia or clumsiness. Developmental coordination disorder is a diagnosis made when other neurological and muscle diseases have been excluded, usually on the basis of history and examination. Although uncommon, it is important to consider mild forms of cerebral palsy, cerebellar disorders including progressive spinocerebellar disorders or tumour, and neuromuscular conditions in the differential diagnosis. There is an association with learning difficulty, especially problems with writing, and with behavioural disorders, including attention-deficit/hyperactivity disorder and Asperger syndrome (see Chapter 4.3).

## Learning difficulty

The largest group of children likely to experience learning difficulty is the approximately 14% of children who are slow learners, with intellectual abilities in the borderline range of 70–85 IQ points. Generally, all subject areas are affected.

Specific learning disorders occur in particular subject areas where there is an unexplained discrepancy between intellectual ability and the level of academic attainment in that subject. The DSM-IV describes specific learning difficulties in reading, maths and writing. The medical term dyslexia describes a specific language-based reading disorder, usually with problems in mastering phonetics. Dyscalculia is a medical term describing difficulties with calculation and mathematics. Dysgraphia is difficulty with writing. Behavioural problems are common in children with learning difficulty particularly attention-deficit/hyperactivity disorder, anxiety and loss of self-esteem or 'learned helplessness' where the child 'gives up'. As in all developmental disorders, learning and behaviour may also be affected by the educational environment, family stress and ill-health in the child.

Although physical and neurological examination are generally normal, it is important to ensure that the child is in good health, with normal hearing and vision, that there are no associated co-morbidities, and that other family and environmental factors are not adversely affecting opportunities for learning. It is also important to advocate for educational assessment and support within the school including, if needed, modification of the curriculum, and to maintain a focus on the child's strengths and their social–emotional development.

# 3.9 Child abuse

Terence Donald

## Development of current concepts

The sanctity and privacy of the Western family and its unfettered authority over its children was not challenged by society as a whole until the late 19th and the first half of the 20th century. For example, in Australia, legislation against neglect of children was enacted in the early 1920s.

Subsequently, state child welfare departments were created and their officers authorized to intervene on behalf of neglected children through the state Children's Courts. The action often led to children being removed from their family, being made state wards and placed in state institutions.

The impetus for the introduction of specific child protection legislation was led by US paediatrician Henry Kempe, who coined the term 'battered baby syndrome' to describe the physically abused infant. Such legislative provisions, related initially to physical or psychological harm and subsequently to sexual abuse, were introduced first in the USA and then, beginning in the 1970s, in other Western countries including Australia, New Zealand and the UK.

Child protection legislation asserts the right of children to be free of harm from abuse or neglect caused by their parents or carers. Most child protection legislation states that the safety of children in their family environment is of paramount importance and must always be considered above the rights or opinions of the parents or carers.

A web link to the various Australian states' child protection legislation is: http://www.aifs.gov.au/nch/pubs/issues/issues22/issues22.html.

- Child abuse is physical or psychological harm from acts of commission by parents or carers.
- Harm from omission occurs when nutrition, hygiene, health and housing needs are neglected.
- Between 50% and 70% of parents who harm their children were harmed when they were children.

Significant psychosocial adversity is present in all families where abuse occurs. The adversity includes poor education, poverty, young parental age, single parenthood, mental ill-health, intellectual disability, substance abuse and intrafamilial violence. Premature and complicated birth is also over-represented in abused or neglected children, as well as poor development of the primary attachment relationship between infant and carer (usually the mother).

The concept of the 'continuum of child protection' has been developed to incorporate the prevention, early intervention, recognition and management of children who might need child protection or who have been harmed through abuse or neglect. The 'continuum of child protection' links together families who are experiencing adversity (which implies there is a potential for abuse to occur) with those in which abuse or neglect has been established. Therefore, even though there is no predictable causal relationship between the presence of adversity and the occurrence of abuse or neglect, the population of families suffering significant adversity will contain the majority of children who will experience such harm. Consequently, child protection from the health professional's perspective begins with the identification of family adversity in pregnancy or early childhood leading into the provision of services to assist in the eradication of the adversity or the minimizing of its effects. Such services are generally community-based and are equivalent to secondary prevention strategies. Their focus is to lessen a family's social isolation, strengthen the interpersonal relationships of the parents, assist the parents' understanding of the developmental demands of young children and provide practical home-based parenting advice. There is evidence to support the efficacy of such preventative programmes in families where adversity is present but abuse has not occurred, but no clear evidence that indicates similar programmes reduce the recurrence of incidents of abuse or neglect once they have occurred. Hence, to maximize successful intervention, it is critical to identify and address adversity before children are harmed.

Once children have been harmed through abuse or neglect, tertiary level services must become involved; these include statutory welfare agencies, the police and often tertiary forensic health services.

This primary, secondary and tertiary approach to child protection has been called the public health model of child protection intervention.

Similar patterns of psychosocial adversity are prevalent in families whether or not abuse has occurred. There is no reliable way of predicting which children are likely to become victims of abuse or neglect; therefore,

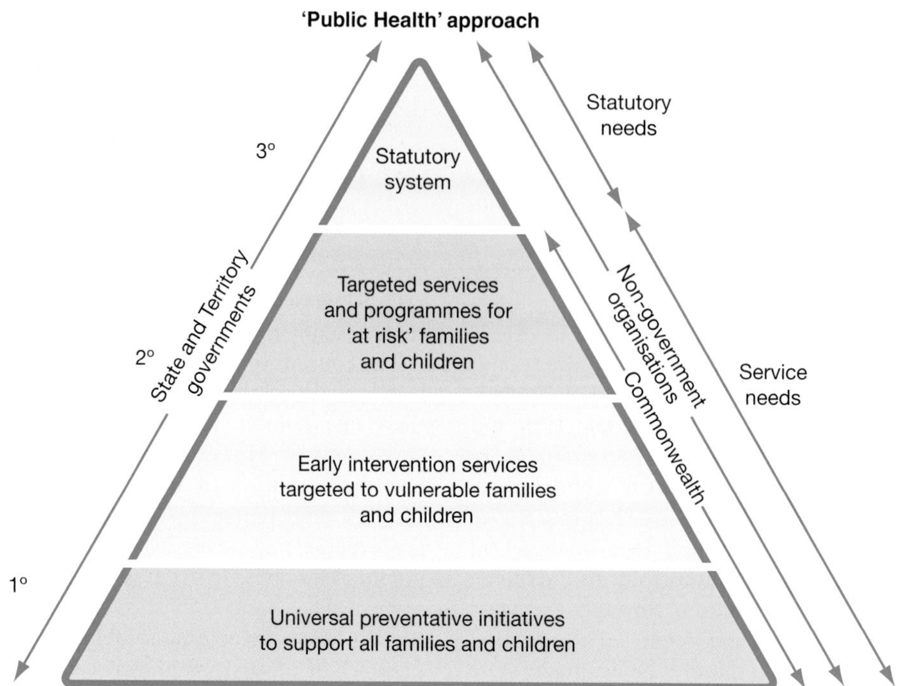


Fig. 3.9.1 Pyramid approach to public health.

the early identification of adversity, even in the antenatal period, is an important strategy. Identification of family adversity can lead to the provision of services to address and ameliorate its presence and effects. This is a child abuse primary prevention strategy.

The Australian National Child Protection Framework represents the public health approach as a pyramid (Fig. 3.9.1).

## Child protection and the concept of mandatory reporting

When child protection legislation was introduced in the USA, Canada and Australia it contained the requirement for mandatory reporting, which refers to the legal requirement placed on specified individuals to notify the designated statutory authority (usually the statutory welfare authority) when the individual has reasonable grounds to suspect that a child has been harmed by abuse or neglect.

Each state in the USA and each of the Canadian provinces has the mandatory reporting requirement. Each Australian state and territory has some level of legislation requiring mandatory reporting to the state or territory statutory agency of a suspicion of harm owing to child abuse or neglect. The breadth of professionals mandated to report varies widely across the states and territories in Australia; medical practitioners are always specified as mandated notifiers.

There is no mandatory reporting requirement in the UK or in New Zealand, but an expectation that the authorities will be informed of children suspected of being abused. The mandatory reporting requirement varies throughout continental Europe; generally, reporting is not mandatory.

Mandatory reporting was introduced when child abuse was considered to be manifest primarily as physical abuse. It was reasoned that physically abused children would usually be brought to medical attention and the abuse would be suspected by the doctor. It allowed a doctor to make a notification to the statutory authority and not be in breach of patient confidentiality, and when a doctor suspected abuse then the legal requirement for notification did not require the doctor specifically to challenge the responsibility of the parents in relation to the suspicion.

Most child protection legislation requires that the anonymity of notifiers be maintained and provides protection of notifiers against legal action that might be initiated by parents or carers.

The value of mandatory reporting in the management of suspected child abuse is still debated. Those regions in which it is not present argue against its introduction. No region that has mandatory reporting has withdrawn it.

A useful summary of the issues related to the mandatory reporting of child abuse was published by the Australian Institute of Family Studies in 2005 (web reference: http://www.aifs.gov.au/nch/pubs/sheets/rs3/rs3.html).

## Physical, sexual and psychological abuse: a general overview

*Physical abuse* is injury inflicted on a child by a caregiver, including injury from physical discipline. The intent to injure is not relevant when considering physical abuse.

*Psychological abuse* is a repeated pattern of caregiver behaviour or extreme incidents that convey to children that they are worthless, flawed, unloved, unwanted, endangered or of value only in meeting another's needs. Such behaviour has significant effects on the developing brains of children, its consequences being manifest in behaviour and developmental problems in preschool children, learning problems in older children, and antisocial and criminal behaviour in adolescents.

*Sexual abuse* has occurred whenever dependent, developmentally immature, children and adolescents are involved in any sexual activities that they do not fully comprehend, to which they are unable to give informed consent or that violate social taboos or family roles.

Sexually abusive behaviour may have serious psychological consequences for the child. It is particularly harmful when it occurs on multiple occasions over a period of time, when it is associated with physical injury, threats of physical harm if others are told, bribery or coercion, or when family members become aware of the allegations but don't believe the child.

Psychological harm is of primary concern as a consequence of both physical and sexual abuse. For example, it can cause problems in children's personality development, their ability to self-regulate their behaviour and to interact socially.

## Prevalence of child abuse in Australia

The Australian Institute of Health and Welfare (www.aihw.gov.au) is responsible for collecting and collating child protection data from throughout Australia. The total number of notifications made nationally, reflecting the number of children in whom child abuse or neglect is suspected, has increased annually from 107 134 in 1999–2000 to 339 454 in 2008–2009. New South Wales contributed 63% of the total notifications. The increase reflects changes in child protection policies and practices, and an increased public awareness of child abuse. It is not clear whether the increased rate of notification is due to an increase in child abuse. In Australia, estimates of the current incidence of child abuse range between 10 and 20 cases per 1000 live births.

In Australia a large proportion of investigations of suspected child abuse are not substantiated. The proportion of finalized investigations that were substantiated varied from 29% in New South Wales to 62% in Victoria. Overall, emotional abuse was the most common type of substantiated abuse, and sexual abuse the least common.

Accurate national data on death due to child abuse are not available in Australia. The most vulnerable are those less than 2 years of age, with most deaths occurring in infants aged under 12 months.

## Child protection systems – the interagency child protection process

This refers to the systems and the services contained within them that are specifically responsible for child protection at either a state or country level.

The provision of services to children anywhere on the child protection continuum (as described above) occurs through the cooperation and collaboration of different agencies, within both the government and non-government sectors. No single professional or agency can adequately provide fully comprehensive services across the whole continuum.

## Principles of interagency practice in relation to the management of suspected child abuse or neglect

This refers to the tertiary level statutory system that is responsible for the management of children who enter the child protection system because of a suspicion that they have been abused or neglected and in whom abuse or neglect is established.

The agencies that comprise the tertiary level system are the statutory welfare agency, the police and, often, tertiary forensic health services. The important principles that support and enable tertiary interagency practice are:

- the presence of policies, procedures and guidelines to address roles, responsibilities, referral practices, timeframes for assessments
- a process for the exchange of information in relation to children who are suspected of having been abused in the context of what is legally appropriate and professionally ethical

- a joint decision-making process between tertiary agencies specifically related to the outcomes and interpretations of assessments, the types of intervention and the provision of treatment to abused children.

The health services, community services and the police have specific roles and responsibilities in managing suspected child abuse and neglect.

### Health

- Recognition of adversity in families and ensuring its active resolution
- Recognition of children in whom abuse/neglect may have occurred
- Ensuring that the child's situation is properly assessed in relation to health and safety needs
- Complying with local legal notification requirements for suspected abuse/neglect
- Determining the ongoing role of the health agency according to agreed interagency practice
- Working to maintain an ongoing professional relationship with families after abuse has been suspected
- Provision of specialist forensic health services to children suspected of having been abused or neglected, complementing community services and the police. These include forensic medical and psychosocial assessment and therapeutic services.

### Community services

- Investigation of notifications/reports of suspected child abuse/neglect
- Coordination with health units and police of each agency's respective role
- Facilitation of the assessment of children in whom abuse/neglect is suspected
- Establishment of the level of danger/safety of children who have been abused or neglected
- Seeking of court child protection orders, when considered necessary, for abused/neglected children, particularly for those who remain in unsafe circumstances
- Optimal placement of children removed from their families because of abuse/neglect
- Ensuring that adequate therapy is provided to children in whom abuse/neglect has been substantiated.

### Police

- Investigation of the criminal aspects of child abuse/ neglect
- Coordination with community services and health units through agreed interagency practices
- Prosecution, when appropriate, of those who have abused, molested or neglected a child.



## Clinical management of suspected child abuse and neglect

A. Recognition of the child who may have been abused or neglected
B. Initiation of the interagency process to ensure optimal assessment of the suspicion
C. The forensic medical assessment
D. Establishment of the ongoing management needs of the child when abuse or neglect is confirmed
E. The health professional's ongoing responsibility to the child in whom abuse or neglect is suspected and to their family.

### A. Recognition by health professionals of children who may have been abused or neglected

Suspicion of abuse/neglect in a child should be reported to the local statutory child protection agency, whether or not there are local mandatory reporting requirements. Reports will bring to light any previous, similar concerns either in the family or involving current family members, ensure a coordinated response and facilitate the optimal assessment and investigation of the suspicions. An optimal assessment will enable informed decisions to be made in relation to the child's need for ongoing protection and therapy.

The suspicion that a child may have been abused or neglected arises in one or more of three ways.

#### 1. An allegation is made on behalf of a child to a professional by another person

These allegations are most often made by one parent against another (from whom they are estranged) or by a family member against a parent. They are often in the context of Family Court proceedings relating to the residency and visitation arrangement of the child. The role of the doctor in such situations is to:

- facilitate a notification of suspected child abuse to the appropriate statutory authority
- establish what, if any, clinical findings are present that support or refute the allegations; for example, when a suspicion of sexual interference has arisen based solely on dysuria, the suspicion may be resolved if a urinary tract infection is confirmed
- ensure that if the child has any other medical problems they are understood in relation to the allegations of abuse (e.g. Henoch–Schönlein purpura and the appearance of 'bruising').

The doctor should never discount the allegations on the basis of a lack of supportive physical findings. All suspicions should be reported and assessed optimally through the interagency process.

When allegations relate to sexual abuse it is necessary for the doctor to conduct only a superficial genital examination to check for external genital inflammation, discharge or bleeding. The definitive examination must be undertaken by an experienced paediatric forensic physician and will occur as part of the forensic medical assessment, which will be initiated by the interagency process.

When there are physical findings present that may support the allegations, they must be documented carefully and thoroughly. For example, superficial or genital injury must be recorded photographically. Normally, this is the responsibility of a paediatric forensic physician and is part of the forensic medical assessment.

### 2. An allegation is made directly to a professional by a child or young person

This may occur as part of a clinical presentation related to the allegation or may arise during an apparently unrelated consultation. For example, in the process of assessing a child for behaviour disturbance an allegation of physical abuse or emotionally harmful parenting may be made. When allegations arise in this way, they must always be notified.

When the complainant is an older child or adolescent it is critical that they are informed of the doctor's obligation to notify. In addition, they must be assisted to deal with the issues that subsequently arise, particularly whether or not they are safe to return home when they have made an allegation against a parent. The role of the doctor in these situations is to establish whether there are any clinical findings that support or refute the allegations.

A forensic medical assessment may be organized after the notification has been made and the interagency process begins.

### 3. The suspicion arises out of a clinical assessment undertaken for other reasons

Concerns may arise in the context of a consultation and be related to non-specific presentations, presentations that raise suspicions, and the injury history.

*Non-specific presentations*

These include sexualized behaviour in young children; aggressive or antisocial behaviour in preschool and primary school children; adolescents who are self-harming or manifesting dangerous and repetitive risk-taking behaviour. None of these behaviours is specifically indicative of abuse having occurred, but it should be considered.

Engagement of such children and adolescents in a counselling process may lead to an allegation of harm being made. The allegation must then be notified.

*Presentations that of themselves should raise suspicions*

- *Injury in infancy and early childhood that is either unexplained* (e.g. a skull fracture with no history of blunt trauma) *or inadequately explained* (e.g. a spiral fracture of the femur in a 6-month-old noticed when she was having her nappy changed).

The younger the injured child, the lower the threshold for suspecting the injury may have been inflicted. It is rare for infants who are not independently mobile to sustain any significant injury. Adequate independent mobility is rare before 14 months of age.

Infants who injure themselves manifest patterns of injury that reflect their mobility, for instance bruising and abrasions over bony prominences of the forehead, chin, knees and shins. Facial bruising over soft areas and bruising over muscle masses (thighs, calves, upper arms), the anterior trunk or abdomen are all rare in young children, especially if not mobile. When bruising occurs in any of these sites in infancy, inflicted injury should be suspected.

Fractures in normal infants are rare and the forces necessary for their production are able to be self-generated only when young children are able to run and climb or when another person, usually an adult, is involved (e.g. young infants may sustain skull fractures from being dropped from the carrying height of a parent).

Fractures of the femur, tibia, humerus (from grabbing, twisting or bending) and ribs (from direct impact or extreme chest compression) in infants should always raise suspicions and be assessed thoroughly. The torsional forces necessary to produce a spiral fracture in either the femur or tibia are able to be self-imposed only by young children who are able to run and climb.

Scalds are the commonest heat injury in infants and young children. Most often the scalds involve children pulling down cups of hot drinks or containers of hot liquids on to themselves. Sometimes these incidents of self-injury are indicative of poor parental supervision or neglect.

Immersion scalds occur when a child is immersed in hot liquid or the liquid surrounding a child becomes hot. The circumstances surrounding immersion scalds require careful and thorough evaluation. Often there is a suspicion that a scald may have been inflicted or occurred through parental neglect. When such suspicions arise they should be reported to the statutory agency.

### Clinical example

A 2-month-old baby girl, one of twins, was brought into the emergency department in the early evening by her mother, who said she became concerned when she took off her baby's nappy and found that the 'skin was peeling off'. She said there had been no signs of any abnormality earlier in the day. The children had been in her care for the whole day; her grandmother had been helping her with the babies during the afternoon.

The doctor considered that the finding was a scald and, because there was no explanation, he considered that it may have been inflicted, so made a notification. A forensic medical assessment was undertaken and confirmed that the abnormality was an immersion scald.

The great grandmother of the baby was interviewed. She said she had changed the baby's nappy in the mid-afternoon. The baby had passed a large amount of faeces and the grandmother had had to wash her buttocks. She described filling a bowl with water straight from the hot tap, lowering the baby into the water without testing the temperature. She said the baby was crying at the time and difficult to settle afterwards. She put another nappy on the child.

When this explanation was discussed with the mother, she confirmed that the hot water was at a high temperature and she had not warned her grandmother of that fact.

The assessment was that the great grandmother's explanation adequately accounted for the scald and the suspicion was resolved.

The features of the scald that indicate it was caused by immersion are:

- the 'tide-mark line' that demarcates the scald from normal skin
- the sparing of the skin in the creases from the hot water.

See Figures 3.9.2 and 3.9.3.

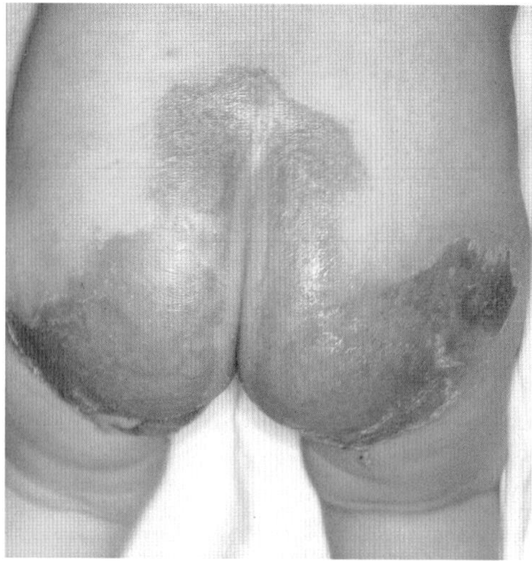

Fig. 3.9.2 Recent immersion scald.

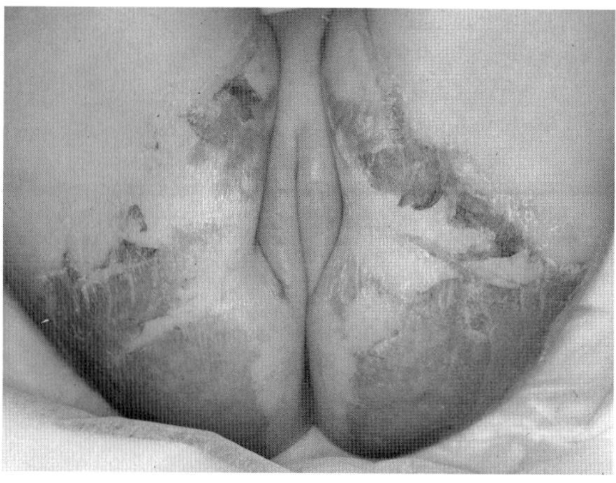

Fig. 3.9.3 Recent immersion scald.

The sequence of events leading to any serious injury in infancy should be easily ascertainable by speaking with the infant's carers. Serious injuries include head injury, abdominal injury, chest injury or widespread multiple injuries. When no adequate history is available, a report of the suspicious nature of the injury/injuries should be made to the statutory welfare agency. Subsequently, a comprehensive forensic medical assessment will ensure that the best informed opinion in relation to the injury mechanism is able to be formulated.

The threshold for suspicion of abuse in such infants, particularly when head injury is the presenting problem, must be low. Head injury in infancy may be manifest as blunt trauma to the cranium with or without intracranial haemorrhage, or may present solely as intracranial haemorrhage without any obvious external signs of injury. Such head injury is most likely to be a manifestation of intracranial acceleration/deceleration injury, which may occur from such harmful behaviours as violent shaking, and is often associated with severe blunt trauma as well.

### Clinical example

A baby boy of 2.5 months was presented by his parents after reportedly having vomited and having a seizure in his father's arms. There was no external sign of injury on examination.

Computed tomography scan of the baby's head (Fig. 3.9.4) showed a recent right-sided subdural haemorrhage that was suspicious of inflicted injury because there was no history of trauma.

A skeletal survey showed healing fractures of the posterior aspects of the 4th to 7th left ribs (Fig. 3.9.5).

After initially denying any incidents of trauma, the father said he had forcibly grabbed the baby around the chest and thrown him into his cot 8 days before presentation and, on the early evening of his presentation, had got angry with the baby and thrown him on to the couch. The seizure and vomiting occurred soon after.

The father was charged and given a suspended sentence. He received psychological treatment.

The child remained with his mother.

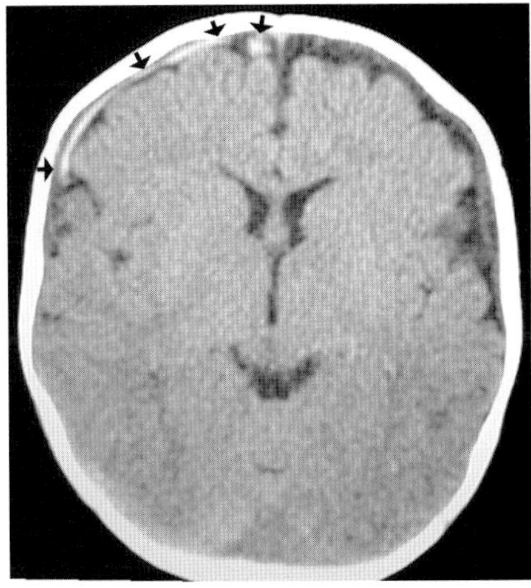

Fig. 3.9.4 Recent subdural haematoma (arrows).

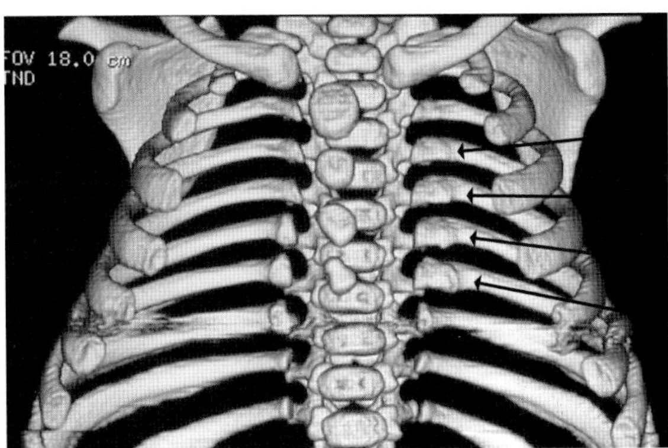


Fig. 3.9.5 Healing rib fractures.

A systematic, structured approach to the taking of an 'injury history' assists in evaluating the adequacy of the provided history and therefore in deciding whether the injury should be considered suspicious.

- *Injuries where the mechanism is apparent* and indicates that the injury has been inflicted (e.g. a patterned bruise to the face indicating a slap mark or punch).
- *Infections that are normally considered to be transmitted by sexual contact* (e.g. gonorrhoea, syphilis, human immunodeficiency virus) or that may be transmitted by sexual contact (e.g. herpes simplex virus, genital warts from human papilloma virus).
- *Infants with unexplained poor growth* who gain weight quickly in an environment where their intake is normal and controlled (e.g. in hospital or out-of-home care).

Each of these presentations should be reported to the appropriate statutory agency. Interagency discussions will then lead to a comprehensive forensic medical and psychosocial assessment being undertaken. A forensic psychosocial assessment in this context involves the interviewing of children who are sufficiently developmentally advanced.

*The injury history*

It is not always clear to the doctor who first sees an injury whether or not it is adequately explained. Generally parents of children less than 3 years old will either be aware of how their child was injured (because they witnessed the incident) or will clearly state that they lost visual contact with their child for a period of time and heard but did not see the incident of trauma that caused the injury.

In both of these situations there will be readily available useful detail to help the doctor decide whether the injury has been adequately explained or not. When an injury has not been adequately explained, it should, generally, be considered suspicious.

The following is a useful protocol to follow when assessing injury in a child.

- When did the injury occur? This refers to the date and time.
- Where did the injury occur? This refers to the exact location.
- What actually went wrong? This refers to the detail of what caused the injury.
- Was the incident actually witnessed and, if so, by whom?

Parents who claim that the incident 'must have happened when …' are not providing useful witness information but merely speculating as to the cause of the incident. Such a speculation is not an explanation, and an injury in that context should usually be considered suspicious.

An injury history must always address the developmental capabilities of the child, particularly in relation

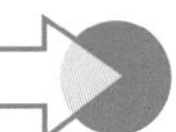

**Practical points**

**The injury history**

When did the injury occur? – This refers to the date and time.
Where did the injury occur? – This refers to the exact location.
What actually went wrong? – This refers to the detail of what caused the injury.
Was the incident actually witnessed and, if so, by whom?
On review of the history, has the child had any previous injuries?
What is the developmental level of the child, particularly in relation to their gross motor abilities (sitting, crawling, walking, running, climbing)?

to gross motor skills, as with independent movement self-caused injury becomes a consideration.

### B. Initiation of the interagency process to ensure optimal assessment of the suspicion

A suspicion of abuse or neglect begins with an interagency response initiated by the child protection notification and involves the statutory welfare agency, the police and the tertiary health service.

At this time, the primary concern of the doctor should generally be the immediate safety and protection of the child. The doctor must decide whether or not to inform the child's parents of the suspicion and will be guided in this decision by factors such as his or her previous relationship with the parents and their behaviour at the time of the presentation of the child.

With infants and young children in whom physical abuse or neglect is suspected, the issue of safety is not always clear and is often best addressed by admission to hospital. This allows the optimal assessment and management of the suspicious injury, the child and the family.

Early discussions must occur between the managing team in the hospital, the statutory welfare agency and the police to clarify roles and responsibilities and to ensure the ongoing safety of the child during the assessment and investigation process.

The statutory agency workers will explain to the parents the 'child protection process' and the immediate plans for the investigation. They will seek the parents' cooperation for the child to remain in hospital.

If there is resistance from the parents to the management plan, the statutory workers may consider applying to court for a child protection order to enable the process to continue.

### C. The forensic assessment in children in whom abuse or neglect is suspected

These assessments are undertaken after a notification of suspicion has been made and the statutory agency has either requested or supports the assessment. There are two components to an optimal forensic assessment: the forensic medical and the forensic psychosocial assessments.

The *forensic medical assessment* establishes the extent of injury in a child and whether or not the injury is considered to have been inflicted. When sexual abuse is suspected, a forensic medical assessment will establish whether or not there is any sign of genital injury or other condition (e.g. a sexually acquired infection) that could support the suspicion.

The *forensic psychosocial assessment* is best undertaken by a psychosocial clinician, a social worker or psychologist, and involves:

- formal interview of a child (when developmentally possible and appropriate) to establish the child's account of events
- evaluation of the child's psychological state in relation to the suspicions or allegations.

The forensic psychosocial assessment is most important in children in whom there are suspicions of sexual abuse because rarely in such cases is there supportive physical evidence or first-hand witnesses to the abuse.

The opinion that is formulated at the completion of the forensic medical assessment is important to the statutory welfare agency and the police, and may influence their ongoing investigation. The outcome of a forensic medical assessment may be that physical evidence supports the suspicion or allegation of abuse. It may conclude that an injury was or was not likely to have been inflicted.

Doctors who are not trained and experienced in forensic paediatric medicine should not undertake forensic medical assessments. A forensic medical assessment is not an extension of a standard paediatric medical assessment, primarily because it is undertaken to enable the formulation of a diagnosis or opinion for potential legal purposes.

Forensic physicians must also ensure that general health and developmental concerns of the children they assess are identified and managed. Forensic medical assessments provide information that may be useful in the statutory agency and police investigation.

The most important forensic principle is the 'chain of evidence'. The chain of evidence is a legal concept which requires that the origin and history of any clinically gathered material that may be presented as evidence in a court must be clearly demonstrated to have followed an unbroken chain from its source to the court, so that there is no chance of its contamination. In the conduct of a forensic medical assessment the 'chain of evidence' relates specifically to:

- documentation (by clinical description and photography) of the physical findings related to the suspicion of abuse or neglect
- accurate recording of the explanation offered (when available) to account for the physical findings
- proper collection of forensic specimens (e.g. swabs of saliva, genital swabs).

There are five steps in a forensic medical assessment:

1. *Determining the extent of obvious injury* (ascertained by physical examination). A complete physical examination is required including neurological assessment and fundoscopy.
2. *Establishing the biomechanics or mechanism of each injury.* This means the types of 'force' involved (tensile or impact, torsional, bending, thermal and combinations) or how the injury was caused (incision, blunt trauma).

3. *Ascertaining the history provided for the injury/injuries.* The explanation(s) must account for the appearance and biomechanics of the suspicious injury in the context of the child's developmental capacity (e.g. if an injury is reported to have occurred by an infant rolling off a flat surface of table height then the infant must be observed to establish that rolling is possible).
4. *Assessing the relevance of additional information*, for example site visit evaluation, witness statements. Site visit evaluation is undertaken by the police to document features of the site where the injury is said to have occurred (e.g. the height of a table, the temperature of hot water, the composition of the reported impact surface). Witness statements are only taken by the police. Their content may assist in establishing an injury timeframe (e.g. the time a neighbour heard an infant scream or whether a facial bruise was present when the child visited the neighbour the day before the suspicion was reported).
5. *Formulating an objective opinion based on the identified injuries.* The forensic opinion must be based solely on the result of the medical evaluation. Factors such as the known level of violence in the child's family and a previous history of physical abuse are critical in the management decisions that will be taken by statutory welfare agencies and the police, but such factors cannot influence the forensic opinion. When they do, the forensic opinion is subjective and of no value in the legal context.

The forensic medical assessment may resolve the suspicion (e.g. the skull fracture was explained adequately); if the possibility that the injury was inflicted remains, further assessments are required to find evidence of any covert skeletal trauma or organ injury or toxic substance administration. The additional assessments include:

- imaging studies (skeletal survey, radionucleotide bone scanning, intracranial imaging), which should be undertaken in infants less than 18 months of age and considered in children aged up to 3 years
- adequate X-rays to attempt the ageing of fractures
- laboratory studies, in particular 'organ enzymes' (liver enzymes, pancreatic enzymes)
- bleeding/clotting studies, including the measurement of the coagulation factors, platelet numbers and function
- toxicology studies to analyse for the presence of drugs and poisons.

The results of these assessments add to the formulation of the forensic medical opinion (Fig. 3.9.6).

## D. The ongoing management needs of the child when abuse or neglect is confirmed

The primary ongoing issues once abuse has been confirmed are:

- The child's safety and any ongoing need for protection.
- If there is a need for protection then legal intervention leading to placement away from the abuser may be necessary.
- The physically injured child may have ongoing medical needs.
- Addressing the psychological effects of abuse as part of a comprehensive therapeutic programme.

## E. The health professional's ongoing responsibility to the child and family when abuse or neglect is suspected

Families involved in the child protection system often isolate themselves from health services because they fear being 'targeted' as abusers. Previous health-care providers should try hard to provide ongoing care to such families from as early as possible in the child protection process.

Health-care providers should ensure that abused/neglected children are provided with therapy and those placed in out-of-home care have their ongoing health needs systematically identified and addressed, because of their high rate of morbidity.

### Practical points

**The five steps of a forensic medical assessment**

1. Determining the extent of obvious injury.
2. Establishing the biomechanics or mechanism of each injury.
3. Ascertaining the history provided for the injury or injuries.
4. Assessing the relevance of additional information – site visit evaluation, witness statements.
5. Formulating an objective opinion based on the identified injuries.

The forensic opinion must be based solely on the result of the medical evaluation.

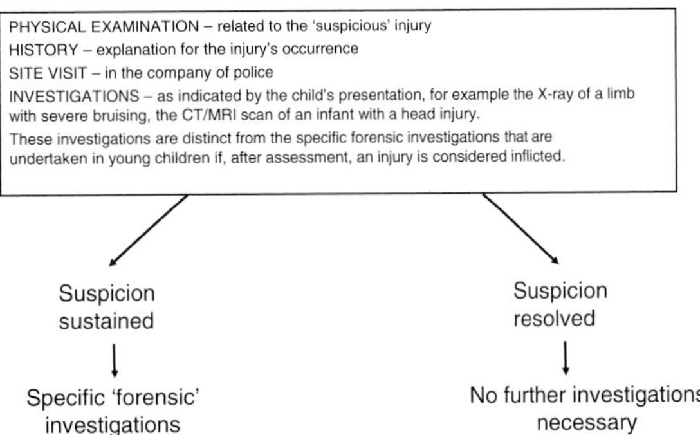
PHYSICAL EXAMINATION – related to the 'suspicious' injury
HISTORY – explanation for the injury's occurrence
SITE VISIT – in the company of police
INVESTIGATIONS – as indicated by the child's presentation, for example the X-ray of a limb with severe bruising, the CT/MRI scan of an infant with a head injury.
These investigations are distinct from the specific forensic investigations that are undertaken in young children if, after assessment, an injury is considered inflicted.
Suspicion sustained
Suspicion resolved
Specific 'forensic' investigations
No further investigations necessary

Fig. 3.9.6 Forensic medical assessment of a 'suspicious' injury. CT, computed tomography; MRI, magnetic resonance imaging.

## The wellbeing of health professionals involved with child protection

Any clinician who deals with children or families may become suspicious that a child has been abused or neglected. An open and honest approach with parents/carers is the best policy, unless there is a possibility of physical danger. It is helpful to assure parents that they are not being accused, but the suspicion needs notification and investigation. It is not good professional practice to offer to make deals with parents when abuse is suspected (e.g. 'If you tell me what happened then I can help sort out this problem quickly').

As a general principle, doctors should have in place a support system that enables them to debrief difficult interactions with patients and should be used when child protection issues arise, and also colleagues with whom they can discuss child protection concerns.

# 3.10 Sudden unexpected death in infancy

Barry Taylor, Dawn Elder

Despite a remarkable increase in knowledge about the aetiology of sudden unexpected death in infancy (SUDI) over the past few decades, it remains a significant clinical problem in Australasia and internationally. This chapter reviews what we currently know about SUDI, how diagnosis and clinical management has changed over time, and how we should assist families who experience the sudden death of an infant.

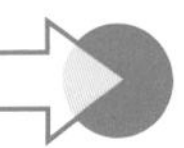

**Practical points**

- A sudden unexpected death in infancy (SUDI) is one not anticipated 24 hours before death occurred.
- All SUDI deaths must be referred to the coroner for investigation.
- After autopsy, an explanation will be found for some SUDI deaths.
- If no explanation is found after examining the circumstances of death, the clinical history and the autopsy findings, the diagnostic label sudden infant death syndrome (SIDS) may be used.
- Parents of SUDI infants should be offered follow-up with a clinician who can discuss the autopsy and other findings in regard to their child's death.
- Advising new parents to sleep their infant supine in a safe sleep space and to avoid smoking in pregnancy are important ways to prevent SUDI.
- A safe sleep space is one designed to make sure that the face is always clear, that there are no risks of wedging or strangulation and that enables a baby to maintain thermal balance.

## Historical perspective

Sudden death in infancy has been reported since the earliest times. In the Book of Kings in the Bible there is a report of an infant being overlain and found dead. From Medieval to Victorian times babies were taken into their parents' beds in the winter to protect them from the cold and some were found dead in the morning. As socioeconomic conditions and the care of newborn infants improved, these types of death became less common. In the 1960s, many babies in newborn intensive care units were nursed prone because of increased stability of the chest wall and better oxygenation in this position, and this sleep position became increasingly used for well babies at home, especially when it was realized that infants went to sleep faster in this position and that it was also associated with less gastro-oesophageal reflux.

In the 1970s and 1980s high rates of sudden infant death were recognized throughout the world and were considered to be so high that a number of large epidemiological studies were set up to try to determine the reason for these deaths. It was usual at this stage for the term 'sudden infant death syndrome', or SIDS, to be applied to these deaths. Both Australia and New Zealand were found to have some of the highest rates of SIDS in the world at this time. The apparent emergence of a new condition was almost certainly mainly related to diagnostic transfer as health professionals and coroners increasingly used the term (recognized with an International Classification of Diseases (ICD) 9 code of 798 in 1977 and an ICD10 code of R95 in 1992). This is strongly suggested because total post-neonatal mortality (within which are almost all SIDS cases) did not increase as SIDS rates rose. Case–control studies identified a number of risk factors associated with SIDS, and the dramatic decrease in SIDS and post-neonatal mortality in countries that intervened around these risk factors (primarily the prone sleep position) strongly suggest a causative relationship. This early research was followed by a plethora of basic science research to try to establish the mechanism by which the risk factors contributed to any individual infant's risk of sudden death.

Despite these efforts there remain a significant number of infants who die suddenly and unexpectedly each year. It has increasingly been recognized that these infants represent a particular group and that many have been found sleeping in an unsafe sleep position or situation. For this reason, terminology has changed over time and this group of deaths is now more commonly discussed under the label 'sudden unexpected death in infancy' (SUDI).

## Definitions

SUDI (sudden unexpected death in infancy), sometimes described as SUD or SUID, is a term used for all unexpected infant deaths, whether the explanation is determined after a thorough investigation or remains unknown. Traditionally all unexplained SUDI deaths have been labelled as sudden infant death syndrome (SIDS), but since the mid-1990s a number of forensic pathologists are becoming increasingly reluctant to use this diagnosis as a cause of death when certain risk factors are present (co-sleeping, prone positioning, issues surrounding appropriate parental care, minor pathological changes, etc.), preferring to use the terms 'unascertained', 'borderline SIDS', 'undetermined', 'unspecified' or 'unknown' when they report their findings to the coroner. The formal definition of SIDS has undergone several revisions since the term was initially coined by Beckwith in 1969, with the broad definition from 1989, '*the sudden death of an infant less than one year of age which remains unexplained after a thorough case assessment, including performance of a complete autopsy, investigation of the death scene, and review of the clinical history*', still being the most widely used. Subsequent suggestions have involved including the need for the death to have occurred during sleep, and also several subclassifications have been suggested, none of which has entered into general usage.

## Incidence and risk factors

As can be deduced from the discussion above, the problems of definition make comparisons over time and between countries problematic! Figure 3.10.1 shows both SIDS mortality and total post-neonatal mortality in 1990 (before risk reduction campaigns in these countries) and in 2005, 15 years later.

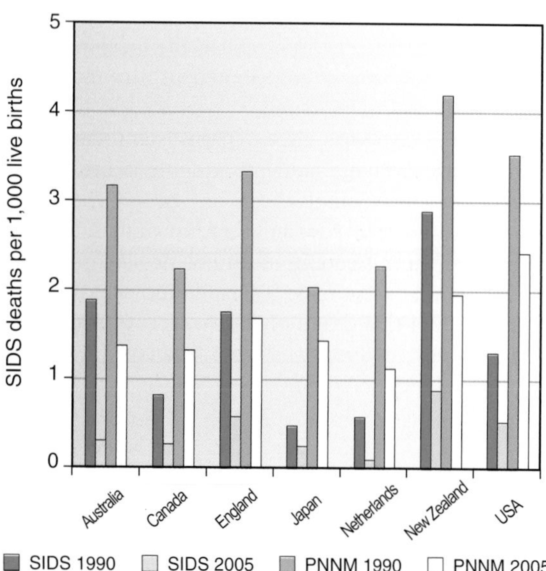


Fig. 3.10.1 SIDS and post-neonatal mortality in selected countries in the years 1990 and 2005.

Many studies have described the characteristics of babies who die from SIDS, and risk factors have been elucidated by a series of case–control studies. There has been much speculation as to why very few babies die in this manner in the first month of life, with the peak age of death at 24 months of age. Other factors such as prematurity and growth restriction at birth are more understandable, as are many risk factors that are difficult to change such as socioeconomic deprivation. More recently there has been concern that these deaths appear to be occurring more frequently in the first month of life.

The focus of much research has been on identifying 'modifiable' risk factors – by comparing the circumstances around the baby who has died with those of babies (matched for age) who have not. The key modifiable risk factors are nicely summarized by the International Society for the Study and Prevention of Perinatal and Infant Death (ISPID) and are:

- prone and side sleep position
- maternal smoking during pregnancy as well as postnatal second-hand smoke
- unsafe sleeping environments – especially parents falling asleep with their baby on the same sleeping surface, or in unusual sleeping places such as sofas
- bedding arrangements that allow the face to become covered.

Two key protective factors have been described – breastfeeding and immunization – with some ongoing discussion over consistent data from many studies suggesting that the use of a pacifier or dummy at the time of going to sleep is also protective.

## Aetiology of sudden death in infancy

Much research has been undertaken in the past few decades to try to find a reason for the death of infants where the clinical history, examination of the scene of death and autopsy has not found a fatal diagnosis. These infants have been labelled as dying from SIDS, and research has indicated that they do have some common characteristics. For 20–30% of infants who appear to have died suddenly and unexpectedly, a clear cause of death is found through either the clinical history, death scene examination or autopsy. These cases can then be considered explained SUDI deaths.

### Explained SUDI

*Infection*

Sudden and overwhelming infection is a possible cause of sudden infant death. Pneumococcal or meningococcal septicaemia or meningitis are often of particularly sudden onset, especially in the young infant. The diagnosis should be clear at autopsy. As evidence of minor infection may be found in infants who have a final diagnosis of SIDS, the pathologist must be convinced that the evidence of infection found is of a degree sufficient to explain the death.

*Homicide*
Homicide must always be kept in mind, especially in the situation where there have been other siblings who have apparently died from SIDS. In general, it is thought that less than 5% of SIDS cases may in fact be homicide. As intentional suffocation is virtually impossible to distinguish from SIDS at autopsy, this diagnosis may not be confirmed unless there are other significant injuries or a confession.

*Accidental asphyxia*
For some infants it is clear at the death scene that death has been due to accidental asphyxia. Some infants have been found dead caught in the bars of their cot or found strangled on a stray piece of cord. It is likely that any infant would die if they got themselves into such a situation. For other infants, the scene may have been suspicious for accidental asphyxia, for example if the infant was found lying under a parent, but it cannot be proven that the infant's airway was completely obstructed at the time of death. The question then arises as to whether the particular infant may have been more vulnerable in a potentially unsafe sleep situation than an otherwise normal infant would be expected to be.

*Cardiac arrhythmias*
Genetic cardiac channelopathies such as prolonged QT syndrome are thought to account for 5–10% of SUDI deaths. A family history of sudden death or deafness should be sought and would suggest that other family members should be screened for these disorders by electrocardiography or 24-hour Holter monitoring. A genetic diagnosis for these disorders can be made after death from stored blood, but this is still not a routine procedure.

*Congenital anomaly*
Occasionally an infant will die suddenly and unexpectedly, and be found at autopsy to have a significant congenital anomaly that has not been recognized in life. Both cardiac and pulmonary anomalies occasionally present for the first time in this way.

*Metabolic*
A small percentage (<1% in the UK) of babies dying from SIDS probably die as a result of medium-chain acetyl coenzyme A deficiency (MCAD). MCAD or another metabolic disorder should be suspected if the baby had decreased oral intake before death or if there was any unusual smell about the baby. An experienced pathologist will usually suspect a metabolic cause of death at autopsy and arrange for the appropriate diagnostic tests to be done. These deaths should be occurring less often as the diagnosis for many of these conditions (including MCAD) can be made by use of tandem mass spectrometry on blood collected on Guthrie cards in the newborn period.

*Other*
Other disease states that have been discovered at autopsy after sudden death include haematological disorders such as leukaemia, gastrointestinal disorders and intracranial haemorrhage.

## Unexplained SUDI

If a specific cause of death is not found after a complete history and thorough post-mortem examination, the death may be labelled as SIDS or the label SUDI–unexplained may be used. Sometimes it will be considered that insufficient information about the circumstances of death is available to rule out a diagnosis of accidental asphyxia, and the death may be labelled as undetermined. Despite using a definition for SIDS that excludes other causes of death and implies that the infant was otherwise healthy prior to death, it has become more apparent over time that the infant who dies suddenly and unexpectedly in seemingly inexplicable circumstances is not completely normal.

The triple risk model provides a useful way to conceptualize the information currently known about the factors that may contribute to risk of sudden death in infancy (Fig. 3.10.2). The model proposes that death occurs when a vulnerable infant is exposed to an external stressor at a critical period of development. It has become apparent over time that more than one final mechanism of death is likely.

### The vulnerable infant

The major epidemiological risk factors for SIDS and SUDI that define the vulnerable infant are exposure to maternal smoking in pregnancy, prematurity, intrauterine growth retardation, lack of breastfeeding and environmental smoke exposure after birth. There are also a number of anatomical and physiological factors that mark the vulnerable infant. Pathological abnormalities present in the central nervous system of SIDS victims include gliosis, delayed central nervous system myelination and arcuate nucleus hypoplasia. The degree of brainstem gliosis varies with the amount of maternal smoking during pregnancy in SIDS infants.

Other findings found at autopsy suggest that SIDS infants may have been exposed to chronic or intermittent hypoxia prior to death. These episodes of hypoxia may be secondary to obstructive apnoea, which is more common in infants who go on to die from SIDS than control infants. A major area of research has been the

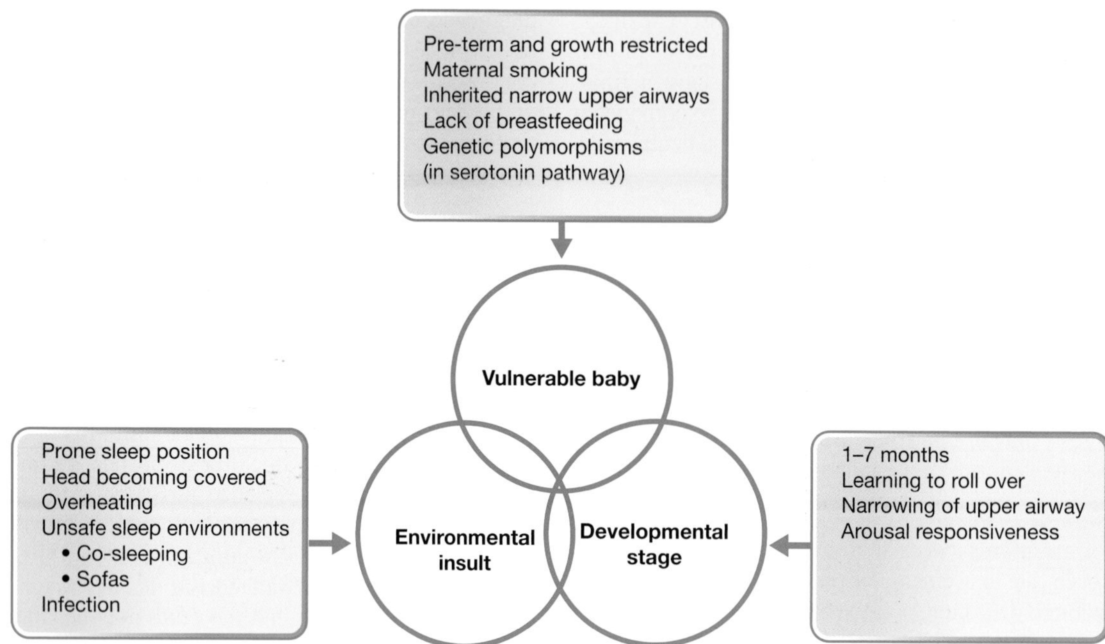


Fig. 3.10.2 The triple risk hypothesis for sudden unexpected death in infancy.

investigation of whether vulnerable infants may have poor arousal responses and are therefore not able to protect themselves in any situation that compromises their breathing in some way. Future SIDS infants also show less arousal during sleep than controls, and infants of smokers have impaired arousal responses. Decreased arousal in quiet sleep has also been shown in infants following infection and in sleep-deprived infants. This may be important as histological and microbiological evidence of recent viral infection has been found in some SIDS infants. Overheating may also contribute to decreased arousability.

Alterations in autonomic function have been found in infants at risk of SIDS, including decreased heart rate variability and diminished heart rate responses after tests of autonomic function. These differences may make it harder for the vulnerable infant to have an appropriate cardiovascular response when stressed by overheating or by an asphyxial episode.

## The contribution of exogenous stressors

It has been established for a number of years that the prone sleep position is a major risk factor for SIDS. Side positioning is also a risk because the infant often falls into the prone position from side sleeping. Other sleep environment factors that have been found to be important are having the head covered, becoming overheated and becoming too cold. Lying on bedding that is too soft or using a pillow are also risk factors, as is having toys around the infant in the cot.

The risks associated with bed-sharing have provoked some controversy. Initially it was thought that bed-sharing with an adult was only a risk when the infant had been exposed to maternal smoking *in utero*. It is now clear that small infants not exposed to smoking are also vulnerable, especially in the first few months of life. In addition, small infants in bed with large adults or adults under the influence of alcohol or drugs are at greater risk. Babies are also very vulnerable if they are on a couch with a sleeping adult, so it is critical that caregivers are alert when they are feeding and holding their infant.

## The contribution of developmental age

The newborn infant has poorly developed muscle tone and poor head control. This means they have very limited physical ability to reposition themselves to improve their airway when it becomes compromised. The airway of immature infants is particularly vulnerable when they are in a car seat, when their head flops forward or to the side, or in a bed-sharing situation. The prone sleep position is particularly dangerous when an immature infant sleeps in this position for the first time, especially if they have not had experience in prone while awake to improve neck muscle control. The 3–5-month age range was previously thought to be the most common time for SIDS deaths, but sudden infant death is increasingly being recognized as occurring in younger infants and even in the first weeks of life.

### Disruption of serotonergic mechanisms and sudden infant death

The areas of the brain that are abnormal histologically in SIDS infants are areas containing serotonergic neurons, and levels of serotonin have been shown to be decreased in these areas. The so-called medullary 5-hydroxytriptamine (5-HT) system is abnormal in at least 50% of SIDS cases. This system is important for central chemoreception and cardiovascular control, and is conceptualized as a 'defence network' that protects against stresses to the vital functions of respiration, blood pressure control, airway patency, thermoregulation, sensory input and arousal. Studies are now reporting that exposure to smoking in pregnancy has a direct effect on serotonin mechanisms.

Gasping is an important autoresuscitation mechanism that appears to fail in some SIDS victims. This may be because serotonin is required for pacemaker generation of respiratory rhythm during hypoxia. Serotonin is also involved in the chemoreceptor response to carbon dioxide. Failure of this response system may be critical for infants exposed to a potential rebreathing situation. Serotonin deficiency may also lead to altered heart rate variability and impaired baroreceptor function. The presence of abnormalities of serotonergic mechanisms in the brain therefore explains some of the physiological findings found in infants at risk of SIDS.

As well as what appear to be acquired lesions in the serotonin network, genetic abnormalities of serotonin metabolism have been described and been associated with an increased risk of SIDS. These include variation in serotonin transporter genes, *FEV* gene mutations, genes associated with a primary cardiac channelopathy, and other genes pertinent to autonomic nervous system development. It is likely that these genetic abnormalities explain some of the ethnic variation in prevalence of SIDS and also why some infants are at risk even when sleeping in the recommended sleep position.

## Classifying SUDI

A proposal for the international classification of SUDI was presented at the 17th Nordic Conference on Forensic Medicine in 2009. The starting point is that all initially unexpected deaths will be labelled as SUDI. An unexpected death is one that was not anticipated as a significant possibility 24 hours before the death occurred or where there was an unexpected major collapse followed by resuscitation and survival for more than 24 hours. The SUDI classification is made when the available information, including history, death scene examination and autopsy, has been assessed and is designed in particular to facilitate research and epidemiological data collection about SUDI deaths internationally. The classification categories are as follows:

- 0 Incomplete investigation (classified SUDI)
- /0 Extension used to denote a potentially important piece of information is missing
- Ia No notable factors identified (classified SIDS)
- Ib Notable factors identified but unlikely to have contributed to death (SIDS)
- IIa Factors(s) identified that possibly contributed to the death (SIDS)
- IIb Factors(s) identified that probably contributed to the death (SIDS)
- III Factors(s) identified that provide a cause of death (classified explained SUDI)

## Procedures when an infant dies suddenly and unexpectedly

When an infant has been found to have died without an apparent cause, a death certificate cannot be written and the local coroner must be notified. It would be usual then for the coroner to direct that a post-mortem examination should be done. The infant autopsy should ideally be undertaken by a paediatric or perinatal pathologist. The police will also investigate the death on behalf of the coroner. Investigation should include careful examination of the scene of death and a review of the events leading up to the death. This is often completed very well by the police, but a medical history is also required to establish whether there are any contributory factors related to the general health and development of the infant, as well as to consider whether there is any risk (environmental or medical) to other children in the household. Where the child that has died is one of twins, it is generally considered essential for the twin to be admitted to hospital for careful review and monitoring for at least 24 hours.

## Parent support after an unexpected infant death

Sudden unexpected death of an infant is devastating to parents, extended family and indeed staff. Empathetic care is needed for all concerned, and dealing with the family in this situation is usually the job of senior and experienced staff. Parents will be reassured if a careful history and examination is done, as they are usually keen to find out why their baby has died. Some parents, often from Indigenous cultures, object to the need for a post-mortem examination, or may ask for a limited autopsy. In this situation careful explanations about why it may be useful for the family to know the cause of death (e.g. to enable genetic counselling and detect possible health threats to other family members), as well as reassurances about the respect and care that will be given to the baby by the pathologist and staff, will lead to acceptance of the need. Ultimately, the coroners of both Australia and New Zealand can direct that a post-mortem examination be done without parental consent.

Parents and family have a complex and difficult grieving task. After initial denial, feelings of guilt can be especially difficult as most babies that die from SUDI have clear risk factors, some of them chosen by the parents. Giving support and clear information is important, and for families that identify as Indigenous, early involvement of a social worker or support person from their own culture is important.

Special attention should be paid to other children in the family and to grandparents. Children who have a sibling die often have 'magical thinking' – they believe that their thoughts and deeds may have caused the death. Clearly telling them that this is not so is an important task for adults in the family to do, often many times over the subsequent months. Grandparents in this situation feel a double loss – the loss of their grandchild, but also the pain of seeing their children suffer. They often feel that they have to support their own children and can have no support or outlet for their own grief. Recognizing this, and talking with them, sometimes separately, can be helpful.

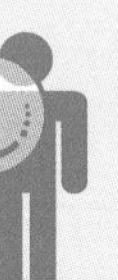

**Clinical example**

A 17-day-old baby was found dead in bed by her mother. She was born at 38 weeks with a birthweight of 2700g. Antenatal ultrasonography had detected intrauterine growth retardation. The mother smoked 20 cigarettes per day, also used marijuana and was obese. The baby was in bed with the mother for a breastfeed. The mother was tired and couldn't remember the baby finishing the feed. The mother was the only adult in the bed, which was a Queen size bed. When the mother awoke the baby was reported to be lying on her back on her mother's arm. There was no sign of life.

No abnormalities were found at post-mortem examination to explain the death. Because the infant was thought to be in an unsafe sleeping environment (in bed with an obese mother who smoked) it was felt a diagnosis of SIDS could not be applied. The cause of death was listed as 'undetermined'. Accidental asphyxia was thought to be the cause, but could not be proven because the only report of how the baby was found came from the mother who was very tired and could not remember all the circumstances clearly. For research purposes this would be classified as SIDS IIb (factors identified that probably contributed to the death).

## Prevention

Increased knowledge about the major risk factors for sudden infant death has lead to prevention programmes being put in place around the world. Because of these programmes, many infant lives have been saved. The main prevention measures are based on the known factors that place infants at risk, which have already been discussed. Efforts at prevention must start early in pregnancy if the risk of maternal smoking in pregnancy is to be decreased. Other times when prevention should be discussed with parents are at the time of birth, prior to discharge from initial maternity care and during well-child checks in the first months of life. The International Society for the Study and Prevention of Perinatal and Infant Death (ISPID) website lists the messages that should be given to parents (http://www.ispid.org/prevention.html):

**Always (day and night) place the baby on his/her back when it's time to sleep**

- The most significant proven risk factor is the sleep position. The risk of SIDS is over three times higher for a baby sleeping on the stomach.
- The practice of always placing the baby on his/her back when its time to sleep should begin at birth. The baby will become accustomed to sleeping on the back and will have no problems falling asleep.
- Make sure every caregiver uses the "back to sleep" position. A caregiver placing a baby to sleep on his/her stomach or side when the baby is accustomed to sleeping on the back raises the risk of SIDS 18-fold.
- Place the baby on the stomach only when he/she is awake and under adult supervision.

**Always keep the baby's environment smoke-free**

- Do not smoke during pregnancy. The more you smoke, the greater the risk for SIDS.
- Second-hand smoke is also a risk factor: stay in a smoke-free environment when pregnant.
- Always maintain a smoke-free environment for the baby.

**Make the sleeping environment as safe as possible and avoid overheating**

- Place the baby to sleep in its own cot next to the parents' bed for the first six months (room sharing).
- Never share a bed with baby if you or your partner smoke. Babies whose parents smoke are at increased risk of SIDS while co-sleeping.
- Never share a bed with baby when you have had alcohol or drugs. (Don't use alcohol or drugs when caring for your baby, especially ANY TIME you may fall asleep.) Babies whose parents have recently used alcohol or drugs are at increased risk of SIDS (and accidental suffocation) while co-sleeping.
- There is a slightly increased risk of SIDS with bed sharing for infants less than 3 months even if they

were not exposed to cigarettes, particularly if the baby was small (less than 2.5kg) at birth or born prematurely.

- In some countries there is a recommendation to avoid all bed sharing, although some disagree and advise avoiding bed sharing only if there are other risk factors present such as smoking or alcohol use.
- Never sleep with baby on a couch or sofa. This increases the risk of SIDS and fatal sleep accidents.
- Keep the cot free of soft objects and anything loose or fluffy (bedding, toys, bumpers, pillows, duvets).
- Do not allow the baby's head to be covered with bedding/blankets.
- Keep the room temperature at 18°C to 22°C and avoid overdressing (i.e. too many layers of clothes; particularly avoid the use of a hat when indoors) when placing the baby to sleep. Overheating has been cited as a risk factor for SIDS in the past, however, it has been shown that thermal factors are less important if the infant sleeps on the back.
- Use a safe, firm mattress that fits the cot properly.
- Use a mattress that is in new or used and in good condition (no tears).

**A word about breast feeding and pacifiers**

- Breast feeding is always recommended for its numerous benefits for babies and mothers (as a source of multiple necessary nutrients, disease protection and as a contributor to mother–baby bonding). Several studies show that breastfeeding also offers a risk reduction for SIDS.
- Research suggests that using a pacifier may reduce the risk of SIDS. Start using a pacifier after one month of age when breast feeding is usually well established. Give a pacifier when you put the baby to sleep, but do not force it. Some but not all studies have shown that pacifiers may have an adverse effect on breast feeding.

**Immunization**

- Infants that are immunized have half the risk of SIDS and are protected against diphtheria, tetanus, whooping cough, etc.

# 3.11 Care of the adolescent

Susan Sawyer, Andrew Kennedy

## What is adolescence?

Adolescence describes the developmental stage between childhood and adulthood. The World Health Organization defines the ages of an adolescent as 10–19 years, and defines youth as 15–24 years. We commonly combine these definitions (10–24 years) and use the encompassing term 'young people'.

The onset of puberty has long been accepted as the starting point of adolescence, whereas key social and role transitions such as completion of education, financial independence, marriage and children have historically marked the end of adolescence. These end-points formerly occurred within the few years from the late teens to the early twenties. As young people now commonly participate longer in education and are marrying and having children later, the end of adolescence has become less distinct.

The majority of adolescents rate their own health, including their mental health, as good. Many adolescents describe the period of adolescence as enjoyable and exciting, and as a time of satisfaction in achieving many milestones such as first relationships, completing school, getting a job and learning to drive. In contrast, adolescence was historically described by adults as a period of turmoil. Certainly, it is a time of increased health risk for healthy young people as well as for those with chronic illness, and there are a significant number of young people for whom adolescence is not 'smooth sailing'. Furthermore, although many health indicators in younger children and older adults have improved (e.g. tobacco use), a wide range of public health indicators in young people has remained static or have declined (e.g. rates of obesity and sexually transmitted infections).

In many parts of the world, specialist children's hospitals still effectively 'end' at 14 years of age, but adolescence is increasingly recognized as an important developmental period within the discipline of paediatrics (which is increasingly referred to as 'child and adolescent health'). Young people up to the age of 18–19 years are now commonly managed in tertiary children's hospitals and paediatric programmes in Australia and New Zealand. The upper age of many community-based children's health and welfare services has also risen. Although many parts of the world also recognize the subspecialty of adolescent health, all doctors must learn the knowledge, attitudes and skills to manage young people's health concerns, regardless of their likely future roles.

## Adolescent development

Just as all paediatricians need sound knowledge of child development, they must also have a sophisticated understanding of adolescent development. The division of adolescent development into the three domains of *physical*, *cognitive* and *psychosocial* can be a helpful framework for monitoring development. An additional approach (if simplistic) is to divide adolescent development into *early*, *middle* and *late* stages. Using this approach, *early* adolescence corresponds to physical development, *middle* relates primarily to cognitive maturation, and *late* to psychosocial aspects.

*Early adolescence* (around 10–14 years old) is characterized by the physical changes of puberty that mark the acquisition of reproductive capacity. It can be a time of increased physical activity and may also be a time where mood changes are noticed by the family. The developmental tasks associated with this period are about establishing a realistic body image and also becoming aware of oneself as a sexual being with a sexual orientation. In response to these hormonal changes, the prepubertal unisex silhouette becomes characterized by a larger, muscular male physique and a more rounded female shape.

*Mid-adolescence* (around 15–19 years old) is characterized by increasing independence, commonly with more time spent with peers outside the home. Education is more demanding of young people's maturing cognitive skills. The developmental tasks of this stage include a stronger sense of oneself as an individual and a greater focus on personal and social values. Neurocognitive maturation is responsible for an increased capacity for abstract thinking, the capacity to think about thoughts. Given how much of health management relates to future health outcomes, understanding young people's cognitive maturation is an important element of the monitoring of adolescent development and of working with young people clinically. Clinical strategies that might influence self-management behaviours in adults who are motivated by future health goals will not be influential in adolescents, who are more motivated by events in the 'here and now'. Neurocognitive maturation is now believed to continue into the early twenties.

*Late adolescence* (20–24 years old) is characterized by a greater focus on vocational goals, the transition between school and work, and a greater enjoyment of intimacy, including sexual intimacy. The developmental tasks are to establish adult roles and responsibilities, including longer-term relationships and less reliance on a peer group. Psychosocial development is characterized by aspects of personal individuation, such as the development of a coherent sense of self and an understanding of individual versus family responsibilities, coming to terms with one's physical self, understanding one's sexuality and being able to provide for oneself financially.

These stages are listed in Table 3.11.1 with an approximate age at which each stage occurs, the main feature of each stage and a key developmental question for young people at this stage.

While there is close association between the different domains of development, adolescent development is characterized by being uneven and complex: like earlier child development, it is influenced by the environment, is mediated by relationships and is triggered by social participation. Chronic illness and disability can affect each of these domains but the effects are inconsistent. For example, although chronic illness and disability may delay the physical changes of the adolescent growth spurt and of pubertal timing, exposure to challenging life decisions or to friends dying can result in earlier engagement with more spiritual elements of life.

The increasing cultural diversity of Australia and New Zealand results in many young people having parents who were born overseas, or who may hold different views of what adolescence is or should be about. Adolescents in these families can sometimes struggle with the discrepancy between the different expectations of their Australian peers and their family about the general aspects of role and identity, as well as specific elements of what is acceptable behaviour at given ages.

Dramatic social changes in the developed world have resulted in young people being generally healthier, wealthier and better educated than previous generations. More young people now complete 12 years of school than previously, with more continuing on with some form of post-secondary training or study. Social roles have widened for females as well as males. In Australia, the mean age of marriage is older than in previous generations, as is the age that women have their first child, which recently exceeded 30 years. In the 1950s most people had left school, got a job, got married and had children by their early twenties. Most contemporary young people achieve these milestones much later. Access to new technologies provides a much larger peer group and virtual community for young people, with uncertain consequences.

These same changes are also occurring for young people in low- and middle-income countries. In these countries, rapid urbanization, rapid social change and a loss of many of the traditional pathways to adult life contribute to many young people in these communities experiencing different pressures during adolescence than previous generations, with consequences for their health.

However, there are still many aspects of adolescence that have not changed over the centuries. Socrates is reported to have written in 450 BC that:

> 'Our youth love luxury. They have bad manners and contempt for authority. They show disrespect for their elders and love idle chatter in place of exercise. Children are now tyrants not the servants of the household. They contradict their parents, chatter before company, gobble up their food and tyrannize their teachers ...'

## Burden of illness in adolescence

Adolescence has long been considered the healthiest time of life. However, dramatic improvements in infant and child mortality globally have brought greater visibility – and concern – about adolescent and young adult mortality, as this age group has experienced far less improvement in mortality than younger children.

**Table 3.11.1 The stages of adolescent development**

| Developmental stage | Age (years) | Main feature | Key question at this stage |
|---|---|---|---|
| Early | 10–14 | Biological | Am I normal? |
| Middle | 15–19 | Cognitive | Who am I? |
| Late | 20–24 | Emotional/Social | Where am I going? |

Worldwide, there are at least 2.6 million deaths in 10–24 year olds annually. There is also a marked rise in mortality from early adolescence (10–14 years) through to young adulthood (20–24 years), with the reasons varying by geographical region and sex. Mortality rates are almost 4-fold higher in low- and middle-income countries than in high-income countries. Importantly, the majority of deaths in adolescence are preventable, with prominent causes being road traffic accidents, violence, self-inflicted injury, human immunodeficiency virus/acquired immune deficiency syndrome (HIV/AIDS) and tuberculosis. Maternal conditions are a leading cause of female death, especially in low-income countries. In 2007, the leading causes of death in 12–24-year-old Australians were injuries (65%), cancer (10%) and diseases of the nervous system, including cerebral palsy and epilepsy (5%).

The burden of illness in adolescents differs greatly from that of infants and young children, who are disproportionately affected by congenital disorders and acute infectious disease respectively, and of adults for whom ischaemic heart disease and cancer predominate. Some 60% of 12–24-year-old Australians have a long-term health condition, and 11% of young Australians have a disability that causes some form of limitation or restriction. Many other causes of ill-health are more commonly psychosocial than biological in adolescence, and tend to reflect unhealthy patterns of risk behaviours and mental disorders.

Thus, the leading causes of mortality and morbidity in the adolescent age group are from accidents and injuries (unintentional and self-inflicted), mental health problems and behavioural problems such as substance use and abuse. Other prominent health issues are unplanned pregnancy and sexually transmitted infections.

Some of the major health issues affecting young people in Australia are summarized in Table 3.11.2. The data refer to 12–24-year-old Australians unless stated otherwise.

## Risk and protective factors

Learning by doing is a normal part of adolescence, but some behaviour can have harmful consequences. The onset of puberty marks a time of growing risk in relationship to certain behaviours and mental health states. Although learning about the harmful effects of alcohol by drinking some alcohol can be considered normal in Australia, binge drinking is associated with many harmful effects such as later regretted sexual activity, alcohol dependence in early adult life and death from road traffic accidents.

Generally, the earlier the onset of these 'risk behaviours', the greater the likelihood of poor health outcomes. For example, although 80% of adult smokers start smoking in adolescence, the onset of smoking at an early age marks a greater risk for continuing smoking as an adult. In other words, the earlier health behaviour is 'learned' the longer it is likely to persist. Young people with one identified health risk behaviour are more likely to have other 'co-morbid' behaviours.

A number of common risk factors predict earlier engagement in many different health risk behaviours and mental health and social outcomes. These include factors within the individual, family, peer and community. There are important additive or synergistic associations between such risk factors. For example, being in a peer group where most of an adolescent's friends smoke increases their later risk of smoking; this risk is even greater if the adolescent is depressed. Lack of family connectedness or support, lack of engagement with friends, bullying at school and poor academic performance are risk factors for a wide range of poor health and social outcomes, such as substance use, poor mental health, early school-leaving and antisocial behaviours. Chronic illness and disability in adolescence is always considered a risk factor.

Identifying risk-taking behaviours and their consequences is an important part of any adolescent health assessment, but protective factors are also important to identify. These are factors that can ameliorate risk factors or increase the likelihood of positive health and social outcomes. Important protective factors are an intact and well functioning family, connectedness with school, community and peers, and participation in enjoyable extracurricular events such as sport or creative activities.

Put simply, the more protective factors in a young person's life, the more likely they are to make healthier choices in adolescence. Although many family factors cannot be changed or 'treated', efforts to alter the school environment can be especially powerful.

Many adolescent health problems are a consequence of health risk behaviours (see Table 3.11.2) and developmental challenges. As a consequence, knowledge and assessment of adolescent development, including exposure to risk and protective behaviours, is the foundation of the clinical approach to working with teenagers. Health problems in adolescents don't occur in isolation; one identified health problem raises the likelihood that there will be other health risk behaviours and various family, peer and community antecedents. Some behavioural concerns in teenagers have their onset in childhood, but others have their onset in adolescence. Once established, there is a greater risk of these behaviours continuing into adult life where they contribute to the adult burden of illness. Early identification and intervention is a desired outcome of any contact by adolescents with the health-care system.

**Table 3.11.2 Some of the key health issues and selected risk factors affecting young Australians**

| Health issue | Burden of illness |
|---|---|
| Emotional distress | 9% of 16–24-year-old Australians had high or very high levels of psychological distress in 2007, and 1 in 4 experienced a mental disorder |
| Obesity and overweight | 35% of young Australians were estimated to be overweight or obese (23% overweight but not obese; 12% obese in 2007–2008) |
| Risky substance use | 11% of young Australians were daily smokers, 30% drank alcohol at risky or high-risk levels for short-term and 12% for long-term harm, and 1 in 5 had used an illicit substance in 2007 |
| Chlamydia notifications | Over the past decade, there has been a large increase in notifications for sexually transmitted infections, particularly chlamydia (5-fold increase) |
| Sexual intercourse in year 10 and 12 students | 27% of year 10 students and 56% of year 12 students had experienced sexual intercourse. Two-thirds of sexually active students (68%) used a condom at their most recent sexual encounter |
| Violence | 7% of young adults were victims of physical or sexual assault and almost half were victims of alcohol- or drug-related violence in 2007 |
| Chronic health condition | 60% of young Australians have a long-term health condition in 2007–2008. The prevalence of long-term conditions has declined since 2001 among 15–24 years from 71% to 64%. |
| Disability | 11% of 12–24-year-old Australians had a disability with specific limitations or restrictions; a quarter of these had profound or severe core activity limitations (2008) |
| Abuse and neglect | 4 in every 1000 young people aged 12–17 years were the subject of a substantiated report of abuse or neglect in 2008–2009. Indigenous young people were over-represented at 5 times the rate of other young people |
| Parent health | 16% of parents living with young people rated their health as fair or poor, and around one-fifth had poor mental health. An estimated 16% of young people lived with a parent with disability |

Source: Australian Institute of Health and Wellbeing (AIHW) 2011 Young Australians: their health and wellbeing 2011. Cat. no. PHE 140. AIHW, Canberra.

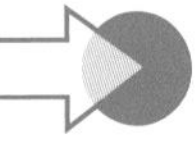

## Practical points

**Teenagers, adolescents, youth and young people**

- Most teenagers are healthy and happy.
- Like younger children, adolescents continue to develop physically, emotionally and cognitively. All consultations with young people should involve an assessment of adolescent development.
- As children mature through adolescence, they are exposed to greater health risks from involvement in behaviours with significant health consequences, such as drugs and alcohol and sexual intercourse.
- The burden of illness in youth differs from younger children and from adults, being disproportionately affected by mental health problems, the consequences of drug and alcohol use, accidents and self-harm, and complications of sexual activity.
- Healthy adolescent development results from complex interactions between risk and protective factors within the individual, family, peers, school and community.

## Medicolegal context and confidentiality

Historically, children were legally viewed as property items of their parents. The law now recognizes the growing maturity of adolescents and their capacity to make independent choices and judgements on matters affecting their future, including their rights to autonomy and privacy in health care, even when they are not legally mature (i.e. under the age of 18 years in Australia). This legal view is consistent with the medical evidence. Studies demonstrate that concerns about confidentiality are a major barrier to young people accessing health services. Once young people have accessed health-care services, they are more willing to disclose honestly important information about health risk behaviours, seek health care and return for follow-up when they understand a service is confidential. Thus, attention to confidentiality should be as much a cornerstone of clinical relationships between doctors and adolescents as it is with adults. Nearly 1 in 10 adolescents report not visiting their health-care provider in the previous year – despite wanting to do so – because of the fear that their parents would find out. However, many adolescents appreciate the opportunity to share sensitive information with their parents (even when it has been obtained confidentially by the doctor), as long as this is handled sensitively, and they are actively engaged in deciding what will (or will not) be shared.

Judgement about whether to maintain confidentiality in consultations with younger adolescents is linked with assessment of maturity. In deciding whether a person is competent or mature enough to consent to medical treatment, a doctor must decide whether the young person is able to understand the nature of the problem, the nature and side-effects of any proposed treatment, and other treatment options.

The doctor can accept consent provided that the treatment is in the young person's best interests and the treatment is not likely to have serious consequences. For more complex or contentious procedures, doctors must balance several factors in making a decision, including the age, maturity and characteristics of the adolescent, the gravity of the presenting illness and treatment, and family issues. It is important to remember that all doctors have a legal and ethical duty of confidentiality to competent young people. This duty should be breached only in serious situations such as risk of self-harm or suicide, or in cases of suspected abuse, as well as some other exceptions discussed below. Doctors should become familiar with the specific laws on this issue in the state or region where they practise. In all Australian states and territories, anyone over the age of 15 years can have their own Medicare card, and a doctor may bulk-bill a consultation without advising the parents.

**Clinical example**

Jennifer, a 15-year-old girl, was taken to her general practitioner by her mother because she had been moody and tearful for the last few weeks. She had also been missing school regularly and often complained of an 'upset stomach' in the mornings. On direct questioning, Jennifer offered very little information about the nature of her symptoms or possible causes. The doctor then asked Jennifer's mother to leave the room for a short time, after having explained confidentiality and its limitations. After the assurance of confidentiality and by taking a psychosocial history, Jennifer felt comfortable enough to tell the doctor that she had had unprotected sex about 5 weeks ago, had not had a period since, and was worried that she might be pregnant. She had been too fearful to tell her parents, stating 'They would kill me!'

A pregnancy test revealed that Jennifer was indeed pregnant. The doctor had a brief discussion about available options and offered to help Jennifer tell her mother, to discuss briefly the various options with her mother and to arrange for them to come back for a more detailed visit. Jennifer agreed with this plan. Although her mother was very surprised and upset, these discussions were able to take place, as well as discussion about the importance of future contraception. The doctor also asked about Jennifer's partner, because of child protection concerns. Her partner was her 16-year-old boyfriend.

Jennifer and her mother left the surgery relieved that it was 'out in the open' and having been made aware of the various supports and available services. At a later appointment Jennifer said she would never have been able to say anything at the time without seeing the doctor alone. As they went out of the door, Jennifer turned to her mother, saying, 'What are we going to tell Dad?'

## The clinical approach

### Meeting the patient

Many younger adolescents, especially those with chronic illness, will only have consulted doctors together with their parents and may therefore not expect anything else. Doctors can actively promote engagement with medical consultations by reinforcing that the young person, not the parent, is the patient. The doctor should introduce themselves to the young person first, then ask them to introduce the accompanying adult. This immediately signals to the young person that they have some control in the consultation. First impressions matter.

### Confidentiality

Following introductions, an important step is to explain the confidential nature of health consultations as it cannot be assumed that young people understand or expect this. We encourage a confidentiality statement to be made when parents are also in the room – as they also need to know. A brief discussion of the limits of confidentiality is also encouraged (the main limitations are risk of suicide or self-harm, risk of homicide or harm to others, and any disclosure of abuse). With practice, this only takes a minute or so:

> 'What we talk about is confidential, which means I won't discuss it with anyone else without your permission. There are three exceptions to this, which are if I am worried that you are at risk of harming yourself, at risk of harming others, or are being abused and are not safe. If these things come up we will deal with them together. I will involve you in any decisions that need to be made around who we need to talk to.'

### Negotiating for time alone

Seeing doctors alone for at least part of the consultation is a mechanism by which, over time, young people can develop the confidence to speak for themselves. The metaphor of 'bicycle training wheels' can be helpful to highlight to parents and young people alike that adolescents need practice consulting with doctors by themselves. The adolescent years are an ideal time to practise, when there is still 'back-up support' available from parents. When framed this way, most parents appreciate the opportunity for young people to spend time alone with the doctor and value the opportunity for their son or daughter to discuss sensitive issues. It is important, however, not to undermine the role of parents and to make sure that they are actively included. This is commonly done by inviting them back at the end of the consultation to discuss the diagnosis and management, having previously negotiated with the young person whether anything needs to be kept confidential.

This is generally not difficult for new consultations. However, it can be harder where a family doctor or paediatrician has seen a child together with the parent for many years. There is no set age to start seeing young people alone within medical consultations. However, it is generally appropriate to offer some time alone from about the age of 13–14 years. Initially, the young person may be seen alone for only a short time. Gradually, however, more time will be spent with the young person alone and less time with the parents and young person together, as young people develop the skills that enable them to be more independent within consultations and more capable of managing their health condition.

### Psychosocial screening (HEADSS)

Health risk screening is an important component of the clinical care of all adolescents. One approach to health risk screening has become known by its mnemonic, HEADSS. This approach, first described in the USA in the early 1980s, helps clinicians to remember the key aspects of the psychosocial history that are important to assess:

H – Home
E – Education/Employment, Exercise and Eating
A – Activities (peer-related)
D – Drug Use
S – Sexual Health and Sexuality
S – Suicide, Self-harm and Safety

The HEADSS mnemonic has been consistently added to, with an extra 'E for eating and exercise' in recognition of increasing rates of overweight and disordered eating, for example.

The HEADSS framework for psychosocial assessment facilitates a holistic approach in which the doctor can engage the young person in discussing a range of behaviours and mental health states that have significant health implications. This approach to taking a psychosocial history extends the consultation beyond treatment of the presenting complaint to a greater focus on more preventative and health-promotional aspects of common behaviours. Thus, in addition to being a framework for psychosocial assessment, it is equally useful as a method of engaging adolescents in the medical consultation, a mechanism for identifying both risk and protective factors, and a framework for delivering relevant anticipatory counselling.

This approach to psychosocial assessment should be explained to the young person, as it may be confusing to be asked about personal behaviours such as drug use when seeing a doctor for asthma. One approach is to say:

> 'When doctors do check-ups with older people they measure physical things like blood pressure. Younger people are more likely to be physically healthy, but their health can be affected by different behaviours, which I'm now going to ask you about. This is something we do with all young people.'

There is no need for the HEADSS topics to be discussed in any particular order, although generally clinicians prefer to start with less sensitive questions and proceed to more personal topics. For this reason, many clinicians actually start with questions about education, as questions about home can be challenging when young people have complex family arrangements. At times, it will not be possible to complete a full HEADSS assessment at the first consultation. It is, however, important to ensure that the issues are discussed at a later date, and recurrently over time.

Most doctors discuss the presenting complaint first and then move on to the psychosocial assessment using the HEADSS framework. It is often useful to remind young people about confidentiality again at this stage and to also let them know that they don't have to answer questions if they feel uncomfortable.

It is important to remember to ask about and discuss protective as well as risk factors. The use of open-ended questions is encouraged to engage young people more actively beyond simple 'yes or no' responses. One of the main reasons for the success of the HEADSS approach is that, when used sensitively, it empowers adolescents to discuss their health seriously with a professional. It also provides opportunities for questions that would not usually be asked of doctors. Discussions such as this are uncommonly initiated by young people, but the majority participate willingly when given the opportunity to do so confidentially. This approach gives the doctor an important opportunity to frame what is going well with young people, to identify areas of concern, to engage in anticipatory counselling and to develop a plan of action.

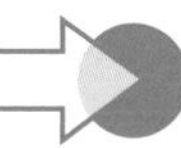

**Practical points**

**A summary of psychosocial screening (HEADSS)**

- **Home**
- Where do you live?
- Who lives with you?
- Who are you closest to at home?
- Is there anyone at home you can talk about personal issues with?
- **Education and Employment**
- Do you go to school? What year are you in?
- What are your grades like?
- Have you changed schools recently?
- Do you have many friends at school?
- Do you have any problems with bullying at school?
- Do you work?
- How many hours a week?
- **Eating/Exercise**
- Has your weight changed recently?
- Have you dieted in the last 12 months?
- Does your eating ever seem out of control?
- How much exercise do you do per week?
- **Activities**
- What do you and your friends do for fun?
- Do you play sport?
- Are you in any clubs or groups?
- What are your hobbies?
- **Drugs**
- Do you smoke cigarettes?
- Do you drink alcohol?
- Do you use any other drugs?

(If yes to any of the above then need to quantify)

- **Sexuality**
- Do you have a partner currently? OR Are you in a relationship currently?
- Have you been sexually active?
- Have you been pressured into sex?
- What do you understand by the term 'safe sex'?
- **Suicide and depression**
- How would you describe your mood lately? (Can ask for score out of 10)
- Are you ever sad or tearful for no reason?
- Do you have any trouble sleeping?
- Have you lost interest in things you used to enjoy?
- Have you ever felt like hurting yourself?
- Have you had any suicidal thoughts?
- Have you ever made a suicide plan?
- Have you previously attempted suicide?
- **Safety**
- Have you ever been seriously injured?
- Do you ever drive with people who have been drinking or taking drugs?
- Is there any violence at home?
- Have you ever been physically or sexually abused?

In consultations with young people, doctors are urged to be respectful, unhurried and non-judgemental. It is not a good idea to try to use current slang or to be 'chummy' with adolescents. Young people, like all patients, are more concerned that their doctors are professional and skilled rather than being 'cool' or acting like a friend.

It is important to ask questions in a way that makes no assumptions. 'Who lives at home with you?' and 'Are you in a relationship?' are preferable to questions that may assume a nuclear family and heterosexuality. It is also best to avoid questions that can be answered yes or no. Asking 'What year are you in at school?' is better than 'Do you go to school?'

Questions about activities are a good opportunity to focus on peer relationships. Questions about future life and career goals are a useful approach to exploring cognitive maturation. In questioning about drug use it is important to normalize experimentation with drugs without condoning drug use. Reference to the third person can be a helpful technique, such as: 'Some young people your age try drugs. What have been the experiences in your group of friends? And what about you?' Most clinicians start by asking about cigarettes and alcohol. Questions about what sexuality education the young person has received at school can be a helpful starting point for this sensitive topic, or about whether a teenage girl has been vaccinated against human papillomavirus (HPV). Other approaches include normalizing statements, such as: 'Many young people your age are starting to develop more meaningful relationships. Are you in a relationship at the moment?' A brief reminder of confidentiality and a reiteration that your interest is health-related sometimes puts nervous teenagers at ease when moving to questions about drugs and sexuality.

Without being judgemental, it is reasonable to comment supportively on healthy choices that the young person may describe. Some young people report that they would simply prefer to be asked directly about issues like sexual activity and safe sex (contraceptive and condom use). A degree of judgement is always required as to an adolescent's maturity and stage of development.

The final S in HEADSS refers to suicidality and safety. It is perhaps better thought of as a depression screen but it is important to ask directly about suicidal ideation and plans, and to act promptly if there are concerns. Contrary to claims that discussing such issues 'puts ideas into their heads', talking about suicide does not increase suicidal behaviour in young people who are not suicidal but can be protective in those who have been thinking of it but have not discussed it with anyone. Questions about safety from abuse of any sort, particularly sexual abuse or violence, should also be asked. Even if no disclosure is made, it is suggested that the young person be informed that sharing this information with others is important and that you would always be available to talk to them about this and any other issues they would like to raise in the future.

### Physical examination

Adolescence is a time of increased sensitivity about one's body and appearance in general. Thus, even a 'routine' physical examination may be a confronting prospect for a young person. It should therefore be conducted in a professional, respectful and sensitive manner.

This must obviously be balanced with the need for a thorough clinical examination. In all cases, measurements of height, weight and pubertal assessment are recommended. Ensure that the patient will not be exposed if someone else enters the room by using curtains or screens. Avoid unnecessary exposure of the body. When a particular area must be examined, the judicious use of clothing and sheets is recommended to keep other areas covered. A screening test of pubertal assessment can be made by adolescent self-report of the standard pictures of Tanner staging on growth charts and confirmed clinically if there are specific concerns.

Although not a legal requirement, the use of chaperones for a physical examination is increasingly recommended, especially when male doctors are examining female adolescents, in order to make the patient feel more comfortable and reduce allegations of misconduct.

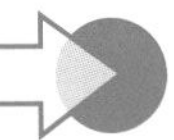

**Practical points**

**Engaging young people in clinical consultations**

- Introduce yourself to the young person and then the parent.
- Explain confidentiality, including limitations, to all adolescents and families.
- Be relaxed and non-judgemental.
- Avoid jargon or slang but use simple language that the young person will understand.
- See the young person alone for part of each consultation.
- Psychosocial screening should start with less sensitive questions before proceeding to more personal questions.
- Be sensitive and respectful during physical examinations.

## Chronic illness

Children and adolescents with special health care needs have been defined as those who 'have or are at increased risk for a chronic physical, developmental, behavioural or emotional condition requiring health and related services of a type beyond those required by children generally'. According to this definition, 15–20% of children and adolescents have a significant, ongoing health-care need. The prevalence of special health-care needs is higher in adolescents than in younger children.

There is a greater prevalence of young people with chronic illness in our community because of improved survival rates from various paediatric illnesses that, as recently as 20 years ago, were associated with extremely poor prognoses. Examples include childhood leukaemia and other cancers, congenital heart disease and cystic fibrosis. Improved medical technologies result in the survival of more young people with complex and severe health-care needs who are reliant on advanced technology and multifaceted health-care support. In addition to improved survival, most developed countries have experienced a true increase in the incidence of certain conditions, such as asthma and allergy, diabetes, obesity, mental disorders and leukaemia.

It is important to remember that young people with chronic illness are first and foremost adolescents. Thus, while it might be assumed that adolescents with chronic illness would not add further risks to their health profile by engaging in risky behaviours, there is no evidence that this is the case. Instead, there is some evidence that young people with chronic illness might be even more likely to participate in health risk behaviours than their otherwise healthy peers.

Furthermore, many young people with chronic illness have a greater attributable risk from these behaviours. For example, in addition to the universal risks of smoking, smoking in young people with asthma, cystic fibrosis or diabetes mellitus can be readily conceptualized as being 'more risky' in terms of their underlying health condition. Another example is the greater attributable risk from alcohol use in young people with diabetes mellitus or epilepsy.

Adolescent development is not a simple linear journey but is a dynamic process that is experienced differently by each individual. Thus, chronic illness and disability can affect adolescents in diverse and complex ways. Physical growth and pubertal development can be delayed, although pubertal development can also commence earlier (precocious puberty) in other conditions (e.g. spina bifida). In addition to these universal elements of adolescent growth and development, adolescence is a time where various physical changes commonly become more significant (e.g. scars from previous surgery such as cleft lip repair or infant bowel obstruction, longstanding clubbing or scoliosis, or the more acute side-effects of steroids) as cognitive maturation brings greater capacity for both the imagination of an ideal body as well as critical comparison with one's peers. This sense of physical inadequacy can be associated with complex adjustment problems in terms of body image, self-esteem, bullying, peer relationships and mental disorder.

Some adolescents with chronic illness and disability may be less well developed socially because of extended hospital admissions over many years, reduced parent expectations or reduced opportunity for normal peer relationships. More specifically, certain chronic illnesses or disabilities can be associated with reduced cognitive or intellectual functioning. As a result, these young people may be relatively more reliant on their parents. Regardless of the explanation, poor peer relationships and fragile educational engagement can reduce educational achievement and limit career opportunities and future socioeconomic status.

Chronic illness in adolescents can also affect wider family functioning, including sibling experiences and parent marital relationships. Attention to the wider family and its functioning is an important part of looking after adolescents with chronic illness and disability.

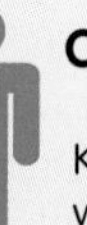

### Clinical example

Karen, a 19-year-old woman with cystic fibrosis, was soon to be transferred to a specialist adult cystic fibrosis centre for ongoing care. However, during the last few admissions, concerns had been raised about her mental state as well as the fact that she had twice discharged herself early against medical advice. The adolescent team was informed that her usual treating team felt her mood was 'pretty flat'.

In taking a detailed psychosocial history, the adolescent team identified that Karen had discharged herself against advice as she had a part-time job and an active social life. These were more important to her than her health, as another few days 'never made any difference'. It emerged that Karen had told no one outside of her immediate family of her illness, including her current boyfriend. Her workplace was also unaware she had cystic fibrosis or had been admitted to hospital. Until recently, she had not required hospitalization for some years. She had hidden the recent admissions by keeping in touch with friends by mobile phone. She finally revealed that the main reason for keeping her illness secret was that a previous boyfriend had broken up with her when she had told him about her cystic fibrosis.

Karen's depressed mood was confirmed and was thought in most part to be due to the stress of living a 'double life'. Although, at least superficially, she denied the severity of her respiratory status, it was considered that the implications of her lung disease (there had recently been discussions about the role of lung transplantation) were likely to have contributed to her depressed mood. She was very poorly adherent with physiotherapy and regular clinic review, but had better adherence with antibiotics.

As a result of these and other discussions, Karen was supported in revealing her illness to some close friends and work colleagues, who were relieved there was an explanation for her significant coughing and supportive of her taking time off for treatment. There was further frank discussion about the severity of her illness, and Karen felt gradually more able to discuss aspects of day-to-day care, including adherence with treatment and transfer to the adult clinic, as well as the possible need for transplantation. Her lung function stabilized.

## Towards self-management

Adolescents with chronic illness and disability are naturally interested in and able to play a greater role in looking after themselves as they mature. However, the skills for self-care do not develop magically but must be practised by young people and supported by their parents and health professionals.

Little is known about the age at which adolescents begin to take on more responsibility for different elements of self-care (such as taking medications, making appointments or seeking care when unwell). Further, it is not known what effect disease severity or intellectual capacity has on these practices. In practical terms, health professionals should encourage parents to support the emerging capacity for self-care in their children as they mature through adolescence. Health professionals can do this by educating the family about adolescent development. For example, many parents can become frustrated when their teenager no longer simply 'does what they are told' in relation to adherence with requests by parents and doctors to 'take their medicine'. Informing parents of the developmental appropriateness of this behaviour and of ways of making it more likely that young people will adhere to treatment regimens is an important educational role for health professionals. Promoting greater self-management in young people with chronic illness is a specific part of the broader 'package' of working with young people that includes understanding adolescent development, health risk screening, appreciation of the value of confidential health care, and understanding the transition to adult health care. This can be summarized as the provision of developmentally appropriate health care to adolescents.

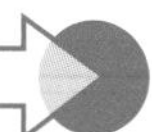

### Practical points

**Self-management in adolescents with chronic illness**

- Ensure parents appreciate that, although their love shouldn't change, their role in managing their teenager's health will change gradually with time.
- As young people mature, they should be encouraged to take on more responsibility for managing their health, with less reliance on their parents for day-to-day care.
- Seeing young people alone for at least part of the consultation will help build young people's confidence and skills in communication with doctors and health professionals.
- Normalize the challenges of adherence in adolescents. Have realistic expectations.
- Rather than focusing on problems, work with the young person to develop practical solutions.
- Short-term adolescent-focused goals are more likely to motivate self-care than longer-term health-orientated goals.
- Development of self-management skills is an important part of young people's transition towards adult health care.

## Adherence with treatment

The terms 'adherence' and 'compliance' are often used interchangeably, but there are subtle distinctions between them. Compliance is defined as the extent to which a patient is obedient and follows the instructions and prescriptions of health professionals. In contrast, adherence is defined as a more active, voluntary and collaborative involvement of the patient in a mutually acceptable course of behaviour aimed at producing a therapeutic or preventative outcome. Most adolescents, like adults, wish to be included in the decision-making process regarding treatment options. The main practical implication of using the term 'adherence' denotes that adherence behaviours are not exclusively the responsibility of patients but are a reflection of the doctor–patient relationship and the support that young people receive from their families.

Adolescents are commonly conceptualized (and judged) as being 'non-compliant'. Like adults, many adolescents struggle to achieve sufficient adherence with treatment. However, there is little evidence that adherence in adolescents is substantially worse than in adults. Indeed, it is worth remembering that many studies show that adherence to treatment in adults with chronic illness is as low as 50%. Young adults can find adherence behaviours especially challenging as parents by this stage are generally less actively involved.

Strategies to improve adherence in adolescents need to take into account the challenge of adolescent development and the ways in which parents can both support and hinder adherence behaviours. Young people are less influenced than adults by the concept of health as a general life goal, or by specific longer-term health risks. For example, adults with diabetes may be concerned about long-term complications, but young people are generally more influenced by things in the 'here and now'. For adolescents, rather than threats to long-term health, development of routines and a focus on short-term goals are more likely to be influential.

Questioning adherence behaviours in a normalizing and non-judgemental way is helpful. The phrasing 'Many people I see your age have trouble fitting their … (medication/treatment/monitoring) into their day. Firstly, are you taking any? … Great.…Tell me, which dose do you find hardest to remember, the morning or the evening dose?' can readily lead to greater discussion about the medication itself, and about routines that they have or do not have around different medication. This approach can help young people find their own solutions. Questions need to be specific for each different aspect of the treatment regimen.

Many young people feel that their parents constantly 'nag' them about their medication. Notwithstanding that the young person might need parental support with their medication, some young people report that parent 'nagging' makes them less likely to want to take their medication responsibly! Negotiating a short period of 'no nagging', especially when combined with strategies to promote the development of treatment routines (consider a diary chart for a week, or mobile phone reminders), can be helpful. Following such approaches, some young people are sobered into understanding how much they need their parents to assist them, and some parents realize that their teenagers can actually manage quite well!

Attention to adherence should be part of every consultation with teenagers.

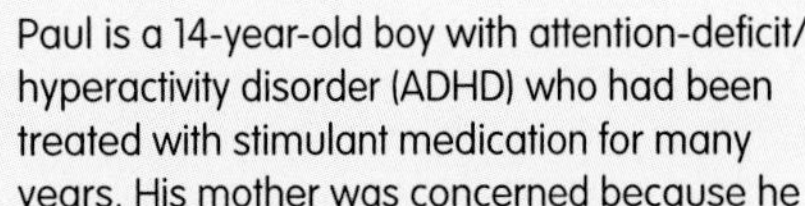

### Clinical example

Paul is a 14-year-old boy with attention-deficit/hyperactivity disorder (ADHD) who had been treated with stimulant medication for many years. His mother was concerned because he had recently stopped taking his medication and his school marks were deteriorating quite rapidly. She said that Paul was impossible to talk to about it, as he just shouted at her when she tried to broach the subject. Paul somewhat reluctantly admitted that the medication helped his concentration but he didn't care about educational success so he didn't feel there was much point in taking it.

Paul was referred to an adolescent specialist, who saw him alone. The specialist identified that Paul was being teased and bullied at school, particularly about his ADHD, which had contributed to him stopping taking the lunchtime dose at school. He also hated the way his mother nagged him in the morning to take his tablets as though he were a 'stupid little kid'. Paul revealed that his mood was very low and that during the last few months he had occasionally wished he was dead. He had no active suicidal plan. After a discussion with Paul and his mother, he was changed to a long-acting form of the medication that had to be taken only in the morning. Discussions were held about how Paul could take greater responsibility for remembering to take the medication, which included a conversation about medication routines, reminder charts and 'dosettes'.

After a few months of regular follow-up, Paul's mood and school performance gradually improved. Initially he was still a bit forgetful about taking the medication but, with the help of his mother, he developed a morning bathroom routine that included his medication. His mother no longer 'nagged' him but instead 'checked in' now and then to monitor the situation. Paul and his mother were communicating much better about this and other issues.

## Transition to adult health care

An important component of self-management for those young people who will continue to require specialist health care as young adults is that their care is transferred from a paediatric to an adult health-care setting. Managing young adults in an adult setting promotes their ongoing development and independence, whereas retaining their care in a paediatric setting is likely to have the opposite effect.

In relation to the provision of health care to adolescents with special health-care needs, transition is defined as 'the purposeful, planned movement of young people with chronic physical and medical conditions from child-centred to adult-oriented health-care systems'. Thus, the physical *transfer* of care from one setting to another is part of a broader process of *transition* to adult health care, which builds on supporting the young person to gain the requisite self-management skills.

There are many barriers to transition to adult health care, with a significant proportion being *attitudinal*. The young person may fear the unknown and be reluctant to leave the security of a system and a group of health professionals that they have come to know and trust. Parents may be concerned that they will be 'shut out' of the decision-making process in the adult setting. This fear may be more acute if parents have continued to be very actively involved in medical consultations without the young person starting to take on greater responsibility.

Some paediatricians (and parents) fear that the young person will receive less optimal care in the adult setting. Others have trouble 'letting go', especially if they have looked after the young person for many years. Some adult physicians may fear taking on 'paediatric' patients, as they may be uncomfortable communicating with patients in this age group.

Other barriers are more *structural*, such as the lack of specific expertise (e.g. congenital heart disease, metabolic disorders, intellectual disability) or the lack of multidisciplinary services within the adult health-care setting. Funding may perversely reduce the desire to transfer care, for example if elements of health care such as total parenteral nutrition or dressings are funded within the paediatric but not the adult setting. Lack of established communication channels between facilities and health-care providers may be another barrier to transferring care.

There is no single model or ideal transition model to follow. Rather, a set of principles has been developed that promote timely transfer to adult settings. Preparation is a key component of transition planning, which should start years before any planned physical move. Each individual should have a health professional in the paediatric setting who has the primary responsibility for developing a transition plan. The family doctor or primary health-care provider is an important link for continuity for the patient and family, and should be actively involved.

Although it has been argued that transfer to adult settings should not occur until the young person has the skills to function in an adult service, it can be equally argued that young people may develop the required skills only once they experience a more challenging environment. If possible the transfer should occur when the adolescent's health is in a relatively stable phase.

There is no correct age for transfer, and different approaches have developed in different countries. In Australasia, most children's hospitals plan to transfer young people to the adult setting once they have completed their secondary education, commonly in their 18th or 19th year.

# Gynaecology 3.12

Sonia R. Grover

Gynaecological problems in childhood are usually minor but not infrequent.

Congenital anomalies affecting the genital tract can be seen in association with endocrine and congenital anomalies, although quite a number do not present until the girl fails to go through puberty, menarche does not occur, or she develops significant atypical period pain. Although surgical correction to reproductive tract anomalies may be undertaken as part of the correction of these anomalies, for example in girls with congenital adrenal hyperplasia, bladder extrophy or cloacal anomalies, follow-up and possible intervention from the genital tract perspective may be required at the onset of puberty, when referral to a gynaecologist with experience with these anomalies may be appropriate.

Gynaecological problems in adolescence have some similarity to adult problems, although the approach to examination, investigation and management are often very different.

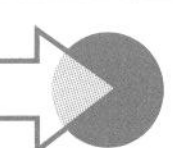

### Practical points

- Vaginal examination is inappropriate in paediatric patients. Ultrasonography or examination under anaesthesia (depending on the clinical problem) will provide the required information.
- For adolescent patients, vaginal examination is infrequently undertaken unless they are sexually active and have given consent for this examination.
- Transabdominal ultrasonography will almost always provide the necessary information in the adolescent population.

## Gynaecological problems in neonates

- Vaginal bleeding – the decline in maternal oestrogens within the first week or 2 of birth – may result in a small vaginal bleed. No investigations are required.
- An imperforate hymen, may present as a perineal lump. The hydrocolpos can be drained and corrected with surgical incision of the hymen.

## Common gynaecological problems in pre-pubescent girls

### Labial fusion or adhesions

Labial fusion or labial adhesions are:

- not present at birth but may develop within a few months; the onset correlates with the decline in maternal oestrogen effects on the skin of the newborn and infant
- thought to occur secondary to skin irritation
- relatively common in childhood
- often first noted by the maternal and child health nurse.

As persistent labial adhesions are not seen in adolescent girls, it can be safely presumed that the natural history of labial adhesions is spontaneous resolution. In the past, the use of lateral traction, surgical division, or the use of topical oestrogen cream was recommended, but there is a high relapse rate with these approaches. As labial adhesions rarely cause any significant symptoms apart from occasional dribbling post-micturition, no intervention is necessary and parents should be reassured.

### Clinical example

A 3-year-old girl was noted by the maternal and child health nurse to have an 'abnormal perineum'. The possibility of an absent vagina was raised, and the mother was advised to take her daughter to the doctor.

On examination of the perineum, the urethral and vaginal openings could not be visualized, as the labia appeared to be joined in the midline. A midline stripe was visible and the general practitioner was able to reassure the parents that the diagnosis was labial adhesions, which would resolve spontaneously. Her parents requested further reassurance that the vagina was actually present, as they had been reading about vaginal agenesis on the internet. Further reassurance was given that vaginal agenesis is a rare problem – and that investigations by any imaging technology to identify a vagina in this age group were unreliable. Instead arrangements were made to review the girl when she was older.

Review 3 years later revealed that the adhesions had almost completely resolved, and the urethral and vaginal opening with hymenal edge were now visible.

### Vulvovaginitis

- Occurs in the context of low oestrogens, with thin, atrophic vaginal and vulval skin.
- Is seen in girls from early childhood through to the establishment of puberty.
- The normal flora in the vagina of young girls is mixed bowel flora (candida is not found in the non-oestrogenized young girl).
- Overgrowth of the bowel flora in the vagina is thought to irritate the atrophic skin, causing a discharge which then irritates the vulval skin.
- The affected skin is primarily the contact surfaces between the labia.

Symptoms are usually intermittent and consist of:

- offensive vaginal discharge
- skin irritation
- burning with micturition.

The possibility of sexual abuse needs to be considered in a child with vulvovaginitis, but other symptoms or problems are usually present (see Chapter 3.9).

*Investigations*

- Swabs are rarely required as no specific organism is found, only mixed bowel flora.
- Take swabs when there is a profuse discharge or skin erythema extends beyond the contact surfaces of the labia majora. In these cases a single organism may be responsible for the problems and specific antibiotics may be required.

*Management*

- Application of a simple barrier cream (such as zinc–castor oil or Vaseline).
- Bathing – the addition of vinegar (half a cup to a shallow bath) is often advocated.
- Parents need reassurance that the natural history is intermittent recurrence until puberty.
- In the presence of this skin irritation it is advisable to avoid other potential irritants such as bubble baths and soaps.
- Faecal soiling as a consequence of poor toileting habits may also be an issue.
- When the skin irritation extends beyond the contact surfaces of the labia, additional irritants such as prolonged periods in wet bathers may have an aetiological role.

### Blood-stained vaginal discharge

Vaginal foreign body needs to be considered in the presence of a persistent vaginal discharge, particularly if blood stained. Vaginal foreign bodies are most often found to be a small amount of toilet tissue, although occasionally there may be beads and other small objects that can be seen on ultrasonography.

Occasionally, small foreign bodies can be flushed from the lower vagina using a syringe and saline, but usually a general anaesthetic to enable a careful examination is required.

If itch is a significant component of the symptoms:

- *pinworms* need to be excluded
- *eczema* superimposed on the vulvovaginitis may be present. Look for evidence of generalized eczema. The approach to management is the same as for vulvovaginitis, with the addition of topical steroids to settle the eczematous component.
- *lichen sclerosis*, with whitened skin changes and superficial splitting of skin, may be present, secondary to the vulvovaginitis but can also be due to a relatively uncommon autoimmune skin problem. In the presence of vulvovaginitis symptoms and findings, the management of lichen sclerosis is as for vulvovaginitis, with the addition of topical steroid cream. A more potent steroid may be required for a short duration. Betamethasone (Diprosone) and methylprednisolone (Advantan) cream are often best tolerated, with others having irritant components in the cream or ointment base.

### Vaginal bleeding

- Foreign body (see above)
- Precocious puberty as a result of the ovarian activity (see Chapter 19.1)
- Rare childhood lower genital tract malignancy – rhabdosarcomas (sarcoma botryoides); may also present as sultana-like polyps at the vaginal introitus.

### Vaginal pain

Distressing vaginal pain waking a pre-pubertal girl at night is likely to be worms. The worms get 'lost' in the vagina and when they crawl on the hymen, which is very sensitive in this age group, they cause significant pain.

Treatment is as for worms – but additional courses, usually once weekly for 3 weeks, are required.

## Adolescent gynaecology

### Overview of puberty, adolescence and the menstrual cycle

- The average age of menarche is 12.5 years.
- Although breast bud development is usually the first sign of puberty, followed by pubic and axillary hair, variations to this can occur (see Chapter 19.1).
- Breast development may be asymmetrical initially and may be mistaken for a 'breast lump'.

- In general, the time from commencement of breast development to first menses is less than 4 years.
- Absence of menses at age 16 years is suggestive of the need for further investigation.
- With the onset of puberty, multiple (15 to 20) follicles can be seen on ultrasonography; this is normal.
- An ovulation cyst or follicle can be 3–4 cm in diameter. On ultrasonography this will appear as a simple 'cyst', which can be expected to resolve and disappear during the next 2–6 weeks. It is important to reassure young women that this cyst is normal and demonstrates that the reproductive system is functioning normally.
- Ovulation can be associated with some pain (Mittelschmerz or mid-cycle pain). Occasionally, haemorrhage into an ovulation cyst can occur, giving rise to a more complex appearance of the cyst on ultrasonography (haemorrhagic corpus luteum).
- Irregular menses in the first 2–3 years is common and normal because of anovulation.

Consultation with young teenage girls needs to be undertaken with careful consideration for their developmental and cognitive stage, recognizing that consultation *without* a parent may be essential to explore relevant issues (see Chapter 3.11).

Adolescent health risk behaviours need to be identified, as they can impact on reproductive health. Eating disorders may be responsible for menstrual problems (amenorrhoea and infrequent menses); smoking may influence choice of medications; sexual activity raises concerns regarding the need for contraception and risk of sexually transmitted infections; and drug and alcohol intake significantly impacts on the chances of risky, unsafe sexual activity.

## Delayed onset of menses – primary amenorrhoea

The onset of periods usually correlates with exposure to oestrogens over some months, during which time breast development, pubic hair and axillary hair growth have occurred. Assessment of the time of onset of breast development and onset of pubic and axillary hair growth is useful to assess whether progression through puberty has been normal. It is important to establish the general health of the young woman as well as the activities in which she participates.

If the young woman has no secondary sexual characteristics, the investigations are guided by the potential causes of delayed puberty (see Chapter 19.1).

Assessment of the presence and extent of hair growth can give valuable clues to the diagnosis (see hirsutism; see Chapter 21.2). Excess hair can be familial and may be related to ethnic origin or due to hormonal causes, with polycystic ovary syndrome being the commonest. Scant pubic and axillary hair in the presence of good breast development is seen in complete androgen insensitivity syndrome. Palpable gonads (testes) may be found in the groin or labia, but they may also be intra-abdominal.

The presence of normal secondary sexual characteristics and intermittent abdominal pain suggests that menstruation may be occurring but an obstruction is present. The commonest cause is an imperforate hymen, which can be confirmed simply by viewing the perineum while applying gentle pressure to the abdominal mass. Pelvic ultrasonography can assist in confirming the presence of cryptomenorrhoea and in clarifying the level of the obstruction. The obstruction can involve a transverse vaginal septum or segmental vaginal atresia, which will require referral to a centre with some expertise in these uncommon anomalies.

Uterovaginal agenesis is absence of the vagina and uterus. Ovarian function is normal, as are all secondary sexual characteristics. The creation of a vagina is most often achieved with the use of dilators (and sexual activity). In the absence of a uterus, carrying a pregnancy is clearly impossible, although surrogacy can now be offered, as ovarian function is normal.

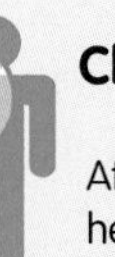

### Clinical example

At the age of 16 years, Tanya was brought to see her general practitioner because of delay in the onset of menses. Her breast development began at the age of 12 years. She was a state champion gymnast and trained intensively 7 days a week. She was of slight build. Examination revealed normal breast development at Tanner stage 3, and pubic hair at Tanner stage 3.

The provisional diagnosis was hypothalamic hypogonadism secondary to the level of physical activity. Follicle stimulating hormone (FSH), luteinizing hormone (LH) and oestrogen concentrations were found to be low. Thyroid stimulating hormone (TSH) and prolactin concentrations were normal. Pelvic ultrasonography demonstrated a small normal uterus.

Tanya was reassured that there was no significant underlying problem and that her relatively low weight combined with her exercise level was the cause for the delay.

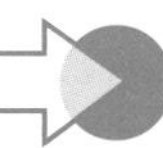

### Practical points

- In the presence of a problem that has an impact on the long-term reproductive health of the young woman, care and sensitivity with respect to the impact of this diagnosis on her self-esteem are critical.
- Careful use of appropriate language, open discussion and disclosure, psychological support, and the opportunity to become involved in a support group are all considered important components in care.

## Irregular periods

The pattern of the periods can be quite irregular during the first few years after the onset of menarche. This can be attributed to an immature hypothalamic–pituitary–ovarian axis. Unless the irregularity is the cause of significant problems, simple reassurance is all that is required. Multiple follicles (15 to 20) may be seen on ultrasonography, but this is a normal finding in over 20% of young women. Unless there is evidence of hyperandrogenism (i.e. significant acne or hirsutism), the term 'polycystic ovary syndrome' should not be used.

## Polycystic ovary syndrome

The diagnostic criteria for this condition are for adults and have serious limitations when applied to teenagers because of the common findings of irregular menstrual cycles and mild acne in this younger population. Classically there is evidence of the metabolic syndrome (see Chapter 3.4) and hyperandrogenism (excess hair and acne). The investigation findings may demonstrate a raised FSH to LH ratio; ultrasonography may show 20 to 30 follicles with increased ovarian stromal density; glucose tolerance test results may be abnormal.

Management consists of improving the diet and increasing the amount of exercise. Additional approaches such as hormonal treatment to regulate irregular and heavy periods, and cyproterone acetate or spironolactone to reduce hair growth, may be added in some cases.

## Heavy periods

Heavy menses in teenagers is often the result of anovulatory bleeding. The possibility of a bleeding disorder also needs to be considered; 10–15% of girls with menorrhagia (in a population without known bleeding disorders, and without predisposing factors such as chemotherapy or warfarin usage) may have an underlying bleeding disorder such as von Willebrand disease or platelet dysfunction (see Chapter 16.2 on bleeding disorders and Box 3.12.1).

*Assessment*

- Care needs to be taken when taking a history of menses as what is 'normal' or 'heavy' may vary with different individuals and in different families.
- Changing soaked super pads (or tampons) 2-hourly is probably a reasonably heavy period.
- Anaemia (in the absence of other dietary or gastrointestinal problems) is supportive evidence.
- Having flooding or 'disasters' regularly is suggestive of heavy loss.
- The presence of clots is usually not significant unless the clots are large (>4–6 cm). Small clots are normal and simply mean that there is adequate time between blood leaving the endometrial surface and reaching the perineum to allow coagulation to occur.

**Box 3.12.1 Useful investigations in menorrhagia**

- Full blood examination, iron studies
- Prothrombin time, activated partial thromboplastin time
- Von Willebrand antigen/factor VIII studies
- Platelet aggregometry or platelet function assays

*Management options*

- Non-steroidal anti-inflammatory drugs (NSAIDs) – reduce menstrual loss by 30%. Where there is concern about a potential bleeding disorder it would be wise to avoid NSAIDs in the first instance.
- Tranexamic acid (500 mg, two tablets q.i.d. p.r.n.) on days of heavy bleeding – reduces loss by 50%.
- Oral contraceptive pill (OCP) – used cyclically or continuously.
- Depot medroxyprogesterone acetate.
- Levonorgestrel intrauterine system has an important place for significant, but difficult to control, heavy menses.
- Acute heavy bleeding – tranexamic acid (as above) combined with progestogens may be helpful in stopping a heavy period. Provera 10 mg b.d. to t.d.s., or norethisterone acetate (NEA) 5–10 mg b.d. to t.d.s. but up to 2-hourly, can be used and then tapered during the next week. Complete withdrawal of progestogens is usually associated with a withdrawal bleed, so continuation for a total of 3 weeks is advised. Ongoing use of cyclic progestogens at a lower dose (Provera 10 mg daily, or NEA 5 mg daily, for 21 days with a 7-day break to allow a withdrawal bleed), or alternatively the OCP can be used as a follow-up for the next 3–6 months.
- Acute, very heavy, bleeding (metrostaxis) – resuscitation including blood transfusion may be required. High-dose oestrogen may be necessary (estradiol valerate 2–4 mg 6-hourly), combined with tranexamic acid. This can be followed by the OCP, commencing 48 hours later.

## Secondary amenorrhoea

Periods can stop for a range of reasons other than pregnancy – from central (hypothalamic) causes to pituitary and ovarian abnormalities. A careful history will correctly identify several of these underlying causes of secondary amenorrhoea.

Useful investigations for secondary amenorrhoea are presented in Table 3.12.1.

**Table 3.12.1 Investigation of secondary amenorrhoea**

| Cause of amenorrhoea | Investigation result |
|---|---|
| Central (hypothalamic) | Low FSH, low LH, normal TSH, low oestrogen, normal prolactin |
| Pituitary | |
| Thyroid disease | Abnormal TSH |
| Prolactinoma | Raised prolactin (needs to be increased on more than one occasion) |
| Ovarian/gonadal failure | FSH and LH very high, oestrogen low |
| Pregnancy | Raised bHCG |

bHCG, β-human chorionic gonadotrophin; FSH, follicle stimulating hormone; LH, luteinizing hormone; TSH, thyroid stimulating hormone.

### Hypothalamic causes

In a slim young woman, having established a good rapport while using HEADSS as a screening tool (see Chapter 3.11) to explore the young woman's physical activities and self-perception, the young woman who is undertaking a great deal of exercise or the teenager with the eating disorder should be identified. Weight loss associated with other medical conditions can also be responsible for central causes of amenorrhoea.

### Pituitary causes

Pituitary problems related to prolactinoma or thyroid disease can cause secondary amenorrhoea.

### Polycystic ovary syndrome

Weight gain and associated insulin resistance and evidence of acne or hirsutism make up the syndrome of polycystic ovary syndrome, which can be responsible for amenorrhoea or oligomenorrhoea (see above).

### Ovarian causes

Ovarian failure can be due to gonadal dysgenesis (most commonly Turner syndrome (see Chapter 10.3) or premature ovarian insufficiency.

### Pregnancy

The sexually active teenager is at risk of secondary amenorrhoea related to pregnancy.

## Pelvic pain

### Dysmenorrhoea

- Primary or prostaglandin-induced dysmenorrhoea is usually not present during the first menses but may begin within a few periods.
- It may occur in ovulatory or anovulatory cycles.

*Symptoms*
- May precede the menses by a few days, or occur on the first or second day of bleeding.
- Are usually absent by the final days of the bleeding.
- May be exacerbated by stress.
- Consist of:
  - cramping lower abdominal pain and low back pain
  - nausea (present in >30% of girls with dysmenorrhoea)
  - vomiting
  - diarrhoea or constipation
  - headaches, dizziness, fainting
  - pallor, lethargy and generalized aches.

These symptoms are generally attributed to prostaglandins, which play a role in coordinating the onset of menstruation.

*Management*
- General approaches, such as exercise, reduce stresses.
- NSAIDs, optimally commenced prior to onset of symptoms.
- Oral contraceptive pill.

Retrograde menstruation occurs in almost all women. This is menstrual flow upwards through the fallopian tubes and into the peritoneal cavity. The presence of free fluid in the peritoneal cavity causes a variable amount of pain. It can cause pain with defaecation and micturition as well as pain on movement. Reducing the menstrual loss by the use of NSAIDs or tranexamic acid usually reduces this amount of retrograde loss and hence lessens the pain.

### Endometriosis

Endometriosis is the presence of ectopic endometrium in the peritoneal cavity. As endometrial cells are present in the retrograde menses it is likely that most endometriosis can be attributed to this origin. Endometriosis can vary in severity from a few small spots to extensive endometriosis with adhesions and cyst formation (endometriomas). It is now generally agreed that mild endometriosis is a physiological finding. Endometriosis can be found in adolescents. Care needs to be taken to exclude or adequately manage other causes of period and pelvic pain, and to ensure that menstrual loss is reduced, as heavy and/or frequent periods are known to be risk factors for endometriosis. Consideration of other factors that may be contributing to the symptoms also needs to be given (careful screening using HEADSS is valuable).

Pelvic ultrasonography should be done prior to considering a diagnostic laparoscopy if symptoms are not controlled by other interventions.

### Atypical dysmenorrhoea

Dysmenorrhoea that progressively worsens through menstruation and lasts beyond the end of bleeding is atypical and an obstructive müllerian (reproductive tract) anomaly needs to be considered. Pelvic ultrasonography can often be more helpful in diagnosis than laparoscopy. Assessment for an absent kidney can also give useful supporting evidence for the likelihood of a müllerian anomaly.

## Ovarian cysts

Ovarian cysts can be physiological (see above), occurring in the context of normal ovarian activity, or they can be pathological. Benign dermoid cysts are the most common non-physiological cysts, although even these are relatively uncommon in the paediatric and adolescent setting. Many ovarian cysts are asymptomatic even when they are very large, and may be found incidentally at the time of other investigations. They may cause vague lower abdominal pain or may present more acutely if torsion of the ovary occurs.

### Ovarian torsion

(See also Chapter 20.1.)

This can be a difficult diagnosis because of the relatively non-specific nature of the symptoms. Failure to consider this diagnosis can lead to loss of an ovary.

- Ovarian torsion is more common in childhood and adolescence than in adulthood.
- There is abdominal pain, often colicky.
- There is associated vomiting and dizziness.
- The ovarian cyst/ mass may not be palpable; it is essential to consider the diagnosis if there is significant and persistent localized tenderness.
- Pelvic ultrasonography demonstrating an enlarged ovary corresponding to the side of maximal tenderness is supportive evidence.
- Exploration with laparoscopy may be the only way to clarify the diagnosis and is necessary if the ovary is to be preserved.

In the post-menarchal adolescent a history of regular menses with onset of pain occurring approximately mid-cycle may be adequate to diagnose mid-cycle pain, or Mittelschmerz. However, consideration of the diagnosis of torsion needs to be made if there is significant tenderness.

## Pelvic inflammatory disease

Sexual activity (or a gynaecological surgical procedure) enabling pathogens to access the upper genital tract is the prerequisite for the development of pelvic inflammatory disease (PID).

The commonest pathogen causing PID is chlamydia. Tubal disease and damage as a consequence of PID is a significant cause of infertility, and early diagnosis and adequate treatment are important. For the young woman who is sexually active and is febrile with significant pelvic tenderness, intravenous antibiotics should be used to cover the possibility of polymicrobial infection. The antibiotics chosen should cover chlamydia, *Neisseria gonorrhoeae* and other anaerobic and aerobic organisms.

Screening for chlamydia in sexually active young woman under the age of 25 years is recommended due to reported rates of asymptomatic infection in up to 15% of young women. Treatment with a single dose of azithromycin is effective and ensures good compliance. Identification of young women with silent carriage should lead to contact tracing of partners. Follow-up should be offered, and further discussion regarding contraception and safe sex is essential.

## Contraception

Discussing and providing contraceptives to teenagers requires careful consultation. The need for contraception will often not be raised by teenagers, but if part of the consultation has occurred without parents and has utilized a careful assessment of social activities and relationships, the young woman who is sexually active should be readily identifiable.

Ideally, involvement of an adult in the decision-making process regarding contraception is preferred, but the younger teenager who demonstrates a clear understanding of the risks and benefits can be provided with contraception. Careful documentation and assessment of the competency of the teenager in demonstrating their understanding is essential (a House of Lords ruling in 1984 on this issue has given rise to the expression 'Gillick competence' for this assessment).

Ensure the teenager is aware of the need for condoms for 'safe sex' to reduce her risk of acquiring a sexually transmitted infection.

### Options for contraception

*Emergency contraception*

This form of contraception is now usually provided as a single-dose progestogen, and is used as soon as possible after unprotected intercourse. The success of this contraception method correlates with the time interval since unprotected intercourse. It is important to do a pregnancy test prior to use.

*Oral contraceptive pill (OCP)*

- A wide variety of OCPs are available.
- For simplicity, be familiar with two or three variations.
- A standard monophasic pill (which allows the possibility of altering the time of the withdrawal bleeds and allows the option of skipping menses for several months at a time) using ethinylestradiol and levonorgestrel is a good first-line contraceptive pill.
- If acne is a major concern, an OCP-containing cyproterone acetate can be valuable.
- For young women on anticonvulsants, use an OCP with a higher oestrogen content (using ethinylestradiol 50 mg) as liver enzymes are induced and metabolism of the OCP is accelerated.

*Progestogen-only pills*

These pills contain low-dose progestogen only and require greater reliability in use, with the pills needing to be taken at the same time every day (±1 hour) This is usually difficult for teenagers to manage in their daily routine and hence is usually not considered a good or reliable choice for contraception for this age group.

*Injectable – depot medroxyprogesterone acetate (Depo-Provera)*

This is a very reliable contraceptive and is usually administered every 3 months as an intramuscular injection. Measurement of β-human chorionic gonadotrophin (bHCG) must be carried out if an injection is overdue, as ongoing amenorrhoea may be due to a pregnancy rather than to effective menstrual suppression.

*Etonogestrel*

This is a subcutaneous hormone released from a filament inserted into the upper arm, which provides contraception for 3 years. It is a very reliable form of contraception but causes irregular bleeding in up to 30% of young women, resulting in requests for removal. An alternative approach, where there are concerns regarding the reliability in taking the OCP, is to leave the etonogestrel in place (as a reliable contraceptive) but to add a low-dose OCP to correct the irregular bleeding. In this context, if the pill-taking is erratic the consequences are breakthrough bleeding rather than pregnancy.

*Progestogen-releasing intrauterine device (IUD)*

The levonorgestrel intrauterine system is a very reliable contraceptive. It is effective for 5 years and causes a 98% reduction in menstrual loss. It has an important place in some specific adolescent populations, including those with heavy periods and those unable to use oestrogens.

## Teen pregnancy

Teenagers often present late with their unplanned pregnancy. If the presentation is early in pregnancy, the opportunity to explore choices with respect to the pregnancy needs to be offered. Young women who are part of a positive educational environment with career plans are more likely to decide to terminate a pregnancy.

For teenagers who are pregnant, antenatal care in a young women's clinic offers the opportunity to address their specific needs, using a multidisciplinary team. Careful assessment is required to identify their housing and financial support requirements. Dietitian involvement is valuable to ensure that eating disorders or poor nutrition secondary to lifestyle and poverty do not impact on the health of the young woman and the fetus.

Alcohol, smoking and illicit drug-taking need to be explored, with links made to appropriate services. Screening for sexually transmitted infections needs to be offered to all pregnant young women as the prevalence, particularly of chlamydia, in the under 25-year-old age group is significant. Exploration of possible past physical or sexual abuse should be undertaken as their sexual activity may be a result of this trauma.

It should not be presumed that any of the preceding issues will be volunteered spontaneously. A positive rapport is essential to gain the confidence of the young woman. Linking the pregnant young woman to educational resources and opportunities may be required, as limited education is a significant factor in lifelong poverty.

Pregnancy in teenagers is generally low risk although gastroschisis occurs more frequently in the babies of teenage mothers.

Parenting as a teenager poses real challenges because of the conflicts between adolescent and parenting tasks. The developmental tasks of adolescence include seeking independence, risk-taking, being part of a peer group and participating in peer activities. As a parent, provision of a stable environment with responsible and committed time to the care of a baby is clearly in contrast to adolescent tasks.

## Intellectual disability – menstrual and contraceptive management

With the onset of puberty, parents and carers of young women with an intellectual disability often become acutely concerned by the further challenges that this sexual development may pose. Although concerns regarding the capacity of the young woman to cope with menstruation itself are often the reason for presentation, underlying worries about the need for contraception, and risks of pregnancy and sexual abuse, are usually also present.

It is impossible to predict exactly when menstruation will begin. Likewise it is impossible to know what problems, if any, the young woman will experience. As for other young women without disabilities, a range of options is available to assist in the management of menstrual difficulties, and these need to be used in response to the specific problems and issues for the individual. Assistance with menstrual management results in positive benefits to the quality of life of these young women.

Identification of associated medical problems will assist in management decisions. All young women with chronic illness have an increased risk of vitamin D deficiency and the subsequent potential negative impact on bone density. The young woman with reduced mobility has additional risks for osteoporosis. In young women already at risk of negative bone influences, any technique that lowers oestrogen levels, such as the use of depot medroxyprogesterone acetate, should be avoided or used only if replacement oestrogen is also provided. For the young woman with unstable epilepsy, seizures may occur cyclically, and achieving a stable hormonal state may be helpful in reducing frequency of seizures.

Menstrual and contraceptive management in the young woman with intellectual disability is summarized in Table 3.12.2.

**Table 3.12.2 Menstrual and contraceptive management in the young woman with intellectual disability**

| Management | Clinical effects | Additional comments |
|---|---|---|
| Non-steroidal anti-inflammatory drugs | Reduce dysmenorrhoea<br>Reduce menstrual loss | No contraceptive effect |
| Tranexamic acid | Reduces menstrual loss | No contraceptive effect |
| Cyclic progestogens | May reduce dysmenorrhoea<br>Regulate bleeding pattern<br>May reduce menstrual loss | No contraceptive effect |
| Oral contraceptive pill | Reduces dysmenorrhoea<br>Reduces menstrual loss | Contraceptive |
| Continuous oral contraceptive pill | May eliminate menses<br>May reduce cyclic seizures | Contraceptive |
| Depot medroxyprogesterone acetate (Depo-Provera) | May eliminate menses<br>May reduce cyclic seizures<br>May have a negative effect on bone density and require replacement oestrogen | Contraceptive |
| Etonogestrel | May reduce menstrual bleeding but significant risk of irregular bleeding | Contraceptive |
| Levonorgestrel IUD | Significantly reduces menstrual loss (often achieves amenorrhoea) | Contraceptive |
| Tubal ligation | No impact on menstrual symptoms | Contraceptive<br>In Australia requires Family Court of Australia approval for those less than 18 years of age |
| Hysterectomy | Eliminates menses and dysmenorrhoea | Contraceptive<br>In Australia, requires Family Court of Australia approval for those less than 18 years of age |
| Endometrial ablation | Reduces menstrual loss (may achieve amenorrhoea) | Not contraceptive<br>In Australia, requires Family Court of Australia approval for those less than 18 years of age |

IUD, intrauterine device.

# Sleep problems 3.13

Sadasivam Suresh, Helen Heussler

## Introduction

Sleep is a universal phenomenon in the animal kingdom. The role of sleep in human beings has been studied with increasing interest over the last 60 years. This has resulted in increased awareness of sleep medicine as a separate entity. This chapter focuses on some of the aspects of paediatric sleep medicine: the physiology and function of sleep, development and maturity of sleep, parasomnias, behavioural aspects of children's sleep, the spectrum of paediatric sleep disorders and its role in future morbidity of the individuals.

> 'If sleep does not serve an absolutely vital function, then it is the biggest mistake the evolutionary process ever made.'
>
> *Dr Alan Rechtshaffen, Sleep Research Pioneer*

## The physiology and function of sleep

Sleep is defined as 'a natural and periodic state of rest during which consciousness of the world is suspended'. This is brought about by complex interactions between the reticular activating system and the diffuse set of neuronal centres that facilitate different aspects of sleep. The most important factor appears to be the desynchronization with the cortical centres that are related to consciousness. Sleep has been further differentiated with the help of electroencephalography (EEG) and the current convention for staging of sleep is EEG based. In infancy it is differentiated as active and quiet sleep, and as the development progresses characteristic features are noted and the sleep is broadly divided as rapid eye movement (REM) and non-rapid eye movement (NREM) sleep. The usual pattern is to cycle through these stages throughout the night and to arouse (often at stage changes) a number of times during the night. This structure is often referred to as sleep architecture. The total amount of sleep from birth to adolescence is shown in Figures 3.13.1 and 3.13.2.

Although sleep has been studied extensively over the past few decades, the exact function of sleep has not been fully discerned. However, there is a reasonable amount of information available to attribute the following functions to sleep:

- Sleep is noted to restore and recuperate the human body to optimal daytime functioning (restoration theory). NREM sleep is thought to function in reparation of body tissue and REM sleep in restoration of brain tissue.
- Sleep is considered important in the process of learning and memory (learning theory). The unlearning theory complements this process by handling the clutter of information and removing non-essential information in an orderly fashion, thereby facilitating enhanced learning.
- Sleep is considered a facet of evolutionary development, and complexity of sleep is attributed to the complex nature of the human physiological system.

## Development and maturity of sleep

Similar to many aspects of development, sleep also undergoes changes with age. The physiological aspects that evolve during the early years are maturation of the EEG, development of cardiorespiratory reflexes, establishment of the circadian rhythm and consolidation of sleep architecture. Some 95% of infants cry with a night awakening that requires a parental response. By the age of 1 year, 60–70% of these infants are able to go back to sleep on their own. The ability to self-soothe and return to sleep is the most important aspect for consolidated sleep as awakenings are a normal part of a night sleep, even in adulthood. Self-sleep initiation is a learned phenomenon and is essential for establishment of sleep continuity ('sleeping through'). Minor arousals will continue to be seen, but will not require external intervention. Sleep maturation is linked to intellectual development in children.

## Behavioural aspects of children's sleep

Unlike adults, infants and young children do not often present with problems in their sleep. The parents present their problem. It is important to evaluate the symptoms properly and assess whether there is a sleep

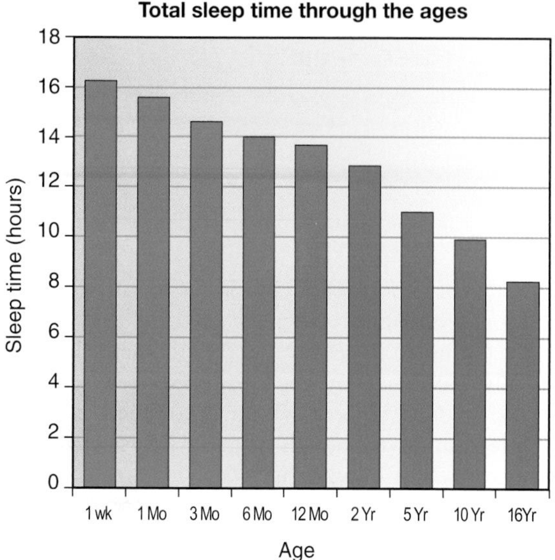


Fig. 3.13.1 Total sleep time through the ages.

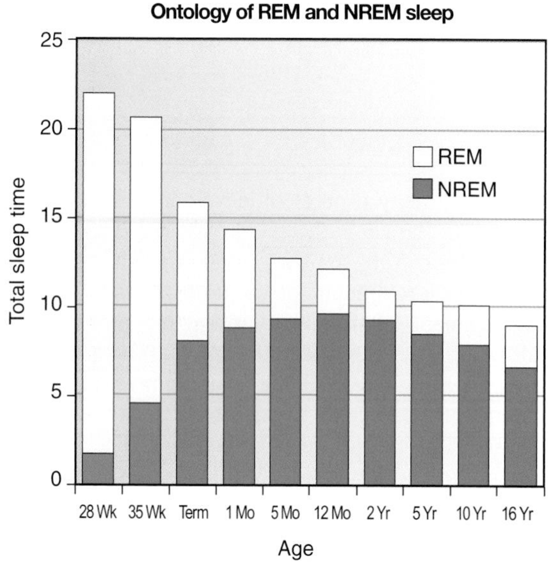


Fig. 3.13.2 Total sleep time with a rapid eye movement (REM)/non-rapid eye movement (NREM) split.

disorder present or just a variation of the normal. The treatment, if any, should be for the child primarily and not necessarily to fulfil parental desire. Age-specific common non-respiratory sleep problems are shown in Table 3.13.1.

Common problems encountered are those of difficulties with sleep initiation, sleep maintenance and circadian scheduling problems. Sleep initiation problems often are related to not being able to self-settle and are common in children with attention-deficit/hyperactivity disorder (ADHD) or autistic spectrum disorders, as well as in some typically developing children. They can also relate to poor routines, limit-setting problems and anxiety issues inherent in the child. It is important, as with adult insomnia, to address what is going on at this time and predisposing factors that may contribute to the difficulty settling. A sleep initiation problem will often lead to a circadian shift and thus to difficulties in getting up in the morning. Practical issues need to be addressed and can be done so with:

- a stable routine that helps with entrainment (external factors that help keep circadian scheduling in a regular pattern)
- settling procedures/relief of anxiety
- entrainment of circadian schedule with regular and stable wake-up and bedtimes
- comfortable non-stimulatory environment
- removal of technology from the bedroom (e.g. televisions, mobile phones, game equipment).

Children will generally need to learn how to self-settle. Methods such as controlled crying work but are often difficult for tired parents to implement. Often, focusing on the sleep initiation and utilizing a camping-out technique are more acceptable to parents.

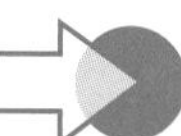

**Practical point**

- Camping out involves a parent sleeping on a mattress or chair in the child's room until the child is going to sleep in his/her own bed and then gradual removal of the parent from the room.

## Sleep phenomena or parasomnias in children

Parasomnias are undesirable motor, autonomic or experiential phenomena that occur exclusively or predominantly during the sleep state. Parasomnias have sleep state-related features and most of them are benign. The majority of these decrease in frequency as the child gets older. Some of them exhibit familial links and may change with time. The predominant management issue is safety. Parents should be alerted if a child is sleepwalking; this can usually be managed by bells or alarms placed on a child's doors or windows. Night terrors can be particularly alarming for some, but the child usually remains unaware of the problem – unlike nightmares, where a child will awaken after a bad dream and have good recall of the dream. Night terrors usually occur earlier in the night and, like most parasomnias, can become worse if the

| Table 3.13.1 Commonest non-respiratory sleep disorders | | | |
|---|---|---|---|
| Infant/toddler (1–2 years) | Preschool child (3–5 years) | Primary school child (6–12 years) | Adolescent (13–18 years) |
| Behavioural insomnia of childhood | Behavioural insomnia of childhood | Insufficient sleep | Insufficient sleep |
| Rhythmic movement | Sleep terrors<br>Rhythmic movement | Bedtime resistance<br>Sleepwalking | Narcolepsy |
| Source: Moore M, Allison D, Rosen CL 2006 A review of pediatric non-respiratory sleep disorders. Chest 130:1252–1262. | | | |

child is woken. They are often also worse if a child is tired; hence many children present with night terrors as they begin to give up their daytime sleep.

Table 3.13.2 gives a simplified summary of parasomnias with prevalence rates from a large population study.

### Clinical example

James is a 5-year-old boy who presents with a story of frequent night waking with screaming. He has trouble getting off to sleep and has been very tired, often falling asleep on the drive home from school, but when it comes to time for bed he won't sleep unless his mother lies down with him. He will then wake frequently during the night with two types of episode – one usually before his parents go to bed and others later in the night. The first ones are the worst, where he is so upset he cannot be comforted. In the later ones during the night, James wakes crying and comes to get a parent but then won't go back to bed unless they are with him.

**What other information might you like?**
Family history is important, as these problems tend to have a familial pattern. Children usually have no daytime nap by the age of 5 years and continuation of daytime napping will have impact on night sleep patterns. The dietary intake of children could have an impact on sleep routine. Habituation of sleep patterns are important and exactly what his mother does at each wake time will have an impact on either exacerbating or reducing the problem.

**What three processes are going on here?**
1. Night terrors.
2. Nightmares.
3. Sleep association and maintenance issues.

**How would you manage this child?**
- Reassure that the waking and parasomnias are normal phenomena that are often worse when tired.
- Normalize James' sleep onset associations (he needs to be able to get off to sleep on his own). The camping out technique may be useful but requires an individual approach.
- Consider organizing with the school an early afternoon or late morning nap, as James has just given this up in his first year of full-time school.

## Polysomnography in children

The main investigative tool in children with suspected sleep disorder is polysomnography (PSG). Like other investigations in medicine, PSG should be performed only after obtaining a proper clinical history and examination. PSG comprises multiple channels and would traditionally include EEG, electro-oculogram (EOG), electromyogram (EMG), thorax and abdominal respiratory bands, oronasal flow sensor, oxyhaemoglobin saturations, transcutaneous/end-tidal carbon dioxide sensor ± video monitoring (Fig. 3.13.3). This helps in ascertaining sleep stages accurately and the nature and severity of sleep related breathing disorder, if any. Children are significantly different from adults, and criteria for scoring vary with modified definition for abnormal thresholds. Various forms of limited-channel PSG have been used and, when carefully planned, the information obtained is beneficial in managing paediatric sleep problems. If seizures in sleep are suspected, full EEG leads will be required. Most sleep studies have limited EEG channels, which are used primarily for sleep staging and not for assessment of seizures.

## Spectrum of paediatric sleep disorders

The general physiological patterns seen as part of various sleep disorders in children for the most part are similar to those in adults. Some differences exist, mainly reflecting aspects of behaviour, psychology and development. The International Classification of Diseases (ICD) includes paediatric sleep disorders in its most recent version. Children experience a broad range of sleep disturbances including obstructive sleep apnoea (OSA), insomnia, parasomnia, delayed sleep phase, narcolepsy and restless legs, but their clinical presentation, evaluation and management may differ from those in adults. Although snoring and sleep apnoea may be the most common indication for an overnight sleep study in a child, one-quarter of children presenting to a sleep clinic

**Table 3.13.2 Parasomnias with population prevalence**

| | NREM related | REM related | Sleep state independent |
|---|---|---|---|
| Normal | Hypnogogic imagery<br>Sleep starts<br>Confusional arousals 17% | Dreams<br>Nightmare 10–50% | Bruxism 28%<br>Rhythmic movement disorder 17%<br>Sleep-talking 55% |
| Abnormal | Night terrors 17%<br>Sleepwalking 14% | Sleep paralysis<br>REM behaviour disorder | Periodic leg movement |

NREM, non-rapid eye movement; REM, rapid eye movement.
Source: Moore M, Allison D, Rosen CL 2006 A review of pediatric non-respiratory sleep disorders. Chest 130:1252–1262.

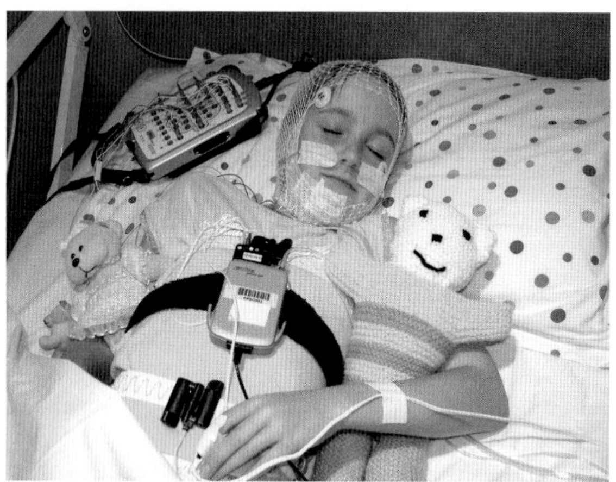

Fig. 3.13.3 Child in the sleep laboratory undergoing polysomnography.

for evaluation will have a second sleep diagnosis, which is often non-respiratory in nature. Especially in children, ruling out OSA is rarely the endpoint of the sleep evaluation. Clinicians involved in sleep medicine must be prepared to recognize, evaluate and manage plans for sleep disorders across the lifespan of the patient.

## Snoring and obstructive sleep apnoea syndrome

Snoring and OSA is one of the outstanding examples of the seamless transition from normal phenomenon to an abnormal pathology. Snoring is noted in at least 20% of the paediatric population at any one stage and is considered benign when it is not associated with any other sleep symptomatology. This is called primary snoring or habitual snoring. William Osler in 1892 stated: 'At night the child's sleep is greatly disturbed, the respirations are loud and snorting, and there are sometimes prolonged pauses, followed by deep, noisy inspirations' in a textbook of paediatrics describing clinical features of tonsillar enlargement. In spite of such a lucid description, the importance of OSA in children has been recognized only in the last 30 years.

The American Academy of Pediatrics has published a consensus guideline regarding the diagnosis and management of paediatric OSA. The main clinical presentation is that of snoring, witnessed pauses, sleep disturbance and poor performance at school. A detailed sleep history supplemented by clinical examination and assessment of breathing during sleep will help in diagnosing OSA. Full PSG remains the 'gold standard' for diagnosis; however, overnight oximetry, when performed and analysed by experienced staff, hastens the clinical diagnosis in view of its very high positive predictive value (97%).

The mainstay of treatment in the paediatric age group is adenotonsillectomy, with a resolution rate close to 90%. In a small proportion of children OSA persists and requires further investigation and treatment. Treatment of any underlying medical condition and control of weight gain contribute significantly in reducing the severity of OSA. Supportive therapy during sleep in the form of continuous positive airway pressure (CPAP) therapy has been proven to be beneficial similar to that in adult patients with OSA.

## Complications of untreated OSA

Severe forms of untreated OSA have been associated with cor pulmonale, developmental delay, failure to thrive or death. Over the last decade there has been increased understanding of the morbidity from untreated OSA, even when the OSA is in the mild to moderate category. There is also evidence emerging that primary snoring might not be as benign as thought previously, and might also be associated with some sequelae. Neurocognitive and learning deficits have been associated with OSA, and early diagnosis

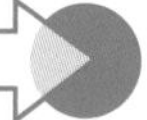

**Practical points**

- Snoring is a very common symptom in childhood with a prevalence of 10–15% .
- Obstructive sleep apnoea occurs in 2–5% of children.
- Early recognition and treatment can have an impact on sleep quality, growth and neurocognitive development.

and appropriate treatment appears to reverse some of these. However, in some children the changes appear irreversible and it is postulated that the older the child at treatment institution the lesser the chance of reversing the deficits. Untreated OSA in adulthood is associated with increased cardiovascular and cerebrovascular morbidity, and it is likely that some of the changes have their origins in childhood.

### Clinical example

Ricky is a 4-year-old boy with a history of snoring and sleep disturbance, as well as recurrent upper respiratory tract infections.

**What further details in clinical history are needed?**
The daily sleep routine needs to be ascertained. The nature of snoring, timing of snoring, variability with posture, time or intercurrent illnesses need to be established. Associated features of snoring such as witnessed pauses or gasps need to be enquired about. The nature and frequency of upper respiratory infections will need further exploration. A history of tonsillitis with difficulty in handling solids/chunky food points to tonsillar hypertrophy. A history of mouth breathing with bad breath may be found in some preschoolers. Symptoms of nasal obstruction and seasonal variation need to be enquired about.

**What are the important features of clinical examination?**
Anthropometric measures of height and weight are important to assess the impact and chronicity of the problem. Examination should include a complete ear, nose and throat (ENT) assessment, including checking for nasal passages, oropharyngeal space and tonsillar size. Auscultation should be performed for a loud second heart sound, which might be present in severe cases of OSA. Blood pressure measurement should be performed.

**What further investigations are appropriate?**
X-ray of the lateral neck to assess adenoidal pad could be a useful investigation in the outpatient setting. PSG is the 'gold standard' for diagnosing OSA. Screening oximetry could be performed to 'rule in' OSA, to expedite further management.

**PSG findings and the next management step**
**PSG demonstrated obstructed breathing with a respiratory disturbance index (RDI) of 10/hour, more marked in REM sleep with an RDI of 22/hour (normal rate <5/hour in young children and <1/hour in older children). What would be the next management step?**

The first line of treatment for OSA would be assessment by an ENT surgeon with a view to considering adenotonsillectomy. Ricky went on to have this operation. His snoring symptoms resolved, with improvement in quality of sleep without sleep fragmentation. His appetite improved and he was able to manage a wide variety of foods, including chunky food.

**After the management step what follow-up arrangements are needed?**
Provided the symptoms resolve completely, no further medical follow-up is warranted. However, with a proven diagnosis of OSA there is a chance that the symptoms might return either with significant weight gain or during pubertal years; Ricky and his family should be advised to seek medical help if this occurs.

### Central hypoventilation and respiratory failure

Congenital central hypoventilation (Ondine's curse) is a rare disorder wherein the respiratory drive in sleep is absent or significantly blunted. This results in significant hypoventilation and respiratory failure. A defect in the homeobox gene *PHOX2B* is found in this condition. Early diagnosis in the neonatal period and institution of ventilatory support via tracheostomy is needed to manage the condition.

Sleep-related hypoventilation is more commonly noted in neuromuscular conditions, and usually presents in the second decade of life with worsening weakness. Poor sleep quality followed by increasing hypoxia and hypercapnia are noted on PSG. Vital capacity below 40% predicted is usually associated with onset of sleep-related hypoventilation. Diagnosis is by demonstrating hypercapnic respiratory failure on PSG, and treatment is usually by non-invasive mask ventilatory (NIV) support. Treatment has demonstrated improved life expectancy and quality of life in patients, especially those with Duchenne muscular dystrophy (DMD).

The increasing epidemic of obesity in childhood has also resulted in another subgroup of patients who present with significant sleep-disordered breathing and need either CPAP or NIV to correct this.

Children with the following specific syndromes are at risk of sleep-disordered breathing, both OSA and hypoventilation: trisomy 21, craniosynostosis syndromes, achondroplasia, spina bifida and Prader–Willi syndrome (amongst others).

### Complications of insufficient sleep

Research in this area in children has been limited; however, there is now emerging evidence that as little as 1 hour less a day can have significant impact on a child's performance at school, particularly in areas of vigilance and sustained attention, as well as working memory.

## Rare conditions

Some disorders that present in sleep include nocturnal epilepsies. These occur rarely and are often associated with repetitive and stereotypical movements, often associated with an intermittent decrease in daytime performance.

Other disorders to be aware of include:

- *Narcolepsy* – a triad of hypersomnolence with an uncontrollable urge to sleep, cataplexy and short REM latency. This commonly presents in early adulthood, adolescence or late childhood, but most people with the diagnosis may have had symptoms for up to 10 years.

- *Klein–Levin syndrome* – a disorder that presents mostly in adolescent males and involves hypersomnolence, hyperphagia and hypersexuality. The condition is episodic, often for periods of 10–14 days, where the patients describe it as 'like being in a dream'. Most adolescents will 'grow out of this', although mild cognitive/memory deficits have been noted in some.

### Clinical example

Keith is a 13-year-old boy with DMD who complains of sleep difficulty. He has been wheelchair-bound since the age of 11 years and has developed a mild scoliosis. His parents are concerned, as he appears very tired during the day and does not appear to have energy to go beyond 2 p.m.

**What clinical features would you elicit to assess Keith's sleep-disordered breathing?**
The sleep routine for Keith, including his daytime resting pattern, needs to be ascertained. A history of daytime somnolence is reflective of poor overnight sleep quality. A history of snoring, multiple wakenings, early morning headaches and increased sweating during sleep all point towards sleep-disordered breathing and hypoventilation in an adolescent with DMD. A history of weight gain (secondary to reduced activity) or loss (secondary to incipient respiratory failure) is also relevant.

**What investigations would you plan?**
Spirometry performed in the outpatient setting will help in assessing the respiratory reserves. Vital capacity below 40% predicted is usually associated with nocturnal hypoventilation and respiratory failure. PSG performed in a sleep laboratory will give information on overall sleep quality, sleep architecture, adequacy of gas exchange and severity of respiratory failure, if any.

**What will be your management strategy?**
Given the history, it is highly likely that Keith will have chronic hypercapnic respiratory failure and, after confirmation with a sleep study, treatment options including initiation of non-invasive mask ventilation (NIV) during sleep-time need to be discussed with Keith and his family. NIV is well tolerated and shown to improve respiratory failure with symptomatic improvement and improved quality of life.

**What other specialists might need to assess Keith?**
In addition to the neurologist and respiratory and sleep pediatrician, Keith would benefit from an assessment by paediatric cardiologist to assess his right ventricular function and the extent of cardiomyopathy, if any, and appropriate treatment commenced. With the increased risk of scoliosis in this group of patients, Keith would benefit from a spinal assessment and correction of scoliosis if that was considered as a reasonable treatment option.

## Conclusion

Sleep is a widespread biological phenomenon and its scientific study is proceeding at multiple levels. Marked progress is being made in answering three fundamental questions: what is sleep? what are its mechanisms? and what are its functions? Sleep is critical for health and is undervalued both in our 24-hour society and in paediatric clinical practice. Sleep problems are extremely common during childhood, from infancy to adolescence. Childhood sleep disorders are often under-recognized and undiagnosed, despite being either preventable or treatable. Sleep impacts on almost all aspects of a child's functioning, and thus the increased recognition and treatment of sleep disorders will have a positive effect on a child's well-being.

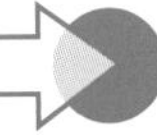

### Practical points

- Sleep is a short- and long-term health investment.
- Do not forget to obtain sleep history as part of a routine paediatric clinical history.

# Refugee health 3.14

Georgia Paxton, David Burgner

## Introduction

This chapter highlights some of the key health issues commonly encountered in refugee children and their families. The focus is on refugee health in Australia, but the concepts are relevant to refugee children and their families settling in other countries.

The protection of people who have been forced to leave their homes due to armed conflict and human rights abuses is a major global challenge. In 2009, there were approximately 15 million refugees worldwide, 1 million people seeking asylum and 27 million people displaced within their own countries because of conflict. The majority of refugees remain in their area of origin. Only about 1% of all refugees are resettled in a third country, and only about 1% of these are resettled in Australia.

Annually, Australia currently accepts 13750 people under its humanitarian programme, and New Zealand accepts 750 refugees. In total, more than 140000 people of a refugee background have arrived in Australia since the mid-1990s, representing a significant population group, with unique health needs. The current Australian humanitarian intake is mainly from Burma (Myanmar), Iraq, Afghanistan, sub-Saharan Africa and Bhutan. Refugee arrivals include a high proportion of children and young people; over half the intake is less than 25 years of age. Families are often large, with women heading the household, and there may be many children within a family group. Some children and young people arrive as unaccompanied humanitarian minors, defined as those aged less than 18 years with no parent to care for them.

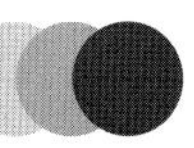

### Definition of refugee and asylum seeker

A *refugee* is a person who:

'Owing to a well-founded fear of being persecuted for reasons of race, religion, nationality, membership of a particular social group, or political opinion, is outside the country of his nationality, and is unable to or, owing to such fear, is unwilling to avail himself of the protection of that country.'

*Article 1, The 1951 Convention Relating to the Status of Refugees*

An *asylum seeker* is a person who has left their country of origin, has applied for recognition as a refugee in another country, and is awaiting a decision on their application.

**Refugee children, young people and families:**

- are usually resourceful and resilient
- will have experienced major transitions with migration and settlement, affecting their family, education and community structure
- may have had inadequate food, water, shelter and safety
- may have spent a prolonged period in refugee camps
- are likely to have come from situations where health care is inadequate
- will have health conditions reflecting their area of origin and country of refuge, with exposure to communicable and vaccine-preventable diseases
- will need catch-up immunization
- may have an incorrect birth date on their paperwork
- are likely to have disrupted education
- may have been separated from their family, or lost family members
- may have experienced physical or sexual violence, including torture and severe human rights violations
- may have mental health problems
- may not be familiar with preventative health care
- may also have more familiar paediatric health issues.

## Refugee health assessments

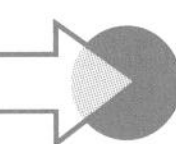

### Practical points

- Refugee children have usually not had pre-departure health screening in their country of origin.
- Health assessment for refugee children/young people is recommended after they settle in a new country; including an assessment of general health, nutrition, immunization status, infectious diseases (malaria, parasites, hepatitis, tuberculosis risk) and mental health.
- There are additional diagnoses to consider for common presentations in refugee children/young people.

Refugees settling in developed countries should be offered voluntary health screening. Screening protocols vary depending on countries of origin and settlement, and may also vary with refugee/asylum seeker status. Health screening may be completed 'offshore' (before leaving the source country) or after arrival in the new country, and may include presumptive treatment for infectious diseases. Many countries use a combination of offshore and post-arrival screening.

### Pre-departure screening

In Australia, health screening and treatment prior to departure is limited for children and younger adolescents. The visa health assessment, completed for any permanent arrival to Australia, not just refugee entrants, is directed at excluding active tuberculosis (TB), and includes a physical examination, urine ward test (age ≥5 years), chest X-ray (age ≥11 years) and human immunodeficiency virus (HIV) serology (age ≥15 years). There are no other routine screening tests. Humanitarian entrants may have additional offshore pre-departure medical screening (PDMS). This varies with port of departure, but may include malaria screening (and treatment if needed), empiric antihelminth treatment and a single mumps, measles, rubella (MMR) vaccination (age from 9 months to 30 years). PDMS is a voluntary process and uptake is not complete.

### Post-arrival health assessment

It is important to explain the concepts of health assessment, screening and disease prevention; families (and adolescents individually) need to understand the importance and implications of health screening and give informed consent. A professional health interpreter will be needed in the majority of consultations. It is never appropriate to use a family member or friend as an interpreter. It is important to explain the bounds of confidentiality for both the medical consultation and working with an interpreter, and this may help families feel more comfortable. One of the simplest clinical points – often forgotten – is that working with an interpreter takes twice as long: everything is said twice and this needs to be factored into appointment times.

**Assessment of newly arrived refugee children and adolescents should focus on:**

- parent (or self-identified) concerns
- excluding acute illness
- confirming the reported birth date
- immunization status and catch-up
- screening for TB
- symptoms of parasite infection, including malaria
- nutritional status and growth
- significant developmental issues, including vision and hearing
- dental health
- mental health issues, particularly features of post-traumatic stress disorder (PTSD)
- issues arising during resettlement (housing, financial stress, education).

It is important to take a routine background history, as for any patient, although there are different factors to consider in children from a refugee background. Access to antenatal and perinatal care may have been limited, and child health screening (neonatal, vision, hearing screening) may have been limited or non-existent. Access to health care, dental care and education varies widely. We have found it helpful to ask specifically about chronic diarrhoea and malnutrition in infancy, hospital admissions overseas, episodes of malaria and/or coma, and trauma, as it is surprising how frequently these issues are not revealed initially.

Understanding the migration pathway, together with the language and education transitions, is important in appreciating the child's and family's experiences and the effects on health and development. This must be handled sensitively, as there may have been significant trauma. It is not usually appropriate to ask about this directly on the initial visit (unless the family volunteers this history). Useful questions include, '*Who is in your family in Australia*?' and '*Do you still have family overseas*?', rather than asking specifically about family members. It is also helpful to ask what people did overseas, recognizing the breadth of occupations/educational levels within refugee cohorts, and acknowledging that people are not simply defined by their refugee experience.

Key points in history and examination related to screening investigations are shown in Table 3.14.1.

Some groups may need additional screening investigations based on prevalence data from their country of origin, or conditions prior to departure. In addition, children with clinical symptoms may require additional investigations. Other differential diagnoses to consider in refugee children are shown in Table 3.14.2.

## Specific health issues

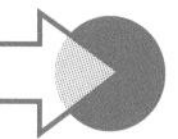

**Practical points**

- Low vitamin D levels are common in refugee children/young people, who may have multiple and ongoing risk factors for vitamin D deficiency and may need long-term treatment.
- Refugee children and young people have high rates of parasites, positive tuberculosis screening test results, and hepatitis, reflecting the prevalence of these health issues in their country of origin.
- Refugee children/young people need an assessment of their immunization status and will all require catch-up vaccinations.

**Table 3.14.1 Key points in history and examination related to screening investigations**

| History | Examination | Suggested initial post-arrival screening investigations |
|---|---|---|
| • Fever (malaria, TB, other infections)<br>• Night sweats/malaise/weight loss/poor growth/chronic cough/ contact and family history, health undertakings (TB)<br>• Low-grade bony and muscular pain, pain with exercise, dairy intake, symptoms of low calcium (muscle cramps), access to outside spaces/ time spent outside, skin colour, covering (vitamin D)<br>• Tiredness, diet (excessive milk, weaning, solids, meat), food access, family history, blood loss (anaemia, iron deficiency)<br>• Jaundice, RUQ pain, family history, transfusion, shared needles (hepatitis)<br>• Abdominal pain, diarrhoea, blood PR, macroscopic worms, rashes, skin nodules (parasites)<br>• BCG status, history of chickenpox, immunization documentation and PDMS (immunization status)<br>• Epigastric pain, early satiety, poor appetite, family history of ulcer disease (*Helicobacter pylori*)<br>• Pregnancy, genital pain, discharge, ulcers, lumps and contact history (STI screening) | A thorough physical examination of all systems is required:<br>• Growth parameters<br>• Nutritional status<br>• BCG scar<br>• Pallor (anaemia, haemoglobinopathies)<br>• Oral health (dentition, periodontal disease)<br>• ENT (chronic middle ear disease)<br>• Goitre (unscreened thyroid disease)<br>• Features of rickets (swelling of wrists/ ankles, deformity (which reflects the age/growth of child when low vitamin D status occurred), delayed dentition, late closure of anterior fontanelle, bossing<br>• Skin, hair, nails (dermatophytes)<br>• Hepatosplenomegaly (e.g. malaria, *Schistosoma*, HIV)<br>• Conditions that would usually be assessed during childhood and may have been missed (e.g. cardiac murmurs, inguinal hernia, undescended testes)<br>• Culturally specific findings (e.g. uvulectomy, teeth removal, scarification) | • FBE and film<br>• Ferritin<br>• Vitamin D, calcium, phosphate, ALP<br>• Vitamin A<br>• Malaria screen (thick and thin films, and rapid diagnostic test)<br>• Hepatitis B screen (HBsAg, HBsAb and HBcAb)<br>• Hepatitis C serology<br>• *Schistosoma* serology<br>• *Strongyloides* serology<br>• Faecal specimen (ideally fixed)<br>• Mantoux test<br>• STI screen (*Neisseria gonorrhoeae* and *Chlamydia trachomatis* urine nucleic acid detection; syphilis serology (TPHA) - consider in all children, to exclude congenital infection) in sexually active adolescents or if there is a history of sexual violence<br>• HIV screening - Consider in all children, should be completed in sexually active adolescents, if there is a history of sexual violence, or where parents are deceased/missing/known to be HIV positive, or if clinical symptoms/signs<br>• *Helicobacter pylori* faecal antigen testing if suggestive symptoms |

ALP, alkaline phosphatase; BCG, bacille Calmette–Guérin; ENT, ear, nose and throat; FBE, full blood examination; HIV, human immunodeficiency virus; HBcAb; hepatitis B core antibody; HBsAb, hepatitis B surface antibody; HBsAg, hepatitis B surface antigen; PDMS, pre-departure medical screening; PR, per rectum; RUQ, right upper quadrant; STI, sexually transmitted infection; TB, tuberculosis; TPHA, Treponema pallidum haemagglutination assay.

## Nutrition and growth

Nutritional issues are common in children from a refugee background. Fussy eating and concerns about weight gain (too little or too much) are often a family priority. Specific issues include low weight and/or height for age, low vitamin D status, other vitamin deficiencies, iron deficiency and anaemia. Several studies suggest the rate of overweight/obesity is low in recently arrived cohorts of refugee children/adolescents; however, immigrant cohorts are observed to have an increased prevalence of overweight/obesity after settlement and in subsequent generations. There are limited data on the prevalence of vitamin deficiencies: low vitamin A levels have been found in up to 40% of African refugee children in Australia; an early history (overseas) suggesting thiamine deficiency is sometimes seen in Burmese children; and $B_{12}$ and folate deficiency have been noted in Afghani refugees.

It is important to take a good dietary and general history, and to ascertain access to and quantity/quality of food overseas and after settlement. Clarify the correct age/birth date, and chart growth parameters. Linear growth is similar in children aged under 5 years worldwide, although growth must be considered in the context of parent height (which should be measured accurately), ethnicity (Australian growth charts are derived from American and European data) and pubertal status. Children may have different parameters to their Australian born peers and still have normal growth; it is important to remember the Australian prevalence of childhood overweight/obesity is above 20%.

An early severe nutritional insult or chronic disease during infancy will affect final height (stunting); this history is usually easily elicited. Consider organic disease early in a refugee child with poor growth or

**Table 3.14.2 Common presentations and differential diagnoses to consider in refugee children**

| Presentation | Common causes | Additional considerations |
|---|---|---|
| Fever | Common viral and bacterial infections (check for localizing features, etc.) | • Malaria*<br>• Dengue and other arboviral infections*<br>• Typhoid*<br>• Dysentery*<br>• TB in any site, especially if prolonged<br>• Dental disease (often missed) |
| Respiratory symptoms | Consider the usual causes of respiratory symptoms relevant to the age group, such as viral respiratory tract infection, pneumonia, asthma, bronchiolitis and croup | • Whooping cough – pertussis vaccination may not have been available in country of origin<br>• TB should be considered in children with cough > 2 weeks<br>• Sickle cell disease may present with acute chest syndrome<br>• Parasite infections may (very rarely) cause wheeze/ respiratory symptoms |
| Abdominal pain | Consider the usual causes, such as acute infection, constipation, surgical or gynaecological problems | • Parasite infection – diarrhoea, rectal bleeding, constipation, hepatic symptoms, haematuria<br>• *Helicobacter pylori* gastritis – early satiety, anorexia, family history of similar symptoms, nausea/vomiting<br>• Hepatitis |
| Diarrhoea | Consider the usual causes of viral and bacterial gastroenteritis | • Bacillary* and amoebic dysentery are common in the developing world<br>• Parasitic infections are common<br>• Lactose intolerance may be more common in some racial groups |
| Rashes | Eczema; dermatophyte (*Tinea*) infections | • *Strongyloides* infection may cause an intermittent urticarial rash lasting a few days (larva currens); this may be located anywhere but is most typically on the buttocks/perianal region<br>• Skin nodules or a depigmented rash on the lower shins suggest parasite infections; specialist consultation is required |
| Continence issues | Typical nocturnal or diurnal enuresis, bladder irritability | • Chronic urinary tract infection may not have been detected/treated<br>• Consider mental health issues as a cause of secondary enuresis<br>• Consider female genital mutilation (FGM) as an additional possibility/contributor in girls (seek advice on how to broach this) |
| Musculoskeletal pain | Low vitamin D status is an extremely common cause in refugee children/ young people with risk factors | |
| Fussy eating | Behavioural issues; excess milk intake | • Food insecurity (not being able to afford/access adequate food) is well documented in refugee families after resettlement<br>• *Helicobacter pylori* gastritis is a common cause of poor appetite and fussy eating<br>• Other gastrointestinal infections<br>• Dental disease – pain with chewing may restrict food intake |

*More likely shortly after arrival.
TB, tuberculosis.

reduced appetite, including gastrointestinal infections (*Helicobacter pylori* gastritis, *Giardia intestinalis*, other parasites), other infections (including TB), low vitamin D levels/rickets and dental disease. Mental health issues may also be a cause of poor intake/growth.

Iron deficiency may affect appetite and compound poor intake. Excessive cow's milk intake is a common cause of iron deficiency. Tea drinking may contribute to iron deficiency in older children as tea chelates iron and reduces absorption.

Fussy eating is often due to high calorie intake in the form of drinks/juice at the expense of solids/mealtimes. It may also be due to a mismatch between food the child is used to and food offered at childcare/school.

Once an initial screen has been completed and treatment initiated as necessary, a period of monitoring growth is often appropriate. The principles of healthy eating are universal and should be discussed with families; essentially this is an opportunity for health promotion in the post-arrival screen. Referral to a local dietitian may be appropriate. Breastfeeding should be promoted. Encourage introduction of solids at 4–6 months, introduction of meat before 12 months, and an appropriate diet containing vegetables, legumes, fruit, cereals, meat and dairy products. Milk should be limited to less than 600 mL daily after 12 months; in children with lactose intolerance, regular yoghurt and cheese are appropriate sources of calcium. Adequate calcium intake is essential for all children, but has additional implications in groups at risk of low vitamin D status. Home-cooked food and maintaining families' cultural food preferences is usually healthier and more economical.

### Vitamin D deficiency and insufficiency

Vitamin D is essential for bone and muscle health (see Chapter 19.5). Groups at risk of low vitamin D include:

- people with naturally dark skin colour
- people with limited sun exposure/excessive time indoors (this should be considered in complex disability/chronic illness), covering clothing
- people with conditions affecting the metabolism of vitamin D (end-stage liver disease, renal failure, some medications, e.g. isoniazid, anticonvulsants)
- babies born to women with low vitamin D
- breastfed babies with other risk factors.

Up to 90% of African Australians living at low latitude have low vitamin D levels, and rickets has re-emerged as a paediatric health issue (Fig. 3.14.1). Low vitamin D levels are also seen commonly in refugee cohorts that wear covering clothing (Afghani, Iraqi), and are increasingly recognized in other population groups.

#### Screening

- Measure vitamin D levels, calcium, phosphate and alkaline phosphatase (ALP) in all children with risk factors. If the initial vitamin D level is normal, repeat at the end of the first winter in Australia.
- Also measure PTH in children with low calcium intake, symptoms/signs or multiple risk factors.
- Children with hypocalcaemia or rickets need urgent specialist assessment and will require further investigations.
- Levels at the start and end of winter can be useful to judge the frequency of dosing. Clinical photography is useful to monitor bony deformity.

A

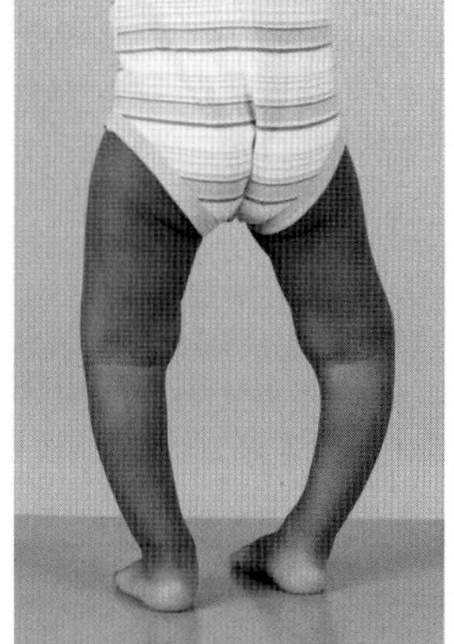

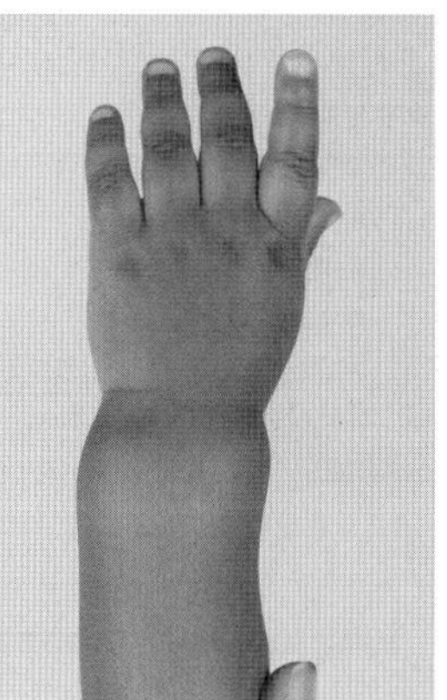

B

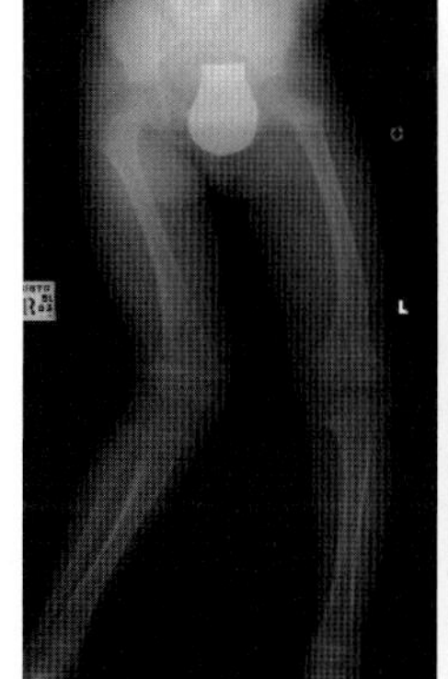

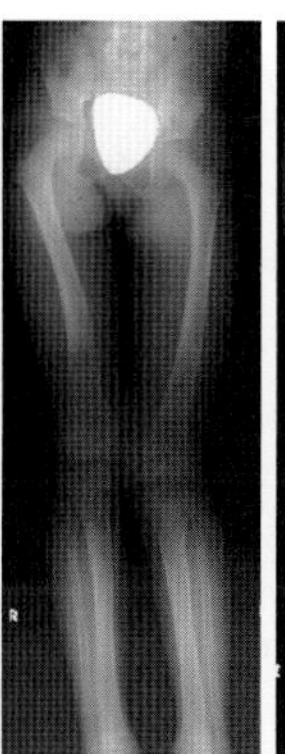

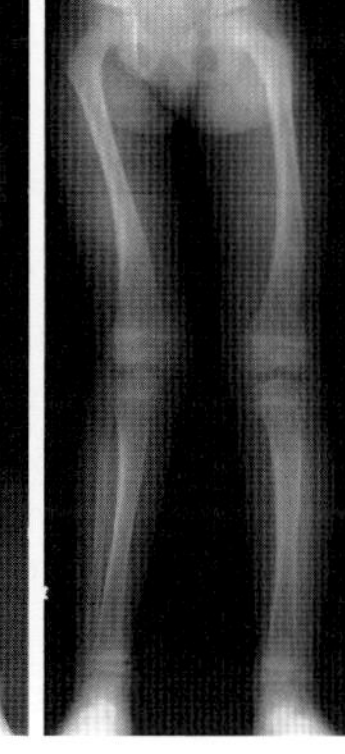

Fig. 3.14.1 **(A)** Rickets at age 2 years, caused by a combination of low vitamin D and low calcium intake in the setting of cow milk allergy. **(B)** Radiographic improvement (in a different child) of severe vitamin D deficiency with vitamin D therapy.

### Management

Prevention is key, so attention to pregnancy and maternal vitamin D status and screening children/adolescents at risk is important. Promote breastfeeding and recommend daily multivitamin supplements containing vitamin D until 12 months of age for all breastfed infants at risk of low vitamin D levels.

- Symptomatic rickets/hypocalcaemia (including tetany, stridor, seizures – more likely in infants) requires hospital assessment, with or without admission. These children may require an intravenous calcium infusion. High doses of vitamin D can worsen hypocalcaemia (by promoting deposition into bones) if there are inadequate calcium stores.
- Low vitamin D status can be treated with either daily dosing (1000–2000 IU orally daily) or a single high dose (up to 150 000 IU stat orally in children aged over 12 months, sometimes called 'Stoss therapy'). Children with levels below 25 nmol/L may require a repeat high dose in 6 weeks. In the longer term, children on high-dose therapy will require repeat dosing every 3–12 months depending on levels/clinical situation.
- Ensure an adequate dietary calcium intake after administration of vitamin D. Calcium supplements may be needed in patients with a low dairy intake.
- Repeat bloods 3 months after starting treatment.

Children with ongoing risk factors require ongoing surveillance/management. Although it is worthwhile recommending time outside, this may not ensure adequate levels during winter at low latitude. There is no single public health message for sun exposure in children that can account for skin colour/latitude; in practice, encourage full sun protection during September to April and encourage play outside before, during and after school. Children with naturally very dark skin have a much lower risk of skin cancer, and can tolerate intermittent sun exposure without sunscreen throughout the year, but should still wear a hat and sunglasses.

## Haematology issues

The prevalence of anaemia in resettled paediatric refugee cohorts is 10–30%; higher rates are reported in studies of children in refugee camps. Iron deficiency affects a similar proportion. Vitamin $B_{12}$ and folate deficiency have been reported in refugees from Afghanistan and Sri Lanka. Haemoglobinopathies are more common in African, Asian and Middle Eastern populations. This means many children will be carriers with mild anaemia (actual disease is uncommon). Lead toxicity has been reported in refugee children.

Anaemia is usually multifactorial in refugee children and young people. Contributors include iron deficiency, malaria and parasite infection/infestation. Iron deficiency is usually nutritional, but may be due to gastrointestinal loss or possibly associated with *H. pylori* infection.

## Immunization catch-up

Vaccine-preventable diseases are endemic and/or epidemic in humanitarian countries of origin, and disruptions to health care may affect vaccine quality and access to immunization. Most refugees do not have written documentation of immunization, and immunization records are not a pre-departure requirement. If present, written records are considered reliable evidence of vaccination status. Serological testing for vaccine-preventable disease is not recommended; there is no significant cost benefit, it requires additional blood sampling, and combination vaccines mean that the same vaccine will be required if there is inadequate immunity to any of the vaccine components.

Specific information on catch-up vaccination information is available from national resources, such as the *Australian Immunisation Handbook*. Key principles include:

- No-one arriving as a refugee will be vaccinated and up to date according to the Australian or New Zealand immunization schedule, owing to differences in country of origin immunization schedules.
- People of a refugee background should be vaccinated so that they are up to date according to the national immunization schedule equivalent to a local born person of the same age.
- Post-vaccination serology is recommended for household contacts of hepatitis B.
- Consider bacille Calmette–Guérin (BCG) vaccination in children aged 16 years or less, if not given previously, and TB screening tests are negative, including for Australian-born siblings.
- Enter immunization data into national registries where available.
- Provide a written record and a clear plan for ongoing immunizations.
- Remind families to plan early for travel immunizations (many families travel, and may be at increased risk when visiting friends and relatives in their country of origin).
- Translated health information sheets are available.

## Tuberculosis screening

TB is due to infection with *Mycobacterium tuberculosis* (MTB) complex. Transmission occurs by exposure to aerosolized droplets from people with respiratory infection. Approximately one-third of the world's population is infected, but only 5–10% of people with infection develop TB disease. Latent TB infection (LTBI) refers to the presence of TB infection (i.e. positive screening test for exposure to MTB) without evidence of active disease on history, examination and chest X-ray. People with LTBI are, by definition, asymptomatic and non-infectious.

TB disease may be either primary or reactivation of LTBI. Primary disease develops as a consequence of initial infection, reactivation disease occurs after a latent period, which may be many years. The risk of progression from TB infection to TB disease is highest in young children, relatively high in adolescents, and increased in the first years after migration. Up to 50% of infants and 15% of older children with LTBI will develop TB disease within 2 years of being infected, hence the importance of TB screening and treatment of both TB disease and LTBI.

BCG vaccine has been used to vaccinate against tuberculosis since 1921, and worldwide coverage is 80%. Protection varies: meta-analysis shows that BCG is about 50% protective against respiratory TB, but more protective against meningitis (64–85%) or death (70–85%). BCG vaccination leaves a scar in 75–99% of recipients. In Australia, BCG is given in the left deltoid; however, it is given in different sites overseas, and scars may be located on the deltoid, forearm, scapula or thigh (either side).

Positive TB screening tests are found in 35–55% of resettled paediatric refugee cohorts. This reflects the prevalence of TB in their countries of origin/transit; however, children may also be infected after settlement through contact with adults with TB disease, including visiting friends and relatives. Active disease is uncommon in refugee children; respiratory disease is the most common form, although non-pulmonary or disseminated/severe disease is more frequent in children than in adults. Younger children with pulmonary TB disease are rarely infectious owing to their pattern of disease (lack of cavitating lesions, low bacterial load) and lack of tussive force.

The Mantoux test remains an appropriate first-line screening test and can be used at any age. The Mantoux test is administered as an intradermal injection, and induration (not erythema) is measured 48–72 hours later. BCG status affects interpretation of the Mantoux test, but does not preclude its use. Essentially a Mantoux test induration $\geq 10$ mm is considered positive in children from endemic areas, and $\geq 5$ mm is considered positive for household contacts of TB cases. Interferon-$\gamma$ release assays are an alternative screening test in adolescents and adults. Children and adolescents with a positive TB screening test and normal history and examination require a chest X-ray. If they have symptoms or signs suggesting active disease, further investigations may be needed. Children with LTBI have a lifetime risk of 5–15% of developing TB, although the risk is higher in recently infected infants and younger children. Isoniazid preventative treatment for 6 months reduces the risk of TB disease by 50–90%. Children with TB disease require specialist management.

## Parasites

### Malaria

Malaria is caused by infection with protozoan parasites transmitted by mosquitoes. Most severe malaria and cerebral malaria is caused by *Plasmodium falciparum* and the highest burden of disease is in young children. Patients with *P. falciparum* disease can deteriorate rapidly. People living in endemic areas typically develop immunity during childhood and may be infected but asymptomatic. They are at increased risk of symptomatic infection after migration as their immunity wanes. The prevalence of malaria was 5–10% in Australian paediatric refugee cohorts from Africa; this has reduced since the introduction of PDMS. Malaria screening is a priority in any recently arrived, febrile refugee. Children with malaria always require hospital assessment, and usually hospital admission.

### Schistosomiasis

Schistosomiasis affects 200 million people worldwide and is endemic in Africa, but is also found in Asia and the Middle East. It is often called 'bilharzia', and families may know this name. The prevalence of *Schistosoma* infection is 12–38% in African refugee cohorts.

Schistosomiasis is caused by infection with one of five species of trematodes (flukes) through contact with infected fresh water. The manifestations of chronic infection depend on the species causing infection; end-stage pathology occurs as a result of granulomatous inflammation in response to the flukes. *S. haematobium* is associated with haematuria and long-term bladder pathology, whereas *S. mansoni* causes gastrointestinal symptoms (pain, diarrhoea/blood per rectum) and portal hypertension. Schistosomiasis is treated with praziquantel.

### *Strongyloides* infection

Strongyloidiasis is a nematode (worm) infection transmitted through contact with infected soil. Humans are the host for *Strongyloides* and the infection can last for decades through a cycle of autoinfection. The prevalence of *Strongyloides* in recent Australian refugee cohorts is 1–9%, although a higher prevalence is reported internationally in African refugees

(23–49%). Most people with *Strongyloides* infection are asymptomatic; however, in the setting of immunosuppression (including steroids) it can cause a hyperinfection syndrome that has a high case fatality rate. Children from *Strongyloides* endemic areas should have screening prior to starting immunosuppression. Treatment is with ivermectin.

### Faecal parasites

Pathogenic faecal parasites are common in refugee children, and are found in 15–40% of children on post-arrival health screening. Some refugee services give empiric antihelminth therapy, which treats many, but not all, parasites. Specific therapy is needed for *Giardia*; *Schistosoma*, *Strongyloides*, amoebiasis, *Taenia* spp and *Hymenolepis nana* (dwarf tapeworm).

*Giardia intestinalis* is the most common pathogen identified, with a prevalence of 10–20%. Pathogenic faecal parasites are found in refugee cohorts from all areas, including Europe and the Middle East, as well as Africa and South Asia. Macroscopically visible worms are likely to be tapeworms or ascarids. Parasite infections may last for years and can affect for nutrition, growth and function. In general, treatment is usually a short course (often single dose) and well tolerated. Table 3.14.3 shows pathogenic parasites requiring treatment and parasites generally considered to be non-pathogenic.

## Other infections

### Hepatitis B

Hepatitis B is a viral infection affecting the liver that is transmitted through exposure to infected body fluids (usually bloodborne or sexual). Horizontal transmission is important in young children and household contacts of people with hepatitis B virus (HBV) infection. Clinical manifestations depend on age of acquisition, viral load and host immune response. Infected children are less likely to have acute symptoms and more likely to develop chronic infection, which is associated with cirrhosis, liver failure and liver cancer. Adolescents and adults usually develop acute symptoms, but clear the infection. Chronic HBV is found in approximately 5–8% of refugee children/young people and requires specialist follow-up and lifelong monitoring. HBV is a vaccine-preventable disease, and immunization of household contacts is a priority.

### Other viral hepatitis

There are limited data on the prevalence of hepatitis C virus (HCV) infection in refugee children, although HCV is common in adults from Egypt, and other parts of Africa and Asia. Hepatitis delta screening is important in children with chronic hepatitis B from Africa and the Middle East. Many refugee children have evidence of past infection with hepatitis A, although few have a history of an acute illness with jaundice/cholestasis.

### *Helicobacter pylori*

*H. pylori* infection is common in refugee children with a prevalence of over 80% in recently arrived African groups. The infection is usually asymptomatic, and its significance is unclear, although *H. pylori* is classed as a carcinogen and treatment is recommended in adults. In practice, it is practical to treat children with symptoms, and the effect is usually dramatic.

## Dental issues

Refugee children have high rates of dental disease, with over half having dental caries or other problems. Access to dental services may be problematic.

**Table 3.14.3 Pathogenic and non-pathogenic parasites**

| Pathogenic parasites requiring treatment | Non-pathogenic parasites (no treatment required) |
|---|---|
| *Entamoeba histolytica* | *Entamoeba coli* |
| *Ascaris lumbricoides* | *Entamoeba hartmanii* |
| *Giardia intestinalis* | *Entamoeba gingivalis* |
| *Ancylostoma or Necator* (hookworm) | *Endolimax nana* |
| *Strongyloides stercoralis* | *Iodamoeba butschlii* |
| *Schistosoma* spp. | *Dientamoeba fragilis** |
| *Taenia solium or T. saginata* (tapeworm) | *Blastocystis hominis** |
| *Trichuris trichiuria* (whipworm) | *Chilomastix mesnili* |
| *Hymenolepis nana* (dwarf tapeworm) | *Trichomonas hominis* |

*Rarely implicated as a pathogen.

## Mental health

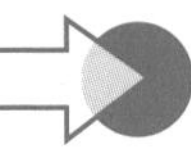

### Practical points

- Refugee children and young people may have witnessed or experienced significant trauma, although this history may not be given offered until a therapeutic relationship is established.
- Refugee children and young people are at high risk for mental health problems, although the reported prevalence of conditions such as PTSD, depression and anxiety varies.
- Most refugee children grow up to be well-adjusted adults.

Children and adolescents of a refugee background will, by definition, have experienced conflict, significant upheaval and transitions with migration and resettlement that may affect their mental health. They may have witnessed or experienced physical or sexual violence and been exposed to life-threatening situations. They may have witnessed significant trauma, including seeing family members killed. Other experiences may include bereavement, being separated from family and community, disruption to schooling or routines, and prolonged periods of dislocation with uncertainty around the future. A history of these profoundly traumatic events is unlikely to be given during the initial assessment; it may emerge once a therapeutic relationship has developed.

Responses to trauma include depression, anxiety, post-traumatic stress, low self-esteem and guilt. These may manifest in a variety of ways including behavioural problems, problems with sleeping and eating, poor school performance, difficulty making friends, enuresis and psychosomatic symptoms. Mental health should be considered in the broader family context; parents with mental health issues often have reduced coping and parenting skills.

There are difficulties with diagnosis and measurement of mental health issues across cultures. Studies of refugee children and young people report widely varying prevalence figures for mental health problems in different groups, partly because of different rating scales are used. Figures range from 3% to 94% for PTSD, 4% to 47% for depression and 3% to 93% for anxiety problems. The largest pooled analysis of mental health problems in people of a refugee background found that the prevalence of PTSD was 11% in children. Unaccompanied minors and people with uncertain visa status are at higher risk of mental health problems.

Although refugees may have experienced significant trauma, there is good evidence that they often have great resilience and positive social adjustment. Experience of trauma does not always predict worse mental health outcomes, and mental health symptoms may not result in functional impairment. The majority of refugee children grow up to be well-adjusted adults and make significant contributions to their countries of resettlement.

## Assessment of development and learning

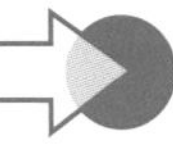

### Practical points

- Refugee children often have additional risk factors for developmental problems, including disrupted or inadequate education, language transitions, mental health and trauma issues and severe medical problems.
- Refugee children and young people may not have had screening for vision or hearing impairment.
- Consider migration, language and environment transitions when establishing a child's developmental milestones.
- Refugee children and young people may have an incorrect birth date on their paperwork; this history may not be given, but has significant effects on development assessment, school placement and using age-standardized testing.

Development may be affected by any combination of biological, environmental, social and emotional factors. Considerations in children of a refugee background include:

- *Biological*: malnutrition, chronic disease, severe infection (including meningitis and cerebral malaria), hearing impairment, visual impairment, family history, prematurity
- *Environmental*: living conditions, access to schooling, access to food, exposure to communicable diseases, migration and language transitions (and the age at which they occurred)
- *Social*: loss of parents, parenting roles, family disruption, roles and responsibilities
- *Emotional*: stress, trauma experiences, displacement, uncertainty around future, mental health problems.

Parental concern about a child's development is highly predictive of developmental delay/disability; however, absence of concern is not necessarily reassuring. Families with multiple children will usually readily identify if one child's development is different to that of their siblings.

Completing a thorough developmental and educational assessment in refugee children/adolescents presents challenges. Like any other child, a developmental and family history is essential; however, migration, education and language transitions in relation to development should be considered. There are different aetiologies to consider in developmental/learning problems in refugee children, and basic screening for contributors such as vision, hearing and mental health problems is frequently missed. There are many issues regarding the timing and validity of formal language or intelligence testing in a child's second language. Incorrect birth dates create additional complexity. A detailed assessment takes time and requires close liaison with the family, and the help of a skilled interpreter.

### Incorrect birth date

Refugee children may have an incorrect birth date on their visa paperwork, which becomes the basis for all the official documentation in the country of settlement. This issue is not uncommon and may have significant effects on school placement, developmental assessment (including formal assessments such as IQ testing) and access to welfare. The reasons for an incorrect birth date are often complex; it may be unknown, due to error, or changed owing to family circumstances/conditions in the country of origin. Any child with a birth date of 01/01/(year) is almost certainly younger. Families may be reluctant to raise this as an issue, and fearful of losing their visa, and it often emerges as an issue some years after settlement. Correcting a birth date requires an assessment of the family narrative, documenting any existing paperwork or known milestones, and an assessment of the child's age and development. A bone age X-ray may be helpful.

### Second language acquisition

Immigrants usually achieve conversational proficiency 2–3 years after starting a new language; however, it takes much longer to achieve academic success in a new language, especially when schooling occurs in the new language. Large international studies in advantaged children with age-appropriate schooling show that children aged 8–12 years when they migrate achieve academic language more quickly than other age groups; however, they take 5–7 years to reach the standard of native-born speakers. Students from a refugee background are likely to have additional risk factors for educational disadvantage, including interrupted or inadequate schooling, financial hardship, mental health issues, cultural transitions and family stressors.

## Settlement considerations

Health assessment is only one part of settlement for refugee children and families, who also need to establish housing, education, employment and the usual routines of daily life in a new country, as well as make friends and community connections. There may be a tension in prioritizing settlement needs, and families may have multiple conflicting appointments, which should be considered when organizing referrals and follow-up. Settlement is an ongoing process, which takes time, sometimes many years; however, people stop being a refugee as soon as they get off the plane – they are Australians, or New Zealanders, of a refugee background.

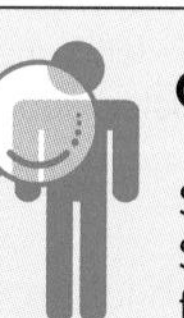

### Clinical example

Sar Po Lay, an 18-month-old child from Karen State in Burma arrived in Australia 4 months ago from a refugee camp on the Thai–Burma border. He has been referred because his height and weight are below the third percentile. His background history includes an uncomplicated pregnancy, delivery at home, and he was noted to be a small baby (birth weight unknown). He breastfed well, but had chronic diarrhoea from the age of 2 months until arrival in Australia. He had one set of immunizations at 6 weeks of age. He is still breastfed, and eats two small bowls of rice porridge daily.

Sar Po Lay's mother is 18 years old; she is 148 cm tall and weighs 38 kg. She has no print literacy and is very shy. They are living with friends and have limited settlement support; they are spending most of their time inside.

Physical examination shows a symmetrically small boy, with reduced subcutaneous fat stores, pale conjunctivae, delayed dentition and a scar on the right shoulder. Sar Po Lay has not had a refugee health check and needs blood tests, a Mantoux test and a faecal specimen, with initial additional investigations including folate, vitamin $B_{12}$ and thyroid function testing because of his poor growth.

These tests reveal *Giardia intestinalis* and a collection of (non-pathogenic) protozoa (likely reflecting water contamination), low vitamin D and raised ALP levels, microcytic anaemia, undetectable ferritin, hepatitis B infection, and a Mantoux test of 20 mm. A subsequent chest X-ray is normal.

Sar Po Lay is treated with metronidazole and high-dose vitamin D, and starts iron supplements. He is given his first set of catch-up immunizations and a plan is devised for introducing an increased range of solid food, including meat, dairy, vegetables and grain, after discussing how his mother could access and afford these foods in Australia. He has another visit organized in 2 weeks to discuss starting isoniazid prevention treatment for latent TB infection (6 months' duration, with vitamin $B_6$ because of his poor growth and monitoring liver function tests because of hepatitis B). The family is referred for case management support, with a plan to access housing support, local maternal and child health, community support groups, a community dietitian, English classes, and a health/mental health assessment for his mother. Sar Po Lay's poor growth is likely a combination of familial factors, low birth weight, chronic diarrhoea, malnutrition, prolonged breastfeeding and delayed introduction of solids. He has severe iron deficiency and is at risk of other micronutrient deficiencies. He will need long-term follow-up for his hepatitis B, and monitoring of his growth.

PART 4

# BEHAVIOUR AND MENTAL HEALTH NEEDS

# 4.1 Life events of normal children

Gehan Roberts, Harriett Hiscock

Although every child follows his or her own individual developmental trajectory, most children achieve developmental milestones at predictable ages (see Chapter 2.2). These anticipated milestones provide an important yardstick against which to assess the individual child's development. A departure from these expected developmental milestones, usually presenting as a developmental delay or behavioural problem, should prompt concerns that development is not proceeding normally.

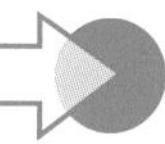

**Practical points**

- Organic causes of infant crying are uncommon but should be suspected if there is associated atopic disease (such as eczema), poor weight gain, frequent (more than three times per day) vomiting or blood/mucus in the infant's bowel actions.
- In toddlers, low-priority misbehaviours (e.g. tantrums, whining) are best managed by ignoring or distraction.
- High-priority misbehaviours (e.g. hitting, kicking) are best managed by asking the child to stop and, if they do not, by putting them in 'time out'.
- A child with unexplained school-based behaviour or learning problems usually needs a multidisciplinary assessment, including vision and hearing testing and, where possible, cognitive testing by an educational psychologist.
- Up to one in five adolescents will experience significant physical or emotional problems. Screening questionnaires that encompass home, school, recreational drug use, sexuality and suicide/depression issues can help to detect these problems.

The development of infants and young children is determined by their genetic potential as expressed by their interaction with the environment. In the early years it is the parents, most often the mother, who shape the infant's environment. Research in recent years has served to re-emphasize the importance of the caretaking environment on the developing brain, which in turn impacts on functioning later in life.

A key requirement for optimal child development is secure attachment to a nurturing and responsive caregiver, with consistent affection and caring. A child's and subsequently an adult's emotional health are significantly influenced by these early relationships. Early development in the context of secure early relationships lays the foundations for future developmental competence.

The child's behaviour and development are always the result of a complex series of transactions between the child and the environment. Assessment of the child's environmental context therefore, is a critical part of behavioural and developmental assessment.

## Risk and resilience

There are well-documented risk factors that make the child vulnerable to a less than optimal outcome. Similarly, there are protective factors that increase the resilience of the child and increase the likelihood of a good outcome. Some of the risk and protective factors are:

- Child factors (e.g. prematurity or chronic illness versus good language or social skills)
- Family factors (e.g. parental mental illness versus stable income or family cohesion)
- Community factors (e.g. inadequate housing versus participation in community activities)
- Broader environmental influences (e.g. drought versus universally available health care).

Parent and family relationships are some of the most important protective factors in promoting optimal development. Recent research suggests the initial 'map' for brain development provided by genes is shaped and sculpted by the caretaking environment. The development of neural connections in early childhood is determined largely by environmental inputs.

Risk and protective factors tend to be cumulative, so that combinations of risk or protective factors are more powerful than individual factors.

## Developmental stages

In the course of the child's development there are certain important transition stages. Each stage is associated with predictable developmental events and behaviours, stresses and challenges. The negotiation of each of these transitions is an important milestone that allows the child and the family to proceed to the next level of development. Stresses and challenges that are commonly encountered during these transitions but not managed appropriately may result in negative influences on the child's developmental trajectory.

Important developmental stages are considered below. Risk factors and professional interventions that may be of assistance are outlined.

## Pregnancy and birth

The goal is to produce a healthy, full-term infant, together with a healthy mother who can cope with the inevitable stresses and change in lifestyle that comes with a newborn baby.

*Risk factors* include maternal factors such as physical and mental illness, substance abuse, smoking, inadequate folate intake, low maternal age, single parenthood and poverty. Infant risk factors include genetic defects, birth trauma and prematurity.

*Professional intervention.* Regular antenatal care enables early detection and intervention for maternal and fetal complications. During labour the presence of a supportive partner or friend has been shown to decrease time in labour and reduce complications. Early mother–baby contact facilitates breastfeeding and sets the stage for a positive mother–infant relationship. While in hospital it is important to establish links with postnatal services such as maternal and child nurses, general practitioners and home visiting services.

## Early infancy (0–6 months)

This is often a challenging time for the family. Parents and family aim to establish a routine incorporating the needs and demands of the new infant. Parents bring to this transaction their own beliefs and experiences, with varying levels of confidence and competence, and skills at handling stress, uncertainty and fatigue. Parents begin to understand their baby's visual, motor and verbal cues, and respond appropriately. This is the beginning of a reciprocal relationship or 'dance' that shapes the baby's brain development. If things do not go smoothly, and the mother perceives the infant as difficult and demanding, the long-term mother–child relationship can be compromised, setting the stage for possible future parenting and behaviour difficulties.

Establishing appropriate feeding patterns, preferably breastfeeding as this has many advantages, is another crucial task. Another important task is the introduction of solids, with many mothers beginning to think about weaning between 4 and 6 months of age.

*Risk factors* include maternal factors such as an unwanted child, prenatal complications, problems with bonding and attachment, maternal depression, social isolation, few or no identified supports, and a stressful family situation. Infant risk factors include difficult temperament, excessive crying and irritability, sleep problems and difficulty feeding.

*Professional intervention.* Providing support to parents is essential. Assisting parents with realistic expectations and understanding of their baby's developmental needs and linking them up with a network of family and professional supports are crucial interventions. Medication and frequent formula changes are usually inappropriate for sleeping and crying problems. Rather, parents need reassurance that their infant is healthy and does not have any underlying medical condition. They should aim to settle their infant with a consistent approach that enables the infant to fall asleep on his or her own rather than being held, rocked or fed to sleep. Some families find a routine of feeding the baby followed by a short play and then sleep helps. Mothers experiencing problems with breastfeeding should be managed by an experienced community nurse or lactation consultant. Sometimes there are early clues as to serious dysfunction, such as maternal depression or major difficulties in the mother–child relationship, so that more intensive intervention may be required. All parents need to learn how to manage the following inevitable issues:

- *Crying*. All infants cry. This is now understood to be a normal part of development. However, some infants are difficult to console and their crying causes major stress for parents. About 10% of infants cry for more than 3 hours per day, 3 or more days per week for 3 or more weeks. These infants are often labelled 'colicky'. Underlying medical causes for crying are uncommon (<5%) and include cow's milk protein allergy, lactose intolerance and possibly gastro-oesophageal reflux disease. Most crying abates by age 3–4 months, and crying persisting after this raises the possibility of organic illness or concerns in the mother–baby relationship.
- *Feeding*. Most mothers want to breastfeed their infant but not all mothers find breastfeeding easy. Problems with incorrect attachment to the breast are common and may lead to difficult and painful breastfeeding and early weaning.
- *Sleeping issues*. Most infants establish a sleep pattern after 3 months of age, although they may not begin to sleep through the night until 6 months. Common parental complaints include difficulties settling their infant and frequent night waking.

**Clinical example**

A mother presented with her 7-week-old baby boy. She said he was crying for 2–3 hours a day and appeared hungry. She was breastfeeding her baby every $1^1/_2$ hours and said she had no milk so she wanted to wean to formula. Her baby vomited a small amount after most feeds and her general practitioner had prescribed a medication for reflux. After a careful examination to exclude a physical cause of the crying, it was explained to her that all babies cry, and that crying reaches a peak around 6–7 weeks of age and then decreases by age 3–4 months. She was shown the PURPLE crying website (http://www.purplecrying.info/), which emphasizes that crying is part of normal development and that not all infant crying can be soothed. She was encouraged to keep breastfeeding and to space the feeds to every 2–3 hours so that her baby had a good feed and was not snack-feeding. Tiredness signs in babies were discussed, and strategies for settling her baby when he was tired were explained. She was asked to keep a feed/cry diary and to stop the reflux medication. Two weeks later, her baby was crying less and was settling to sleep better. He was feeding every 3 hours and seemed content.

### Late infancy (6–12 months)

This is a time of rapidly emerging cognitive, developmental and social competencies in the infant. The baby is interested in the environment and will very often initiate interaction with caregivers, wanting to play and to be stimulated in appropriate ways. Paradoxically, during this time the first signs of stranger anxiety and separation protest appear. The infant becomes anxious around strangers and is no longer willing to be picked up by an unfamiliar person. The infant also may become distressed when the parent is out of sight, for instance at bedtime or if left in the care of a babysitter or in childcare.

During this time, food issues become increasingly important, with most mothers completing weaning and moving towards a varied diet with regular meals.

*Risk factors* include maternal and family stress, inappropriate responses to increasing infant needs for stimulation and social interaction, difficulty changing from breast/bottle-feeding to a solid diet, and sleep difficulties.

*Professional intervention.* Continued support for parents, provision of accurate information about developmental and other needs of their rapidly developing infant, and ensuring that there is a 'goodness of fit' between the infant and his or her parents are essential. Parents should realize that much of their infant's behaviour is exploratory and that the infant is not being deliberately naughty. Sleep problems can be managed with behavioural interventions such as 'controlled crying', where parents leave their infant for increasing periods of time to enable them to fall asleep on their own, or 'camping out' whereby a parent gradually withdraws their presence from a baby's bedroom over a number of nights (see http://www.raisingchildren.net.au). Good eating habits can be established with regular mealtimes of a short duration (typically 20 minutes or less) and encouraging the older infant to finger-feed. Parents should offer a variety of foods, understanding that their infant may try a food many times before finally accepting it.

### Toddler period (1–3 years)

This is a major transition time, as the child moves from being an infant to being an active, curious toddler with an increasingly complex set of developmental competencies, including language. One of the normal developmental tasks in this age group is to develop autonomy and independence. Parents often perceive these 'terrible twos' as a challenging time when their child becomes oppositional and stubborn, seems always to be testing boundaries and likes to get his or her own way.

*Risk factors*, such as the child having a difficult temperament or the use of inconsistent or harsh parenting strategies, make these issues more likely.

#### Common problems in the toddler period

*Temper tantrums* are common, especially when the child is frustrated at being unable to master a task, or restrictions are placed on his or her autonomy. Sleep problems and problems around mealtimes also are very common. Most children will begin, and some will complete, toilet training during this time period, and this sometimes becomes a symbol of the struggle between the parents and the child regarding the child's autonomy. Signs of developmental delay, including language problems, may also become evident during this time period.

*Professional intervention.* The primary goal of intervention is to teach parents to understand their child better and to change maladaptive parenting strategies into consistent, warm and logical strategies. Parents also need to understand what is developmentally normal at this age. For example, temper tantrums can be managed by:

- staying calm
- walking away
- ignoring the behaviour until the tantrum stops
- praising the child when appropriate behaviour begins again.

Most tantrum behaviour will escalate initially and then will decline with this approach. For more aggressive behaviour, 'time out' may be used. This involves placing a child in a quiet room or corner for a maximum of 1 minute per year of age whenever the undesired behaviour occurs. The child is allowed out from the 'time out' place when he or she is quiet. This is effective in children over 18 months of age and its use should be limited to only the two or three most problematic behaviours.

## Preschool period (3–5 years)

During this period, there continues to be a rapid expansion in language, cognitive ability and social skills. Enriching early learning settings such as kindergarten allow the child's natural curiosity to be stimulated by systematic input from trained preschool teachers and by exposure to same-age peers. Language continues to develop rapidly, as do the child's cognitive ability and social–emotional skills.

*Risk factors* in children include language or other developmental delay, poor social skills, difficulty focusing attention, separation difficulties from parents and behaviour problems (especially aggression). Family risk factors include low maternal educational levels, poverty and being a single parent.

At the end of this period the child makes the very important and symbolic transition to school, so issues of school readiness become apparent. There is an emerging understanding that 'school readiness' is not a threshold of skills that a child needs to achieve in order to start school, but rather an assessment framework for better understanding the child's unique profiles of strengths and vulnerabilities, and risk and resilience factors. School readiness has the following three key dimensions:

- Children who are ready to learn
- Schools that are ready for children
- Parents and communities who are able to support the child's development.

Readiness to learn is further divided into five skill areas

- Health and physical development
- Emotional wellbeing and social competence
- Approaches to learning
- Communication skills
- Cognitive skills and general knowledge.

A number of tests assess school readiness but none is sufficient in isolation. The decision to send a child to school should be made by the parents, with input from those involved with the child, especially the preschool and primary teachers. The rate of maturation during the preschool period may be uneven and is certainly not linear. The child who appears 'immature' at the age of 4 years, for example, may mature rapidly during the following 6 months.

### Common problems presenting in preschool

*Hitting and biting* are common in the preschool setting. Occasional biting is usually experimental. Repeated hitting or biting may occur when a child is frustrated, stressed, or feels powerless. The key to management is identifying the cause of the frustration or stress (e.g. not wanting to share a toy) then removing, redirecting or distracting the child away from the cause. Parents should respond promptly and calmly, telling their child not to hit or bite when they remove the child from the situation. As for toddlers, 'time out' is also an effective strategy.

*Tantrums* are very common (see Toddler section above).

*Language delay* affects around 10% of preschool children (see Chapter 2.2). Causes include simple language delay (expressive and/or receptive), deafness, autism spectrum disorder, global developmental delay and social–emotional deprivation. Referral for a speech therapy assessment is recommended if a child uses fewer than 50 words at 2 years of age or has no two-word combinations at 2½ years of age, or does not understand simple instructions without gesture. Any child with a language delay needs to be referred for audiology testing to exclude hearing problems.

A delay in *toilet training* may be due to a global developmental delay or may reflect a toddler's 'battle' with parents as the toddler tries to establish autonomy. A programme of regular toileting together with frequent praise and rewards (e.g. stickers) will often achieve continence. Most children are toilet trained by 4 years of age.

*Professional intervention:* Parents of preschool children often seek professional help for concerns about language or developmental delay, behaviour problems, delayed toilet training, or questions about school readiness. Feedback to families about the results of assessments at this age needs to be cautious because of the great variability in maturation rates. Providing parents with information about realistic expectations in this age group and teaching basic skills in behaviour modification is often very helpful. Many problems are minor and are often transient, and simple, short-term interventions are often effective. However, in some children there are emerging signs of more serious problems, including developmental delay, communication problems, attention difficulties or more serious behaviour problems. These children may require vision and hearing testing, a speech assessment and, where an autism spectrum disorder is suspected, a multidisciplinary assessment.

## School years (over 5 years)

School is an important formative experience for all children. Children who have difficulty functioning at school, because of learning difficulties, attention or behaviour problems, or social difficulties, will almost always experience adverse outcomes beyond school. Children who struggle academically or socially have been shown to be at major risk in adolescence and later life for delinquency, unemployment and depression.

The early years of school are particularly important. Children who have difficulty reading from the outset and who are not established readers by the end of grade 2 are likely to continue to have problems throughout their school career.

*Risk factors* include chronic health problems, vision and hearing deficits, problems with concentration and subtle developmental weaknesses in the areas of motor function, visual–motor integration, temporal sequential organization (problems remembering the order of information) and language. Risk factors in the family include low parental education, low expectations of school achievement, parenting difficulties and other family dysfunction. Other risk factors include a poor match between the child's temperament and preferred style of learning, and classroom placement or teacher expectations and teaching style.

### Common problems presenting at school

*Attention difficulties* may manifest in many ways, including poor concentration, 'day-dreaming', quiet withdrawal or disruptive behaviour. Causes include attention-deficit/hyperactivity disorder (ADHD), learning difficulties, intellectual disability, language delay, absence seizures, hearing and vision problems, and depression/anxiety. Each of these can affect a child's learning. Treatment depends on the underlying cause and health professionals need to liaise with the child's teacher to ensure that the teacher understands the child's difficulties and how they may affect learning (see Chapter 4.3).

*Learning difficulties* occur when a child's academic achievement in areas such as reading, spelling, writing or mathematics is substantially below the level predicted by their intellectual abilities. Learning difficulties affect 10–15% of schoolchildren. Early recognition, diagnosis and remedial teaching are vital to ensure that the child does not lose confidence and become angry, depressed or frustrated. Children with learning difficulties should also have their vision (see Chapter 22.2) and hearing assessed and any problems treated so that their ability to learn in the classroom is optimized. Children with learning difficulties are unlikely to 'grow out of' their difficulties, so reassurances that the child will improve with maturity are usually inappropriate.

*Bullying* is the deliberate desire to hurt someone with words or actions. Children who are bullied may refuse to go to school, be very tense and unhappy after school, or show other signs of unhappiness such as difficulty sleeping. Children who bully may be physically punished at home and are more likely to grow up to hit their own partners and children. Managing bullying involves the whole school, with increased awareness, teaching students about conflict resolution and assertiveness training, peer counselling and improved adult supervision.

*Professional intervention.* It is important to identify school learning and behavioural difficulties as soon as possible so that appropriate interventions can be put in place. The longer this is delayed, the greater the chance of a poor outcome. Assessment should involve close evaluation of biological, developmental, behavioural and environmental factors that may be contributing to problems. Hearing and vision should be assessed. Often in this age group a multidisciplinary evaluation that includes a special educational assessment is the most appropriate. Where possible, a child should be referred to an educational psychologist for formal cognitive testing, including tests of intelligence. A detailed and comprehensive assessment will often point to the need for specific developmental and educational interventions that address the individual needs of the child. These may include remedial classes at school and/or tutoring outside school.

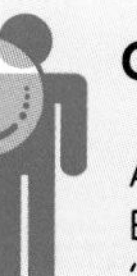

**Clinical example**

A mother presented with her 8-year-old son, Ed. His teachers had complained that he was 'mucking around' in class and was disruptive. He had problems with spelling and writing. His father had had similar problems at school and left in year 10. His mother said that Ed was fine at home and tended to play computer games or ride his bike. He was noted to be quiet during the consultation and he said he had few friends at school. His vision and hearing were assessed and they were normal. A neurodevelopmental assessment was performed, which revealed weaknesses in auditory sequencing and language processing. The school psychologist performed a cognitive assessment, which revealed that Ed had normal intelligence but a specific learning difficulty involving reading, writing and spelling. This was discussed with his teachers, who arranged remedial teaching and more computer time for Ed's class work.

## Adolescence

Adolescence is a time of immense change (see Chapter 3.11). The young person needs to adjust to physical and emotional change, acquire an appropriate gender role, join peer groups, become emotionally independent of parents and other adults, and prepare for career and relationships in life. Although most adolescents negotiate this period successfully, up to one in five will experience significant physical or emotional problems. Adolescents often experiment with drugs, alcohol and cigarettes, and nicotine addiction usually begins in adolescence.

*Risk factors* include chronic health problems, learning disability, social isolation, parental physical or mental illness, and family dysfunction.

*Professional intervention.* Health professionals need to address the concerns of the young person as well as the parents. Clarifying the professional obligation of confidentiality at the start of a consultation will reassure and facilitate rapport. In addition to addressing specific problems, screening questionnaires that encompass home, school, recreation, drug use, sexual activity and suicide/depression issues enable a full picture of the adolescent to emerge (see Chapter 3.11). Parents need to know what is normal during adolescence and be given effective strategies for both communicating with their adolescent and managing common problems.

## Conclusion

Development, the progression from a newborn to a socially, physically and intellectually competent adult, involves a complex interplay of genes and environmental influences. Helping parents to understand the normal life events, developmental stages and transition points in a child's life can help promote optimal developmental outcomes for their child.

# 4.2 Common mental health problems

Michael Sawyer, Brian Graetz

Child and adolescent mental health problems are common in the community. They have a significant impact on the lives of children and parents, and also impose a substantial financial burden on families and communities. In Australia, the National Survey of Mental Health and Wellbeing estimated that 14% of children and adolescents experience significant mental health problems (Table 4.2.1). Adolescents with mental health problems frequently exhibit other health risk behaviours, including smoking, drinking and drug abuse (see Chapter 3.11). They also report much higher rates of suicidal ideation and behaviour than other adolescents in the community. A minority of children and adolescents with mental health problems receive professional help.

This chapter describes common mental health problems experienced by children (for brevity, the term 'children' will be used to refer to children and adolescents). It also describes practical steps that can be taken to help children, parents and families. The chapter is divided into three components. The first describes the features of common mental health problems, the second describes general approaches to the assessment and management of these problems, and the third provides information about some specific problems experienced by children.

## Features of mental health problems

Two approaches are used to describe childhood mental health problems. One approach views childhood problems as lying on a continuum from those with very few problems to those with a large number of problems. Children identified as having a very large number of problems are considered to fall in the 'clinical range' of the continuum and to be in need of help. Typically, problems are divided into two broad groups called externalizing problems and internalizing problems.

Externalizing problems include over-activity, aggressive and antisocial behaviour. Internalizing problems include anxiety, depression and shyness. Questionnaires completed by children, parents and teachers can be used to assess the level of problems experienced by children. When a continuum approach is used, it is possible to compare the number of problems reported for an individual child with the number typically reported for others of the same age and sex in the community. It is also possible to assess treatment effectiveness by evaluating whether there is a reduction in problems.

The second approach divides childhood mental health problems into a range of different mental disorders. Each mental disorder consists of a different group of symptoms. There are two main diagnostic classification systems that identify these symptom groups. One is the International Classification of Diseases developed by the World Health Organization (ICD-10), and the other is the *Diagnostic and Statistical Manual* developed by the American Psychiatric Association (DSM-IV; Table 4.2.2). This categorical approach is used widely in mental health services to describe children's problems. A common feature of both of these approaches is their focus on observable features of children's problems rather than on their presumed aetiology. This has facilitated a broad investigation of the aetiology of children's problems during the last three decades. Both the DSM and ICD classification systems are currently being revised, with DSM-V scheduled for release in 2013.

### Features of internalizing problems

Many children experience anxiety or sadness. However, when these problems are severe, persist over time, and are associated with significant problems with daily functioning, they may indicate the presence of a mental disorder and the need for professional help. Children with high levels of internalizing problems should be assessed for the presence of depressive disorders or anxiety disorders, and for the presence of suicidal ideation.

Children with depressive disorders feel sad, lack interest in activities they previously enjoyed, criticize themselves, and are pessimistic or hopeless about the future. DSM-IV identifies two types of depressive disorder. *Major depressive disorder* consists of acute episodes of depressed mood, loss of interest and pleasure in activities, reduced appetite, sleep disturbance, low energy, low self-esteem, poor concentration and feelings of hopelessness. Children with *dysthymic disorder* will experience similar problems,

**Table 4.2.1 Prevalence of mental health problems among children and adolescents aged 4–17 years in Australia**

| Child Behaviour Checklist Scale | Prevalence (%)* |
|---|---|
| **General areas** | |
| Total problems | 14.1 |
| All externalizing problems | 12.9 |
| All internalizing problems | 12.8 |
| **Specific areas** | |
| Somatic complaints | 7.3 |
| Delinquent behaviour | 7.1 |
| Attention problems | 6.1 |
| Aggressive behaviour | 5.2 |
| Social problems | 4.6 |
| Withdrawn | 4.3 |
| Anxious/depression | 3.5 |
| Thought problems | 3.1 |

Problem areas are not mutually exclusive, and thus 'Total problems' does not equal the sum of externalizing and internalizing problems.
*Percentage of children scoring in the clinical range on the Child Behaviour Checklist Scales in Sawyer MG, Arney FM, Baghurst PA et al 2000 Child and Adolescent Component of the Australian National Survey of Mental Health and Wellbeing. Commonwealth Department of Health and Aged Care, Canberra.

**Table 4.2.2 Important DSM-IV disorders among children and adolescents**

| DSM-IV category | Specific disorders |
|---|---|
| Disruptive behaviour disorders | Attention-deficit/hyperactivity disorder<br>Conduct disorder |
| Mood disorders | Major depressive disorder<br>Dysthymic disorder<br>Bipolar disorder |
| Anxiety disorders | Separation anxiety disorder<br>Social phobia<br>Obsessive–compulsive disorder<br>Post-traumatic stress disorder |
| Learning disorders | Reading disorders<br>Written expression disorders |
| Pervasive developmental disorders | Autistic spectrum disorders |
| Elimination disorders | Enuresis<br>Encopresis |

with the distinction being that their symptoms are less severe but more chronic. Children experiencing depression may think that life is not worth living and they may contemplate suicide. It is essential that all children exhibiting depressive symptoms be carefully evaluated for suicidal risk (see Chapter 4.4).

Fear and anxiety are common to the human condition, but some children experience anxiety that is well beyond that which occurs during normal development. These children suffer personal distress and their anxiety interferes with their daily functioning. Children with anxiety disorders exhibit physiological symptoms (e.g. tremors, sweating and palpitations), maladaptive behaviours (e.g. avoidance of feared situations) and maladaptive thinking (e.g. 'I cannot talk in front of the class because people will think I'm stupid').

DSM-IV identifies a number of different types of anxiety disorder. One of the most common among children is *separation anxiety disorder*, which is defined as excessive and developmentally inappropriate anxiety regarding separation from home or from major attachment figures. Separation anxiety disorder is a common cause of persistent school refusal.

*Obsessive–compulsive disorder* is characterized by obsessions (persistent thoughts, impulses or images that are intrusive and distressing) and compulsions (repetitive behaviours or mental acts employed to reduce anxiety or distress). This disorder causes considerable distress for children and parents. It is important for medical practitioners to be familiar with the typical symptoms of this disorder, because effective interventions are available to provide help. These include both psychotropic medications and behavioural treatments.

*Social phobia*, which typically begins during the teenage years, comprises fear of social or performance situations in which embarrassment can occur. This condition can adversely affect the development of social skills and can also hinder academic progress at school. Adolescents with this disorder may be reluctant to attend professional services because of their insecurity and fear of social embarrassment.

## Features of externalizing problems

Externalizing problems refer to problems such as temper tantrums, aggressive behaviour, stealing and truancy. Boys are more frequently identified as having externalizing problems than girls. Problems in this area, particularly those involving aggressive behaviour, can persist over long periods of time. For example, infants with a difficult temperament may exhibit oppositional and defiant behaviour as preschoolers, and may subsequently develop behavioural disorders during later primary school or high school.

Two common mental disorders in this area are *conduct disorder* and *attention-deficit/hyperactivity disorder (ADHD)*. The typical behaviour of those with conduct disorder includes bullying, frequent physical fights, deliberate destruction of other people's property, breaking into houses or cars, staying out late at night despite parental prohibitions, running away from home and frequent truancy from school.

ADHD is defined as a persistent pattern of inattentive behaviour and/or hyperactivity/impulsivity that is more frequent and severe than is typically observed in individuals of the same age. Children with inattentive behaviour problems make careless mistakes with schoolwork, find it hard to persist with tasks and are distracted easily. Those with problems in the area of hyperactivity/impulsivity often fidget and talk excessively, interrupt others, and are described as constantly being 'on the go' (see Chapter 4.3).

Young people attending clinical services often have co-morbid conditions. For example, children with behavioural problems may also have problems with anxiety or depression.

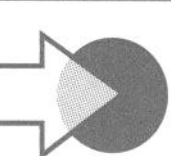

### Practical points

**Assessment of mental health problems**

- Careful assessment is essential before initiating any treatment programme for mental health problems.
- Assessment requires knowledge and understanding of children's presenting problems, developmental history, family and social environment.
- Information must be obtained from multiple informants (children, parents and teachers).
- Aetiological factors can be divided into predisposing, precipitating, perpetuating or protective factors.

## Assessment and management of mental health problems

### Assessment

The onset of childhood disorders is usually due to the combined influence of several biological, psychological and social factors. A careful assessment of children's problems and the factors giving rise to their onset is an essential prerequisite to effective treatment. This should include information about the child's current problems, a developmental history, and relevant information about the child's family and social environment. It is important to develop a clear understanding of the nature of a child's presenting problems and the factors that have given rise to these problems. One way of organizing these factors is shown below:

- Predisposing factors
- Precipitating factors
- Perpetuating factors
- Protecting factors.

Information about children's problems should be obtained from children, parents and teachers. Children are the key source of information about their internal state, including their experience of subjective feelings such as anxiety and depression. Parents can provide information about more readily observed behaviour such as sibling conflict or school refusal, and are an important source of information about the child's early development and the chronicity and severity of the problems. Teachers can report on academic progress and peer relationships. The assessment and treatment of ADHD relies heavily on reports from teachers.

### Clinical example

Peter, a 12-year-old boy, lived with his single mother. Peter's mother had a history of depression and his father had been treated for alcohol abuse. Peter's mother sought advice about how to manage his defiant and aggressive behaviour. She said that, from the time he was born, she had struggled to cope with Peter's difficult temperament and behaviour. This problem had greatly worsened since she divorced Peter's father last year. Since the divorce Peter had had little recent contact with his father and he was suspended from school on one occasion after damaging property in the school science centre. Peter's teacher described him as being easily distracted and impulsive during the past year. Despite these problems, Peter had continued to maintain satisfactory academic progress and his teacher believed that Peter's intelligence was above average.

The following factors were important in this problem:

- Predisposing factor: family history of psychiatric disorder
- Precipitating factor: divorce of parents
- Perpetuating factor: rejection by father
- Protecting factor: child's intelligence.

### Management

To manage childhood mental disorders effectively it is necessary to address as many relevant biological, psychological and social factors as possible that are giving rise to their onset and persistence. Many disorders persist over long periods of time (e.g. ADHD) or tend to recur (e.g. major depressive disorder). In the light of this, the development of long-term management plans for these disorders is important. The development of such plans requires consideration of several key issues.

Firstly, it is important to recognize that specific interventions are now available for many disorders. Medical practitioners need to be familiar with these interventions and to avoid 'one size fits all' methods of counselling. Secondly, the management of children's problems often involves the use of a combination of biological (e.g. psychotropic medications), psychological (e.g. cognitive–behavioural therapy) and social interventions (e.g. peer relationship programmes). Finally, the management of children's problems requires the cooperation of children, parents and teachers. It is important to involve all of these groups when treating children with mental health problems.

Psychological interventions available to help those with mental disorders include:

- Individual psychotherapy, which focuses on helping children
- Family therapy, which focuses on relationships between all family members
- Behaviour modification, which focuses on the antecedents and consequences of children's behaviour
- Cognitive therapy to address maladaptive thinking styles.

Recent reviews have drawn attention to the importance of implementing these interventions correctly. It appears that failure to do this may explain why their effectiveness, when delivered in clinic settings, is often less than that achieved in the university or research environments where they were developed.

A wide range of medications is used to treat children with mental disorders. However, although many of these medications have the potential to provide help, evidence of their effectiveness is often based on studies of adults. There has been particular concern with antidepressant medications, which appear less effective for treating children and adolescents than for adults. Several national authorities have advised medical practitioners to be cautious when using antidepressant medications with children and adolescents, because they increase the risk of suicidal thinking.

When psychotropic medications are used to help children, very clear treatment goals should be identified, along with careful monitoring of effectiveness and adverse effects. Pharmacological treatment should always be used as part of a broader management plan developed in conjunction with children and parents. Only one psychotropic medication should be prescribed at a time. If a medication is ineffective after an appropriate trial, an alternative may be selected. Only after consultation with a child psychiatrist or paediatrician experienced in paediatric psychopharmacology should multiple psychotropic medications be used concurrently to treat a child with a mental disorder.

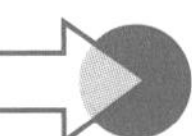

**Practical points**

**Treatment of mental health problems**

- Treatment plans need to be individualized.
- It is important to obtain cooperation from children, parents and teachers.
- Psychological interventions should generally be employed before the use of medication.
- In general, only medical practitioners with specialist knowledge should initiate treatment of child and adolescent mental health disorders with psychotropic medications.

## Problems of infancy

Infant mental health is a rapidly developing field. Debates about nature versus nurture have been superseded by interactional models that link the styles of parenting to an infant's psychological and physical health, developmental maturity and evolving personality. This is set in a cultural and extended family context. Attachment theory describes the relationships that occur between infants and parents. There is increasing evidence that these interactional styles, already measurable by 12 months of age, predict children's interactional patterns later in life.

Recent work has also shown that early experiences have a measurable effect on infant's brains. It is believed that tract and synapse development is significantly conditioned by the style of parenting. An infant's brain has the potential to develop and mature, and this potential can best be achieved by parenting that is attuned to the needs of the infant. Thus, appropriate parenting in which love and limits are evident, along with a focus on helping with developmental stages, is likely to promote neural tract development.

It is known that a wide range of parent and infant issues can interfere with optimal parenting. These include postnatal depression and anxiety, troubled marital relationships, and compromised role models of parenting and prematurity. Physical or emotional abuse has particular and longlasting consequences. A growing number of interventions are being developed to address these problems in the early years. There is also a growing body of knowledge about the benefits of early (e.g. antenatal) identification of parent risk factors, and the potential for health promotion and early intervention at this early stage of an infant's development.

## Special issues

### Suicidal ideation and behaviour

All suicide attempts should be treated seriously. Although suicidal ideation and behaviour are relatively rare before the age of 12 years, they become more frequent during adolescence (see Chapter 3.11). In the Child and Adolescent Component of the Australian National Survey of Mental Health and Wellbeing, 4% of adolescents reported a suicide attempt in the previous 12 months. Furthermore, adolescents with more emotional and behavioural problems reported substantially more suicidal ideation and behaviour (Fig. 4.2.1). Completed suicide is less common. Adolescent males have higher rates than females (9–10 per 100 000 annually for males, compared with 3–5 per 100 000 for females).

Suicidal ideation and behaviour is often associated with symptoms of a depressive disorder along with a history of abuse of alcohol or other drugs. Many young people who attempt suicide live in families where there is a high level of interpersonal conflict and where parents have a history of mental disorder or drug and alcohol abuse. As well as a history of chronic adversity, many young people report an immediate precipitant to their suicide attempt. This may involve an argument over parental or school discipline, or a difficulty in a relationship with a friend.

All children who report thoughts of suicide or who attempt suicide should be assessed carefully. This should include assessment of the mental state of the child and the seriousness of the suicidal attempt. Characteristics that suggest that a suicide attempt was serious include:

- Family history of suicide attempts
- Previous history of suicide attempts
- Presence of a mental disorder (e.g. major depressive disorder)
- Evidence of premeditation and planning
- An expectation by the young person that the attempt would result in death
- A suicide attempt made while alone or isolated
- Precautions taken to make discovery unlikely during or after the suicide attempt.

During the period of time that a young person remains at high risk for suicide, it is important that they be in a safe environment where their behaviour can be monitored. During this time their mental status should be assessed and help provided to address personal or family problems. In some circumstances, such as when a young person has a serious mental disorder or where they have no secure place of residence, it is necessary to arrange hospital admission.

It is important to provide appropriate treatment for depressive disorders experienced by young people who make suicide attempts. This should include the use of specific counselling techniques such as cognitive–behavioural therapy and, where appropriate, the use of antidepressant medication. Every effort should be made to reduce the impact of ongoing stressors, such as family conflict, that may precipitate further suicide attempts. When appropriate treatment methods are employed, a high rate of recovery can be achieved. However, major depressive disorder often recurs, and it is important that young people and their parents are advised of the continuing risk of further episodes and the symptoms that may signal the onset of a recurrence.

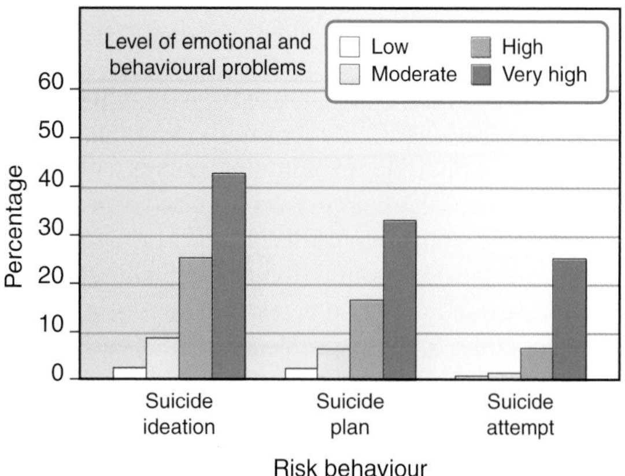


Fig. 4.2.1 Suicide ideation and suicidal behaviour.

### Attention-deficit/hyperactivity disorder

This is covered in Chapter 4.3.

### School refusal due to anxiety problems

A small number of children exhibit high levels of distress when they first commence school, and this may be associated with temper tantrums, excessive fearfulness and complaints of somatic symptoms (e.g. stomach aches or headaches) for which no biological cause can be identified. In some children, this pattern persists and it may give rise to a situation where children do not attend school for long periods of time. School refusal adversely affects these children in two ways. Firstly, they are at increased risk of receiving an inadequate education. Secondly, they miss out on important socializing experiences. As a result, they may enter later life lacking important social skills. For these reasons, school refusal is a very serious problem that requires urgent and effective management. Often, it will be necessary to provide help to children and parents over long periods of time.

Among younger children who refuse to attend school there may be a history of separation anxiety disorder. Children with this disorder have a history of anxiety when separated from their primary caregiver, may insist on sleeping in their parents' bedroom at night, and may refuse to stay overnight with friends. In primary school, the children will describe their fear of separation from parents, describe worrying at school about their parents, and may be excessively anxious if their parents are late to collect them from school. They may also express fear of punishment from teachers or concern about bullying by peers.

Adolescents who refuse to attend school may be suffering from social phobia. Adolescents with this condition experience marked fear of social or performance situations. As a result, they are reluctant to attend school where they have to mix socially with peers and demonstrate adequate academic progress.

Assessment should be initially broad-based and aimed at understanding the cause of children's problems. A developmental history should be obtained with a particular focus on symptoms of anxiety. Information should be obtained about the child's environment both at home and at school. This should include information about family functioning, the classroom and school environment, and peer relationships. It is important to determine whether bullying by peers at school is a significant precipitant or perpetuating factor for school refusal, and to be aware that it can take multiple forms (e.g. verbal, physical, social, psychological or cyber bullying). It is essential that contact be made with children's teachers to obtain information about these last issues, with parents being encouraged to raise any concerns about bullying with school staff. Information should also be obtained about the severity, duration and pervasiveness of school non-attendance, noting possible antecedents of the problem and consequences that may be responsible for maintaining the behaviour.

A number of specific approaches can be used to help children with school refusal due to anxiety problems. Implementing these requires the combined efforts of children, parents and teachers. Children need help to manage their anxiety better. This should include the use of techniques such as:

- Relaxation training
- Systematic desensitization
- Cognitive restructuring
- Shaping and contingency management
- Life skills training.

Parents need to be taught how they can manage children's temper tantrums and how to help children who report somatic complaints. In two-parent families, it is important that both parents participate in treatment programmes. In situations of chronic school refusal, assessing the significance of children's somatic complaints can be helped by close liaison with a general practitioner, who can quickly assess a child and advise parents whether the presence of a physical illness precludes school attendance. This support can reduce the pressure on parents, who must decide whether or not to allow their child to miss further schooling. Where there is no evidence of a physical illness, every effort should be made to ensure that children return to school at the earliest possible opportunity. Teachers can play a vital role supporting the child's return to school after an absence and helping to reduce anxiety at school due to bullying or performance pressure.

## Enuresis and encopresis

### Nocturnal enuresis

Although most children have achieved bladder control by the age of 5 years, a significant number continue to have problems with nocturnal enuresis. This is embarrassing for children and is a burden for their parents.

In the absence of physical causes, such as a urinary tract infection, nocturnal enuresis is generally not a serious problem. Indeed, it may simply reflect normal variation in the development of bladder control, where there is a familial tendency to later maturation of bladder control. Discussing this familial pattern with parents may help them better understand the nature of their child's problem. Exposure to stressful events may also induce children with previously good bladder control to recommence bed-wetting.

For younger children, management consists of reassurance and the establishment of a convenient pattern of hygienic care of bed and clothing. Simple procedures such as fluid restriction at night or getting children to empty their bladder when the parents are ready to retire may help. Incentive systems can be put in place to assist children's motivation to remain dry. One method is to reward children for achieving a given number of consecutive dry nights, with the number of nights gradually extended over time.

For more persistent cases of bed-wetting, an enuresis alarm has been shown to be an effective treatment in the majority of cases. The alarm consists of a detector mat placed on a child's mattress. The mat is connected to an alarm and when the child begins to urinate during sleep, a circuit is completed and the alarm sounds. The procedure (often called a 'bell and pad') uses simple conditioning rules to train children to achieve better bladder control. Many children's hospitals or chemists have such devices available for hire. However, it is important to ensure that the mat and alarm both function properly, or they will not condition children to achieve better bladder control. Children who are not easily awoken by the alarm will initially require parental assistance to finish voiding in the toilet. This is important in ensuring that the conditioning treatment achieves success.

In recent years, desmopressin has been used as a short-term treatment for children with nocturnal enuresis. It is administered orally or as a nasal spray and acts to decrease urine production at night. Studies report varying success rates but relapse is high and side-effects such as headache and abdominal pain have been noted. A Food and Drug Administration warning about the risk of hyponatraemic seizures should be noted (http://www.fda.gov/Drugs/DrugSafety/PostmarketDrugSafetyInformationforPatientsandProviders/ucm125561.htm). Tricyclic antidepressants such as imipramine should no longer be used to treat enuresis because of high relapse rates, possible cardiac adverse effects, and the risk of severe morbidity or even death from overdose.

## Encopresis

Encopresis affects between 2% and 8% of primary school children. It is more common among boys and a high proportion of children with encopresis have concomitant constipation. The problem is distressing for children and may be associated with conflict between parents and children. Several types of encopresis have been described:

- Constipation with overflow
- Failed toilet training
- Toilet phobia
- Stress-induced loss of control
- Provocative soiling.

Considerable overlap occurs between these different types of encopresis. However, the descriptions provide a general indication of the types of issue that must be considered when assessing children with encopresis. Before treatment is commenced, it is important to identify the causes of the child's encopresis. This should include a physical examination to identify whether the child has constipation.

There are three elements to the treatment of encopresis. Firstly, it is important to treat constipation when this is present. This can generally be achieved through the use of laxatives or microenemas. Less commonly, it will be necessary to employ a bowel washout. Secondly, it is important to ensure that the diet contains adequate fibre to reduce the likelihood of future constipation. Finally, it is important to establish a routine of regular toilet use, which can be difficult with children. There may be a history of conflict between parents and children about toilet use. Children may also be unclear about the linkage between irregular toilet use and encopresis, particularly if previous interventions have focused largely on punishing children who soil their clothes. Children may also be upset or embarrassed by their problem and may refuse to participate in treatment programmes.

It is important to ensure that children understand why they are experiencing constipation and soiling. A simple schematic diagram showing the key features of the gastrointestinal system can be used to help children understand the nature of their problem. Children need to understand that constipation occurs when there is a build up of faeces because of a failure to empty the bowel regularly. Once they understand this, it is easier to work with them to plan a programme of regular toilet use.

Small rewards given after each use of the toilet can be helpful with young children. In children with toilet phobia, rewards may be given initially for simply sitting on the toilet for a few minutes, progressing to rewards provided when the child empties their bowel in the toilet. To achieve maximum effect, rewards need to be given immediately after children use the toilet, they need to be inexpensive (because of the need to reward each use of the toilet) and must be given consistently when the child uses the toilet. Jointly identifying appropriate rewards can be used to build a therapeutic alliance with children and encourage their cooperation with the treatment programme. Seeking children's active involvement in treatment planning can also be used to reduce the conflict between children and their parents, with the latter taking on a more supportive and advisory role.

# 4.3 Hyperactivity and inattention

Jill Sewell

Hyperactive and inattentive behaviours are common in children, ranging in a continuum from normal behaviours, especially in young children, to developmentally inappropriate behaviours that impair daily activities at home and at school.

Developmentally inappropriate levels of hyperactivity and inattention may be the result of many factors, both intrinsic and environmental. These risk factors (Box 4.3.1) must all be considered in the assessment of children with difficult behaviour, especially when considering the diagnosis of attention-deficit/hyperactivity disorder (ADHD).

## Definition of attention-deficit/ hyperactivity disorder

ADHD is considered to be a developmental disorder of self-regulation, characterized by inattention and hyperactivity/impulsivity. The underlying neurobiological pathway involves the frontal–striatal–cerebellar networks, with deficits occurring in executive functioning, particularly response inhibition, vigilance, working memory and planning.

The diagnosis of ADHD is made using DSM-IV criteria. It is a descriptive diagnosis without implying cause, as it is not a discrete entity and has multiple causes. There must be developmentally inappropriate symptoms of inattention (Box 4.3.2) and/or hyperactivity/impulsivity (Box 4.3.3) with onset before 7 years of age, impairing social, academic or occupational functioning across multiple settings, and these symptoms are not a result of pervasive developmental disorder, psychosis or severe emotional disorders. Subtypes include mainly inattentive, mainly hyperactive or combined.

ADHD is common. The prevalence in the school-aged population generally is considered to be 3–5%. Boys are affected more commonly, particularly with hyperactivity. There is a higher incidence in disrupted families and in those with low incomes, again particularly with hyperactivity. There is a strong genetic factor, with about 30% of siblings, 25% of parents and 80% of identical twins affected. Molecular genetic studies have focused on chromosomes that regulate dopamine, the neurotransmitter most associated with learning, motivation, goals and movement, and noradrenaline (norepinephrine), involved in maintaining alertness and attention, particularly with novel stimuli. Two candidate genes, the dopamine transporter and dopamine receptor genes, are reported to be associated with ADHD.

**Clinical example**

Sammy, aged 6 years, was in his second year of school. His teacher complained that he never sat still, did not complete tasks, talked too much, interrupted, and was well behind with reading.

His mother recalled that he had been 'on the go' since about 2 years of age, always preferred playing outdoors rather than settling to games inside, never seemed to remember instructions or the house rules, and acted without thinking about the consequences. He hated homework and 'often forgot' to bring home his school reader.

Sammy's problems are consistent with a diagnosis of ADHD and learning difficulties. Stimulant medication and consistent structure at home and at school helped his behavioural symptoms, but he also required educational assessment and specific reading support in the classroom.

Many children with ADHD have associated neurodevelopmental or mental health problems (co-morbidities) (Box 4.3.4). Because of overlapping features, separation into these diagnostic categories is complex; however, it is helpful when completing a descriptive assessment and recommending specific management programmes.

## Assessment

The assessment of children for ADHD with its multiple risk factors and co-morbidities requires skilled interpretation of information from the child, family and teachers. Relevant factors include:

- medical
- developmental
- family history
- family, social and cultural environment
- the school setting
- academic progress
- socialization skills.

**Box 4.3.1 Risk factors for hyperactivity and inattention**

- Difficult temperament
- Poor parenting skills
- Family dysfunction
- Child abuse, particularly deprivation
- Developmental delay
- Language disorders
- Learning difficulties
- Anxiety/mood disorders
- Sleep disorders
- Medical conditions, e.g.
  - very low birth weight or small for gestational age
  - fetal alcohol syndrome
  - prenatal exposure to smoking and stress
  - lead poisoning
  - acquired brain syndrome (head injury)
  - chromosomal abnormalities (e.g. fragile X, velocardiofacial syndrome)
  - food intolerance (rare)

**Box 4.3.2 DSM-IV: Symptoms of inattention**

- Poor attention to detail, careless mistakes
- Difficulty sustaining attention
- Seems not to listen
- Seems not to follow through
- Difficulty with organization
- Avoids tasks requiring sustained attention
- Loses things
- Easily distracted
- Forgetful

**Box 4.3.3 DSM-IV: Symptoms of hyperactivity/impulsivity**

- Fidgets
- Often leaves seat
- Runs, climbs excessively
- Difficulty playing quietly
- 'On the go'
- Talks excessively
- Blurts out answers
- Difficulty awaiting turn
- Interrupts others

**Box 4.3.4 Co-morbidities with attention-deficit/hyperactivity disorder**

- Learning difficulties (10–30%)
- Language disorder (30–50%)
- Oppositional defiant disorder (30–50%)
- Conduct disorder (16–20%)
- Anxiety, mood disorders
- Developmental coordination disorder
- Tics, Tourette syndrome

General family functioning, behavioural patterns over time, antecedents and consequences of behaviours, and family and school management of behaviours must be understood. Standardized behavioural rating scales completed by parents, teachers and adolescents help to put the behaviours into a normal community context. Thorough physical examination helps to exclude the rare associated medical conditions. Neurodevelopmental assessment provides information on motor skills and auditory and visual processing. Many children require formal assessment of auditory, cognitive, language and educational function. Neuroimaging, quantitative electroencephalography and neurophysiological tests, for example of continuous performance, are research tools only at this stage and are not yet ready for use in clinical diagnosis.

The diagnosis of ADHD can be made only against a thorough understanding of normal patterns of development and behaviour. This is particularly important when considering the diagnosis in a preschool-aged child, with wide variations expected in normal behaviour, development and temperament, and vulnerability to adverse family and social circumstances.

**Clinical example**

Byron, aged 3½ years, was extremely active, aggressive and oppositional, and had a mild language delay. Recently, his mother had separated from Byron's father and begun a new relationship. The family had moved several times and had been involved with a number of family support agencies. His mother wanted Byron to go on stimulant medication, like his older half-brother.

Byron was diagnosed with oppositional defiant disorder and language delay, in the context of a dysfunctional but committed family. He could also have been diagnosed with ADHD on DSM-IV criteria, but such a diagnosis at this age might be misleading and could shift focus away from the critical issue of effective family support.

## Management

ADHD is a chronic condition requiring long-term management based on partnership with the child, the family and the child's teachers from year to year. Counselling on the nature, causes, risk factors and course of ADHD, setting realistic expectations in the light of such understanding, and making accommodations at home and at school will help the child maintain confidence and self-esteem.

Multimodal management includes:

- Stimulant medication
- Parental behaviour management
- Classroom behaviour management
- Management of co-morbidities, e.g.
  - special education support for learning difficulties
  - treatment of anxiety, depression
- Structured parenting programmes, parent support groups.

## Stimulant medication

Stimulant medications, which increase dopamine levels in the brain (methylphenidate and dexamfetamine), are the most effective treatments for ADHD and improve target symptoms in about 75% of children with the condition. Improved concentration and decreased hyperactivity, impulsivity and distractibility lead to enhanced task completion, academic progress and social interaction, sustained over time.

These medications are safe and have a low profile of adverse effects, which either subside spontaneously within the first 2–3 weeks of treatment or can be managed by altering the dose or timing of medication. Insomnia, appetite suppression and headache can be troublesome in some children. There is some evidence that height growth may be suppressed initially, particularly with younger children and with higher doses, and growth must therefore be monitored carefully.

Extended-release preparations of methylphenidate enable morning-only dosage. Atomoxetine, a noradrenergic reuptake inhibitor, is used in those intolerant of stimulant medication.

There is considerable community concern that too many children are taking stimulants and other psychotropic drugs, with over-diagnosis and medicalization of social problems. There is community concern also about a perceived risk of psychological dependence on drugs instead of developing self-responsibility. The reality is that ADHD is a developmental disorder with significant long-term risk factors in educational, social and vocational outcomes, and only 2% of school-aged children in Australia have been prescribed stimulant medication, despite the prevalence of ADHD of at least 3–5%. There is very good scientific evidence for the long-term safety of these drugs. There is also clear evidence that effective treatment with stimulants of adolescents with ADHD protects against substance abuse.

Medication treatment is only one of the treatment modalities for ADHD. It is also critically important for health professionals to advocate community services and family support for children who are at risk for adverse developmental, behavioural and social outcomes, whether or not they have ADHD.

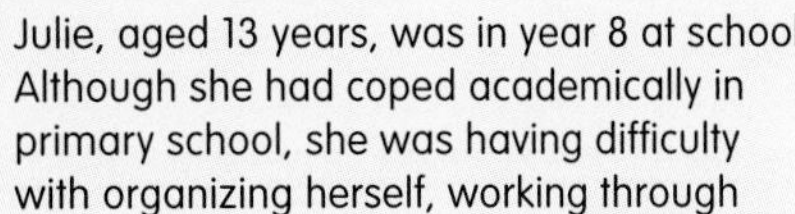

**Clinical example**

Julie, aged 13 years, was in year 8 at school. Although she had coped academically in primary school, she was having difficulty with organizing herself, working through assignments and getting homework completed on time. Her written work was messy, she was distracted easily and she daydreamed in the classroom. She was worried that she would not do well enough at school to go to university.

Julie's assessment indicated long-term problems with attention, distractibility and impulsivity. She commenced stimulant medication for her ADHD (inattentive type) and developed better organization, task completion and interest in work, and neater handwriting. She began to feel that she was much closer to reaching her academic potential.

## Behaviour management

Behaviour management programmes use a structured setting to promote behavioural control, reinforcing appropriate behaviours and reducing negative behaviours with specific strategies. Emphasis should be on antecedent support and control, rather than on consequences (i.e. anticipation of the difficulties and plan/teach to avoid) (Box 4.3.5).

In the classroom, additional techniques include seating the child close to the teacher, breaking tasks down into small units, frequent exercise breaks (preferably productive and responsible, such as taking a message to the office), structured teaching materials adapted to the child's needs, and unrelenting positive encouragement.

Behavioural therapies are particularly important when conditions such as persistent oppositional behaviour and parent–child discord coexist with ADHD.

## Alternative/complementary therapies

A small number of children react to synthetic food colours with severe irritability and restlessness. These children, who are very few in number, are helped by

**Box 4.3.5 Behavioural strategies**

**To reinforce**: 'catch 'em being good'; use verbal praise and concrete rewards

- Teach listening skills
- Teach problem-solving skills (e.g. 'game plan')

**To reduce**: ignore unwanted behaviours

- 'Act, don't speak' (i.e. clear discipline with minimal reprimands and discussion)
- Logical consequences

dietary restriction. There is no evidence that a sugar-free diet, megavitamins, sensory integration training or neuro-feedback are of therapeutic benefit.

## Outcome

Hyperactivity tends to diminish in adolescence, although physical restlessness may continue. Inattention, impulsivity and distractibility can continue into adulthood, although self-awareness and self-regulation improve with developmental, cognitive and emotional maturation. Co-morbidities, such as learning difficulties, subtle language disorders and conduct disorders, and associated risk factors, such as family dysfunction and poor educational opportunity, can contribute to adverse outcomes, including poor school retention, a limited vocational outlook, and risk-taking behaviours in adolescence and early adulthood.

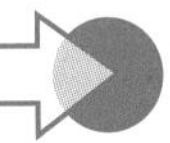

### Practical points

- Not all children with hyperactivity and inattention have ADHD.
- Genetic and environmental influences contribute to the diagnosis.
- Assessment is complex – consider risk factors and co-morbidities.
- Stimulant medication is safe and effective.
- Long-term behavioural, family and educational support is required.
- Adverse outcomes in adolescence and early adulthood are common, particularly in association with reading difficulty and aggressive behaviour.

## Prevention

Externalizing behaviour problems such as hyperactivity, oppositional defiance and aggression are very common in young children, some of whom will go on to a diagnosis of ADHD in the future. Group parenting programmes can help established externalizing behaviour problems by improving nurturing and responsiveness, and diminishing harsh discipline. Evidence is now building regarding the prevention of externalizing behaviour problems by using effective parenting programmes that start in infancy, raising the possibility of universal prevention in primary care settings.

From the above, it is clear that there are many reasons why children have hyperactive and inattentive behaviours. These behaviours must be interpreted with an understanding of normal development and behaviour, and how these interact with family and community function. When such behaviours are excessive and pervasive, a diagnosis of ADHD may be made, paying attention to causes, risk factors and co-morbidities.

Treatment of ADHD is multimodal, with stimulant medications being safe and most effective, but adjunctive behavioural management and family support are essential. Understanding and adjustment in the school setting, with appropriate educational support, are paramount for the child's long-term wellbeing.

Universal prevention and targeted early intervention of externalizing behaviour problems may help more children to start school with better self-regulation and capacity to learn, both academically and socially.

# Major psychiatric disorders 4.4

Brett McDermott

The major psychiatric disorders are characterized by relatively specific symptomatology and functional impairment in the family, social and educational domains. The primary care physician's role in the management of these disorders is early recognition, baseline risk assessment, diagnostic clarification if warranted, collaboration in shared care, and ensuring maintenance of the patient's general health. A contemporary conceptualization is that individuals are on developmental trajectories and, although variability in functioning and achievement over time is typical, nevertheless the individual shows steady improvement in ability and mastery of their environment across childhood and adolescence. Disorders can be developmental continuities: a child, although progressing, is doing so on an impaired trajectory compared with their peers – the child more rapidly develops symptoms and impairment. Examples of developmental discontinuities include the onset of major depression disorder or obsessive compulsive disorder.

The following symptoms should alert the primary physician to the possibility of a serious psychiatric disorder:

- Infancy and early childhood:
  - failure to thrive without physical cause
  - delay in spoken language
  - failure to respond normally to parental physical contact or voice
  - stereotyped, repetitive movements (e.g. hand-flapping)
  - concern by experienced parents that behaviour is unusual or bizarre.
- Middle childhood:
  - severe, persistent oppositional and/or aggressive behaviour
  - persistent stealing
  - developmentally inappropriate sexual behaviour
  - persistent fire-setting
  - cruelty to animals
  - truancy and/or unexplained absences from school
  - persistent unexplained physical symptoms (e.g. abdominal or limb pain)
  - severe, persistent separation anxiety (e.g. on leaving home to go to school)
  - failure to speak outside the home
  - obsessions and compulsions
  - persistent low or irritable mood
  - deterioration in school performance
  - failure to make friends, solitary interests.
- Adolescence:
  - unexplained loss of weight, uncontrolled dieting
  - secretive bingeing and vomiting
  - deterioration in school performance
  - social withdrawal and cessation of sporting/ recreational activities
  - disorganized thought processes, hallucinations, delusions
  - persistent or recurrent depressive mood
  - suicidal ideation or attempted suicide
  - panic attacks
  - excessive risk-taking, running away from home, sexual promiscuity
  - recent gravitation toward 'bad companions'
  - unexplained school absences/truancy
  - frequent fighting/explosive rage
  - persistent, unexplained physical symptoms.

In this chapter we describe some of the major psychiatric disorders that may occur at various ages in childhood and adolescence.

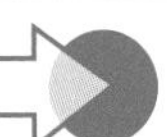

**Practical points**

**The role of the primary care physician**

- Recognize as early as possible the signs of a major psychiatric disorder.
- Exclude as quickly as possible non-psychiatric causes of the symptoms.
- Refer as soon as possible to mental health consultant.
- Explain the nature of the problem and the reason for referral to the patient and family.
- Collaborate with the psychiatrist in the shared extended care of the patient.
- Support the patient and family in adhering to the treatment plan.
- Maintain the patient's general health.

## Infancy and early childhood

### Reactive attachment disorders

Both infant and parent contribute to attachment. However, attachment is best conceptualized as the quality of the relationship between the two. Attachment disorders do not include disorders with a biological (proven or presumed) substrate. Hence impaired emotional reciprocity seen in autism is not a feature of a reactive attachment disorder. Occasionally, the distinction between pervasive development disorders and attachment disorders can be difficult. Typically, the infant fails to initiate or to respond appropriately to social interaction, exhibiting social withdrawal, inhibition, avoidance or, conversely, a superficial, undiscriminating sociability.

Attachment disorders develop as a result of parent depression, psychosis, personality disorder or severe psychosocial stress; the parent has failed to attend to the infant's basic needs for affection, contact comfort and stimulation, or there have been so many changes of caregiver that the infant has not been able to develop a stable attachment. Attachment disorder should be distinguished from pervasive developmental disorder, intellectual retardation and developmental language disorder.

Non-organic failure to thrive is arrested physical and psychosocial development secondary to severe attachment disorder, and should be differentiated from physical causes of failure to thrive. It is usually encountered in children from 18 months to 7 years of age. Typically, during hospital admission the child develops greater language and/or social ability as well as gaining weight, only to stall after returning home. The prognosis for intellectual and social development is poor unless adequate surrogate care is provided or the primary caregiver's parental capacity can be addressed.

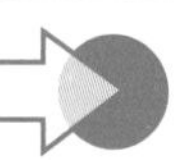

**Practical points**

**Reactive attachment disorder**

- Caused by defect in infant's capacity to elicit parental care and/or by failure of the parent to provide adequate or consistent care
- Reflected in the infant's failure to initiate or respond to social contact
- Can lead to stunting of physical or intellectual growth
- Must be differentiated from organic failure to thrive
- Treatment involves the provision of adequate surrogate parental care while the mother–child unit is treated

## Pervasive developmental disorders

This group of conditions is characterized by a developmental continuity in delayed intellectual, communicative and social development, together with stereotyped behaviour and circumscribed interests.

*Autistic disorder* occurs in about 1 in 1000 children, with a male to female ratio of 3:1. The features of autistic disorder are shown in Box 4.4.1.

**Box 4.4.1 Clinical features of autistic disorder**

- Marked impairment of eye-to-eye gaze and communicative gestures
- Failure to develop peer relationships
- Lack of socio-emotional reciprocity
- Impaired capacity for joint attention
- Incapacity for make-believe play
- Failure to imitate others
- Delay of language development
- Unusual use of language (e.g. for self-enchantment rather than communication)
- Stereotyped, restricted interests and rituals
- Motor mannerisms (e.g. finger-flicking or hand-flapping)

The incidence of all *autistic spectrum disorders* may be as high as 3–6 per 1000 children. A major cause of varying prevalence is inconsistency in diagnostic approaches. In approximately 50% of autistic children, a physical cause can be diagnosed (e.g. congenital rubella, fragile X syndrome, neurofibromatosis, phenylketonuria, tuberous sclerosis). There are numerous causal theories for pervasive developmental disorders of unknown aetiology, such as deficits of interneuron communication, possibly dendritic spine morphological change, more so in males. However, definitive statements about causation are not currently possible.

The child suspected of autistic disorder should be assessed as follows:

- Physical examination
- Dental examination
- Assessment of hearing and vision
- Psychological testing for cognitive level and pattern of intellectual abilities
- Speech and language assessment
- Genetic and metabolic testing to exclude known genetic and biological causes
- Electroencephalography.

Autistic disorder should be differentiated from:

- Developmental language disorder
- Intellectual retardation
- Sensory impairment (e.g. deafness)
- Selective mutism (see below)
- Severe psychosocial deprivation
- Mild forms of pervasive developmental disorder (see below).

Although many parents become concerned that their child is abnormal by the age of 6–12 months, autistic disorder is often not diagnosed until much later in childhood. This is regrettable because the earlier the diagnosis, the sooner effective treatment can be provided. In a minority of cases, the child is described as developing normally at first, only to regress into an autistic state when 2 or 3 years old.

**Clinical example**

John, aged 4 years, was referred because his preschool teacher was concerned about his poor language and lack of interest in other children. His mother said John had always been 'different'. He did not seek or give affection. He did not play with toys like other children but preferred to line them up or watch them falling, one by one, off a table. If anyone interrupted this game, he would scream. He was fascinated by light switches and electric fans, and liked to parrot television commercials. John avoided looking at people by averting his gaze to one side. He did not respond to the doctor's questions. At one point, he suddenly became upset and began to run around the office on tiptoes, flicking his fingertips. He was referred to a developmental paediatrician for a full diagnostic work-up for suspected autistic disorder.

The best predictors of outcome are IQ and the presence of functional speech at 5 years of age. Epilepsy occurs in approximately 20%, usually in adolescence. Treatment may be specific if a known disorder is diagnosed (e.g. fragile X syndrome). In all cases, diagnosis is multidisciplinary and involves a comprehensive behavioural analysis that establishes targets for behavioural interventions. Often behaviour is slowly shaped towards the desired outcome. Specific augmentation and communication strategies are effective, especially if commenced early in life. Pharmacotherapy has a limited role, and is of use mainly in children who exhibit severe hyperactivity, aggressiveness or self-harm.

Parents are not usually concerned about children with *Asperger's disorder* until the child is 2–4 years old. By middle childhood, the child exhibits the following characteristics:

- impairment of non-verbal communication (e.g. impaired eye contact, lack of facial expression and gesture, and monotonous vocal intonation but intact language development otherwise)
- average or above average intelligence
- lack of interest in peer relationships
- lack of social reciprocity, shared enjoyment and humour
- circumscribed interests (e.g. fixated on earthquakes) and inflexible routines
- mannerisms (e.g. hand-flapping) and motor clumsiness.

It is unclear whether Asperger's disorder is a variant of, or different from, autistic disorder, and whether it is distinct from non-verbal language disability, semantic pragmatic processing disorder or related to later schizoid personality disorder. Because of uncertainty about the boundaries of this condition, its prevalence is unclear. A useful approximation is an Asperger's to autism ratio of 5:1. Like autism, this condition is more common in males. By adolescence, many children with this condition become frustrated by their lack of friends and the teasing or social rejection to which they are prone. Treatment involves social–cognitive language programming in the educational mainstream. As adults, people with Asperger's disorder are more effective in jobs that make few social demands.

## Middle childhood

### Disruptive behaviour disorder

*Oppositional defiant disorder* and *attention-deficit/hyperactivity disorder* (ADHD) are described in Chapters 4.2 and 4.3 respectively. *Conduct disorder* refers to a group of children characterized by some or all of the features listed in Box 4.4.2.

Conduct disorder can emerge first in adolescence but the more serious variant is continuity from oppositional defiant disorder of middle childhood. The prevalence is 3% in Australian children and adolescents, with a male to female ratio of about 3:1. Conduct disorder is commonly associated with other problems, particularly ADHD (see Chapter 4.3), alcohol and substance use, mood disorder, post-traumatic stress disorder (PTSD) and learning disorder. In the clinical setting, much of the most severe aggressive behaviour is displayed by children under child protection orders, often with multiple past abuse histories, dysregulated mood and impulses, as well as significant self-harm. These adolescents may meet criteria for conduct disorder, but the presentations are best conceptualized as either a complex PTSD or a reactive attachment disorder.

The genetic background of conduct disorder is unclear, but twin and adoption studies suggest there is an inherited component. Current aetiological models of conduct disorder highlight necessary (but not sufficient) vulnerability factors, including genetic factors such as a functional polymorphism of the monoamine oxidase gene, early life exposure to coercive parenting and/or early abusive and neglected parenting. Later contact with deviant peers is often important. Significant associations include (early)

**Box 4.4.2 Features of conduct disorder**

- Persistently aggressive behaviour (bullying, intimidation, frequent fighting, cruelty, coercive sexual behaviour, use of a weapon)
- Destructiveness (fire-setting, vandalism)
- Deceitfulness (breaking and entering, stealing, lying, trickery)
- Rule violation (truancy, staying out late at night, running away from home, refusal to accept rules at home or school)

lack of empathy, relative school failure and early initiation into smoking, sexual activity, and alcohol or drug taking.

If conduct problems do not first appear until adolescence, and few risk factors are operative, the individual will probably not go on to become antisocial as an adult. When behaviour problems begin at an early age and many of the cumulative risk factors apply, it is more likely that the individual will become an adult criminal. Children with conduct problems are usually referred for evaluation during late childhood or adolescence. It would be preferable if this serious disorder could be detected and treated earlier. The combination of early educational intervention with parenting programmes (e.g. triple P) designed to alter coercive childrearing have an increasing evidence base. Recently multisystemic therapy involving goal-directed strategic/behavioural family therapy aimed at promoting effective parenting, along with individual counselling and environmental interventions, has produced good results. The placement of offenders in therapeutic foster homes has also shown promise. In foster home programmes, the house parents are trained to be firm and consistent in their discipline and to ensure that the adolescent does not associate with antisocial peers. Foster care without input from an evidence-based programme is not effective for this group. It is also ineffective to treat children with conduct disorder in community or institutional groups composed of like-minded peers. 'Boot camps' and 'scaring then straight' programmes have no evidence of effect.

## Anxiety disorders

*Separation anxiety disorder* is described in Chapter 4.2. *Generalized anxiety disorder* is characterized by persistent, excessive worrying about life events (e.g. school performance, dating) accompanied by physical symptoms (e.g. abdominal pains, headaches, fatigue, diarrhoea, urinary frequency). Children with this disorder are likely to have been behaviourally inhibited as preschoolers and to have a parent with an anxiety disorder or high trait anxiety. Generalized anxiety disorder overlaps with *social phobia*, in which the child is particularly fearful of performance situations that incur the scrutiny of others (e.g. reading in front of the class, athletic competition). School phobia (or "school refusal") can be a severe anxiety disorder that requires multidisciplinary intervention; indeed, 20% of school refusing children never return to the general classroom.

*Panic disorder* involves repeated attacks of sudden, disabling anxiety, often without any apparent precipitant, associated with the physiological concomitants of anxiety (e.g. hyperventilation, racing heart, cold sweaty hands, choking sensations, dizziness, fainting) and a fear of dying. The onset of panic disorder is most often in mid-adolescence; it is rare in middle childhood. *Selective mutism* often coexists with panic disorder or social phobia. The child, more often a girl, fails to speak in social situations outside the home or to strangers. The average age of onset is 2–5 years. In about 30% of cases there has been a premorbid speech or language problem. Selective mutism should be differentiated from deafness, intellectual disability, developmental language disorder, aphonia and the inability of a migrant child to understand English.

Anxiety disorders frequently coincide with attention-deficit disorder and depressive disorder. Given that parental anxiety (especially separation or social anxiety) is highly contagious, treatment must therefore involve the parents.

*Obsessive compulsive disorder* (OCD) has the features listed in Box 4.4.3. OCD has a 6-month prevalence of 0.5–1%. The onset is usually between 6 and 11 years, with bimodal peaks, the latter being in the early twenties. The male to female ratio is probably equal, although males predominate in the younger age group. Neuroimaging, neuropsychological and genetic studies support the concept that the disorder is neuropsychiatric in nature. A subgroup of patients may have sustained an autoimmune reaction and are positive for antibodies to β-haemolytic streptococci. OCD should be distinguished from:

- transient benign habits and rituals such as 'not stepping on the crack' (no impairment)
- worries associated with generalized anxiety disorder (e.g. worries about daily events)
- Tourette disorder (associated with tics)
- pervasive developmental disorder (rituals are not distressing and there is marked social impairment).

OCD is commonly co-morbid with other anxiety disorders, mood disorder, tic disorder and disruptive behaviour disorders. It often persists into adulthood.

Anxiolytic drugs (e.g. benzodiazepines) should be avoided in the treatment of anxiety disorders because they have addictive and sedative potential. Further,

**Box 4.4.3 Features of obsessive compulsive disorder**

- Recurrent, distressing thoughts about such matters as germs, contamination or harming the self or others, or preoccupation with excessive moralization or religiosity (obsessions)
- Recurrent distressing rituals involving excessive washing, repeating, checking, touching, counting or ordering (compulsions)
- These thoughts or actions are regarded by the patient as abnormal and are resisted, but the patient is forced to continue to think thus, or to continue the actions
- Symptom exacerbation in times of stress (e.g. starting at a new school)
- Impairment of functioning (e.g. completing chores, getting ready for bed, finishing schoolwork, relating to other family members)

**Clinical example**

Barbara's mother reported that she was worried because Barbara, aged 10 years, had begun to behave in an odd manner. She would touch doorknobs again and again, and spent ages getting to bed because she had to arrange her teddy bears just so around her pillows and at the foot of the bed. She had reluctantly admitted to her mother that she arranged the teddy bears in that way in order to control a fear of being abducted at night. She would wriggle her toes and clench her jaw in a special way, but did not know why she did so. When she tried to resist wriggling her toes, she became very anxious and had to give in and do it.

they prevent habituation to anxiety and may therefore perpetuate the condition. The most effective treatment is cognitive–behavioural therapy (CBT). As parental anxiety is commonly associated with childhood anxiety disorder, parent involvement is always indicated. In OCD, CBT involving exposure to anxiety-provoking situations, systematic desensitization and the prevention of compulsive responses to anxiety-provoking stimuli has been found to be effective. For OCD specifically and other anxiety presentations with an inadequate response to CBT, selective serotonin-reuptake inhibitors (SSRIs) are often effective and well tolerated. Family therapy is aimed at educating the family and disentangling the parent's from the child's rituals.

## Adolescence

### Major depressive disorder

The prevalence of major depressive disorder rapidly increases during adolescence. The characteristic symptoms are listed in Box 4.4.4.

Depressive symptoms are commonly associated with anxiety, conduct problems, post-traumatic symptomatology, eating disorders, learning disability, substance abuse and school refusal. A recent Australian population survey found the 6-month prevalence of depression to be 3% in childhood and adolescence. Typically, there is an increased prevalence of depression in the families of depressed children. However, the genetic background of the disorder is still unclear, as is the nature of the interaction between genetic propensity and the adverse life events that often precede depressive episodes.

**Box 4.4.4 Symptoms of major depressive disorder**

- Persistent depressed or irritable mood
- Feelings of worthlessness and hopelessness
- Suicidal ideation
- Loss of pleasure in activities that were formerly enjoyed
- Social withdrawal and cessation of sporting and recreational activities
- Insomnia or hypersomnia
- Loss or gain of weight
- Loss of concentration and deterioration in school performance
- Lack of energy, ready fatigue

Depression often presents as a discontinuity from the previous developmental trajectory and so the clinician should be alerted to the possibility whenever school performance inexplicably drops or there is a change in mood, control of temper, social involvement or sleep patterns. Information is needed from both parent and child with regard to the clinical features and contemporary psychosocial stressors. The child should be assessed for risk of suicide; clinicians are reminded that talking about suicide will not introduce the adolescent to this possibility. A differential diagnosis is an emerging personality disorder, often typified by chronic mood dyscontrol as well as impulsivity, relationship instability, self-harm and an unstable sense of self (see Chapter 4.2). The 2011 Australian Clinical Practice Guidelines for Adolescent and Youth Depression advise CBT or interpersonal psychotherapy as the treatment of first choice. There is evidence for the effectiveness of the SSRI fluoxetine, but SSRIs are associated with a small rise in emergent suicide thinking and behaviour from approximately 2% (placebo rate) to 4%. There is no evidence that tricyclic or heterocyclic antidepressant drugs are effective in child/adolescent major depression. Furthermore, they can have serious side-effects. There is evidence that CBT combined with an SSRI modifies the danger of emergent suicidal thinking. Although most depressed adolescents recover from depression within a year, many relapse and the risk of subsequent episodes continues into adulthood.

**Clinical example**

Bill, aged 14 years, was referred because the school had become concerned about his surliness, rebelliousness and tendency to submit class assignments with macabre content. His mother said that Bill would do nothing to help her at home and spent most of his time in his bedroom listening to 'heavy metal' rock music. Bill's father had left the family several years before to live in a distant city and start a new family. Bill presented as a slim adolescent, dressed in black, with close-cropped hair and a nose ring. After initially sparring verbally, he admitted that he hated his life. He said that he slept poorly and was too tired to concentrate in school. He had recently begun to smoke marijuana. He had no friends he could rely on except, maybe, other 'stoners'. He reported that he thought often about committing suicide, probably by jumping from a bridge. A mood disorder was diagnosed and Bill was referred for psychiatric evaluation.

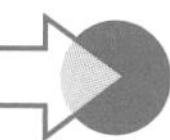

### Practical points

**Depressive disorder**

- Presents in adolescence with physical symptoms, irritability, social withdrawal, deterioration in school performance.
- Have a high index of suspicion for this disorder because of the potential for suicide.
- Usually associated with environmental stress (e.g. parental divorce, abuse, bullying) or loss.
- Refer early if condition is severe or patient is suicidal.
- Psychotherapy is the first treatment choice.
- Selective serotonin receptor inhibitor (SSRI) medication should be used only in moderate/severe cases.
- SSRIs are associated with emergent suicide thinking and behaviour.

## Bipolar disorder

There is controversy over the validity of the diagnosis of bipolar disorder in childhood, and its prevalence. It is clear, on the other hand, that bipolar disorder is underdiagnosed in adolescence and many young people with early-onset psychosis are later reclassified as having bipolar disorder. In bipolar I disorder, the patient has experienced at least one manic or mixed manic–depressive episode. In bipolar II disorder, the patient has experienced at least one episode of both major depression and hypomania, but no manic or mixed episodes. Mania is characterized by the following symptoms:

- abnormally elevated mood persisting for at least 1 week
- grandiose thinking
- pressured speech, racing thoughts and distractibility
- increased activity and recklessness
- marked deterioration in functioning at school, with peers and at home.

Hypomania is characterized by similar but less intense symptoms, and less functional deterioration. In a mixed episode, manic and major depressive symptoms coincide. Adolescents with mania often have hallucinations, paranoid ideas and marked lability of mood, causing the aforementioned diagnostic confusion with schizophrenia. The risk of suicide is increased in bipolar disorder, especially during depressive phases.

Bipolar disorder is familial, although the mode of genetic transmission has not been elucidated. Bipolar disorder should be differentiated from schizophrenia, major depression with agitation, PTSD, disruptive behaviour disorder, and disorder of mood or delirium secondary to a medical condition (e.g. hyperthyroidism, porphyria) or intoxication with illicit or prescribed drugs (e.g. amphetamines, phencyclidine).

The treatment of bipolar disorder is primarily pharmacological. Acute mania can be a medical emergency requiring a rapid-acting antipsychotic and/or a benzodiazepine. Rapidly dissolving wafer forms of antipsychotic medication (e.g. olanzapine) are preferable. Treatment of less acute presentations and ongoing maintenance are with mood stabilizers (lithium, valproate, carbamazepine) and atypical antipsychotics. In adolescent women, valproate is not advised given its risk of major birth defects. Adjunctive psychosocial interventions improve functioning and medication compliance.

## Schizophrenia

Psychoses in general are heterogeneous in origin and in paediatrics may be seen in individuals with velocardiofacial syndrome, Prader–Willi syndrome or other rare developmental presentations. Schizophrenia is predominantly a disorder of late adolescence and early adulthood. Schizophrenia may be acute or subacute in onset, especially if triggered by illicit drug use. For many individuals there is a prodrome phase that is more insidious and typified by:

- social isolation or withdrawal
- deterioration in functioning at home, at school, and in grooming and personal hygiene
- vague conversation with poverty of content
- odd, overvalued beliefs (e.g. of telepathy), rituals or magical thinking.

Symptoms typical of acute schizophrenia include:

- hallucinations (most commonly auditory)
- delusions (e.g. of persecution, thought insertion, thought loss)
- thought disorder with disorganized or incoherent conversation
- disorganized behaviour (e.g. posturing, catatonic stiffness, agitation)
- flattening of affect, poverty of speech, anergia.

Schizophrenia is a familial disorder with a complex mode of genetic transmission and variable expression. Schizophrenia should be differentiated from:

- mood disorder (especially bipolar I disorder)
- psychosis due to medical disease (e.g. epilepsy, brain tumour, porphyria, acquired immune deficiency syndrome [AIDS]) or substance abuse (e.g. stimulants, cocaine, hallucinogens, phencyclidine)
- psychosis associated with developmental disorders
- other psychoses (complex PTSD with dissociative hallucinations, schizophreniform disorder).

Patients with below-average IQ, premorbid signs of Asperger's disorder or pervasive developmental disorder, speech disorders or cardiac disorders should undergo genetic testing for known behavioural phenotypes.

Acute schizophrenia conveys a risk of suicide or, more rarely, danger to others. Acute presentations usually require hospitalization for diagnosis and stabilization. Patients are usually treated initially with an atypical antipsychotic medication, such as risperidone, olanzapine and quetiapine, which are associated with relatively few side-effects other than weight gain, sedation and, in some cases, sexual dysfunction. Adjunctive benzodiazepines may be useful in highly aroused distressed individuals, especially as antipsychotic medication may take 2–6 weeks for significant symptom reduction. Psychoeducation for parents is essential in order to foster compliance and independent living skills, and to counteract the high levels of emotional expression between family members that increase the likelihood of relapse. Liaison with the school is necessary. A poor prognosis is associated with early or insidious onset, low socioeconomic status, family history of schizophrenia, absence of precipitating stress and severe negative symptoms.

**Clinical example**

Annabelle, aged 15 years, had always been an emotionally fragile child who tended to have intense, dependent relationships with her peers. However, recently she had become withdrawn and self-absorbed, telling her mother that she wanted to drop out of school and pursue religious studies. At interview, she was fearful and apparently distracted. She asked whether the interview was being videotaped. After some time she revealed that she had been 'chosen' to do something very important in the world. She had become aware of this as a result of a revelation, recently, when the Earth shone and she 'knew' her destiny. Her conversation meandered and was often difficult to follow. Several times during the interview she stopped talking and smiled to herself. Physical examination was normal. Annabelle was referred to a psychiatrist, who confirmed the diagnosis of schizophrenia, admitted Annabelle to hospital, excluded organic pathology and commenced antipsychotic medication. After Annabelle's discharge, her medication was monitored by her family doctor, and appointments were made for her to see the psychiatrist every 6 weeks.

### Post-traumatic stress disorder

PTSD occurs in response to the personal experience of overwhelming, terrifying, potentially fatal stress directed toward the child or someone with whom the child has a close attachment. In childhood and adolescence, the commonest kinds of threat causing PTSD are motor vehicle accidents, burn injury, natural or man-made disasters, animal attack, criminal assault, observation of parental homicide or suicide, and war. A particularly pathogenic stress or threat involves repeated exposure to coercive intrafamilial physical or sexual abuse when the child is unable to disclose or escape the abuse and when, after disclosure, the non-abusive caregiver fails to provide adequate support. The clinical features of PTSD in childhood are very similar to those in adulthood:

- persistent intrusive imagery concerning the traumatic event (e.g. flashbacks, nightmares)
- repetitious play representing the event
- generalized nightmares and trauma nightmares
- the conviction that one is destined for an early death and that there were omens before the trauma
- avoidance of things, people or situations that remind one of the event
- persistent autonomic arousal with an exaggerated startle response.

When PTSD is caused by repeated physical or sexual abuse, dissociative symptoms may be seen, for example:

- amnesia for all or part of the event or events
- vagueness, daydreaming and the sense of being estranged from others
- trance-like states
- audiovisual hallucinations that represent fragmentary memories of the abuse
- bodily symptoms (such as pseudoseizures or pelvic pain) that represent somatic memories of the abuse.

PTSD is likely to be co-morbid with, or to be succeeded by:

- mood disorder
- anxiety disorder
- hyperactivity, especially in boys
- alcohol/drug use
- dissociative and somatoform disorders.

Recent clinical research suggests that children under the age at which sequential, narrative, autobiographical memory can be encoded and recounted (i.e. below 3 years of age) can also manifest a form of PTSD. The outcome of acute stress is affected adversely if the child is separated from parents, if the parents die, if the parents develop psychiatric symptoms or if there is a contagion of symptoms between children.

Interventions firstly emphasize hierarchy of needs, hence immediate attention to physical and psychological safety. This is the case for all causes of emotional trauma. In this early stage, critical incident debriefing is no longer recommended. Psychoeducation is appropriate. Children who continue to manifest symptoms after 1 month should be referred for individual treatment. In PTSD associated with child maltreatment, CBT and family therapy have proved helpful. CBT must be trauma-focused. If medication is required, an SSRI such as fluoxetine may be useful in alleviating some anxiety symptoms.

## Somatoform disorders

This group of disorders is characterized by physical symptoms that suggest an underlying physical disease but for which either no such basis can be found, or the symptoms are disproportionate in intensity or duration to a known physical disorder. *Somatization disorder* and *hypochondriasis* involve the conviction that physical symptoms have a physical cause and the tendency to present repeatedly for medical care even though no physical cause can be found. The commonest presentations are abdominal pain, headaches, or fatigue and muscle weakness. This kind of problem is generally associated with other family psychopathology such as parental anxiety, depression or somatization, and may be based on the parent's conviction that the child has a physical disease such as chronic fatigue syndrome. It is frequently encountered in sexually abused children. In conversion disorder, the dramatic symptoms suggest a physical disease but no such disease can be found, and the symptoms are distributed or displayed in accordance with a naive view of bodily functioning (e.g. glove-and-stocking anaesthesia). The commonest conversion symptoms are paralysis, paresis, seizures, anaesthesia, paraesthesia, vomiting, aphonia, headaches, blindness and deafness. Conversion disorder typically follows or accompanies a severe psychosocial stress such as sexual abuse, bereavement or family conflict.

The prevalence of somatoform disorders is probably high. They are closely related to the emotional climate of the family and to parental psychopathology. The primary physician should investigate thoroughly to rule out organic pathology, avoiding interminable testing lest the symptoms become chronic and irreversible. Psychiatric consultation should be sought as early as possible. In conversion disorder, once the hidden stressor is disclosed, symptoms usually dissipate with suggestive therapy such as graduated exercises. In somatization syndromes, the family can be helped to interpret the symptoms as signs of stress and to manage stress, for example with relaxation exercises.

## Eating disorders

*Anorexia nervosa* is characterized by:

- an intense fear of becoming fat or losing control of eating
- a relentless pursuit of thinness
- secretive food refusal, dieting and exercise causing marked loss of weight (below 85% of weight expected)
- the perception of being overweight despite extreme thinness
- amenorrhoea.

*Bulimia nervosa* is characterized by:

- binge-eating with a sense of loss of control
- self-induced vomiting
- the use of dieting, laxatives, diuretics, enemas and exercise to control or reverse weight gain.

Both eating disorders are much more common in girls than in boys; ballet dancers, gymnasts and athletes are particularly at risk. It is likely the prevalence of anorexia peaked during the 1980s; however, recent trends include presentation of patients at a younger age and more boys are presenting with anorexia. In the 15–25-year-old group, bulimia is more common than anorexia nervosa. The onset of anorexia occurs during mid-adolescence. Bulimia usually begins in late adolescence and may be a sequel of earlier anorexia nervosa. The adolescent who develops anorexia nervosa is likely to have been a compliant, conscientious child who had enmeshed family relationships. Secretive dieting and exercise often begin after a minor precipitant, such as being told that one is overweight. The child hides the amount of weight loss from her parents. Menses cease. The child becomes moody, irritable and withdrawn. Eventually, the physical signs of starvation appear:

- emaciated facies and body
- fine body hair growth
- dry hair
- cold hands
- slow pulse
- low blood pressure.

The individual often resists medical help and is unable to appreciate how emaciated she has become. The adolescent with bulimia nervosa has dramatic weight fluctuations and develops swollen salivary glands, abraded knuckles and dental caries. Eventually, as a result of chronic metabolic alkalosis, kidney function may be compromised.

Eating disorders are psychological conditions, often with marked physical complications. A useful conceptualization is that initial dieting is a reinforced solution to the individual feeling distressed and out of control. It is likely that a more enduring problem occurs in individuals with perfectionist personality traits with over-regulated effect. Excessive dieting may represent the pursuit of an idealized body image and self-control by a child who perceives herself as helpless to direct her own life. Eating disorders must be differentiated from other disorders that can cause weight loss, such as malabsorption disorders, chronic infection, occult malignancy, substance abuse, chronic depression, paranoid schizophrenia and psychogenic vomiting.

Hospitalization and paediatric/psychiatric collaboration are required if the patient is metabolically unstable, as evidenced by dehydration, inanition, electrolyte imbalance, bradycardia and low blood pressure, if she resists treatment, or if outpatient treatment has failed. Nasogastric feeding is required in extreme cases. The patient is not discharged from hospital until a reasonable target weight has been attained. Treatment plans should be individualized and goal-directed. For patients aged 18 years and younger, family therapy has the most rigorous evidence base. Bulimic patients, who are usually older, generally respond best to CBT. Long-term follow-up studies have revealed that patients with anorexia have a variable course; 80% respond initially to family therapy, although relapse and symptom chronicity also occur. The mortality rate associated with anorexia is 3–5%, 50% of which is by suicide. Chronic anorexia and significant co-morbid depression can be a psychiatric emergency.

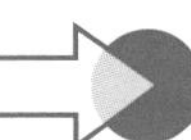

**Practical points**

**Eating disorder**

- Adolescents with eating disorders are skilled in their ability to conceal loss of weight and failure to eat.
- Exclude other causes of weight loss as soon as possible.
- Hospitalize if the child is metabolically unstable (electrolytes, heart rate, blood pressure, dehydration).
- Otherwise, the child should be treated as an outpatient with family and individual psychotherapy.
- The older the patient at presentation, the worse the prognosis.

PART 5

# PAEDIATRIC EMERGENCIES

# 5.1 Emergencies: causes and assessment

Jeremy Raftos

There are many causes of collapse leading to the need for emergency medical intervention in the child. Table 5.1.1 lists some of the causes of common paediatric emergencies.

The following information outlines the requirements for early assessment and reassessment in paediatric emergencies. Details of the emergency care of the collapsed child are provided in the next chapter.

In approaching the critically ill child, the diagnosis is of secondary importance to:

- *primary assessment*, which is a structured activity, and
- *timely resuscitation procedures*.

The *primary assessment,* sometimes also known as the primary survey, follows progression through the following A, B, C, D, E steps:

- **A**irway
- **B**reathing
- **C**irculation
- **D**isability (deficiency of cerebral function), with attention to
- **E**xposure.

This structured approach is based on the knowledge that the brain requires a continual supply of its two main metabolites: oxygen and glucose. An airway problem, by depriving the brain of its oxygen supply, will lead rapidly to death and therefore must be corrected first. A breathing problem preventing oxygen moving into the lung and carbon dioxide out of the lung is the next priority. A circulatory problem preventing the oxygen being carried to the brain is next, and so on.

The resuscitation measures required and management of the collapsed child are described in detail in Chapter 5.2.

## The primary assessment

### Airway

Child and infant airways, compared with those of the adult, present particular anatomical and physiological differences that increase their susceptibility to compromise. Infants are obligate nose-breathers. Infants and small children have smaller airways and a smaller mandible, a proportionately larger tongue, and more floppy epiglottis and soft palate. The narrowest portion of their airway is below the cords at the level of the cricoid ring, in contrast to adults, where the narrowest portion is at the level of the vocal cords. The trachea is short and soft, and hyperextension or flexion of the neck may cause obstruction.

Ensuring that the patient has a patent airway is of the highest priority. In evaluating the airway a look, listen and feel approach is used.

Look carefully for movement of the chest wall and the abdomen. Note the degree to which intercostal and other accessory muscles are being used to overcome obstruction. Paradoxical movement of the abdomen may occur if there is upper airway obstruction.

Listen over the mouth and nose for air movement. Particular note should be made of inspiratory stridor, which is a sign of tracheal, laryngeal or other upper airway obstruction. In severe obstruction, expiratory sounds may also be heard but inspiratory noises will still predominate. A stethoscope should be used to listen over the trachea and in the axillae for air movement.

Finally the examiner, by placing his or her face close to the child's mouth, may feel evidence of air movement.

### Breathing

In childhood, conditions that result in respiratory compromise are the most common reason for emergency intervention, and are the major cause of a poor outcome.

As with the airway, there are important differences between the child and the adult. Children have a higher metabolic requirement. They have more immature musculature, with easy fatigability of the diaphragm, which is the major muscle of respiration. The chest wall is more compliant and the ribs are more horizontal, decreasing the efficiency of the bellows effect.

The airways in the child are proportionally smaller and therefore produce an increased resistance to air flow, especially when traumatized or inflamed. Resistance (R) across an airway is inversely proportional to the fourth power of the radius ($r$):

$$R = 1/r^4$$

Thus, halving the radius increases the resistance very significantly.

**Table 5.1.1 Causes of paediatric emergencies**

| Airway | Breathing | Circulation | Disability | Exposure |
|---|---|---|---|---|
| Croup | Asthma | Congenital heart disease | Seizure | Hypothermia |
| Epiglottitis | Bronchiolitis | Duct dependent lesions: | Meningitis | Hyperthermia |
| Laryngeal foreign body | Pneumonia | Critical aortic stenosis | Encephalitis | Inflicted injury |
| Bacterial tracheitis | Foreign body | Hypoplastic left heart | Head injury | |
| Trauma | Congestive heart failure | Coarctation | Raised intracranial pressure | |
| Angioneurotic oedema | Neuromuscular diseases | Dysrhythmias: | Hypoglycaemia | |
| Retropharyngeal abscess | Trauma: | Bradycardia | Metabolic disorder | |
| | Pneumothorax | Tachycardia | Poisoning | |
| | Haemothorax | Supraventricular | Envenomation | |
| | Lung contusion | Ventricular | | |
| | Flail chest | Torsade de pointes | | |
| | Near drowning | Fibrillation | | |
| | Smoke inhalation | Pulseless electrical activity | | |
| | Metabolic acidosis: | Shock: | | |
| | Diabetic ketoacidosis | Cardiogenic | | |
| | Poisoning | Cardiomyopathy | | |
| | Salicylates | Heart failure | | |
| | Methanol | Myocardial contusion | | |
| | | Hypovolaemic | | |
| | | Haemorrhage | | |
| | | Vomiting/diarrhoea | | |
| | | Burns | | |
| | | Distributive | | |
| | | Septicaemia | | |
| | | Anaphylaxis | | |
| | | Spinal cord injury | | |
| | | Obstructive | | |
| | | Cardiac tamponade | | |
| | | Hypertension | | |
| | | Dissociative | | |

Having established patency of the airway, evaluation for the presence and adequacy of breathing should follow. It is helpful to divide this into three aspects:

- effort of breathing
- efficacy of breathing
- effects of respiratory inadequacy on other organs.

## Effort of breathing

Respiratory rate is age-dependent (Table 5.1.2). Tachypnoea is an early response to respiratory failure. Increased depth of respiration may occur later as respiratory failure progresses. However, it should be noted that tachypnoea does not always have a respiratory cause and may occur in response, for example, to metabolic acidosis. As the intercostal muscles and diaphragm increase their contraction, intercostal and subcostal recession develop. In the infant, sternal retraction may also occur.

The ribs are horizontal in young children, in contrast to the downward slanting in older children and adults. This reduces the 'bellows' effect that the intercostal muscles give to the latter. In the child, the sternomastoid muscles must be recruited to raise the upper ribs further to increase ventilation.

In infants and small children, flaring of the alae nasi may be seen. It must be remembered that, in this age group, 50% of airway resistance occurs in the upper airway and flaring is an attempt to reduce this resistance. This is a late sign and is indicative of severe respiratory distress.

The effort of breathing is diminished in three clinical circumstances. These must be recognized, because urgent intervention may be required. Firstly, exhaustion may develop as a result of the increased respiratory demands. The younger child is even more prone to this due to immature musculature. Secondly, respiration requires an intact central respiratory drive centre. Conditions such as trauma, meningitis and poisoning may depress the respiratory centre. Thirdly, neuromuscular conditions that cause paralysis, such as muscular dystrophy and Guillain–Barré syndrome, may result in respiratory failure without increased effort.

Symmetrical movement of the chest should be confirmed. In the younger child the diaphragm is the

**Table 5.1.2 Vital signs by age**

| Age (years) | Respiratory rate (breaths/min) | Heart rate (beats/min) | Systolic blood pressure (mmHg) |
|---|---|---|---|
| <1 | 30–40 | 110–160 | 70–90 |
| 1–2 | 25–35 | 100–150 | 80–95 |
| 2–5 | 25–30 | 95–140 | 80–100 |
| 5–12 | 20–25 | 80–120 | 90–110 |
| >12 | 15–20 | 60–100 | 100–120 |

main muscle of respiration; therefore, one should also look for movement of the upper abdomen.

Inspiratory and expiratory noises should be noted. Wheezing is heard with lower airway narrowing, as in asthma, often with a prolonged expiratory phase. Crepitations may be heard with pneumonia and heart failure.

### Efficacy of breathing

Auscultation of both sides of the chest will confirm air movement. Beware the silent chest! Oximetry is useful for providing a measure of arterial oxygen saturation ($S_ao_2$), which reflects the efficacy of breathing, but oximetry readings may be difficult to obtain in the cold or shocked child because of poor perfusion, and are less accurate when the $S_ao_2$ is less than 70%.

### Effects of respiratory inadequacy on other organs

The impact of hypoxia on the cardiovascular system is to cause tachycardia, but pre-terminally it may cause bradycardia.

Cyanosis is also a pre-terminal sign. Hypoxia may also cause peripheral shutdown and pallor secondary to sympathetic stimulation.

The effect of hypoxia on the brain is to cause initial agitation and irritability in infants, followed by increasing loss of consciousness.

**Clinical example**

A 1-week-old infant presented after a 3-day illness, cyanosed and with marked tachypnoea. He was severely ill.

In this situation, rapid systematic assessment and resuscitation measures must go hand in hand. The airway and breathing must be assessed first. This infant was breathing fast and was cyanosed. Points that have to be considered urgently are: Is there intercostal, sternal or subcostal recession, or use of accessory muscles indicating increased effort of breathing? Are there inspiratory or expiratory noises? Is grunting or flaring of the alae nasi present? Efficacy of breathing needs to be assessed by assessing the degree of chest expansion, breath sounds and oximetry. The effect of respiratory inadequacy can be seen in an increased heart rate, change in skin colour and mental status.

The infant was found to have a marked increase in effort of breathing, flaring of the alae nasi, bilateral crepitations and tachycardia. In addition to the cyanosis, he was drowsy.

Assessment of the cardiovascular system showed normal pulse volume, capillary return and blood pressure. A search for evidence of heart failure revealed no gallop or heart murmur, no liver enlargement and the presence of femoral pulses.

With high flow oxygen his colour improved, as did his mental status. A diagnosis of severe bronchiolitis was made.

To complete the assessment the infant was found to have no rash, his initial temperature was 35°C, and with appropriate warming his temperature rapidly reached 36°C.

## Circulation

Cardiac output is the product of stroke volume and heart rate. The normal heart rate decreases with age (see Table 5.1.2). Infants have a small, relatively fixed, cardiac stroke volume; thus they must increase their heart rate to respond to increased demand.

Infants have a relatively larger intravascular volume (85 mL/kg) that decreases with age to 60 mL/kg in the teenager. The normal ranges for blood pressure increase with age (see Table 5.1.2 and Chapter 18.2), because systemic vascular resistance increases as the child gets older.

### Assessment of circulation

An increase in heart rate is the earliest response to any reduction in intravascular volume. As shock progresses, bradycardia may develop as a pre-terminal sign. It is important to assess pulse volume both peripherally and centrally. Weak central pulses indicate severe shock. Capillary refill can be a sensitive indicator of vascular status. To assess this, light pressure should be applied to the skin over the sternum for 5 seconds. In the normal individual, capillary return of blood, seen as a slight flush of the pallid area where pressure was applied, will occur in less than 3 seconds. Caution should be used in interpreting this sign in the child who has been exposed to a cold environment.

In the shocked child, hypotension is a late pre-terminal sign.

### Effects of circulatory inadequacy on other organs

Circulatory inadequacy leads to poor tissue perfusion, which in turn leads to metabolic acidosis. Tachypnoea occurs to compensate for the acidosis.

Initial sympathetic stimulation may cause agitation, but later poor cerebral perfusion causes increasing drowsiness and coma in the pre-terminal phase.

Pre-renal failure develops with hypovolaemia and hypotension, with reduction of urine output. Normal urine output is greater than 1 mL per kg per h in the child and more than 2 mL per kg per h in the infant.

### Signs of cardiac failure

The signs of cardiac failure should be sought. This is critical to assessment, because the finding of cardiac failure will influence the approach to resuscitation discussed in the next chapter. Raised jugular venous pulse height is important in the older child but may be difficult to determine in the younger child because of the relatively short, often chubby, neck. Listen for a gallop rhythm and for lung crepitations. Palpation of the abdomen may reveal an enlarged liver.

## Disability

The assessment of neurological function as part of the primary assessment has three main aims:

- to determine rapidly the level of consciousness
- to find localizing intracranial lesions
- to determine whether there is raised intracranial pressure.

It must be remembered that respiratory and cardiovascular failure can cause decreased consciousness and must be dealt with first.

### Conscious level

Conscious level can be rapidly assessed using the AVPU method:

- *A* Alert
- *V* responds to Voice
- *P* responds to Pain
- *U* Unresponsive.

The child who is unresponsive or who responds only to pain has a Glasgow Coma Scale (GCS) score of 8 or less. The GCS has no place in the primary survey, but is a useful tool for monitoring changes in neurological status after initial stabilization (Table 5.1.3).

**Table 5.1.3 Glasgow Coma Scale and Children's Coma Scale**

| Glasgow Coma Scale (4–15 years) | | Child's Glasgow Coma Scale (<4 years) | |
|---|---|---|---|
| Response | Score | Response | Score |
| **Eye opening** | | **Eye opening** | |
| Spontaneously | 4 | Spontaneously | 4 |
| To verbal stimuli | 3 | To verbal stimuli | 3 |
| To pain | 2 | To pain | 2 |
| No response to pain | 1 | No response to pain | 1 |
| **Best motor response** | | **Best motor response** | |
| Obeys verbal command | 6 | Spontaneous or obeys verbal command | 6 |
| Localizes to pain | 5 | Localizes to pain or withdraws to touch | 5 |
| Withdraws from pain | 4 | Withdraws from pain | 4 |
| Abnormal flexion to pain (decorticate) | 3 | Abnormal flexion to pain (decorticate) | 3 |
| Abnormal extension to pain (decerebrate) | 2 | Abnormal extension to pain (decerebrate) | 2 |
| No response to pain | 1 | No response to pain | 1 |
| **Best verbal response** | | **Best verbal response** | |
| Orientated and converses | 5 | Alert; babbles, coos, words to usual ability | 5 |
| Disorientated and converses | 4 | Less than usual words, spontaneous irritable cry | 4 |
| Inappropriate words | 3 | Cries only to pain | 3 |
| Incomprehensible sounds | 2 | Moans to pain | 2 |
| No response to pain | 1 | No response to pain | 1 |

### Posture and tone

Hypotonia may be seen in the seriously ill child no matter what the underlying diagnosis. Hypertonia and posturing should be observed, if present, and any asymmetry noted. Decorticate posturing is evidenced by flexed upper limbs and extended lower limbs, whereas in decerebrate posturing both the upper and lower limbs are extended. These are both pre-terminal signs and must be acted on immediately.

### Pupil size and reactivity

Examination of the pupils can give valuable information. It is important to determine whether there is dilatation, non-reactivity or inequality. Most importantly, unequal pupils may indicate tentorial herniation or a rapidly expanding lesion on one side of the brain. Small, reactive pupils may indicate a metabolic disorder or medullary lesion.

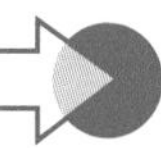

**Practical points**

- In the collapsed child, a careful and orderly primary assessment and timely resuscitation measures are of more importance than the diagnosis.
- Children differ from adults physiologically and anatomically.
- Conditions affecting respiration are a common pathway to collapse in the child.
- Cyanosis and hypotension are pre-terminal signs.
- Decerebrate and decorticate posturing are pre-terminal signs.

### Respiratory patterns in neurological failure

Raised intracranial pressure can lead to a number of abnormal breathing patterns, ranging from hyperventilation to apnoea.

### Circulatory changes in neurological failure

Hypertension, bradycardia and hypoventilation form the Cushing triad. These are late signs of raised intracranial pressure and must be acted on immediately. Hypotension is a pre-terminal event.

### Exposure

Infants and small children have a proportionately greater surface area and therefore lose heat more rapidly than older children and adults. Infants are also less able to respond to hypothermia. Early measurement of core temperature is therefore important, and appropriate warming during resuscitation should be maintained.

Fever may indicate infection.

It is important to expose the child fully for the primary assessment, as valuable clues such as rashes in meningococcal disease or bruises in inflicted injury may be missed.

The child may respond with fear or embarrassment to exposure and therefore it must be undertaken sensitively.

## Reassessment

Frequent reassessment should be undertaken, especially if there is any deterioration during the resuscitation. A search for a definitive diagnosis should now be completed.

## Putting it all together

Table 5.1.4 summarizes the components of the primary assessment in table format.

**Table 5.1.4 Putting it all together: the primary assessment**

| **Airway – Assess patency** | | |
|---|---|---|
| Look for | Listen for | Feel for |
| Movement of the chest wall<br>Intercostal and accessory muscle use | Air movement<br>Abnormal sounds – stridor | Air movement |
| **Breathing – Assess adequacy of breathing** | | |
| Effort of breathing | Effectiveness of breathing | Effects of inadequate respiration |
| Recession<br>Respiratory rate<br>Inspiration or expiration noises<br>Grunting<br>Accessory muscle use<br>Flare of the alae nasi | Breath sounds<br>Chest expansion<br>Abdominal excursion | Heart rate<br>Skin colour<br>Mental status |
| **Circulation – Assess adequacy of circulation** | | |
| Cardiovascular status | Effects of circulatory inadequacy on other organs | Signs of cardiac failure |
| Heart rate<br>Pulse volume<br>Capillary refill<br>Blood pressure | Raised jugular venous pulse height (not in infancy)<br>Respiratory rate and character<br>Skin appearance and temperature<br>Mental status<br>Urinary output | Gallop rhythm<br>Crepitations in lungs<br>Enlarged liver |
| **Disability – Assess neurological function**<br>A rapid measure of level of consciousness should be recorded – AVPU method<br>Note the child's posture and tone – especially any lateralizing features<br>Check pupils for size, equality and reactivity<br>Note the presence of convulsive movements | | |
| **Exposure**<br>Take the child's core temperature<br>Look for a rash or injury | | |
| **Reassessment**<br>Should be performed regularly, especially if there is deterioration | | |
| AVPU: Alert, Voice, Pain, Unresponsive. | | |

# 5.2 Resuscitation

Ed Oakley, Mike South

The term 'collapse' is used here to describe a state in which a child's neurological and/or cardiorespiratory function is acutely and severely impaired.

## Diagnosis

Collapse may occur because of: a primary neurological process; loss or reduction of oxygen supply to the brain; or a metabolic disturbance or toxins affecting brain function. Collapse may be the result of many different disease processes, some examples of which are shown in Table 5.2.1. A more thorough differential diagnosis and approach to assessment of the collapsed child is presented in Chapter 5.1.

### Clinical example

David, a 2$^1/_2$-year-old boy, was found collapsed in the bedroom while visiting his grandmother's house. He was taken immediately to a local hospital where he was noted to be floppy and poorly responsive to voice or physical stimulation. He had an adequate airway, his breathing was a little shallow and slow, and he was slightly dusky in colour. His limbs were pink and felt warm, and he had strong pulses.

David was placed on his side and oxygen was administered by facemask; his colour improved immediately. He was afebrile, with normal blood glucose on bedside testing, and no other physical abnormalities were found.

A careful history showed that he had been very well all day. He had been playing unobserved in his grandmother's house for about an hour before he was found. His grandmother kept some sedative drugs (nitrazepam) in the bedside cabinet, and a telephone call back to the house revealed that the tablet bottle was lying open on the bedroom floor.

David continued to receive oxygen and close observation, and his clinical condition improved steadily over the next 12 hours. He was discharged home well the following day.

Sometimes the cause of collapse is immediately obvious, as in head injury or drowning, but sometimes it may be a diagnostic problem initially (e.g. sepsis or drug ingestion). In this latter setting, resuscitation usually has to take priority over obtaining a complete history, examination and investigation. With sufficient personnel available, diagnostic and resuscitative procedures may progress in parallel. One important investigation to consider early when the cause of collapse is unknown is a blood glucose estimation.

## Resuscitation

If you find yourself responsible for the immediate care of a collapsed child, you should be familiar with at least the procedures used in basic life support. The general principles may be the same as those used in the resuscitation of adults, but specific techniques are required in children.

The primary aim is to restore an adequate supply of oxygenated blood to the brain – to prevent secondary brain damage. The resuscitation procedures required will vary, depending on the degree of physiological impairment, from simple ones, such as application of an oxygen facemask or administration of a bolus of intravenous fluid, through basic cardiopulmonary resuscitation (CPR) to advanced life support measures including endotracheal intubation, mechanical ventilation and the use of vasoactive drugs.

Resuscitation techniques for newborn infants are discussed in detail in Chapter 11.1.

### Life support

The environment is important: make sure you are in a safe situation – you will be of no value to the collapsed child if you, the rescuer, become a second victim (e.g. at a road accident scene). Get someone to summon sufficient extra help.

Quickly evaluate the degree of collapse:

- Assess the child's response to verbal or physical arousal (e.g. gentle shaking)
- Colour – pale or blue
- Temperature – cool peripheries.

Then move quickly to the ABC. The term ABC is a useful reminder of not only the manoeuvres required (Airway, Breathing, Circulation) but also of the correct sequence in which to apply them. **Assessment of the airway and breathing should be**

**Table 5.2.1 Some causes of collapse in children**

| Category | Diagnosis |
|---|---|
| Primary neurological process | Meningitis<br>Head injury<br>Encephalitis<br>Seizures |
| Failure of oxygen supply to brain | Acute asphyxia (e.g. drowning, birth asphyxia)<br>Respiratory causes (e.g. severe asthma, croup)<br>Cardiac causes (e.g. arrhythmias, myocarditis)<br>Hypovolaemia (e.g. dehydration, haemorrhage)<br>Sepsis<br>Anaphylaxis |
| Metabolic disturbance or toxins | Hypoglycaemia<br>Hyponatraemia<br>Drug or other toxic ingestion<br>Envenomation<br>Bacterial toxins |

**performed quickly, with emphasis on rapid progression to the circulation.**

In obviously more advanced states of collapse, do not waste time on assessment but commence CPR immediately.

### Clinical example

Jodie, a 6-year-old girl, was a rear seat passenger when her family's car was involved in an accident while travelling at around 60 km/h. She was not wearing a seat belt.

On arrival at hospital, she was awake but agitated with multiple superficial abrasions to her face, trunk and limbs. Within 20 minutes her state of consciousness deteriorated, she developed increasing tachycardia and her blood pressure had fallen.

Jodie was intubated to protect her airway; during the procedure careful attention was paid to prevent excessive movement of her cervical spine. The doctor had already inserted a large-bore cannula into a vein in her antecubital fossa, and through this she was given 40 mL/kg saline. She was re-examined for possible sites of hidden bleeding, including the abdomen and limbs (especially fractured femur). Her abdomen was noted to be distended and she underwent computed tomography (CT), which showed small lacerations of the liver and spleen. CT of her brain, performed at the same time, was normal. Jodie was managed with supportive care, including mechanical ventilation and blood transfusion. Surgical exploration of the abdomen to control bleeding was considered but not performed, as she stabilized with medical treatment. She was discharged from the intensive care unit 4 days later.

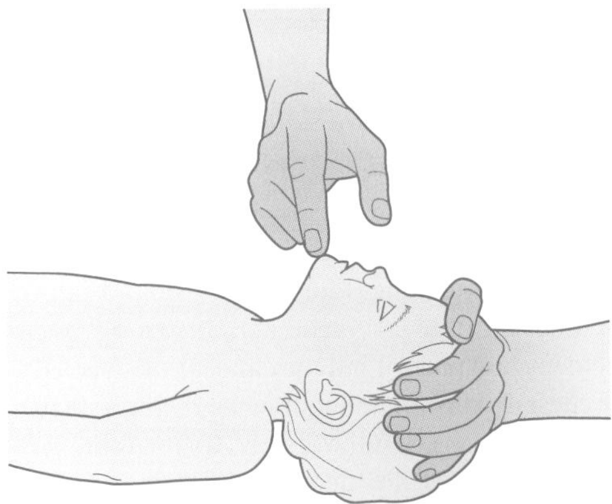

Fig. 5.2.1 Optimal head and neck position for airway protection in an infant. Do not overextend the neck. This head and neck position may be used with the child on its side or lying on its back.

## Airway

If conscious, the child will usually adopt the best posture to maintain his or her own airway: don't force the child to lie down.

In an unconscious child, assess the adequacy of the airway by observing the degree of chest movement and by listening and feeling for breath at the mouth (place your ear close to the child's mouth).

An unconscious child with a patent airway should be placed on the side: this improves the size of the airway (gravity pulls the jaw and tongue forward), allows saliva and other secretions to drain from the mouth, and reduces the risk of aspiration of gastric contents should they be regurgitated. Moving the child in this way may be harmful if there is a possibility of cervical spine injury (e.g. following road trauma); in this case, work to obtain an optimal airway in the existing position without excessive rotation, flexion or extension of the neck.

If the airway is completely or partially obstructed, it may be further improved by extending the neck to the neutral, or slightly extended, position, and supporting the jaw in a forward position; this is easiest done with the child on their back (Fig. 5.2.1). This may be done by placing your fingers behind the angle of the mandible and applying gentle forward pressure. If secretions, gastric contents or food may be obstructing the airway, suck them out, preferably with a wide-bore rigid sucker.

If the airway is still not optimal, an oropharyngeal airway device may be tried. It must be of the correct size and inserted appropriately. If too large, it may increase airway obstruction and induce laryngospasm; it may also stimulate vomiting if the patient is partially conscious. The best size may be approximated by laying the airway beside the face: select a size that reaches from the front teeth to the angle of the mandible.

If it is not possible to secure an adequate airway by these means, endotracheal intubation will be required (see below).

## Breathing

Once you are sure that the airway is patent, assess the adequacy of breathing: look at the rise and fall of the chest and the rate of breathing. If strong breathing movements are present but they appear obstructed (with poor chest expansion and indrawing of the soft tissues), recheck and reposition the airway. If breathing remains inadequate or you are uncertain, commence artificial respiration. Do not delay, as ongoing hypoxaemia and hypercarbia are dangerous to a child whose brain is likely to be already compromised by the primary problem.

Artificial respiration may be given to assist existing breathing efforts, or as the sole source of gas exchange. If you are assisting the patient's existing but inadequate breathing efforts, you should attempt to synchronize artificial breaths with any taken by the patient. Additional breaths may also be required.

Respiratory support may take various forms: expired-air breathing; bag and facemask breathing; or endotracheal intubation and mechanical ventilation by machine or bag. The choice will depend on the state of the child, the availability of equipment and your experience. If inexperienced with endotracheal intubation, do not attempt this unless it is not possible to provide adequate respiration by other means (this is unusual in children). Appropriate sizes of endotracheal tube are given in Table 5.2.2.

In children less than 1 year of age, expired-air resuscitation should be administered with the rescuer's mouth covering the entire mouth and nose of the infant; in older children, mouth to mouth respiration is used (pinching the nose shut), as for adults.

Facemask and bag resuscitation may be performed with a variety of systems. Those with self-inflating bags are easiest to use.

**Table 5.2.2 Resuscitation card**

| Age | Weight (kg) | Min. sys. BP (mmHg) | HR (bpm) | RR (bpm) | Adrenaline 1:10 000 (mL) | Adrenaline 1:1000 (mL) | ETT int. diameter (mm) | ETT lip/ nose (cm) | DC shock 4 J/kg (J) | Fluid bolus 20 mL/kg (mL) |
|---|---|---|---|---|---|---|---|---|---|---|
| Term | 3.5 | 50 | 100–170 | 40–60 | 0.4 | – | 3.0/3.5 | 8.5/10.5 | 14 | 70 |
| 3 months | 6 | 50 | 100–170 | 30–50 | 0.6 | – | 3.5 | 9.5/11 | 24 | 120 |
| 6 months | 8 | 60 | 100–170 | 30–50 | 0.8 | – | 4.0 | 13/10 | 32 | 160 |
| 1 year | 10 | 65 | 100–170 | 30–40 | 1.0 | 0.1 | 4.0 | 14/11 | 40 | 200 |
| 2 years | 13 | 65 | 100–160 | 20–30 | 1.5 | 0.15 | 4.5 | 15/12 | 52 | 260 |
| 4 years | 15 | 70 | 80–130 | 20 | 1.5 | 0.15 | 5.0 | 14/17 | 60 | 300 |
| 6 years | 20 | 75 | 70–115 | 16 | 2.0 | 0.2 | 5.5 | 15/19 | 80 | 400 |
| 8 years | 25 | 80 | 70–110 | 16 | 2.5 | 0.25 | 6.0 | 16/20 | 100 | 500 |
| 10 years | 30 | 85 | 60–105 | 16 | 3.0 | 0.3 | 6.5 | 17/21 | 120 | 600 |
| 12 years | 40 | 90 | 60–100 | 16 | 4.0 | 0.4 | 7.0 | 18/22 | 160 | 800 |
| 14 years | 50 | 90 | 60–100 | 16 | 5.0 | 0.5 | 7.5 | 19/23 | 200 | 1000 |
| 17+ years | 70 | 90 | 60–100 | 16 | 10 | 0.5 | 7.5/8.0 | 19/23 | 300 | 1000 |

Adrenaline 1:1000, volume of 1:1000 adrenaline (epinephrine) to give a dose of 10 μg/kg; adrenaline 1:10 000, volume of 1:10 000 adrenaline (epinephrine) to give a dose of 10 ∝g/kg.

bpm, Beats or breaths per minute; ETT int. diameter, endotracheal tube size (internal diameter); ETT lip/nose, depth of endotracheal tube for fixation at lip (oral tubes) or nose (nasal tubes) – always verify that tube is in mid-trachea by clinical examination and X-ray; DC 4, direct current shock energy in joules for 4 J/kg – use same values for both monophasic and biphasic defibrillators (exact settings may have to be modified according to those available on the specific defibrillator); fluid bolus (saline), volume of saline for 20 mL/kg; HR, heart rate normal range; min. sys. BP, minimum acceptable systolic blood pressure; RR, respiratory rate normal range; term, term newborn infant.

Ideally, any collapsed child should receive high concentrations of inspired oxygen. This may be by simple facemask or through the circuit of the resuscitating bag. It is important to recognize that with most self-inflating bag systems a flow of oxygen is supplied to the patient only when the bag is squeezed. The appropriate delivery system for administering oxygen to a spontaneously breathing child is a simple facemask. Choose a facemask that covers the child's mouth and nose.

Assess the effectiveness of delivered breaths by watching the chest move. Ensure the administered breaths are of sufficient volume, but try not to blow excessively hard as this can lead to gastric distension. If there is no adequate chest movement, try re-establishing the airway as described above. Move on to manage the circulation, but quickly return to artificial breathing unless adequate spontaneous respiration has commenced.

**If there is difficulty with airway or breathing, or concern about performing mouth to mouth ventilation, move quickly to the circulation and return to the airway and breathing after 1 minute of external cardiac compressions.**

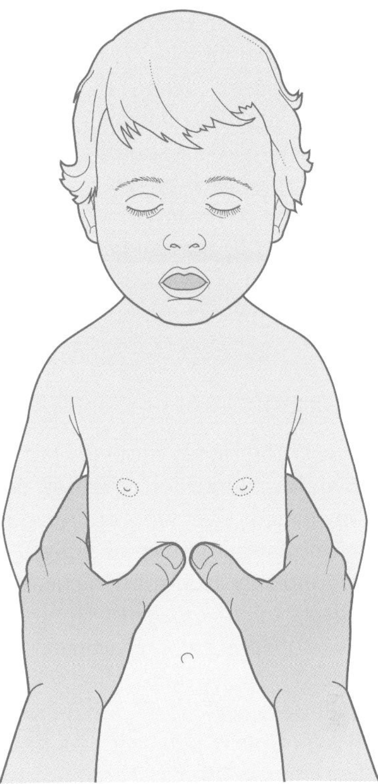

Fig. 5.2.2 In an infant, the chest may be compressed effectively by encircling the chest with your hands, with the thumbs over the lower sternum. This technique is not very suitable for solo rescuers as it is time-consuming to re-establish the position after administering a breath; in this situation, compress the chest with two fingers of one hand over the lower sternum.

## Circulation

The circulation is inadequate if:

- no central pulses (e.g. carotid or femoral) are palpable
- the heart rate is less than 60 in a collapsed child, or
- the pulses are weak, with other signs of poor tissue perfusion (pallor, coldness, poor capillary refill).

Cardiac compression is indicated for a child with no pulses, weak pulses, bradycardia, or if there is any uncertainty.

**The pulse can be difficult to assess in an emergency situation. If in doubt, commence compressions – you will be unlikely to do any harm.**

The optimal technique for chest compression varies with age:

- *Infant.* Encircle the chest with the hands, with the thumbs over the lower sternum (Fig. 5.2.2). This technique is not very suitable for solo rescuers as it is time consuming to re-establish the position after administering a breath; in this situation, compress the chest with two fingers of one hand over the lower sternum.
- *Small child.* Use the heel of one hand, centred one fingerbreadth above the xiphisternum.
- *Larger child.* Use the heels of both hands (one atop the other), centred two fingerbreadths above the xiphisternum.

The aim for all ages is to compress the lower half of the sternum.

### Clinical example

Marco, a 2-year-old boy, was found at the bottom of his uncle's unfenced swimming pool during a family barbecue. No one knew how long he had been missing. When the ambulance arrived, his father was giving CPR and Marco was floppy and unresponsive, with no spontaneous respiration or palpable pulses. The ECG monitor showed asystole. Marco was intubated by a paramedic and an intraosseous needle was inserted. He received continuing CPR and multiple doses of intraosseous adrenaline (epinephrine) during transfer to hospital. Despite 30 minutes of further resuscitation efforts in hospital, he remained in asystole. It was clear that the prognosis for survival was hopeless and resuscitation was discontinued.

For children of all sizes, the chest should be compressed around 100 times/minute, depressing the anterior chest wall about one-third of the anteroposterior diameter. Push hard and fast.

Any child who requires chest compressions will also require artificial respiratory support; the converse is usually true also. For a single rescuer, chest compression and artificial respiration should be given at a ratio of approximately 30:2, whereas with two or more rescuers the ratio should be 15:2. Chest compressions should be resumed towards the end of the child's expiration. Once the child has an endotracheal tube in place, chest compressions should not be interrupted during the delivery of each breath.

Once CPR has commenced, a cardiac monitor should be connected to the child as soon as it is available. The rhythm should be assessed as VF/VT or non-VF/VT and management continued as in Figure 5.2.5A and B below.

## Fluid administration

Hypovolaemia is commonly an important factor in a collapsed child. Rapid infusion of a fluid bolus should be tried in any patient with signs of an inadequate circulation. Again, if in doubt go ahead and give some fluid: you are unlikely to do any harm and you can assess the effects on the patient's circulation. Initial boluses of 10–20 mL/kg are appropriate; these may be repeated as necessary. Normal saline is usually used, but colloid solutions such as 5% albumin may also be used. Avoid hypotonic fluids, such as dextrose solutions with low concentrations of sodium.

### *Vascular access*

A collapsed child will need vascular access for the administration of fluids and drugs.

Cannulation of a peripheral vein will provide adequate initial access. Try to place a large cannula if possible, or more than one cannula, particularly if you suspect that the collapse is related to haemorrhage.

Cannulation of a peripheral vein can be very difficult in a collapsed child; do not waste time trying for more than a few minutes. Central venous catheterization is an option but can be very difficult in this setting, even for experienced operators; it also takes a significant amount of time. A better alternative is the insertion of an intraosseous needle, whereby a needle is inserted into the bone marrow (which is a vascular space that cannot collapse because of the surrounding bone cortex). This technique is simple, quick and provides access for the administration of fluids and drugs that will reach the central circulation as quickly as if administered into a peripheral vein.

Commercially available intraosseous needles that include a stylet and handle are most commonly used, but a wide-bore lumbar puncture needle is a satisfactory alternative. With the stylet in place, insert the needle through the skin, perpendicular to the surface of the bone in all directions. Local anaesthesia is not required unless the patient is conscious. Twist the needle back and forth along its long axis while firmly pushing it into the bone. Do not rock it from side to side. A 'give' is usually felt as the needle tip enters the marrow cavity. Once you feel this, or once the needle has been inserted 1–2 cm into the bone, remove the stylet and aspirate the needle with a small syringe. Aspiration of dark, blood-like fluid confirms you are in the correct spot. Commercially available needles usually come with a plastic fixation device. If using a lumbar puncture needle, you can fashion a suitable fixation from plaster of Paris. The aim is for the needle to be well supported, to prevent it being dislodged and to prevent sideways movement and enlargement of the entry hole in the bone. Administration of fluid may require pressure on the infusion bag or the use of a syringe and three-way tap.

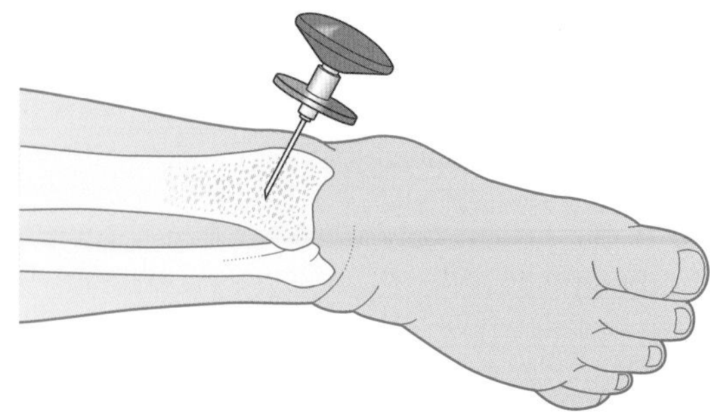

Fig. 5.2.3 Insertion of a needle into the bone marrow at the distal end of the tibia. The black handle facilitates the twisting motion and application of steady pressure as the needle is inserted. The handle, along with the attached stylet, is removed once the needle is in place.

Appropriate sites for intraosseous needle insertion include:

- the distal tibia (the medial aspect where the shaft of the tibia meets the malleolus; Fig. 5.2.3)
- the proximal tibia, about one-third of the way down from the knee to the ankle (on the flat part of the anteromedial aspect of the tibial shaft)
- the anterior iliac crest.

The tibia is most suitable for children under 5 years of age.

## Putting it all together

The basic life support approach to a collapsed child and the advanced management of established paediatric arrest are summarized in Figures 5.2.4 and 5.2.5.

It is important that life support measures (**especially external cardiac compressions**) are applied *continuously*. They should be interrupted only very briefly to assess response, heart rhythm, etc. They should not be terminated until stability has been clearly achieved or the decision to abandon further attempts has been made definitively.

## Ongoing resuscitation

If the child has persistently poor circulation despite the presence of sinus rhythm, and after 40–60 mL/kg intravenous fluid has been given, look for causes of

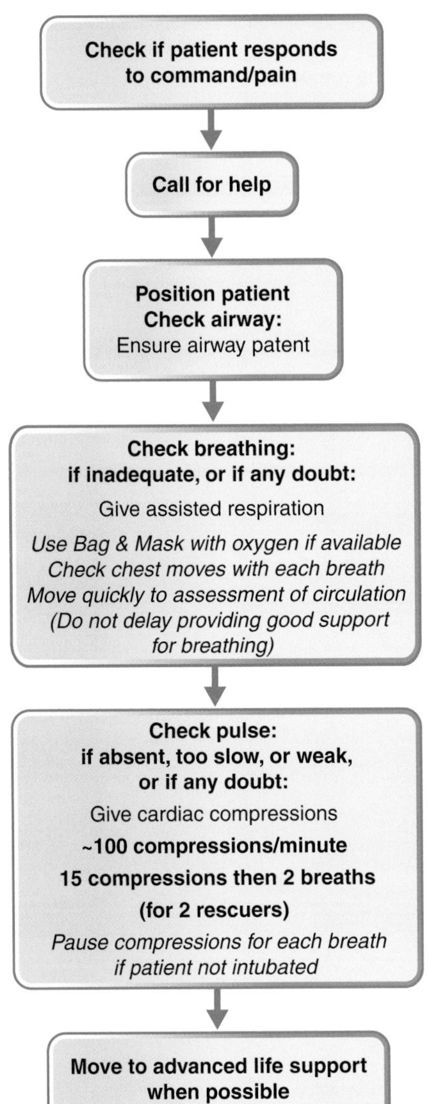


**Fig. 5.2.4** Basic life support.

hidden bleeding (especially abdomen, chest and fractured femur); also consider the use of an inotropic infusion such as dobutamine (10 ∝g per kg per min – put 15 mg/kg of the drug into 50 mL saline and run at 2 mL/h).

If the child is successfully resuscitated, careful ongoing monitoring and treatment will be required. It is a mistake to terminate intubation and mechanical ventilation too soon. Ensuing brain swelling may lead to a secondary deterioration.

It is important to know when to stop if resuscitation efforts are producing no effect. Except in cases of extreme hypothermia, as occur in drowning in near freezing water, persisting cardiac arrest after 20–30 minutes of good resuscitation is an indication of a hopeless prognosis. When hypoxia or hypovolaemia has resulted in cardiac arrest with asystole, particularly in an out-of-hospital setting, the prognosis for recovery or survival is very poor.

Temperature control following resuscitation is an area of controversy. Traditional teaching was to maintain normal body temperature using blankets and overhead heaters. There is now animal research, and some human studies, that suggest improved neurological outcome after cardiac arrest, or head trauma, if body temperature is quickly lowered to around 32–33 °C for a period of 48–72 hours following the insult. More research is needed before firm conclusions can be drawn regarding the use of therapeutic hypothermia in resuscitation of children.

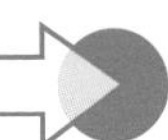

**Practical points**

- Learn the basics of paediatric life support before you need them – you won't have time to consult a textbook in an emergency.
- Do not waste time assessing the adequacy of breathing and circulation in a collapsed child. Assessment can be misleading and time-consuming.
- If the circulation or breathing are inadequate or you are uncertain, administer cardiac compressions and artificial respiration.
- Never hesitate to give a trial of an intravenous fluid bolus to a collapsed child.
- Learn the technique of intraosseous needle placement – this simple technique can be life-saving.
- Call for extra assistance early.

## Appendix

### Resuscitation guide A

Table 5.2.2 provides a summary of acceptable physiological parameters for children according to age, along with endotracheal tube sizes, DC shocks and doses of adrenaline (epinephrine) used in resuscitation. This table can be photocopied (or downloaded and printed from the internet at http://www.rch.org.au/clinicalguide/forms/resusCard.cfm). If folded horizontally at the centre, it can be laminated and punched to attach conveniently to a hospital ID badge, so making it readily available for reference in the clinical setting. It is also available for download to display on an iPhone, iPad, PDA and other smart phones.

### Resuscitation guide B

Another useful aid to resuscitation can be downloaded from the internet at http://www.rch.org.au/clinicalguide/cpg.cfm?doc_id=5137. It will run as a utility with any recent internet browser. It produces a table of appropriate drug doses, DC shocks and endotracheal tube sizes according to the age and weight of the patient.

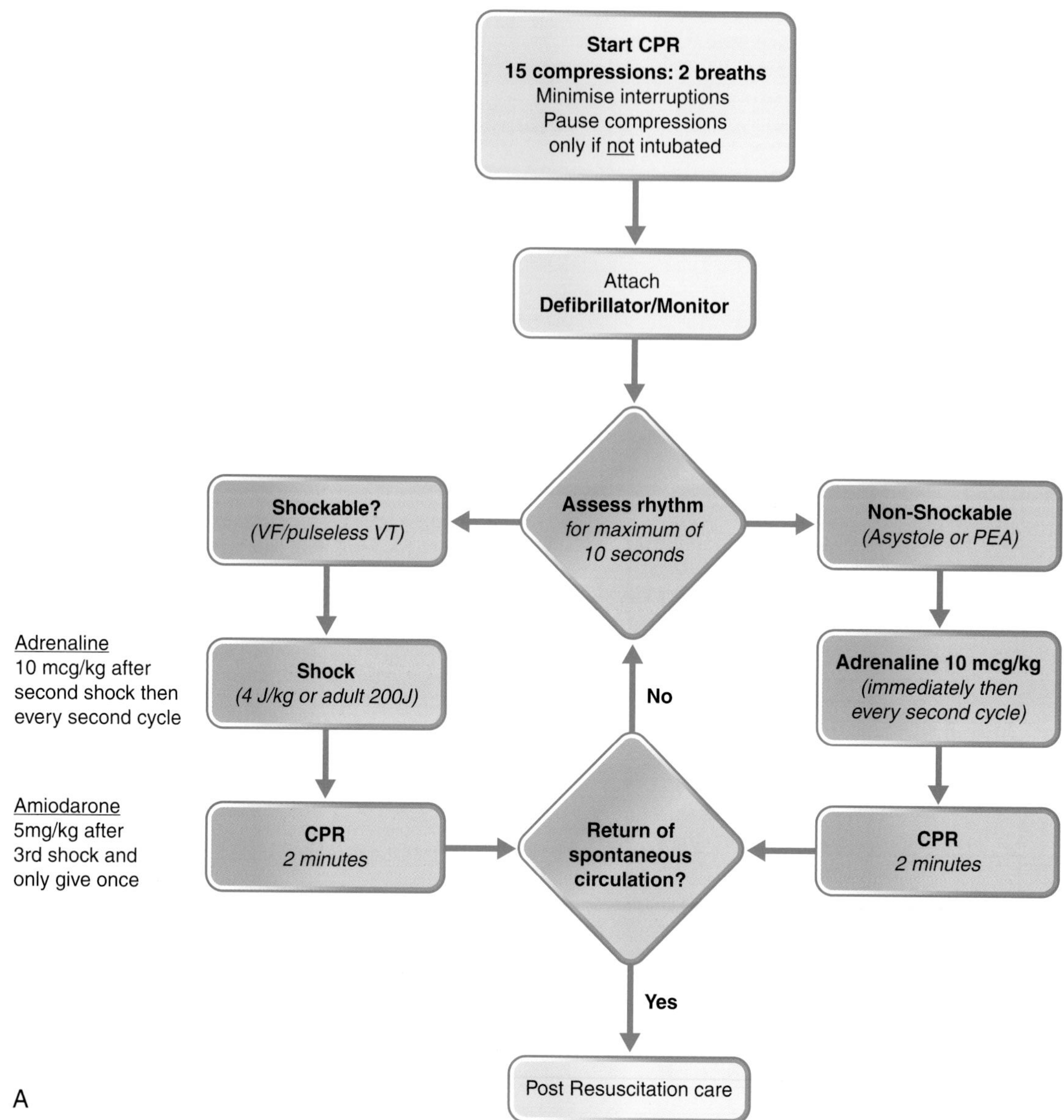


**Fig. 5.2.5A** Advanced life support. CPR, cardiopulmonary resuscitation; DC, direct current; IO, intraosseous; IV, intravenous; VF, ventribular fibrillation; VT, ventricular tachycardia.

**Double check:**
- ETT position
- Oxygen supply
- Function of self-inflating bag
- ECG leads in contact
- Defibrillator paddles in contact
- IV or IO access is secure

**Cardiac compression is tiring**
- Monitor technique
- Change operators every few minutes if possible

**Do not waste time when cardiac compressions might be given**
- Commence CPR immediately.
- If in doubt about circulation – give CPR.
- No prolonged attempts at intubation without CPR.
- During resuscitation cycles, do not check for pulse unless ECG shows an organized rhythm.
- Do not check rhythm immediately after DC shock – give CPR for 2 min then check.

**Correct treatable causes**
- Hypoxaemia
- Hypovolaemia
- Hypo/hyperthermia
- Hypo/hyperkalaemia
- Tamponade
- Tension pneumothorax
- Toxins/poisons/drugs
- Thrombosis

**Other drugs to consider**

***Atropine***
For persistent / bradycardia (20 µg/kg)
(min 100 µg, max 600 µg)

***Amiodarone***
If VF or pulseless VT persists after 3–4 DC shocks.
(5 mg/kg, max 300 mg) by bolus injection if patient unstable, or over 40 min if stable.
Flush IV line well afterwards.

***Lidocaine***
Same indications as amiodarone (1 mg/kg)
(0.1 mL/kg of 1%)
Amiodarone is the preferred agent; use lidocaine only if unavailable. Never give lidocaine after amiodarone.

***Magnesium sulphate***
For hypomagnesaemia
or for polymorphic VT (torsade de pointes)
50% solution: 0.05–0.1 mL/kg
(0.1–0.2 mmol/kg) (max 2 g) by intravascular infusion over 5 mins.

Sodium bicarbonate, calcium, and doses of adrenaline > 10 µg/kg have no place in routine resuscitation.

**Other issues**

***Blood gas analysis***
Arterial (and to some extent venous) blood gas analysis can help determine degree of hypoxaemia, adequacy of ventilation, degree of acidosis, and presence of electrolyte abnormalities such as hyopmagnesaemia. It is not a priority in initial resuscitation attempts, and obtaining a sample should not distract from other resuscitation manoeuvres.

B

Fig. 5.2.5B Advanced life support – notes. CPR, cardiopulmonary resuscitation; DC, direct current; ECG, electrocardiography; ETT, endotracheal tube; IO, intraosseous; IV, intravenous; VF, ventribular fibrillation; VT, ventricular tachycardia.

# 5.3 Poisoning and envenomation

James Tibballs, Ed Oakley, Ken Winkel

Poisoning and envenomation are two important areas of emergency care that should be familiar to any health practitioner involved with acute care of children and young people.

## Poisoning

Poisoning is a common health problem among children. It is responsible for numerous attendances to emergency departments of children's hospitals. Over 3500 children aged 0–4 years are admitted annually to Australian hospitals as a result of poisoning incidents. Worldwide, poisoning is the third most common cause of death among young children. A great deal of effort is expended upon a problem that is largely preventable. A Poisons Information Centre serving a population of 5 million receives approximately 40000–50000 telephone enquiries per annum; two-thirds concern actual poisoning and, of those, 60–70% concern children aged 4 years and younger.

### Epidemiology

The nature of poisoning varies for different age groups in children. Although poisoning in childhood is usually unintentional, the possibility of deliberate poisoning in the younger child as part of child abuse should not be forgotten. Pharmaceutical substances are involved in 70% of poisonings. In hospitals, errors in drug administration are frequent causes of poisoning.

#### Newborns

Poisoning is almost always iatrogenic in this age group. For example, newborns are at risk at delivery, when they may be given ergometrine instead of vitamin K, causing severe hypertension, convulsions and coagulopathy. In intensive care units, the frequent use of potent cardiovascular drugs, gentamicin, barbiturates, phenytoin, theophylline, digoxin, furosemide and opiates predispose the infant to poisoning.

It is not acceptable to perform noxious procedures without analgesia and sedation, and it is commendable that opiates are used in the newborn, but great care should be taken to ensure that overdose does not cause cardiorespiratory failure. Repeated doses or infusions of opiates should be confined to newborns who are mechanically ventilated, and, wherever possible, local or regional anaesthesia should be employed for surgical procedures. Local anaesthetic agents or opiates administered to the mother during labour may poison the newborn.

Care should be exercised with the use of topical antiseptics. Mercurochrome, commonly applied to the umbilical stump, may cause mercury poisoning if used in excess. Hexachlorophene should not be used as a regular bathing solution because it is readily absorbed percutaneously, causing neurotoxicity. If used in excess, iodinated compounds may cause hypothyroidism. Occasionally, mistakes in the preparation of artificial foods may cause serum electrolyte disorders and dehydration.

#### Age 1–5 years

Poisoning occurs most frequently in this age group. Most instances are said to be accidental, in which the young child discovers a drug or a household cleaning or chemical agent. The majority of serious poisonings occur with prescribed drugs or with over-the-counter drugs. Parents are often unaware that drugs must be stored safely and they underestimate the capabilities of young children who, at this age, become increasingly mobile and curious. They eat substances that are not palatable to adults, and tablets and capsules that resemble lollies (sweets).

The incidence and severity of accidental poisoning from drugs has been reduced markedly by the use of blister packs and containers with child-resistant lids. Poisoning in the home often occurs between 10 am and noon or between 6 pm and 8 pm when the child is active or hungry and when supervision has lapsed because the parent is involved in other household activities.

#### Age 6–12 years

Poisoning is relatively uncommon in this age group but it may be truly accidental, such as drinking a poison from a bottle that has been labelled wrongly, or when toxic agents have been stored inappropriately. A common example is storage of potentially toxic liquids in soft-drink containers in garden sheds.

Although uncommon, deliberate self-poisoning in this age group may occur as drug abuse or manipulative behaviour, or, less commonly still, genuine suicidal intent.

### Age 13–17 years

Emotionally disturbed adolescents and young adults may poison themselves deliberately, usually by ingestion, to manipulate their environment, or they may harbour a genuine suicidal intent. They may seek the thrill of drug abuse by inhalation or injection, sometimes as group behaviour. The peak incidence of teenage poisoning is at 14–16 years of age. Repeated episodes occur more frequently among girls but boys' suicide attempts tend to be more successful.

## Management

The immediate aim in the management of poisoning, whether serious or not, is to attend to the effects of the poison on the patient. Later, attention should be given to the circumstances with the aim of preventing a recurrence. There are innumerable poisons. All medicines and many household substances are poisonous if taken in sufficient quantity. Upon presentation, the action to be taken, if any, will be determined by the substance involved, its amount, the interval between ingestion and presentation, and the effect of the poison. The following principles of management may be applied universally.

In adolescents with intentional ingestions all medications should be removed from their person on arrival at hospital to prevent further ingestion.

### Support vital functions

It is imperative to maintain and support vital functions if these are depressed. Many poisons are excreted adequately or metabolized by the body if the vital functions are maintained. If the patient is unconscious, the airway, the depth and frequency of breathing, and the circulation should be examined for adequacy. Chapter 5.2 provides a full discussion on the management of deficiencies of the airway, breathing and circulation.

Loss of consciousness due to poisoning may be associated with cardiorespiratory failure and require endotracheal intubation and mechanical ventilation, preferably given by experienced personnel.

### Establish the diagnosis

It is important to establish:
- what poisons are involved
- in what quantity
- when exposure occurred.

Often the diagnosis of poisoning is self-evident, but at times the diagnosis is not obvious. When a poison has been identified, it should never be assumed that other poisons could not be involved. The symptoms and signs of poisoning are diverse but dangerous drugs threaten vital functions. Seriously poisoned patients present commonly with:
- unconsciousness
- cardiorespiratory failure
- convulsions.

If any of these are present and the cause is otherwise not known, poisoning should be high on the list of differential diagnoses. A meticulous physical examination and history provides invaluable help in diagnosis and treatment. Laboratory investigations may be necessary to establish a diagnosis, determine the amount of poison in the body, and help determine specific treatment for certain poisons.

### Prevent absorption

Some poisons contaminate the skin, conjunctivae and mucous membranes, and other poisons are inhaled as gases. Surface contamination requires copious irrigation with water, whereas inhalational poisoning may require oxygen therapy and mechanical ventilation. The great majority of poisons are ingested, for which the options for therapy include induced emesis (rarely), oral or gastric administration of activated charcoal, gastric lavage and whole bowel irrigation. If the poison has been absorbed already and has reached the vascular compartment, invasive techniques such as the following may be required:
- plasmafiltration
- haemofiltration
- charcoal haemoperfusion
- haemodialysis
- peritoneal dialysis
- exchange transfusion.

The poison, its amount and the seriousness of its effects determine the treatment of the poisoned patient. These must be weighed against the hazards of removal. Unconscious or drowsy patients, or patients who cannot protect their own airway, should not undergo induced emesis or gastric lavage or be given activated charcoal or colonic washout solutions. The consequences of aspirating gastric contents during vomiting or regurgitation in a less than fully conscious state far outweigh the dangers of many untreated poisons, as the mortality rate from severe pneumonitis is approximately 50%. However, it is appropriate to remove a wide variety of ingested poisons with either:
- activated charcoal
- whole bowel irrigation
- gastric lavage, or
- a combination of these techniques.

Circumstances of presentation and ingestion dictate the choice of technique.

Induced emesis, using ipecacuanha, was a commonly applied form of therapy but has now been largely abandoned because of limited effectiveness, the development of more effective techniques (e.g. activated charcoal) and risk of aspiration of gastric contents.

Activated charcoal is probably the most appropriate therapy in the emergency department, although whole bowel irrigation may be preferable for some agents. Gastric lavage should be reserved for a recent (within 1 hour) serious life-threatening ingestion in a conscious patient or for serious poisoning in a less than fully conscious patient who has airway protection. It is preferable that all patients undergoing gastric lavage have the airway protected with endotracheal intubation. The circumstances for the employment of each technique are summarized in Figure 5.3.1.

*Activated charcoal*

Activated charcoal is itself not absorbable but it adsorbs many different poisons in the gastrointestinal tract and thus prevents absorption of poison into the circulation. However, activated charcoal does not adsorb some poisons, including some elemental metals, some pesticides, ferrous sulphate, ethanol, corrosives and petrochemicals. There are many different preparations of activated charcoal, some with sorbitol as a laxative, but with these excessive diarrhoea and hypernatraemic dehydration may result.

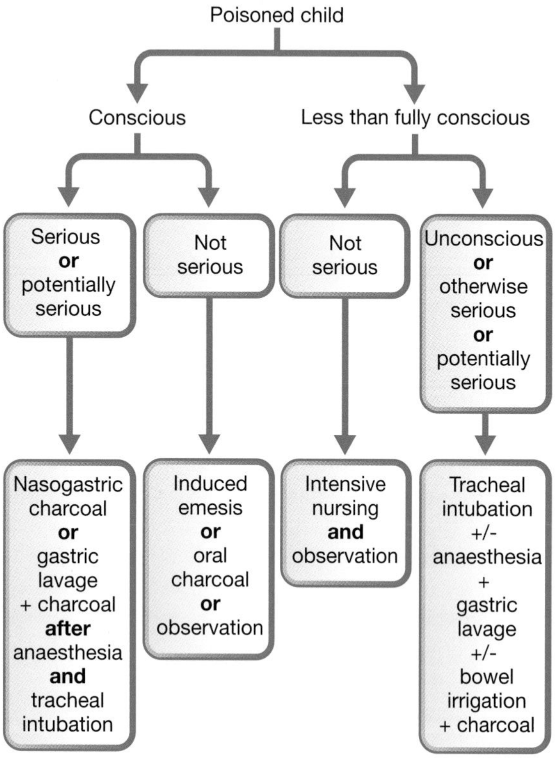

To be effective, activated charcoal should be administered within 1 hour of ingestion by mouth or by a nasogastric tube in a fully conscious patient, or by gastric tube in a less than fully conscious patient after the airway has been secured with an endotracheal tube. Children may be more likely to drink it if it is cooled and offered in an opaque paper cup with a lid and a black straw. The dose of activated charcoal is 10 times the ingested poison by weight or 1–2 g/kg of the child's body weight. Continued or repeated doses of activated charcoal, at doses of 0.25 g/kg 4–6-hourly, are useful if the poison is in a sustained-release preparation or if the charcoal is known to increase the total body clearance of the poison by interruption of its enterohepatic circulation or by leaching it from the circulation of the gastrointestinal mucosa. An alternative dosage regimen is 0.25 g/kg hourly for 12–24 hours. Activated charcoal should not be administered if gastrointestinal ileus is present, as this may cause regurgitation. Aspiration of activated charcoal may have a fatal outcome.

Activated charcoal is often administered, probably unnecessarily, with a laxative, notably magnesium sulphate, to prevent constipation. If magnesium sulphate is used, care should be taken to avoid hypermagnesaemia, a potential risk with repeated doses. Activated charcoal does not adsorb ipecacuanha and thus there is nothing to be gained by administering it to the patient whose induced emesis is excessive.



Fig. 5.3.1 Management of poisoning.

*Gastric lavage*

Gastric lavage was a commonly applied form of therapy but has now been largely abandoned. It is an invasive procedure and is justified only for significant recent poisoning when other techniques are contraindicated or are unreliable. It may also be indicated when the poison delays gastric emptying or forms concretions in the stomach. To be effective, however, it must be performed well and care must be taken to prevent complications. It is preferable to protect the airway with endotracheal intubation in all patients. Endotracheal intubation should be performed only by a person experienced in rapid sequence intubation and resuscitation.

Gastric lavage should not be performed after the ingestion of a corrosive substance because additional damage to the oesophagus (perforation, mediastinitis) and stomach (perforation) may occur. It is also unwise to perform gastric lavage after ingestion of petrochemicals or hydrocarbons as these substances have a very low surface tension and cause severe pneumonitis, even after minor contamination of the oropharynx, which may occur after the passage of the lavage tube renders the gastro-oesophageal sphincter incompetent. The risk of causing or exacerbating chemical pneumonitis exceeds the benefit of poison removal, despite the depression of central nervous system function that may follow. Such patients recover if vital functions are preserved.

Gastric lavage is a potentially traumatic procedure, particularly to the oropharynx, even when indicated. Occasionally the oesophagus and stomach have been perforated. It is psychologically as well as physically traumatic. For physical safety, the child must be restrained: this is best achieved by wrapping the child in a sheet with the arms pinned by the side. The child must be held in a lateral head-down position. For gastric lavage to be performed well, safely and atraumatically, it should be preceded by induction of general anaesthesia with endotracheal intubation.

*Whole bowel irrigation*

This is an effective technique to limit absorption of a poison. It is the preferred technique when the poison has passed beyond the pylorus and therefore cannot be removed by gastric lavage and when the substance is a drug or substance not adsorbed by activated charcoal. Slow-release drug preparations may also be removed with this technique.

The agent used is a mixture of polyethylene glycol and electrolytes that flushes out the contents of the bowel without disturbing the serum volume, osmolality or electrolytes. It is administered via nasogastric tube at a rate of 30 mL per kg per h for 4–8 hours until the rectal effluent is clear. It should not be administered to a less than fully conscious patient or when gastrointestinal ileus is present. Concomitant administration of activated charcoal is counterproductive.

*Removal from the circulation*

If the poison reaches the circulation, an invasive extracorporeal technique may be necessary to achieve removal. Usual techniques include forced diuresis, haemodialysis, plasmapheresis and charcoal haemoperfusion. These techniques are usually reserved for recognized circumstances when there is deterioration of vital functions despite maximal therapy (mechanical ventilation, inotropic/vasopressor therapy and artificial renal therapy) or the lack or failure of an adequate excretory or metabolic pathway (renal, hepatic) to eliminate the poison. For these techniques to be effective, however, the poison must have a relatively small volume of distribution. Peritoneal dialysis is not an efficient technique to remove poisons from the blood. Occasionally, the small size of a patient and the properties of a poison permit its removal by exchange blood transfusion.

## Administer an antidote

Only relatively few poisons have antidotes, but knowledge and use of these can be life-saving. The appropriate dose of each is determined by the amount of poison and its effects. A list of common important antidotes is given in Table 5.3.1.

**Table 5.3.1 Antidotes to some serious poisons**

| Poison | Antidotes | Comments |
|---|---|---|
| Amphetamines | Esmolol i.v. 500 µg/kg over 1 min, then 25–200 µg/kg/min | Treatment for tachyarrhythmia |
| | Labetalol i.v. 0.15–0.3 mg/kg or phentolamine i.v. 0.05–0.1 mg/kg every 10 min | Treatment for hypertension |
| | Diazepam 0.2 mg/kg i.v. | Controls agitation, aggression |
| Benzodiazepines | Flumazenil i.v. 3–10 µg/kg, repeat 1 min, then 3–10 µg/kg/h | Specific receptor antagonist |
| Beta-blockers | Glucagon i.v. 140 µg/kg, then 0.2–1 µg/kg/min | Stimulates non-catecholamine cAMP, preferred antidote |
| | Isoprenaline i.v. 0.05–3 mg/kg/min | |
| | Noradrenaline (norepinephrine) i.v. 0.05–1 µg/kg/min | Beware hypotension |
| Calcium channel blocker | Calcium chloride i.v. 10%, 0.2 mL/kg | |
| Carbon monoxide | Oxygen 100% | Decreases carboxyhaemoglobin. May need hyperbaric oxygen |
| Cyanide | Dicobalt edetate i.v. 7.5 µg/kg (max 300 mg) over 1 min, then 300 mg at 5 min | Give 50 mL 50% glucose after each dose |
| | Sodium nitrite 3% i.v. 0.33 mL/kg over 4 min, then sodium thiosulphate 25% i.v. 1.65 mL/kg (max 50 mL) at 3–5 min | Nitrites form methaemoglobin–cyanide complex. Beware excess methaemoglobin >20% Thiosulphate forms non-toxic thiocyanate from methaemoglobin–cyanide |

*Continued*

**Table 5.3.1 Antidotes to some serious poisons—cont'd**

| Poison | Antidotes | Comments |
|---|---|---|
| Digoxin | Magnesium sulphate i.v. 25–50 mg/kg (0.1–0.2 mmol/kg)<br>Digoxin Fab i.v: acute – 10 vials per 25 tablets (0.25 mg each), 10 vials per 5 mg elixir; steady state – vials = serum digoxin (ng/mL) × BW (kg)/100 | |
| Ergotamine | Sodium nitroprusside infusion 0.5–5.0 µg/kg/min<br>Heparin i.v. 100 units/kg then 10 30 units/kg/h | Treats vasoconstriction. Monitor BP continuously<br>Monitor partial thromboplastin time |
| Heparin | Protamine 1 mg/100 units heparin | |
| Iron | Desferrioxamine 15 mg/kg/h over 12–24 h if serum iron > 90 or > 63 µmol/L and symptomatic | Give slowly; beware anaphylaxis |
| Lead | Dimercaprol (BAL) i.m. 75 mg/m² 4-hourly for 6 doses then i.v. $CaNa_2$ edetate (EDTA) 1500 mg/m² over 5 days if blood level > 3.38 µmol/L. If asymptomatic and blood level 2.65–3.3 µmol/L, infuse $CaNa_2$ EDTA 1000 mg/m²/day over 5 days or oral succimer 350 mg/m² 8-hourly over 5 days, then 12-hourly over 14 days | |
| Methaemoglobinaemia | Methylene blue i.v. 1–2 mg/kg over several minutes | |
| Methanol, ethylene glycol, glycol ethers | Ethanol i.v. loading dose 10 mL/kg 10% diluted in glucose 5%, then 0.15 mL/kg/h to maintain blood level 0.1% (100 mg/dL) | |
| Opiates | Naloxone i.v. 0.01–0.1 mg/kg, then 0.01 mg/kg/h as needed | |
| Organophosphates and carbamates | Atropine i.v. 20–50 µg/kg every 15 min until secretions dry<br>Pralidoxime i.v. 25 mg/kg over 15–30 min then 10–20 mg/kg/h for 18 h or more. Not for carbamates | Blocks muscarinic effects<br>Reactivates cholinesterase |
| Paracetamol | *N*-acetylcysteine i.v. 150 mg/kg over 60 min then 10 mg/kg/h for 20–72 h or oral 140 mg/kg, then 17 doses of 70 mg/kg 4-hourly (total 1330 mg/kg over 68 h) | Restores glutathione, inhibits metabolites. Give within 18 h according to serum paracetamol level |
| Phenothiazine dystonia | Benztropine i.v or i.m. 0.01–0.03 mg/kg | Blocks dopamine reuptake |
| Potassium | Glucose i.v. 0.5 g/kg plus insulin i.v. 0.05 units/kg<br>Salbutamol aerosol 0.25 mg/kg<br>Sodium bicarbonate i.v. 1 mmol/kg<br>Calcium chloride 10% i.v. 0.2 mL/kg<br>Resonium oral or rectal 0.5–1 g/kg | Decreases serum potassium rapidly. Monitor serum glucose levels<br>Decreases serum potassium rapidly<br>Decreases serum potassium slightly; beware hypocalcaemia<br>Antagonizes cardiac effects<br>Adsorbs potassium slowly |
| Tricyclic antidepressants | Sodium bicarbonate i.v. 1 mmol/kg to maintain blood pH > 7.45 | Reduces cardiotoxicity |

BW, body weight; cAMP, cyclic adenosine monophosphate; EDTA, ethylenediamine tetra-acetic acid.

## Recognition of poisons

There are literally thousands of poisons and no one person can be expected to be familiar with them all. However, it is vital to recognize that any substance that has effects, or side-effects, on the central nervous system, cardiovascular system and respiratory system is a potential serious poison. It is prudent to be familiar with serious poisons that are ingested commonly (Box 5.3.1) and those that have delayed actions, such as colchicine, paracetamol and paraquat. The content of unfamiliar proprietary preparations should be sought, as effects may not be obvious from common usage. For example, the antidiarrhoeal drug Lomotil contains atropine and the opiate diphenoxylate, which may cause respiratory depression. Swallowed disc or 'button batteries' that impact in the oesophagus may cause ulceration into surrounding structures (trachea, aorta), whether by release of corrosive chemicals or by electrochemical activity, and must be removed urgently by endoscopy.

It is important to have access to a Poisons Information Centre by telephone, fax or e-mail. These centres maintain a vast store of up-to-date information and are usually accessible on a 24-hour basis. While Poison Information Centres provide an invaluable service, the management of the poisoned patient is the responsibility of the treating physician.

**Clinical example**

Simon, a 15-month-old toddler, was noted by his mother to be irritable, drooling saliva and to have inflamed lips after tasting the residue of the powder in their automatic dishwasher door. On examination, oropharyngeal ulceration was observed. An intravenous cannula was inserted for fluid and nutrition therapy, and endoscopy of the upper gastrointestinal tract was performed. Significant burns to the mid-oesophagus were discovered; these healed with stricture formation, necessitating repeated dilatation with bougies.

### Prevention

Too many poisonings are so called 'accidents', particularly among young children. Every opportunity should be taken to educate parents about the dangers of drugs and toxic substances in the home. A warning should be issued whenever a drug is prescribed and counselling given whenever poisoning occurs. It is erroneous to believe that young children cannot open drawers, cupboards and handbags or gain access to benchtops.

All drugs, however common and easily available, should be stored in a locked, childproof cabinet. Out-of-date drugs should be discarded safely. Household cleaning substances, fuels, and garden and workshop chemicals should be stored in truly inaccessible places. This applies particularly to automatic dishwasher powders and detergents, and to sink and oven cleaners, all of which are highly caustic and corrosive to the gastrointestinal tract. Corrosive poisoning occurs most often when small children have access to dishwashing powder or its residue in the receptacle of an open automatic dishwasher door.

Older children should be taught at home and at school of the dangers of drug abuse, including those of 'street' and pharmaceutical drugs, and that sniffing glue or hydrocarbons may cause a fatal dysrhythmia. In the case of self-poisoning by adolescents, the provocation is often the result of complex social and

**Box 5.3.1 Common lethal/serious poisons and substances**

- Antihistamines
- Aspirin
- Barbiturates
- Carbamazepine
- Carbon monoxide
- Caustic soda
- Chloral hydrate
- Clonidine
- Digoxin
- Disc batteries
- Dishwashing powder
- Hydrochloric acid (spirit of salts)
- Iron
- Major tranquillizers
- Opiates
- Paracetamol
- Theophylline
- Tricyclic antidepressants
- Verapamil
- Volatile substances

In rural areas/developing countries: paraquat, chloroquine, organophosphate insecticides

**Clinical example**

Amanda, a 3-year-old girl, was brought to the emergency department by her parents. Two hours previously she had been perfectly well when they were visiting friends, but since that time had become progressively drowsy and was unconscious on presentation. On examination, her respiration was shallow and her blood pressure was low. No signs of external trauma or infection were obvious. Mechanical ventilation, intravascular volume support and vasopressor therapy were necessary. In spite of the parents' denial of drug ingestion, a high level of amylobarbital was discovered in her urine, and the next day it was revealed that an opened bottle of tablets had been found in their friends' house. Amanda recovered completely.

**Clinical example**

Mario, a 13-year-old boy in previous good health but known to have experimented with drugs, collapsed while in the garage of a friend's house. The parents of the friend found him unconscious and summoned an ambulance, whose officers diagnosed ventricular fibrillation. They attempted to resuscitate him with mechanical ventilation and DC shock but were unsuccessful. External cardiac compression was continued, and on arrival at the hospital's emergency department he was still in refractory ventricular fibrillation. Numerous additional attempts at defibrillation using 4 J/kg DC shock administered with amiodarone and adrenaline (epinephrine) over 45 minutes failed to achieve sinus rhythm. Eventually asystole occurred. Post-mortem blood samples revealed high levels of *N*-butane and isobutane, constituents of cigarette lighter fluid, which presumably had been inhaled.

psychological disharmony, making remedial action lengthy and difficult (see Chapter 3.11).

All age groups are subject to iatrogenic poisoning at home and in hospital. Most iatrogenic errors result from mistakes in prescription (i.e. the dose of a drug and its interval). It is particularly important for doctors to refer always to a recognized prescription manual for children rather than relying upon memory or extrapolation from adult dosages, especially when dealing with infrequently used potent drugs. Prescriptions must be clearly written and, if abbreviations are employed, such as 'μg' or 'mcg' for microgram, they must be recognized by all staff. If in doubt, longhand printing should be used. Care should be taken with a decimal point. Equally, interpretation of a prescription must be with care, and the preparation checked before administration. All too often in hospitals, wrong drugs or wrong doses are given to the wrong patients.

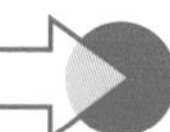

**Practical points**

- Childhood poison exposure is very common.
- Most exposures carry minimal morbidity but some are serious and can be fatal.
- You should know the general principles of management for poisoning.
- Poison Information Centres can provide detailed management advice.

## Envenomation

Australia harbours a wide variety of terrestrial and marine creatures. Of these, those that cause the most frequent or serious envenomation are species of snakes, spiders and jellyfish (Table 5.3.2).

**Table 5.3.2 Effects of Australian venomous animals and their treatments**

| Animal | Main effects | Main treatments |
|---|---|---|
| Snakes (many terrestrial and marine species) | Paralysis (rapid)<br>Haemorrhage | Pressure–immobilization bandage<br>Antivenom with premedication<br>Endotracheal intubation and mechanical ventilation<br>Clotting factors if haemorrhaging |
| Funnel-web spiders | Paralysis (rapid) | Pressure–immobilization bandage<br>Antivenom<br>Endotracheal intubation and mechanical ventilation |
| Redback spider | Pain<br>Paralysis (slow) | Antivenom |
| Australian paralysis tick | Paralysis (slow) | Remove tick<br>Endotracheal intubation and mechanical ventilation |
| Bees, wasps, ants | Anaphylaxis | Adrenaline (epinephrine) |
| Australian Box jellyfish | Paralysis<br>Hypotension<br>Pain | Douse with vinegar<br>Antivenom<br>Endotracheal intubation and mechanical ventilation |
| Blue-ringed octopuses | Paralysis (rapid) | Pressure–immobilization bandage<br>Endotracheal intubation and mechanical ventilation |
| Stone fish | Pain | Antivenom |

## Snake bite

Australia has over 100 species of snake, of which a dozen are among the world's most deadly. The average mortality rate from snake bite in Australia is two to three deaths per annum, approximately equal to the mortality rate from bee-sting anaphylaxis. The species that have caused mortality and significant morbidity belong to the genera of:

- Tiger snakes (*Notechis*)
- Brown snakes (*Pseudonaja*)
- Death adders (*Acanthophis*)
- Taipans (*Oxyuranus*)
- Black snakes (*Pseudechis*)
- Copperhead snakes (*Austrelaps*)
- Rough-scaled snake (*Tropidechis*).

Tiger snakes and Brown snakes account for most envenomations. All Australian snakes are elapids, whose venoms do not cause severe local effects.

The main components of venoms are:

- presynaptic and postsynaptic neurotoxins, which cause paralysis
- prothrombin activators, which cause disseminated intravascular coagulation and haemorrhage
- anticoagulants, which cause haemorrhage
- rhabdomyolysins, which may cause weakness and renal failure.

Different species have different effects, but the two most common acute threats to life are neuromuscular paralysis causing respiratory failure and coagulopathy causing bleeding. The combined effect is cardiorespiratory failure.

## Management

Snakes may bite but fail to inject venom on approximately 40–50% of occasions. In young children, particularly, snake bite is suspected even though a snake was not observed. In only 17–20% of such presentations has both a bite and envenomation occurred. Thus, one of the difficulties in the management of snake bite is to determine whether envenomation has actually occurred, irrespective of whether or not a bite by a snake was observed.

The syndrome of envenomation is characterized by a rapid onset of paralysis accompanied by coagulopathy over many minutes to several hours. However, an early diagnosis may be dependent upon subtle clinical signs and symptoms, abnormal laboratory tests of coagulation and a positive test for venom in the patient's urine or blood. The early reliable symptoms of envenomation are:

- headache
- abdominal pain
- vomiting.

Abnormal laboratory tests of coagulation are also very sensitive and reliable after bite by a species with coagulopathic effects. Most species can cause serious coagulopathy with the exception of Death adders. The onset of paralysis of large muscles, including respiratory muscles, is preceded by paralysis of the bulbar muscles, so that it is imperative to enquire and seek evidence of dysfunction of the external ocular muscles (double vision, ophthalmoplegia), facial muscles (ptosis), and the muscles of speech and swallowing (dysphonia, dysphagia).

The clinical diagnosis of envenomation may be confirmed with the snake venom detection kit test (CSL Diagnostics, Australia). This is a rapid enzyme immunoassay designed for clinical use. It gives a result in approximately 25 minutes and is capable of detecting venom in a concentration of as little as 10 ng/mL. The test can be applied to a swab of the bite site or to the victim's blood or urine. A positive result does not necessarily identify the snake but it stipulates which antivenom to administer, if clinically indicated.

The principles of treatment for snake bite are:

- to prevent rapid absorption of the venom from the subcutaneous tissue into the circulation by application of a pressure–immobilization bandage
- to neutralize the venom by the administration of antivenom
- to treat the effects of the venom, principally respiratory failure and bleeding.

The management of suspected and definite envenomation is summarized in Figure 5.3.2.

*Pressure–immobilization first aid*

Limbs sustain 95% of all bites. Snake venoms gain access from the subcutaneous tissue to the circulation via the lymphatics. These channels can be effectively occluded by the application of a firm crepe (or crepe-like) or elasticized bandage applied over the bite site and whole of the limb (Fig. 5.3.3). The application of a splint that includes joints on either side of the bite prevents the use of surrounding muscle groups and hence decreases lymph flow. Although the technique is a first-aid measure that should be applied at the scene of the snake bite to prevent initial absorption of venom, it is also used in established envenomation in hospital to prevent additional absorption of venom while preparations are being made to administer antivenom.

The bandage can be left in place indefinitely as it should be no tighter than a bandage for a sprained ankle. However, the bandage does not allow substantial inactivation of venom in the tissues and should be removed once the asymptomatic patient reaches a hospital that has a stock of antivenom, or after the envenomated patient has been given antivenom. It is dangerous to remove a bandage from an envenomated patient before administration of antivenom because its release allows a substantial additional quantity of venom to gain rapid access to the circulation. The splint and bandage should not be removed solely to allow inspection of the bite site of an envenomated patient; instead, the splint should be removed temporarily and a window should be cut in the bandage to allow a swab of the bite site to be taken for

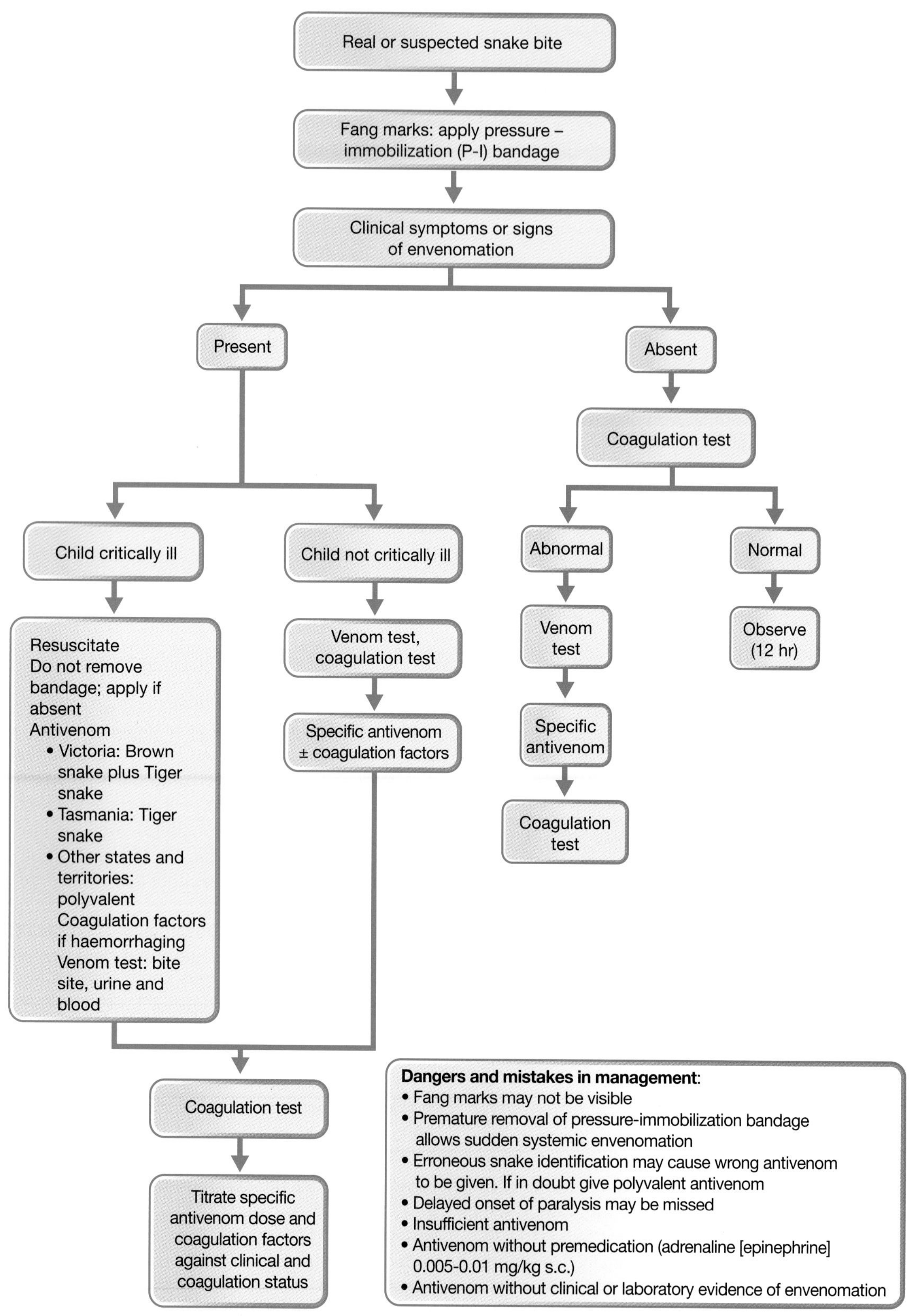


Fig. 5.3.2 Management of snake bite.

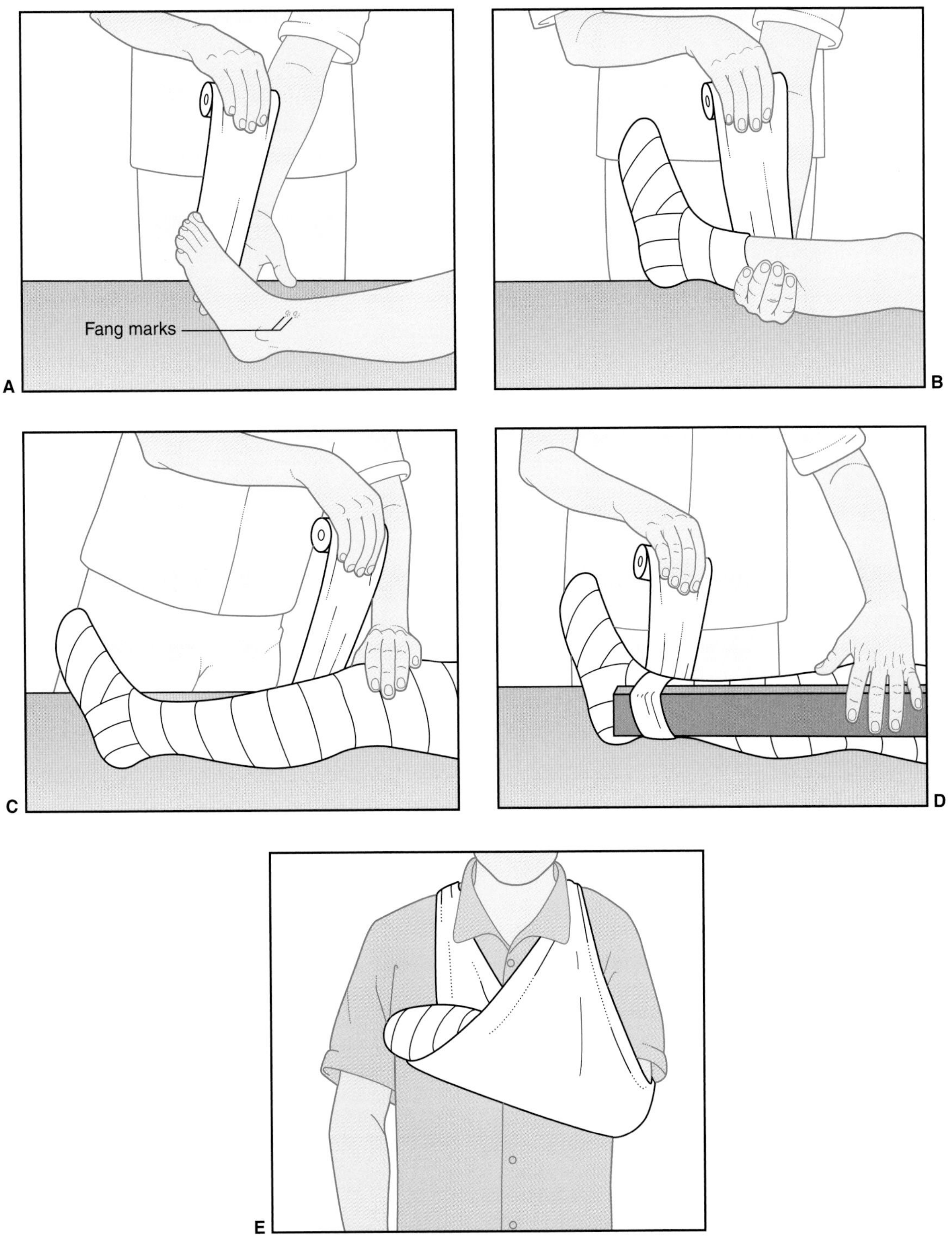


Fig. 5.3.3 Technique for applying pressure–immobilization first-aid bandage. **A–D**, Lower limb; **E**, upper limb.

venom testing, then the bandage should be reinforced and the splint reapplied. Bites are usually visible as scratches or puncture wounds, but their presence and appearance, or absence, does not prove or disprove envenomation and does not allow identification of the snake involved.

*Antivenom*

Specific monovalent antivenoms (Commonwealth Serum Laboratories, Melbourne) are manufactured against Tiger, Brown, Taipan, Black, Death adder and Beaked sea snake (*Enhydrina schistosa*) venoms. These are effective against all known snakes in Australia and

Papua New Guinea. A mixture of the five terrestrial antivenoms is available as a polyvalent preparation. The antivenoms are highly purified equine immunoglobulins. Cross-reactivity between species is limited, so it is essential to administer the correct antivenom according to the identity of the snake.

If the identity of the snake is not known or uncertain, the type of antivenom to be administered is based on the known geographical snake distribution or according to the result of a venom detection kit test (Commonwealth Serum Laboratories). In Tasmania, Australia, where dangerous snakes are a Tiger snake and a Copperhead species, the appropriate antivenom is Tiger snake antivenom. In Victoria, Australia, where the dangerous species are Tiger, Brown, Black and Copperhead snakes, the appropriate antivenom therapy is Tiger snake plus Brown snake antivenom. Everywhere else in Australia additional species exist and the polyvalent preparation should be chosen.

Although essential and life-saving, antivenoms are foreign (equine) proteins that may cause a life-threatening anaphylactoid reaction. However, this may be prevented by premedication with subcutaneous (not intravenous or intramuscular) adrenaline (epinephrine) 0.005–0.01 mg/kg. Additional protective agents such as a steroid (hydrocortisone) and an antihistamine may be indicated if the patient has a known allergic history. Only one premedication dose of adrenaline is required. The antivenom should be administered intravenously, diluted with a crystalloid solution, over approximately 30 minutes. However, for severe envenomation it may be delivered rapidly. If polyvalent antivenom or multiple doses of monovalent antivenom are required, a course of steroid therapy (prednisolone 1–2 mg/kg daily for 5 days) should be given to prevent serum sickness.

The dose of antivenom is never certain at the beginning of treatment because the amount of venom injected is unknown. Each vial of antivenom contains enough to neutralize the average yield from 'milking' – a process whereby venom is collected by inducing a snake to bite a membrane stretched tautly over a receptacle. However, the venom injected on biting is highly variable and bites may be multiple. Children are more susceptible than adults because of the larger venom:body mass ratio. The majority of envenomations are treated adequately with one to three vials, but this dose should never be relied upon; many more vials are usually required in life-threatening envenomations.

Antivenom should not be withheld if indicated, as there is no other satisfactory treatment. Antivenom should be administered either if there are clinical signs or symptoms of envenomation after snake bite or if in their absence a substantial coagulopathy is present. Occasionally, venom can be detected in the urine but there is no clinical evidence of envenomation or only a very mild coagulopathy. In this case antivenom may be withheld, but the patient's clinical and coagulation status should be checked regularly.

*Life support*

Bulbar and respiratory muscle paralysis in the severely envenomated patient requires endotracheal intubation and mechanical ventilation. If antivenom therapy is delayed, mechanical ventilation may be required for many days.

Coagulopathy may cause massive haemorrhage from mucosal surfaces and subsequent peripheral circulatory failure. Haemorrhage may occur into a vital organ, particularly the brain. It is essential to restore the circulatory volume with blood transfusion and to normalize coagulation with antivenom and coagulation factors (fresh frozen plasma). Antivenom neutralizes venom but it does not, *per se*, restore coagulation. Hepatic regeneration of clotting factors requires at least 6 hours after neutralization of venom with antivenom. Repeated laboratory tests of coagulation (prothrombin time, activated partial thromboplastin time, serum fibrinogen and fibrin degradation products) or a bedside test of whole-blood clotting time should be performed repeatedly to determine the need for more antivenom and coagulation factors. The coagulation status is the most sensitive guide to the need for additional antivenom after bite by coagulopathic species.

**Clinical example**

Martina, a $2^1/_2$-year-old child, collapsed with weakness, shallow respiration and weak pulses soon after playing in long grass where Tiger snakes had been observed. Mechanical ventilation was necessary. A test of coagulation revealed prolonged prothrombin and activated partial thromboplastin times, a depleted serum fibrinogen level, a low platelet count and a high level of fibrin degradation products. Haematuria and melaena were observed. Venom was detected in the child's urine and blood, and from scratch and puncture marks on the child's foot. Eight vials of Tiger snake antivenom and transfusions of platelets, packed cells and fresh frozen plasma were required before her coagulation status returned to normal. Adequate spontaneous respiration was resumed after 48 hours.

## Spider bite

Several thousand species of spiders exist in Australia. However, only Funnel-web spiders and the Redback spider are known to be potentially lethal or to cause significant illness. However, all spiders have venom and a few species may cause severe local injury. The White-tailed spider is often suspected of causing local tissue damage, but the number of cases where it has been clearly identified as the responsible spider is very small.

### Funnel-web spider bite

Several species of the genera *Atrax* and *Hadronyche* cause significant illness and are potentially lethal.

The most well-known species, *Atrax robustus* (Sydney funnel-web spider), is a large, aggressive spider that has caused the deaths of more than a dozen people inhabiting an area within an approximate 160 km radius of Sydney, Australia. The male is more dangerous than the female, in contrast to other species, and is inclined to roam after rainfall. In doing so it may enter houses and seek shelter among clothes or bedding and give a painful bite when disturbed.

Bites do not always result in envenomation, but envenomation may be rapidly fatal. The early features of the envenomation syndrome include nausea, vomiting, profuse sweating, salivation and abdominal pain. Life-threatening features are usually heralded by the appearance of muscle fasciculation at the bite site, which quickly involves distant muscle groups. Hypertension, tachyarrhythmias and vasoconstriction occur. The victim may lapse into coma, develop hypoventilation and have difficulty maintaining an airway free of saliva. Finally, respiratory failure and severe hypotension culminate in hypoxaemia of the brain and heart. The syndrome may develop within several hours, but it can be more rapid. Several children have died within 90 minutes of envenomation, and one died within 15 minutes. The active component in the venom is a polypeptide that stimulates the release of acetylcholine at neuromuscular junctions and catecholamines within the autonomic nervous system.

Treatment consists of the application of a pressure–immobilization bandage, intravenous administration of antivenom and support of vital functions, which may include artificial airway support and mechanical ventilation. No deaths or serious morbidity have been reported since introduction of the antivenom in the early 1980s.

### Redback spider bite

This spider is distributed all over Australia and is to be found outdoors in household gardens in suburban and rural areas. Redback spider bite is the most common cause for antivenom administration in Australia. The adult female is easily identified. Its body is about 1 cm in size and it has a distinct red or orange dorsal stripe over its abdomen. When disturbed, it gives a painful pinprick-like bite. The site becomes inflamed and may be surrounded by local swelling. During the following minutes to several hours, severe pain, exacerbated by movement, commences locally and may extend up the limb or radiate elsewhere. The pain may be accompanied by:

- profuse sweating
- headache
- nausea
- vomiting
- abdominal pain
- fever
- hypertension
- paraesthesias
- rashes.

In a small percentage of cases, when treatment is delayed, progressive muscle paralysis may occur over many hours and will require mechanical ventilation. Muscle weakness and spasm may persist for months after the bite. Death has not occurred since the introduction of an antivenom in the 1950s. If the effects of a bite are minor and confined to the bite site, antivenom may be withheld, but otherwise antivenom should be given intramuscularly or intravenously. In contrast to a bite from a snake or Funnel-web spider, a bite from a Redback spider is not immediately life-threatening, but inadequate initial treatment may result in long-term disability. There is no effective first aid, but application of a cold pack or ice may relieve the pain.

## Jellyfish stings

The most venomous animal in the world is the Australian Box jellyfish (*Chironex fleckeri*) and related species. It has caused at least 70 deaths in the waters off the north Australian coast. Other jellyfish species, notably numerous carybdeid species, may cause a significant illness known as the 'Irukandji syndrome'.

### Box jellyfish

This large jellyfish has a cuboid body up to 30 cm in diameter, and multiple tentacles that trail several metres. It is semitransparent and difficult to see by anyone wading or swimming in shallow water, where stings usually occur. The tentacles are lined with millions of nematocysts that, on contact, discharge tubules (barbs) coated with venom. The tubules pierce subcutaneous tissue, including small blood vessels allowing intravascular envenomation. Contact with the tentacles causes severe pain and, if envenomation is severe by contact with metre lengths of tentacles, it may cause death within several minutes. Death is probably due to both neurotoxic effects causing apnoea and direct cardiotoxicity. The protein venoms probably act by forming pores in cellular membranes. Although many stings are minor, the skin that sustains the injury may heal with disfiguring scars.

First aid, which must be administered on the beach, consists of dousing the skin with acetic acid (vinegar), to inactivate undischarged nematocysts. Adherent tentacles can then be removed safely. Cardiopulmonary resuscitation may be required on the beach. An ovine antivenom is available but prevention is of paramount importance. Water must not be entered when this jellyfish is known to be close inshore. Wetsuits, clothing and 'stinger suits' offer protection.

**Clinical example**

A 12-year-old boy sustained a massive jellyfish sting to his legs while wading in water close to the shore. Immediately he experienced excruciating pain but managed to reach the shore, where he became apnoeic. His father gave mouth-to-mouth breathing. Vinegar was poured over the wounds, typical Box jellyfish tentacles were removed and an ambulance was summoned. Shortly before arrival at hospital the boy became pulseless. Bag–mask ventilation with oxygen, external cardiac compression and intravenous adrenaline (epinephrine) were given. Spontaneous circulation was restored and he recommenced spontaneous respiration. In hospital, Box jellyfish antivenom was infused. Thereafter the boy made a slow recovery, but pulmonary oedema necessitated oxygen therapy and diuretic and inotropic infusion for several days. The boy recovered fully, but the stings healed with disfiguring scars.

### Irukandji syndrome

This is caused by the stings of some jellyfish belonging to the order Carybdeidae, including *Carukia barnesi* (Barnes' jellyfish). These are jellyfish with only four tentacles; they are small, transparent and very difficult to see in the water. A sting is usually very minor, but after some 30 minutes the victim experiences severe muscle pains, especially of the lower back, muscle cramps, vomiting, sweating, agitation, vasoconstriction, prostration and hypertension. The syndrome is in part due to release of catecholamines. Heart failure and hypertensive stroke may occur. Treatment is parenteral analgesia, control of hypertension and cardiorespiratory support in severe cases.

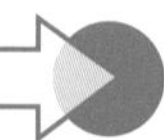

**Practical points**

- Envenomation is a serious and potentially fatal problem.
- Do not remove the pressure–immobilization bandage from a child bitten by a snake until the child is in a facility with resuscitation equipment, skilled staff and a supply of antivenom.
- Many cases of suspected or confirmed snake-bite will not require antivenom.
- Only give antivenom to symptomatic patients or those with significant coagulopathy.
- Very large doses of antivenom may be needed for massively envenomated children.

PART 6

# FLUID REPLACEMENT

# 6.1 Fluid replacement therapy

Trevor Duke, Sarah McNab

Safe management of the fluid and electrolyte needs of unwell children requires knowledge of body water and electrolyte composition, fluid requirements during health and illness, an ability to recognize signs of dehydration and overhydration, an understanding of composition of fluid replacement, and monitoring.

## Body fluid composition

Body fluids are separated into two main compartments, intracellular (ICF) and extracellular (ECF) fluid. ECF is further separated into intravascular and interstitial fluid. The proportion of body weight that is water falls from about 78% in a term newborn to 60% in adults (Table 6.1.1). Intracellular water accounts for about 40% of body weight. Intravascular fluid (plasma) accounts for only about 5% of body weight. Interstitial fluid is proportionately higher than intravascular fluid in infants, with an interstitial to plasma volume ratio of 5 : 1, compared with 3 : 1 in adults. Large changes in body weight over 24 hours or less usually reflect changes in total body water (TBW), because it takes a much longer period for substantial weight change due to growth or subcutaneous tissue wasting. In the first few days of life, there is a shift of water from ECF to ICF, accompanied by a 7% loss of TBW, so this is a very vulnerable period for dehydration with illness. Body fat contains only 20% water, so obesity implies a relative reduction in percentage of body weight as water. Conversely, malnourished children may have up to 80% of body weight as water. The clinical consequences are that:

- the severity of dehydration may be underestimated in obese children
- nutritional wasting is easily confused with dehydration as the clinical signs are similar
- fluid loads are poorly tolerated in severe malnutrition.

Water balance depends on intake, output and usage for metabolism. Water is normally lost from skin, lung, intestine and kidney. Fluid and energy requirements as a proportion of body weight decrease from infancy to adult life, so infants and children have higher metabolic requirements than adults and smaller absolute fluid stores, making them more vulnerable to dehydration.

ECF has relatively high sodium and chloride content. ICF has high potassium, phosphate, magnesium and protein concentrations (Fig. 6.1.1). Small intestinal secretions are high in sodium, diarrhoea fluid is high in potassium, gastric fluid is high in chloride and pancreatic secretions are high in bicarbonate (Table 6.1.2).

Cell membranes are relatively permeable to water, potassium and chloride, and relatively impermeable to sodium, phosphate and protein. Sodium is actively transported out of cells by energy-dependent sodium pumps. There is equilibrium in tonicity, hydrostatic and colloid osmotic pressure between plasma and interstitial fluid. Water leaves the arterial end of the capillary under hydrostatic pressure and is drawn into the venous end of capillary beds by plasma oncotic pressure.

### Regulation of extracellular fluids

The plasma osmolality, being the concentration of solute particles, remains almost constant between 285 and 300 mOsmol per kg $H_2O$. The osmolality of plasma is controlled through a finely regulated feedback system in the hypothalamus, the posterior pituitary and the collecting duct of the nephron, which contain osmoreceptors and volume receptors.

In health, the intake of water is regulated by thirst. This is controlled by a centre in the mid-hypothalamus, which responds to changes in circulating blood volume, via stretch and baroreceptors in the cardiovascular system, or small changes (as little as 1–2%) in plasma osmolality.

In the kidney, nephrons regulate water and electrolyte excretion. The nephron comprises the proximal tubule, the hypertonic medulla and ascending loop of Henle, the distal tubule and the collecting duct. The precise regulation of fluids and electrolytes in the ECF occurs by reabsorption of the glomerular filtrate into capillaries, secretion into the tubule lumen and eventual excretion in the urine.

Each day normal adult kidneys filter 180 litres water, 25 000 mmol sodium, 5000 mmol bicarbonate and 700 mmol potassium. Under normal circumstances

**Table 6.1.1 Body water distribution**

| Age group | Total body water (% of body weight) | ICF (% of body weight) | ECF (% of body weight) | ECF : ICF ratio | Blood (mL/kg) |
|---|---|---|---|---|---|
| Newborn | 79 | 35 | 44 | 1.25 | 100 |
| Infant | 60 | 33 | 27 | 0.82 | 80 |
| Child | 62 | 41 | 21 | 0.51 | 70 |
| Adult | 58 | 39 | 19 | 0.49 | 60 |

ECF, extracellular fluid; ICF, intracellular fluid.

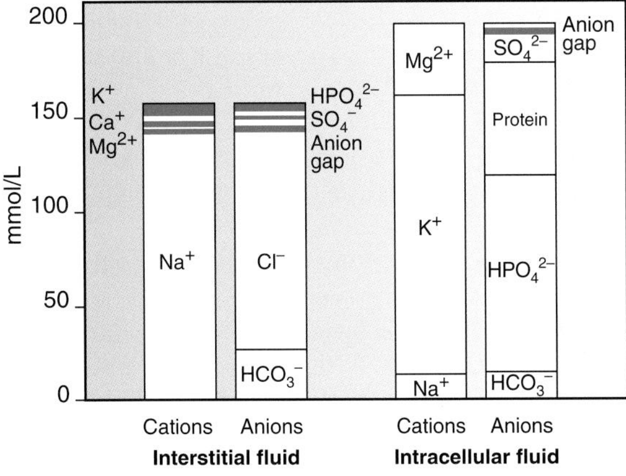


**Fig. 6.1.1** Electrolytes in body fluids.

**Table 6.1.2 Typical composition of body fluids in children (mmol/L)**

| Source | $Na^+$ | $K^+$ | $Cl^-$ | $HCO_3^-$ |
|---|---|---|---|---|
| Blood | 140 | 4 | 100 | 25 |
| Normal sweat | 22 | 9 | 18 | 0 |
| Bile | 150 | 10 | 100 | 20 |
| Gastric | 50 | 15 | 125 | 0 |
| Pancreatic | 140 | 10 | 100 | 45 |
| Small bowel | 140 | 8 | 60 | 70 |
| Diarrhoeal stool | 40 | 50 | 25 | 65 |

These are illustrative mid-range values but there is considerable variation in individual values.

most of this is reabsorbed. Approximately two-thirds of the filtered sodium is reabsorbed in the proximal convoluted tubule. Another 25% is reabsorbed in the loop of Henle, which is used to create a concentration gradient for the countercurrent multiplier system, allowing the production of concentrated urine. In adults, urine osmolality can vary from a maximal dilution of 100 mOsmol/kg to a maximal concentration of 1400 mOsmol/kg; newborns and young children have a more limited ability to concentrate and dilute urine. The distal tubule reabsorbs only 5% of the filtered sodium, but the electrical gradient generated is used for potassium and hydrogen ion excretion into the distal tubule. Renal sodium retention also occurs via the renin–angiotensin–aldosterone system.

Water retention is regulated via antidiuretic hormone (ADH) released from the posterior pituitary. The primary action of ADH is to increase the permeability of the renal collecting ducts to water. A rise in plasma osmolality is corrected by increased ADH secretion, resulting in a reduced volume of urine, which is concentrated. This allows the body to conserve free water to reduce plasma osmolality. Conversely, a fall in plasma osmolality inhibits ADH secretion, resulting in excretion of an increased volume of dilute urine.

Circulating blood volume is contained in arteries (10%), the venous system (55%), and heart, lungs and capillary bed (35%). The volume and distribution within the circulation is controlled by rapid feedback loops. Baroreceptors and stretch receptors in the heart and large vessels detect changes in venous tone and stimulate ADH secretion or inhibition and changes in venous tone, cardiac output and arteriolar resistance via the autonomic nervous system. Volume depletion is the dominant stimuli to thirst and ADH release, and so may stimulate water retention and oral intake at the expense of hypotonicity.

There are also non-osmotic drivers of ADH secretion, which allows ADH to be released despite normal or low plasma osmolality. Many of these stimuli are present in sick children and include intracranial pathology (e.g. meningitis, head injury), respiratory disease (pneumonia), surgery and pain. The potential for non-osmotic ADH stimuli must be considered when prescribing fluid replacement. ADH reduces the body's ability to excrete free water and may lead to hyponatraemia if an inappropriately hypotonic fluid is given.

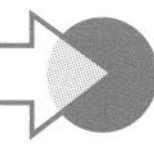

**Practical points**

- Antidiuretic hormone (ADH) helps maintain intravascular volume and osmolality.
- In unwell children, ADH secretion may occur despite normal or low osmolality. This decreases water excretion, further decreasing plasma osmolality.
- This must be taken into consideration when considering the volume and composition of fluid replacement.

### Oedema

Oedema is increased interstitial fluid and occurs by several mechanisms:

- increased hydrostatic pressure in the capillaries: venous obstruction, congestive heart failure
- decreased plasma oncotic pressure: hypoproteinaemic states such as nephrotic syndrome, protein-losing enteropathy, severe liver disease, and severe protein-energy malnutrition or kwashiorkor
- increased capillary permeability: this can occur locally from insect bites, or in one organ, such as cerebral oedema from traumatic brain injury, brain infection or other brain injury, or generally as in capillary leak syndrome from severe septicaemia.

Oedema may also occur if interstitial lymphatic vessels are poorly developed (Turner syndrome) or obstructed (e.g. filariasis, lymph node obstruction from tuberculosis).

## Assessment of dehydration

### Clinical history and examination

A detailed history and examination is essential for the assessment of any child with suspected dehydration, overhydration or electrolyte imbalances. The symptoms listed below are relevant to different cases, although they may not always be available or reliably elicited on history-taking.

#### History

- *Diarrhoea*: duration, frequency, basic estimate of volume (small, large, profuse), presence of blood, mucus
- *Vomiting*: duration, frequency, volume, presence of bile or blood, whether projectile
- *Eating and drinking*: frequency, thirst, type of fluid intake (e.g. breast milk, oral rehydration solution, cordials, hypercaloric feed supplements)
- *Urine output*: frequency, number of wet nappies
- *Associated symptoms*: fever, cough, shortness of breath, abdominal pain, seizures, rashes, etc.
- *Nutritional status*: view the child's growth chart including trend in values. Check skin folds on triceps and buttocks for presence of wasting. Also check weight for height, and height for age (low height for age in a malnourished child is stunting, which suggests chronic undernutrition).

#### Examination

- *General condition*: drowsy, restless or irritable
- *Vital signs*: temperature, pulse volume and heart rate, respiratory rate, blood pressure
- *Eyes*: sunken, no tears on crying
- *Mouth and tongue*: dry mucous membranes
- *Skin*: skin turgor reduced or central capillary refill time increased
- *Muscle tone*: weak, floppy or unable to hold head up
- *Chest*: deep acidotic breathing
- *Abdomen*: distended or tender, palpable masses.

The signs of dehydration are listed in Table 6.1.3. Precise estimation of percentage of dehydration is not possible using clinical signs, but an indication of the degree of dehydration, sufficient for formulating a plan for fluid management, is possible. Combinations of these signs are more specific than any individual sign. Clinical signs may be combined to classify a child as having mild (3–5%) dehydration (usually accompanied by few, if any, clinical signs), moderate (6–9%) dehydration, or severe (>10%) dehydration.

### Weight change

When available, weight change from the immediate premorbid state is the most accurate way of estimating the degree of dehydration. If the child has been weighed accurately in the last few days, the percentage weight loss will be approximately equal to the percentage dehydration. Another way of thinking of this is that the weight loss in grams is approximately equal to the fluid deficit in millilitres. However, the weights (premorbid and when sick) should be done using a comparable method: similar scale accuracy, unclothed, etc. If the premorbid weight was recorded more than a couple of weeks previously in young infants, the interpretation is less reliable and must take account of the weight gain expected because of growth.

**Table 6.1.3 Signs of dehydration**

| Degree of dehydration (approximate deficit)* | Mild, 3–5% (30–50 mL/kg) | Moderate, 6–9% (60–90 mL/kg) | Severe, ≥10% (100–150 mL/kg) |
|---|---|---|---|
| **Validated signs** | | | |
| General appearance | Well, alert | Thirsty, restless, irritable | Drowsy, floppy, limp ± comatose |
| Eyes | Normal | Slightly sunken | Very sunken |
| Mucous membranes | Moist tongue | Sticky tongue | Dry tongue |
| Tears on crying | Present | Decreased | Absent |
| Capillary return | Normal | Sluggish (2–3 s) | Slow (>3 s) |
| Respiratory rate | Normal | Increased | Fast |
| Skin pinch | Goes back quickly | Goes back slowly | Goes back very slowly |
| **Other signs** | | | |
| Thirst | Drinks normally, but may refuse ORS | Thirsty, drinks eagerly | Drinks poorly or not able to drink |
| Pulse | Normal | Fast | Fast, weak |
| Hands and feet | Normal | Normal | Cool, blue nail-beds |

*In young children.

ORS, oral rehydration solution.

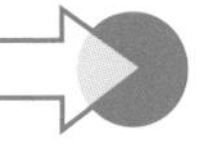

### Practical points

**Clinical evidence on assessing dehydration**

- A change in weight, where available, is the most accurate way to assess the degree of dehydration.
- Clinical signs will allow an estimation of dehydration, with combinations of signs performing better than individual signs.
- This classification is most reliable:
  - no signs of dehydration (usually less than 5% dehydrated)
  - some signs of dehydration (typically 6–9% dehydrated)
  - many signs of dehydration/signs of severe dehydration (10% dehydrated or more).
- Additional history and laboratory tests (e.g. bicarbonate) may be helpful in selected cases.

## Fluid requirements

Before administering fluid replacement, five questions need to be addressed:

1. Why am I giving fluid?
   Reasons for giving fluid can be broadly grouped into:
   - resuscitation
   - deficit
   - maintenance
   - ongoing losses.
2. How will I give the fluid?
   Options include:
   - oral
   - nasogastric/percutaneous endoscopic gastrostomy (PEG) tube
   - intravenous.
3. What type of fluid should I use?
4. How much fluid should I give?
5. How will I monitor the child receiving fluid replacement?

The fluid requirements of acutely unwell children are dynamic, and frequent monitoring of clinical signs, weight, urine output and some laboratory tests are essential so that appropriate modifications to fluid administration can be made.

### Resuscitation for shock

Fluid resuscitation involves the rapid restoration of intravascular volume and is needed where shock is present. The clinical signs of shock are poor peripheral perfusion, cool pale extremities, tachycardia with low-volume pulses, low blood pressure, high blood lactate levels or large base deficit. *Although hypotension is a sign of shock, this is usually a late sign in children; the absence of hypotension should not delay appropriate treatment.* Children with more than one of these cardiovascular signs require intravenous fluid resuscitation. If an intravenous cannula cannot be inserted in a child needing fluid resuscitation, use the intraosseous route to the circulation. A volume of 20 mL/kg of an isotonic fluid should be administered as a bolus (i.e. run through as rapidly as possible). As this fluid will replace intravascular volume, its osmolality should be similar to that of plasma. Examples of appropriate fluids are: 0.9% sodium chloride (also known as normal saline) or Hartmann's solution (also known as Ringer's lactate solution) (Table 6.1.4). In severe septic shock in adults and in severe malaria in children, there is some evidence that outcomes are better when

**Table 6.1.4 Types of intravenous fluid available**

| | $Na^+$ (mmol/L) | $Cl^-$ (mmol/L) | $K^+$ (mmol/L) | $Mg^{2+}$ (mmol/L) | Calcium (mmol/L) | Lactate (mmol/L) | Acetate (mmol/L) | Gluconate (mmol/L) | Glucose (g/L) |
|---|---|---|---|---|---|---|---|---|---|
| 0.18% sodium chloride (N/5) with 4% dextrose (hypotonic) | 30 | 30 | – | – | – | – | – | – | 40 |
| 0.45% (N/2) sodium chloride with 5% dextrose (hypotonic) | 77 | 77 | – | – | – | – | – | – | 50 |
| Plasmalyte148 solution (isotonic) | 140 | 98 | 5 | 1.5 | – | – | 27 | 23 | – |
| 0.9% sodium chloride (isotonic) | 154 | 154 | – | – | – | – | – | – | – |
| Hartmann's solution (similar in ionic composition to Ringer's lactate) (isotonic) | 131 | 111 | 5 | – | 2 | 29 | – | – | – |

Many pre-manufactured fluids are available in Australia, some examples of which are listed above. When listing a fluid as hypotonic, isotonic or hypertonic, we are referring to the *in vivo* tonicity. Given that dextrose metabolizes rapidly to free water, the *in vivo* tonicity of fluids containing dextrose differs from the *in vitro* tonicity or osmolarity. The *in vitro* osmolarity refers to the number of osmoles of solute per litre of solution, whereas the *in vivo* tonicity is the total concentration of solutes available to exert an osmotic force across the cell membrane. For example, the *in vitro* osmolarity of 0.18% sodium chloride with 4% dextrose is 286 mOsm/L $H_2O$, which is the same osmolarity as plasma. However, 5% dextrose is rapidly metabolized to free water. This results in an *in vivo* tonicity of 60 mOsm/L $H_2O$, which is markedly hypotonic.

albumin is used compared with crystalloids. If there is no improvement, a further 20 mL/kg should be administered. Any child receiving fluid resuscitation should be monitored closely and reassessed immediately after giving the fluid. If signs of hypovolaemia persist despite two 20 mL/kg boluses of fluid, the child should be monitored in an intensive care unit. Check for signs that are suggestive of an underlying cause of shock (e.g. sepsis, cardiogenic, metabolic, diabetic ketoacidosis, intussusception, poisoning).

## Replacing the fluid deficit

A patient's fluid deficit refers to the degree of dehydration at the time of presentation (see assessment of dehydration above and Table 6.1.3). If shock is present, this should be corrected first as described above.

If a recent premorbid weight is available, the volume of fluid deficit in millilitres is equal to the weight lost in grams. When a recent weight is unavailable, the percentage of dehydration must be approximated using the guidelines for assessment outlined above. The volume of fluid deficit may then be calculated using the following formula:

$$\text{Calculated fluid deficit}(\text{mL}) = \%\text{dehydration} \times \text{weight}(\text{kg}) \times 10$$

(e.g. 7% dehydration in a 12 kg child = $7 \times 12 \times 10 = 840$ mL deficit).

Deficits can be replaced either orally, via a nasogastric (or PEG, where there is one present) tube or intravenously, depending on the severity of illness and other factors.

Oral rehydration salts are the mainstay of treatment of dehydration from gastroenteritis for the majority of children. Specific oral rehydration solutions (ORS) can be suggested (for further information on ORS, see Fluid and electrolyte problems in specific illnesses – gastroenteritis, below). Where vomiting is present, oral rehydration is best achieved by offering small volumes of fluid frequently. This may be achieved by offering fluid via a syringe every 10 min or by using ORS icy-poles, which are available commercially. In general, aim for 10 mL/kg every hour.

ORS can be given via a nasogastric tube where adequate oral fluid is not tolerated and the child has moderate to severe dehydration, even if the child is vomiting. Nasogastric tubes can be unpleasant and carry a risk of pulmonary aspiration. After insertion, the position of a nasogastric tube needs to be checked. This is indicated by the presence of acidic gastric fluid aspirated from the nasogastric tube. Deficit can be rapidly replaced with ORS via a nasogastric fluid running at 25 mL per kg per h for up to 4 h or until the deficit is replaced. Where there is significant vomiting, the rate of nasogastric replacement may be reduced and, if the vomiting is due to gastroenteritis, ondansetron, an antiemetic, may be considered. A deficit should be replaced more slowly (over approximately 6–8 h) in young infants or those with significant abdominal pain.

Where oral or nasogastric fluid replacement is not tolerated or is contraindicated (e.g. suspected appendicitis), intravenous fluids are used. A fluid deficit primarily involves loss of extracellular fluid and, as such, should be replaced with an intravenous fluid with a similar osmolality to the extracellular space (e.g. Hartmann's solution or 0.9% sodium chloride). Hypotonic fluids (containing significantly less sodium than plasma) such as 4% dextrose with 0.18% sodium chloride should never be used. These fluids can lead to hyponatraemia, seizures and cerebral oedema.

When replacing a deficit intravenously, the rate of administration depends on the underlying condition. In general, where the deficit has occurred rapidly (e.g. acute gastroenteritis, appendicitis), it may be replaced rapidly (over approximately 4–8 h). Where the deficit has occurred over a longer period of time or there is significant electrolyte imbalance, the volume should be replaced more cautiously (over 24–48 h). In these circumstances, the ongoing requirement for maintenance hydration must also be taken into consideration (i.e. the maintenance requirement should be given in addition to the deficit replacement), plus additional fluid if there are ongoing abnormal losses such as persisting diarrhoea or vomiting.

Any child receiving fluid rehydration for a pre-existing deficit should be monitored closely. They should be weighed and clinically assessed prior to commencing therapy and after 6 h of rehydration. Those who are severely dehydrated should be assessed prior to this. Where the deficit is being replaced intravenously, serum electrolytes should be repeated after 6 h of therapy (sooner if there is an electrolyte imbalance). See "Assessment of dehydration" for important features to note on clinical assessment. Examining a child for signs of fluid overload is also important once fluid therapy has been instituted. All children should be reassessed after the deficit therapy is replaced to determine their ongoing fluid requirements.

## Maintenance fluids

Maintenance requirements involve replacement of normal losses from urine, sweat, lungs and faeces, and assume that any fluid deficit (dehydration) has been replaced.

The usual daily maintenance requirement can be calculated from the following formula:

- first 10 kg body weight: 100 mL/kg per day
- 11–20 kg: (100 mL/kg for the first 10 kg = 1000 mL) + 50 mL/kg for every kilogram above 10 kg
- above 20 kg: (100 mL/kg for the first 10 kg = 1000 mL) + (50 mL/kg for the second 10 kg = 500 mL) + 20 mL/kg for every kilogram above 20 kg.

The hourly maintenance requirement can be calculated from the following formula:

- first 10 kg body weight: 4 mL/kg per h
- 11–20 kg: (4 mL/kg for the first 10 kg = 40 mL) + 2 mL/kg for every kilogram above 10 kg
- above 20 kg: (4 mL/kg for the first 10 kg = 40 mL) + (2 mL/kg for the second 10 kg = 20 mL) + 1 mL/kg for every kilogram above 20 kg.

This is summarized in Table 6.1.5.

These volumes represent the water that is required, under normal physiological conditions, to excrete the daily production of nitrogenous wastes the body produces as urine that is isosmotic with plasma (i.e. that is neither overconcentrated nor overdiluted). These maintenance volumes are only a guide, and they cannot be applied directly to all seriously ill children, where water balance may be very different from normal physiology (Table 6.1.6).

Reduced free-water excretion is common in several conditions, including meningitis, encephalitis, bronchiolitis, pneumonia, perioperative states, burns, nausea and vomiting, where ADH release is stimulated by a variety of non-osmotic stimuli. In the past, hypotonic saline solutions (such as 0.18% saline plus 4% dextrose) (see Table 6.1.4) were often used as maintenance fluid for hospitalized children. However, administration of such hypotonic solutions, which have a markedly lower sodium concentration than the intravascular space, can lead to hyponatraemia, especially where free-water excretion is reduced or when large fluid volumes are administered. This can shift water intracellularly, causing seizures, cerebral oedema and death in some patients. To avoid these complications, solutions with a higher content of sodium (such as Hartmann's solution, normal 0.9% saline or half-normal 0.45% saline) should be the intravenous maintenance fluids of choice, and the volumes

**Table 6.1.5 Daily and hourly maintenance fluid requirements**

| Weight | Maintenance fluid requirement for 24 h | Maintenance fluid requirement per hour |
|---|---|---|
| First 10 kg | 100 mL/kg | 4 mL/kg |
| Second 10 kg | 50 mL/kg | 2 mL/kg |
| Subsequent kilograms | 20 mL/kg | 1 mL/kg |

**Table 6.1.6 Conditions affecting normal fluid requirements**

| Condition | Response in terms of fluid requirements |
|---|---|
| Non-osmotic ADH production | (a) Decrease fluid requirements for bacterial meningitis, acute pneumonia, head injury<br>(b) Decrease fluid requirements in stress (pain, surgery, emesis)<br>(c) Decrease fluid requirements with certain drugs (opiates, NSAIDs, vincristine) |
| Physical activity | Increase if active, decrease if inactive |
| Body temperature | Increase for fever, decrease for hypothermia |
| Metabolic rate | Increase if high, decrease if low |
| Respiratory rate | Increase for fast breathing |
| Humidity | Decrease for high humidity |
| Environmental temperature | Increase for sweating |

ADH, antidiuretic hormone; NSAID, non-steroidal anti-inflammatory drug.

administered should take account of the reduced free-water excretion that is common in many serious childhood conditions.

Although there is insufficient evidence from clinical trials to be certain how to avoid iatrogenic hyponatraemia and its serious consequences, after correction of signs of dehydration with isotonic saline it is essential to avoid rapid or excessive infusion of hypotonic fluids, to avoid overhydration and to monitor serum sodium regularly in children on intravenous fluids, particularly in conditions associated with increased ADH release.

Potassium is usually added to maintenance fluids unless the patient is in the immediate postoperative period, has renal impairment or is hyperkalaemic. Potassium requirements are around 2 mmol/kg daily, which equates to approximately 20 mmol/L running at standard maintenance rates.

Dextrose should be added to intravenous maintenance hydration. Current practice differs between institutions, but ranges between 2.5% and 5%, and sometimes up to 10% in neonates.

## Ongoing losses

Ongoing loss most frequently refers to diarrhoea and vomiting, although it also includes losses from stomas, drains, etc. Losses are often difficult to quantify, so it is better to review fluid balance, weight changes and clinical signs frequently, and adjust fluid rates accordingly. Ongoing losses should be replaced in addition to deficit replacement and maintenance hydration. A rough estimate for the additional volume lost in any diarrhoeal stool is:

- children under 2 years of age: 50–100 mL (¼ to ½ cup)
- children aged from 2 up to 10 years: 100–200 mL (½ to 1 cup).

Run the fluid rate as calculated for rehydration over 4 h, then review: weight, clinical examination including vital signs, ongoing losses, urine output and fluid intake (including breast milk). Be prepared to change the rate of administration depending on the above findings.

### Clinical example

Lucy is a 15-month-old girl who presented to the emergency department with a 24-hour history of decreased oral intake, profuse watery diarrhoea and one or two vomits (clear liquid). She was diagnosed with gastroenteritis. Her weight was 10.5 kg. No recent premorbid weight was available. Based on clinical signs, she was assessed as being moderately dehydrated. Her fluid deficit was calculated assuming a 7% deficit, which equated to approximately 735 mL ($7 \times 10 \times 10.5$ kg = 735 mL).

Her family had attempted oral fluid replacement at home using a bottle. However, every time she was offered the bottle, Lucy drank a large volume rapidly, which exacerbated her vomiting.

In the emergency department, it was explained that the most successful way to facilitate oral rehydration is by giving small volumes of oral rehydration solution (ORS) frequently. Her parents were given a cup of ORS and a 10-mL syringe, and instructed to give Lucy 10–20 mL ORS every 10 min. This was well tolerated and her parents slowly increased the volume offered. Lucy was also given an ORS icy-pole, which she enjoyed.

Lucy's parents felt well able to continue her fluid management at home. She was discharged following a period of observation.

## Clinical example

How would you manage the first 24 h of fluid replacement for a 2-year-old child weighing 12 kg who is assessed to be 7% dehydrated, has normal electrolytes and is unable to tolerate oral or nasogastric fluid?

**Fluids: deficit calculation**

| Intravenous rehydration | Maintenance (24-h requirement) | Total fluid (24-h requirement) | Total fluid (hourly requirement) |
|---|---|---|---|
| 7 × 10 × 12 kg = 840 mL | (10 kg × 100) + (2 kg × 50) = 1100 mL | 840 + 1100 mL = 1950 mL + ongoing losses | 1950/24 = 81 mL/h |

- This child requires 1950 mL fluid replacement over the first 24 h, which equates to approximately 81 mL/h.
- The deficit may be replaced over 24 h in conjunction with maintenance replacement. Given the large deficit, it would be appropriate to use an isotonic fluid for fluid replacement (see Table 6.1.4).
- The patient should be monitored clinically and have electrolytes determined after 6 h therapy. Ongoing losses should be measured and replaced.

## Electrolyte disturbances

Severe electrolyte disturbances occur in a significant proportion of hospitalized children in whom electrolytes are measured. Infants less than 6 months of age and children with severe dehydration are affected disproportionately. Derangements of acid–base, sodium and potassium are the most common abnormalities. In Aboriginal children with acute gastroenteritis in northern Australia, two-thirds have metabolic acidosis and/or hypokalaemia at the time of presentation. Children with diabetes, infants with pyloric stenosis, burns and adrenal insufficiency pose particular challenges.

### Hypokalaemia

Potassium can be lost from the extracellular space in diarrhoeal stools, especially with osmotic diarrhoea. In severe dehydration, rehydration and correction of metabolic acidosis may worsen hypokalaemia as ECF potassium moves intracellularly. With high aldosterone levels in dehydration, sodium and water retention by the kidney may also lead to potassium loss. Hypokalaemia may be manifest as hypotonia, irritability, intestinal ileus with abdominal distension, and cardiac arrhythmias with T-wave changes (flattened or inverted T waves or U waves). The serum potassium concentration may not reflect the degree of total body potassium depletion, as most is stored intracellularly (particularly in muscle and brain). Before giving potassium you must ensure that a child does not have renal failure. In view of the cardiac effects of extremes of plasma potassium concentration, electrocardiographic monitoring is important in severe hypokalaemia (<2.5 mmol/L) and with intravenous infusions of potassium in concentrations greater than 40 mmol/L.

#### Management

*Intravenous*

Unless the serum potassium is very low, commence an IV infusion of appropriate fluid including 20 mmol/L potassium. Monitor the serum level and increase to 40 mmol/L if the potassium level remains low. You must always calculate both the $K^+$ infusion rate (mmol per kg per h) and the $K^+$ concentration (mmol/L). Never exceed an infusion rate of 0.4 mmol per kg $K^+$ per h (as cardiac arrhythmias may occur) or an infusion concentration of 40 mmol/L $K^+$ (unless it is given via central vein), as it is irritating to peripheral veins.

*Oral*

Give 8–10 mmol per kg $K^+$ per day in divided doses 4–6-hourly. Large doses of oral potassium may induce vomiting, so each individual dose should not exceed 1.5 mmol/kg.

### Hyponatraemia

The most common causes of hyponatraemia in young children are hypotonic dehydration and iatrogenic water overload. This often occurs where there is ADH secretion (the so-called syndrome of inappropriate ADH secretion: SIADH) (see Table 6.1.6 and Chapter 12.3). Other causes include salt-losing nephropathy and salt wasting in some intracranial pathologies. Hyponatraemia with dehydration often accompanies acute gastroenteritis and is corrected by the standard rehydration protocols, including treatment of the fluid deficit. It is unwise to infuse large volumes of hypotonic solutions in children.

#### Management

- *Reassess for signs of dehydration.* Is hyponatraemia associated with dehydration? If the child is more than 5% dehydrated and the hyponatraemia is

due to gastroenteritis, rehydrate with an isotonic solution (e.g. 0.9% sodium chloride or Hartmann's solution) as above.
- *Assess for signs of fluid overload.* Is hyponatraemia associated with oedema or fluid overload? Look for excessive weight gain, oedema, signs of cardiac failure. If signs of fluid overload are present, decreasing the rate of administering fluid or ceasing IV fluid altogether is often all that is necessary.
- The use of hypertonic saline infusions (such as 3% sodium chloride) to correct hyponatraemia is indicated only in severely symptomatic children (e.g. seizures when the serum sodium is less than 120 mmol/L) and should be given only to correct the sodium to a safe level (such as 5 mmol/L more than the starting level) and until severe symptoms resolve. This should be done only after appropriate consultation.
- After initial correction of any severe symptoms of hyponatraemia (e.g. convulsions), the rate of rise of serum sodium should not exceed 1 mmol/L every 2 h. This is important to avoid causing osmotic demyelination. The longer the child has had hyponatraemia, the slower the correction should be.

Large increases in plasma lipids due to hyperlipidaemia or nephrotic syndrome may reduce the measured plasma sodium concentration, but the overall ECF sodium content may remain within the normal range (artefactual hyponatraemia). In diabetes mellitus, hyperglycaemia increases ECF osmotic pressure and draws water out of cells, causing a decrease in the plasma sodium concentration (see Diabetic ketoacidosis, below).

### Hypernatraemia

Hypernatraemia ($Na^+$ >150 mmol/L) may occur with moderate or severe dehydration, especially if oral fluids too high in solutes have been used for rehydration. This occurred frequently when boiled skim milk and homemade salt–sugar solutions were used to treat diarrhoea, and unmodified cow's milk was used for infant feeding. Fortunately this is now relatively uncommon. More recently hypernatraemic dehydration has occurred when hyperosmolar feeds (e.g. Poly-Joule) are continued in children with diarrhoea; this can lead to persistence of osmotic diarrhoea and hypernatraemia.

In children with hypernatraemia, the degree of dehydration is often underestimated because fluid shifts from the intracellular to the extracellular space, maintaining plasma and interstitial fluid volumes; therefore, the common clinical signs of intravascular dehydration (tachycardia, weak thready pulse) occur only when a child has very severe dehydration. Children with hypernatraemic dehydration may have marked irritability and a 'doughy feeling' to the skin over their abdomen, due to loss of intracellular water in the brain and soft tissues respectively. As the intravascular space is relatively well preserved, shock usually occurs late and may be sudden. Cerebrovascular thrombosis may occur because of hyperosmolarity.

#### Management

- Avoid rapid correction of hypernatraemia, as rapidly falling serum sodium may shift fluid from the extracellular into the intracellular space (following an osmotic gradient), causing cerebral oedema or seizures. Adjust fluid volume and composition to return the serum sodium to normal slowly (no more than 1 mmol/L every 2 h, or 10–12 mmol/L per 24 h). Do not use hypotonic maintenance intravenous fluids such as 4% + 0.18% saline, as this is likely to drop the serum sodium level too rapidly. Use Hartmann's solution, 0.9% NaCl (normal saline) or 0.45% NaCl (half-normal saline) if intravenous fluids are necessary.
- Rehydration with oral fluids is a good alternative, correcting the fluid deficit over 24 h.
- Regardless of the method of rehydration, the child's electrolytes and clinical signs need to be monitored frequently.

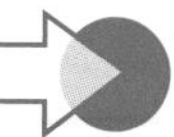

**Practical points**

**Electrolyte calculations**
- NaCl contains 17 mmol sodium and chloride per gram
- KCl contains 13 mmol potassium and chloride per gram, 0.75 g/10 mL = 1 mmol/mL $K^+$
- Sodium bicarbonate contains 12 mmol sodium and bicarbonate per gram, and 8.4% $NaHCO_3^-$ contains 1 mmol/mL sodium and bicarbonate per millilitre
- Osmolality of serum = $2Na^+$ + glucose + urea (in mmol/L), which is normally 270–295 mOsmol/kg
- Anion gap = $Na^+ + K^+ - (HCO_3^- + Cl^-)$, which is normally less than 12 mmol/L.

## Acid–base balance

### Metabolic acidosis

Metabolic acidosis commonly complicates severe illness but will usually correct with treatment of the primary disorder, provided there is normal renal function and bicarbonate production. Acidosis warrants specific treatment only if the low pH is interfering with normal cellular function, often considered as pH <7.15 (normal range 7.35–7.45). In severe sepsis, asphyxia, multi-trauma and cardiovascular collapse, tissue oxygen delivery or cellular oxygen utilization are impaired.

To produce sufficient energy for cell metabolism, adenosine triphosphate (ATP) is produced through anaerobic glycolysis. Excess hydrogen ions ($H^+$) in the form of lactate are produced in this process. These are initially buffered by red cells, plasma proteins or bicarbonate, or compensated for by increased removal of carbon dioxide by the respiratory system. The latter is manifest by tachypnoea, and sometimes by Kussmaul (deep sighing) respiration. Bicarbonate reacts with hydrogen ions to produce water and carbon dioxide: $H^+ + HCO_3^- \rightarrow H_2O + CO_2$.

When buffers become limited, blood pH falls, causing metabolic acidosis. pH and $H^+$ have a logarithmic relationship, such that a fall in the pH to 7.1 means the $H^+$ level has doubled from 40 to 80 nmol/L (Table 6.1.7).

Metabolic acidosis often accompanies diarrhoea with dehydration. There are a number of causes of acidosis in diarrhoea, including:

- bicarbonate loss in stool – the most common mechanism
- starvation ketosis
- lactic acidosis – this is rare in diarrhoea and occurs only in severe dehydration with decreased tissue oxygen delivery
- diminished renal function.

Acidosis is corrected by fluid replacement, correction of hypoxaemia, provision of calories and treatment of any infection. Intravenous sodium bicarbonate is rarely indicated in acidosis associated with diarrhoea and has the disadvantage of transiently worsening the hypokalaemia. Persisting metabolic acidosis with diarrhoeal disease may indicate the need for further rehydration (i.e. the degree of dehydration has been underestimated).

### Anion gap

Measurement of serum chloride and the anion gap (see Practical points: Electrolyte calculations) may be useful in determining the cause of metabolic acidosis:

Causes of metabolic acidosis with normal anion gap (8–12 mmol/L)

- Gastrointestinal loss of bicarbonate (diarrhoea)
- Renal loss of bicarbonate (renal tubular acidosis).

Note that the urine anion gap will be negative with gastrointestinal causes of acidosis and positive with renal causes of acidosis (decreased ammonia excretion)

Causes of metabolic acidosis with increased anion gap (>12 mmol/L)

- Increased organic acid production (e.g. lactic acidosis, diabetic ketoacidosis, organic acidaemias)
- Ingestion of toxic substances (e.g. salicylates, methyl alcohol, ethylene glycol)
- Decreased excretion of acid (e.g. acute and chronic renal failure).

### Alkalosis

Although much less common than acidosis, there are a few conditions where alkalosis occurs in children. Metabolic alkalosis occurs with recurrent vomiting in pyloric stenosis and diuretic use, and respiratory alkalosis occurs in hyperventilation.

## Fluid replacement in specific illnesses

### Gastroenteritis

Gastroenteritis is a common cause of dehydration worldwide. In mild to moderate dehydration due to gastroenteritis, rehydration with ORS is usually successful. Oral rehydration salt is a powder containing a specific balance of electrolytes and glucose, formulated for use in children with diarrhoea. ORS is based on the principle of glucose-facilitated intestinal sodium absorption. Soft drinks, sports beverages

**Table 6.1.7 Acidosis and alkalosis**

| Acid–base status | Clinical example | pH | Primary | Compensatory | Clinical feature |
|---|---|---|---|---|---|
| Metabolic acidosis | Diabetic ketoacidosis | ↓ | ↓ $HCO_3^-$ | ↓ $P_{CO_2}$ | Deep breathing |
| Metabolic alkalosis | Pyloric stenosis | ↑ | ↑ $HCO_3^-$ | ↑ $P_{CO_2}$ | Decreased respiration |
| Respiratory acidosis | Severe asthma | ↓ | ↑ $P_{CO_2}$ | ↑ $HCO_3^-$ | Respiratory distress, chest in-drawing |
| Respiratory alkalosis | Hysterical hyperventilation | ↑ | ↓ $P_{CO_2}$ | ↓ $HCO_3^-$ * | Tetany |

*May take several hours to develop, so is often not present initially.
$P_{CO_2}$, partial pressure of carbon dioxide.

and fruit juices are not appropriately constituted to be an effective ORS to treat dehydration, and may cause osmotic diarrhoea and hypernatraemic dehydration. Cereal-based solutions (e.g. rice ORS) have no advantage over glucose solutions in non-cholera diarrhoea.

The World Health Organization (WHO) ORS solution composition has been improved in recent years (now 75 mmol/L $Na^+$, compared with 90 mmol/L $Na^+$ in the solution that was used formerly). Reduced osmolarity ORS results in a decreased need for intravenous therapy and no increased risk of hyponatraemia compared with the ORS containing 90 mmol/L. Commercial solutions that have even lower sodium content (60 mmol/L) are more widely used in developed countries (Table 6.1.8). Continuation of feeding, particularly in breastfed infants, is important in the management of gastroenteritis. Continued breastfeeding, or early semisolid feeding, within 4 h reduces weight loss during illness and does not worsen diarrhoea or vomiting.

The failure rate of oral rehydration when used for gastroenteritis is low, at less than 5%. The main reasons for failure of oral rehydration are persistent vomiting, high purging rates (stool output), electrolyte disturbance (e.g. hypokalaemia), excessive drowsiness and shock.

In gastroenteritis, the use of antiemetics (e.g. ondansetron – available in wafers) has been shown in randomized controlled trials to reduce episodes of vomiting, and may facilitate oral or nasogastric fluid replacement.

Probiotics may be a useful adjunct to ORS in treating acute viral gastroenteritis, but may not benefit subgroups such as partially breastfed children or those with bacterial or parasitic causes of diarrhoea. Antidiarrhoeal drugs (such as opioids and binding agents) and antimicrobials have no place in the management of acute watery diarrhoea.

In young children, rotavirus is the most common cause of acute gastroenteritis. Since mid-2007, the rotavirus vaccine has been on the immunization schedule for all Australian children at 2, 4 and 6 months of age. This vaccine has been proven markedly to reduce episodes of severe gastroenteritis.

## Pyloric stenosis

Severe or protracted vomiting causes a hypochloraemic hypokalaemic metabolic alkalosis. Hydrochloric acid is expelled in gastric juice. The kidneys aim to correct the systemic alkalosis that results by retaining hydrogen ions at the expense of potassium ions. Infants with severe vomiting may have a serum chloride concentration below 80 mmol/L and bicarbonate above 40 mmol/L. In view of the alkalosis, Hartmann's solution is not an ideal rehydration fluid in pyloric stenosis as it contains lactate as a bicarbonate precursor. Normal saline with additional potassium can be used to replace the deficit, followed by normal maintenance fluids. It is important to correct dehydration and alkalosis before surgery, as severe alkalosis can result in postanaesthetic apnoea.

## Burns

For children with a burn requiring fluid resuscitation (usually more than 10% body surface area burned), an appropriate starting formula is intravenous Hartmann's solution 4 mL per kg per 1% burned surface area. Half of this fluid is given in the first 8 h and the remainder over the next 16 h, adjusting the rate according to the patient's response, best measured by the urine output. For adequate fluid resuscitation, children with burns may need to gain more than their preburn weight because of intracellular and interstitial oedema. During the second day after the burn, oedema fluid starts to be reabsorbed and urine output

**Table 6.1.8 Oral rehydration solutions (mmol/L of made-up solution)**

| Solution | $Na^+$ | $K^+$ | $Cl^-$ | Citrate (base) | Glucose | Osmolality |
|---|---|---|---|---|---|---|
| WHO (standard) | 90 | 20 | 80 | 10 | 111 | 310 |
| WHO (hypo-osmolar) | 75 | 20 | 65 | 10 | 75 | 245 |
| Gastrolyte-R | 60 | 20 | 50 | 10 | (111 as rice*) | 226 |
| Repalyte | 60 | 20 | 60 | 10 | 90 | 240 |
| Pedialyte | 45 | 20 | 35 | 10 | 126 | 250 |

*80% amylopectin, 20% amylose.
WHO, World Health Organization.

should increase. A rough guide to fluid requirements on day 2 is half of the first day's requirement, but as Hartmann's solution with 5% glucose. There is still controversy about whether colloid should be provided in the early period of burns resuscitation. Children with extensive burns or those involving the face or airway should be managed in specialized units.

## Bacterial meningitis

Careful management of fluid and electrolyte balance is important in the treatment of meningitis since overhydration or underhydration is associated with an adverse outcome. Many children have increased ADH secretion, and some have dehydration due to vomiting, poor fluid intake or septic shock. Hyponatraemia occurs in about one-third of children with meningitis and is variously as a result of increased ADH secretion, increased urine sodium losses and excessive electrolyte-free water administration. Children with meningitis require careful and regular monitoring of clinical signs of hydration state, including signs of overhydration, serum sodium and laboratory markers of hypovolaemia, and the total fluid intake adjusted accordingly. The fluid rates suggested in Table 6.1.9 are starting rates only. Enteral feeds should be started

**Table 6.1.9 Recommended total fluid intake (mL/h for the first 24–48 h) for children with suspected or confirmed meningitis, divided into four groups**

| Weight (kg) | A. Normal serum $Na^+$ and no dehydration, oedema or raised ICP | B. Serum $Na^+$ <135 mmol/L and no dehydration, oedema or raised ICP | C. Signs of dehydration or hypovolaemia | D. Signs of raised ICP or generalized oedema |
|---|---|---|---|---|
| 3 | 9 | 6 | 9 | 5 |
| 4 | 12 | 8 | 12 | 6 |
| 5 | 15 | 10 | 15 | 7 |
| 6 | 18 | 12 | 18 | 9 |
| 7 | 21 | 14 | 21 | 11 |
| 8 | 24 | 16 | 24 | 12 |
| 9 | 27 | 18 | 27 | 14 |
| 10 | 30 | 20 | 30 | 15 |
| 11 | 32 | 21 | 32 | 17 |
| 12 | 33 | 22 | 33 | 18 |
| 15 | 38 | 25 | 38 | 20 |
| 20 | 45 | 30 | 45 | 22 |
| 30 | 53 | 35 | 53 | 27 |

**Group A. Normal serum $Na^+$ and no signs of hypovolaemia, dehydration or raised intracranial pressure (ICP).** Fluid guideline based on giving 3 mL per kg per h up to a weight of 10 kg (about 70% of 'maintenance fluid requirements') as normal saline + 5% dextrose.

**Group B. Hyponatraemia ($Na^+$ <135 mmol/L) but no signs of hypovolaemia, dehydration or raised intracranial pressure.** Fluid guideline based on giving 2 mL per kg per h up to a weight of 10 kg (about 50% of 'maintenance fluid requirements') as normal saline + 5% dextrose. If the serum $[Na^+]$ is very low (<130 mmol/L) refer to the intensive care unit (ICU).

**Group C. Signs of dehydration or hypovolaemia at presentation.** Give repeated boluses of 10–20 mL/kg normal saline until hypovolaemia is corrected. Refer to ICU if signs of hypovolaemia persist. Ongoing fluid guideline based on giving 3 mL per kg per h up to a weight of 10 kg as normal saline + 5% dextrose.

**Group D. Signs of raised intracranial pressure or generalized oedema.** Fluid guideline based on giving 1–2 mL per kg per h up to 10 kg (about 25–50% of 'maintenance fluid requirements') as normal saline + 5% dextrose. A child with any clinical signs of raised intracranial pressure (e.g. very bulging fontanelle, unresponsiveness to painful stimuli or papilloedema) or of overhydration (e.g. facial or generalized oedema) should have fluids restricted and be monitored in an ICU. Development of generalized oedema is a major risk factor for serious adverse outcomes in meningitis, due, at least in part, to excessive fluid administration.

when the child is stable, but should be withheld in children who are poorly conscious, vomiting or having frequent convulsions. Children who are drinking well should have intravenous fluids running very slowly or the cannula capped.

### Diabetic ketoacidosis

Children with diabetic ketoacidosis (DKA) are at risk of cerebral oedema. After initiation of insulin therapy, glucose moves into cells and serum osmolarity falls, causing fluid to shift from the extracellular to the intracellular space. This can be exacerbated if hypotonic fluids are used for rehydration. Therefore, an isotonic fluid (e.g. 0.9% sodium chloride) should be used and any fluid deficit should be replaced slowly (over approximately 48 h). Potassium should be added to the fluid as insulin will drive potassium intracellularly, resulting in hypokalaemia.

Patients should be monitored frequently (1–2 hourly) with a clinical assessment (including neurological), fluid balance and venous blood gas (including sodium, potassium and glucose). In treating children with DKA, the serum glucose should fall slowly and the serum sodium and osmolarity should rise; this protects against cerebral oedema.

Cerebral oedema should be suspected if there is severe headache or any decrease in conscious state. Measures to reduce intracranial pressure (such as mannitol) should be started, computed tomography performed, and the child managed in the intensive care unit.

#### Clinical example

A 15-month-old Aboriginal boy presented with diarrhoea, floppiness and fast breathing. His mother said that he had had many watery bowel movements over a short period of time. On examination, he appeared unwell and was lethargic with sunken eyes. His vital signs were: temperature 37.5°C, heart rate 120/min, respiratory rate 60/min and blood pressure 86/53 mmHg. Although alert and responsive, he was noted to be floppy, with a dry mouth, absent tears on crying, weak radial pulses, a capillary refill time of over 2 seconds and slow skin pinch recoil. On auscultation, his heart sounds were normal and his lung fields were clear. His abdomen was soft and slightly distended with no tenderness, masses or visceromegaly. Bowel sounds were present. Neurological examination was normal except for mild hypotonia.

His weight on admission was 6.1 kg and his height 68 cm. These are all below the third centile. His head circumference was 43.6 cm, well below the second centile for age (Z-score −3.0).

He was given a bolus intravenous infusion of 120 mL (20 mL/kg) 0.9% sodium chloride solution, and blood was taken for full blood count and urea and electrolyte estimation.

The laboratory findings were as follows (reference ranges in parentheses):

**Blood tests**

***Full blood count***

Haemoglobin (g/L): 82 (105–135)
Mean corpuscular volume (MCV) (fL): 53.9 (75–85)
Red cell distribution width (RDW) (%): 24.1 (11.5–14.5)
Platelets ($\times 10^9$/L): 724 (150–450)
White cells ($\times 10^9$/L): 15.6 (6.0–11.0)
Blood film report: Marked microcytosis and hypochromia, moderate anisocytosis and poikilocytosis, neutrophil leukocytosis with no toxic changes and moderate eosinophilia.

***Electrolytes***

Sodium (mmol/L): 138 (132–144)
Potassium (mmol/L): 2.0 (3.2–4.8)
Chloride (mmol/L): 111 (98–106)
Bicarbonate (mmol/L): 6 (18–27)
Anion gap (mmol/L): 23 (8–12)
Urea (mmol/L): 5.3 (1.4–5.4)
Creatinine (mmol/L): 44 (0–55)

***Blood gases***

pH: 7.12 (7.35–7.4)
$P\text{CO}_2$ (mmHg): 20.3 (35–45)
Base excess: −18 (−4 to +3)
Blood lactate (mmol/L): 1.6 (0.8–1.8)

The boy was rehydrated with 600 mL Hartmann's solution with 1 g/L KCl added (17.4 mmol/L) over 4 h, followed by maintenance fluids at 24 mL/h with breastfeeding. By 24 h after admission he had been given 1200 mL fluids and his condition had much improved. His weight was now 6.7 kg, which implied that he had been about 9% dehydrated on admission ($6.7 - 6.1 = 0.6$ kg; $0.6 \div 6.7 \times 100 = 8.96\%$). His diarrhoea was settling and he was passing dilute urine.

Over the next 24 h, however, he had six foul, watery stools containing large amounts of reducing substances. There was also a decrease in his pH, bicarbonate and magnesium levels compared with 24 h previously. This relapse of osmotic diarrhoea was due to breast milk lactose overcoming the lactase threshold in the small intestinal mucosal brush border. He improved on oral lactase drops (β-D-galactosidase) with breastfeeds. The stool microscopy result reported ova of *Strongyloides stercoralis*.

This is a fairly typical case of acute gastroenteritis in an Aboriginal child from northern Australia, whose illness is frequently complicated by osmotic diarrhoea, hypokalaemia, acidosis and iron deficiency. The underlying small bowel damage could be prevented by improving hygiene, reducing overcrowding, and prompt treatment of micronutrient deficiencies, which would then make community oral rehydration therapy more effective.

PART 7

# PRINCIPLES OF IMAGING

# 7.1 Imaging

Rita L. Teele, Helen L.M. Bird

## Introduction

The tools of the radiologist include plain radiography, fluoroscopy (screening), intravenous, intracavity and gastrointestinal contrast media, angiography, nuclear medicine, ultrasonography, computed tomography (CT) and magnetic resonance imaging (MRI). Interventional radiology uses imaging for procedures such as abscess drainage, sclerosis of vascular malformations, biopsy and intravenous access.

There are many differences between imaging the child and imaging the adult. Radiologists rely heavily on the expertise of medical radiation technologists and sonographers in acquiring diagnostic images in sick or injured children. The child's physical and psychological welfare during diagnostic imaging must be considered. Imagine how the typical 2-year-old child, scheduled to have a micturating cysto-urethrogram, would react when introduced to a stranger wielding a catheter. Cooperation from young children is not possible when procedures are long and/or invasive; sedation is needed for many.

Paediatric ailments often differ from those of the adult. Congenital disease as well as acquired disease must be considered in the differential list of diagnoses. History-taking and clinical examination of infants and children is not easy; thus, information from imaging is crucial in certain situations. Radiation protection is important both for the child and for society as a whole; a child is 2 to 10 times more radiosensitive than an adult. Some specific disease states and syndromes are associated with increased susceptibility to injury from radiation (e.g. ataxia telangiectasia).

Radiation protection is provided by the following measures:

1. Limiting examinations to those that are likely to provide diagnostic help and influence treatment decisions
2. Using optimal technical factors in order to provide the lowest dose of X-rays for a diagnostic study
3. Limiting fluoroscopic time and using 'last image hold' techniques when possible
4. Using shielding whenever possible.

Measures 2–4 are the responsibility of the radiologist and radiographer, but the clinician is responsible for choosing imaging studies carefully. The radiologist should be available for discussion of appropriate imaging for a given diagnostic consideration.

The equipment in the department of radiology should be calibrated to provide images requiring low-dose irradiation but still provide good diagnostic detail. Factors for image production from CT should be modified to suit the size and age of the patient. Dose measurements are expressed in units termed gray (Gy) (absorbed dose; 1 Gy equals 100 rad) or sievert (Sv) (equivalent dose; 1 Sv equals 100 rem in the old terminology).

Every person is exposed to background radiation from the world around them and from cosmic rays. Radon gas provides the major source of background dose. Total annual background dose, per person, therefore depends heavily on the geographical location, and is estimated to be 2–3 mSv (Table 7.1.1). This does not include medical exposure, predominantly from CT, which in the USA has recently doubled the average per person background dose to 4–6 mSv. For comparison, two radiographs of the chest give 0.02–0.08 mSv – less radiation than received on a round trip by air across the Pacific Ocean.

Conversely, advances in imaging have made diagnosis far more accurate and safe than in the past. Radiologists can often demonstrate the likely cause(s) for a child's symptoms and signs, enabling timely medical or surgical treatment.

Paediatric radiologists play an important intermediary role between paediatrics and radiology, in both the conduct and the interpretation of an examination. They are the clinician's friend and the patient's advocate. Imaging has to be problem-oriented. The most important information on a requisition form, apart from the child's name and age, is the question to be answered. The next most important items are the legible name and contact number of the person asking the question. In this age of computerization, conversation on the telephone or, better still, face to face is invaluable when a complicated situation arises. The paediatric radiologist should do the least investigation to achieve the most information about a child's condition.

In concluding this introductory section, we note that reliable evidence-based information, to support many of the recommendations that are in print regarding appropriate algorithms for paediatric imaging, is difficult to access. There are few clinical situations and ethical guidelines that allow performance of several studies on a child simply to compare their utility. Clinical information is frequently incomplete; 'comparable' studies are rarely comparable. Furthermore, local traditions, practitioners in the area, available facilities and economic conditions

| Table 7.1.1 Estimated equivalent background radiation for various imaging procedures | |
|---|---|
| Study | Estimated equivalent background assuming background of 2.5 mSv/year |
| Chest X-ray, 2 views | 3 days |
| Abdominal X-ray, 2 views | 1 week |
| Extremity X-ray, 2–3 views | 5 hours |
| Skull series X-ray, 3 views* | 3 weeks |
| Upper gastrointestinal series* | 6–12 months |
| Barium enema* | 8–16 months |
| MCU (VCUG) | 1–7 weeks |
| Chest CT | 12–18 months |
| Abdominal CT | 2 years |
| Cranial CT | 8–12 months |

CT, computed tomography; MCU, micturating cystourethrography; VCUG, voiding cystourethrography.
*From adult data.

usually prevail in decision-making. If you have any question about the appropriate imaging for your patient, ask for help from a radiologist who is experienced in paediatric diagnosis. With these caveats, and encouragement to you, the reader, to challenge algorithms when they seem less than sensible, the following sections outline appropriate imaging considerations for particular situations, and are arranged anatomically, for easy reference.

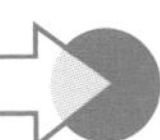

**Practical points**

- Find out whether there are clinical guidelines for your department/institution. They may include guidelines for imaging.
- Generally, in a complicated case, it is best to begin with uncomplicated imaging, such as plain radiographs. They may provide the diagnosis; if not, they can help point the way to other studies.
- Provide relevant clinical information to the radiologist when requesting examinations.
- Consult a paediatric radiologist, or one experienced in paediatric diagnosis, when you have questions about the imaging of a specific clinical problem.
- Be prepared to answer questions from parents regarding ionizing radiation and know whom to ask for more information.
- Be familiar with the preparation, immediate complications and sequelae of invasive imaging procedures.

## Neurology

### Acute head trauma, all ages

See Chapter 3.6.

- CT of the brain following the CHALICE (Children's Head injury ALgorithm for the prediction of Important Clinical Events) rule (Fig. 7.1.1).

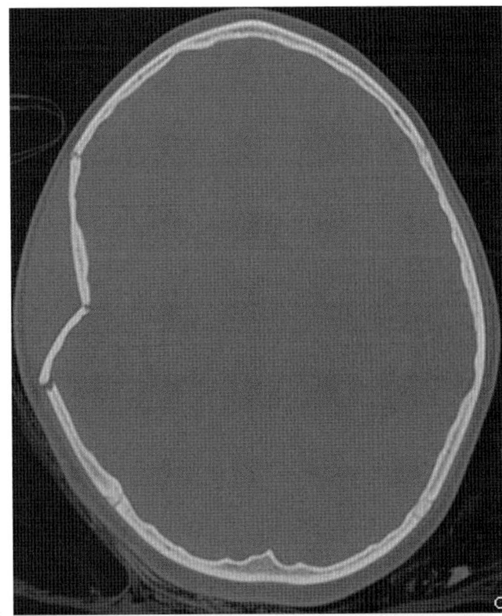

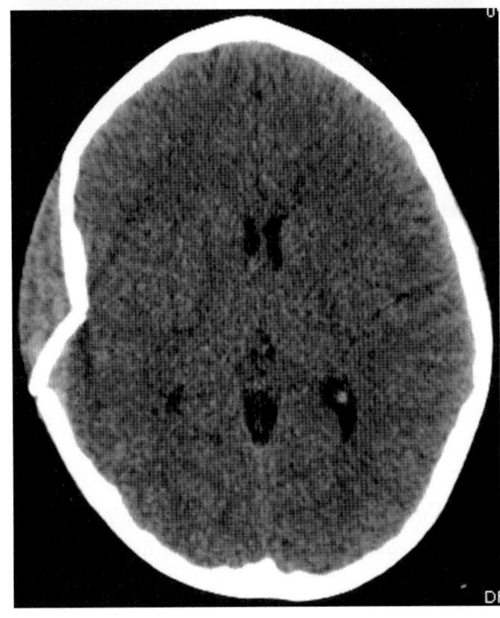

Fig. 7.1.1 Axial computed tomograms of the brain in an 8-year-old involved in a high-speed motor vehicle accident: **(A)** bone window; **(B)** brain window. The Glasgow Coma Scale score on arrival in the emergency department was 7/15. The scan reveals a large comminuted and depressed skull fracture involving right frontal and temporal bones with a small underlying extra-axial haematoma and midline shift to the left.

- Use NEXUS clinical prediction rule (altered neurological function, intoxication, midline posterior spinal tenderness, and/or distracting injury) to identify which children and adolescents should have imaging of the cervical spine.
- MRI when CT findings are negative in an infant or child with persisting abnormal neurological signs.

#### Notes

Radiographs of the skull are poorly predictive of intracranial pathology. They are of use in the situation of suspected inflicted injury (non-accidental injury) where multiple fractures or fractures of different ages are helpful in establishing the diagnosis.

For suspected injury to the neck, a lateral radiograph, in collar, can be followed by anteroposterior (AP) view of the cervical spine and odontoid view. Plain radiography can detect 94% of fractures. In infants and young children, the immature anatomy of the cervical spine along with the head being relatively large in proportion to the neck, results in the upper cervical spine (C1–C3 vertebral bodies) being more commonly injured than the lower spine, as seen in older children and adults. For this reason, careful scrutiny of the upper cervical spine on plain radiographs is needed. In some centres, the upper cervical spine is scanned at the time of brain imaging in the setting of significantly altered conscious state and major trauma. CT of the entire cervical spine, often routinely acquired in adults, includes the thyroid gland and is used in children only when there is credible utility.

### Newborn

- Portable ultrasonography when screening for germinal matrix/intraventricular and intraparenchymal haemorrhage in the premature infant.
- CT for suspected acute extra-axial collections (bleeding, infection).
- MRI for suspected non-haemorrhagic parenchymal disease (e.g. hypoxic–ischaemic insult, neuronal migrational disorders).

#### Notes

Follow local protocols for timing/frequency of ultrasonographic screening for premature infants. Generally, a scan is performed at 3–4 days of age in infants who weigh less than 1500 g unless there is clinical concern that prompts an earlier study.

Timing of MRI for hypoxic–ischaemic insult depends on the availability of resources. One scan at 24–48 hours of life followed by a scan at 7–10 days of life is ideal for both assessment of timing of injury and severity of injury; a compromise is one scan at 3–4 days.

### Seizures

See Chapter 17.1.

For *acute non-febrile seizure*:

- MRI or, if not available, CT (clinically significant yield of 3–8%).

#### Notes

Because of the variable availability of MRI, local protocols should be consulted for neurological diagnostic work-up. Imaging following a single generalized non-febrile seizure in children is an area of controversy. Focal non-febrile seizures will usually be investigated by electroencephalography (EEG) and cerebral imaging. Temporal lobe lesions are more likely to be shown on MRI than CT.

Simple febrile seizure (single or recurrent) does not usually warrant imaging.

### Altered conscious state, suspected tumour and stroke

- MRI
- CT (if MRI not available).

MRI is the preferred diagnostic test for a child presenting with acute neurological signs (Fig. 7.1.2). If MRI is not available, CT can diagnose established infarction, haemorrhage and most tumours. MRI is the preferred test as it detects infarction earlier, can provide perfusion imaging in the setting of stroke and angiographic sequences in the setting of vascular disease. It also provides more detailed imaging (in multiple planes) for surgical planning in the setting of tumour.

### Developmental delay

- MRI.

MRI is the preferred examination as it can assess white-matter volume and distribution along with grey-matter abnormalities (sulcation, heterotopias and other migration anomalies) better than CT. Timing for the examination needs to be considered, with children under 2 years undergoing progressive myelination (sometimes making white-matter signal assessment more difficult) and most children below 6–7 years (and often later when developmentally delayed) requiring general anaesthesia for the examination.

### Spinal cord and cauda equina symptomatology

- MRI is the diagnostic test of choice in all age groups.

### Spinal dysraphism

- Ultrasonography in neonates (first month of life; can be later if prematurely born)
- MRI in older children.

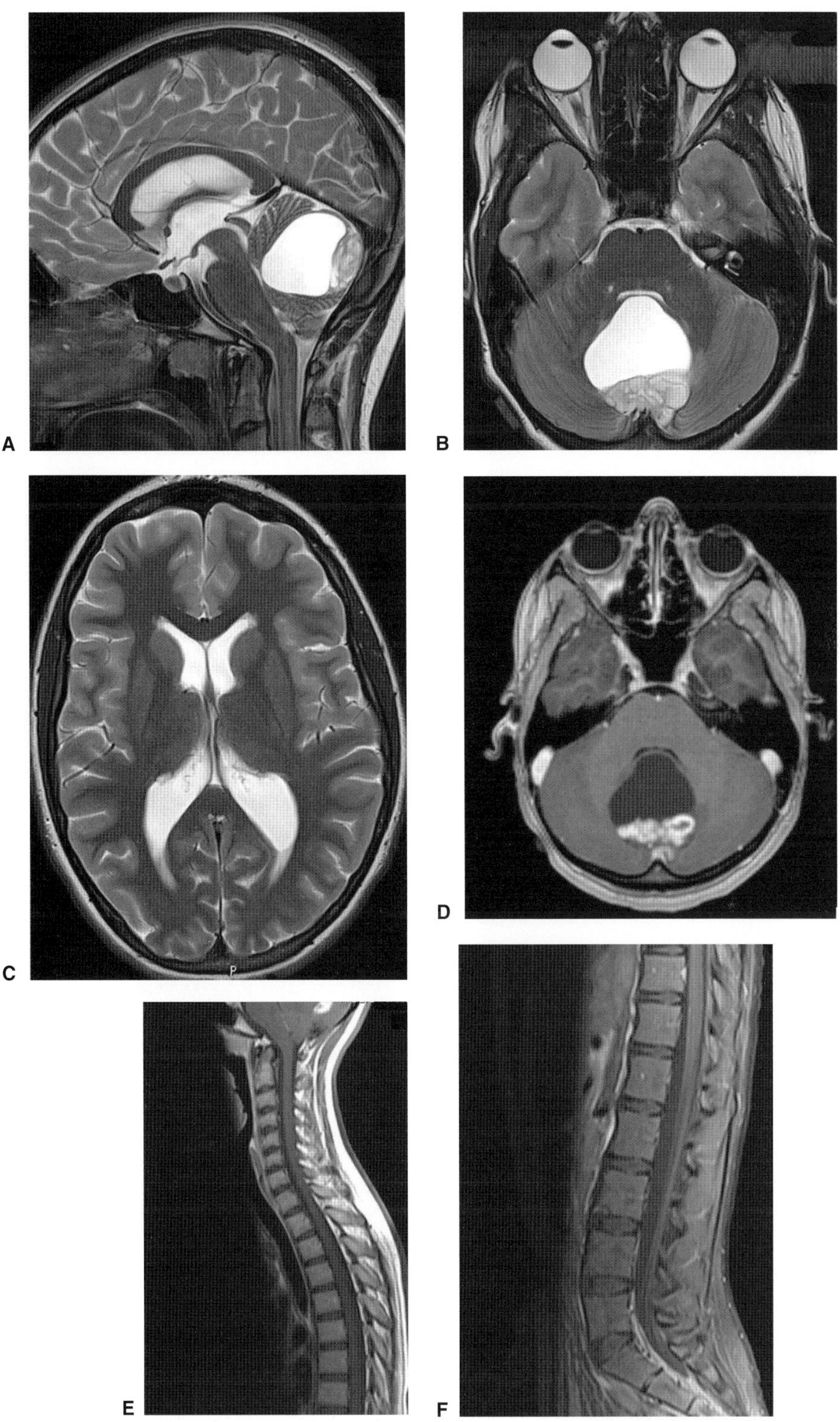

Fig. 7.1.2 Magnetic resonance images of brain and spine in this 15-year-old shows a large tumour in the posterior fossa. Sagittal T2 **(A)**, axial T2 **(B)**, axial T2 level with the lateral ventricles **(C)**, axial T1 post-contrast **(D)** and sagittal T1 post-contrast through the spine **(E, F)** are representative images from the study. On the T2 (water) weighted images, the tumour is predominantly bright in keeping with 'fluid' contents; soft tissue is present along the posterior surface. This soft tissue enhances on the contrast sequences, in keeping with mural nodules. The axial image at the level of the lateral ventricles reveals early ventricular dilatation and transependymal flow of cerebrospinal fluid, in keeping with early obstruction (due to pressure from the tumour on the cerebral aqueduct and fourth ventricle). No spinal metastases are identified. The tumour was a pilocytic astrocytoma.

Notes

Spinal ultrasonography is unnecessary in cases of classical myelomeningocele; however, the accompanying Chiari II malformation of the brain can be assessed with ultrasonography or MRI, and the degree of ventricular dilatation after shunt placement or third ventriculostomy can be monitored.

For neonates with midline dermal abnormality, mass, abnormal sacral cleft/dimple, sacral agenesis, anorectal malformation or vertebral anomaly on plain radiographs, ultrasonography can assess the spinal canal, spinal cord and cauda equina. Ossification of posterior elements as the child grows obscures the sonographic window and, when this occurs, MRI is used to assess the anatomy.

## Cardiology

See Chapter 15.1.

### Suspected congenital heart disease

(E.g. abnormal prenatal ultrasonography, cyanosis, murmur, unexplained oxygen requirement.)

- Posteroanterior (PA) and lateral chest radiographs to include upper abdomen (Fig. 7.1.3)
- CT or MRI for anatomical detail of vascular rings as necessary.

(Cardiac angiography/interventional procedures are arranged by paediatric cardiologists in most centres.)

### Central/cardiac pain

- Posteroanterior (PA) and lateral chest radiographs to include upper abdomen.

Notes

Plain radiography is not an accurate screening test for presence or absence of structural cardiac disease, but has a role in the identification of coexistent airway and/or pulmonary abnormality, skeletal anomaly that may direct investigation of other systems, and as a baseline study, particularly in regard to the state of the pulmonary vasculature in neonates. Echocardiography, in most centres related to the department of cardiology, is the 'gold standard' for all patients in whom structural cardiac abnormality is suspected. Most echocardiographic examinations are time-consuming; sedation may be needed for transthoracic scanning and is always required for transoesophageal scans.

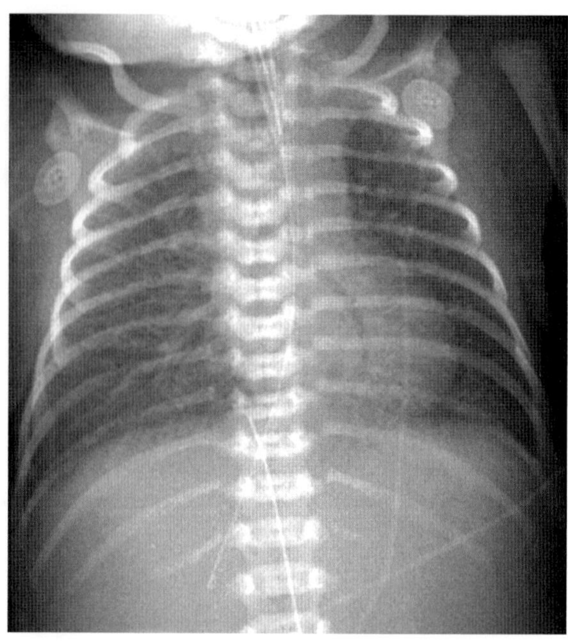

**Fig. 7.1.3** The anteroposterior radiograph of this newborn, who presented in severe respiratory distress, has features that identify cardiac abnormality as the likely aetiology, although the heart is normal in size. Note that the nasogastric tube is entering a right-sided stomach, whereas the apex of the heart is left-sided. The tracheostomy tube is deviated leftward by a right-sided aortic arch and the umbilical artery catheter is in a right-sided descending aorta. This infant had heterotaxy syndrome with multiple cardiac anomalies. The venous congestion that is apparent in the lungs is from obstructed anomalous pulmonary venous return, the major cause of the respiratory distress.

## Pulmonary/airway

See Chapter 14.5.

### Cough and fever

- PA and lateral chest radiography.

### Pleuritic pain

- PA and lateral chest radiography.

### Suspected sepsis in a neonate

- PA and lateral chest radiography.

### First episode of wheezing

See Chapter 14.3.

- PA and lateral chest radiography
- Fluoroscopy/screening if foreign body is suspected.

Imaging is usually indicated only when the history is suggestive of inhaled or ingested foreign body, the child has no coryzal illness, or the child does not respond as expected to treatment for bronchiolitis/asthma.

## Unexplained stridor

See Chapter 14.2.

- PA and lateral chest radiography
- Lateral radiograph of the neck
- Fluoroscopy/screening/barium swallow depending on plain radiographic findings.

## Trauma to the chest

- AP supine chest radiography
- Computed tomographic angiography (CTA) with intravenous contrast if mediastinal, vascular and/or major airway injury suspected.

## Thoracic mass

- PA and lateral radiography (Fig. 7.1.4)
- CT or MRI or, occasionally, both, depending on the organ(s) of origin and involvement
- Echocardiography for mass related to the heart.

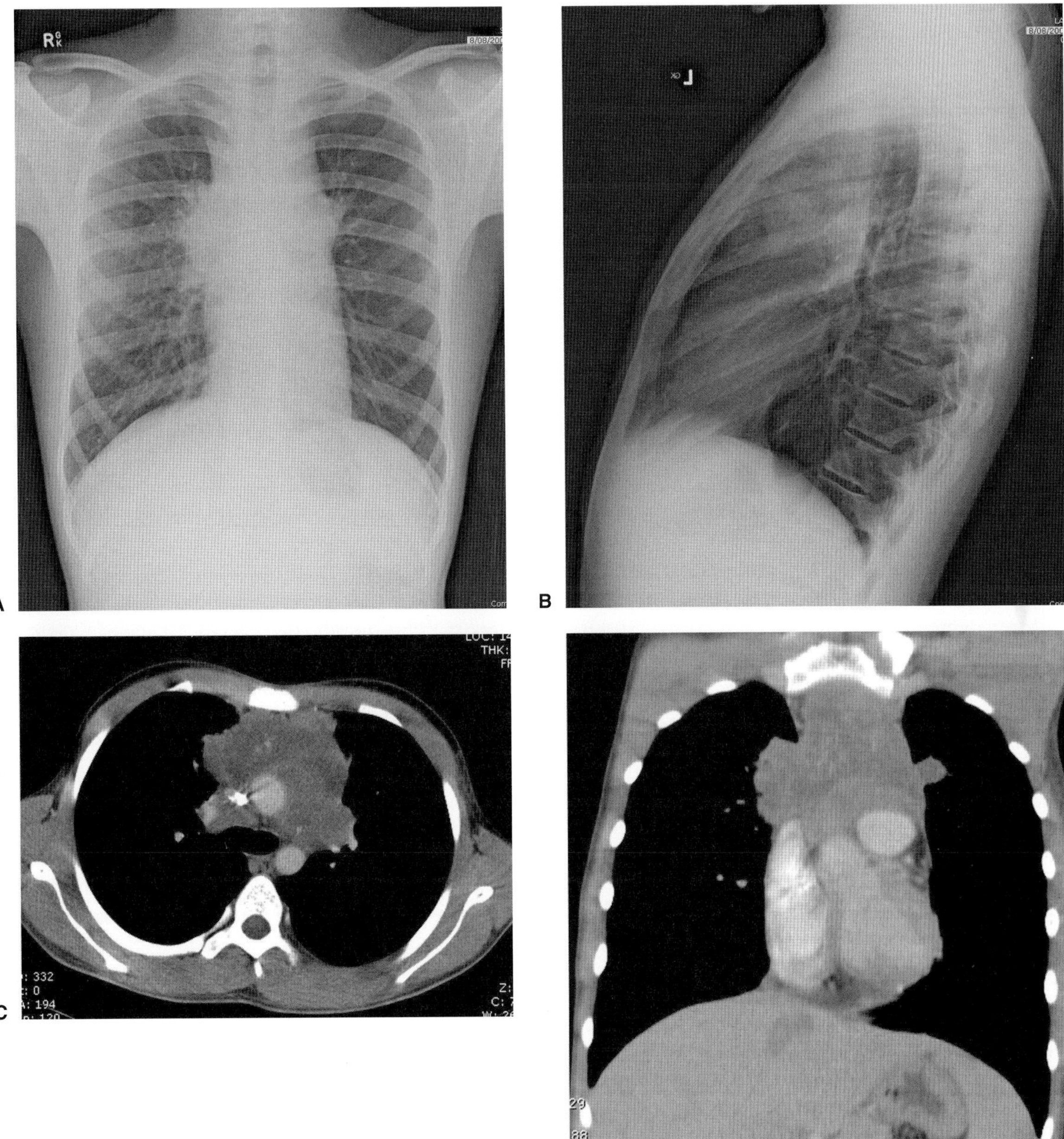

Fig. 7.1.4 **(A)** Posteroanterior (PA) and **(B)** lateral radiograph of the chest in an adolescent boy shows mediastinal widening and bulky hilar regions on the PA view with a retrosternal mass on the lateral view. Axial **(C)** and coronal **(D)** computed tomography (CT) after intravenous contrast confirms a large soft tissue mass involving the anterior and middle mediastinum, with areas of calcification. B-cell lymphoma was the diagnosis after a CT-guided biopsy of the mass.

### Notes

There is great debate as to whether a previously well child who has clinical symptoms and signs of pneumonia requires radiography at all. Likewise, there is argument as to whether the workup of sepsis in an infant, and the first episode of wheezing (without history of aspiration of foreign body), requires imaging. Normal radiographs and fluoroscopy do not rule out the presence of an endobronchial foreign body: there has to be enough obstruction of an airway to provide radiographic evidence of its presence. Bronchoscopy should follow if there is a good history of aspiration.

Some centres perform a single PA radiograph for indications such as suspected pneumonia as it halves the radiation dose and often provides the diagnosis in clinical settings such as sepsis/pneumonia. There is no good prospective study that compares the utility of the PA-only radiography with PA and lateral views of the chest. There is anecdotal evidence that supports the acquisition of both views. In many cases, lower lobe pneumonia is difficult to diagnose from the PA view alone. The cardiac size is easier to judge when the shape of the chest is defined by two views. When both radiographs are normal, the radiologist can state with certainty that the chest is normal to radiographic examination. In some situations, it is just as important to document normality as to find an abnormality.

There is general consensus that follow-up radiography for uncomplicated pneumonia is unnecessary. Follow-up radiographs are reserved for children who have persisting symptoms of chest disease or who have had unusual radiographs on presentation.

Stridulous breathing implies narrowing of the trachea. A vascular ring, endotracheal haemangioma, tracheitis or epiglottitis are all possible causes. If a vascular ring is obvious on plain radiography, MRI or CT should follow. Imaging is not needed in children with classical croup and can be dangerous in children who are suspected of having epiglottitis. No child or infant with respiratory compromise should be sent for imaging without adequate safeguards for provision of an airway.

A chest mass may be diagnosed on radiography after a child presents with pain, cough, respiratory compromise, etc. It may also be an incidental finding; a posterior mediastinal mass may be clinically silent. The diagnostic approach is tailored to the clinical situation. As examples, an anterior mediastinal mass in the setting of T-cell leukaemia needs no further imaging. A posterior mass with vertebral involvement will require further cross-sectional imaging.

## Abdomen/gastroenterology

### Abdominal pain

See Chapter 20.1.

- Supine and upright or decubitus radiographs for acute abdominal pain
- No imaging, or ultrasonography only, for non-specific periumbilical abdominal pain.

### Constipation

- No imaging or single plain radiograph of the abdomen
- Plain radiography then contrast enema for the neonate who fails to pass meconium.

### Notes

Constipation/encopresis is a clinical diagnosis but some clinicians order a plain radiograph for the initial evaluation of a child who has constipation. The radiograph is used for assessment of the degree of distension of bowel, but this has poor repeatability and does not alter treatment or predict response to therapy. It can be useful for examining the lumbosacral spine for occult dysraphism, but this has a very low yield in children with isolated constipation and no neurological signs. Rarely do plain radiographs reveal a specific cause for chronic constipation, and many question their value in this setting. There is no correlation between plain abdominal radiographs and intestinal transit time. Evaluation of transit time through the gastrointestinal tract can be performed with sequential radiographs following ingestion of radio-opaque markers or by nuclear medicine studies following ingestion of an isotopic marker. For the child who has chronic periumbilical abdominal pain, ultrasonography is often used as a means of reassuring parents, child and clinician that there is no anatomical abnormality of the liver, spleen, pancreas and kidneys, but again this has a very low yield. Limiting radiographic imaging to patients who have had previous abdominal surgery, suspected ingestion of foreign body, abnormal bowel sounds, abdominal distension or peritoneal signs identifies virtually all patients with significant disease.

The evaluation of a child suspected of having appendicitis (Fig. 7.1.5) is heavily reliant on the clinical practice guidelines established at the point of care. Many institutions rely on an approach that limits CT to those with negative findings on ultrasonography or those suspected of rupture/abscess. Ultrasonography requires competent practitioners and good equipment, and is far easier to perform and interpret in children who are not obese. CT requires injection of contrast media, irradiation and good interpretation of the resultant images.

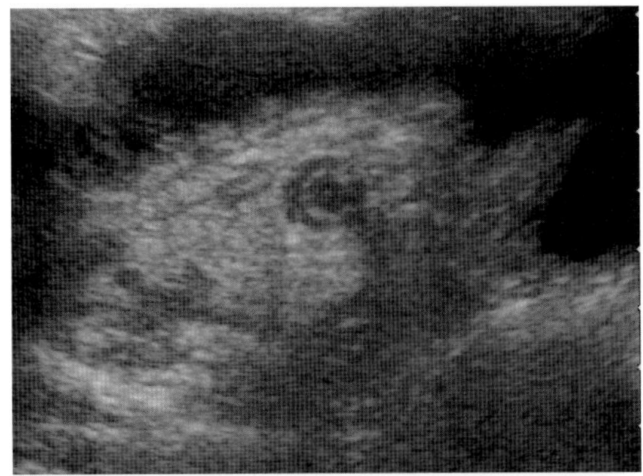

A

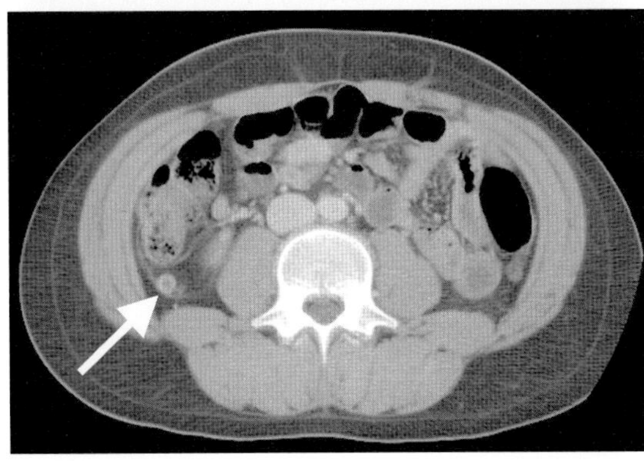

B

Fig. 7.1.5 Appendicitis is diagnosed with ultrasonography **(A)** when a non compressible, blind ending tubular structure is contiguous with the caecum and measures 6 mm or greater in diameter. There is often surrounding inflammatory change within the fat, as shown in this scan. The presence of a shadowing appendicolith, although helpful in the diagnosis, is not a necessary feature. In another case **(B)**, retrocaecal appendicitis is evident on this slice from a computed tomogram after intravenous contrast. The appendix (arrow) is thick-walled, measures 8 mm in diameter and has adjacent inflammation, including thickening of the posterior peritoneum.

## Abdominal mass

- Plain radiography of abdomen when aetiology of the mass is in doubt, except for a female with a pelvic mass
- Ultrasonography
- CT if necessary (Fig. 7.1.6)
- MRI for neurogenic tumour, soft tissue tumour, bony involvement by tumour, choledochal cyst or an unusual mass.

### Notes

Besides usually demonstrating the mass and its locale, plain radiography also provides information regarding the bases of the lungs, presence of calcification, effects of the mass on contiguous organs, bones and/or gastrointestinal tract. Most abdominal masses in childhood are related to the retroperitoneum and, in particular, the kidney. Examples are obstructive hydronephrosis, multicystic dysplastic kidney and Wilms tumour. A mass that is gastrointestinal in origin (e.g. intussusception) requires a different approach from a mass that is hepatobiliary, such as a choledochal cyst. When intussusception is diagnosed, air enema for reduction is the first therapeutic method of choice. Remember to consider pregnancy in an adolescent female who has a pelvic mass! If a malignant tumour is diagnosed, the affected child may be enrolled in treatment protocols that have very specific requirements in terms of imaging at staging and follow-up.

## Abdominal trauma

- Supine radiography, with decubitus if possible
- Cross-table lateral view of lumbar spine if there has been hyperflexion of the spine, such as with a lapbelt injury
- CT with intravenous contrast (Fig. 7.1.7).

### Notes

Many trauma protocols for evaluating the severely injured child have been based on the approach to adults, who have different mechanisms and types of abdominal injury. For example, a screening pelvic radiograph is part of the 'adult' trauma series. Its use in children has not been proved to be helpful. If any screening view is considered, it should be an abdominal radiograph, which will include the pelvis. Peritoneal lavage is not a helpful diagnostic test in paediatric trauma. Major organ injury can occur without there being free intra-abdominal fluid. Ultrasonography is not as sensitive a method of diagnosis as CT, but in some remote areas may be the only tool available to search for free fluid, intraparenchymal laceration/haematoma and renal perfusion (with Doppler).

A child should be stabilized before being moved to a CT scanner. Craniospinal imaging can occur at the same time if needed. Oral contrast medium is not usually used for the following reasons: risk of aspiration; time needed to allow contrast to pass through intestinal tract; and relative ileus in the situation of severe injury. However, some centres use positive contrast and some instill water through a nasogastric tube to outline the duodenum.

## Non-bilious vomiting

See Chapter 20.1.

- Ultrasonography when pyloric stenosis is suspected but a pyloric mass is not palpated (Fig. 7.1.8)
- Upper gastrointestinal series with barium.

## Bilious vomiting

- Plain radiographs
- Upper gastrointestinal series with barium if the obstruction seems proximal.

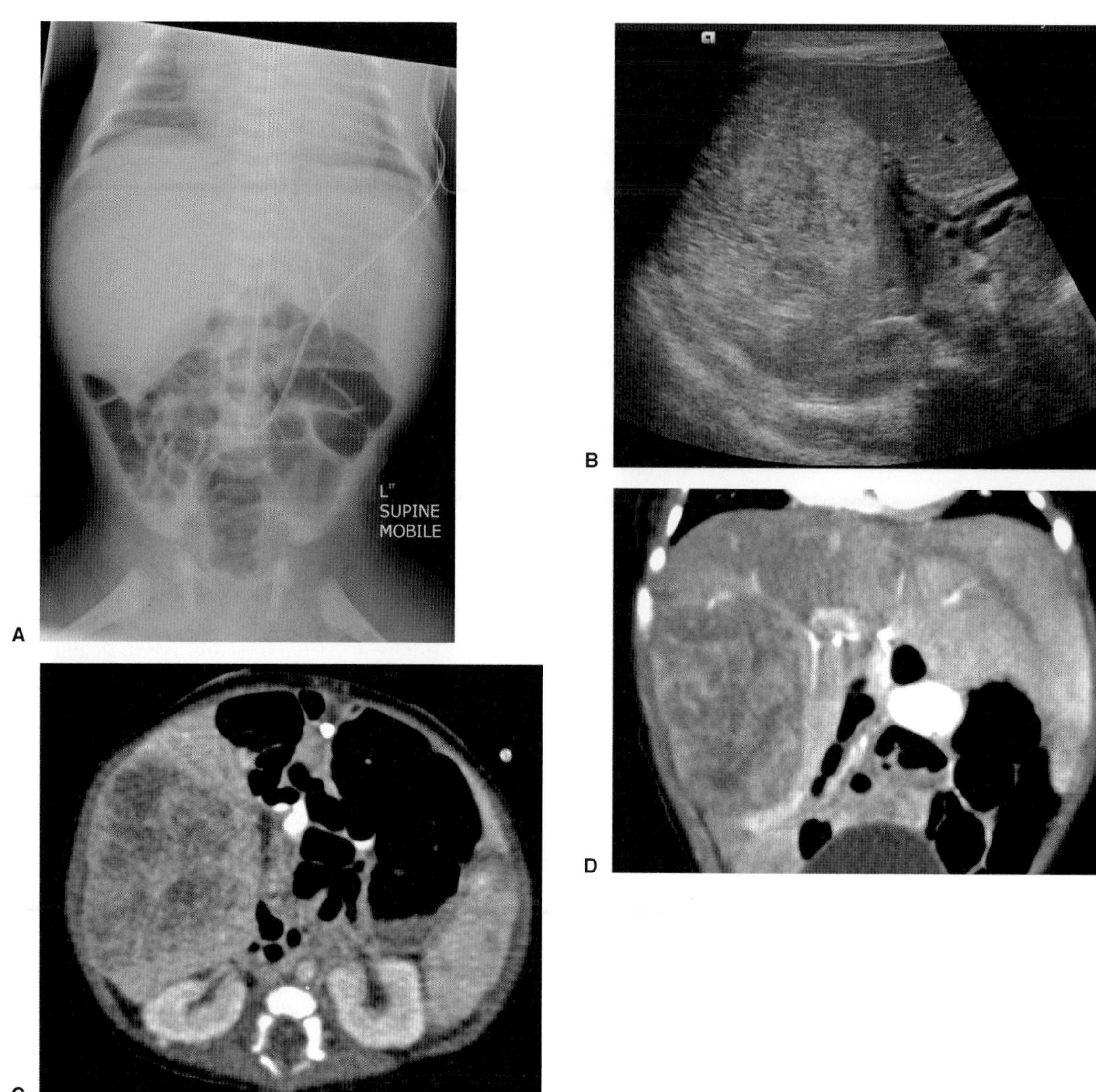


Fig. 7.1.6 Four-day-old neonate with a liver mass that had been diagnosed antenatally. The plain radiograph **(A)** suggests hepatic enlargement. The longitudinal sonographic view **(B)** reveals a large heterogeneous mass within the right lobe of liver. Axial **(C)** and coronal **(D)** computed tomograms though the abdomen, after intravenous contrast, reveal the large hypo-attenuating mass in the liver. Non-uniform splenic enhancement on the axial image reflects the arterial timing of the scan. Biopsy of the hepatic mass revealed hepatoblastoma.

### Chronic diarrhoea

- Upper gastrointestinal series with follow-through examination of small bowel when the cause is not obvious from clinical and laboratory data, cultures and small bowel biopsy. When Crohn's disease is suspected clinically, but not proven, consider MR enterography.

### Subacute small bowel obstruction

- CT after ingestion of water-soluble oral contrast is usually more revealing of the site and source of obstruction than follow-through AP radiographs after the ingestion of barium.

### Gastrointestinal bleeding

- Technetium-99m pertechnetate scintiscan when a Meckel diverticulum is suspected
- Upper gastrointestinal series with follow-through examination of small bowel and antegrade evaluation of colon and/or air-contrast barium enema when all other investigations are unhelpful (e.g. upper gastrointestinal endoscopy, colonoscopy and/or video capsule endoscopy).

#### Notes

The availability of consultants trained in paediatric gastroenterology and their skill in endoscopy is directly

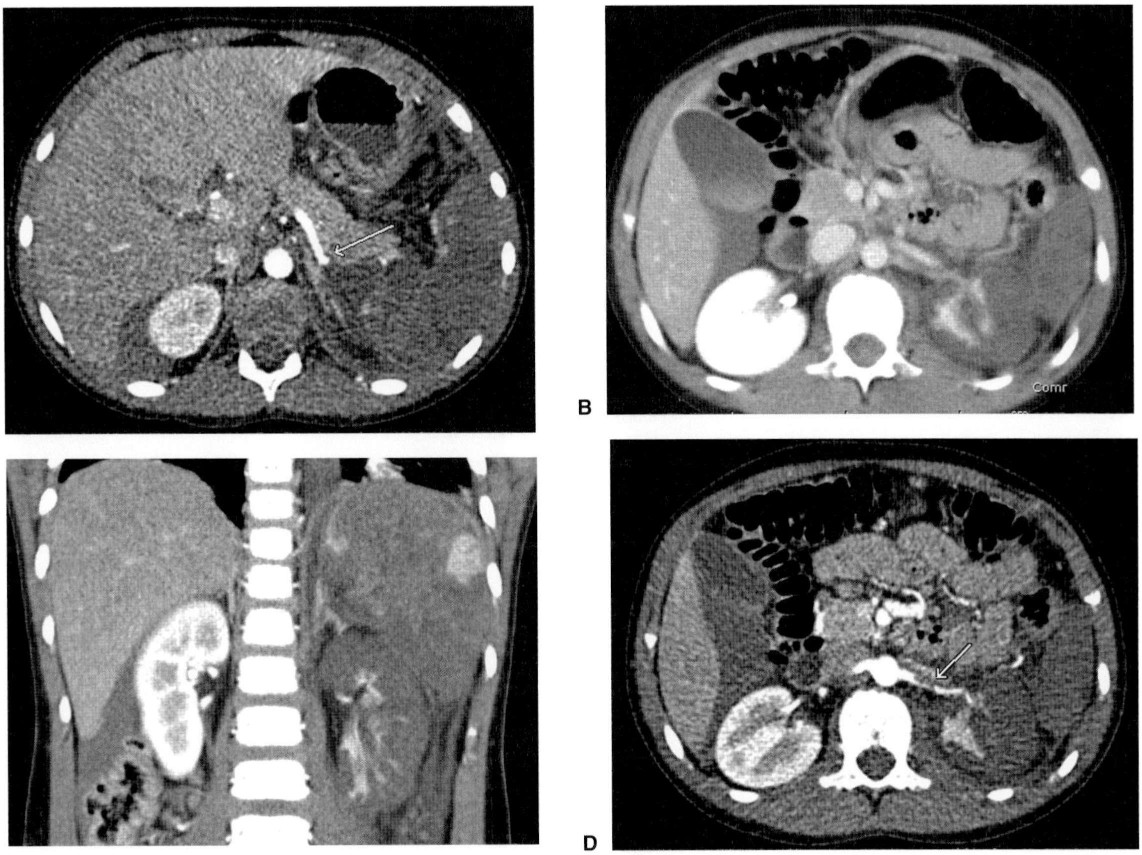

Fig. 7.1.7 This 9-year-old child had suffered severe blunt trauma to the abdomen. Axial arterial **(A)**, axial portal venous **(B)** and coronal **(C)** computed tomograms through the abdomen reveal a largely non-enhancing spleen and only partially enhancing left kidney, indicating lack of vascular perfusion. There is a small volume of enhancing splenic tissue anterosuperiorly (supplied by collateral vessels). The majority of the organ has lost arterial blood supply, owing to traumatic dissection of the splenic artery. Note the abrupt cut off of this vessel (arrow) posterior to the tail of pancreas in **(A)**. The splenic vein remains patent. A dissection has also occurred in the left renal artery **(D)**. Note the free fluid adjacent to the liver edge.

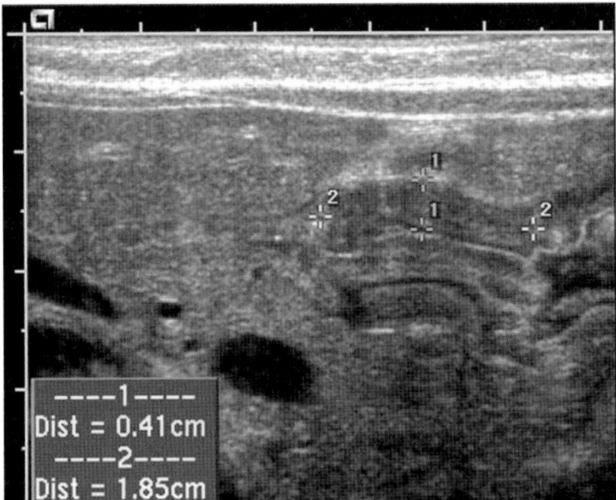


Fig. 7.1.8 Ultrasonography was performed after this 4-week-old infant presented with persistent vomiting. A scan along the long axis of the antropyloric region shows the typical features of pyloric stenosis with thickening of the muscle and elongation of the channel.

related to the need for radiological investigation of gastrointestinal diseases. The use of video capsule endoscopy in paediatrics has also decreased reliance on imaging.

Normal infants regurgitate feeds. If the infant is gaining weight normally, imaging is unnecessary. Projectile vomiting warrants consideration of pyloric stenosis, which can be imaged with ultrasonography (see Fig. 7.1.8). Pulmonary symptomatology, failure to thrive, feeding difficulty and gastrointestinal blood loss are reasons to consider upper gastrointestinal series.

Problems in the neonatal period, such as failure to pass meconium, bilious vomiting and distension, tend to be congenital in origin and the appropriate sequence of imaging requires close cooperation between paediatric surgery and radiology. Bilious vomiting may occur with distal obstruction. One cannot rely on ultrasonography to confirm or exclude malrotation: a contrast study of the upper gastrointestinal tract is the current 'gold standard'.

# Hepatobiliary

## Neonatal jaundice

See Chapter 11.2.

- Ultrasonography to establish anatomy
- Magnetic resonance cholangiopancreatography (MRCP) and/or radionuclide study with technetium-99 m iminodiacetic acid derivative when choledochal cyst, biliary hypoplasia or atresia is a consideration (Fig. 7.1.9).

## Right upper abdominal pain

- Plain radiography and, often, the addition of ultrasonography.

### Notes

Right lower lobe pneumonia may present as severe right upper abdominal pain; therefore, always look at the bases of the lungs on abdominal radiographs. Gallstones in childhood are more likely to be pigment stones than cholesterol stones and may contain enough calcium to be visible on radiography.

## Juvenile/adolescent jaundice

- Ultrasonography of liver, biliary tract, pancreas and spleen
- CT or MRI, depending on the results of ultrasonography.

## Abnormal hepatic function

- Ultrasonography when the clinical situation is atypical for hepatitis
- Ultrasound-guided biopsy if the diagnosis is uncertain.

# Nephrology/urology

## Urinary infection

See Chapter 18.1.

- Ultrasonography of the urinary tract in neonates, at the time of infection, to rule out an obvious surgical problem, such as obstruction
- Ultrasonography and micturating cystourethrography (MCU) in some infants and children who have had a documented urinary tract infection (Fig. 7.1.10)
- Technetium-99m diethylenetriamine penta-acetic acid (DTPA) or Mag3 scans, with furosemide, for evaluation of the child with possible obstruction at the pelviureteric junction or ureterovesical junction

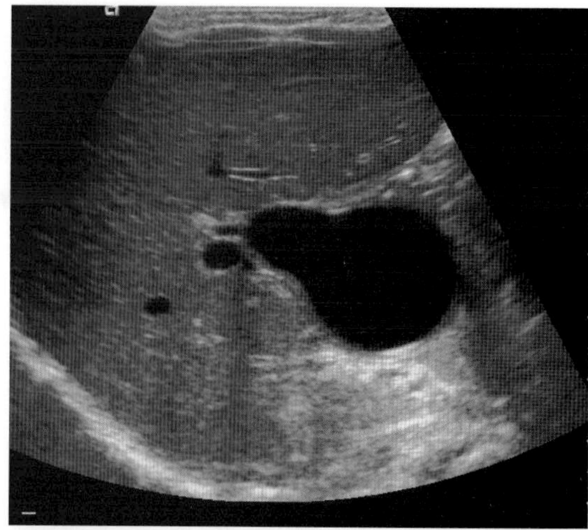

A

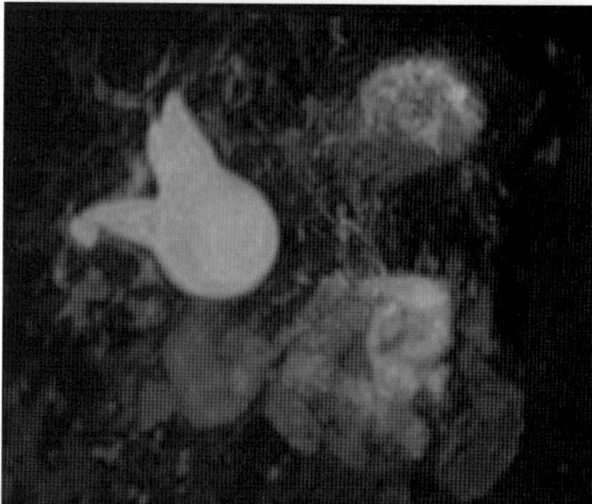

B

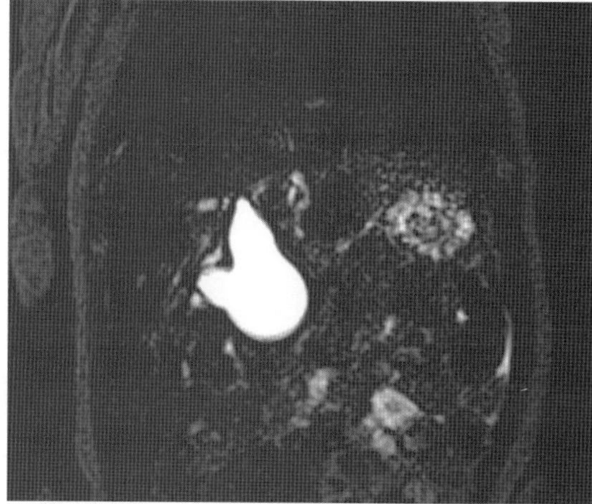

C

Fig. 7.1.9 Ultrasonographic **(A)** and magnetic resonance cholangiopancreatography (MRCP) **(B, C)** images show a type 1 choledochal cyst. The cyst is separate from the collapsed gallbladder and there is no dilatation of intrahepatic bile ducts.

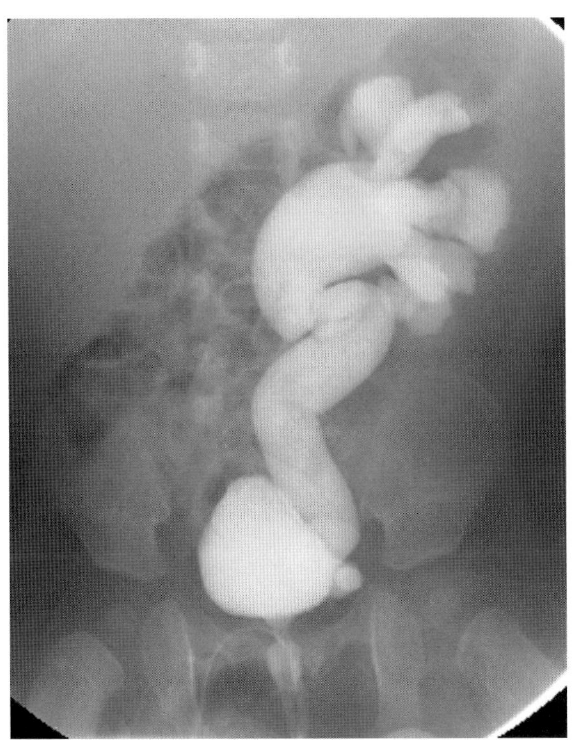

Fig. 7.1.10 Micturating cystourethrography reveals severe reflux into the left kidney in this infant who presented acutely ill with infection. This reflux is classified as Grade 5, due to the degree of distension of the collecting system.

- Technetium-99m dimercaptosuccinic acid (DMSA) or Mag3 scans during the acute illness can support the diagnosis of pyelonephritis, and/or after infection has cleared can document renal scars.

### Renal failure

- Ultrasonography of urinary tract
- Ultrasound-guided biopsy of kidney, if necessary for diagnosis.

#### Note

Ultrasonography, which does not rely on renal function for images, can usually aid in triage of the patient by determining a surgical or medical cause for renal failure.

### Hypertension

See Chapter 18.2.

- Ultrasonography of urinary tract and adrenal glands
- Nuclear medicine for quantitative, divided renal vascular flow and function
- CTA/angiography in the rare situation of suspected renal vascular disease
- MRI or CT with intravenous contrast if an endocrine tumour such as phaeochromocytoma is suspected from laboratory data. Most phaeochromocytomas are intra-abdominal and adrenal in location.

#### Note

Examination of the kidneys with Doppler is difficult, time-consuming and often insensitive to subtle vascular narrowing. Accessory renal vessels may be overlooked. Mid-aortic syndrome and neurofibromatosis are rare and, when present, typically have other signs and symptoms. A 'negative' examination does not rule out renal vascular disease.

CTA can define renal vascularity with greater clarity than ultrasonography.

### Haematuria unrelated to trauma

- Ultrasonography of urinary tract
- CT if there is a strong likelihood of renal/ureteral stone that has not been identified with ultrasonography
- CT or MRI if a renal tumour is suspected
- MCU or retrograde urethrography if a distal site of bleeding is suspected and cystoscopy is not available.

## Musculoskeletal

### Trauma

See Chapters 3.6 and 8.1.

- Two orthogonal radiographic views of the bone or joint that has been injured (Fig. 7.1.11). Oblique/special views as needed of areas such as scaphoid, radial head, shoulder
- CT for special cases such as intra-articular fractures of ankle, pelvic fracture.

### Fever/pain/swelling related to the musculoskeletal system

See Figure 7.1.12.

- Two orthogonal radiographic views of the symptomatic bone or joint
- Nuclear medicine technetium-99 m diphosphonate bone scan
- MRI for difficult diagnoses, tumour, occult infection
- Ultrasonography for specific questions: localization of collection of fluid, joint effusion.

#### Notes

MRI is fast replacing radionuclide studies in cases where there is localized pain or swelling and clinical concern regarding a single septic joint or focus of osteomyelitis. Follow-up studies of children with diagnosed bone tumour should be performed with MRI

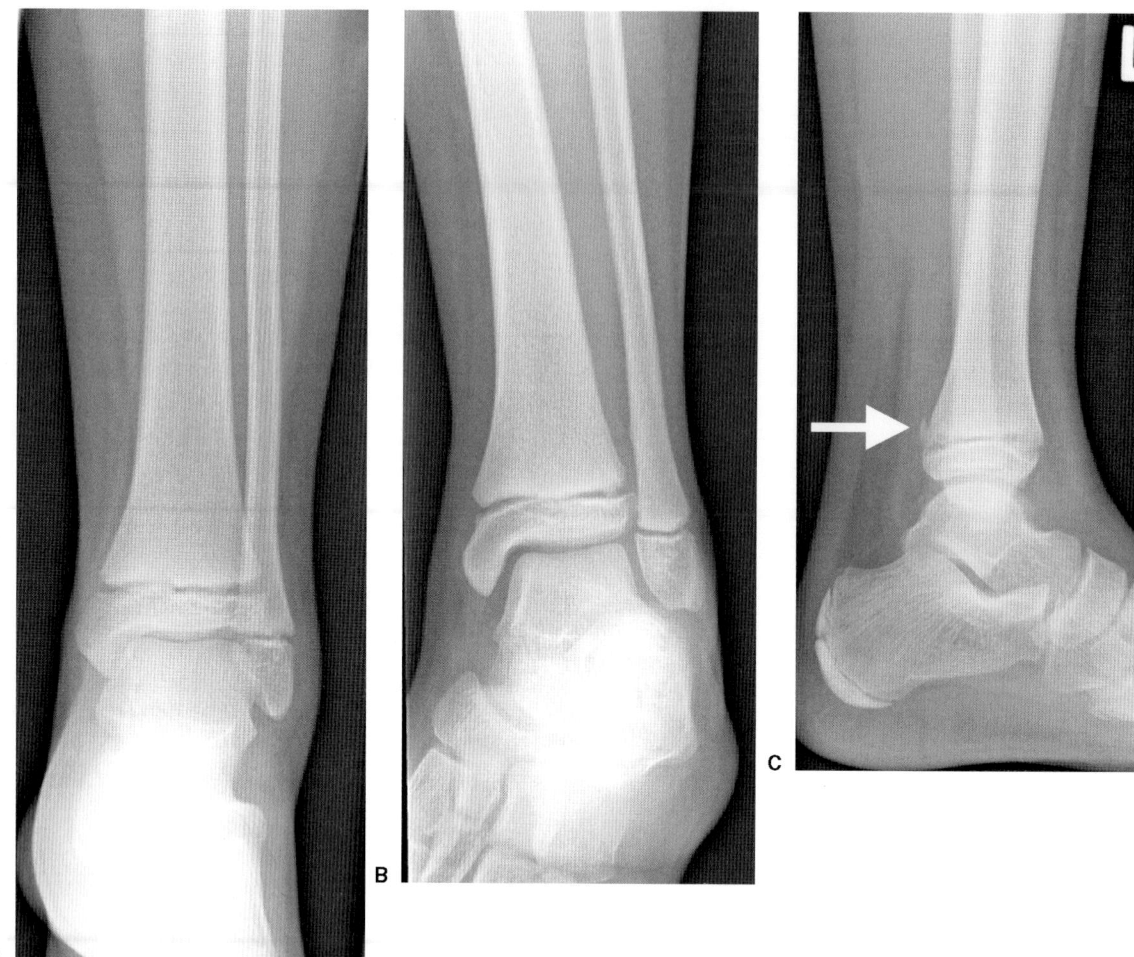


Fig. 7.1.11 Anteroposterior **(A)**, mortise **(B)** and lateral **(C)** views of the ankle were obtained in this girl who had tripped while running. Note that the fracture of the posterior malleolus (arrow) can be identified only on the lateral view. Views in two or more planes are necessary for adequate diagnosis of bony injury.

rather than CT; MRI gives far more information regarding adjacent soft tissues and bone marrow.

### Metabolic disease

- AP plain radiograph of wrist and/or knee.

#### Notes

Because metabolic disease such as rickets is more obvious in areas of rapid bone growth, the wrists and knees are more revealing of abnormality than other sites. Other views (hands, clavicles) may show changes of secondary hyperparathyroidism in those with renal failure.

### Syndrome with potential skeletal involvement

- Plain radiography of chest, spine, pelvis, skull, one leg and left arm to include hand for determination of bone age. If patient has asymmetrical limbs, the other arm and/or leg should also be imaged.

### Developmental dysplasia of the hip

See Chapter 8.1.

- Ultrasonography at 4–6 weeks of age if developmental dysplasia of the hip (DDH) suspected but not obvious on physical examination, or if risk factors (female, breech, positive family history) present, *or*
- Plain radiography at 4–6 months of age if DDH suspected but not obvious on physical examination.

#### Notes

This is another area of contention. Ultrasonography of the infant's hips requires training and practice. Early radiography of neonates is unhelpful because

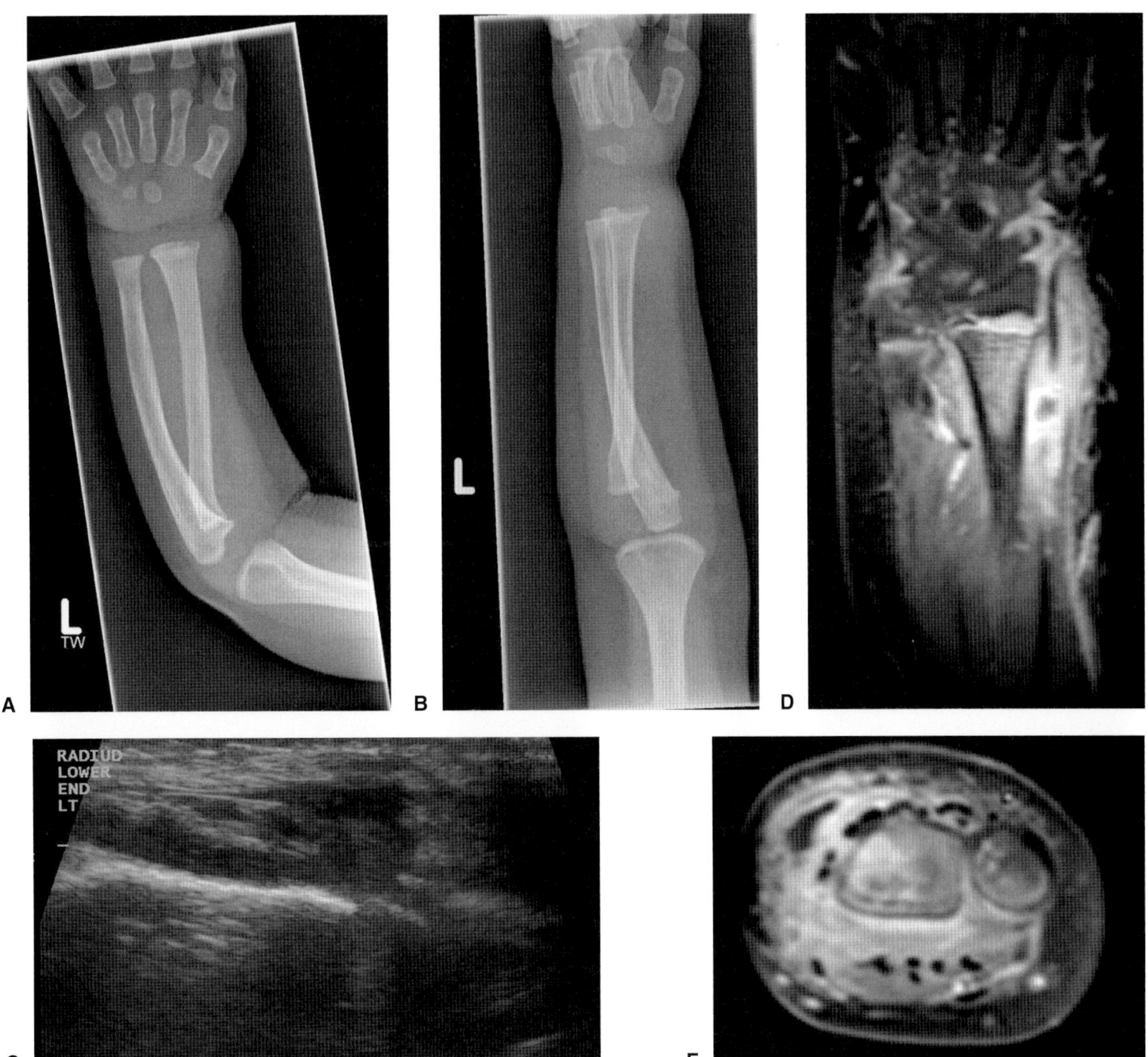


Fig. 7.1.12 This 8-month-old infant presented with a 10-day history of swelling around the distal forearm. Plain radiographs **(A, B)** show marked soft tissue swelling about the distal radius with focal osteopenia involving the lateral aspect of the distal radial metaphysis. A sonogram **(C)** shows the extent of the soft tissue swelling with several focal small fluid collections. Post-contrast T1 weighted coronal **(D)** and axial **(E)** magnetic resonance images show the full extent of the infection. The distal radial metaphysis demonstrates contrast enhancement and there is significant enhancement with several small fluid pockets in the surrounding soft tissue. The child had established osteomyelitis with several small abscesses.

so much of the anatomy is cartilaginous. Radiographs at 4–6 months are more informative and still allow intervention if necessary. In some areas of Europe, ultrasonography is used to screen all newborns. Such studies have a high false-positive rate of diagnosis of DDH. Repeated physical examination is the cornerstone of diagnosis. Infants may not have an obvious problem until after the neonatal period; hence the change in name from CDH (congenital dysplasia of the hip) to DDH. The availability of experienced paediatric orthopaedic surgeons has an effect on the local imaging protocols.

### Inflicted injury (non-accidental injury)

See Chapter 3.9.

- CT (in acute situation of cranial injury) or MRI of brain to assess extra-axial spaces, parenchymal injury
- Complete skeletal survey (infants) with high-detail images to search for evidence of fracture
- Follow-up skeletal survey (infants) 2 weeks after acute admission depending on original findings
- Nuclear medicine technetium-99 m diphosphonate bone scan
- CT of abdomen, with intravenous contrast, if evidence of abdominal trauma.

Notes

Some centres use nuclear medicine in imaging protocols for infants and young children if there is availability and local expertise in interpretation.

Often a follow-up skeletal survey or limited survey may be very revealing. Periosteal reaction takes about 7–10 days to appear. The acute fracture may be occult. The radiology department needs a close relationship with child protection services within the hospital to make sure that the appropriate studies, appropriately timed, are performed.

## Acknowledgements

The support of the Paediatric Radiologists at Starship Children's Hospital, Auckland, New Zealand, during the preparation of this manuscript is gratefully acknowledged. Radiation dose estimates were kindly provided by Keith J. Strauss.

## Abbreviations

The following abbreviations are in common use in imaging:

**AP,** anteroposterior
**PA,** posteroanterior

These terms relate to the course of the X-ray beam through the body. Anteroposterior, supine chest radiographs are much easier to accomplish in infants who cannot sit without support. Magnification of the heart is not as significant an issue as it is in adults.

**CT,** computed tomography
**CTA,** computed tomographic angiography (rapid injection of contrast with imaging in the arterial phase)
**MCU,** micturating cystourethrography
**MRCP,** magnetic resonance cholangiopancreatography
**MRI,** magnetic resonance imaging
**US,** ultrasound or ultrasonography

# PART 8

# COMMON ORTHOPAEDIC PROBLEMS AND FRACTURES

# 8.1 Orthopaedic problems

Peter Cundy

See Chapter 12.2 for Bone and joint infections.

## Skeletal variations during growth

Parents can be anxious about whether their child is normal. They refer to adult posture, which is different to that of infants and children. These 'developmental' postures can be due to:

- *intrauterine posture*, sometimes described as 'packaging'
- *developmental variants* – not present at birth, but may appear during growth and then disappear spontaneously. These include the common conditions of bow legs, knock knees, flat feet and in-toeing. These conditions seldom require active treatment but parents do need informed reassurance, which must be based on accurate knowledge of the natural history of these variations of posture in infants and children.

### Intrauterine posture

The position of the child before birth is normally one of flexion. The spine is flexed so that it forms a long curve with a concavity forward, the arms and legs are flexed, and the feet may assume a variety of postures. In the newborn the intrauterine posture can be readily reconstructed by 'folding' the baby into his or her most comfortable position, and this may indicate any postural abnormality present.

Two common foot postures are seen in newborns.

#### Talipes calcaneovalgus

Many babies are born with the foot turned upwards at the ankle so that the toes lie close to the front of the shin: this is known as talipes calcaneovalgus (Fig. 8.1.1). This posture can be corrected passively so that the foot can be brought down to a plantigrade position or even into equinus. The condition has a strong tendency to correct itself spontaneously over a period of 2–3 months.

#### Postural talipes equinovarus

Some babies are born with one or both feet in a position of plantar flexion at the ankles, and inversion of the remainder of the foot, so that the sole of the foot faces the opposite foot. This is postural talipes equinovarus and may be distinguished from true talipes equinovarus, known as clubfoot deformity (which is rigid and not passively correctable). Postural talipes equinovarus resolves spontaneously with assistance of simple stretches and rarely a cast, if not improved at 6 weeks.

#### Bow legs

Bow legs (Fig. 8.1.2) are common up to 2 years of age; the parents will often be concerned that the legs are bowed and the feet turn in. The condition is not caused by bulky nappies, because the bowing is in the tibiae. It is a normal developmental process and does not require treatment apart from parental reassurance. If the bowing is in one leg only, you should investigate with plain X-rays to exclude pathological causes such as a bone dysplasia or growth abnormality.

#### Knock knees

A large proportion of the population between the ages of 2 and 7 years have knock knees (Fig. 8.1.3). This condition has a strong tendency to correct itself by the age of 7 years and as a rule the only management necessary is parental reassurance that improvement will occur. There is a rare form of knock knees (adolescent tibia vara) that presents in overweight children around the age of 12 years and which may require treatment by staple epiphysiodesis.

#### Rolling in of ankles

Parents will frequently mention this, especially after it has been noticed by a concerned grandparent or shoefitter. The rolling of the hind foot into valgus is due to physiological joint laxity and requires no treatment. The clinician can show the parents how the hind foot straightens when the child stands up on high tiptoes. This is the tiptoe test, which also demonstrates development of the medial longitudinal arch (Fig. 8.1.4). Orthotics for 'rolling in' are not required (see below).

#### Flat feet

Flat feet in children are a frequent cause for parental concern. Usually this concern is unwarranted and the child's foot is normal for age (Fig. 8.1.5). Often parents

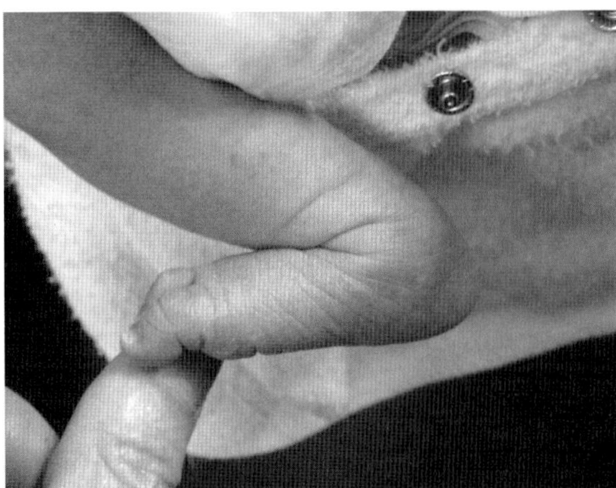

Fig. 8.1.1 Calcaneovalgus foot in a newborn – this will correct spontaneously.

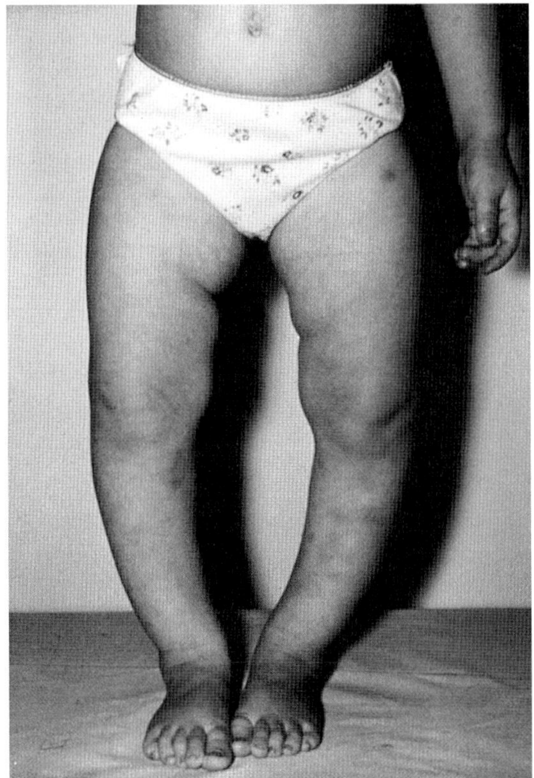

Fig. 8.1.2 Bow legs in a toddler: a normal phenomenon.

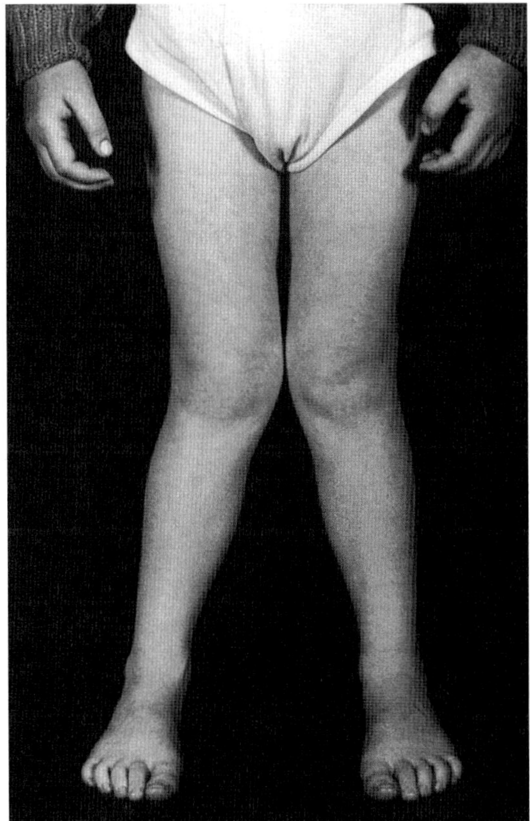

Fig. 8.1.3 A 5-year-old child with pronounced knock knees.

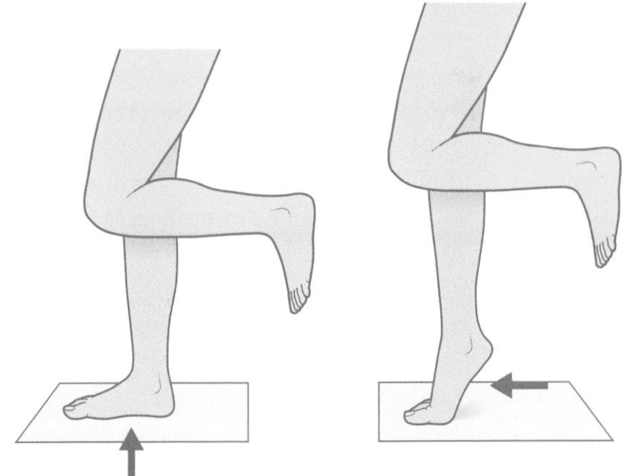

Fig. 8.1.4 If the arch appears when standing on tiptoe, the feet are flexible. The flat arch is of no significance and requires no treatment apart from explanation.

notice that their child's foot appears flat. Sometimes the attendant fitter at the shoe shop may comment on the shape of the child's foot. Children usually have low arches because they are loose-jointed and flexible. The arch flattens when they are standing. However, the arch can be better seen when the feet are hanging free or the child stands on tiptoes (the tiptoe test; see Fig. 8.1.4).

When a child first learns to walk, the stance is usually wide to assist balance, and the feet roll. As the child grows and ankle muscles strengthen, the foot gradually develops its mature shape with some medial arch. Flat feet are common in preschoolers and are present in over 10% of teenagers. The final shape of the foot may also be influenced genetically, in that one or both parents may have low arches.

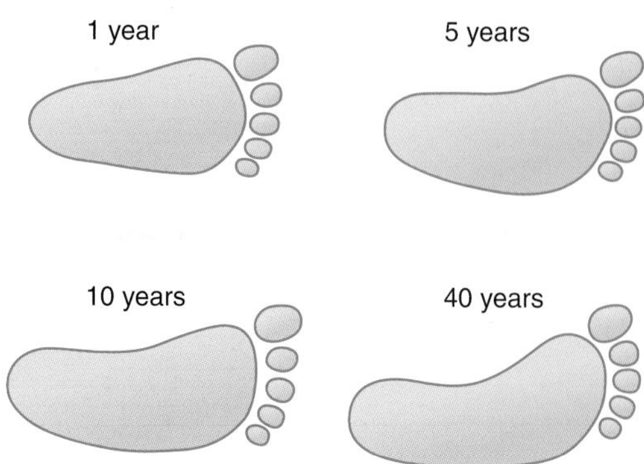


Fig. 8.1.5 Flexible flat feet are normal in infants and children. The arch develops whether the child wears shoes or goes barefoot.

Between the ages of 2 and 8 years, parents are often concerned because a 'second ankle bone' appears on the medial aspect of the foot. They are referring to prominence of the navicular bone, which is present in most children who have flat feet. Unless the prominence of this bone is causing symptoms, it can be ignored.

Children with flat feet generally have some valgus deformity of the heel; when viewed from behind the heels do not point straight up and down, but tend to slope outwards and downwards. The heels will correct and even swing into varus during the tiptoe test. This seldom persists into adult life.

During the first 7 or 8 years of life the majority of children develop a medial longitudinal arch, but approximately 15% do not. Clearly, the results of any form of treatment for flat feet are excellent, as some 85% improve whether or not they are treated. Sometimes treatment with shoe inserts (orthotics) or other forms of arch support/shoe modification are recommended by therapists. These may satisfy concerned parents but do little, if anything, to correct the 'flat foot' and certainly do not make an arch where one is not present. Orthotics for flexible flat feet are not necessary for children.

Other treatments, such as splints, massage or special shoes may be offered but there is little evidence that these interventions alter the foot for the better.

*Shoes*

The only essential is that children's shoes should be roomy enough. Shoes themselves are not necessary to promote normal foot growth and development; they are worn only for protection and need not be worn until activities demand this protection. Boots are no better than shoes, although parents may prefer boots for toddlers in that they are less likely to fall off or be taken off.

It is not harmful to use 'handed down' shoes in good condition from older children in the family, provided they are roomy enough. There is no evidence that sandals, thongs or sneakers have any harmful influence on the feet. If the child has excessive wear on the inner side of the sole of the shoes, advise parents to look for shoes that have a stiffer heel area. Some children with flexible flat feet are rather hard on their shoes and this can be dealt with by selecting shoes of stronger construction. This is usually much less expensive than elaborate and unnecessary orthotics.

## Accessory navicular bone

The child with a prominent accessory navicular may have some temporary discomfort, which may be relieved by wearing arch supports for a year or two. Frequently the ossicle either unites with the main navicular bone or just becomes asymptomatic. Excision of the accessory navicular bone is required only rarely.

## Curly middle toe

Sometimes the third toe curls inwards under the second toe so that the second toe tends to lie above the level of the first and third toes. Parents generally notice the abnormal posture of the second toe, but it is the third toe that is the cause of the problem. This can be safely ignored until the child is at least 2 years old. Occasionally a flexor tenotomy is required and provides excellent correction (Fig. 8.1.6).

## In-toe gait (pigeon toeing)

In-toeing in childhood is common. It may appear worse when the child is running or tired. It does not cause arthritis or back problems later in life. It can be due to one or more of the following:

- inset hips
- internal torsion of the tibia
- metatarsus adductus.

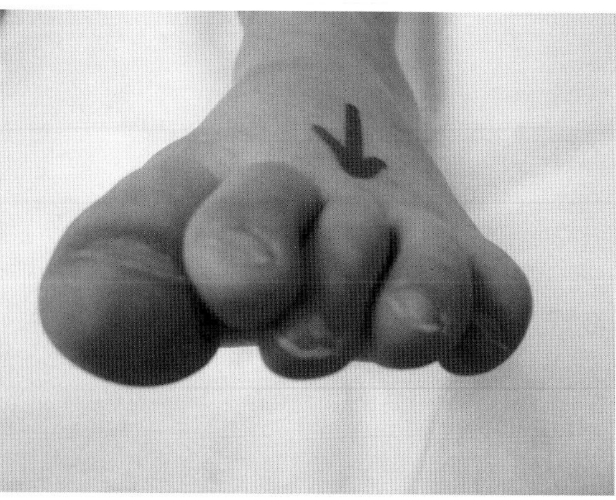

Fig. 8.1.6 Curly middle toes – flexor tenotomy is sometimes needed for severe cases.

*Inset hips (persistent femoral neck anteversion)* have internal rotation in excess of the range of external rotation. The condition is more common in girls and the feet seem to fly out sideways when running. The pathology lies in the top of the femur where there is a normal twist of 30° at birth, which unwinds gradually by the age of 7 years. In severe cases, when there is a major cosmetic problem unresolved by about 10 years, derotation femoral osteotomy can be performed, but this is rarely required.

Children with inset hips commonly sit between their feet with their hips in full internal rotation, the knees flexed and the legs splayed outwards (the 'W' position) (Fig. 8.1.7). This is the only way they can sit comfortably as they cannot externally rotate their hips sufficiently to sit in a cross-legged fashion. It is almost unknown for an adult to present with a complaint of in-toeing, which tells us that the natural history is spontaneous resolution.

*Internal tibial torsion* (a twist in the shin bone) is usually due to intrauterine pressure and can persist up to the age of 3 years and then spontaneously corrects.

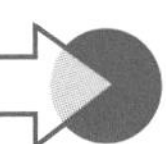

**Practical points**

- Bow legs and knock knees are common normal variants.
- Flexible flat feet are normal and need no treatment.
- Examine the child with in-toe gait to decide cause (metatarsus adductus, tibial torsion or inset hips).
- Provide brochure information to reassure.

*Metatarsus adductus* (Fig. 8.1.8) is a condition in which the feet are banana-shaped, with the convexity of the banana outwards and the toes directed towards each other. This may be due to intrauterine pressure; however, if it persists it is called metatarsus adductus. It is passively correctable and slowly rights itself, especially after walking commences. Very rarely, manipulation and plaster immobilization is necessary.

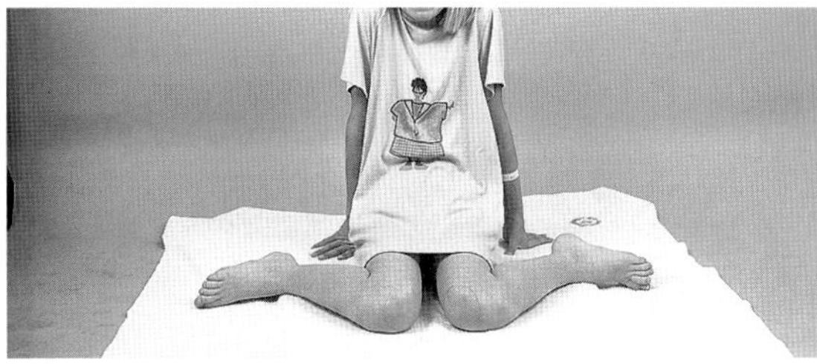

**Fig. 8.1.7** 'W' sitting is easy for the child with inset hips.

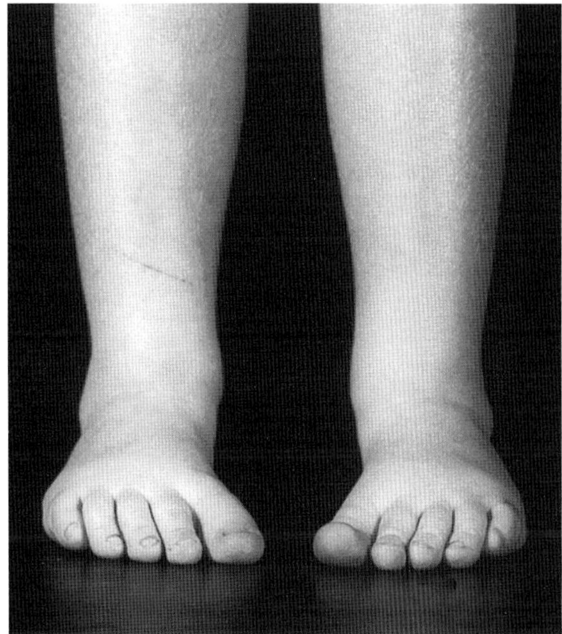

**Fig. 8.1.8** A 3-year-old child with metatarsus adductus. Note the metatarsals and toes curving inwards.

## Congenital abnormalities

### Developmental dysplasia of the hip

This condition was previously called congenital dislocation of the hip (CDH); however, developmental dysplasia of the hip (DDH) is now the preferred term as it tells us that some of these hip problems develop after birth. DDH is the most common musculoskeletal abnormality in neonates. The incidence of this condition in Australia and North America is 7 per 1000 live births. In some regions of Europe it is more common.

#### Clinical classification

DDH can be classified clinically as follows:

- stable
- subluxatable
- dislocatable
- dislocated, reducible
- dislocated, irreducible
- teratological.

#### Main risk factors

Some of the important risk factors for DDH (with the degree of increased risk) are:

- breech presentation (10×)
- female baby (4×)
- oligohydramnios (4×)

- big baby >4 kg (2×)
- first-born baby (2×)
- family history.

When diagnosed and treated from birth, it is possible to produce a normal hip joint after a few months of treatment in an abduction splint. However, if the diagnosis is not made until after the child begins to walk, the treatment is long and tedious, and often ends with an imperfect joint.

## Diagnosis in the newborn

The Barlow and Ortolani tests are used for diagnosis (Fig. 8.1.9). Every baby should be examined for hip dislocation during the first day of life and again at discharge from the maternity ward, and at ages 6 weeks, 3 months, 6 months and 1 year. The baby must be relaxed for the examination to be meaningful. If the baby is crying, a bottle or pacifier is offered or the baby is examined later when relaxed. With the legs extended, any asymmetry of the legs or thigh creases is noted. The examiner then holds the leg to be examined. With the knee flexed, the thumb is placed over the lesser trochanter and the middle finger over the greater trochanter. The pelvis is steadied by the other hand and the flexed thigh is abducted and adducted, and any clunk or jerk is noted.

It is very important to note that frequently a fine click can be felt in the hip joint without any laxity or abnormal movement. Sometimes the click comes from the knee joint. This is very common and is of no significance. Also, it is common in the first 2 or 3 days of life for the hip to be felt to subluxate smoothly without any clunk. This is especially felt in premature babies and requires repeated examination; frequently the hip becomes normal without treatment but it must be followed carefully.

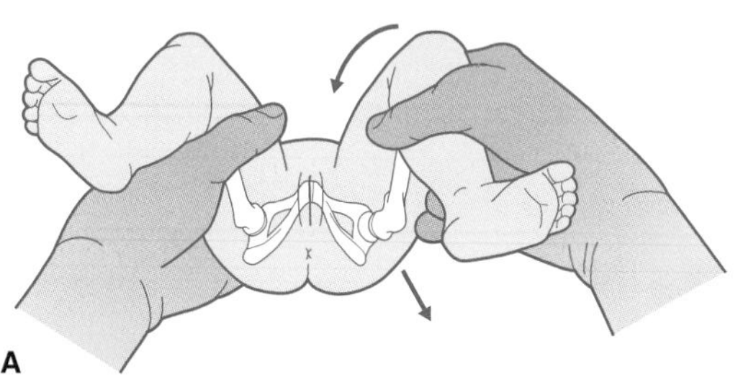


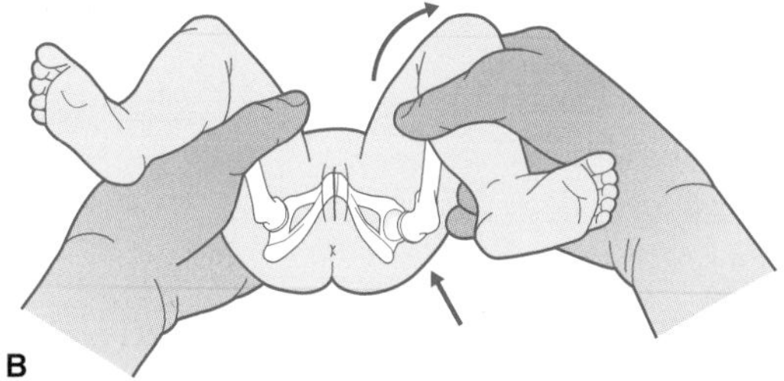


Fig. 8.1.9 **(A)** The Barlow test is positive if the hip can be manually dislocated. **(B)** The Ortolani test is positive if the hip is lying in a dislocated position and is manually reducible.

Radiography has no place in the diagnosis of developmental dysplasia of the hip in the neonatal period (see Chapter 7.1). Ultrasound examination of the hips gives the clinician useful information as to the relationship of the femoral head to the acetabulum and the existence of any acetabular dysplasia during the first 6 months of life. Be aware that ultrasonography has a high false-positive rate in babies under 6 weeks of age and scans should only be performed under 6 weeks either to check whether a hip is 'in joint' while in a splint or to check a 'doubtful' hip when the Barlow or Ortolani tests are equivocal. Over the age of 4 months, the degree of ossification of the upper femur and acetabulum enables X-rays to be of value.

If the dislocatable or dislocated hip is held in a flexed and abducted position for 8–12 weeks, it will usually develop normally. The Pavlik harness or Denis Browne splint is used to maintain this position. Subluxatable hips can be observed with a later ultrasound examination after 6 weeks or radiography at 4 months. The use of double nappies is not recommended.

All abnormal or treated hips require follow-up until normal hip morphology is ascertained.

*Teratological hip*

If there is considerable restriction of abduction in flexion and the 'clunk' sign cannot be elicited, this usually means that the hips are dislocated and irreducible. These hips require paediatric orthopaedic surgical assessment and probably operative reduction at a later date.

*Swaddling/wrapping*

This has been popularized recently to help a baby settle. However, swaddling infants with the hips and knees in an extended position increases the risk of hip dysplasia and dislocation. Hips should be positioned in flexion and abduction, knees should be maintained in slight flexion, and free movement in the direction of hip flexion and abduction may have some benefit.

## Diagnosis in the older infant

The Barlow and Ortolani tests become more difficult to elicit after 3 months of age. In the abnormal hip, a new sign of limited abduction appears due to tightness of the adductor tendons. This sign is not diagnostic but an X-ray is indicated when there is asymmetry in the range of the abduction of the hips or when the range of abduction of both hips is inappropriate for the age of the child. In the first year of life the range of abduction in flexion is usually 60–90°; this arc normally lessens with age.

The physical signs of late presenting dislocation include:

- higher greater trochanter
- wide perineum
- asymmetrical gluteal buttock crease
- short leg
- abnormal gait.

If a dislocation presents after walking age, an open reduction operation is usually required and these hips are rarely normal, with an increased risk of early hip osteoarthritis. Hence early diagnosis and treatment of DDH is the best way to prevent hip arthritis.

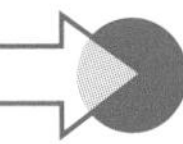

**Practical points**

- All babies should be assumed to have dislocated hips until proven otherwise.
- Re-examine babies' hips at every well-baby check.
- If in doubt, do an ultrasound examination when 6 weeks of age.
- Ensure that the sonographer is experienced in babies' hips.
- Swaddling/wrapping increases the risk of hip dysplasia.

## Congenital talipes equinovarus (club foot)

Congenital talipes equinovarus is the commonest congenital abnormality of the foot, occurring in about 1 per 1000 live births. The male : female ratio is 2 : 1. The condition is bilateral in 40% of cases and there is a 2% chance of a subsequent child being affected if there is a positive family history.

The deformity is a combination of:

- equinus of the hind foot
- varus of the hind foot
- adductus of the midfoot
- cavus of the medial arch.

The degree of each deformity is variable, but all are rigid and are incapable of being fully corrected manually (Fig. 8.1.10). This is distinct from the 'postural club foot', which is due to intrauterine pressure and is fully passively correctable and resolves without treatment, as described above.

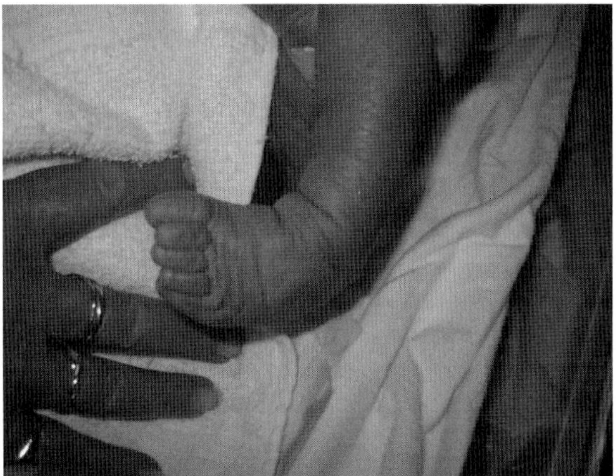

Fig. 8.1.10 Club foot deformity is rigid and cannot be corrected passively.

Club feet should start treatment in the first week of life. Treatment involves serial plaster casting by Ponseti method for 6 weeks, and then Achilles tenotomy followed by a cast for a further 3 weeks followed by 'boots and bars' until the age of 4 years. Sometimes later tendon surgery is required.

## Congenital muscular torticollis

Torticollis usually presents in the first few months of life when some tilt of the head and limited lateral flexion is noted. Sometimes it can remain undetected for 1–2 years. The head is held with a lateral flexion toward the shoulder and with rotation of the face towards the opposite side. The face on that side is smaller and the eye is lower on the side of the tight sternomastoid. Most patients will have presented in the first few months of life with a sternomastoid tumour – a palpable lump in the middle of the sternomastoid muscle.

The cause of this condition is unknown. Treatment in the first 6 months of life with a stretching programme supervised by a physiotherapist is usually effective, with full resolution. If the condition does not resolve, surgical correction at 2–4 years of age is required. At operation, the muscle is divided transversely and the corrected position maintained by the use of a collar.

Alexander the Great (354 BC) is reported to have had this condition, with statues showing a persistent head tilt.

## Trigger thumb

This presents with the parents suddenly noticing that their 1–3-year-old child has a bent thumb. At this age children start to handle objects and the thumb deformity becomes obvious. The thumb is bent about 30° at the interphalangeal joint and cannot be straightened passively (Fig. 8.1.11).

It is due to a constriction in the flexor tendon sheath and a nodule on the tendon itself. The cause is unknown and the treatment is surgical release of the tendon sheath under general anaesthesia. Surgery should be performed around the age of 2 years to prevent permanent joint changes.

## Scoliosis

Scoliosis (lateral curvature of the spine) is most commonly seen in its adolescent idiopathic form (Fig. 8.1.12). However, there are other forms of scoliosis. The common ones are:

- *Congenital* – vertebral anomalies are responsible for the curvature. Usually the deformity is minor and

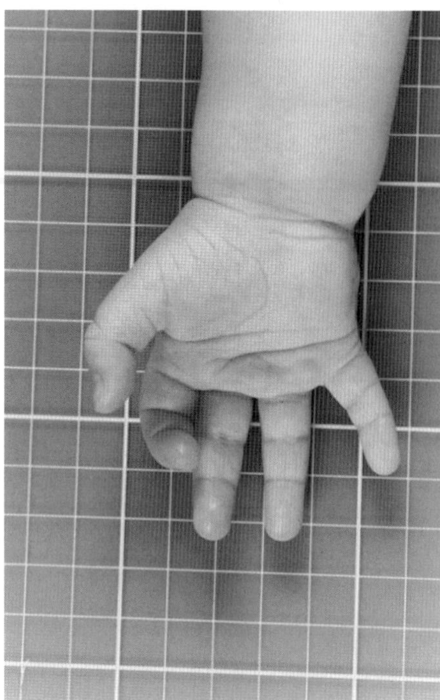

Fig. 8.1.11 Trigger thumb (left hand) showing 30° flexion deformity at the interphalangeal joint. Palpate a nodule at the level of the metacarpophalangeal joint.

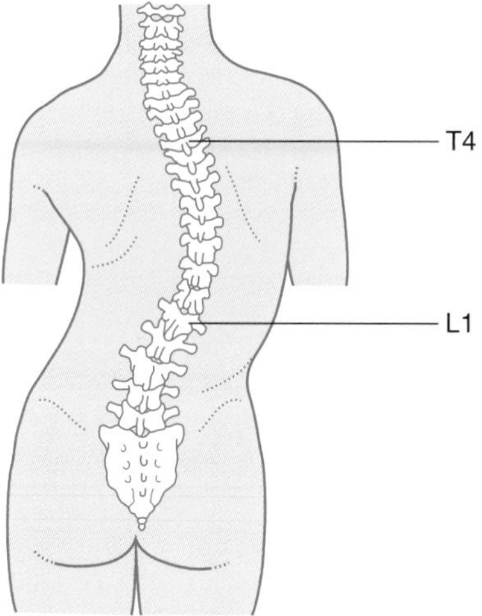


Fig. 8.1.12 Adolescent idiopathic scoliosis; the curve is usually convex to the right side.

may be present at birth or develop during growth. In only 5% is the deformity progressive.

- *Neuromuscular* – such as Duchenne muscular dystrophy, cerebral palsy or spina bifida.
- *Idiopathic* – mostly *adolescent idiopathic scoliosis*. Sometimes in younger children as:
  - *infantile idiopathic scoliosis* – most commonly seen in males and may be seen in association with DDH and other congenital anomalies. The natural history is for the curve to resolve in a high proportion of cases.
  - *early-onset idiopathic scoliosis* – a curve diagnosed under the age of 10 years.

## Adolescent idiopathic scoliosis

Some 90% of cases are in girls and the scoliosis progresses during the rapid growth spurt years.

For diagnosis, the child must remove all clothing above the waist and stand with the back facing the examiner (Fig. 8.1.13). In all but very minor curves, the deformity will be readily apparent. Signs to look for are:

- uneven shoulders
- waist (flank) asymmetry
- a unilateral rib prominence when the child bends forward (Fig. 8.1.14).

If the curve disappears completely when the child bends forward, it can be labelled 'postural' and treatment is not required. Should a rib hump become visible (due to rotation of the vertebrae and consequent rib deformity; see Fig. 8.1.14) the curve is labelled 'structural'.

There are three main treatment options:

- observation for curves of less than 20°
- bracing for curves of 20–40°
- surgery for curves greater than 50° (due to high risk of continued progression in adult life).

These are broad guidelines only. Larger curves may not be treated if proven to be non-progressive in a skeletally mature patient. There is no scientific evidence that exercises or physiotherapy/chiropractic treatments alter the natural history of the curve.

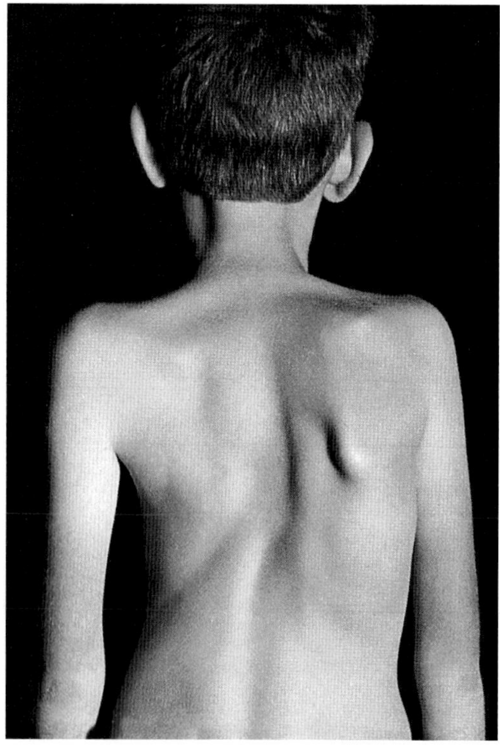

Fig. 8.1.13 Adolescent scoliosis in a male; 90% occur in females.

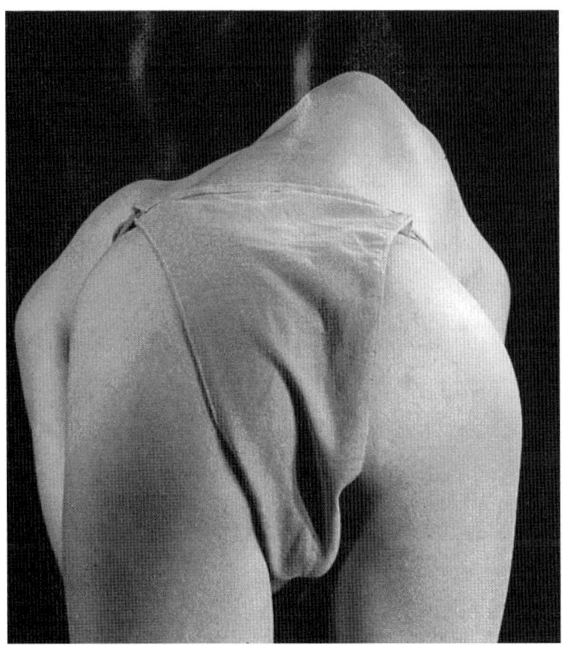

Fig. 8.1.14 On flexion, a rib hump becomes readily visible.

## Osteochondroses (osteochondritis)

These conditions involve the epiphysis. The pathology consists of localized areas of ischaemic bone necrosis and sometimes oedema of adjacent soft tissues. The tendency is for healing to occur but this is dependent on a number of factors, including age, the site of the lesion, its blood supply and perhaps the method of treatment. The aetiology is uncertain.

The common osteochondroses are:

- Sever's condition of the heel: 10–12 years
- Osgood–Schlatter's condition of the tibial tubercle: 10–14 years
- Chondromalacia patellae: 10–20 years
- Slipped capital femoral epiphysis of the hip: 10–15 years
- Scheuermann's condition of the thoracic spine: 12–16 years.

### Sever's condition

This is an apophysitis of the os calcis (heel) bone where the Achilles tendon attaches. It is seen in children aged between 10 and 12 years. It resolves over 12 months and is best treated by reassurance, calf stretches and sometimes a simple rubber heel raise. Sport is allowed within the child's level of comfort.

### Osgood–Schlatter's condition

This is an apophysitis of the tibial tubercle and presents with pain and swelling (Fig. 8.1.15). Children notice the pain and then an adult sees the swelling and can be concerned about a sinister cause such as malignancy. The common age of presentation is 10–14 years and the natural history is resolution over a 12–18-month period. Warn the parents that a lump will remain permanently but that it will be smaller than when first seen. Normal activities within the limits of the child's comfort are allowed. The tibial tubercle does not detach or pull off. Radiography is not necessary for diagnosis. Simple measures such as quadriceps stretches and massage with a liniment can provide some symptomatic relief. Rarely, a small loose ossicle remains and can be excised after the child reaches 15 years.

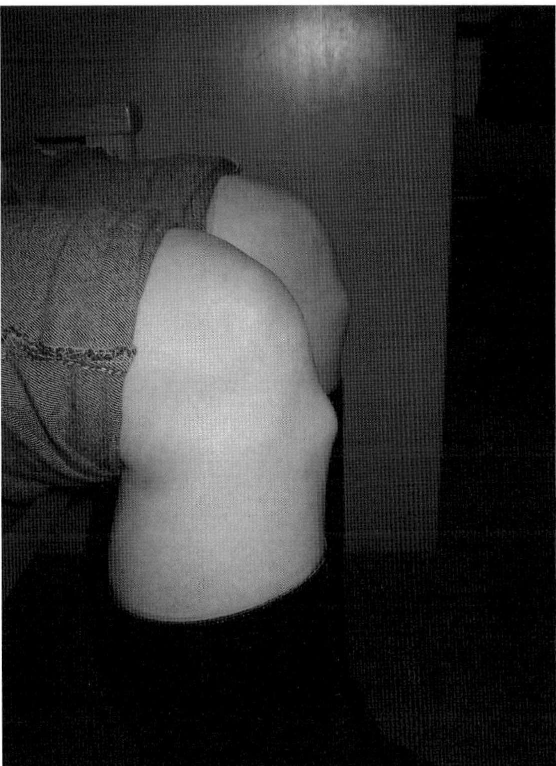

Fig. 8.1.15 Osgood–Schlatter's condition presents with painful enlarged tibial tubercles.

### Chondromalacia patellae

This condition has a number of other names, including:

- anterior knee pain
- lateral pressure syndrome
- maltracking of the patella.

It is particularly common over the age of 10 years. It is characterized by pain in the knee after activities that involve flexing the knee and quadriceps contraction. The child complains of aching around the patella during or especially after exercise. Stairs precipitate discomfort, particularly walking downstairs. It is more common in adolescent females, both in those who enjoy sport and in those who wish to avoid physical education lessons at school.

Clinically there is little to find, although occasionally there is some patellofemoral crepitus and rarely an effusion in the knee. Ensure that the hips are normal and the symptoms do not relate to a slipped hip. The diagnosis is based upon obtaining the relevant history.

Treatment involves education of the child and concerned parents (explain that the 'back of the knee cap is soft' and will toughen up with time), some limitation of flexed knee/jumping activities, quadriceps stretches, elastic knee support and tincture of time. Frequently, children tolerate their symptoms and continue with their sport. The natural history suggests spontaneous resolution of symptoms over 1–2 years in 90% of patients.

Some children are point tender at the inferior pole of patella (apophysis) and have a condition called Jumper's knee. Treatment is massage with anti-inflammatory gels, quadriceps stretches and the expectation that symptoms will resolve over 18 months.

### Slipped capital femoral epiphysis

This is primarily a disorder of adolescents between the ages of 10 and 15 years. Approximately 40% of cases are bilateral. Its aetiology is unknown but recent reports suggest that hormonal factors may be of importance. Most cases present with pain and limp; pain is often referred to the knee and it is important to consider hip radiography when children present with distal thigh or knee pain.

Types of slip:

- *Acute* – the child feels the hip 'collapse' and is unable to walk. This is uncommon and needs urgent treatment.
- *Acute on chronic* – the child has months of discomfort and then a worsening over a few weeks with a pronounced limp.
- *Chronic* – many months of thigh ache and a mild limp.

Examination reveals limited internal rotation of the hip compared with the other side and some joint irritability. The diagnosis is confirmed radiologically, especially with a frog lateral view (Fig. 8.1.16).

All cases of slipped capital femoral epiphysis require surgery with screw fixation across the physis to prevent further slip.

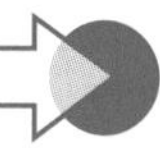

**Practical points**

- Knee/distal thigh pain often comes from the hip.
- Always think of a slipped hip in adolescents with a limp or knee/thigh pain.
- Know the various apophysitis pains in children.
- Anterior knee pain is common in teenagers.

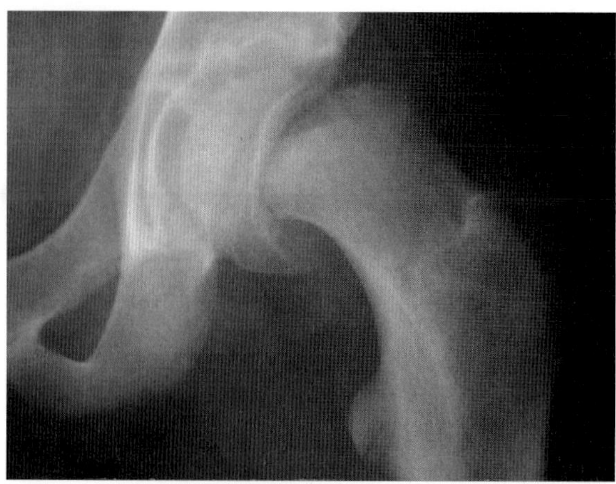

**Fig. 8.1.16** Slipped capital femoral epiphysis often presents with thigh or knee pain – always exclude hip pathology when a child presents with knee/thigh pain.

### Scheuermann's condition

The adolescent is noted to have an increased kyphosis (round back) and complains of mid to low thoracic back pain. The physis of the vertebral bodies is involved. Usually the condition is seen in the thoracic vertebrae but occasionally in the lumbar spine. Most merely require observation, encouragement to exercise and stand straight, and to be instructed in exercises by a physiotherapist. Some progress rapidly and require management in a brace. Rarely is surgery required.

The condition is frequently 'overdiagnosed' in radiology reports and causes anxiety in families, especially when the radiological changes are described as Scheuermann's 'disease'. The term 'condition' is preferred.

## Injuries in infancy and childhood

Children are susceptible to injury because of their carefree play habits, and skeletal injuries are common. For practical purposes, sprains do not occur in children: 'children break bones and adults tear ligaments'. Post-trauma pain, swelling and loss of function are nearly always the result of a fracture or growth plate separation; therefore X-rays are obligatory.

Dislocations are rare in childhood, although shoulder and patella dislocations are seen in adolescents. The type of injury that may produce dislocation of an adult joint usually gives rise to a fracture or growth plate separation in a child.

Fractures are the commonest type of skeletal injury in childhood; they generally unite in less than half the time the equivalent injury would take to heal in an adult, and non-union is almost unknown. Childhood fractures may unite in a position of deformity, with the deformity correcting itself spontaneously over the ensuing 6–12 months, especially if the fracture is near the ends of the bone where there is most growth. Some shortening of bones also can be expected to correct spontaneously due to growth stimulation of the physis from prolonged increased vascularity to heal the fracture.

Child abuse is an important cause of childhood injury; it is important because, if unrecognized, further abuse is likely to occur and might even be fatal. When assessing a child after trauma, ensure that you check the whole child, using the principles of emergency management of severe trauma (EMST), and look for hidden injuries.

### Clavicle fractures

These are the most common fractures seen in children. The fracture is usually midshaft and of greenstick type. Complete fractures with overlap of the ends are seen in older children and unite well. It is important to warn the parents at the beginning that they must expect to see a large lump develop: this is healing callus, which will remodel over 6–12 months without any cosmetic or functional deficit.

Treatment is with a triangular sling inside the clothes to support the elbow, regular analgesia and rest. The clavicle will start to join within a week and the sling can usually be discarded by 4 weeks.

### Forearm fractures

Children's bones can break in several ways, namely:
- bend
- buckle
- greenstick
- complete, with/without displacement and overlap.

Most forearm fractures are of the buckle or greenstick variety, and if there is minimal tilt or deformity they can be treated in an above-elbow cast for 5 weeks. It is important to perform check radiography after 7–10 days to ensure that the fracture has not tilted more. If it has tilted to an unacceptable position, the fracture can still undergo a closed reduction before firm union occurs.

Fractures with visible deformity or significant tilt/displacement (Fig. 8.1.17) require closed reduction and a similar time of cast immobilization.

Ensure that you complete and document a neurovascular examination of the limb initially. Provide the parents with written instructions for neurovascular observations at home and with emergency contact details if excessive swelling or symptoms develop. Look for the five Ps:
- *Pain* in excess of that expected
- *Paraesthesia* (compression of the sensory nerves)
- *Paleness* of the fingers
- *Plum*-coloured (venous congestion)
- *Pulseless.*

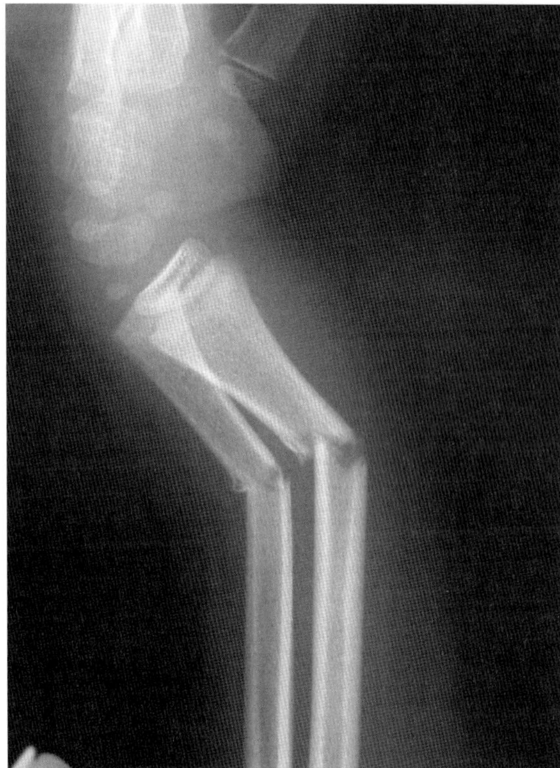

Fig. 8.1.17 Forearm fractures usually have dorsal tilt.

Approximately 30% of children's fractures involve the growth plate (physis). If the physis suffers permanent damage, the bone can end up:
- short (all growth of physis stops), or
- angulated (one side of the physis stops growing).

The Salter–Harris classification is used for growth plate fractures (Fig. 8.1.18). Type I is often seen in the distal fibula as the childhood equivalent of the adult ankle sprain. Type II is the commonest variety and frequent in the distal radius. Types III and IV have a much higher risk of growth disturbance and usually require accurate reduction and internal fixation to minimize the risk of growth arrest.

### Supracondylar fracture of the humerus

This fracture is often seen in children aged 4–10 years after a fall from a height, such as from monkey bars, or when running. Usually caused by hyperextension of the elbow joint with the olecranon acting as a fulcrum lever to cause the fracture.

Neuropraxia of the radial, median or ulna nerve is common. Occasionally displaced fractures cause damage to the brachial artery. Neurovascular assessment is mandatory. Minimally tilted fractures can be treated in a collar and cuff under the clothes for the first 2 weeks,

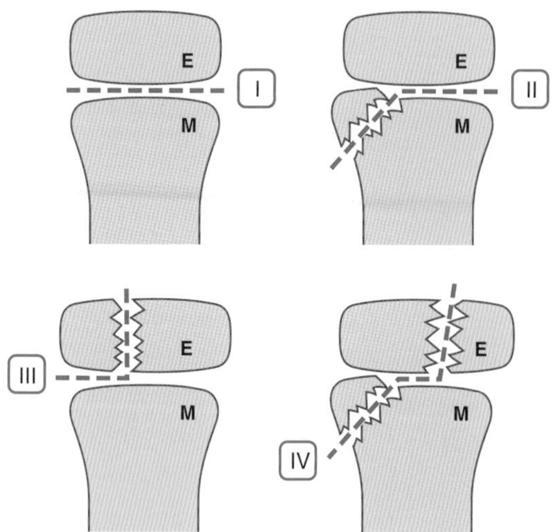


Fig. 8.1.18 Salter–Harris fracture: type I, the fracture passes directly through the physis; type II, a corner of the metaphysis (M) is broken off; type III, the fracture passes through the physis and the epiphysis (E); type IV, the fracture passes through the epiphysis and the metaphysis, causing a high risk of growth arrest.

then outside the clothes for a further 2 weeks. Warn the parents to expect elbow stiffness, especially loss of elbow extension for several months.

Displaced fractures require accurate reduction to avoid later deformity. Often the fracture will be held with K wires, which are removed at 4 weeks (Fig. 8.1.19).

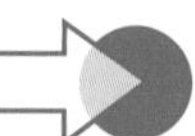

**Practical points**

**Rules of 2 for fractures**

- 2 views (anteroposterior and lateral X-ray)
- 2 joints (X-ray the joint above and joint below to exclude dislocation)
- 2 joints (immobilize the joint above and below the fracture in a cast)
- 2 times (ensure the fracture has not shifted after 1 week)
- 2 sides (you can X-ray the contralateral side for comparison if needed)

### Toddler fracture of the tibia

This distal shaft fracture may not be visible on initial radiographs and often perplexes clinicians faced with a toddler who refuses to walk for days after a seemingly minor trauma. The fracture can be diagnosed clinically by twisting the good leg first and then noting the cry or facial expression when twisting the affected side. Warn the parents what you are going to do first!

Treat the fracture in an above-knee cast and allow weight-bearing as the child dictates. Most will walk after 1 week in the cast, and the cast can be removed at 3 weeks. Warn the parents to expect a limp for 1–2 months; the limp will resolve spontaneously.

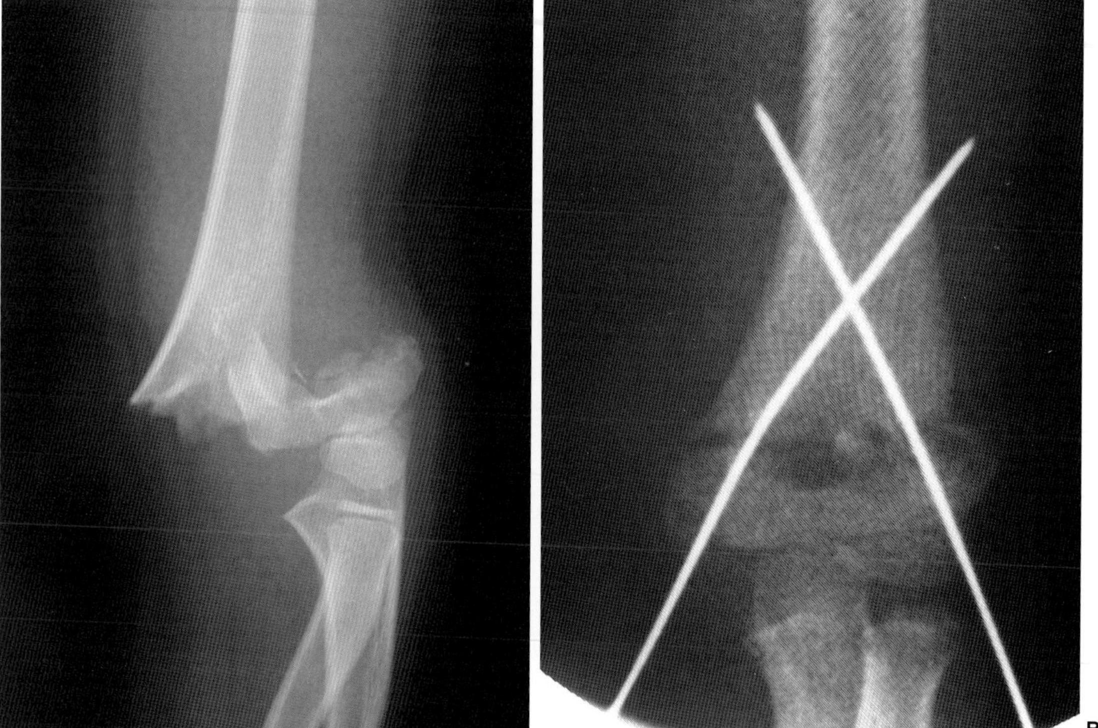


Fig. 8.1.19 **(A)** Supracondylar fracture of the humerus may have a nerve injury. **(B)** Displaced fractures require reduction and K-wire fixation.

### Pulled elbow

The patient is usually a child aged 1–4 years who has been pulled along or up by the hand or treated to a 'whizzy'. The child presents with 'pseudo-paralysis' of the upper limb, with the limb held by the side with the elbow extended and pronated. (Note that most elbow fractures present differently, with the elbow flexed and held across the body.)

The history is typical in all cases. The pathology is believed to be a minor stretch of the annular ligament around the radial head. It is treated by forced full flexion and simultaneous full supination of the elbow. Sometimes a satisfying click can be felt. A collar and cuff sling in flexion is worn overnight with the expectation of ready return to full function. Warn parents that it can recur and that it is best to avoid pulling on the hand.

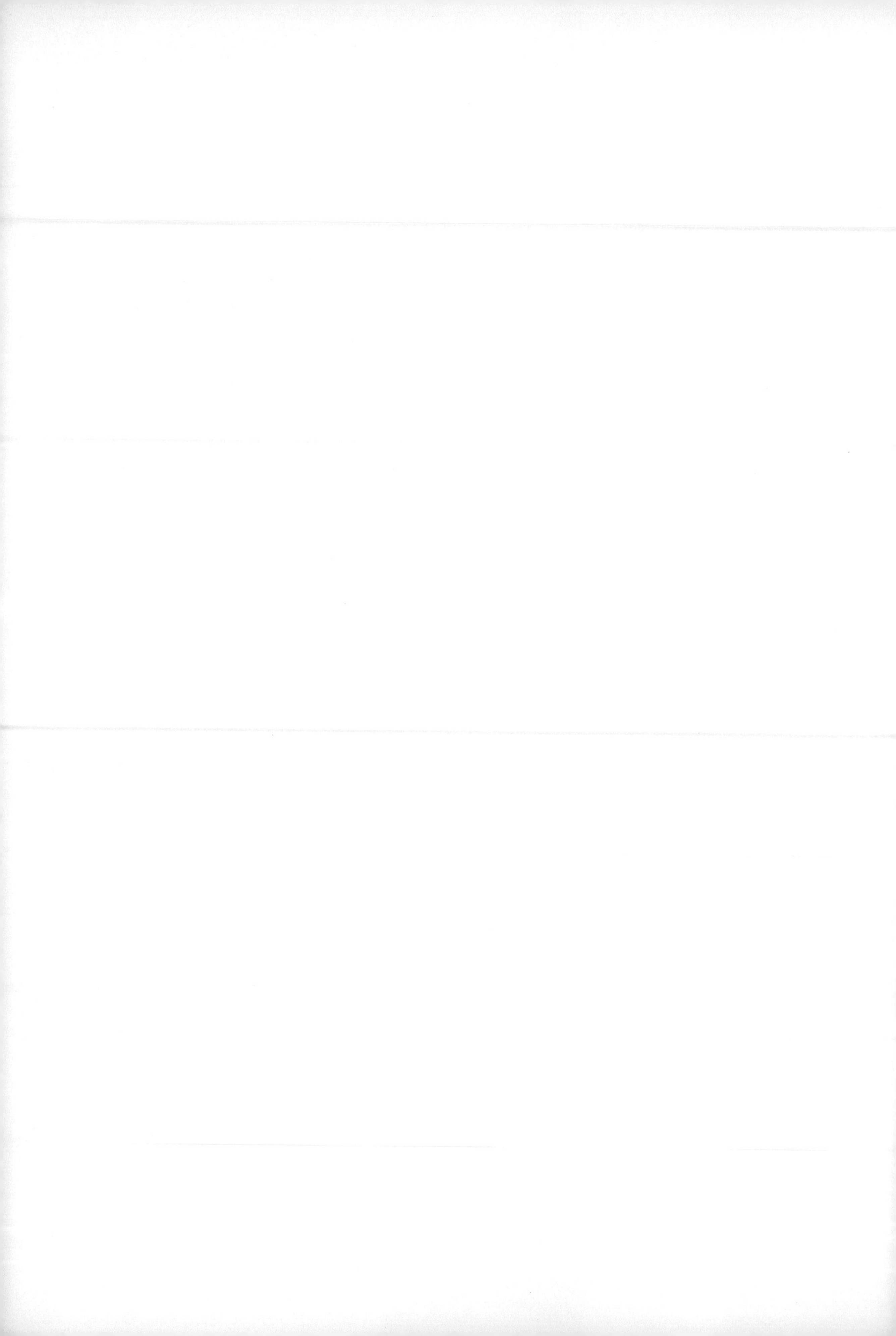

PART 9

# COMMON PAEDIATRIC SURGICAL PROBLEMS

# 9.1 Surgical conditions in older children

Sebastian K. King, Spencer W. Beasley

## The penis and foreskin

The glans of the uncircumcised penis is protected by a layer of loose skin called the foreskin or prepuce. The amount of foreskin present varies widely among boys. At birth, and for many years afterwards, it is normal for part or all of the undersurface of the foreskin to be adherent to the glans. This adherence slowly separates during childhood. Forcible retraction of the foreskin before it is ready can damage the glans and may cause secondary phimosis. Therefore, the foreskin should not be retracted forcibly. Spontaneous separation of these adhesions is normally complete by puberty.

### Smegma

Smegma is formed from desquamated cells and accumulates beneath the adherent foreskin. It appears as asymmetrical accumulations of yellow-tinged material, predominantly in the coronal groove beneath the foreskin (Fig. 9.1.1). There may be sufficient smegma to produce a noticeable swelling, which may be misdiagnosed as a dermoid cyst or tumour. It is often misinterpreted as being mid-shaft because a small child's coronal groove may be a long way from the tip of the foreskin. Smegma is normal, and is released spontaneously as the foreskin separates from the glans. When it is released, it may be associated with some redness and irritation of the foreskin for a day or so; this, too, is a normal process.

### Balanitis

Infection can develop beneath the foreskin and, if severe, pus may appear from the end of the foreskin. Balanitis is often associated with phimosis. Infection may cause considerable redness and swelling of the penile shaft, necessitating treatment with either topical or oral antibiotics.

### Phimosis

In phimosis the opening at the tip of the foreskin has narrowed down to such a degree that the foreskin cannot be retracted (Fig. 9.1.2). The external urethral meatus is not visible. Phimosis must be distinguished from the normal adherence of the foreskin to the glans. In most boys, phimosis can be treated by topical application of steroid ointment (e.g. betamethasone valerate ointment) to the tight, shiny part of the partially retracted foreskin. This usually obviates the need for circumcision. However, marked previous inflammation, infection, skin splitting and balanitis xerotica obliterans (BXO) can lead to marked scarring of the foreskin and phimosis, and in many of these children the only reasonable treatment is circumcision. Sometimes the severity of phimosis is such that there is ballooning of the foreskin on micturition, and on rare occasions it may even cause urinary retention with a distended bladder. A degree of phimosis is common in infancy but tends to resolve spontaneously in the first few years of life, and is not considered abnormal in this age group.

### Paraphimosis

Paraphimosis occurs when a mildly phimotic foreskin has been retracted over the glans and has become stuck behind the coronal groove, causing oedema of itself and the glans (Fig. 9.1.3). It is a painful and progressive process. Treatment involves gentle manipulation of the foreskin forwards; this may require a general anaesthetic. Circumcision is not performed at this time, but a few children may need it subsequently if the phimosis does not respond to topical application of steroid ointment.

### Hypospadias

It is important to recognize hypospadias when it is present (Fig. 9.1.4). The dorsal foreskin looks square and hangs off the penis, whereas the ventral foreskin is deficient, and the shaft of the penis is bent ventrally. The two main problems in hypospadias are:

- the location of the urethra (which can be found on the ventral side of the shaft of the penis, proximal to its correct position)
- chordee (ventral angulation of the shaft and glans) – correction of chordee to straighten the penis is required to allow later successful sexual function. The operation is usually performed as

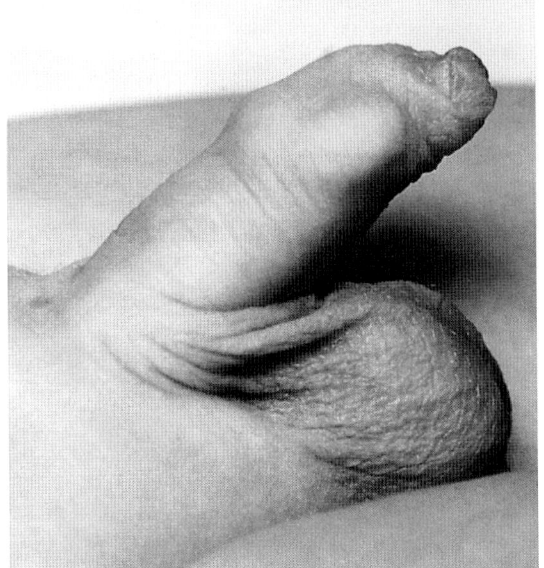

A

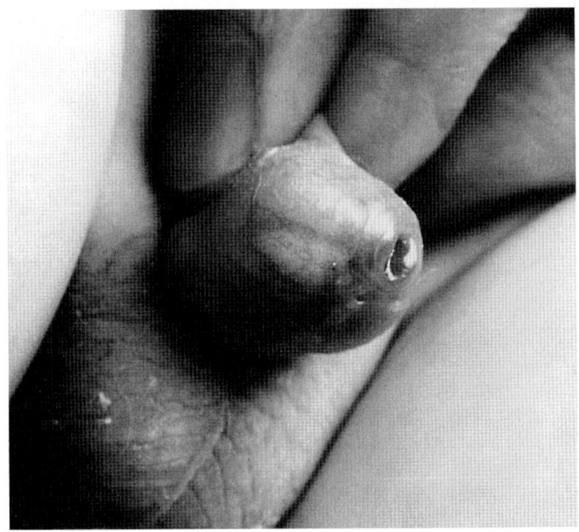

B

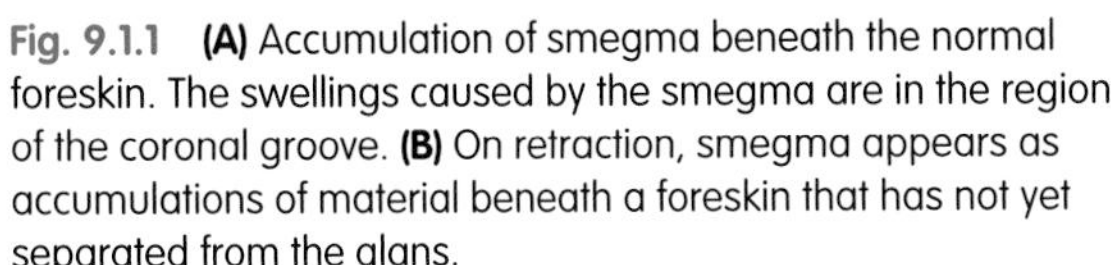

Fig. 9.1.1 **(A)** Accumulation of smegma beneath the normal foreskin. The swellings caused by the smegma are in the region of the coronal groove. **(B)** On retraction, smegma appears as accumulations of material beneath a foreskin that has not yet separated from the glans.

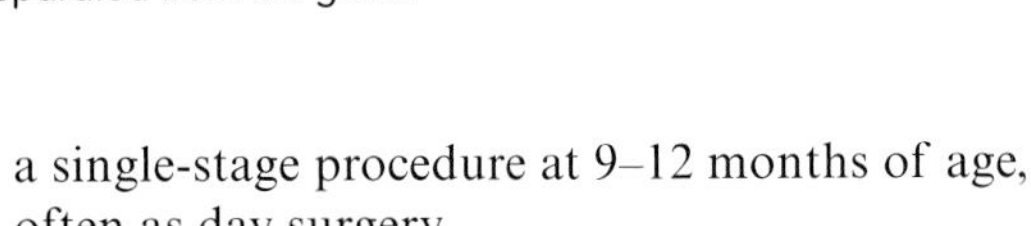

a single-stage procedure at 9–12 months of age, often as day surgery.

Circumcision is absolutely contraindicated in hypospadias because the skin of the foreskin is used during the hypospadias repair. Severe hypospadias may be indicative of an intersex abnormality. For example, when there is penoscrotal hypospadias and a bifid scrotum, the scrotum should be examined carefully for testes, as some of these children may be females with congenital adrenal hyperplasia; the labioscrotal folds are labia rather than scrota, and the presumed urethral opening may in fact be the entrance to the vagina (see Chapter 19.3).

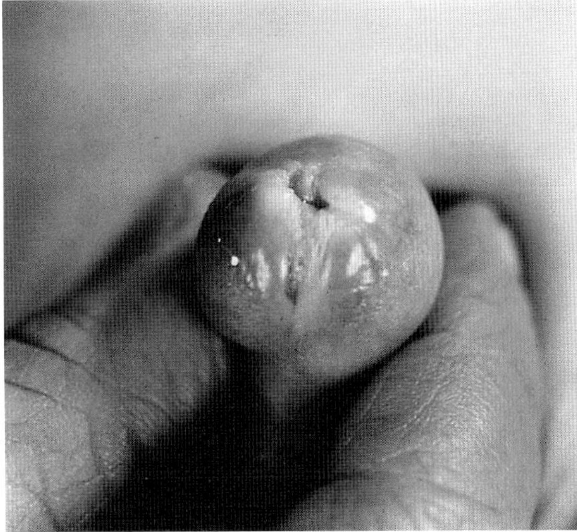

Fig. 9.1.2 In phimosis, the foreskin is narrowed and cannot be retracted.

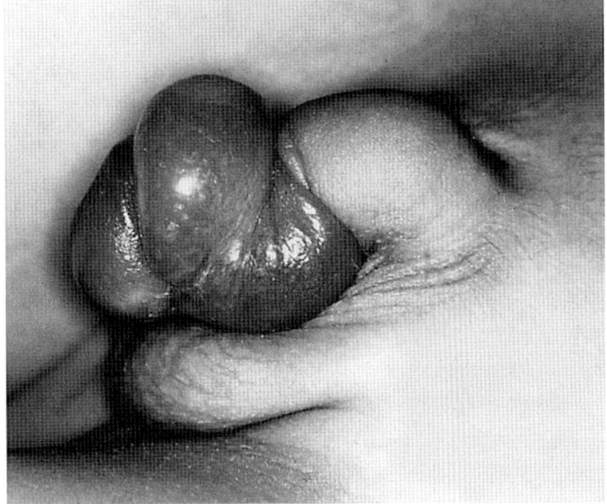

Fig. 9.1.3 In paraphimosis, the foreskin is stuck behind the coronal groove.

## Circumcision

The indications for circumcision remain controversial. Phimosis resulting from balanitis xerotica obliterans (see above) is the only undisputed indication. In many countries, circumcision has been abandoned in the neonatal period because of its relatively high complication rate. Apart from the risk of septicaemia and meningitis when performed in the relatively immunologically immature neonate, there are a number of problems that may occur during circumcision at any age. These include removal of too much or too little foreskin, postoperative bleeding and infection. Haemorrhage postoperatively occasionally requires surgical reintervention. The most troublesome and common complication of circumcision is abrasion and

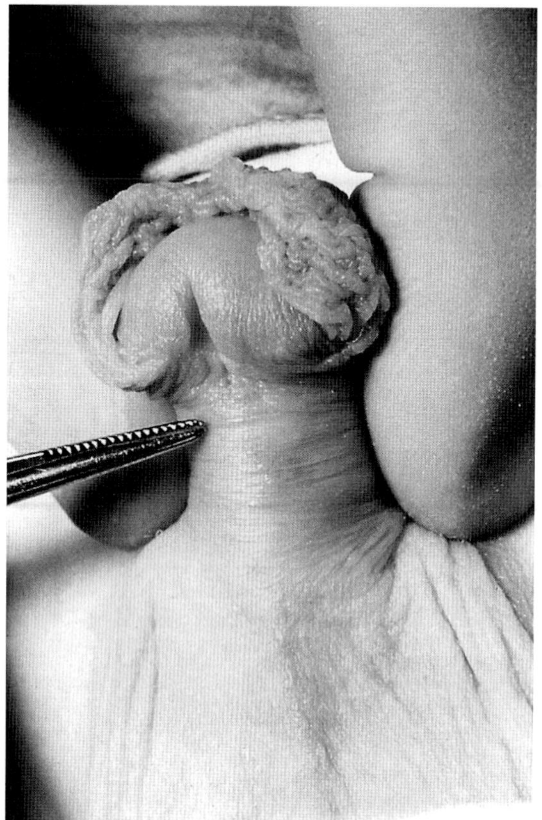

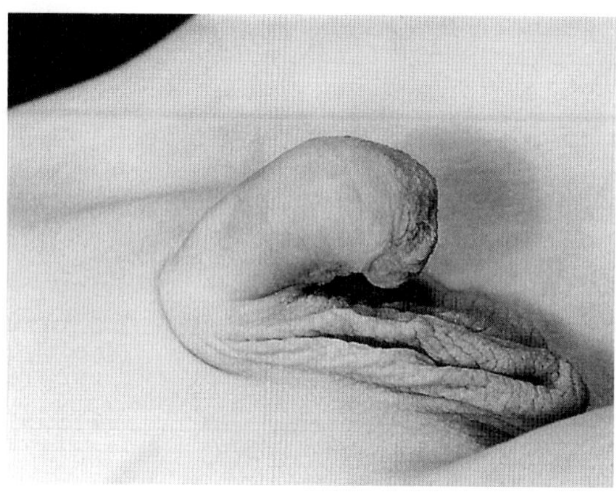

Fig. 9.1.4 In hypospadias, the ventral shaft of the penis is angulated and shortened (chordee), the urethral meatus is ventrally placed and the foreskin is deficient on the underside. **(A)** Ventral aspect; **(B)** lateral aspect.

ulceration of the sensitive glans, particularly near the urethral meatus. As the meatal ulceration heals it may produce meatal stenosis and require a meatotomy to re-establish an adequate urinary stream.

### Epispadias

Epispadias is a very rare condition in which the urethra opens on to the dorsal aspect of the base of the penis. Epispadias is part of a spectrum of lower abdominal wall defects in which ectopia vesicae (bladder exstrophy) and cloacal exstrophy are the most severe forms. Boys with epispadias are often incontinent of urine because the sphincter of the bladder neck is also deficient.

> **Clinical example**
>
> James was a 7-year-old boy who presented following two episodes of balanitis. He also complained of discomfort on micturition. Examination revealed a tight foreskin that could not be retracted; the urethral meatus could not be seen. After 1 month of topical application of betamethasone ointment four times a day to the tight part of the foreskin, he was able to retract it fully. Circumcision was not necessary.

## The inguinoscrotal region

### Inguinal hernia

After the testis has descended into the scrotum during the seventh month of pregnancy, the canal down which it migrates, the processus vaginalis, should obliterate. Failure of obliteration of the processus vaginalis may produce an inguinal hernia, a hydrocele or an encysted hydrocele of the cord.

A widely patent proximal processus vaginalis allows bowel (and, in girls, the ovary as well) to enter the inguinal canal, producing a reducible lump in the groin called an indirect inguinal hernia (Fig. 9.1.5). This occurs in about 2% of infant boys but is less frequent in girls. The greatest incidence is in the first year of life.

The usual presentation is that of an intermittent swelling, overlying the external inguinal ring, that has been noticed by a parent. At times it may appear to cause discomfort. It is most likely to be obvious during an episode of crying or straining, and in infants may be seen during nappy changes. Inguinal herniae should be repaired as soon as practicable.

Strangulation of inguinal herniae is common, particularly during the first 6 months of life. Strangulation can be recognized when the groin swelling becomes irreducible. If left untreated, a strangulated hernia may damage the trapped bowel and, occasionally, by compressing the testicular vessels, may lead to testicular atrophy. For this reason, an immediate attempt should be made to reduce the hernia manually. This is done by first manoeuvring the hernial contents through the external inguinal ring, and then reducing them along the line of the inguinal canal. Fortunately, most herniae that become stuck can be reduced manually; the hernia can then be repaired as an elective procedure within a few days. This is best done in a specialist paediatric surgical centre.

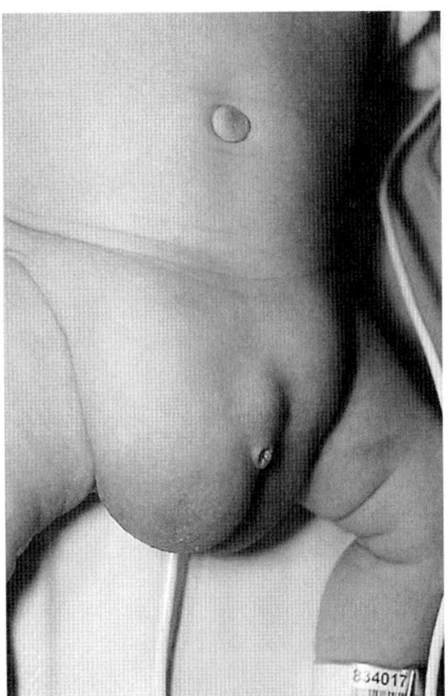

Fig. 9.1.5 Large bilateral inguinal herniae.

## Hydrocele

A hydrocele presents as a painless cystic swelling around the testis in the scrotum (Fig. 9.1.6). It contains peritoneal fluid that has tracked down a narrow but patent processus vaginalis. It transilluminates brilliantly. When the hydrocele is lax, the testis can be

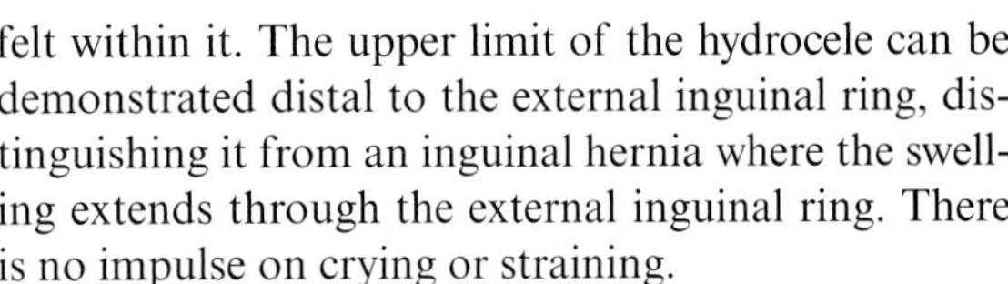

felt within it. The upper limit of the hydrocele can be demonstrated distal to the external inguinal ring, distinguishing it from an inguinal hernia where the swelling extends through the external inguinal ring. There is no impulse on crying or straining.

Hydroceles are common in the first few months of life, do not cause discomfort and usually disappear spontaneously within a year. Surgery involves an inguinal herniotomy and is indicated only if the hydrocele persists beyond 2 years of age.

## Undescended testis

Undescended testis (or cryptorchidism) is a term used to describe the testis that does not reside spontaneously in the scrotum. Cryptorchidism occurs in about 2% of boys, being more common in premature infants. Spontaneous descent of the testis is unlikely beyond 3 months post-term. Cryptorchidism is important to detect because it can result in reduced fertility if left untreated. It is suspected that the higher temperature to which an undescended testis is subject impairs spermatogenesis.

The diagnosis is made by examining the inguinoscrotal region. Normally, the testis should be found within the scrotal sac. In cryptorchidism the scrotum looks empty (Fig. 9.1.7). The testis is 'milked' down the line of the inguinal canal towards the scrotum with

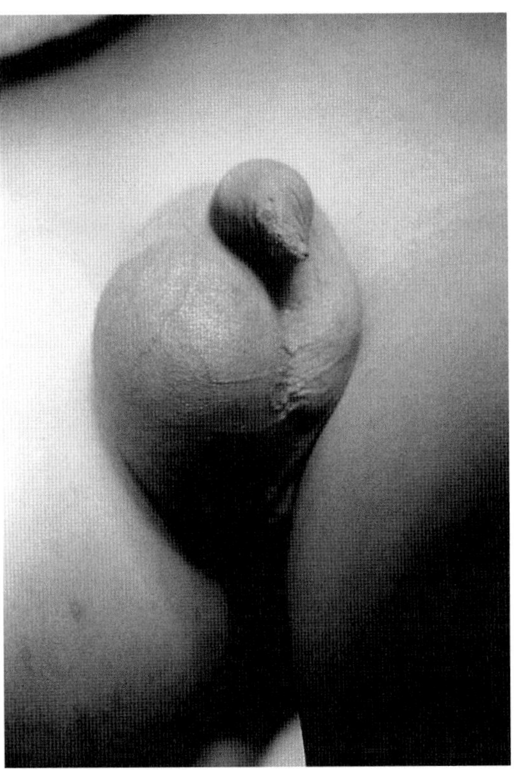

Fig. 9.1.6 Right hydrocele.

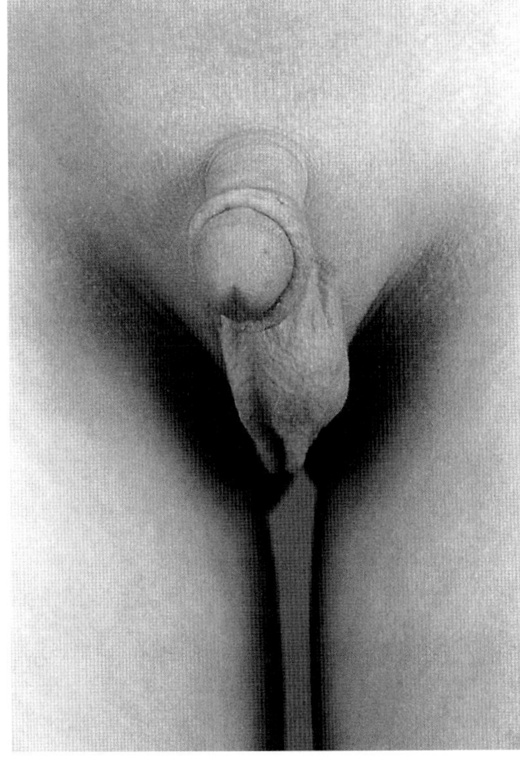

Fig. 9.1.7 Right undescended testis.

the left hand and pulled gently towards the scrotum with the right hand. If the testis cannot be brought into the scrotum, or will not remain there spontaneously, it is considered undescended.

Clinically, it may be difficult to distinguish a retractile testis from an undescended testis. In most normal boys the testis resides in the bottom of the scrotum, but the cremasteric reflex, which is prominent during mid-childhood, may cause it to move upwards, sometimes completely out of the scrotum. A retractile testis found outside the scrotum initially can be brought down into the normal position and should stay there spontaneously, at least until the cremasteric reflex is stimulated (Table 9.1.1). An undescended testis will not stay in the scrotum spontaneously and usually cannot even be coerced beyond the neck of the scrotum. It is often smaller than the normal testis on the other side.

Undescended testes should be brought down into the scrotum surgically between 9 and 12 months of age. Unfortunately, in many boys the diagnosis is not made until the child is older. The later the testis is brought down, the more likely it is that there will be damage to spermatogenesis. Orchidopexy is performed as a day case procedure. In general, the results are excellent when the procedure is performed by a specialist paediatric surgeon.

## The acutely painful scrotum

There are a number of conditions that cause an acutely painful or enlarged scrotum (Fig. 9.1.8). Whilst torsion of a testicular appendage is the most common, torsion of the testis itself is the most important (Table 9.1.2). In both conditions the boy complains of severe pain in the scrotum. In the early stages of torsion of a testicular appendage, a blue–black 'pea-sized' swelling which is extremely tender to touch may be seen through the skin of the scrotum near the upper pole of the testis. Palpation of the testis itself causes no or little discomfort. Later, a reactive hydrocele develops, the tenderness becomes more generalized and the clinical features may make it difficult to distinguish from torsion of the testis.

If torsion of the testis has occurred, both the testis and the epididymis are exquisitely tender (unless

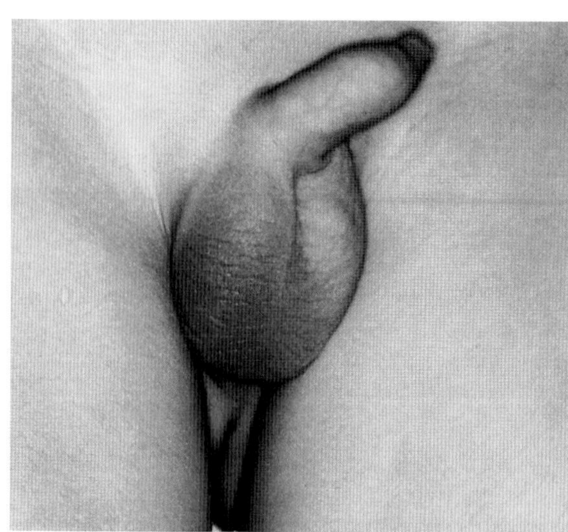

Fig. 9.1.8 An acutely painful scrotum in a child is most likely to be caused by torsion of an appendix testis or torsion of the testis.

necrosis has already occurred) and the testis may be lying high within the scrotum. In older boys the pain radiates to the ipsilateral iliac fossa and may be associated with nausea and vomiting, producing symptoms similar to those of appendicitis. This association highlights the importance of always examining the scrotum in boys presenting with lower abdominal pain.

### Treatment

Urgent surgical exploration of the scrotum is required to untwist the testis and epididymis and to suture both testes to prevent subsequent torsion. A completely necrotic testis should be removed. A torted and infarcted testicular appendix should be removed. In this situation the testis should be checked to make sure that it has not twisted but otherwise it requires no treatment.

## Other causes of scrotal pathology

Epididymo-orchitis is unusual in children; it is most often seen during the first year of life, where it may signify an underlying structural abnormality of the

**Table 9.1.1 Comparison of undescended and retractile testes**

| Feature | Undescended testis | Retractile testis |
|---|---|---|
| Can be brought fully to bottom of scrotum | No | Yes |
| Remains in scrotum spontaneously for a period before retracting | No | Yes |
| Resides spontaneously in scrotum at times | No | Yes |
| Testicular size | Normal or small | Normal |

**Table 9.1.2 Causes of an acutely painful scrotum**

| Condition | Comment | Frequency |
|---|---|---|
| Torsion of testicular appendix | Peak age 11 years<br>Unilateral tenderness | >75% |
| Torsion of testis | Peaks in neonatal and adolescent age groups<br>Surgical emergency | 20% |
| Epididymo-orchitis | Usually in infancy<br>Association with urinary tract abnormalities | Rare |
| Idiopathic scrotal oedema | Usually in young child<br>Bilateral oedema<br>Testes not tender | Rare |

genitourinary tract. For this reason investigation involves renal ultrasonography and micturating cystourethrography. Examination of the urine may show leukocytes and bacteria. Mumps orchitis is extremely rare prior to puberty. In idiopathic scrotal oedema there is painless boggy oedema of the whole scrotum and the testes are completely non-tender. Testicular malignancy is occasionally seen in leukaemia and lymphoma, or with a primary testicular neoplasm.

## Abnormalities of the umbilicus

The umbilical cord desiccates and separates several days after birth, allowing the umbilical ring to close. Sometimes the stump of the cord may become infected, the umbilical ring may not close, or there may be remnants of the embryonic channels that pass through the umbilicus before birth (Table 9.1.3).

### Umbilical hernia

Failure of the umbilical ring to close after birth produces an umbilical hernia (Fig. 9.1.9). Umbilical herniae are common in neonates but most close spontaneously in the first year of life. The skin overlying the umbilical hernia never ruptures and strangulation of the contents is virtually unknown. Parents may be concerned about the swelling, which will become tense when the infant cries or strains. Umbilical herniae normally do not cause pain. If the hernia is still present after the age of 3 years, it can be repaired as a day surgical procedure.

### Discharge from the umbilicus

Discharge from the umbilicus may be pus, mucus, faeces or urine. An umbilical granuloma is a common lesion that first becomes evident after separation of the umbilical cord. There is a small accumulation

**Table 9.1.3 Abnormalities of the umbilicus**

| Abnormality | Comment |
|---|---|
| Exomphalos | See Chapter 11.5 |
| Gastroschisis | See Chapter 11.5 |
| Umbilical hernia | Common (most resolve)<br>Asymptomatic<br>Skin covered |
| Umbilical sepsis ('omphalitis') | Neonatal<br>Serious condition |
| Umbilical granuloma | Common<br>Often pedunculated<br>Treat with silver nitrate |
| Ectopic bowel mucosa | Treat with silver nitrate |
| Patent vitellointestinal duct | Sinus opening at umbilicus<br>Communication with ileum<br>Discharges faecal fluid and gas |
| Patent urachus | Communication with bladder<br>Discharges urine |

of granulation tissue in the umbilicus, accompanied by a seropurulent discharge. If it has a definite stalk it can be ligated without anaesthesia, but most often it is treated by topical application of silver nitrate. Ectopic bowel mucosa has a similar appearance but has a smooth, red, glistening surface and discharges mucus. Topical application of silver nitrate in patients with ectopic bowel mucosa is typically less effective than in those with an umbilical granuloma.

Persistence of part or all of the vitellointestinal (omphalomesenteric) duct produces one of a number of abnormalities, which usually present in early infancy but may not be evident for some years. Complete

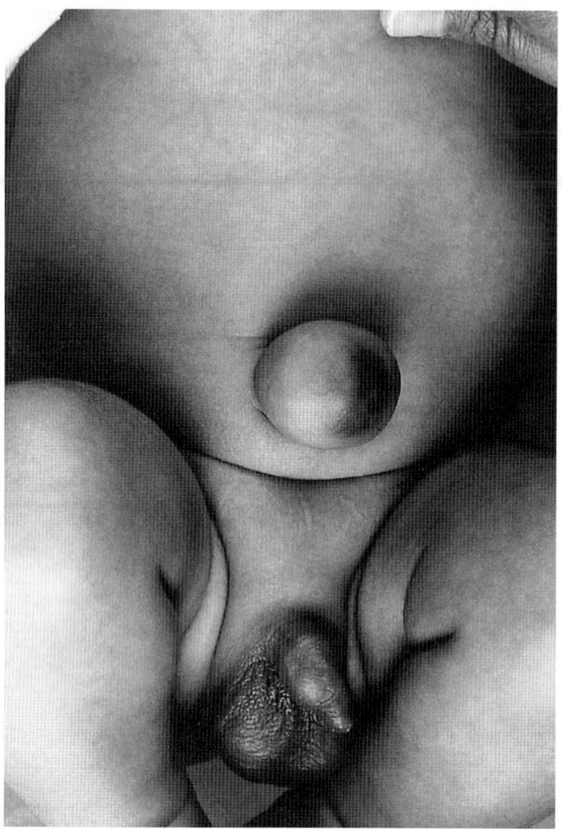

Fig. 9.1.9 Umbilical hernia.

patency of the duct allows ileal fluid and air to discharge from the umbilicus. Persistence of one part produces a sinus or cyst, which may become infected to form an abscess and may discharge pus. A vitellointestinal band attaching the ileum to the deep surface of the umbilicus may cause intestinal obstruction. A Meckel's diverticulum represents persistence of the ileal part of the duct. Vitellointestinal duct remnants are excised.

Urinary discharge from the umbilicus suggests a persistent communication with the bladder in the form of a patent urachus. Sometimes it may produce a cystic mass or abscess in the midline just below the umbilicus. Urachal remnants should be excised.

## The anus and perineum

A variety of unrelated conditions affect the anus and perineum in children.

### Anal fissure

This is usually seen in infants and toddlers when passage of a hard stool splits the anal mucosa, causing sharp pain and often a few drops of bright blood. The condition is of little consequence and the fissure usually heals within days. Examination of the anal margin shows a split in the epithelium anteriorly or posteriorly in the midline. Occasionally an anal fissure may occur in an older child, and is usually related to constipation. The child experiences severe pain on defaecation and becomes reluctant to defaecate, further worsening the constipation. Treatment is directed at overcoming the underlying constipation. A stool softener and lubricant (e.g. paraffin oil) may be helpful. A chronic indolent, often non-painful, fissure away from the midline may indicate inflammatory bowel disease, such as Crohn's disease.

### Perianal abscess

This is most likely to occur in the first year of life from infection of an anal gland. The abscess points superficially, a centimetre or two from the anal canal. The abscess should be drained and the fistula between the abscess and the anal canal laid open during the same operation to reduce the likelihood of recurrence.

### Rectal prolapse

Rectal prolapse tends to occur in the second and third years of life in otherwise normal children. The rectum prolapses during defaecation and returns spontaneously afterwards. In some, manual reduction is required. The prolapsed mucosa may become congested and bleed, but causes little discomfort. Clinically, it needs to be distinguished from prolapse of a benign rectal polyp (a benign hamartomatous lesion seen in children) and the apex of an intussusception (the child would have other symptoms of intussusception). The passage of time, and treatment of any underlying constipation, is all that is required in the majority of toddlers. Rarely, for persistent cases, a sclerosant is injected into the submucosal plane of the rectum.

In a few patients there is an underlying organic cause for the rectal prolapse. Usually the reason is obvious, as in paralysis of anal sphincters in spina bifida and sacral agenesis, undernourished hypotonic infants, bladder exstrophy, cloacal exstrophy, following surgery for imperforate anus, or malabsorption.

## The neck

Lesions of the neck fall into two broad groups: developmental anomalies and acquired lesions. The exact location of the lesion will usually provide a clue as to its nature.

### Midline neck swellings

The most common midline neck swelling in children is a thyroglossal cyst (Table 9.1.4). Typically, there is a swelling overlying and attached to the hyoid bone

**Table 9.1.4 Midline neck swellings**

| Cause of swelling | Comment |
|---|---|
| Thyroglossal cyst | Most common (80% of midline neck swellings)<br>Moves with tongue protrusion and swallowing<br>Attached to hyoid bone |
| Ectopic thyroid | May be only thyroid tissue present<br>Do thyroid isotope scan |
| Submental lymph node/abscess | Check inside mouth for primary infection<br>Other cervical lymph nodes may be enlarged |
| Dermoid cyst | Small, mobile, non tender<br>Yellow tinge through skin<br>In subcutaneous layer |
| Goitre | Lower neck |
| Cystic hygroma | Hamartoma<br>Usually evident from birth<br>May be extensive |

that moves on swallowing and tongue protrusion. It can become infected to form an abscess with overlying erythema of the skin. The thyroglossal cyst and the entire thyroglossal tract are best excised before the cyst becomes infected. Excision must include the middle third of the hyoid bone (Sistrunk operation), otherwise recurrence is common. Ectopic thyroid tissue is a less common cause of a midline neck swelling. Clinically, it can be difficult to distinguish from a thyroglossal cyst. If suspected preoperatively, a thyroid isotope scan will clarify the distribution of all functioning thyroid tissue.

Congenital dermoid cysts can occur along any line of fusion, including the neck where they are situated in the midline. A midline cervical dermoid cyst is occasionally mistaken for a thyroglossal cyst. It contains sebaceous material surrounded by squamous epithelium. Dermoid cysts enlarge slowly. The most common congenital dermoid cyst is the external angular dermoid, which is found at the orbital margin. They are usually removed.

## Lateral neck swellings

Most lateral neck swellings are acquired, being due to infection of one or more of the cervical lymph nodes. Persistently enlarged cervical lymph nodes are normal in children with frequent upper respiratory infections: they represent a normal response to infection (i.e. reactive hyperplasia) and require no treatment. Lymph nodes can enlarge rapidly and become tender during active infection, but usually settle with rest, analgesia and antibiotics as required. In children aged 6 months to 3 years, lateral cervical lymphadenitis can progress to abscess formation: the lymph nodes enlarge over 4–5 days and become fluctuant, although deeper nodes may not exhibit fluctuation. The overlying skin becomes red. Treatment involves incision and drainage of the abscess under general anaesthesia.

Cystic hygromas are congenital hamartomas of the lymphatic system (Fig. 9.1.10). They vary greatly in size and can involve the front of the neck or one or other sides asymmetrically. Complex cystic hygromas can contain cavernous haemangiomatous elements and can extend into the floor of the mouth or the thoracic cavity. They can enlarge rapidly from viral or bacterial infection, or from haemorrhage. Depending on their extent and location, the airway can be compromised, leading to life-threatening respiratory obstruction. Surgery involves excision or debulking of the lesion. In some situations they are injected with sclerosants.

### MAIS lymphadenitis

Cervical lymphadenitis due to atypical mycobacterial infection is seen in preschool children. Infection with MAIS (*Mycobacterium avium, intracellulare, scrofulaceum*) may also be referred to as MAC (*Mycobacterium avium* complex). It produces chronic cervical lymphadenitis and usually affects the jugulodigastric, submandibular or preauricular lymph nodes. The involved lymph node increases in size over several weeks before erupting into the subcutaneous tissue as a collar-stud 'cold' abscess. Eventually, if untreated, it may cause purple discoloration of the overlying skin and will ulcerate through the skin to produce a chronic discharging sinus. MAIS infections respond poorly to antibiotics. Treatment involves surgical removal of the collar-stud abscess and excision of the underlying infected lymph nodes.

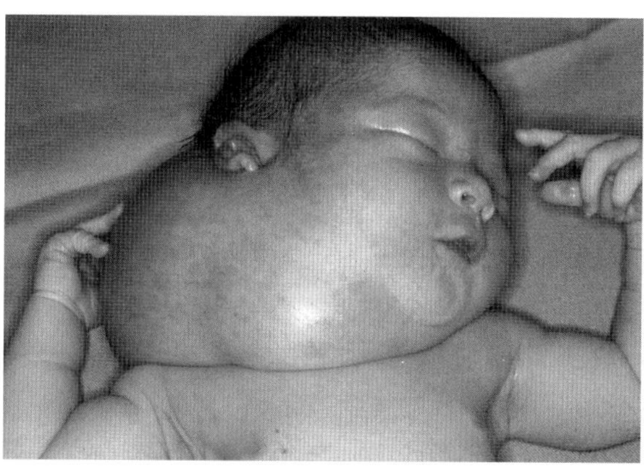

Fig. 9.1.10 Cystic hygroma in a neonate.

### Lymph node tumours

Primary tumours involving the lymph nodes tend to occur in older children. Both Hodgkin and non-Hodgkin lymphomas may involve cervical lymph nodes. Rarely, other tumours may metastasize to the cervical lymph nodes (e.g. neuroblastomas and nasopharyngeal tumours).

## Branchial remnants

Branchial remnants arise from the branchial arch system. A variety of abnormalities occur, including branchial cysts, branchial sinuses, branchial fistulae and persistent cartilaginous remnants. Branchial fistulae are present from birth but, because the opening is so tiny, they may not be noticed for some years. A drop of mucus or saliva may be observed leaking from the external orifice near the anterior border of the sternomastoid muscle at the junction of its middle and lower thirds. Branchial cysts present later in childhood with a mass beneath the anterior border of the sternomastoid near its upper third. They may become infected and should be removed. Sinuses or fistulae usually arise from the second branchial cleft, although sometimes the first and third clefts are responsible.

## Torticollis

Torticollis, or wry neck, has many causes in childhood (Table 9.1.5). The most common cause is a sternomastoid tumour that presents in the third week of life with a hard lump in the neck and an inability to turn the head to one side. The head is flexed slightly to the side of the shortened sternomastoid muscle, but turned to the contralateral side. There may be a history of breech delivery or forceps delivery. There is a hard, painless swelling, usually 2–3 cm long, in the shortened sternomastoid muscle (Fig. 9.1.11). Sometimes the whole muscle may be involved. Rotation of the head to the side of the tumour is limited. Plagiocephaly and hemihypoplasia of the face may develop in subsequent months. The 'tumour' disappears within 9–12 months in the vast majority of affected infants without treatment. If fibrosis persists and causes permanent shortening of the muscle with persistent torticollis, the sternomastoid muscle should be divided. Occasionally, older children present with torticollis due to a short, tight and fibrous sternomastoid muscle; the ipsilateral shoulder is elevated, there may be compensatory scoliosis, and the child has difficulty rotating the head towards the affected side. These children also require surgical division of the muscle.

**Table 9.1.5 Causes of torticollis**

| Cause | Comment |
|---|---|
| Sternomastoid tumour | Not evident at birth<br>Present at 3 weeks of age<br>Tight, shortened sternomastoid muscle<br>Most resolve without treatment |
| Postural torticollis | Present at birth<br>Disappears in months<br>From intrauterine position |
| Cervical hemivertebrae<br>Imbalance of ocular muscles (strabismus)<br>Lateral cervical lymphadenitis<br>Tumours<br>Atlanto-occipital subluxation<br>Benign paroxysmal torticollis of infancy | |

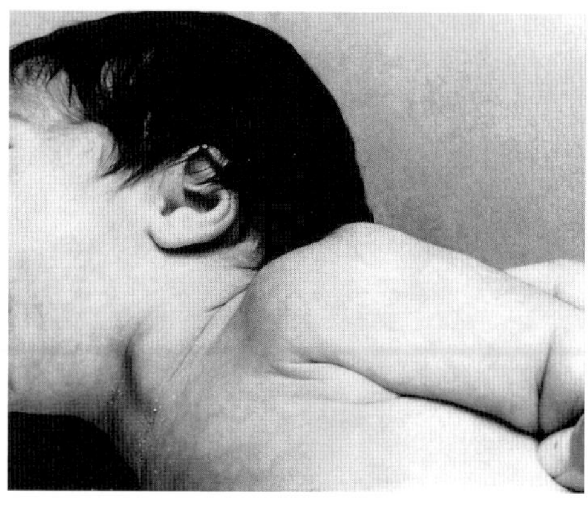

Fig. 9.1.11 Sternomastoid tumour in torticollis.

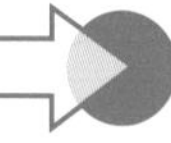

**Practical points**

- A degree of narrowing of the foreskin ('physiological phimosis') is common in many boys during the first years of life and usually resolves spontaneously without intervention.
- Inguinal herniae are common in boys (2%), and if they become strangulated should be reduced urgently.
- The most important cause of an acutely painful scrotum is testicular torsion, which requires urgent surgical exploration to untwist and salvage the testis.
- Umbilical herniae are common, but most resolve spontaneously in the first years of life, and require surgical repair only if they persist.
- A thyroglossal cyst is the most common cause of a midline neck lump.

# PART 10

# INHERITED AND METABOLIC PROBLEMS

# 10.1 Birth defects, prenatal diagnosis and teratogens

Jan Liebelt, Neil Hotham

## Birth defects

A birth defect is any abnormality, structural or functional, identified at any age, that began before birth, or the cause of which was present before birth. Examples of structural birth defects include spina bifida and cleft lip. Duchenne muscular dystrophy and Huntington disease are examples of functional birth defects.

With continued advances in obstetric and paediatric medicine, birth defects have become the most important cause of perinatal and post-neonatal mortality in developed countries.

Birth defects:

- are the leading cause of perinatal death (20–25% of deaths)
- are now the leading cause of post-neonatal deaths (25–30%), as deaths due to sudden infant death syndrome continue to decline
- are responsible for a major proportion of the morbidity and disability experienced by children and young adults
- are the cause for 20–30% of the admissions to a tertiary paediatric hospital
- have an immense impact on the emotional and physical wellbeing of the children and their families
- have a significant financial cost for the community.

### Types of structural birth defect

Classified on the basis of the mechanism by which they arise:

- *Malformations* arise during the initial formation of the embryo and fetus as a result of genetic and/or environmental factors during organogenesis (2–8 weeks post-conception). Malformations may include failure of formation, incomplete formation or abnormal configuration. Examples include spina bifida, cleft palate and hypospadias.
- *Disruptions* result from a destructive process that alters structures after formation. Examples include early amnion rupture causing amputation defects of digits, and vasoconstriction defects caused by cocaine.
- *Deformations* result from moulding of a part by mechanical forces, usually acting over a prolonged period. Examples include talipes, congenital hip dislocations and plagiocephaly associated with oligohydramnios.

### Causes

Birth defects can be caused by a wide variety of mechanisms including:

- genetic abnormalities, both monogenic and polygenic
- chance events within the developing embryo (e.g. vascular accidents)
- environmental factors:
  - teratogens generated by the mother (e.g. maternal phenylketonuria and maternal diabetes)
  - teratogens originating outside the fetomaternal unit (e.g. medications and infectious agents).

Table 10.1.1 provides a framework for thinking about causes of birth defects. Most have a multifactorial basis, reflecting interaction between genes, environment and chance events within the developing embryo and fetus.

### Genes

Early human development from fertilized ovum to fetus involves numerous processes controlled by genes, expressed sequentially in a defined cascade. The processes and developmental phases include:

- definition of polarity
- cell division
- formation of the germ layers
- segmentation of the embryo
- cell migration
- organ formation
- cell differentiation
- interactions between cells, tissues and organs
- programmed cell death.

There has been a recent, rapid increase in knowledge of the genes that determine or predispose to birth defects. This has resulted from technological advances in molecular genetics, in phenotype delineation, gene mapping and gene discovery in humans and other species, and

**Table 10.1.1 Causes of birth defects**

| Mechanism | Example | Cause |
|---|---|---|
| Whole chromosome missing or duplicated | Down syndrome<br>Turner syndrome | Trisomy 21<br>Monosomy X (XO) |
| Part of chromosome deleted or duplicated | *Cri du chat* syndrome<br>Cat eye syndrome | Deletion 5p<br>Duplication 22q |
| Sub-microscopic deletion or duplication of chromosome material | Williams syndrome<br>Velocardiofacial syndrome<br>Charcot–Marie–Tooth disease 1A | Deletion 7q<br>Deletion 22q<br>Duplication 17p |
| Mutation in single gene | Smith–Lemli–Opitz syndrome<br>Holt–Oram syndrome<br>Apert–Crouzon–Pfeiffer syndrome | 7-Dehydrocholesterol reductase<br>TBX5<br>Fibroblast growth factor receptor 2 |
| Consequence of normal imprinting | Prader–Willi syndrome | Maternal uniparental disomy or paternal deletion for 15q12 |
| Imprinting errors | Beckwith–Wiedemann syndrome<br>Angelman syndrome | Multiple mechanisms resulting in overexpression of IGF-2<br>Mutations in *UBE3A* gene |
| Multifactorial/polygenic: one or more genes and environmental factors | Isolated heart malformations, neural tube defects and facial clefts | Complex interactions between genes and environment |
| Non-genetic vascular and other 'accidents during development' | Poland anomaly<br>Oculoauriculovertebral dysplasia | Subclavian artery ischaemia<br>Stapedial artery ischaemia |
| Uterine environment | Talipes, hip dysplasia,<br>Plagiocephaly | Oligohydramnios, twins<br>Bicornuate uterus |
| Maternal environment | Mental retardation<br>Caudal regression | Maternal phenylketonuria<br>Maternal diabetes mellitus |
| Wider environment | Fetal rubella syndrome<br>Fetal alcohol syndrome<br>Microcephaly<br>Limb deficiency | Rubella infection in pregnancy<br>Maternal alcohol ingestion<br>High-dose X-irradiation<br>Thalidomide |

IGF-2, insulin-like growth factor 2; TBX5, T-box transcription factor 5.

an understanding of the cascade of sequential gene expression during embryonic development in other species.

An example of these genes is the homeotic (*HOX*) gene family. *HOX* genes are involved in the formation of structures developing from specific segments of the embryo.

## Frequency

Major birth defects:

- are those with medical and social consequences
- are present with the highest prevalence among miscarriages, intermediate in stillbirths and lowest among live-born infants
- are recognized at birth in 2–3% of live-born infants.

The birth prevalences of the more common birth defects are shown in Table 10.1.2. They represent the frequency with which the defect occurred during development (its incidence), less the spontaneous loss of affected fetuses during pregnancy. An almost equal number of additional major abnormalities, particularly of the heart and urinary tract, will be recognized by 5 years of age during clinical examinations or because of symptoms.

Minor birth defects:

- are relatively frequent, but pose no significant health or social burden
- are recognized in approximately 15% of newborns
- are important to recognize, because their presence prompts a search for coexistent, more important, abnormalities.

**Table 10.1.2 Prevalence of some common birth defects**

| Defect | Rate per 1000 births* |
|---|---|
| Malformations of heart and great vessels | 12.0 |
| Developmental hip dysplasia | 6.9 |
| Hypospadias | 3.7 |
| Talipes equinovarus | 2.2 |
| Hypertrophic pyloric stenosis | 1.9 |
| Down syndrome | 1.8 |
| Cleft lip with or without cleft palate | 1.1 |
| Spina bifida | 0.9 |
| Anencephaly | 0.7 |
| Renal agenesis and dysgenesis | 0.6 |
| Tracheo-oesophageal fistula, oesophageal atresia and stenosis | 0.4 |
| Abdominal wall defects: exomphalos and gastroschisis | 0.6 |

* Rate per 1000 births including terminations of pregnancy, stillbirths and live-births.
Source: South Australian Birth Defects Register 1986–2003.

Infants free of minor defects have a low incidence of major malformations, approximately 1%. Those with one, two or three minor defects have risks of major malformations of 3%, 10% and 20%, respectively.

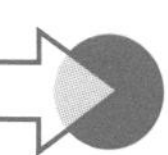

**Practical points**

**Birth defects**

- Birth defects are the leading cause of perinatal and post-neonatal deaths, and result in substantial morbidity and disability in developed countries.
- There is a wide variety of mechanisms including genetic, environmental and multifactorial.
- Major birth defects affect 2–3% of live-borns, and minor birth defects affect 15%.
- Preventative strategies remain limited, but include maternal folic acid supplementation, reduction in teratogen exposure, alternative reproductive options, prenatal detection and neonatal screening.

## Multiple birth defects

Various terms have been used to classify multiple birth defects in the hope that the terminology will convey information about aetiology, pathogenesis and the relationship between the birth defects. However, no system of naming meets all these criteria or is able to meet all the situations encountered in clinical practice. Some commonly used terms are *syndrome*, *association*, *sequence* and *developmental field defect*; these are defined in Chapter 10.3. *Phenotype* is a useful general term that makes no assumptions about aetiology or pathogenesis but registers the fact that multiple birth defects are present and are related in some way. *Complex* and *spectrum* are alternative terms that have been used in this context.

## Diagnosis

Hundreds of patterns of multiple birth defects have been defined and the diagnosis for a child with multiple birth defects is often not obvious.

The primary reasons for pursuing a diagnosis are that a specific diagnosis allows:

- discussion with the parents about the prognosis for their child
- parents to develop an understanding of how the birth defect arose
- counselling of the parents regarding recurrence risk and possibilities for reduction of this risk.

Thorough investigation, including autopsy if the child dies, may lead to a diagnosis, and referral to a clinical geneticist should be considered. Diagnosis is aided by computerized syndrome identification systems such as POSSUM (Physiological and Operative Severity Score for the enUmeration of Mortality and morbidity) and the London Dysmorphology Database. In spite of the large number of known syndromes, clinicians continue to encounter many children with birth defects the cause of which cannot be diagnosed or ascertained.

## Birth defect/congenital malformation registers

Birth defects registers were established in many countries following the 'thalidomide tragedy' in which hundreds of children were born with a range of anomalies following maternal use of thalidomide in pregnancy as an antiemetic.

Registers serve a number of purposes, including:

- early warning of new environmental teratogens
- identifying precise prevalence figures for individual birth defects and syndromes
- identifying geographical and temporal trends in birth defects

### Clinical example

Susan and Craig's first child, Anna, was diagnosed soon after birth with a significant congenital heart defect (tetralogy of Fallot) that required surgery. No concerns had been raised at the mid-trimester ultrasound. Anna was also noted to have a number of minor birth defects, including unusually shaped ears, and a hemivertebra in the thoracic spine, seen on chest X-ray.

The family was referred to a clinical geneticist for an opinion regarding the possibility of an underlying genetic condition to account for Anna's health issues. The geneticist also noted that Anna had relatively long, slender fingers and that her mother reported frequent nasal regurgitation of milk during feeds, suggesting palatal dysfunction. This combination of issues raised the possibility of a condition called velocardiofacial syndrome, caused by a microdeletion on chromosome 22q. A chromosome array was arranged, which confirmed the diagnosis.

Some 90% of children with this condition are the first person in their family to be affected. However, 10% have inherited the condition from an undiagnosed, mildly affected parent. The recurrence risk for further pregnancies differs significantly between these two situations. Craig was found also to have the microdeletion on chromosome 22q and, when his medical history was taken, he reported having required serial plastering for talipes as an infant, had struggled academically at school and was now being treated for depression, all of which can be features of this condition.

Given the wide variability of potential medical issues associated with velocardiofacial syndrome, a number of screening tests were arranged for Anna and Craig to detect any previously unrecognized birth defects. This included renal ultrasonography, immune function tests, serum calcium levels, thyroid function tests, eye and hearing reviews, and spine X-rays and cardiology review for Craig. The potential long-term consequences of the condition were discussed with the family and they were put in touch with the local support group. Anna was referred to a general paediatrician for ongoing medical and developmental follow-up. It was discussed with the family that there would be a 50% chance that any further children they conceived would also inherit the condition, but that they might experience more or less severe medical issues.

A range of reproductive options was discussed with the couple, including sperm donation, prenatal diagnosis and pre-implantation genetic diagnosis. Anna required multiple hospitalizations in the first few years of life related to her condition, which placed a great deal of stress on the family. Subsequently, in the couple's second pregnancy, they chose to have chorionic villus sampling (CVS) with testing for the microdeletion to assess whether the fetus had inherited velocardiofacial syndrome. The results showed that the fetus had not inherited the condition and a healthy boy was subsequently born.

- assessment of the impact of population-based prevention strategies and prenatal diagnosis
- collecting data for research into the epidemiology of birth defects.

### Prevention

Despite considerable research efforts there are very few preventative strategies that effectively reduce the incidence of birth defects. Some effective population-based examples include:

- oral folic acid supplementation at least 1 month prior to and in the early months of pregnancy can reduce the incidence of neural tube defects by up to 70%
- education and legislation to reduce potential exposure to teratogens:
  - public health policy on rubella immunization
  - restrictions on prescribing of known teratogens such as thalidomide and retinoids
- education about avoidance of foods in pregnancy that may predispose to maternal infection with known teratogenic agents (e.g. toxoplasmosis and uncooked meat)
- genetic counselling and the development of alternative reproductive options, including donor gametes and embryos, to allow avoidance of the risk of conception of a child with a birth defect related to a specific genetic condition
- neonatal screening to detect children with those types of birth defect that do not cause permanent damage before birth, with a view to early treatment and improved prognosis. Neonatal screening for phenylketonuria, hypothyroidism and cystic fibrosis, and clinical examination for hip dislocation are examples of highly successful screening programmes.

At present, the primary approach to the prevention of the birth of children affected by birth defects is prenatal diagnosis.

## Prenatal diagnosis

Prenatal diagnosis refers to testing performed in pregnancy aimed at the detection of birth defects in the fetus. Depending on the type of birth defect identified, the gestation of the pregnancy and the perceptions of the parents, prenatal detection of a birth defect may allow:

- the option of termination of an affected fetus
- potential treatment *in utero* or postnatally to improve prognosis related to the defect
- preparation for the birth of a child with a specific medical condition.

The number of prenatal tests available and the range of birth defects that may be detected are expanding rapidly. Many chromosome abnormalities, structural anomalies, enzymatic and single-gene defects are already potentially detectable prenatally. Advances in knowledge regarding the aetiology of birth defects and technical aspects of testing will expand this range further. Despite these advances, the majority of birth defects remain undetected until after birth.

In our society, it is an individual decision whether or not to utilize prenatal testing in a pregnancy. The provision of antenatal care must therefore ensure that parents are able to make informed decisions about testing and are supported throughout the testing process.

## Types of prenatal test

Prenatal tests fall into two main categories:

- screening tests
- diagnostic tests.

These are discussed further below.

## Screening tests

Prenatal screening tests:

- are aimed at all pregnant women
- assess whether an individual pregnancy is at increased or low risk of a particular birth defect
- generally pose no risk to maternal or fetal wellbeing
- are followed by an offer of a diagnostic test if an increased risk is identified
- are aimed primarily at the detection of structural anomalies and chromosomal abnormalities, in particular Down syndrome.

Screening tests in pregnancy are evolving rapidly, with the aim being earlier, more accurate and more accessible tests.

## Screening tests available

Currently, screening tests are performed on a serum sample from the mother, or utilize ultrasonography.

### Maternal serum screening

- Maternal serum screening (MSS) is aimed primarily at the detection of Down syndrome and, in some programmes, trisomy 18.
- MSS involves measuring the levels of a number of different analytes produced by the fetus in a blood sample from the mother.
- The analytes have been selected on the basis that large population studies have shown the levels of the analytes in maternal serum to differ significantly between pregnancies in which the fetus does or does not have Down syndrome.
- MSS can be offered in the second trimester (around 15–18 weeks) using various combinations of three or four analytes. These may include oestriol, α-fetoprotein (AFP), inhibin and the α and β subunits of human chorionic gonadotrophin (hCG), or in the first trimester using analytes such as inhibin and pregnancy-associated plasma protein A (PAPP-A).
- A computer-based algorithm, which takes into account the mother's age-related risk, the gestation of the pregnancy and the analyte levels, is used to calculate a risk figure for Down syndrome in that pregnancy.
- If the risk value is greater than a predetermined 'cut-off' value, the risk is considered to be increased and a diagnostic test is offered to clarify the situation.
- Most programmes are designed so that 5% of women having the test will receive an increased risk result. The majority of these women will go on to have healthy babies.
- If all of these women chose to have a diagnostic test, the screening programme would be expected to detect up to 80% of cases of Down syndrome.
- If AFP is one of the analytes used in second-trimester MSS, the test can also be used to screen for open neural tube defects, as AFP levels are increased when neural tissue is exposed to the amniotic fluid. If the level is raised, the diagnostic test is tertiary-level ultrasonography to examine the fetal spine.

### Ultrasonography

Ultrasonography uses sonar waves to allow real-time, two-dimensional visualization of the fetus *in utero*. The fetus can be examined in different views and fetal movements studied. Improved technology and training allow excellent views to be obtained to allow detection of many specific structural anomalies. Most antenatal care programmes now offer ultrasonography between 18 and 20 weeks of gestation to screen for fetal anomalies.

Ultrasonography is usually considered a screening rather than a diagnostic test, because:

- some structural anomalies may not be readily detected (e.g. transposition of the great vessels)
- interpretation of a possible anomaly and its impact on fetal development may be limited
- the detection rate of anomalies is dependent on the skill of the operator, equipment and fetal views obtained.

More recent advances that may enhance the value of fetal imaging as a screening test in pregnancy include three-dimensional ultrasonography and alternative imaging techniques such as fetal magnetic resonance imaging (MRI).

### Nuchal translucency screening

During the past two decades, a new form of ultrasound-based screening for Down syndrome in the first trimester has been developed, based on the MSS model. This depends on the assessment of the nuchal (posterior neck) region of the fetus:

- All fetuses have a collection of fluid in the nuchal region that can be visualized as a translucent area and can be measured by ultrasonography at the end of the first trimester (11–13 weeks' gestation).
- Large population studies have shown that on average this nuchal translucency measurement is increased in pregnancies in which the fetus has Down syndrome.
- As with MSS, a computer algorithm that takes into account the mother's age-related risk, the gestation and the thickness of the nuchal translucency measurement is used to calculate a risk for that individual pregnancy.
- If the risk is above a predetermined 'cut-off risk', a diagnostic test is offered.
- The detection rate of a nuchal translucency screening programme is dependent on the skill of the operator; however, detection rates of up to 70–80% of cases of Down syndrome have been reported.
- Other chromosome abnormalities, in particular Turner syndrome (45,XO) and triploidy, are also often associated with an increased nuchal translucency measurement.
- An increased nuchal translucency measurement in the presence of normal chromosomes may be an indicator of other types of fetal anomaly, such as cardiac malformations or skeletal dysplasias. Detailed ultrasound follow-up is then recommended.

### Combined screening

In order to increase the detection rates of screening tests, combinations of the different tests are being explored. The most commonly utilized is the combination of a nuchal translucency measurement with the measurement of two first-trimester maternal serum analytes to give a combined first-trimester risk. This allows increased detection rates for Down syndrome of up to 90%, with a 5% false-positive rate, and is increasingly replacing second-trimester maternal serum screening as the screening test of first choice, with the added advantage of allowing an earlier diagnostic test to be offered. The best combination of screening tests is continually being assessed by large multicentre trials that are in progress to address this issue.

## Diagnostic tests

Prenatal diagnostic tests:

- are aimed at pregnant women who have been identified to be at increased risk of having a baby with a particular birth defect (see below)
- allow accurate clarification of whether an individual fetus is affected or not
- usually pose a small risk of fetal loss; this risk relates to the need to sample fetal tissue for testing
- are aimed primarily at the detection of chromosomal abnormalities, enzymatic and single-gene defects.

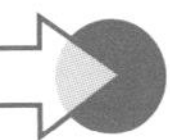

**Practical points**

**Prenatal diagnosis**

- Prenatal diagnosis is aimed at detection of birth defects prior to birth to allow options for parents.
- There are two main categories: diagnostic and screening.
- There is a move towards earlier, less invasive, testing options such as pre-implantation genetic diagnosis and combined screening tests.
- The majority of birth defects remain undetected by current prenatal diagnostic methods.
- Prenatal diagnosis for specific genetic conditions usually requires significant pre-pregnancy workup.

New diagnostic tests continue to be developed, with the principal aim of increasing both the safety of the tests and the range of conditions that may be tested for.

## Indications for diagnostic prenatal tests

Although all women are at risk of conceiving a baby with a birth defect, for an individual woman there are a number of risk factors that increase the risk above the background population risk. In general, diagnostic prenatal tests are offered to women whose risk of conceiving a baby with a specific birth defect is considered to be above an arbitrary level. This 'cut-off' level takes into account the risk of fetal loss related to the test and economic issues relating to the number of women who would be offered testing.

Some of the reasons why a woman may be offered a prenatal diagnostic test include:

- advanced maternal age (see below)
- increased risk identified by a screening test (e.g. maternal serum screening)
- a previous child with a birth defect for which a prenatal test is available and an increased risk of recurrence is recognized (e.g. chromosome abnormality, neural tube defect, single-gene disorder such as cystic fibrosis)
- a parent or couple known to carry a genetic mutation for which testing is available and that poses a risk of abnormality in offspring (e.g. chromosome translocation or single-gene defects)

- other factors known to increase the risk of birth defects (e.g. exposure to teratogens such as maternal infection).

### Advanced maternal age

As maternal age increases, there is an increased risk of conception of a fetus with some specific chromosomal anomalies, primarily trisomies (an additional copy of a single chromosome). Most fetuses conceived with a trisomy miscarry. However, trisomy 21, 13 and 18 are potentially viable chromosomal anomalies leading to the potential birth of a baby with specific constellations of birth defects (see Chapter 10.3). Maternal age is not associated with an increased risk of other birth defects.

Trisomy 21 (Down syndrome) is the most common chromosome abnormality seen at live birth in our population. Many screening and diagnostic prenatal tests are therefore aimed at detection of this condition. Population data exist that can be used to counsel women regarding their 'age-related' risk in order that they may make informed decisions about prenatal testing (Table 10.1.3).

**Table 10.1.3 Age-specific risks for a live-born child with Down syndrome**

| Maternal age (years) | Risk (1 in) at expected time of delivery |
|---|---|
| 20 | 1441 |
| 25 | 1383 |
| 30 | 959 |
| 34 | 430 |
| 35 | 338 |
| 36 | 259 |
| 37 | 201 |
| 38 | 162 |
| 39 | 113 |
| 40 | 84 |
| 42 | 52 |
| 44 | 38 |
| 46 | 31 |

The risk of any chromosome abnormality is approximately double these risks.
After Gardner RJM, Sutherland GR 2004 Chromosome abnormalities and genetic counseling (3rd edn). Oxford University Press, New York.

### Diagnostic tests available

Most diagnostic tests involve sampling of fetally derived tissue, which can then be directly analysed for abnormalities. The most common test performed is chromosomal analysis. However, tissue may also be used as a source of DNA for molecular genetic tests, for metabolic tests or, more rarely, to look for evidence of fetal infection or histological confirmation of abnormality of a specific tissue (e.g. the skin for the diagnosis of epidermolysis bullosa).

Amniocentesis and chorionic villus sampling (CVS) are the two principal diagnostic tests used. However, fetal blood samples, skin, liver or kidney biopsies may be required in very specific, rare circumstances. Amniocentesis, CVS and fetal blood sampling are performed as outpatient procedures under ultrasound guidance (Fig. 10.1.1). Each of these tests has advantages and disadvantages in certain situations (Table 10.1.4).

### Imaging techniques

In some circumstances, ultrasonography or other forms of fetal imaging such as MRI, or even plain X-rays, are considered diagnostic and may be the only tool available for diagnosis of genetic conditions that do not have a chromosomal, enzymatic or known molecular basis. Examples include neural tube defects, skeletal dysplasias and congenital heart defects. Imaging techniques, however, are dependent on gaining adequate views and appropriate interpretation of the views, and are limited by the gestation at which some defects may be identifiable; for example, hydrocephalus may not become apparent in a fetus until the third trimester.

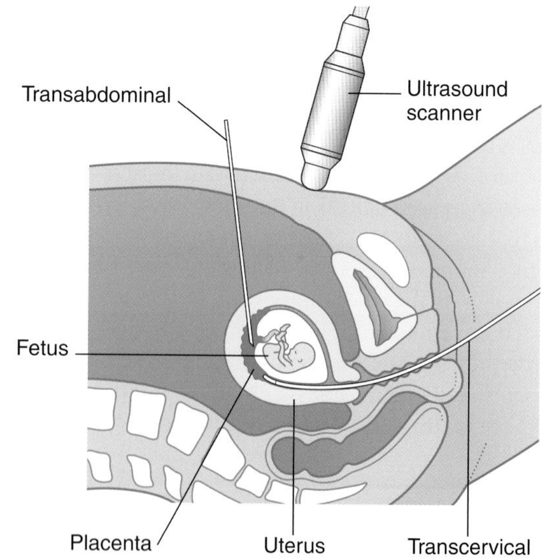


Fig. 10.1.1 Schematic representation of chorionic villus sampling showing transabdominal and transcervical routes. (Courtesy of Ultrasound Department, Royal Women's Hospital, Melbourne.)

**Table 10.1.4 Prenatal diagnostic tests**

| | CVS | Amniocentesis | Fetal blood sampling or fetal biopsies |
|---|---|---|---|
| Tissue sampled | Chorionic villi derived from the same initial fertilized ovum as the fetus | Amniotic fluid containing fetal cells | Fetal blood, liver or skin |
| Indications for test when | Increased risk of fetal chromosomal anomaly<br>Increased risk of specific genetic conditions for which a molecular or enzymatic test exists | As for CVS<br>Increased risk of fetal infection<br>Other less common indications, AFP measurements to assist in diagnosis of neural tube defects | Increased risk of fetal chromosome anomaly when rapid results are required<br>Diagnosis of fetal haemoglobinopathy<br>Diagnosis of fetal conditions by tissue histology (e.g. some skin disorders) |
| Gestation at which test is performed | Can be performed safely after 10 weeks' gestation; most often done between 11 and 13 weeks' gestation | Can be performed safely after 15 weeks' gestation; most often done at 16–18 weeks' gestation | Can be performed after 18 weeks' gestation |
| Risks | 0.5–1% rate of miscarriage related to the test | 0.5% rate of miscarriage related to the test | 1–5% rate of miscarriage related to the test, depending on the indication for the test |
| Other issues | 1% risk of a discrepant result between fetal and placental tissue (confined placental mosaicism), requiring amniocentesis to clarify | 1% risk of failure of amniocytes to culture, requiring a repeat test | Potentially difficult access |
| Timing of results | Rapid chromosome analysis by FISH 24–48 hours*<br>Final chromosome, DNA or enzyme test results 7–21 days | As for CVS | Dependent on test performed |

*FISH (fluorescence *in situ* hybridization) involves the use of labelled DNA probes designed to bind to specific regions of individual chromosomes. This allows the number of a specific chromosome in an interphase cell to be ascertained within 24–48 hours.
AFP, α-fetoprotein; CVS, chorionic villus sampling.

### Future options

Hope for 'non-invasive' diagnostic testing previously rested on the concept of isolation of fetal cells found within the maternal circulation during pregnancy. More recently, recognition of 'free fetal DNA' within the maternal circulation during pregnancy, and the fact that fetal cells can be isolated from cervical swabs during pregnancy, has raised the potential for future options that would allow collection of fetal tissue for the purpose of testing without risk to fetal wellbeing. Current techniques do not yet allow this option to be used widely in a clinical setting; however, research continues.

## Prenatal diagnosis for specific genetic conditions

Rapid progress in knowledge of the underlying molecular genetic aetiology of specific conditions allows an increasing number of genetic conditions to be diagnosed prenatally by utilizing specific DNA-based technology. In order that this can occur for any individual couple known to have an increased risk of conceiving a child with such a disorder, a number of conditions must be satisfied:

- accurate diagnosis of the condition in the affected family member

- confirmation of the aetiology of the condition by identification of a mutation in the causative gene or an enzymatic defect that can be tested for accurately in fetal tissue (a process that may take many months and may not be possible in some cases)
- appropriate pre-test (preferably pre-pregnancy) counselling regarding the process of testing and implications and options relating to the potential results of testing
- appropriate support throughout the process.

Prenatal diagnosis in these circumstances is best provided by an experienced multidisciplinary team consisting of an obstetrician, clinical geneticist, genetic counsellor and experienced laboratory staff. CVS is usually the preferred method for DNA-based and enzymatic prenatal tests, as it often allows direct testing rather than a need for culturing of tissue prior to testing. Examples of conditions that DNA-based prenatal diagnosis may be available for include: Duchenne and Becker muscular dystrophy, fragile X syndrome, cystic fibrosis and haemoglobinopathies.

In some families, although the specific mutation causing the condition in the family has not been identified, linkage studies using polymorphic DNA markers close to or within the gene may be possible. This requires further testing of family members and has a margin of error related to the possibility of genetic recombination. For X-linked conditions in which the gene has not yet been identified or a mutation cannot be identified, identification of the sex of the fetus by chromosome analysis and termination of males (50% of whom would be unaffected) may be the only available option.

### Pre-implantation genetic diagnosis

Prenatal diagnosis with termination of affected pregnancies may not be an option for some couples, for ethical and moral reasons. Following advances during the last two decades in both reproductive and molecular genetic technology, the technique of pre-implantation genetic diagnosis (PGD) has become an alternative option.

The principle of this technique is the genetic analysis of an embryo produced by *in vitro* fertilization (IVF) technology, in order to select those embryos free from a specific genetic condition for transfer to the woman's uterus to establish a pregnancy.

A single cell can be removed for genetic analysis on day 3 to day 5 post-conception from an embryo cultured *in vitro*. Genetic analysis may consist of specific mutation detection or a limited analysis of chromosomes. The limited amount of material and the limited timeframe available for analysis have provided the impetus for the development of specialized techniques to prevent misdiagnosis. Thousands of babies have now been born worldwide following PGD in a number of highly specialized centres. Continual improvements in genetic techniques and pregnancy rates following IVF will mean that PGD will continue to become a more common alternative to the well established methods of CVS and amniocentesis.

## Teratogens

A teratogen is an environmental agent that can cause abnormalities of form or function in an exposed embryo or fetus. It is estimated that between 1% and 3% of birth defects may be related to teratogenic exposure.

A teratogen may cause its effect by a number of different pathophysiological mechanisms, including:

- cell death
- alteration of cell division and tissue growth, including cell migration
- interference with cellular differentiation.

Examples include, alcohol and sodium valproate, which are believed to cause underdevelopment of the mid-face and philtrum due to cell death in these areas, whereas syndactyly can result from failure of programmed death of cells between the digits.

### Requirements of a teratogen

In theory, to produce a malformation a teratogen must be present in a sufficient amount, at the appropriate time, in a genetically susceptible individual, where other conditions do not prevent the effects from occurring.

Factors that can modify the effects of a teratogen include:

- timing of exposure
- dose to the fetus
- genetic susceptibility
- access of the drug to the fetus
- interaction between teratogens
- maternal folic acid supplementation.

#### Timing of exposure

The effect of an environmental agent may differ depending on the gestational age at which exposure occurs:

- Exposure very early in embryogenesis, prior to organogenesis (less than 2 weeks after conception) is likely to cause embryonic death rather than malformations. This is seen as an 'all or nothing' effect.
- During organogenesis (2–8 weeks after conception), malformations may occur if the exposure is not fatal.

- Each organ develops during a specific time period and will be susceptible to the malforming effects of teratogens only during that critical period.
- During fetal development (after organogenesis), although malformations can still occur in slowly forming organs such as the brain and kidney, this is the time when functional effects, such as cognitive impairment, or behavioural effects are more likely. Teratogens such as vasoactive drugs (e.g. cocaine) may also damage structures that have already formed.

Classical examples include thalidomide, which affects limb development only at the time when limb buds are developing (between 27 and 41 days), and doxycycline, which causes staining of teeth if there is fetal exposure after 18 weeks' gestation.

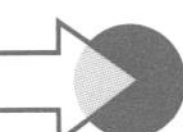

**Practical points**

**Teratogens**

- Timing of exposure to teratogens is important: there may be an 'all or nothing effect'.
- The 'dose' received by the fetus may be critical. All teratogens have a threshold dose, after which abnormalities increase.
- Risk–benefit ratios need to be considered (e.g. maternal wellbeing versus teratogenic risk).
- Genetic susceptibility may be important in exposure to some teratogens.
- Access of the drug to the fetus should be considered. Is it absorbed by the mother? Does it cross the placenta?
- Interaction between teratogens may increase risk (e.g. polypharmacy of antiepileptic drugs).

### Dose

The harmful effects of teratogens are dose-dependent. A dose threshold is where the rate of abnormalities rises. For example, there is no observed effect of X-rays at doses routinely used in diagnostic radiology, whereas doses associated with nuclear explosions cause microcephaly, mental retardation and growth failure.

### Genetic susceptibility

There are marked differences in genetic susceptibility to environmental agents, both between species and between individuals of one species. It is likely that the susceptibility to the harmful effects of many teratogens depends on the genetically determined efficiency of detoxifying metabolic pathways in both the mother and the fetus. Thalidomide, again, forms an example of this, in that it is not teratogenic in a large number of species but is teratogenic in some rabbits and some primates, including humans. Phenytoin metabolism by a fetus with low epoxide hydrolase activity may put the fetus at risk of fetal phenytoin syndrome.

### Access

A teratogen must gain access to the fetus. Some potentially harmful agents are not teratogens because their molecular size, means of transport or binding properties prevent or restrict them from crossing the placenta. Examples include heparin and pancuronium.

### Interaction between teratogens

Ingestion of multiple medications can have additive effects. An example is that the risk of fetal effects is greater if a mother with epilepsy is taking multiple anticonvulsants (polypharmacy) rather than a single one.

## Some important teratogens

Selected teratogens that cause common clinical issues are discussed below; a more extensive list is provided in Box 10.1.1.

### Rubella virus

Infection of the fetus by the rubella virus in the first trimester can cause devastating birth defects, including mental retardation, short stature, deafness, blindness and congenital heart defects.

- The risk is greatly reduced if the mother has been immunized prior to pregnancy.
- As immunity may wane, the immune status of women planning pregnancy should be reviewed.

### Alcohol

The harmful effects of ethanol on the developing human are well documented:

- Teratogenic effects of alcohol are dose-related, ranging from clinically inapparent effects to the fetal alcohol syndrome (FAS): prenatal and postnatal growth failure, microcephaly, intellectual disability, a characteristic facial appearance, cleft palate, microphthalmia and heart defects.
- Heavy drinking throughout pregnancy is associated with a 10% risk of FAS and a 30% risk of observable fetal alcohol effects (FAEs).
- No threshold dose has been defined; therefore women should be advised to avoid alcohol during pregnancy.

### Antiepileptic medication

Women with epilepsy receiving treatment with anticonvulsant medication have a 2–3-fold increased risk of giving birth to a child with a birth defect.

**Box 10.1.1 Environmental agents that can adversely affect human development**

**Infectious agents**

**Viruses:** rubella, cytomegalovirus, varicella-zoster, Venezuelan equine encephalitis, herpes simplex, [parvovirus B19]
**Bacteria:** syphilis, [*Listeria*]
**Parasites:** toxoplasmosis

**Physical agents**
Ionizing radiation, carbon monoxide, (heat)

**Drugs and chemicals**
**Environmental chemicals:** organic mercury compounds, (polychlorinated biphenyls; PCBs)
**Non-prescription drugs:** ethanol, cocaine, (amphetamines), [tobacco smoking, marijuana smoking]

**Prescription drugs:**
*Anticancer drugs:* aminopterin, busulfan, chlorambucil, cyclophosphamide, plicamycin, methotrexate, cytarabine, (dacarbazine, fluorouracil, procarbazine)
*Anticonvulsants:* phenytoin, sodium valproate, carbamazepine, trimethadione, (primidone, phenobarbital, lamotrigine)
*Hormones:* diethylstilbestrol, male sex hormones, strongly androgenic progestogens
*Antibacterials:* tetracyclines, streptomycin, (gentamicin, quinolones, fluconazole (high doses 400–800 mg daily), trimethoprim)
*Antivirals:* ribavirin, (ganciclovir, zalcitabine)
*Anthelmintics:* (albendazole)
*Antimalarials:* (chloroquine when used to treat malaria but not when used for prophylaxis)
*Retinoids:* systemic isotretinoin, acetretin, (vitamin A, topical tretinoin and isotretinoin)
*Immunomodifiers:* (methotrexate), [interferon-β1b]
*Miscellaneous:* thalidomide, misoprostol, penicillamine, warfarin, phenindione, lithium, intra-amniotic methylthioninium chloride {methylene blue}, (diazepam, antithyroid drugs, statins, mycophenolate, ACE inhibitors, angiotensin II receptor antagonists)

**Maternal disorders**
Insulin-dependent diabetes mellitus, maternal phenylketonuria

The above list should be considered illustrative only and may change in the light of new knowledge.
No brackets, teratogen; ( ), possible teratogen; [ ], not known to be teratogenic but may cause other effects, including embryonic/fetal death and/or growth retardation.
ACE, angiotensin-converting enzyme.

- Most anticonvulsants have not been shown to be safe in pregnancy, and specific teratogenic effects have been defined for phenytoin, sodium valproate, carbamazepine and trimethadione, particularly for neural tube defects.
- Periconceptional folic acid supplementation at a dose of 5 mg daily should be recommended for women on anticonvulsant medication because of this.
- The risk to the fetus increases if multiple anticonvulsants are needed to prevent seizures.
- It is likely that individual susceptibility exists, based on pharmacogenomics.
- Epileptic women must accept some additional risk of birth defects in their infants, but the risk can be minimized if epileptic control can be achieved with a single drug at the lowest possible dose.

### Vitamin A analogues: isotretinoin and acetretin

These highly potent analogues of vitamin A are extremely teratogenic – even more so than thalidomide.

- Their systemic use in early pregnancy is associated with a high (greater than 35%) risk of birth defects, including serious abnormalities of brain development, with microcephaly, hydrocephalus, cortical blindness and intellectual disability, cranial nerve palsies, dysmorphic facial features, microtia, cleft palate, heart defects, thymic hypoplasia and genitourinary abnormalities.
- No 'safe' period or threshold dose has been determined for these drugs.

#### Clinical example

Kylie, a 25-year-old woman, has just found out that she is 4 weeks' pregnant. She has an artificial heart valve and has taken warfarin for the past 6 months. She had been advised not to become pregnant and had used medroxyprogesterone depot for contraception. However, she had not recently renewed it because of side-effects experienced after her first dose 4 months ago. Now condoms had failed. Kylie also has a urinary tract infection and treatment with trimethoprim was being considered. Her partner, Adam, had taken large doses of vitamins, including vitamin A, prior to conception and had read that vitamin A can be harmful in pregnancy. They sought advice about risks to their unborn baby.

Firstly, reassurance was given about the paternal exposure to vitamin A. Drugs and chemicals taken by men have not been proven to increase the incidence of abnormalities in their offspring (http://www.otispregnancy.org). Vitamin A analogues are potent teratogens when used by the mother.

It was important to treat the urinary tract infection; however, trimethoprim, an antifolate antimicrobial, is not suitable in the first trimester. Another agent was recommended.

Warfarin treatment for Kylie was of concern. Four weeks of pregnancy (4/40) is earlier than the time of warfarin's greatest teratogenic susceptibility, at 6–9 weeks of gestation (6–9/40). However, Kylie's medical condition required anticoagulation with warfarin, which crosses the placenta, and she was counselled that there was approximately a 5% chance of fetal warfarin syndrome. Heparin does not cross the placenta and is not teratogenic, but unfortunately is inadequate prophylaxis for pregnant patients with artificial heart valves.

In spite of negative product information, the medroxyprogesterone depot was not a cause for concern, even if Kylie had received the dose while in early pregnancy.

- Many countries have restricted the prescribing of these drugs to particular groups of doctors: women should use effective contraception for 1 month before and throughout treatment, and for a time after treatment stops. They should have a pregnancy test before commencing treatment.
- Isotretinoin is used orally and topically to treat severe cystic acne. Although it has a short elimination half-life, it is recommended that pregnancy should be avoided for at least 1 month after the last dose.
- Acetretin is used to treat psoriasis and other disorders of keratinization. It has a relatively short half-life, but is converted to etretinate during therapy. Etretinate is readily taken up into adipose tissue, and has a long elimination half-life of 120 days. It is recommended that pregnancy be avoided for 2 years after the last dose.

**Clinical example**

Michelle is a nurse in a paediatric and women's hospital, and is unexpectedly pregnant. As an occupational health and safety issue, she had received a rubella vaccine about 6 weeks prior to conception. A week before her positive pregnancy test she had an oral treatment with a single dose of fluconazole for vaginal thrush.

Concern about the rubella vaccine, which is live-attenuated, and the fluconazole, can be addressed using two facts. Both involve the key words of timing and dose.

No cases of congenital rubella have been proven to be caused by this vaccination given just before or in early pregnancy. The waiting time recommended prior to conception has been reduced from 3 months to 1 month. Fluconazole single-dose therapy does not appear to cause any increase in abnormalities above the background rate. However, repeated doses of 400–800 mg daily have been associated with a consistent pattern of birth defects, similar to those seen in animal studies.

### Warfarin

Warfarin is used in the treatment of thromboembolic disease and for individuals with artificial heart valves.

- Warfarin crosses the placenta, is teratogenic and may cause haemorrhage in the fetus.
- The teratogenic effects appear to result from inhibition of vitamin K and/or arylsulphatase E activity during skeletal development.
- The fetal warfarin syndrome comprises nasal hypoplasia, short fingers with hypoplastic nails, low birth weight, stippling of epiphyses on X-ray and intellectual disability.
- The risk of fetal warfarin syndrome in the babies of women who require warfarin throughout pregnancy is low, around 5%.
- The period of greatest embryonic susceptibility is between 4 and 7 weeks after conception, although it is recommended that the drug should be avoided throughout the first trimester.
- Warfarin exposure limited to the second and third trimesters has a low risk of causing brain and eye damage, presumably as a result of haemorrhage.
- Heparin is not a teratogen as it does not cross the placenta.
- Use of heparin instead of warfarin may be appropriate when the indication is venous thrombosis, but not when it is used for artificial heart valves. Low-dose heparin carries a significant risk of valve thrombosis, and high-dose heparin in the outpatient setting carries a risk of serious maternal and retroplacental haemorrhage.

### Ionizing radiation

- Risks to the fetus are very low when performing diagnostic radiology in pregnancy.
- Women inadvertently exposed to diagnostic X-rays in early pregnancy can usually be reassured, although they may find it hard to understand that, although public health policy strongly recommends avoidance in pregnancy, the absolute risk to the baby is negligible.
- Doses delivered to the appropriately shielded uterus by modern X-ray equipment are well below the level that is teratogenic.
- Very high doses of X-rays can affect the fetus, resulting in growth failure, microcephaly, ocular defects and intellectual disability.
- If an undiagnosed pregnancy was irradiated during radiotherapy, the dose and the risk should be assessed.
- The sensitive period for these effects appears to be between 2 and 4–5 weeks after conception.
- Ionizing radiation is not only potentially teratogenic but also potentially mutagenic and carcinogenic. It is likely that even low-dose irradiation of the fetus, as with the child and adult, does have mutagenic and carcinogenic potential, but the absolute size of the risk increase is very small.

### Diethylstilbestrol (DES)

This drug, widely used in the 1950s and 1960s in the belief that it prevented miscarriage, is both a teratogen and a prenatal carcinogen.

- Exposure, especially before 10 weeks' gestation, can cause cervical abnormalities, uterine malformations and vaginal adenosis in girls. These areas of epithelium have an increased risk of progressing to vaginal adenocarcinoma years later.

- This highlights that there can be a delay of many years before the effects of fetal exposure to environmental agents become apparent, and absence of birth defects in the earliest years of life is not sufficient evidence to declare a drug safe in pregnancy.
- Exposed boys appear to have an increased risk of testicular abnormalities, infertility and possibly testicular malignancy.

## Paternal exposures

To date, there is no convincing evidence that preconception paternal exposure to environmental chemicals is teratogenic, although paternal drugs may affect fertility. For paternal exposure to be teratogenic, it would have to involve mutagenesis of paternal DNA. A mutagenic agent could affect any part of the genome, resulting in the spread of risk of mutation across a very large number of individual genes. Although new dominant and X-linked mutations could potentially occur, one would not expect a consistent pattern of birth defects in the children of exposed men. At present, any teratogenic risk from paternal exposures should be considered negligible, although it is admitted that it would be very hard to see an effect against the significant background prevalence of birth defects in humans. It is theoretically possible that environmentally induced mutations could contribute to the known paternal age-related risk of new dominant mutations, for example for achondroplasia (http://www.otispregnancy.org/files/paternal.pdf).

## Teratogen information services

Understandably, as a result of the thalidomide disaster, there is public concern about possible effects of exposure to environmental agents in pregnancy, and a general uneasiness about environmental agents and health. This has resulted in the establishment of services to provide information to health professionals and the public. Teratogen information services have access to online databases such as TERIS and Reprotox, containing the most recent distillation of information about individual agents. They have experience in assessing the significance of an exposure and counselling skills, and can usually be contacted by phone when the need arises. They are usually located in large public obstetric hospitals.

# Modern genetics 10.2

Nicola Poplawski

A clinical geneticist is a medical specialist who has expert knowledge of human clinical and laboratory genetics. However, because genetic information underlies the development and responses of every individual, an understanding of human genetics is essential for every medical practitioner. This chapter provides a brief overview of the principles of genetics as they pertain to paediatrics, but readers are cautioned that there is much that is both important and fascinating that cannot be covered in the space available. It is strongly recommended that readers utilize other resources that are relevant to this section. Readers should also bear in mind that genetics is a rapidly developing field, and detailed information derived from any source may become outdated within a matter of months.

Many technical terms are used throughout this chapter and readers need to be familiar with these terms. Many will be familiar from courses in genetics or biochemistry.

## Genetic information

### Genetic information is encoded in DNA

Deoxyribonucleic acid (DNA) is a complex molecule located within the nucleus of every cell of a body (Fig. 10.2.1.) It is the biological 'library' of the genetic information needed for a fertilized egg to develop into a complex and functional organism (a person) comprised of a wide variety of cell and tissue types.

- DNA is a linear molecule comprised of subunits called nucleotides.
- There are four different nucleotides; adenosine (A), thymidine (T), cytosine (C) and guanidine (G).
- Each nucleotide is linked to its immediate neighbour by a sugar molecule, deoxyribose, forming a long chain.
- Two chains of nucleotides are linked together by hydrogen bonds.
- Adenosine in one chain pairs with thymidine in the other chain, and cytosine pairs with guanidine.
- The hydrogen bonds between the A–T and C–G pairs are like the rungs on a ladder.
- The entire ladder is twisted along its length into a conformation that is often called a 'double helix'.
- The entire DNA sequence is called the human genome and is encoded by approximately three billion ($3 \times 10^9$) nucleotides.

### DNA is located in two different parts of a cell

The human genome is separated into two parts. The smaller mitochondrial genome (mtDNA) is located in the matrix of mitochondria and encodes just 37 genes. The larger nuclear genome (nuclear DNA) is located in the nucleus of the cell and encodes more than 25 000 genes.

### Nuclear DNA forms tightly coiled lengths of DNA called chromosomes

Nuclear DNA is packaged into 23 fragments of varying length. During mitosis each fragment is visible down a light microscope as a short bundle or chromosome. A *gene* is located at the same point on the same chromosome in all human individuals. A *locus* is the unique chromosome position that defines the location of each individual gene or DNA sequence.

- Human *somatic* ('body') cells have two copies of the nuclear genome, one copy inherited from each parent; this DNA is packaged into 46 chromosomes (23 pairs).
- Sperm and ova (*gametes*) have a single copy of the nuclear genome packaged as 23 unpaired chromosomes.
- Fertilization of an ovum by a sperm restores the usual amount of nuclear DNA in a somatic cell; 46 chromosomes; 23 pairs.
- In a karyotype, chromosome pairs are arranged in a standard format based on their size, banding pattern and centromere position; the first 22 pairs are called autosomes; the 23rd pair are the two sex chromosomes.
- In females there are two equivalent long sex chromosomes called X chromosomes.
- In males there is one long X chromosome and a small Y chromosome.

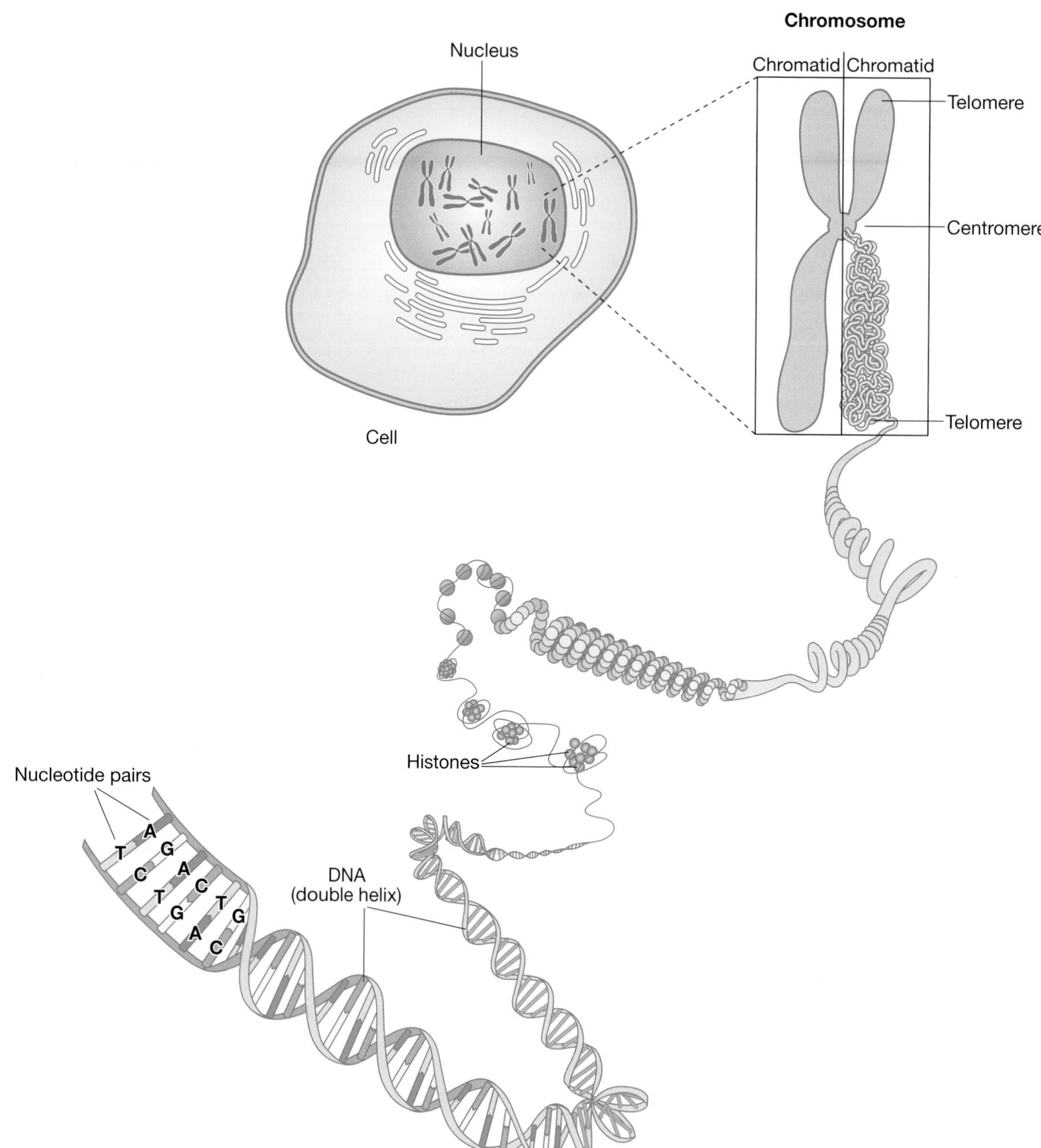


Fig. 10.2.1 Organization of our nuclear genome.

## One X chromosome is inactivated in females

The difference in the number of X chromosomes between males and females represents a profound difference in the amount of genetic information in the cell. Females compensate for the presence of two X chromosomes by inactivating one X chromosome, a process called lyonization.

- At the time of conception both X chromosomes in a female conceptus are active.
- After a few cell divisions, one X chromosome in each cell is inactivated by methylation; the same X chromosome remains inactive in all daughter cells derived from that ancestral cell.
- The result is that both males and females have only one active X chromosome in each cell.

- On average, each of the two X chromosomes will be active in half of the cells of a female's body.
- Because X inactivation is initiated when the conceptus consists of a small number of cells, by chance approximately 10% of females have the same X chromosomes active in 90% or more of cells (skewed X inactivation).

### Mitochondrial DNA is a small, circular, double-stranded DNA

Mitochondria are small organelles within the cell that have an essential role in many metabolic processes including oxidative phosphorylation, the process that generates adenosine triphosphate (ATP) via aerobic metabolism. Mitochondria contain more than 1000 different proteins, including over 60 proteins directly involved in oxidative phosphorylation. Most, *but not all*, of these mitochondrial proteins are encoded by nuclear genes.

- mtDNA is a double-stranded loop, 16 569 nucleotides long, that is joined end-to-end in a circle.
- mtDNA encodes 13 proteins involved in oxidative phosphorylation, as well as 24 non-coding ribonucleic acids (RNAs) important for normal mitochondrial function.
- Each mitochondrion has 5 to 10 copies of mtDNA and, depending on the type of tissue, a single somatic cell may contain as many as 1000 mitochondria.
- Tissues that are highly dependent on oxidative phosphorylation (e.g. neurons) have more mitochondria per cell than tissues that are less dependent (e.g. some epithelial cells).
- Mitochondria and mtDNA are copied independently of the process of copying nuclear DNA.
- Mitochondria are maternally inherited – all the mitochondria in an individual's cells are derived from the original ovum.
- The exclusive maternal inheritance of the mitochondrial DNA is in marked contrast to the bi-parental inheritance of nuclear DNA.

## The function of our genome: DNA, genes and proteins

### Protein-coding genes

A unit of DNA sequence that encodes a protein is called a gene. The genetic information contained in the gene flows from DNA to RNA to protein.

- A gene consists of a sequence of nucleotides.
- Some genes are encoded by several hundreds of nucleotides and others by many thousands.
- The DNA sequence of most nuclear genes is broken up into coding modules (exons), which are separated from each other by regions of non-coding DNA (introns) (Fig. 10.2.2).
- Mitochondrial genes do *not* have introns.
- Specific DNA sequences define the beginning and the end of a gene.
- Exons are usually a few hundred nucleotides long.
- Introns may be many thousands of nucleotides in length.
- Introns have regulatory and evolutionary roles that are poorly understood.

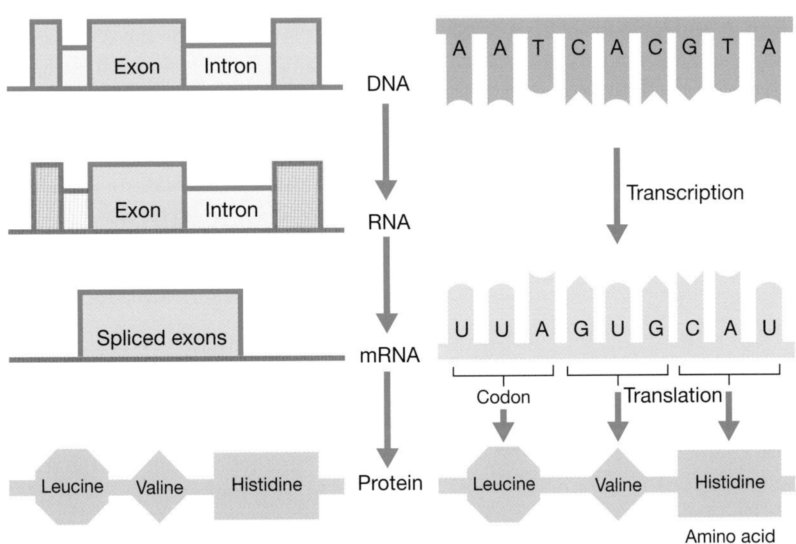


Fig. 10.2.2 Transcription and translation.

### Non-protein-coding genes

A unit of DNA sequence that encodes a functional, non-coding RNA transcript is also called a gene.

- Non-coding RNA transcripts are *not* translated to make a protein polypeptide.
- Non-coding RNA transcripts help regulate the transcription and splicing of one or more genes (i.e. they have a role in the regulation of gene expression).

### The DNA sequence of a gene is transcribed into RNA

To access the genetic information encoded in a gene, the enzyme RNA polymerase uses the gene's nucleotide sequence as a template to synthesize a molecule of RNA, a process called transcription (see Fig. 10.2.2).

- RNA has a structure that is similar to DNA, except it is usually single-stranded and uracil (U) substitutes for thymidine.
- DNA is transcribed to a primary RNA transcript; a series of processing reactions follow, including removal of introns, producing a shorter, mature RNA transcript.
- There are many different types of mature RNA that have a range of different functions, some unknown.
- Protein-coding genes encode a special form of mature RNA, messenger RNA (mRNA), which serves as a template for synthesis of a protein polypeptide.

### mRNA is translated into protein via a triplet nucleotide code

Protein polypeptides are made of many amino acids joined end to end in a long chain with a specific sequence. This chain of amino acids folds to form a three-dimensional shape that is unique to each specific protein polypeptide.

- mRNA is translated (decoded) to make a protein polypeptide at ribosomes.
- The information encoded in the mRNA sequence is interpreted via a triplet nucleotide code (a codon), which determines the exact amino acid sequence of the protein (see Fig. 10.2.2).
- There are also specific stop codons that indicate the end of a gene.

### Our understanding of the function of DNA is changing

Until recently the accepted understanding was that genes occur infrequently along the human genome and that these genes encode RNA, which in turn encodes the amino acid sequence of protein polypeptides. By this view, a gene encodes a single protein polypeptide and is separated from its neighbouring genes by long stretches of intergenic non-coding 'junk' DNA. It is now clear that this is a simplified interpretation of the function of DNA, and of what constitutes a gene. Below is a summary of our current understanding of the function of the genome, but readers are again cautioned that this information will rapidly become outdated and that other resources should be consulted.

- About 5% of the human genome sequence has been highly conserved by evolution, and most of this DNA is functionally important.
- Around one-fifth of this conserved sequence encodes proteins (protein-coding DNA).
  - Some protein-coding genes encode multiple proteins.
  - Some genes overlap other genes, or are embedded within larger genes.
  - Occasionally, parts of the sequence of two or more different genes are spliced together at the RNA level to produce a functional transcript.
- The other four-fifths of this conserved sequence is non-protein-coding DNA which encodes functionally important RNA molecules that are not translated into proteins (i.e. non-coding RNA transcripts).
- Although the remaining 95% of the human genome sequence is less conserved, it is estimated that around 85% is transcribed to non-coding RNA transcripts.
  - Transcription is pervasive and the distinction between a gene and intergenic DNA is becoming blurred.
  - Cells are 'full' of these non-coding RNA transcripts but we have little understanding of their function.

## Gene regulation

### The regulation of human gene expression is incompletely understood

Our understanding of the ways the human genome is regulated and integrated within a cell (or an individual) is rudimentary. It is beyond the scope of this chapter to discuss all that is known or hypothesized about gene regulation, but the reader should be familiar with two important concepts: inactivation of genes by methylation, and imprinting.

Genes are controlled by regulatory DNA sequences. These regulatory sequences can be chemically altered by the addition of methyl groups (–CH3) to the nucleotides of the sequence, this is called methylation.

- Methyl groups interfere with the binding of molecules to the regulatory sequence of a gene.
- The net effect of this methylation is inactivation of the gene.
- Methyl groups may also be removed, activating a gene.
- Methylation provides a means for varying gene activity in normal cells.
- Some genes are inactivated in cells of a specific tissue type(s), resulting in tissue-specific expression of the gene.
- Some genes are inactivated at certain times during development leading to developmental stage-dependent expression.
- X chromosome inactivation in females is an example of gene inactivation due to methylation.

The activation or silencing of a gene is usually independent of whether the gene was inherited paternally or maternally. An exception is genes that are *imprinted*.

- Imprinting is the selective inactivation of a gene according to the sex of the parent who passed on that gene.
- Imprinting is a normal process and results in only one active copy of the gene in a cell.
- Inactivation occurs because of methylation of a regulatory region of the gene.
- Some imprinted genes are selectively inactivated when transmitted by sperm and selectively activated when transmitted by an ovum (they are paternally imprinted).
- Other genes demonstrate the reciprocal pattern and are selectively inactivated when transmitted by an ovum and selectively activated when transmitted by a sperm (they are maternally imprinted).
- Normally the methylation 'imprint' is removed in sperm and ova so that inactivation of the imprinted gene is always determined by the sex of the parent of origin.
- Imprinting is an example of an epigenetic mechanism; a heritable change in gene expression that does not occur because of a change in DNA sequence.

Failure of normal imprinting results in overexpression or underexpression of a gene, which may lead to a clinical disorder.

- Failure to imprint a gene results in there being two *active* copies of the gene, producing a 'functional duplication' of that gene.
- Inappropriate imprinting of a gene results in there being two *inactive* copies of the gene, producing a 'functional deletion' of that gene.
- Examples of imprinting disorders include Prader–Willi syndrome, Angelman syndrome, Russell–Silver syndrome and Beckwith–Wiedermann syndrome.

### Uniparental disomy

Uniparental disomy is the situation where a child inherits two copies of a particular chromosome from one parent and none from the other, rather than having one copy from each parent. The total number of chromosomes is normal, but if any gene(s) on the chromosome is normally imprinted a functional genetic imbalance results.

When the *paternal copy* of the gene is normally imprinted:

- if both copies of the gene are inherited from the father there are zero active copies of the gene instead of the normal single active copy and a 'functional deletion'
- if both copies of the gene are inherited from the mother there are two active copies of the gene and a 'functional duplication'.

When the *maternal copy* of the gene is normally imprinted:

- if both copies of the gene are inherited from the father there are two active copies of the gene and a 'functional duplication'
- if both copies of the gene are inherited from the mother there are zero active copies of the gene instead of the normal single active copy and a 'functional deletion'.

## Genes and networks

A single gene does not produce its effect independent of the action of other genes. All processes within a single cell are regulated by an interacting network of many genes. For example, a network of several hundred different genes is involved in intracellular galactose metabolism. This leads to a degree of biological robustness because a mutation (genetic error) in a single gene will not necessarily result in cellular dysfunction if the remainder of the genetic network is able to compensate for the mutated gene.

This network of genes is embedded within a network of interacting cells within a single tissue or organ, which is embedded in a network of interacting tissues and organs within a single individual. Individuals, in turn, are embedded in social and environmental networks. The interplay and variation within and between these genetic, cellular, biological, social and environmental networks helps explain why the clinical features of a specific disorder can vary from one individual to another.

**Clinical example**

Cystic fibrosis (CF) is a common autosomal recessive disorder:

- It affects approximately 1 in 2500 Caucasian children.
- 1 in 25 healthy Caucasian adults are carriers of a mutation that can cause CF.
- More than 2000 different mutations have been identified in the CF gene (genetic heterogeneity).
- One mutation (deltaF508) accounts for about 80% of all mutations; other mutations are much less common.
- Without treatment, children with classical CF usually die during infancy.
- With treatment, at least 50% of these children are alive in their mid-40s.

The classical clinical expression (phenotype) of CF has three major features:

- Chronic respiratory infections leading to bronchiectasis.
- Malabsorption of fat due to exocrine pancreatic dysfunction.
- Raised sweat sodium and chloride concentrations.

Phenotypic variation (heterogeneity) occurs between affected individuals:

- The survival of affected individuals (including siblings) can vary by years or even decades.
- CF gene mutations are well documented in individuals with non-classical (milder) phenotypes of CF.
- Non-classical CF phenotypes include:
  - typical CF respiratory disease without pancreatic dysfunction
  - milder respiratory disease with no other clinical features of CF
  - male infertility due to congenital bilateral absence of the vas deferens without other clinical features of CF.

Networks help explain the phenotypic heterogeneity:

- Different mutations have different effects; in general, mutations that severely disturb the function of the CF protein are associated with more severe disease.
- Variations in other genes influence disease severity and survival; for example, genes encoding proteins in the immune system may modulate the severity of the respiratory infections.
- Social factors are important; for example, good access to health care and support from family and friends are associated with longer survival.
- Environmental factors such as aerobic fitness, nutritional status, smoking and the colonization of the respiratory tree by certain bacteria can affect disease severity and survival.

## Genetic variation

### What causes genetic variation?

DNA replication consists of accurately replicating both copies of the three billion nucleotide-long genome that are within the nucleus of a cell. The resulting DNA must then be carefully separated into two equivalent portions, one for each daughter cell. The process of copying DNA and dividing it into two equivalent cells is called *mitosis*.

- The enzyme DNA polymerase copies DNA very accurately, having an error rate of only one wrong nucleotide pair per million processed; however, given the size of the genome, this would amount to thousands of new errors every cell division.
- There is a 'proofreading' mechanism that compares the original with the copied DNA strand and corrects any mismatched nucleotides on the new strand; this mechanism reduces the overall new error rate to approximately one wrong nucleotide per billion processed (six new errors per cell division).

The accumulation of new errors is relentless. Each person consists of billions of cells, each of which is derived from the original fertilized egg. Every error that was generated during any cell division will be present in the descendants of that cell.

- By adulthood, every cell in the body has accumulated hundreds of new errors that were not present at the moment of conception.
- Most of these errors occur in non-coding DNA and have no obvious adverse effect on the function of a gene; clinical geneticists often call such a change in the DNA sequence a non-pathogenic variant or *polymorphism*.
- A small number of these errors occur in coding DNA and have an adverse effect on the function of a gene; clinical geneticists usually call a pathogenic change in the DNA sequence a *mutation*.

### Most genetic variations are common and do not cause disease

The genome of different individuals is not exactly the same. There are several different types of variation and most of these variations are non-disease causing.

Single nucleotide polymorphisms (SNPs) are common changes to the nucleotide sequence of an individual's genome, compared to a reference sequence.

- There are about three million SNPs in an individual's genome.
- SNPs are the most numerous variants in the human genome.
- Most SNPs are common and non-pathogenic (benign); they reflect the normal variation in DNA that exists between different individuals.
- SNPs play a central role in identifying and analysing genes because they act as landmarks along the DNA sequence.
- A SNP that is located near a disease-causing gene may be associated (linked) with that disease, but is not disease-causing.
- A rare single nucleotide change within a gene that affects the function of that gene is a mutation.

A copy number variation, or CNV, is a region of DNA with a variable number of copies of that particular DNA sequence compared to a reference genome; either more copies (duplication) or fewer copies (deletion).

- There are about 100 large CNVs (longer than 1 kilobase or 1000 nucleotides) in an individual's genome; there are many more smaller ones.
- Most CNVs are non-pathogenic; they reflect the normal variation in DNA that exists between different individuals.
- Some CNVs cause or predispose to disease, usually by affecting the function of several or many genes.

### Pathogenic CNVs

Chromosome analysis using conventional cytogenetics (a karyotype) can detect large pathogenic CNVs such as gain or loss of a whole chromosome, or gain or loss of a microscopically visible section of a chromosome. However, chromosome analysis has relatively low resolution (5–10 megabases). Microarray is a new technology that can detect deletions and duplication that are below the resolution of conventional cytogenetics but above the single-gene level. Microarray is now commonly used in the assessment of children with developmental disabilities (e.g. autism spectrum disorder, intellectual disability), and detects pathogenic CNVs in 15–20% of these children.

Although it provides a high-resolution scan of both non-pathogenic and pathogenic CNVs across the entire genome, a normal microarray result does not exclude all abnormalities involving DNA.

- Microarray does not detect most single-gene disorders.
- Microarray does not detect very small CNVs beyond the resolution of the microarray.
- Microarray does not reliably detect *mosaicism* (the situation where some but not all cells of the body carry a genetic abnormality).
- Microarray does not detect chromosome alterations that do not involve missing or extra segments of DNA (e.g. balanced translocations).

## Mutations

### What types of mutation cause disease?

It is convenient to divide mutations into groups according to the scale of the mutation:

- small-scale mutations that usually affect a single gene
- large-scale mutations that affect several or many genes.

It is also useful to divide mutations based on whether they:

- primarily affect the structure of the gene(s); or
- primarily affect the function of the gene(s).

In reality these distinctions are somewhat artificial; nevertheless they provide a useful construct for understanding the effects of various mutations. The different types of mutation are summarized in Table 10.2.1.

**Table 10.2.1 Types of mutation**

| Scale and type of mutation | Description and effect | Disease examples* |
|---|---|---|
| **Structural errors of genes** | | |
| Deletion | Loss of all or part of a gene resulting in little or no protein product | Duchenne muscular dystrophy |
| Duplication/insertion | Duplication of all or part of a gene resulting in excess (or deficiency) of protein product | Charcot–Marie–Tooth disease |
| Nonsense (truncating) | Mutation in one or more nucleotides preventing generation of a complete RNA strand | Hurler syndrome |
| Missense | Mutation involving one codon that causes a critical alteration in the protein sequence | Achondroplasia |
| Splicing site mutation | Mutation involving the nucleotides which identify the junction between exons/introns leading to generation of an abnormal RNA strand | |
| **Functional errors of genes** | | |
| Regulatory | Mutation in the regulatory region of a gene causing inappropriate activation or silencing of gene | Thalassaemia |

*Continued*

**Table 10.2.1 Types of mutation—Cont'd**

| Scale and type of mutation | Description and effect | Disease examples* |
|---|---|---|
| Abnormal imprint | Reversal of the normal silencing or activation genes in the maternal or paternal germline | Beckwith–Weidemann syndrome |
| Unstable triplet repeat | Increase in the number of copies of a repeated triplet of nucleotides causing abnormal function of a gene or protein product | Fragile X syndrome |
| **Structural errors of chromosomes†**<br>Monosomy (deletion) | Loss of whole (or part) of a chromosome | Turner syndrome |
| Trisomy (duplication) | Excess of the whole (or part) of a chromosome | Down syndrome |
| Triploidy | Presence of an extra copy of each chromosome | Miscarriage |
| **Functional errors of chromosomes**<br>Uniparental disomy | Both copies of all or part of a chromosome inherited from just one parent | Prader–Willi syndrome |

*Note that different patients with the same genetic disorder may have different types of mutation in the same gene.
†Structural errors of part of a chromosome are often called a copy number variation, or CNV.

## Triplet repeat mutations

Triplet repeat mutations are a special class of mutation. Throughout the genome there are many locations where pairs or triplets of nucleotides are present as multiple adjacent copies. Most of these nucleotide repeats occur in non-coding DNA and are of no clinical consequence. However, some occur within genes or within nearby regulatory regions.

- A number of genes contain the DNA sequence CAG–CAG–CAG repeated many times.
- The codon CAG encodes the amino acid glutamine.
- The proteins synthesized from genes with runs of CAG repeats contain regions of polyglutamine.
- The number of CAG repeats in a gene varies within a certain normal range in the general population.
- If the number of CAG repeats in an *exon* increases outside this normal range, the length of polyglutamine in the protein increases abnormally; this usually interferes with protein function or degradation.
- If the number of CAG repeats in a *regulatory region* expands outside this normal range, a gene may be inactivated.
- Larger degrees of expansion tend to be associated with more severe disruption of the normal function of the gene or protein.

One of the most striking features of these expanded triplet repeat mutations is that they tend to increase in size (expand) during cell division.

- This tendency to expand means a genetic disorder due to a triplet repeat mutation may become more severe when passed from parent to child, a phenomenon called *anticipation*.
- In some cases there is a parent-of-origin effect, and large expansions are seen mainly in the gametes from the parent of one sex; this reflects a difference in the survival of gametes with large expansions (*not* a tendency to expand more in a sperm versus an ovum, or vice versa).

### Clinical example

Four-year-old Andrew has behavioural problems, delayed language development and mild dysmorphic features (large everted ears, an elongated face and hyperflexible joints). His mother had learning difficulties at school, particularly with mathematics. A maternal uncle has a moderate intellectual disability. A molecular test for fragile X syndrome (FRAX) identified a full mutation in the *FMR1* gene.

**Discussion**

FRAX is caused by a triplet repeat mutation in the *FMR1* gene, which is located on the X chromosome. There are two forms of the genetic error: a pre-mutation (55–200 CAG repeats, rather than the normal 5–44) and a full mutation (more than 200 repeats). Males with a full mutation have intellectual impairment, usually in the moderate intellectual disability range. Males with a pre-mutation do not have intellectual disability, but are at risk of developing fragile X-related tremor ataxia syndrome (FXTAS) as adults. Approximately 50% of females with a full mutation have an intellectual disability, which is usually in the mild range. Females with a pre-mutation do not have intellectual disability, but about 20% develop premature ovarian failure.

### Mutations that arise in an egg or sperm can be transmitted to offspring

The majority of the mutations present at conception are new mutations that occurred during the formation of the individual ovum or sperm. The frequency of new mutations in gametes accounts for much of the high failure rate of human conception; three-quarters of all human conceptions fail to survive longer than the first 6 weeks of a pregnancy (most of these miscarriages occur before a woman is aware that she is pregnant).

- A sporadic (new) mutation that occurred during the formation of a gamete cell in one generation can be transmitted to the next generation, and become a familial mutation.

### Mutations occurring during embryogenesis are limited to specific lineages of cells

Embryogenesis encompasses the first 12 weeks of a pregnancy. It is the period when the organs of the body are formed.

- A new mutation that occurs during embryogenesis may affect the structure, function or survival of tissues derived from that cell lineage.
- The other cells of the body that lack this mutation function normally.
- A mixture of normal cells and cells with a mutation is called *somatic mosaicism*.
- If a mosaic mutation is not present in the gonads, it will not be transmitted to the next generation and will not be familial.
- If a new mutation occurs in a cell that contributes to the formation of an ovary or testis, the mature gonad will contain a mixture of gamete cell precursors, some that have and others that do not have the mutation; this situation is called *gonadal mosaicism*.
- Gonadal mosaicism can result in a healthy person having a number of children with the same 'new' mutation.

The focal effects of a mosaic mutation can be mimicked by X inactivation.

- Females inactivate one X chromosome in each cell of the body (lyonization).
- In healthy females there is little to distinguish cells that have inactivated different X chromosomes.
- A mutation on one X chromosome can result in patchy birth defects as the mutation will interfere with the development of cells in which the mutant X chromosome is left active; cells that inactivate the mutant X chromosome will develop normally.
- The cells giving rise to the female's ovaries will also have the mutation, so the mutation may be transmitted to her children.

**Clinical example**

Osteogenesis imperfecta type II is a severe bone dysplasia that is usually fatal in the newborn period.

- Each affected baby has a new mutation that occurred in one of the gamete cells from which the baby developed.
- The parents are at a 5% risk of having a second affected child.
- Familial cases are due to one parent having a mixture of mutant and normal gamete cells in their testes or ovaries (i.e. gonadal mosaicism).
- The mutant gamete cells are derived from a single mutant precursor cell in the parent.

### Mutations occurring after embryogenesis cause many of the features of ageing

After embryogenesis is completed, new mutations continue to be generated and are transmitted to all the progeny of a cell.

- As a person ages, mutations accumulate within a cell's genetic code and eventually interfere with cellular function.
- If the cellular dysfunction results in cell death, the loss of an individual cell will usually go unnoticed.
- If a cell accumulates mutations in a number of growth-limiting genes, the consequence will be failure to regulate cell division; this is clinically evident as cancer.

The progressive accumulation of mutations in the nuclear DNA is compounded by a similar process occurring in mitochondrial genes.

- Mutations accumulate in mtDNA 10–20 times faster than in nuclear genes.
- A number of factors are responsible, including the relatively high exposure of mtDNA to oxygen radicals (a byproduct of ATP synthesis) and the lack of protective proteins and effective DNA repair mechanisms in mitochondria.
- mtDNA is replicated independently of nuclear DNA and, as a result, mitochondrial mutations accumulate in cells (such as neurons) that are not actively dividing.

- As a person ages, mtDNA mutations may be so widespread that energy production in many cells is compromised, which may result in problems such as cardiac failure or dementia.

### How are mutations inherited?

The fact that an individual's genetic code is not static but is accumulating mutations constantly from the moment of conception has been highlighted above.

- Mutations that are present only in somatic cells may account for the development of clinical problems in an individual, but they are not passed to the next generation.
- Mutations that are present in the cells of the gonads may be transmitted to a fertilized egg in the next generation.
- A mutation that is present at conception will be present subsequently in the ovaries or testes of the developing child; if the child survives to have children of their own, the mutation may be transmitted again to the next generation.

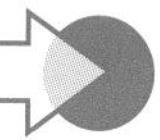

**Practical points**

- Inaccurate DNA copying generates new mutations that are transmitted to all of a cell's progeny.
- New mutations account for many congenital abnormalities and disorders of ageing.
- Mutations that are present only in somatic cells are not inherited.
- Mutations in the ovary or testis may be inherited.

## Patterns of inheritance

Mendelian disorders are those that are explained by mutations in a single nuclear gene. There are five basic patterns of mendelian inheritance (see below). However, most genetic or partially genetic disorders are not caused by mutations in a single gene; they are caused by mutations in genes at multiple loci (oligogenic and polygenic disorders). Environmental factors make an important contribution to the clinical expression or *phenotype* of many polygenic disorders; thus they are often considered to be multifactorial.

### Autosomal recessive inheritance

If a mutation interferes with the function of one copy of a gene, the presence of the other normal copy of the gene may be sufficient to prevent the development of a condition. This type of mutation could be inherited by many family members who remain healthy and are unaware that they are carrying the mutation. This is called an autosomal recessive mutation (Fig. 10.2.3).

### Autosomal dominant inheritance

For certain autosomal genes and mutations, the presence of one abnormal gene may be sufficient to cause a clinical disorder. In this situation, most of the family members who have the mutated gene will be affected. This type of mutation is called an autosomal dominant mutation (Fig. 10.2.4).

**Hallmarks of an autosomal recessive disorders**

- often affect metabolic pathways
- affect both males and females
- affected individuals are usually born to unaffected parents
- other members of the extended family are also unaffected
- vertical transmission (from an affected individual to the next generation) is not usually seen
- an affected individual carries a mutation in both copies of an autosomal gene and is *homozygous* for the disorder
- a person who carries a mutation of one copy of a particular gene is *heterozygous*; they are not affected by the disorder
- the frequency of the disorder is determined by the frequency of carriers in the population
- the carrier frequency of some disorders is increased in certain ethnic groups (e.g. Gaucher disease in Askenazi Jews; cystic fibrosis in Caucasians)
- parental consanguinity increases the chance of having an affected child

Examples

- congenital adrenal hyperplasia
- recessive congenital deafness
- spinal muscular atrophy (SMA)
- hereditary haemochromatosis
- Tay--Sachs disease
- phenylketonuria (PKU)
- beta-thalassaemia
- cystic fibrosis
- sickle cell disease
- MCAD deficiency

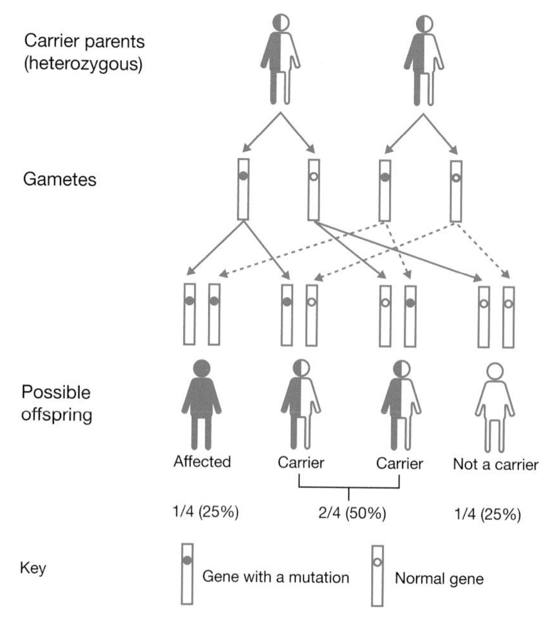


Fig. 10.2.3 Autosomal recessive inheritance. MCAD, medium-chain acyl-CoA dehydrogenase.

**Hallmarks of an autosomal dominant disorders**
- often affect genes coding for structural coding
- affect both males and females
- transmitted by males and females
- vertical transmission is seen; affected parents may have affected children
- other members of the extended family may also be affected
- an affected individual carries a mutation in one copy of a particular gene and is *heterozygous*

**Complexities**
- variable expression; different family members with the same disease-causing mutation show different features of the disease
- non-penetrance; when an individual carries a disease-causing mutation but is unaffected (phenotypically normal)
- gonadal mosaicism (see text)
- lack of family history may be explained by a new mutation, non-penetrance or non-paternity

**Examples**
- Marfan syndrome
- Huntington disease
- familial hypercholesterolaemia
- hypertrophic cardiomyopathy
- neurofibromatosis type 1
- achondroplasia
- long QT syndrome
- familial retinoblastoma

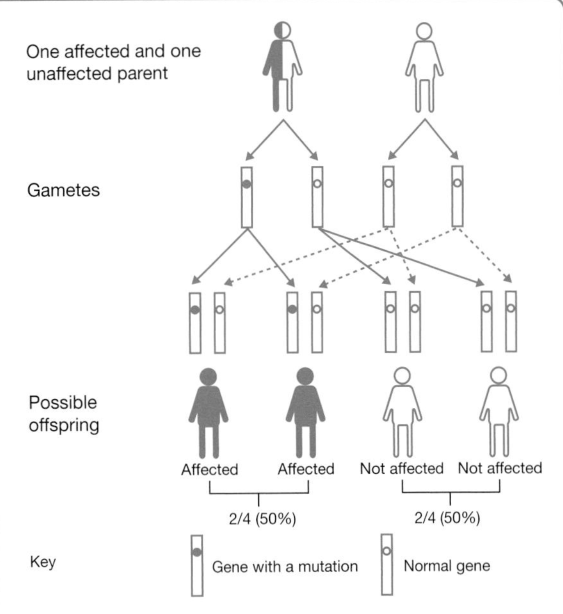


Fig. 10.2.4 Autosomal dominant inheritance.

## X-linked recessive inheritance

If a female has a recessive mutation on one X chromosome, the presence of the normal gene on the other X chromosome usually prevents the development of a severe genetic disorder. A male has just one X chromosome and a mutation in a male's single X chromosome gene results in a genetic disorder (Fig. 10.2.5). Recurrence risk counselling is a major challenge in families with affected male members.

## X-linked dominant inheritance

This pattern of inheritance is usually characterized by a similar disease frequency in males and females, although the female phenotype is often milder than

**Hallmarks of an X-linked recessive disorders**
- affects mainly males
- females unaffected or have very mild disease
- affected males never pass the disease to their sons, but pass the mutated X to all their unaffected daughters, who are obligate carriers
- female carriers pass the mutated X to half their sons (who are affected) and half their daughters (who are carriers)
- an affected male carries a mutation on his only copy of a particular X-linked gene and is *hemizygous*
- a carrier female carries a mutation of one copy of a particular X-linked gene and is *heterozygous*

**Complexities**
- transmission from an affected male to a carrier daughter to an affected male grandchild (the 'knight's move')
- skewed X-inactivation in affected females (see text)
- recurrence risk counselling in families with one affected male is difficult

**Examples**
- Duchenne muscular dystrophy
- red–green colour blindness
- X-linked retinitis pigmentosa
- X-linked mental retardation
- Haemophilia A
- Lesch–Nyhan syndrome
- Fabry disease
- Hunter disease

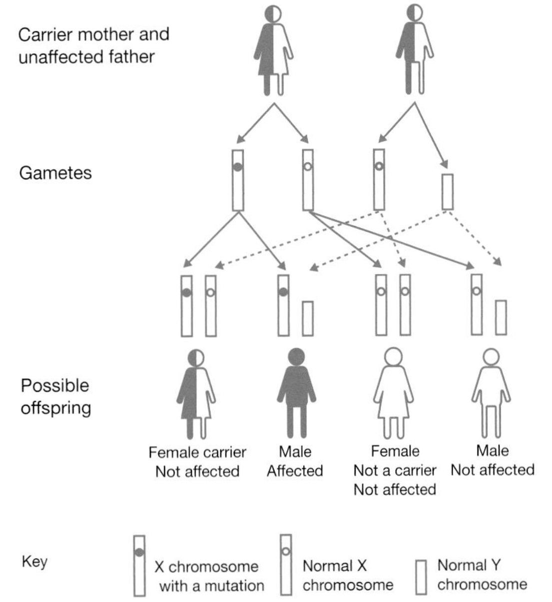


Fig. 10.2.5 X-linked recessive inheritance.

the male phenotype (sex-dependent expression). The absence of male-to-male transmission distinguishes X-linked dominant disorders from autosomal dominant disorders. Regarding X-linked dominant disorders:

- if a male is affected, all of his daughters, but none of his sons, are affected
- if a female is affected, half of her daughters and half of her sons are affected
- X-linked dominant disorders are uncommon
- examples include X-linked dominant forms of Alport syndrome and hypophosphataemic rickets
- Rett syndrome is a rare, progressive, X-linked dominant neurological disorder that almost exclusively affects females, being lethal in affected males.

## Y-linked inheritance

This pattern of inheritance is characterized by exclusively male-to-male transmission of a disorder that only affects males. The Y chromosome has very few genes, most of which are involved in normal male sexual development, so the phenotype of a Y-linked disorder may include infertility.

- Y-linked inheritance is uncommon.
- Affected males pass their Y chromosome to *every* son, who will be affected.
- Females inherit an X chromosome from their fathers, and are *not* affected by a Y-linked disorder.

## Mitochondrial DNA mutations and maternal inheritance

An abnormality of mitochondrial function due to a mutation in a nuclear gene demonstrates autosomal recessive, autosomal dominant or X-linked recessive inheritance (see Figs 10.2.3–10.2.5). Because a nuclear gene mutation affects all the mitochondria in the body, affected individuals in a family tend to have similar problems.

Mitochondrial abnormalities due to a mutation in a mtDNA gene are maternally inherited (Fig. 10.2.6). An affected individual may have a mixture of mutant and non-mutant (wild-type) mitochondria, which is called heteroplasmy. Heteroplasmy leads to marked variability in both the severity and the type of tissue involved within one family.

## Polygenic and multifactorial disorders

Many common genetic disorders cannot be attributed to a mutation in a single gene. They result from the interaction of a number of genes, each of which has a mutation or polymorphism that increases an individual's susceptibility to the disorder (Fig. 10.2.7). Even if an individual has inherited a number of mutations that places them at increased risk of a *polygenic* disorder, non-genetic factors such as nutrition or chance may ultimately determine whether the disorder occurs. A disorder due to the interaction of multiple genes and non-genetic factors is called a *multifactorial* disorder.

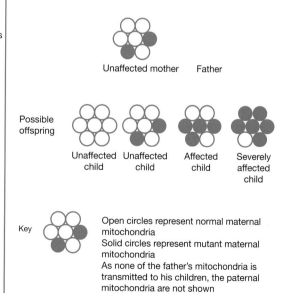

**Hallmarks of disorders with mitochondrial inheritance**

- affect males and females
- affected males never pass the disease to their sons or daughters
- demonstrate marked variability in clinical symptoms within a single family

**Complexities**

- difficult to recognize because of clinical variability
  - if the majority of a person's mitochondria are normal they are unaffected
  - if the majority of a person's mitochondria are mutant they are severely affected
  - if a person has an intermediate proportion of normal and mutant mitochondria the clinical symptoms depend on the proportion of mutant mitochondria in various tissues
  - usually the probabilities of each of these outcomes cannot be predicted
- recurrence risk counselling in families is very complicated

**Examples**

- Leigh syndrome
- MERRF syndrome
- Leber's hereditary optic neuropathy
- MELAS syndrome
- mitochondrial diabetes mellitus with deafness

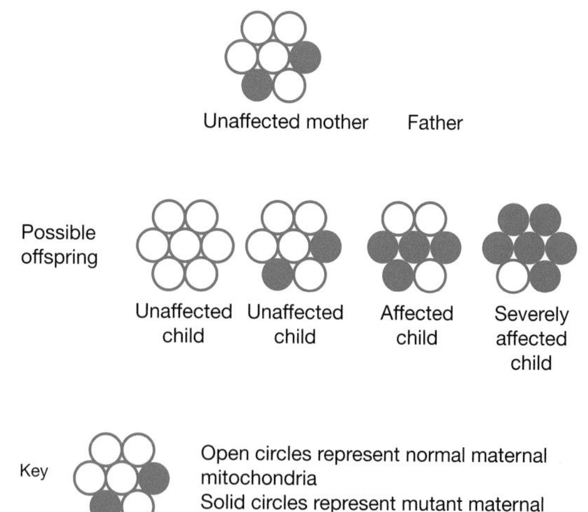


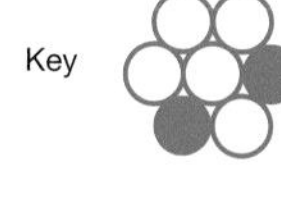


Open circles represent normal maternal mitochondria
Solid circles represent mutant maternal mitochondria
As none of the father's mitochondria is transmitted to his children, the paternal mitochondria are not shown

Fig. 10.2.6 Mitochondrial inheritance. MERRF, myoclonic epilepsy with ragged red fibers; MELAS, mitochondrial encephalomyopathy, lactic acidosis, and stroke-like episodes.

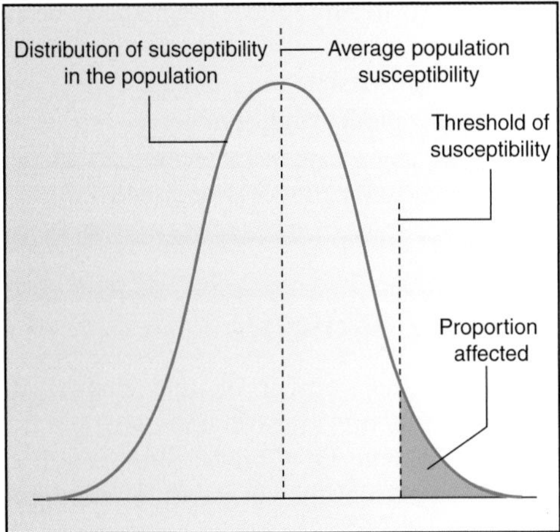


Fig. 10.2.7 Threshold model for multifactorial disorders. Below the threshold of susceptibility the disorder is not expressed. Individuals above the threshold have the disorder.

Over the last 5 years scientists have identified a number of genes that confer susceptibility to polygenic and multifactorial disorders. Identification of additional susceptibility genes remains a major objective in genetic research.

- One mutation or polymorphism is unlikely to cause the disorder on its own.
- As the number of susceptibility genes a person inherits increases, the likelihood of the disorder occurring increases.
- If the number of genes reaches a critical value (the threshold), the susceptibility is so great that the disorder occurs.
- Multifactorial disorders typically affect between 0.1% and 1% of the population.
- The recurrence risk among close relatives is usually 10–20 times higher than the general population risk.
- Examples: some congenital malformations such as cleft lip and neural tube defects, and disorders of later life such as asthma, diabetes and ischaemic heart disease.

### Clinical example

Neural tube defects are a group of related congenital malformations caused by failure of normal closure of the neural tube, and are seen in approximately 1 in 1000 live births.

- Examples include spina bifida, anencephaly and hydranencephaly.
- Deficiency of the vitamin folate and variations in genes responsible for folate metabolism are associated with an increased risk of this group of major malformations.

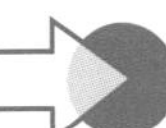

### Practical points

- An autosomal recessive disorder is expressed in an individual who is *homozygous* for a mutation in the disease gene.
- An autosomal dominant disorder is expressed in an individual who is *heterozygous* for a mutation in the disease gene.
- An X-linked disorder is transmitted via the X chromosome; it never displays male-to-male transmission.
- A mitochondrial disorder can be caused by a mutation in nuclear DNA or mtDNA; these disorders may display autosomal dominant, autosomal recessive, X-linked or maternal inheritance.
- Multifactorial disorders result from the interaction of multiple susceptibility genes, environment and chance.
- The pattern of inheritance of a condition provides essential information regarding the recurrence risk among relatives.

### Clinical example

Hereditary haemochromatosis (HH) is an autosomal recessive condition caused by mutations in the *HFE* gene, and there are two common mutations in the Caucasian population.

- HH is characterized by abnormal storage of iron in a range of body tissues.
- Iron overload causes progressive organ damage and complications including cirrhosis of the liver, cardiomyopathy, diabetes mellitus and arthritis.
- The clinical features of HH are usually manifest in adulthood, and are more common in males.
- A significant proportion of people with two abnormal *HFE* genes never develop signs of organ damage.
- Iron overload can be easily prevented by regular phlebotomy.

It has been proposed that all babies born in Caucasian communities be screened for the presence of the common *HFE* mutations. The aim would be to:

- identify individuals with two mutations, and
- prevent the development of iron overload in adult life by regular phlebotomy.

Some arguments in favour are:

- HH is common, life-threatening, yet preventable if regular phlebotomy is initiated before organ damage is established.
- Inclusion of *HFE* gene screening in a newborn screening programme would be straightforward.
- Identification of a single mutation in a baby would trigger investigation of family members and might identify other relatives with two mutations prior to the development of iron overload.

Some arguments against are:

- Neonatal diagnosis is not necessary as treatment is not needed until adult life.
- A newborn infant cannot give consent for testing or retain privacy regarding the test result.
- There may be a risk of discrimination in the long term (e.g. in relation to life or health insurance).
- A significant and ill-defined proportion of those with two mutations never develop iron overload.

## Genetics and ethics

The ability to define a genetic condition, its pattern of inheritance, the gene(s) and the mutation(s) responsible for the condition raises many ethical questions including:

- DNA is 'shared' amongst a family, but who 'owns' genetic information about an individual?
- If a serious genetic condition is identified in a family member, should at-risk relatives be informed when that family member wishes to keep the information private?
- Should children be tested to determine carrier status at a young age so that they can grow up mindful of this knowledge, or should genetic testing be deferred until a child can give informed consent to have the DNA test performed?
- For a couple with an affected child, should prenatal diagnosis in subsequent pregnancies be an option?
- Should a couple be able to terminate a pregnancy affected by a genetic condition?
- Should there be widespread screening for carriers of common autosomal recessive disorders?

## Acknowledgements

The structure and content of this chapter draws heavily from the previous versions written by my friend and colleague Dr Graeme Suthers – I thank and acknowledge him for his clarity of thought and written word.

# The dysmorphic child 10.3

Elizabeth Thompson, Christopher Barnett

Dysmorphic, which literally means 'abnormal form', refers to an unusual appearance, usually of the face. A dysmorphic child may have an underlying diagnosis that could have implications for the health not only of the child but also of other family members if the condition is inherited. With the advent of new genetic testing options such as array comparative genomic hybridization ('microarray') and an upsurge in commercially available tests for single-gene disorders, our understanding of the genetic basis underlying the dysmorphic child is improving all the time. The dysmorphic child may present as a neonate with one or more birth defects (e.g. a missing hand), or later with developmental delay or intellectual disability, failure to thrive or obesity, short or tall stature, a behavioural disturbance or a metabolic problem.

Birth defects can be classified as deformations, disruptions, dysplasias or malformations (see Chapter 10.1). It is important to distinguish between abnormalities and minor variants that are common in the general population. These can, however, appear in syndromes. For example, a unilateral single transverse palmar crease is seen in 4% of normal people but is more common in Down syndrome. Some physical traits, such as an unusually shaped nose, are a harmless family variant but again could be part of an undiagnosed syndrome in the family.

Making an overall diagnosis relies on recognizing a pattern of problems. The types of pattern include:

- *Syndrome*. This is from the Greek 'running together' and refers to a cluster of physical and other features occurring in a consistent pattern, with an implied common specific cause that may be unknown. The word syndrome is often used loosely to describe any of the other diagnostic patterns described below.
- *Association*. This is a group of physical features that tends to occur together but the link is not consistent enough to allow the term syndrome to be used. An example is the VATER association (see below). The distinction between a syndrome and an association may be artificial and, increasingly, associations are being redefined as syndromes as their genetic basis is identified. For example, in 2004 CHARGE association (Coloboma, Heart defects, Atresia choanae, Retardation of growth and development, Genital and Ear anomalies) was identified as being due to mutations in the *CHD7* gene on chromosome 8; with this, CHARGE association became CHARGE syndrome.
- *Sequence*. This refers to a group of abnormalities caused by a cascade of events beginning with one malformation. An example is the Potter sequence, which can result from any cause of severe oligohydramnios. For example, renal agenesis results in no fetal urine, leading to severe oligohydramnios, with the consequence of lung hypoplasia and intrauterine constraint, causing limb deformities, such as talipes, and a compressed facial appearance.
- *Developmental field defect*. This refers to a group of malformations caused by a harmful influence in a particular region of the embryo. Abnormalities of blood flow are thought to underlie many of these. An example is hemifacial microsomia with unilateral facial hypoplasia and ear anomalies relating to an abnormality in development of first and second branchial arch structures.

Why is it necessary to recognize an underlying diagnosis? Some important reasons are:

- avoiding unnecessary investigations
- providing information about prognosis for doctors and family
- recognizing and treating complications that need to be looked for prospectively
- determining the pattern of inheritance and recurrence risk
- enabling support from other families. Individual syndromes are rare and parents become the experts in day-to-day management of the child and can share this with other families.

Are there any pitfalls in making a diagnosis? Some areas for consideration are:

- The diagnosis must be correct: the diagnosis may be based on clinical assessment alone with no confirmatory tests available; diagnosis must not be undertaken lightly as it can be difficult to remove or alter a diagnosis once it has been made, with harmful consequences for the child and family.
- Parents do not wish their child to be labelled, especially if the child is young and they do not yet perceive any problems themselves.
- Doctors may attribute all new problems to the syndrome.

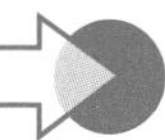

**Practical points**

- Syndromes are individually rare but collectively common.
- Accurate syndrome diagnosis is important to give information about prognosis, associated problems, recurrence risk and support groups for families.
- Diagnoses are made by thorough clinical assessment followed by use of aids such as computerized syndrome databases.
- Even an experienced clinical geneticist may not make a syndrome diagnosis in a child with dysmorphic features.
- It is better to make no syndrome diagnosis than to make an incorrect diagnosis.

## How to assess the dysmorphic child

### Instant recognition

A 'waiting room diagnosis' based on the facial 'gestalt' might be made if the doctor has seen a person with the particular syndrome before, just as most people are able to recognize whether a person in the street has Down syndrome. Often, however, the diagnosis is not apparent initially, and the following approach is recommended.

### History

Special points in the medical history include:

- Antenatal history:
  - teratogens, such as drugs, viruses, maternal diabetes, maternal hyperthermia (see Chapter 10.1)
  - fetal movements – a neuromuscular disorder may cause reduced fetal movements, resulting in arthrogryposis (multiple fixed deformities of joints)
  - prenatal screening and diagnostic tests.
- Perinatal history:
  - weight, length, head circumference and Apgar scores at birth

Growth and development, behaviour, sleep patterns.

Family history – draw a three-generation family tree noting miscarriages, stillbirths and deaths of siblings, any history of intellectual disability, congenital abnormalities or consanguinity (i.e. are the parents related?), and enquire about other family members with the same features.

### Examination

Observe the child before undressing or disturbing her or him. On the other hand, the examination is not complete until the child has been fully undressed. Especially note:

- behaviour and alertness
- height, weight, head circumference and shape, body proportions (e.g. height to arm span ratio, upper and lower body segment length) and any asymmetry
- always plot measurements on standard normal charts. Charts are available for many different body parts (e.g. hand measurements, foot and ear length). Special charts are available for certain disorders (e.g. Down syndrome) and various bone dysplasias (e.g. achondroplasia)
- facial features (Fig. 10.3.1) – careful assessment of facial anatomy often provides clues to the diagnosis
  - spacing of the eyes (hypertelorism or hypotelorism, i.e. wide or closely spaced); slant of the palpebral fissures (up or down)
  - shape and size of the nose and mouth
  - structure and position of the ears
- chest shape and spinal curvature
- proportions of the limbs, muscle bulk and tone, joint contractures and mobility
- structure of hands and feet (shape, length, number of digits, dermal ridges, nails)
- skin pigmentary or vascular markings
- external genitalia
- any birth defects? (e.g. cleft palate)
- auscultate the chest for any cardiac murmurs
- palpate the abdomen for organomegaly.

A photograph (with parental consent) is useful for:

- later comparison to see how the face has changed
- consulting colleagues.

When examining the family of a child with unusual facial features:

- parents and siblings should be examined to see whether this is a family characteristic
- photographs of them at a younger age and of other family members may be helpful
- in the event of a syndrome being diagnosed, the family should also be examined for its specific features.

### Putting it all together

- *Check textbooks of syndromes* (e.g. Smith's Recognizable Patterns of Human Malformation) by trying to match the most important dysmorphic features and comparing the photographs with those of the patient.
- *Consultation*:
  - Referral to a *paediatrician* is often appropriate in the first instance for assessment of a potential syndromic diagnosis.
  - Referral to a *clinical geneticist,* who is a specialist paediatrician, trained in clinical genetics, with experience in identifying many more syndromes. Some have a special interest and expertise in syndrome diagnosis (dysmorphologists).
- *It's not easy!* A skilled dysmorphologist makes a syndrome diagnosis in a dysmorphic child in

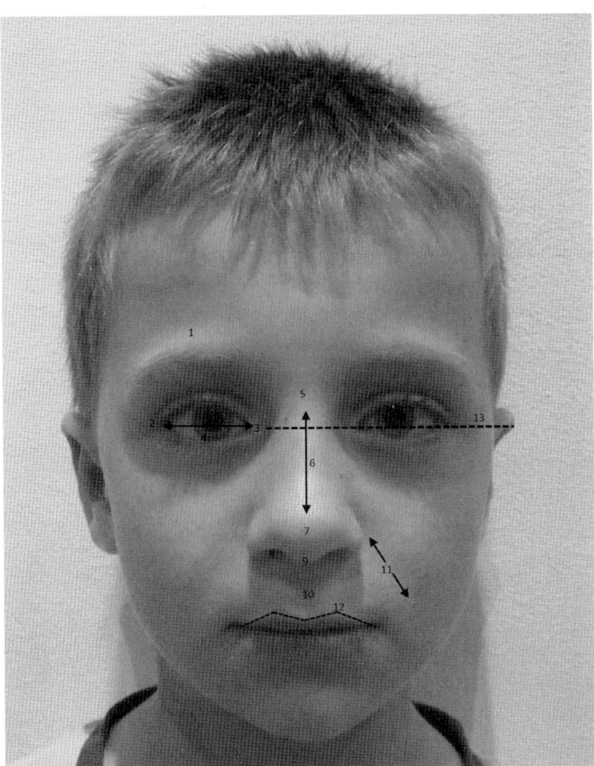


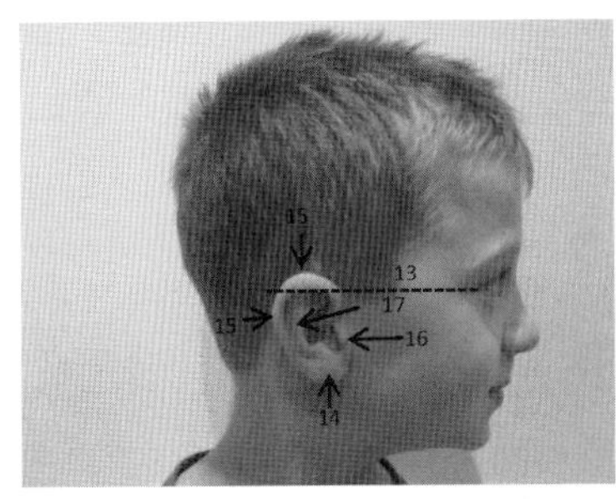


Fig. 10.3.1 Normal human face: list of common terms used in dysmorphology. (**A**) 1, Supraorbital ridge; 2, outer canthus; 3, inner canthus; 4, palpebral fissure (line from inner canthus to outer canthus); 5, nasal root; 6, nasal bridge; 7, nasal tip; 8, naris/nares; 9, columella; 10, philtrum; 11, nasolabial fold; 12, upper vermillion border of lip. (**B**) Lateral view: 13, line indicating normal ear height – the superior attachment of the pinna should lie above an imaginary line drawn through both inner canthi and running posteriorly; 'low-set' ears are below this line; 14, lobule; 15, helix; 16, tragus; 17, antihelix.

about 30% of cases referred by an experienced paediatrician. If an overall diagnosis is not made, the recognized problems must still be managed.

- *Review* in 3–5 years' time is often valuable and may allow a diagnosis to be made as the features of the syndrome evolve over time and new information or laboratory techniques become available.
- *Computerized databases:*
  - Several thousand syndromes are published, and many are individually rare
  - Computerized databases combine pictures and descriptions of syndromes
  - Searches are made using a few key dysmorphic features and a number of possible diagnoses are suggested that can be compared with the patient
  - Success is more likely if relatively rare features are used for the search; for example, a common feature such as hypertelorism (widely spaced eyes) would give a long list of suggested syndromes, whereas imperforate anus would give a more manageable list to consider
  - Training and experience are needed to use these databases effectively.
- Examples of these databases are:
  - POSSUM (Pictures Of Standard Syndromes and Undiagnosed Malformations), developed by the Genetic Health Services, Victoria, Australia
  - London Dysmorphology Database
  - London Neurogenetics Database.

## Investigations

Investigations are a necessary adjunct to the assessment of the dysmorphic child in most cases.

A routine *chromosome study* (karyotype) on blood lymphocytes remains an important test in some circumstances. It is still widely used prenatally and a karyotype is done when there is a high level of clinical suspicion about a known chromosomal disorder such as Down syndrome. A karyotype will detect balanced chromosome arrangements such as balanced translocations. Occasionally translocations interrupt genes and result in syndromes. In the paediatric population, most applications of karyotype have been superseded by microarray.

*Array comparative genomic hybridization* ('microarray') is a new technology that, in many circumstances, has replaced the karyotype as the primary investigation of the dysmorphic child. In simple terms, microarray is a blood test that allows detection of gains or losses of DNA, with much higher resolution than standard karyotyping. In addition to diagnosing well-known syndromes such as Down syndrome (trisomy 21, a gain of chromosome 21) and Williams syndrome (a deletion (loss) involving numerous genes on chromosome 7), microarray has resulted in the diagnosis of a new generation of previously undescribed microdeletions and microduplications, many with distinct facial dysmorphism. A microarray should be done on all children with an intellectual disability or autism, especially when dysmorphic features and birth defects are present. A microarray abnormality is found in 15–20% of such cases. Parental chromosomes may need to be examined if a structural alteration is found, in order to clarify the abnormality and to facilitate genetic counselling in the family.

### Other investigations

Other investigations such as metabolic studies or radiology should be done as clinically indicated.

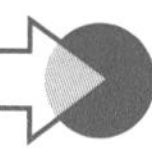

**Practical points**

- Taking a good history is as important as physical examination in the assessment of a dysmorphic child.
- Microarray technology has revolutionized syndrome diagnosis and largely replaced karyotyping as the investigation of choice.
- Examination of other family members (or their photographs) may be required in the assessment of the dysmorphic child.

## Common chromosomal disorders

Children with chromosome disorders, particularly of the autosomes (chromosomes 1–22), tend to be small, dysmorphic and have intellectual impairment.

### Numerical chromosome disorders

#### Trisomy 21 (Down syndrome)

Down syndrome is the commonest chromosome disorder in liveborn babies and is the commonest genetic cause of intellectual disability:

- Birth incidence is about 1 in 1200 live births; the overall incidence rises after maternal age of 35 years.
- Maternal serum screening and ultrasonography can be offered to all pregnant women to identify those at high risk, who may then opt for prenatal diagnosis by amniocentesis (see Chapter 10.1).

Features of Down syndrome include:

- flat midface, flat occiput, upward slanting eyes with medial epicanthic folds, Brushfield spots in the iris, palpebrae 'purse' on laughing or crying, small, downturned mouth and protruding tongue, small ears, excess nuchal skin in the neonatal period
- short fingers, clinodactyly of the fifth fingers (short middle phalanges lead to incurving), single palmar creases, widened gap between first and second toes
- birth defects may be present (e.g. congenital heart disease in 40–50%, duodenal atresia, anal atresia and many others)
- intellectual disability of varying degree, mean IQ less than 50, up to about 70 and declines with age; all have neuropathological changes of Alzheimer disease by 35–40 years with clinical onset in the early 50s; is an important cause of death in adults
- reduced lifespan (around 60 years if no organ defects)
- follow-up is necessary for children with Down syndrome to monitor for cataracts, strabismus (30–40%), leukaemia, hypothyroidism, obesity, infections, constipation, obstructive sleep apnoea, dental problems and atlantoaxial instability, although only a minority develop neurological complications from this
- behaviour: often happy, affectionate, friendly, but anxiety and depression often occur with age.
- Genetics:
  - 95% have trisomy for chromosome 21 with a low recurrence risk
  - the remainder have either a robertsonian translocation (a chromosome 21 attached to another similar chromosome, usually chromosome 14) or mosaicism (some cells with trisomy 21 and some with a normal karyotype)
  - half of the translocation cases are inherited from a parent, so parental chromosomes should be checked only if there is a translocation. An inherited translocation is associated with an increased risk of recurrence.

#### Trisomy 18 (Edwards syndrome)

The birth incidence of trisomy 18 is about 1 in 8000 live births:

- many have prenatal ultrasound abnormalities and are then detected at amniocentesis
- low birth weight, prominent occiput, dysplastic low-set ears, micrognathia (small chin), short palpebral fissures, small mouth
- characteristic clenched hand posture (fifth and second fingers overlap fourth and third); prominent heels

- malformations are common (e.g. heart, brain, exomphalos, kidney)
- behaviour: poor feeding and neurological development, about one-third die in the first month, less than 10% live beyond 1 year.
- Genetics:
  - most have trisomy for chromosome 18, which is associated with advanced maternal age; a few have translocations
  - recurrence risk for trisomy or non-inherited translocation is low and prenatal diagnosis is available for the next pregnancy.

### Trisomy 13 (Patau syndrome)

The birth incidence of trisomy 13 is about 1 in 30000 live births:

- many have prenatal ultrasound abnormalities and are then detected at amniocentesis
- low birth weight, microcephaly with sloping forehead, scalp defects, cleft lip and palate, broad flat nose, polydactyly (extra digits)
- birth defects such as holoprosencephaly and heart defects are common
- very poor neurological status and 50% of babies die within the first month.
- Genetics:
  - most have trisomy 13 associated with advanced maternal age; some have translocations
  - recurrence risk for trisomy is low and prenatal diagnosis is available.

### Turner syndrome

Turner syndrome is one of the commonest chromosome defects at conception but the majority miscarry, usually at an early stage of pregnancy:

- birth incidence is around 1 in 3000 liveborn girls
- lymphoedema of the hands and feet, and redundant nuchal skin are common in neonates
- may present in childhood with short stature, or in adolescence with failure of onset of puberty
- variable features, which include: webbed neck, increased carrying angle of elbows, broad chest, pigmented naevi, narrow, deep-set hyperconvex nails, coarctation of the aorta, idiopathic hypertension, renal anomalies
- intelligence usually normal but specific learning problems are common; 1 in 10 has a generalized learning disability
- most are infertile because the ovaries are dysplastic
- pregnancy has been achieved by *in vitro* fertilization using donor eggs
- the mean untreated adult height is around 140 cm. Refer early for assessment regarding growth hormone treatment.
- Genetics:
  - 60% have 45,X; others have a structural defect in which one X chromosome is missing all or part of the p (short) arm, or there is mosaicism 46,XX/45,X
  - not associated with advanced maternal age; recurrence risk not increased.

### Klinefelter syndrome

Klinefelter syndrome is a disorder of males in which there is an additional X chromosome:

- birth incidence is about 1 in 700 liveborn males
- many present as adolescents with delayed puberty, or as adults with infertility
- occasionally present in childhood with developmental delay, especially of speech or with learning disabilities, often involving reading and mathematics
- overall, IQ is reduced compared with that of siblings, but usually in normal range.
- features: tall stature, long limbs, small testes, undescended testes, gynaecomastia and female fat distribution with age, infertility, behaviour problems
- treatment with testosterone at puberty will bring about a more normal virilization
- early access to reproductive medicine services (i.e. in teenage years) to store sperm enhance reproductive chances.
- Genetics:
  - 47,XXY karyotype; extra X chromosome inherited from either parent
  - recurrence risk is low.

### Triple X syndrome

This is a syndrome in which females have an extra X chromosome:

- birth incidence is about 1 in 1500 liveborn females
- features: tall stature, few dysmorphic features
- intellect: usually in normal range, but overall the IQ is lower than that of siblings. Learning difficulties, delayed speech and motor milestones, poor coordination and behaviour problems are common
- pubertal development and fertility are generally normal.
- Genetics:
  - 46,XXX karyotype; extra X chromosome inherited from mother
  - recurrence risk to siblings and offspring is low.

## Structural chromosome disorders

### Velocardiofacial syndrome

The estimated birth incidence of the velocardiofacial syndrome (VCFS), also called 22q deletion (Fig. 10.3.2, 10.3.3) or DiGeorge syndrome, may be

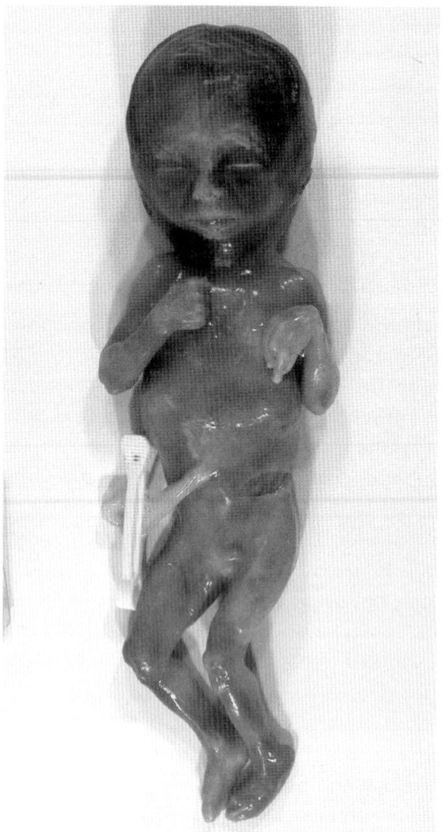

Fig. 10.3.2 22q microdeletion syndrome. Note small mouth and broad nasal bridge with rounded nasal tip.

as high as 1 in 2000. It is a very variable syndrome, with more than 180 clinical features described. The diagnosis should be suspected if a child has the following two features:

- palatal abnormality (cleft palate, bifid uvula, velopharyngeal incompetence) – found in 70% of patients with VCFS; 11% of patients have an overt cleft palate
- conotruncal congenital heart defects (tetralogy of Fallot, aortic arch defects, ventricular septal defect, pulmonary atresia/stenosis, and truncus arteriosus) – found in 70% of patients with VCFS.

The facial appearance is variable but often there is a prominent nasal bridge, narrow nostrils and a bulbous nasal tip. Older children often have developmental delay and learning disabilities, social immaturity, anxiety and phobias. Up to 20% of adults with the syndrome have psychiatric illness:

- Genetics:
  - deletion of 22q11, visible on karyotyping in 15% of cases but detectable by microarray in the remainder
  - up to 5% who clinically appear to have the syndrome have no detectable deletion
  - parents should be tested, as features can be mild and risk to each child of a carrier is 50%.
  - prenatal diagnosis is available.

## Trinucleotide repeat sequence disorders

Fragile X syndrome is one of the commonest causes of intellectual disability (1 in 4000 males and 1 in 10 000 females) and is one of a range of disorders caused by 'unstable triplet repeats' of DNA. In fragile X syndrome, an unstable triplet repeat of DNA next to the *FMR1* gene expands and switches off the *FMR1* gene on the X chromosome (see below).

The features of fragile X syndrome are:

- intellectual disability of varying degree, usually more severe in males than females
- mild dysmorphism with macrocephaly, high forehead, long face, large jaw, big ears, post-pubertal macro-orchidism (large testes)
- soft skin, joint laxity
- shy personality, autistic features.
- Genetics:
  - a normal *FMR1* gene contains a sequence with 5–54 copies of a CCG triplet
  - DNA testing can identify carriers of the pre-mutation and full mutation
  - a pre-mutation contains 55–200 CCG repeats. Male and female carriers of this do not have fragile X syndrome, but females can have a child with fragile X and both males and females are at risk of other health problems (see below)

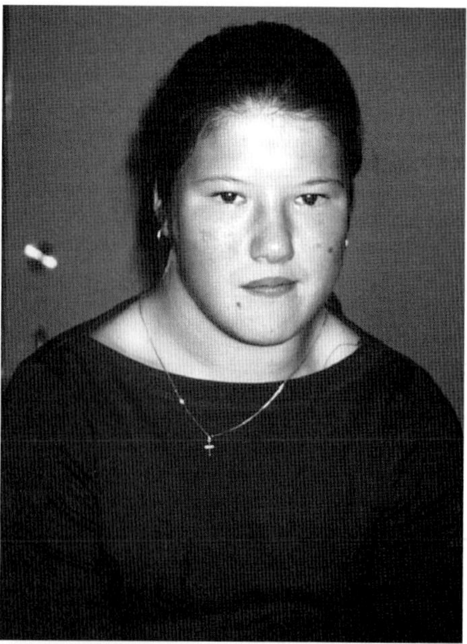

Fig. 10.3.3 Velocardiofacial syndrome. Note long mid-face, prominent nose with a squared-off nasal tip and notched nares.

- a full mutation contains more than 200 CCG repeats. All males and about 60% of females with a full mutation show clinical features of the syndrome. The full mutation in males and some females is associated with the appearance of a 'fragile site' on light microscopy when cells are cultured in folate-deficient medium
- when the CCG repeat is passed from a carrier mother to a child (but not from a carrier father), it is unstable and tends to enlarge
- intellectual impairment increases with CCG repeat number
- female carriers pass the abnormal gene to 50% of their children but only males with the full mutation and 60% of females with the full mutation will be affected with the syndrome
- male pre-mutation carriers pass the pre-mutation unchanged to their daughters
- male pre-mutation carriers (and to a lesser extent females) are at risk after their 50s of the fragile X tremor ataxia syndrome (FXTAS) with ataxia, parkinsonian features and cognitive defects
- female pre-mutation carriers are at risk of premature ovarian failure (menopause before the age of 40 years)
- prenatal diagnosis on chorionic villus sampling or amniocentesis is available but is complicated by the uncertainty of clinical outcome in a female fetus carrying a full mutation.

Another name for fragile X is fragile XA syndrome. There is also a much less common fragile XE syndrome, which is similar clinically and at the DNA level but involves a CCG repeat in the *FMR2* gene on the X chromosome.

## Other common disorders

### VATER association

VATER is an acronym for Vertebral anomalies, Anal malformations, Tracheo-(O)Esophageal fistula with (o)esophageal atresia (American spelling), Radial and Renal anomalies.

- Cardiac and non-radial Limb abnormalities are common and the association is sometimes enlarged to VACTERL
- no particular facial appearance is associated and mental development is usually normal
- cause is unknown
- recurrence risk is low.

### Noonan syndrome

The birth incidence of Noonan syndrome (Fig. 10.3.4) is 1 in 1000–2500 live births. It may present *in utero* with fetal nuchal oedema. The main features are:

- short stature – some have growth hormone deficiency
- short neck with webbing or redundancy of skin
- cardiac defect, especially pulmonary stenosis, atrial septal defect, ventricular septal defect, patent ductus arteriosus, hypertrophic cardiomyopathy
- characteristic chest deformity with pectus carinatum superiorly and pectus excavatum inferiorly
- broad chest with widely spaced nipples
- characteristic facial appearance that changes with age: hypertelorism, broad forehead, ptosis, down-slanting eyes in infancy, epicanthic folds, posteriorly rotated ears; similar facial appearance to Turner syndrome, but affects both sexes and chromosomes are normal

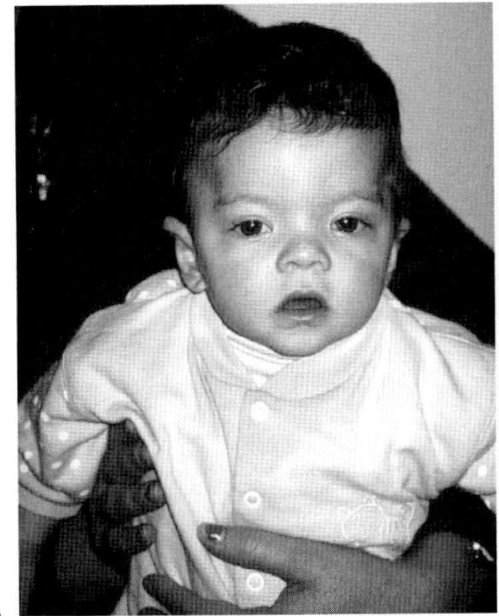
A

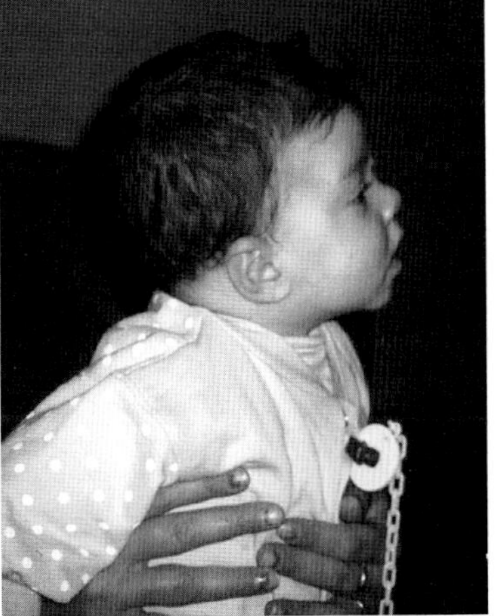
B

Fig. 10.3.4A,B Noonan syndrome. Note droopy eyelids (ptosis), mild hypertelorism and posteriorly-rotated low-set ears.

- developmental delay is common and mild intellectual disability occurs in about one-third of cases.
- Look for:
  - hearing loss (one-third of cases)
  - a bleeding diathesis (one-third of cases)
  - visual problems (in most children with the syndrome).
- Genetics:
  - many are sporadic but transmitted to offspring of affected people as an autosomal dominant
  - mutations in five genes (*PTPN11*, *SOS1*, *KRAS*, *RAF1* and *NRAS*) have been identified in about 75% of patients with Noonan syndrome (other loci may be involved)
  - prenatal diagnosis is possible but not available routinely.

## Marfan syndrome

This is a syndrome associated with tall stature and a number of other features:

- incidence 1–2 in 10 000 individuals
- connective tissue disorder caused by mutations in the fibrillin1 gene (at chromosome 15q21.1)
- diagnosis is clinical and is based on established criteria (the Ghent criteria, 2010).

Features include:

- musculoskeletal:
  - tall stature, long limbs with significantly increased arm span and reduced upper to lower body segment ratio
  - long fingers (arachnodactyly)
  - joint laxity and flat feet
  - chest deformity and kyphoscoliosis
  - long narrow face with deep set eyes, a high narrow palate and dental crowding
- cardiovascular:
  - mitral valve prolapse
  - dilatation of the ascending aorta in 50% of children, which requires drug therapy to prevent or delay development of aortic dissection and rupture
- eye:
  - ectopia lentis (dislocation of the lens, often upward)
  - myopia
  - retinal detachment
- mental development is normal.

Other problems such as spontaneous pneumothorax, striae (stretch marks of the skin) and hernias can occur.

- Genetics:
  - autosomal dominant; 25% of cases are new mutations (i.e. parents are normal)
  - prenatal diagnosis is possible in some families in which the fibrillin1 mutation has been identified.

## Achondroplasia

This is the commonest and most widely recognized skeletal dysplasia, affecting about 1 in 26 000–28 000 newborns.

- Main features:
  - short stature – mean adult height is 130 cm in males and 125 cm in females
  - short limbs, most marked in the upper segments of the limbs (rhizomelic shortening)
  - short fingers with 'trident' hand shape
  - relatively large head, depressed nasal bridge
  - small chest.
- Radiological features are also characteristic and allow a firm diagnosis to be made soon after birth.
- Length can be within the normal range at birth. Occasionally the diagnosis is unrecognized for a few months.
- Guidelines for health supervision include regular follow-up throughout childhood to monitor for complications such as:
  - hydrocephalus
  - constriction of the cervicomedullary junction, mainly in the first 2 years
  - upper airway obstruction, especially during sleep, due to small upper airway size
  - middle ear dysfunction and hearing loss
  - kyphosis
  - lumbosacral spinal stenosis causing symptoms in older children and adults
  - hypermobile joints, knee instability
  - varus deformity (bow legs)
  - dental crowding
  - adverse psychosocial impact of the disorder on the child and family.
- Treatment:
  - growth hormone transiently increases growth velocity but it is not known whether final adult height is increased
  - limb lengthening by cutting and stretching the long bones with an external distractor is controversial. A radio-operated internal distractor device has been developed with a reduced risk of infection compared with the external one. Many families believe it is better to modify the environment rather than the child.
- Genetics:
  - Autosomal dominant inheritance is usual, but most cases result from a new mutation in the *FGRF3* (fibroblast growth factor receptor 3) gene.

# Genetic Counselling 10.4

Zornitza Stark, Martin Delatycki

Genetic counselling involves a health professional talking to an individual, a couple or a family about a medical condition or disease that is, or may be, genetic in origin. Genetic counselling is not always provided by genetic specialists (clinical geneticists or genetic counsellors). It is appropriate for paediatricians and disease-oriented specialists to counsel in their own area of expertise. It may be difficult, however, for the doctor who looks after a child with a genetic condition to challenge a family to look at their feelings in the genetic counselling context. Even when another practitioner provides genetic counselling to the immediate family, the genetic specialists will often be involved in counselling the broader family.

The provider of counselling for any particular condition or situation tends to evolve with time. As new technology arises it is often the genetic specialist who will counsel the family, but with time this often falls to the disease-oriented specialist and general practitioner. An example is counselling for advanced maternal age and tests to diagnose Down syndrome prenatally. In the 1980s medical geneticists and some specialized obstetricians largely undertook this. It is now usually done by obstetricians and general practitioners.

## Genetic specialists

Clinical geneticists are medical practitioners who undertake specialist training in this discipline. Their primary training is usually in paediatrics or adult internal medicine but can be in other areas, such as obstetrics and gynaecology.

Genetic counsellors come from a range of different backgrounds, such as science, nursing and teaching. They undertake a basic training programme in both genetics and counselling, followed by on-the-job training.

Areas that are covered by genetic specialist practice include:

- dysmorphology
- prenatal counselling and testing
- neurogenetics
- cancer genetics
- bone dysplasias
- metabolic diseases.

As can be seen, it covers a wide age range of patients – from pre-conception to autopsy! Traditionally a paediatric specialty, the genetic specialist is increasingly involved in diagnosis and counselling for adult-onset diseases as more and more genes are discovered for these conditions.

## Indications for formal genetic counselling

Anybody who suspects they might be at increased risk of a genetic condition or producing a child with a genetic condition or birth defect may wish to receive formal genetic counselling. This includes:

- individuals who themselves have a genetic disorder
- couples who have had a stillbirth
- couples who have had a child with a birth defect
- couples who have had a child with intellectual disability
- family history of any of the above
- family history of known genetic disorders, such as Huntington disease, muscular dystrophy
- multiple miscarriages
- exposure to radiation or drugs during pregnancy
- advanced maternal age
- consanguinity
- chromosome anomalies, including translocations and inversions
- cancers, particularly where there are multiple affected family members and/or where there is a very young age at disease onset.

## Process of genetic counselling

Genetic counselling is the process by which individuals with or at risk of an inherited disorder are advised of:

- the consequences and nature of the disorder
- the probability of developing or transmitting the disorder, and
- the options open to them in management and family planning in order to prevent, avoid or ameliorate the disorder.

This is a complex process that encompasses both diagnostic and supportive aspects, and genetic specialists need to allow each family sufficient time in quiet surroundings for this to occur.

Diagnostic information is gathered by obtaining detailed histories or records of probands (the affected individual through whom a family with a genetic disorder is ascertained). Medical records and doctors' reports are best obtained before undertaking counselling, as this makes the consultation more efficient. A pedigree is drawn with a minimum of three generations (see below). Probands and other members of the family are examined carefully and investigated as necessary. Only then can counselling be undertaken properly.

Genetic counselling is generally non-directive. A genetic specialist will not tell the family what they should do, but will help them reach an informed and reasoned decision based on the family's own values. Thus, when a family asks, 'Should we have another child?', rather than giving a direct answer the geneticist might ask, 'How would you feel about having another child with cystic fibrosis?' In this way families are encouraged to explore their own feelings. For many families it is possible to be counselled in a single visit, but some families need to return for further discussions.

It is excellent practice to write to all families seen for counselling, restating the advice given to them at the time. This letter should be written in simple, clear language and outline the discussion that has taken place. A copy of this letter is sent to the family doctor and other specialists so that everybody involved has the same information. This document then serves as a valuable family record, can be shown to other professionals and overcomes the problem of selective recall.

## Diagnostic precision

A critical element in genetic counselling is establishing the correct diagnosis. A precise diagnosis may not influence treatment but may dramatically alter the genetic counselling given to the patient and family. An example is muscular dystrophy. There are many different forms of muscular dystrophy. The principles of management are similar for these (e.g. appropriate splints, physiotherapy and occupational therapy). The risk for other family members, however, varies considerably depending on whether the muscular dystrophy is autosomal dominant, autosomal recessive, X-linked recessive or mitochondrial (see Chapter 10.2). To counsel a family appropriately, the exact diagnosis must be known.

A post-mortem examination may be necessary to establish a precise diagnosis. This can be of particular importance in a child with malformations or retardation, and in adults with neurological disorders. Post-mortem examinations need to be planned in advance, so that specific tissues can be obtained for biochemical study, electron microscopy or histochemistry. When death can be anticipated, it is best to raise the issue of an autopsy before death occurs. In practice this works better than asking permission immediately after the death, when families are grieving deeply. When permission for an autopsy has been granted, it is of the greatest importance that the parents return to discuss the autopsy findings fully.

### Clinical example

Thi and her partner Nam were planning to start a family. They sought genetic counselling because Thi's sister had a son with muscular dystrophy. They were told that it is usually an X-linked condition, in which case there would be a significant risk that they could have a son with the same condition. After gaining permission from Thi's sister, a muscle biopsy from the affected child revealed the diagnosis of limb-girdle muscular dystrophy 2B, an autosomal recessive condition. Thi and Nam were counselled that the risk for their own children was low.

Diagnostic precision may require the help of specialists who are expert in differentiating various neuromuscular diseases, retinal dystrophies and other complex problems. Dysmorphic and intellectually disabled children often require investigation before counselling can be given. An underlying chromosomal or metabolic basis should always be excluded and specific dysmorphic syndromes identified where possible (see Chapters 10.1, 10.3 and 10.5).

With advances in DNA technology it has become essential to store samples of DNA from affected family members who are likely to die, as well as from relatives such as grandparents. This enables subsequent family members to benefit from advancing knowledge. Such samples can also be obtained, with permission, at the time of autopsy if not collected earlier. Appropriate samples to allow DNA to be stored include blood and fibroblasts from a small skin biopsy.

## Obtaining and recording a family history

The family history is an essential part of genetic consultations, and is usually recorded graphically as a pedigree (family tree) using a standard set of symbols. The pedigree provides a concise record of both medical data and biological relationships between family members. It serves as a tool in making a diagnosis and establishing the pattern of inheritance. It can be used to identify relatives at risk of a genetic disorder, calculate their risks, and decide on the most

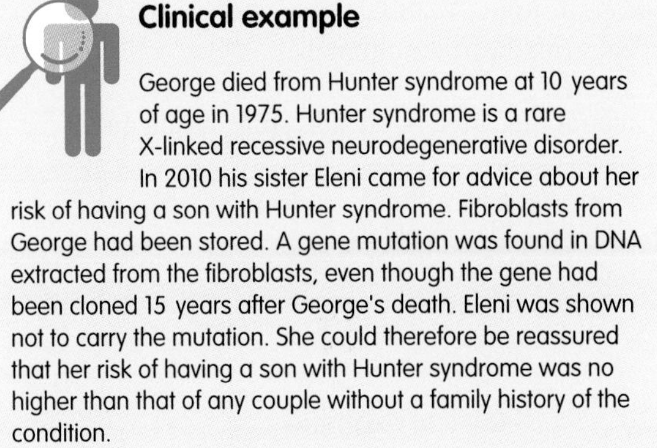

### Clinical example

George died from Hunter syndrome at 10 years of age in 1975. Hunter syndrome is a rare X-linked recessive neurodegenerative disorder. In 2010 his sister Eleni came for advice about her risk of having a son with Hunter syndrome. Fibroblasts from George had been stored. A gene mutation was found in DNA extracted from the fibroblasts, even though the gene had been cloned 15 years after George's death. Eleni was shown not to carry the mutation. She could therefore be reassured that her risk of having a son with Hunter syndrome was no higher than that of any couple without a family history of the condition.

effective cascade testing strategy. The process of taking a family history provides an excellent opportunity to establish rapport with the patient, and can give valuable insights about family dynamics and life experiences that may be influencing decision-making within the family. Reviewing the pedigree with the patient can help explore their understanding of the condition and its inheritance, and clarify misconceptions.

### Clinical example

Giovanna (III:4) sought advice about the risk of having a child with Norrie disease, a rare X-linked retinopathy. She was concerned because her cousin Angelo (III:2) had been born with the condition. The pedigree revealed that Angelo's mother Maria (II:2) was Giovanna's paternal aunt. As Giovanna's father (II:3) was unaffected, Giovanna was not at increased risk of having a boy with Norrie disease (Fig. 10.4.1).

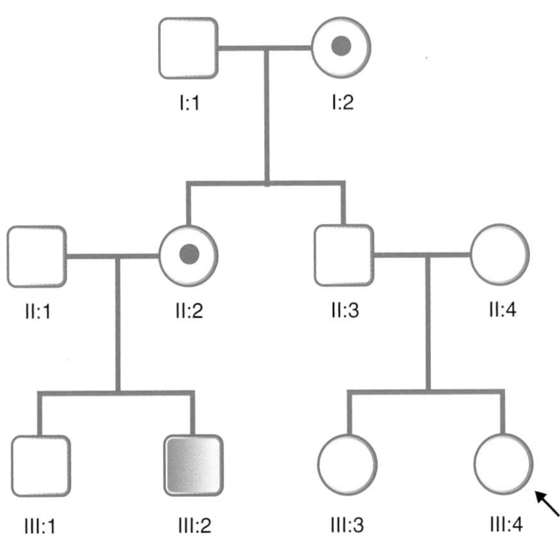


Fig. 10.4.1 Pedigree for Norrie disease (see Clinical example box).

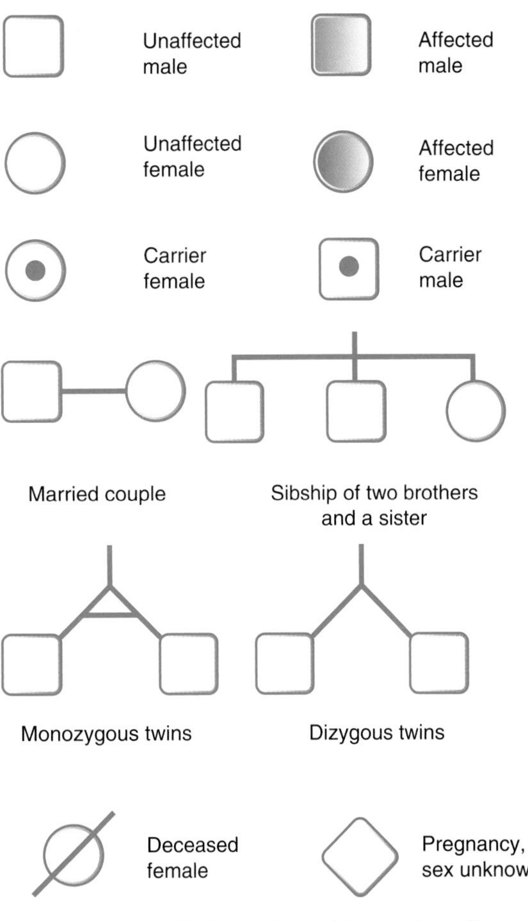


Fig. 10.4.2 Standard symbols used to record a pedigree.

The pedigree should consist of at least three generations. The individuals in each generation are recorded on a single horizontal line. The pedigree starts with the patient and their spouse(s) or partner(s) if any in the middle of the page. Next record their first-degree relatives (children, siblings and parents). Extend the pedigree to include second-degree relatives (nieces and nephews, aunts and uncles, grandparents and grandchildren). Ask systematically about each person, noting their names, dates of birth, dates of death and cause of death if applicable, and any relevant clinical information. Enquire specifically about miscarriages, stillbirths, reproductive problems and consanguinity – information that is not usually volunteered. Different shading or hatching patterns can be used to record the clinical features of each individual, in which case it is essential to include a key or legend with the pedigree. Examples of standard symbols used in pedigrees are provided in Fig. 10.4.2.

## Counselling for risk

Following diagnostic evaluation, an estimate of risk can be made. Risk is a numerical estimate of the likelihood of a particular disorder occurring in a current or future pregnancy.

### Risk in specific situations

#### Mendelian disorders

These are conditions that are autosomal dominant, autosomal recessive or X-linked. Some 6500 mendelian disorders have been described in humans. They are comprehensively catalogued in Online Mendelian Inheritance in Man (OMIM; http://www.ncbi.nlm.nih.gov/entrez/query.fcgi?db=OMIM). Where the disorder follows mendelian inheritance, risk calculation is based on the mode of inheritance and other factors, such as carrier testing. DNA testing has improved the precision of counselling in some cases.

**Clinical example**

Lara's brother James had recently had a child, Craig, who was diagnosed with cystic fibrosis by newborn screening. Lara and her partner Ivan were planning a family and sought advice about their risk of having a child with this condition. Based on a community carrier rate of 1 in 25, Lara and Ivan were informed that their risk was 1 in 200. Mutation testing of the *CFTR* gene revealed that Craig was homozygous for the p.F508del mutation, the commonest mutation that leads to cystic fibrosis. Lara was tested and was shown to carry this mutation. Ivan was then tested and was shown to carry another cystic fibrosis mutation, p.G551D. This meant that they had a 1 in 4 risk of having a child with cystic fibrosis and that it was possible for them to have prenatal or pre-implantation testing by DNA analysis for this condition.

#### Polygenic or multifactorial inheritance

There are many common disorders in which there is a genetic component and where the inheritance pattern cannot be explained simply in terms of mendelian inheritance or chromosomal rearrangement. It appears that these disorders are due to the cumulative action of a number of genes together with environmental influences. This is called polygenic or multifactorial inheritance, and numerically is the commonest pattern of inheritance responsible for the familial tendency or predisposition to various disorders. The recurrence risk of multifactorial disorders after a single affected child or with a single affected parent depends on the condition and can often be estimated from empirical data. The following are examples of conditions that generally follow multifactorial inheritance:

- congenital cardiac anomalies
- asthma
- neural tube defects, such as spina bifida and anencephaly
- coronary artery disease
- cleft lip and cleft palate
- congenital dislocation of the hip
- pyloric stenosis.

**Clinical example**

Tatiana and her partner Boris had a child with anencephaly, a neural tube defect. This is an invariably fatal condition where the skull and brain do not form fully. They sought counselling about the risk of recurrence and what could be done to avoid this, and to detect it if it did recur. They were informed that the risk of a neural tube defect (anencephaly, spina bifida, encephalocele) in Tatiana's next pregnancy was about 1 in 25. This risk could be reduced by Tatiana taking folate 5 mg daily for 3 months prior to conception and during the first 3 months of pregnancy. Tatiana and Boris were told that detailed expert ultrasonography at about 11 and 18 weeks' gestation are the best tests to detect a neural tube defect.

#### Unknown diagnosis

Of children presenting with intellectual disability or dysmorphic features, approximately half will not have a precise diagnosis. There is a large body of empirical data that can be used for counselling in this group. The only caveat is that appropriate examination and investigation should be done by an experienced clinician to exclude known disorders. Although an inability to label a child with a specific diagnosis is disappointing and frustrating for both parents and doctors, it should not disadvantage the affected child, as management can be based on periodic assessment and planning.

The evolution of knowledge and new techniques makes it necessary to look again at old problems. Thus, patient review is of the greatest importance. For example, when the underlying chromosomal fragile site in fragile X syndrome became recognized as a major cause of intellectual disability, many families required further study using new chromosome techniques. This process was repeated again using DNA studies when the triplet repeat abnormality was recognized as the cause. More recently, the advent of microarrays for diagnosing subtle chromosomal deletions and duplications has improved the diagnostic yield for individuals with intellectual disability and congenital anomalies from about 4% from a standard karyotype to about 10%.

### Interpretation of risk

Many families do not have a good grasp of probability, and careful discussion is needed to give meaning to any risk estimate. It is important to emphasize to families that chance has no memory. Simple illustrations and a concrete example such as tossing two coins are often helpful. Describing the risk in more than one way can also be helpful for some people. Thus, some may understand a 25% recurrence risk more readily than 1 in 4.

It can be helpful to put risk into the perspective of how their risk compares with that of other families. There is approximately a 1 in 30 risk that any child will be born with a major defect. This is the risk that any family either accepts or ignores, and is a useful point of comparison. Although genetic counselling does not aim to tell a person what to do, it is important for a counsellor to see that parents understand the meaning of any numbers used.

## From the nuclear to the extended family

Where a disorder is identified in a family that puts other family members at significant risk of either a problem themselves or of having a child with a problem, the extended family needs to be offered the opportunity to discuss this and have testing. An example of this is the clinical example of Lara and Ivan (above), where their risk of having a child with cystic fibrosis came to light only because a child was born in the family with this condition. This form of testing is called cascade testing. Examples of conditions where the extended family may be at risk are: a chromosome translocation, an autosomal dominant disorder such as Marfan syndrome, common recessive disorders such as cystic fibrosis and haemochromatosis, or sex-linked disorders such as Duchenne muscular dystrophy. Where members of the extended family need to be informed that there is a risk to them or their offspring of having a genetic disorder, a letter from the genetic specialist can be very helpful in conveying this sensitive information.

**Clinical example**

Fergus had symptoms of lethargy, joint pain and abdominal pain. Extensive medical evaluation eventually revealed that the underlying cause for this was iron overload due to hereditary haemochromatosis. He was shown to be homozygous for the common C282Y mutation in the *HFE* gene. Fergus had a brother, Patrick. Patrick was found to be C282Y-homozygous, and iron studies showed a moderately raised ferritin and transferrin saturation. He had had no symptoms referable to haemochromatosis. He had regular venesections to return his iron indices to normal. By doing this, Patrick was avoiding the risk of developing symptomatic haemochromatosis.

## Predictive testing

Predictive or pre-symptomatic testing is defined as a test on an asymptomatic person that allows that individual to know whether or not they will go on to develop the condition in question. The test may be genetic (e.g. testing for the CAG triplet repeat expansion in Huntington disease) or may involve other types of investigation (e.g. nerve conduction studies in an asymptomatic person at risk of Charcot–Marie–Tooth disease).

Predictive testing is available mainly for neurodegenerative diseases (e.g. Huntington disease, autosomal dominant spinocerebellar ataxia) and some cancers (familial breast/ovarian cancer, familial bowel cancer). It is conducted in the setting of a counselling protocol to give those undertaking the testing the opportunity to understand what a gene-positive or -negative result would mean for them. Where no preventative treatment is available (e.g. Huntington disease), the majority of those at risk choose not to be tested. Predictive testing for conditions where the onset is generally in adulthood and where no preventative treatment is available is not generally undertaken on minors for ethical reasons (when they grow up, they might not want to be tested), but minors might be tested ethically if there are treatment implications.

**Clinical example**

Sue and David were 12-year-old twins and had a 50% risk of having familial polyposis coli (FAP). FAP results in an affected individual having hundreds or thousands of bowel polyps, and, if untreated, invariably leads to malignant change in one or more polyps. Sue and David's mother, uncle and grandfather, as well as a number of other relatives, had FAP. The causative mutation in the *APC* gene in Sue and David's family was known. Because polyposis and malignant change may occur in the teens, it was recommended that surveillance by lower gastrointestinal tract endoscopy begin in the early teens. Sue and David underwent predictive testing. It was found that Sue did not have the familial mutation but David did. David was therefore recommended to have yearly colonoscopies, but Sue did not need them. Prior to the availability of molecular diagnosis, Sue would have had yearly colonoscopies until she reached her 30s before a confident diagnosis that she did not have FAP could be made.

## The burden

The burden of an actual or possible genetic diagnosis is of great importance in genetic counselling. This can be considered in two contexts: in prenatal diagnosis and diagnosis in a child. Where a diagnosis is made prenatally, the couple needs to be fully informed about the problems a child with that condition may face. This is to allow an informed decision about pregnancy termination, but it also allows couples who choose not to terminate the pregnancy to prepare for the child's birth. Where there is a strong family history of a condition, the couple may be well aware of the burden. An example is a pregnant woman who grew up with a brother with Duchenne muscular dystrophy, and who has prenatal testing that reveals that the male she is carrying has this condition. More difficult is where a diagnosis is made that was not specifically being looked for. An example is the diagnosis of Klinefelter syndrome (47,XXY) on a prenatal chromosome test done to look for Down syndrome. Here much time is often required to help the couple understand what that diagnosis will mean for their child and the rest of the family.

Similar issues exist where a child is diagnosed with a particular condition. For example, parents of a baby recently diagnosed as having cystic fibrosis or intellectual disability may have little idea of what lies ahead for the child and themselves. It is necessary to give parents an understanding of what is going to be involved in the care of the child, including the life expectancy, quality of life, treatment and variability that exist for that disorder. Just as importantly, it is vital that, in situations where the prognosis cannot be predicted, this uncertainty is conveyed to the parents. For instance, an individual with a mutation in one of the two tuberous sclerosis genes may present with severe epilepsy and profound intellectual disability, he or she may be unaffected or may have problems that fall between these two extremes.

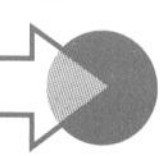

**Practical points**

- Accurate diagnosis is critical to enable the most accurate advice to be provided.
- Thorough assessment and investigation is essential to give the best chance of a specific diagnosis.
- All reproductive options should be discussed so individuals and couples can make an informed choice about the best option for them.
- Sensitivity to the emotional impact of genetic disease is critical and should be sought and addressed in all consultations.

## Alternatives for families at risk

Where a couple have a child or know they are at risk of having a child with a genetic condition, there are a number of reproductive options available to them. These include:

- childless lifestyle
- acceptance of risk
- adoption
- intrauterine diagnosis
- donor gametes
- donor embryo
- pre-implantation genetic diagnosis.

### Childless lifestyle

A family may choose not to have children where there is a risk of a genetic condition or where a child has been born with a genetic condition.

### Acceptance of risk

For some couples the risk of the disorder may be acceptable compared with the burden of other alternatives. This may relate to the perceived severity of the disorder. Thus, prenatal diagnosis is requested much more often when the disorder is fatal in childhood (e.g. Duchenne muscular dystrophy) than when it frequently leads to many years of health before its onset (e.g. Huntington disease) or where its severity is unpredictable and it is often relatively mild (e.g. neurofibromatosis type I). Religious and cultural factors may contribute to this decision.

### Adoption

The number of young babies available for adoption is very limited because of the increase in single-parent families and termination of pregnancies. Thus, adoption is much less common and less easily arranged than in the past.

### Intrauterine diagnosis

Intrauterine diagnosis provides an option for many couples. This can be offered to families who feel that termination of pregnancy is acceptable. The range of disorders that can be recognized by intrauterine diagnosis is constantly increasing (see Chapter 10.2).

### Donor gametes

Artificial insemination by donor (AID) is of limited appeal. Although many couples and ethnic groups find it unacceptable, couples should be informed about the option of AID to determine whether or not it is acceptable to them. AID can provide an alternative when the father has an autosomal dominant disorder, carries a chromosome translocation, or is a carrier for an autosomal recessive disorder.

*In vitro* fertilization (IVF) using donor ova can be offered when a woman is a carrier for an X-linked or autosomal recessive disorder, has an autosomal dominant disorder, carries a chromosome translocation, or has a mitochondrial DNA mutation. Parents may find this more acceptable, as the mother still experiences the pregnancy. However, this option is limited by the shortage of donor ova available.

### Donor embryo

Donor embryos are usually donated by couples who have utilized IVF and have stored residual embryos but do not require them as they have completed their family. Some couples prefer this to donor sperm or ova, because they feel uncomfortable about only one partner being genetically related to their offspring.

### Pre-implantation genetic diagnosis

In pre-implantation genetic diagnosis (PGD), cells from an embryo produced by IVF are tested for the disorder in question. This may be through DNA analysis or chromosome examination by fluorescence *in situ* hybridization (FISH). Only unaffected embryos are returned to the uterus. The advantage of PGD is that termination of pregnancy is not required. The disadvantages are that it is expensive, labour-intensive and often subject to long delays. For each cycle of IVF, the completed pregnancy rate is well below 50%, even in fertile couples.

## Emotional impact of genetic counselling

Patients often feel very vulnerable when referred for genetic counselling. This may be because of the recent birth of a child with a disability, a stillbirth or a neonatal death. People might be concerned about details of their family history and worry that they might be blamed for the problem that led them to seek genetic counselling. It is important to use sensitive language to avoid perpetuating feelings of guilt, shame and stigmatization. For example, a gene may be referred to as being 'changed' or 'altered', rather than 'bad' or 'faulty'. It is also important specifically to reassure couples that a genetic condition is not anyone's fault, and has not been caused by anything they have done before or during the pregnancy.

In counselling, the emotional impact of a birth defect or the risk of producing a child with a birth defect is explored carefully. People need an opportunity to vent their fears and anxieties. Discussions of emotional issues are of equal importance to discussions of risk, burden and alternatives. Families who have recently lost a child may need understanding and reassurance about the process of mourning, and may need to allow time before they are ready for a further pregnancy.

## Acknowledgements

We wish to thank Dr John Rogers for teaching us about the practice of genetic counselling. Dr Rogers was the author of this chapter in the first four editions of *Practical Paediatrics* and the current chapter draws much from that work.

# 10.5 Inborn errors of metabolism

David Coman, Jim McGill

Inborn errors of metabolism (IEM), or metabolic disorders, are clinical conditions that result from a block in one of the metabolic or biochemical pathways in the body. Although individually uncommon, collectively metabolic disorders are frequent. The main forms of presentation are:

- acute decompensations – at any age, usually triggered by an intercurrent illness or dietary changes
- neurodegeneration
- multisystem disorders with organ dysfunction.

IEM, particularly in those presenting acutely, remain underdiagnosed. Diagnostic clues such as:

- hypoglycaemia
- presence or inappropriate absence of ketosis
- metabolic acidosis (usually with a high anion gap)
- lactic acidosis
- respiratory alkalosis

are often overlooked or are misinterpreted as being due to a precipitating infection or dehydration. Investigations often have the highest yield during an acute decompensation. Rapid diagnosis and institution of appropriate therapy are essential to avoid death or permanent neurological damage.

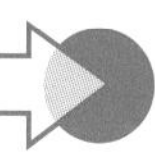

**Practical points**

- Inborn errors of metabolism, particularly those presenting acutely, remain significantly underdiagnosed.
- Presence of hypoglycaemia, presence or inappropriate absence of ketoacidosis, metabolic or lactic acidosis, or respiratory alkalosis should raise suspicion of a disorder of metabolism.
- In a child presenting acutely with a metabolic acidosis or hypoglycaemia, it is essential that the first urine passed is analysed for organic acids, as the diagnostic metabolites can clear quickly once intravenous glucose is given.
- Plasma ammonium values increase markedly if the specimen is allowed to sit around – collect the sample on ice and analyse it quickly.
- Abnormal liver function tests are not always indicative of hepatic pathology; for example, increased levels of aspartate and alanine aminotransferase (AST and ALT) occur in muscle disease also warranting the need to check creatine kinase levels.
- Pan-hypopituitarism can present in the neonatal period with hypoglycaemia plus conjugated hyperbilirubinaemia.



## Acute metabolic decompensation

Acute metabolic decompensations can occur at any age and are generally a result of either accumulation of a specific toxin or an energy deficiency or both.

### Neonatal presentations

Neonates have limited physiological repertoire to deal with stress, and an acutely unwell neonate with an IEM will look similar to that of other neonatal emergencies (e.g. sepsis, duct-dependent cardiac lesion). The placenta acts as an excellent filtration device, so the 'toxin accumulation' decompensations often occur at day 2–5 of life.

The following can act as clues to prompt consideration of an IEM in an acutely unwell neonate:

- Specific pattern of biochemical derangements (Table 10.5.1). (Note that ketosis in a neonate is always abnormal and must prompt consideration of an IEM)
- Multisystem organ involvement
- Specific end-organ involvement
  - hepatic failure
  - cardiomyopathy
  - seizures and aberrations in movement and tone (especially peripheral hypertonia combined with central hypotonia)
- Family history of neonatal deaths or sudden infant death syndrome
- Dietary triggers (e.g. galactose; see Table 10.5.1).

### Older children

Acute metabolic presentations in children beyond the neonatal period are normally precipitated by a viral illness associated with loss of appetite or vomiting. Ingestion of large amounts of protein or deliberately fasting (e.g. for surgery) can also precipitate an acute decompensation in some disorders. Protein aversion in a child warrants consideration of an IEM, especially a urea cycle defect or an organic aciduria.

#### Decreased conscious state

A decreased conscious state may be the result of:

- metabolic encephalopathy
- metabolic strokes

**Table 10.5.1 Biochemical approach to delineating an inborn error of metabolism in an acutely unwell neonate**

| Disease | pH | Ketones | Lactate | $NH_4$ | Glucose |
|---|---|---|---|---|---|
| Maple syrup urine disease | – | ++ | – | – | – |
| Organic acidurias | Acidosis | ++ | ↑/– | ↑/↑↑ | ↑↓ |
| Mitochondrial disorders | Acidosis | ++ | ↑↑ | –/↑ | ↑↓– |
| Urea cycle defects | Alkalosis | – | – | ↑↑ | – |
| Fatty acid oxidation defects | Acidosis | –/+ | ↑ | ↑ | ↓ |
| Seizures | – | – | – | – | – |

- hypoglycaemia
- hyperammonaemia
- aminoacidopathies (e.g. maple syrup urine disease).

## Hyperammonaemia

### Clinical example

Joseph was born at term to non-consanguineous parents. He fed well on the breast initially and was discharged to home on day 2 of life. On day 3 he was noted by his mother to be sleepy and feeding poorly. By that afternoon he could not be roused for feeds and he presented to the emergency department. He was afebrile and a septic workup was negative. Blood gases revealed a respiratory alkalosis and the alert paediatric registrar ordered a plasma ammonium, which was 830 mmol/L (normal <60). He was treated with peritoneal dialysis, sodium benzoate, sodium phenylbutyrate (alternative pathways to excrete nitrogen) and arginine, and his ammonium level gradually returned to normal. Plasma amino acid analysis showed high glutamine and low citrulline concentrations, and his urine was positive for orotic acid. DNA studies confirmed ornithine transcarbamylase deficiency, and testing showed his mother was a carrier.

Hyperammonaemia often causes a respiratory alkalosis. Findings and possible causes of hyperammonaemia may be:

- normal anion gap:
  - urea cycle disorders (e.g. ornithine transcarbamylase (OTC) deficiency)
  - lysinuric protein intolerance
  - transient hyperammonaemia of newborn (premature babies with respiratory distress)
- increased anion gap:
  - liver disease/failure
  - organic acidaemias (e.g. methylmalonic acidaemia, propionic acidaemia).

OTC deficiency is an X-linked disorder, so an extended family pedigree on the maternal side may be useful. Females heterozygous for the gene may be symptomatic. Children with milder or partial deficiencies of urea cycle enzymes, including some females who are heterozygous for OTC deficiency, present later in life, usually after a high protein intake or with catabolism with an intercurrent illness. Abdominal pain and vomiting are early symptoms.

## Hypoglycaemia

### Clinical example

Rebecca, aged 18 months, was noted to have a protuberant abdomen. She had hepatomegaly, but no splenomegaly. Liver function test results were normal. Four months later she was noted not to be using her left arm and further testing revealed a left hemiplegia. Investigations at that time revealed marked hyperlipidaemia and an appropriate diet was introduced. A further 5 months later, she presented acutely with anorexia due to an upper respiratory tract infection. She was tachypnoeic and sweating, but conscious. Her blood glucose level was 0.8 mmol/L and her bicarbonate level was 12 mmol/L (normal range 22–33) with a high anion gap. Further testing showed a lactate of 15.0 mmol/L (normal 0.7–2.5). With correction of the blood glucose, the lactate concentration returned to normal.

Glycogen storage disease was suspected and confirmed by a liver biopsy, which showed glycogen accumulation in the liver and a deficiency of glucose-6-phosphatase (glycogen storage disease type 1b). Hyperlipidaemia is a feature of this disorder. The brain can learn to use lactate as an alternate fuel and that is why Rebecca was conscious with such a low blood glucose value.

Hypoglycaemia is a common issue in general paediatrics; it is always abnormal in children, and must be investigated and managed promptly. See

Figures 10.5.1–10.5.3 for an overview of the practical approaches to refining a differential diagnosis of hypoglycaemia and an investigation pathway and the Practical points box on hypoglycaemia, below.

Tests to be collected at the time of hypoglycaemia are:

- Endocrine:
  - glucose
  - insulin
  - C-peptide
  - growth hormone
  - cortisol
  - adrenocorticotrophic hormone (ACTH)
- Metabolic:
  - acylcarnitine profile
  - lactate
  - ammonium
  - plasma amino acids
  - free fatty acids
  - ketones (β-hydroxybutyrate, acetoacetate)
  - urine organic acids.

## Metabolic acidosis (excluding lactic acidosis)

Common disorders in this group are methylmalonic, propionic and isovaleric acidaemias. The clinical signs in a child with a metabolic acidosis are non-specific; for example, the associated tachypnoea can be mistaken for respiratory disease. The metabolic acidosis has a high anion gap (metabolic acidosis plus normal anion gap can occur with renal tubular acidosis). Associated laboratory abnormalities can include neutropenia, thrombocytopenia, hypoglycaemia or hyperglycaemia, hypocalcaemia and hyperammonaemia. The diagnosis is reached by the examination of urine organic acids or plasma acylcarnitine profile, both of which are most likely to be diagnostic if the specimen is collected during the acute decompensation.

## Lactic acidosis

These patients have an energy deficiency. The main symptoms are due to the high anion gap acidosis. In neonates, ketosis is an important clue and increases

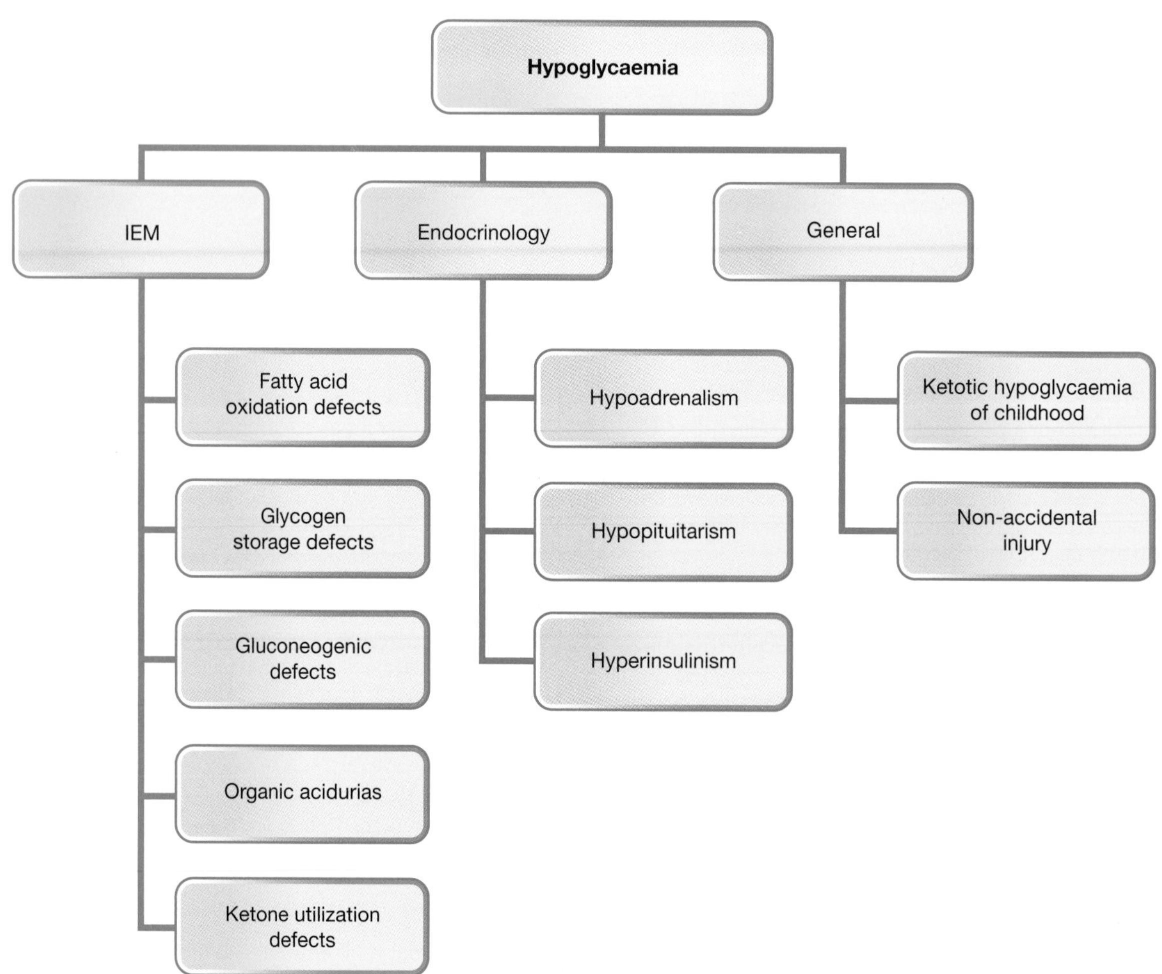


Fig. 10.5.1 Overview of differential diagnosis associated with paediatric hypoglycaemia.

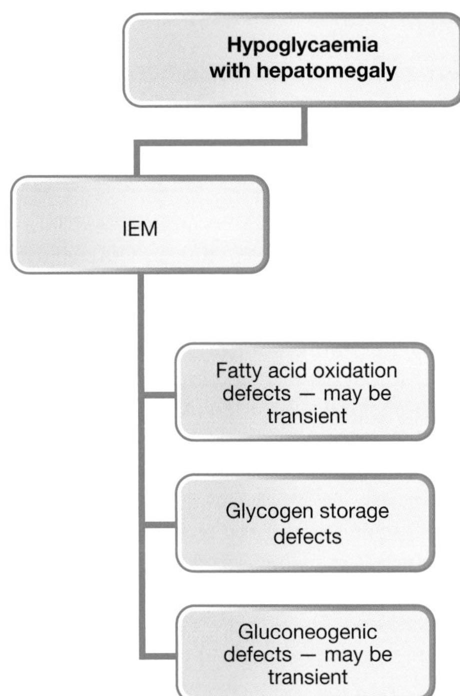


Fig. 10.5.2 Differential diagnoses of hypoglycaemia with hepatomegaly.

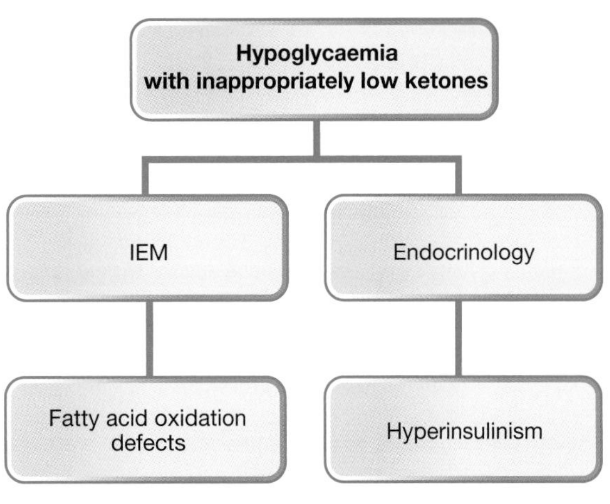


Fig. 10.5.3 Differential diagnoses of hypoglycaemia associated with inappropriately low ketone levels.

the likelihood of a metabolic disease as it is not usually present with hypoxia. Some of the disorders causing lactic acidosis have associated dysmorphic features and malformations. The most common cause for an acutely raised lactate concentration is poor perfusion, for example cardiac decompensation or sepsis (Fig. 10.5.4).

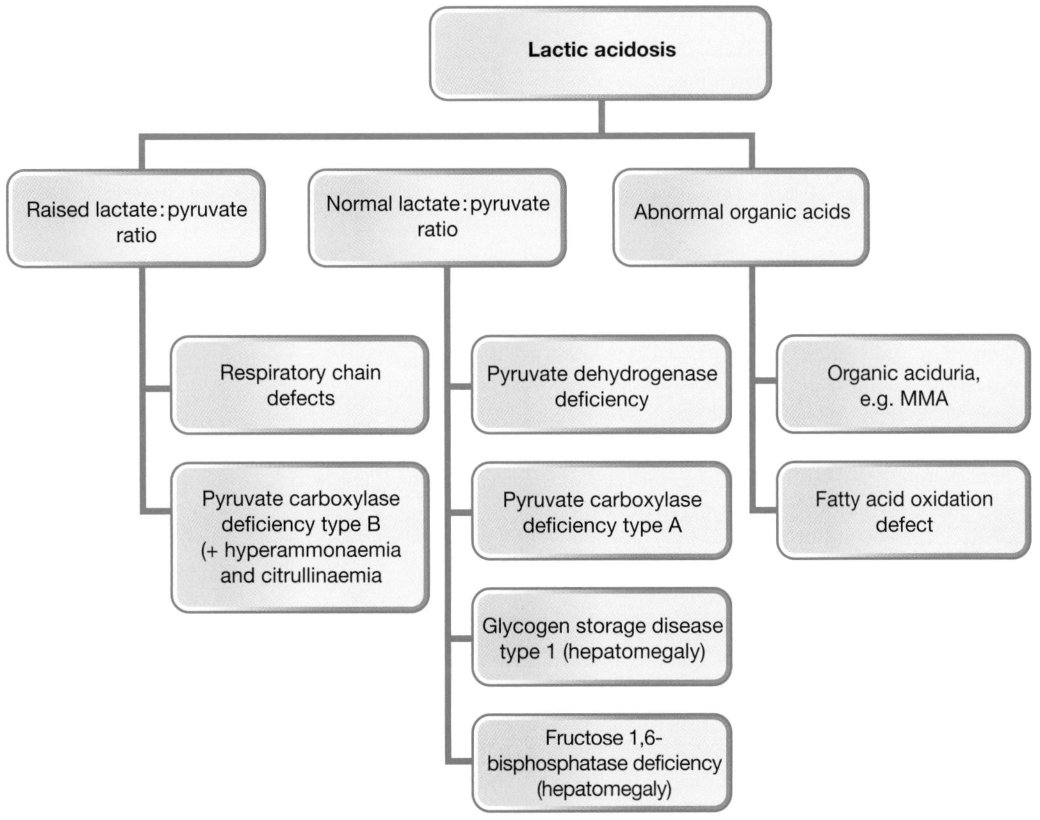


Fig. 10.5.4 Metabolic approach to lactic acidosis. MMA, methylmalonic aciduria.

**Clinical example**

A 2-year-old boy, Gareth, presented with a 2-day history of vomiting and diarrhoea. He had reduced consciousness and was tachypnoeic. Blood gas analysis revealed a compensated metabolic acidosis. His urine had large amounts of ketones on standard urine dipstick testing, and was positive for Phenistix, suggesting aspirin ingestion. His parents denied giving him aspirin but were not believed and were warned of the dangers of aspirin in children. The boy made a good recovery with intravenous fluids and was discharged. Six months later he re-presented after a more severe vomiting illness and was again acidotic with a pH of 7.1, and the anion gap was 28 mmol/L (normal range 4–13). He required ventilation in the intensive care unit, and after recovery was found to have dystonia. Magnetic resonance imaging of his brain showed basal ganglia changes. Urine organic acids showed large amounts of methylmalonic acid. Gareth was not responsive to vitamin $B_{12}$ injections. The positive Phenistix was due to methylmalonic acid, not aspirin. An opportunity had been lost to diagnose methylmalonic aciduria before it caused permanent disability.

### Seizures

Seizures are common in metabolic conditions, especially neonatal seizures. The most common disorders in the group are non-ketotic hyperglycinaemia (diagnosed by a raised cerebrospinal fluid (CSF) : plasma glycine ratio), sulphite oxidase deficiency (diagnosed by urine metabolic screen), disorders of the mitochondrial respiratory chain and peroxisomal disorders (diagnosed by plasma very long-chain fatty acids and phytanic acid). This last group is usually dysmorphic and hypotonic.

Defects in pyridoxine metabolism are an important differential diagnosis in the neonate with seizures. Diagnostic clues to the precise block in pyridoxine metabolism can be elucidated from CSF neurotransmitters and urine α-aminoadipic semi-aldehyde measurements. A trial of pyridoxine and pyridoxal phosphate should not be withheld while awaiting these results. The classical story of the EEG findings and seizures ceasing after administration of pyridoxine is not universal in these conditions.

Glucose transporter 1 deficiency is an important consideration in children with seizures, as it causes reduced transport of glucose across the blood–brain barrier. It is diagnosed by a low CSF : plasma glucose ratio. A ketogenic diet is very effective in controlling the seizures in this disorder. Milder forms of this condition can present with dystonia alone.

Metabolic disorders can cause underlying structural brain malformations as part of their phenotype, for example the peroxisomal biogenesis defects.

### Treatment

The basis of treatment in the disorders of fat and protein metabolism is to reverse the catabolism. This is usually achieved by intravenous 10–20% dextrose with maintenance salts. Sometimes it is necessary to remove the toxins by dialysis or haemoperfusion. Many of the enzymes have vitamin co-factors, and in a small proportion pharmacological doses of the vitamin can overcome the defect (e.g. vitamin $B_{12}$ for methylmalonic acidaemia and biotin for biotinidase deficiency). A secondary carnitine deficiency may develop in many of these disorders and correction of that is essential.

In the long term, disorders of protein metabolism require a low protein diet supplemented by amino acid formulas lacking the amino acid or acids that accumulate proximal to the block and boosted in those amino acids that are deficient distal to the block.

High-glucose infusions may exacerbate disorders of the mitochondrial respiratory chain and pyruvate dehydrogenase deficiency. In these disorders, a high proportion of calories needs to come from fats.

## Diagnosis and genetics

The greatest impediment to diagnosing an IEM is simply not thinking of them in the first place. Collection of appropriate samples during an acute decompensation can hone a diagnosis rapidly (e.g. urine organic acids, plasma acylcarnitine profiles and amino acids). A secure formal diagnosis relies on biochemical clues, but also confirmation at the enzymatic and molecular level. This can be important for accurate genetic counselling for the family. IEM exhibit all modes of genetic transmission, with autosomal recessive being the most common.

## Neurodegeneration

Metabolic disorders are high in the differential diagnosis for children who have a loss of acquired skills following a period of normal development. This is termed regression and the disorders causing it are termed neurodegenerative disorders. Seizures are a frequent associated symptom. Lysosomal storage disorders, peroxisomal disorders and disorders of the mitochondrial respiratory chain can all be associated with neurodegeneration.

## Multisystem disease (Table 10.5.2)

### Lysosomal storage disorders

In these children, the lack of one of the lysosomal enzymes results in the accumulation of the substrate in a variety of tissues. Presenting features include

**Table 10.5.2 Clinical clues prompting consideration of an inborn error of metabolism**

| Clinical feature | Common metabolic causes |
|---|---|
| Cataract | Galactosaemia, galactokinase deficiency, peroxisomal disorders, CDG, pentose pathway defects |
| Dislocated lenses | Homocystinuria, sulphite oxidase deficiency |
| Eye movement disorders | Upward gaze palsy: Gaucher disease, Neimann–Pick disease type C<br>Rotatory nystagmus: Pelizaeus–Merzbacher disease |
| Retinal haemorrhages | Glutaric aciduria type 1 |
| Retinitis pigmentosa | Peroxisomal disorders, NARP, CDG, lysosomal storage defects (especially Batten disease) |
| Cherry red spots | Multiple lysosomal storage diseases |
| Optic atrophy | Panhypopituitarism, mitochondrial respiratory chain defects, organic acidurias |
| Cardiomyopathy | Respiratory chain disorders, CDG, carnitine deficiency, disorders of fatty acid oxidation, Pompe disease, glycogen storage disease, lysosomal storage disease (especially Danon disease), organic acidurias |
| Cardiac arrhythmias | Fatty acid oxidation defects, Pompe disease, Danon disease |
| Strokes | Homocystinuria, CDG, MELAS |
| Movement disorders | Mitochondrial respiratory chain, neurotransmitter disorders, purine and pyrimidine defects, glutaric aciduria type I, iron metabolism defects |
| Brain malformations | Perisylvian polymicrogyria: mitochondrial respiratory chain defects, peroxisomal biogenesis defects<br>Lissencephaly: peroxisomal biogenesis defects, O-glycosylation defects<br>Enlarged sylvian fissures: glutaric aciduria type 1<br>Cerebellar atrophy/hypoplasia: CDG<br>Midline defects: cholesterol biosynthesis defects<br>White matter abnormalities: mitochondrial respiratory chain defects, cerebral organic acidurias, lysosomal disorders<br>Cerebral cysts: cerebral organic acidurias |
| Macrocephaly | Glutaric aciduria, cerebral organic acidurias |
| Microcephaly | Multiple causes |
| Myopathy | Respiratory chain disorders, disorders of fatty acid oxidation, Pompe disease, glycogen storage disease, lysosomal storage disease, channelopathies |
| Behaviour/psychiatry | Autism: purine and pyrimidine defects (Lesh–Nyhan syndrome), cholesterol biosynthesis defects<br>Attention-deficit/hyperactivity disorder: MPSIII<br>Self-mutilation: purine and pyrimidine defects (Lesh–Nyhan syndrome) |
| Liver failure | Galactosaemia, hereditary fructose intolerance, tyrosinaemia type 1, mitochondrial respiratory chain disorders, neonatal haemochromatosis, bile acid synthesis defects, pentose pathway defects, CDG |
| Obstructive jaundice | Panhypopituitarism, peroxisomal disorders, $\alpha_1$-antitrypsin deficiency, bile acid synthesis defects, lysosomal storage disorders (especially Niemann–Pick disease type C), CDG |
| Intestine | Protein-losing enteropathy: CDG<br>Diarrhoea: neurotransmitter defects<br>Motility disorders: mitochondrial defects |
| Respiration and sleep | Respiratory failure: Pompe disease<br>Interstitial lung disease: lysosomal storage diseases<br>Disturbed sleep: MPSIII |
| Immune deficiencies | Congenital disorders of glycosylation |

**Table 10.5.2 Clinical clues prompting consideration of an inborn error of metabolism—Cont'd**

| Clinical feature | Common metabolic causes |
|---|---|
| Renal cysts | Glutaric aciduria II, CDG, peroxisomal disorders, CPT-II |
| Dysmorphic face | Smith–Lemli–Opitz syndrome, peroxisomal disorders, CDG |
| Skin | Ichthyosis: peroxisomal biogenesis defect, cholesterol biosynthesis defect<br>Gaucher disease: collodian baby<br>Acrodermatitis enteropathicia: zinc deficiency, biotinidase deficiency<br>Fungal infections: organic acidurias (T-cell dysfunction) |
| Abnormal hair | Menke syndrome, argininosuccinic aciduria, CDG, biotinidase deficiency (alopecia) |

CDG, congenital disorders of glycosylation; CPT-II, carnitine palmitoyltransferase II; MELAS, mitochondrial encephalomyopathy, lactic acidosis and stroke-like episodes; MPSIII, mucopolysaccharidosis III; NARP, neuropathy, ataxia and retinitis pigmentosa.

developmental regression, hepatomegaly, splenomegaly, coarse facial features, corneal clouding and skeletal involvement (dysostosis multiplex). Not all types have central nervous system (CNS) involvement. Storage bodies may be seen in white blood cells on a blood film. Diagnosis is made by urine screens for mucopolysaccharides and oligosaccharides and confirmed by white cell, plasma or fibroblast lysosomal enzyme analysis.

Enzyme replacement therapy (ERT) is already commercially available for Gaucher disease types I and III, Fabry disease, mucopolysaccharidoses types I, II and VI, and Pompe disease (glycogen storage disease type II). The ERT does not effectively cross the blood–brain barrier and so disorders that involve the CNS need different approaches (intrathecal injections of the enzymes are being trialled).

Cord blood stem cell transplantation is an effective treatment for several lysosomal disorders with CNS involvement. The outcome depends on the neurological status at the time of transplant. The transplanted cells can cross the blood–brain barrier and can therefore stabilize brain pathology. Substrate inhibition therapy is also being trialled for disorders with CNS involvement.

## Mitochondrial respiratory chain disorders

Tissues that most depend on mitochondrial adenosine triphosphate (ATP) production, such as brain, skeletal muscle and heart, are more frequently affected in disorders of the mitochondrial respiratory chain, but the clinical presentations are vast and can occur in any organ at any age. Common presentations in childhood include seizures, developmental delay, regression, strokes, lactic acidosis, myopathy, endocrine disorders, cardiomyopathy, liver failure, renal disorders, ophthalmoplegia, retinitis pigmentosa and deafness. There are mitochondrial mutations that predispose to aminoglycoside toxicity, and many of the patients who developed liver failure after sodium valproate therapy had a mitochondrial disease.

The diagnosis should be suspected in any child with a combination of symptoms, particularly if they are unrelated (e.g. CNS and liver disease or renal tubular acidosis and a neurodegenerative disease). The basal ganglia are often seen to be involved on magnetic resonance imaging (MRI) and are a useful marker for this group of disorders.

Mitochondria have their own DNA and mitochondria are inherited from the mother via the egg (maternal inheritance). Some mitochondrial diseases are inherited as mutations in the mitochondrial DNA, for example MELAS (mitochondrial encephalopathy, lactic acidosis and stroke-like episodes), MERRF (myoclonic epilepsy and ragged red fibres), NARP (neurogenic muscle weakness, ataxia and retinitis pigmentosa) and Leigh disease. Others, such as complex IV and polymerase γ (POLG) deficiencies (mitochondrial depletion syndrome), are inherited from nuclear genes, mainly autosomal recessive. The latter form of inheritance is more common in childhood.

The diagnosis of mitochondrial diseases is difficult. Screening tests include raised lactate levels in the blood or CSF, and histological changes on muscle biopsy including ragged red fibres. Mutations in nuclear genes are more common than mutations of mitochondrial DNA in affected children and may be present only in some tissues, such as muscle. Enzyme complexes of the respiratory chain can be measured in muscle, liver or skin, and may be tissue-specific. It is important to realize that, at present, there is no test that can exclude a disorder of the mitochondrial respiratory chain.

A 'cocktail' of co-factors of the mitochondrial respiratory chain, including coenzyme Q10, thiamine, riboflavin, vitamin C and vitamin K, are usually trialled but are not often of significant benefit in the majority of patients.

## Congenital disorders of glycosylation

Glycoproteins are proteins that require the attachment of specific carbohydrate residues for their function, protein folding, signalling pathways. and receptor and cell membrane integrity. Glycosylation is a biochemical process called post-translational modification, and many new disorders wait to be discovered in this field over time. Clinical presentations include multiorgan failure, neuropathies, strabismus, dysmorphic features (facial changes, inverted nipples, fat pads), coagulation disorders, cardiomyopathy, ataxia, psychomotor retardation, stroke-like episodes, gastrointestinal symptoms and hormonal disorders. Cerebellar hypoplasia is found on cerebral imaging in the common type 1a form. Recently, mild forms have been identified in individuals who are able to participate in the open workforce.

Transferrin isoforms is an easily accessible screening tool for these disorders, but a negative test result does not exclude them. A formal diagnosis is confirmed by enzyme analysis or DNA techniques. Therapy is symptomatic for most forms. Mannose has been successful in the treatment of type 1b.

### Peroxisomal disorders

Peroxisomes are subcellular organelles involved in the metabolism of many compounds including very long-chain fatty acids, phytanic acid, ether lipids and bile acids. Disorders in this pathway often involve assembly problems and therefore affect all the enzymes that normally function within the peroxisomes. Children with these biogenesis defects usually present in infancy. Profound hypotonia is a common problem but other features include seizures, cataracts, retinitis pigmentosa, liver disease, renal cysts and dysfunction, and dysmorphic features.

X-linked adrenoleukodystrophy (XALD) is the most common peroxisomal disorder in older children. It usually presents at 4–10 years of age with behavioural disturbances, motor problems, regression and adrenal insufficiency. It is rapidly progressive over a few years. A milder disorder of the same gene, adrenomyeloneuropathy (AMN), occurs later in life with spasticity and peripheral neuropathy as well as adrenal insufficiency. The adrenal insufficiency, Addison disease, may be the only symptom in some males. The different forms can all occur within the one family. Bone marrow or stem cell transplantation remains the treatment of choice for XALD. The role of Lorenzo's oil in the treatment of this group of disorders remains unclear.

## Newborn screening

Newborn screening is performed from a blood sample collected on to blotting paper at 2–3 days of age. Tests are performed to identify disorders that are difficult to recognize clinically and for which early treatment is beneficial. The first and most successful disorder so diagnosed is phenylketonuria (PKU). Prior to newborn screening, children with PKU were not diagnosed until they presented in childhood with intellectual impairment. With treatment in the neonatal period, intelligence is normal.

All Australian states and New Zealand screen for PKU, cystic fibrosis and hypothyroidism, and most screen for galactosaemia. A new form of screening based on tandem mass spectroscopy has commenced in Australia and New Zealand that allows the diagnosis of organic acidaemias (e.g. methylmalonic acidaemia), aminoacidopathies (e.g. maple syrup urine disease) and disorders of fatty acid oxidation (e.g. medium-chain acyl-CoA dehydrogenase deficiency; MCAD) in addition to the above disorders. Lysosomal storage disorders and congenital adrenal hyperplasia are also likely to be added to newborn screening protocols in the near future.

## Peri-mortem protocol

If the possibility of a metabolic disorder is considered in an infant or child who has a terminal condition, it is important to arrange to collect appropriate samples either before or as soon as possible after death (within 1–2 hours, but the sooner the better). This should be discussed with the parents before death (see Chapter 10.4) and the parents must be allowed some time with their child after death before the procedure occurs.

Samples of blood (plasma and serum), CSF and urine should be collected and frozen. Muscle, liver, skin for fibroblast culture and, if indicated, heart tissue should be collected.

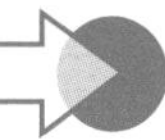

## Practical points

**Hypoglycaemia**

- Ketones are normal in a child with vomiting or starvation from other causes. Their presence in less than expected amounts is abnormal and warrants further investigation, especially considering a fatty acid oxidation defect or hyperinsulinism.
- Glucometers are often unreliable for measuring hypoglycaemia; all children in whom there is a suspicion of hypoglycaemia should have it confirmed by a formal blood glucose measurement.
- The time elapsed from the last meal to the development of hypoglycaemia is an essential aspect of the history and fashions the differential diagnosis list; for example, hypoglycaemia 4 hours after a meal in a 2-year-old infant would prompt consideration of a glycogen storage disease, whereas hypoglycaemia after 24 hours of fasting in a 2-year-old child is more likely to be ketotic hypoglycaemia of childhood.
- Hyperinsulinism creates a voracious glucose requirement to maintain glucose homeostasis at greater than 10 mg/kg/min (normal value usually 3–4 mg/kg/min), and is uncommon outside the neonatal period.
- Beyond the neonatal period, plasma cortisol and urine organic acids at the time of hypoglycaemia are the most useful diagnostic tests.
- Ketotic hypoglycaemia of childhood is a common self-limiting condition (usually 6–8 years of age) of uncertain aetiology, but is a diagnosis of exclusion. Every child with this diagnosis requires an appropriate unwell management plan to maintain glucose homeostasis during intercurrent illness.

## Clinical example

A 3-year-old girl, Roberta, presented to a general paediatrician because her mother was concerned about her gait. She had seen another paediatrician when she was aged 18 months. At that time an ataxic, broad-based gait had been noted but no cause had been found. Her gait had deteriorated and was associated with poor muscle bulk and low tone. There were no fasciculations. MRI showed changes in the basal ganglia and posterior white matter. Her plasma lactate level was 4.2 mmol/L (normal range 0.7–2.5), CSF lactate was 4 mmol/L (normal 0.7–2.5) and the lactate : pyruvate ratio was 24 (10–16).

A disorder of the mitochondrial respiratory chain was confirmed by muscle and liver biopsies, which showed low complex IV activity. By the age of 3½ years Rebecca was unable to walk or crawl and was having swallowing difficulties. Following placement of a gastrostomy allowing improved nutrition, she became stronger but still could not walk.

PART 11

# NEONATAL PROBLEMS

# 11.1 The newborn infant: stabilization and examination

Brian Darlow

Dr Neil Campbell began this Chapter in the fifth edition of this book, thus:

> 'Most babies are born at term gestation (37–42 weeks), following normal pregnancy and labour, and are healthy. Having a baby is for most people one of life's most joyous and enriching experiences. Health professionals should keep these matters in mind and be as unobtrusive as possible with medical interventions, remembering we are, in a way, privileged to share in this special experience.'

## Introduction

Currently, annually, there are approximately 295 000 babies born in Australia and 64 000 born in New Zealand. In both countries the average age of a mother having her first baby has been increasing in recent years and is now around 30 years. Approximately 92% of all births are at term (at least 37 completed weeks of gestation). Around 25% of all births are now by caesarean section, although in many other countries this figure is much lower.

It is worth being aware that the outcome from pregnancy in developed countries does not always conform to parental expectations:

- around 1 in 5 pregnancies ends in an early miscarriage
- about 6%–8% of infants are born preterm (less than 37 completed weeks)
- 1% of infants still die around the time of birth
- up to 5% of infants will have some form of birth defect.

## Neonatal transition

Much of the adaptation of the fetus to life *ex utero* takes place over a few days and may bring to light congenital disorders. If the process is disrupted, serious disease may result.

### Circulation

*In utero* there is high pulmonary vascular resistance such that only 10–15% of the cardiac output goes through the pulmonary circulation. Most of the cardiac output bypasses the lungs by flowing right-to-left across the foramen ovale or through the ductus arteriosus (Fig. 11.1.1). With the infant's first breath the pulmonary vascular resistance falls and blood flows to the lungs; with cord clamping the peripheral vascular resistance rises and the foramen ovale is kept shut; and with the rise in partial pressure of oxygen ($P_ao_2$) and withdrawal of prostaglandins produced by the fetoplacental unit, the ductus closes. In some babies with persistent pulmonary hypertension, these changes do not occur and there continues to be a right-to-left shunt at the atrium and ductus. Such infants are tachypnoeic and remain cyanosed.

### Respiration

The fetal lungs are filled with fluid that has been secreted by the pulmonary epithelium. There is a net outward movement of this fluid into the amniotic fluid with breathing movements during fetal life. Hormonal changes, including a rise in catecholamines, occurring with the onset of labour, lead to the reabsorption of some of this fluid from the alveolar sacs. Most remaining fluid is squeezed out of the lungs during passage of the chest through the birth canal (and can be seen as clear fluid around the nose and mouth at birth). With normal chest recoil the infant's lungs fill with air, surfactant is released from the type II pneumocytes, lowering surface tension in the alveoli, and the residual lung volume is established with the first few breaths. Infants born by caesarean section, prior to labour, are more likely to have retained lung fluid (transient tachypnoea of the newborn; see Chapter 11.3).

### Temperature control

Newborn infants have a larger surface area compared to their weight than do adults and can become cold rapidly. They are wet at birth and lose heat through water evaporation, as well as via radiation, conduction and convection if not clothed. After birth, hormonal changes lead to heat production from non-shivering thermogenesis in the brown adipose tissue. Core temperature is normally maintained at 36.5–37°C. Hypothermia will increase oxygen consumption

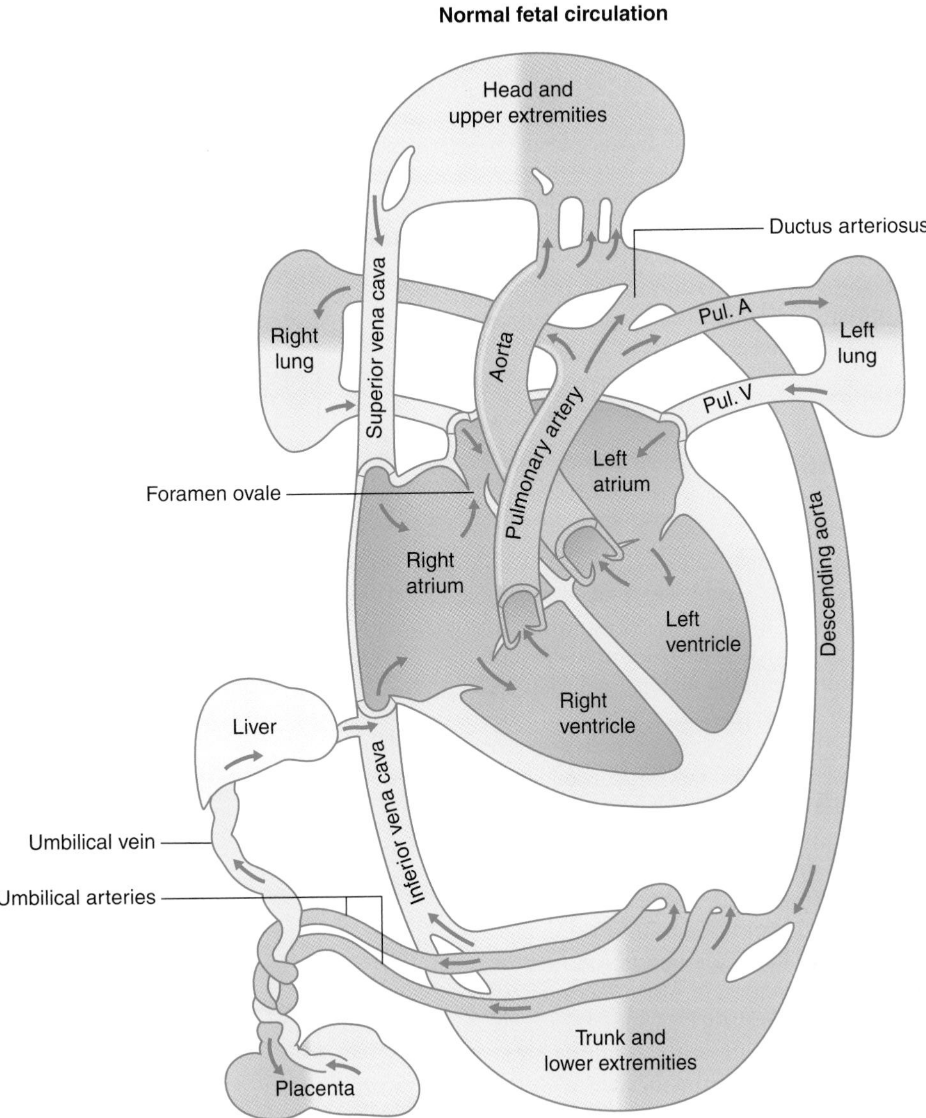


Fig. 11.1.1 The normal fetal circulation. Pul. A, pulmonary artery; Pul.V, pulmonary vein.

required for basal metabolism and is a not uncommon cause of tachypnoea (see Chapter 11.3). Hypothermia may also occur in conditions such as sepsis.

## Metabolism

The fetus is dependent on the maternal supply of glucose via the placenta, and glycogen stores are laid down in the liver, muscle and heart as gestation increases. At birth the maternal glucose supply ceases and the infant's glucose levels fall over the next 1–2 hours before hormonal mechanisms bring about a rise from mobilized stores. Infants who have delay in feeding, preterm, growth retarded and sick infants, as well as infants of diabetic mothers, are all at increased risk of significant hypoglycaemia (see Chapter 11.2).

## Fluid balance

Fetal urine contributes significantly to the amniotic fluid volume. The fetal urine is dilute and the placenta is responsible for fluid and electrolyte haemostasis. After birth a transition is made to water and salt conservation by the kidneys. In the first 2–3 days there is a negative sodium and fluid balance, contributing to much of the infant's weight loss, as well as a shift in fluid from the extracellular to the intracellular compartments.

## Gastrointestinal

The fetus swallows amniotic fluid, which is rich in growth factors. After birth, coordination of sucking and swallowing is readily established on day 1, and healthy term infants demand to feed from the breast eight or more times a day. Meconium should be passed by all infants by 48 hours of age. Before birth, unconjugated bilirubin is excreted by the placenta. During the transition to hepatic conjugation and excretion of bilirubin, all infants have raised serum bilirubin levels to some degree (see Chapter 11.2). All newborn infants have low levels of vitamin K-dependent clotting factors. Intrinsic vitamin K production follows bacterial colonization of the gut. This occurs in the first few days, but the vitamin K deficiency state carries with it a risk of haemorrhage (see below).

## Neonatal stabilization and resuscitation

More than 5 million neonatal deaths occur worldwide every year, with the World Health Organization estimating that 19% of these are from birth asphyxia. In developing countries, nearly 1 in 4 infants who fail to initiate and sustain breathing at birth will die, yet easily acquired skills and simple equipment can help the majority of these babies.

It is estimated that 5–10% of newborns need some stimulation to breathe at birth. However, population-based surveys in developed countries suggest only 1–2% of term or near-term infants need active resuscitation with inflation breaths from a bag and mask. Only 20% of these (2 per 1000 births) progress to intubation.

Resuscitation of the newborn infant follows the same principles as resuscitation at other times (A, B, C, D: Airway, Breathing, Cardiac, Drugs). At the same time there are important differences resulting from the unique physiological changes associated with the infant's transition from *in utero* to *ex utero* existence, as well as pathological states presenting at birth. In most cases it is better to talk of neonatal stabilization rather than resuscitation, and delayed onset of respiration rather than birth asphyxia.

Advanced resuscitation skills can be learned readily with the aid of mannequins and teaching scenarios. There are a number of different neonatal resuscitation guidelines and courses. Because neonatal resuscitation demands a team approach, it is essential to be familiar with local equipment and protocols.

Animal experiments carried out in the 1960s looked at the effects of acute, total asphyxia on heart rate (HR) and breathing (Fig. 11.1.2). At delivery by caesarean section (simply to control the situation), air breathing was prevented totally by occlusion of the airway. There was an initial period of gasping followed by cessation of breathing (*primary apnoea*), then a further period of gasping and finally no breathing (*terminal apnoea*).

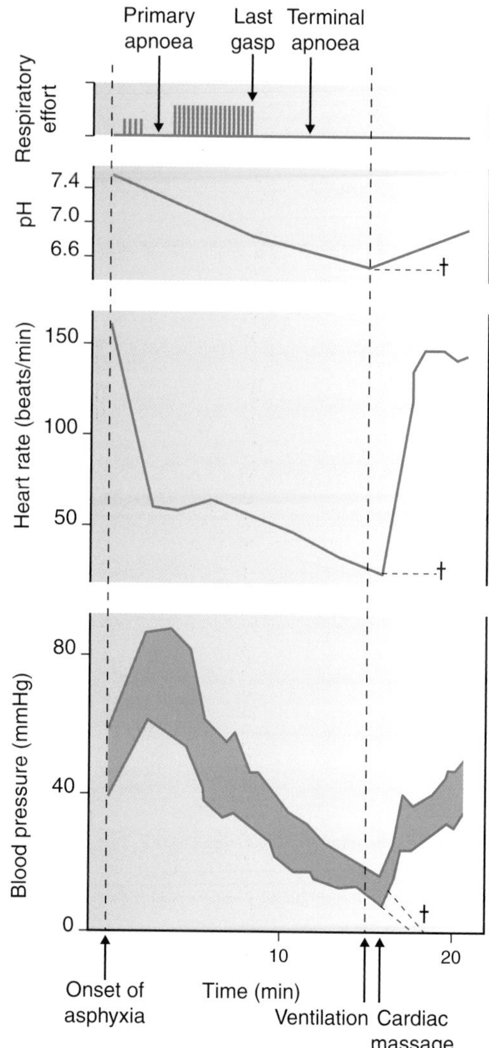


Fig. 11.1.2 Physiological changes after acute asphyxia in a newborn monkey.

Primary apnoea usually lasted for 1–2 min, with HR maintained at 80–120 bpm. It could be prolonged by commonly used obstetric analgesic or anaesthetic agents. Simple tactile stimulation shortened the time to further gasping. In terminal apnoea, the time from the start of active resuscitation (ventilation) to further gasping and regular breathing reflected the degree of acidosis from asphyxia.

In the human situation there is always a chance acute total asphyxia may occur, although it is uncommon, for example with shoulder dystocia and a tight cord around the neck (nuchal cord), placental abruption or cord accidents. However, most peripartum hypoxia is in the context of prolonged, partial insults, and many of these can be predicted by the obstetric situation and fetal monitoring. At birth, most such infants will not have progressed to terminal apnoea and will respond promptly to resuscitation.

Because the extent of the asphyxial insult will be reflected by the pH and lactate in the arterial cord blood, resulting from anaerobic metabolism, a segment of cord can be clamped at each end and sampled up to 20 min later.

## Apgar scores

Since the 1950s the Apgar score (Table 11.1.1) has been used to assess the infant's condition at birth and to differentiate those who are vigorous or depressed. Many health jurisdictions require the Apgar score at 1 and 5 minutes to be recorded.

**Historical note**

Virginia Apgar was an American obstetric anaesthetist. Her score, based on the five signs typically used by anaesthetists to monitor their patients, was first published in 1953 as a method of assessing the effect of obstetrical and maternal anaesthetic management on the newborn.

There are many problems with the Apgar score:

- Different observers will record slightly different scores.
- There are clearly many routes to a score of 5 or 6 (for example), and both this and the infant's condition should be fully described.
- Vigorous infants should not be suctioned (as this may lead to vagus-induced bradycardia or even vocal cord occlusion) and so a score of 2 is awarded for 'reflex irritability' by inference. Such infants will all have scores of 9–10.
- The score is much less satisfactory in very preterm or ventilated infants.
- For an individual infant there is little correlation between the Apgar score and pH or lactate values, and unfortunately neither is good at predicting the long-term outcome.

However, the 1-minute Apgar, if low, does indicate the need for stimulation, and the 5-minute Apgar indicates the response to earlier resuscitation.

### Which births to attend?

All births do need someone capable of looking after the mother and a separate person capable of looking after the infant. Anyone involved in the practice of childbirth has a duty to be competent in neonatal resuscitation and a responsibility to see that the appropriate equipment is available and in working order.

Resuscitators should become familiar with their equipment, or that provided in the health facility in which they practise. The main tools to deliver positive pressure ventilation, short of intubation, are self-inflating bags (Laerdal) or T-piece resuscitators (Neopuff), and appropriately sized face masks. The wearing of gloves is recommended.

### Basic care and stabilization (Fig. 11.1.3)

- Check the maternal and obstetric history.
- Anticipate problems.
- Check the equipment: infant overhead warmer, air and oxygen supply, suction apparatus, self-inflating bag and appropriately sized masks and/or pressure device and T-piece, intubation equipment, umbilical catheter, drugs.
- Start stopwatch when infant's body is free from the mother.
- Assess the infant rapidly, particularly tone, breathing and HR (use stethoscope on chest):

1. *The infant is vigorous and crying.* Leave alone (but dry and wrap, or place in skin to skin contact with mother).
2. *Infant cyanosed, irregular respirations, HR > 100.* Gentle stimulation, check head in neutral position (avoid neck flexion and hyperextension) to open the airway, gentle oropharyngeal suction if obvious obstruction. Most respond.

**Table 11.1.1 The Apgar score**

| | Score | | |
|---|---|---|---|
| | 0 | 1 | 2 |
| **A** Appearance (colour) | Pale or blue | Body pink, extremities blue | Pink |
| **P** Pulse rate | Absent | <100 | >100 |
| **G** Grimace (reflex irritability – the response to nasal suction) | None | Some, e.g. grimace | Vigorous, cry |
| **A** Activity (tone) | Floppy | Some flexion | Good flexion |
| **R** Respiratory rate | Apnoeic | Irregular, weak | Active crying |

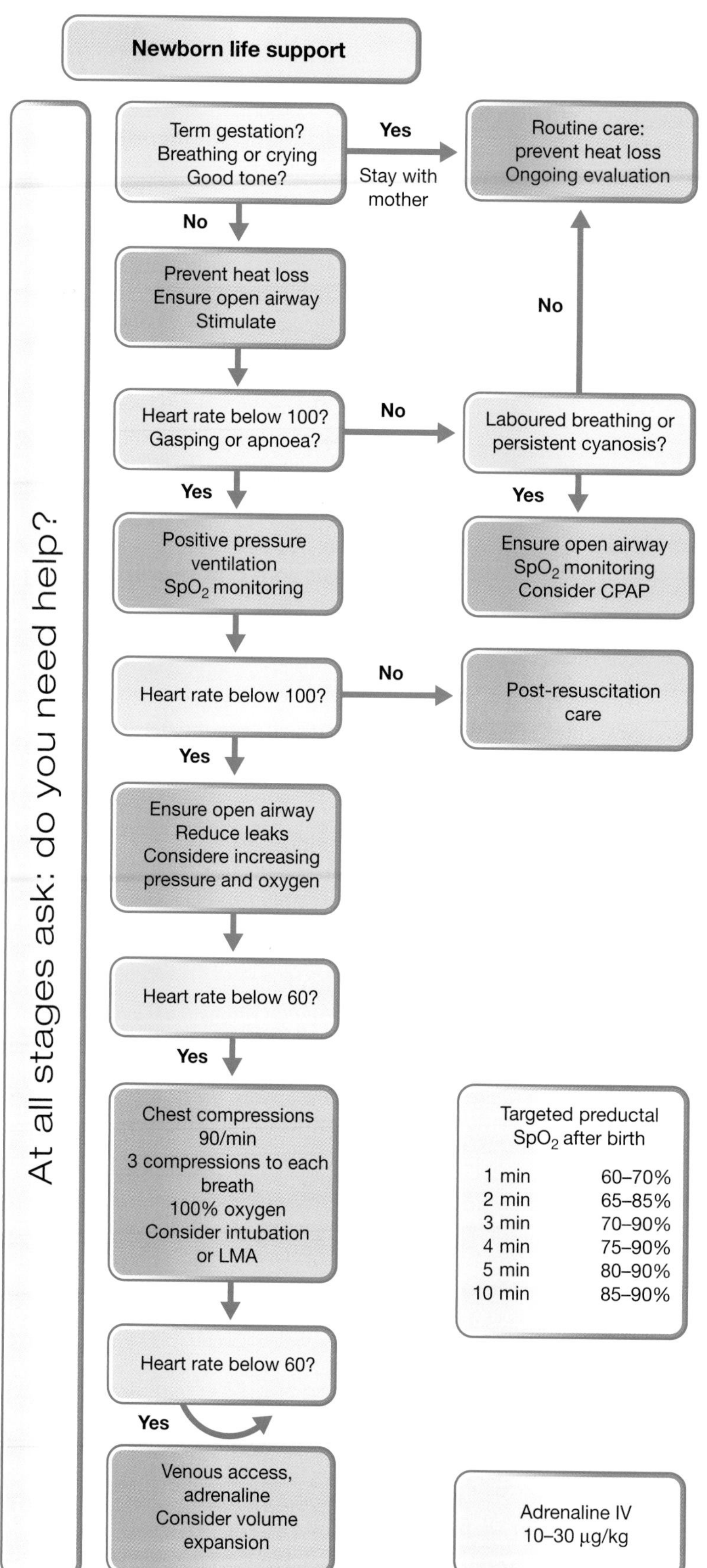


Fig. 11.1.3 Newborn resuscitation algorithm. CPAP, continuous positive airway pressure; LMA, laryngeal mask airway; $SpO_2$, peripheral oxygen saturation Australian Resuscitation Council 2010.

3. *Still inadequate respirations or apnoea, or HR <100: (30 seconds from birth).* Three to five slow (3 seconds) breaths then bag and mask at 40–60 per minute. Have pop-off valve or manometer set at 30 cm$H_2O$, but lower pressures are probably adequate. Check the response: should be visible chest movement and increase in HR.
4. *HR <60 and not increasing, inadequate respirations or apnoea.* Proceed to ADVANCED resuscitation. Call for help. Intubate, if skilled. Otherwise continue with bag and mask, check head in neutral position with jaw thrust, check chest movement and air entry. Give 3 cardiac compressions (see below) to 1 breath. Consider drugs: IV adrenaline (epinephrine).

- Call for help at any time
- Assessment of colour is considered unreliable so oxygenation should be assessed by pulse oximetry. Applying the probe to the right hand or wrist before connecting to the instrument produces faster readings.

Studies have shown the appropriate technique to achieve the most effective use of a face mask during neonatal resuscitation (Fig. 11.1.4).

- Hold the newborn head in a neutral position (A).
- Gently roll the mask on to the face from the tip of the chin (B, C).
- Hold the mask with thumb and index finger at the top where the silicone is thickest (D).

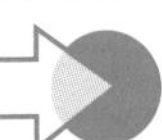

**Practical points**

**Neonatal resuscitation**

- It is essential to be familiar with the equipment in the birthing location and with the local resuscitation protocols.
- The vast majority of term or near-term infants do not need active resuscitation.
- Apgar scores are useful to assess the infant's condition at birth but do not predict long-term outcome or the cause of any future disability.
- Initial resuscitation with air is at least as good as 100% oxygen for term or near-term infants.

- With the thumb and index finger apply even downward pressure on top of the mask (D).
- Do not let the fingers encroach on to the skirt of the mask.
- The other fingers perform a chin lift with upward pressure.

## Additional notes

### The use of supplementary oxygen in newborn resuscitation

The time-honoured practice of using 100% oxygen in neonatal resuscitation has recently been challenged in a number of ways, including trials comparing resuscitation in air or 100% oxygen in term infants. Meta-analyses of these studies have resulted in the recommendation that, for term infants, room air should be used for initial resuscitation with oxygen as backup if resuscitation fails. Ideally blended air and oxygen will be available with the concentration delivered guided by preductal (probe placed on right hand or wrist) pulse oximetry. Note that even in healthy term newborns it may take 5–10 minutes for the preductal oxygen saturation to reach 90%.

### Chest compressions

Newborn infants generally experience bradycardia secondary to respiratory problems rather than primary cardiac arrest:

- It is essential that chest compressions follow a period of adequate lung inflation – which is generally the most effective.
- Chest compressions must not divert attention from ongoing lung inflation, or compromise adequate ventilation.
- The correct method is with hands encircling the chest and thumbs on the lower third of the sternum, compressing about one-third of the depth of the chest.
- One large survey of over 30 000 births suggested that only around 1 per 1000 infants 'need' cardiac compressions. It is likely that chest compressions are overused.

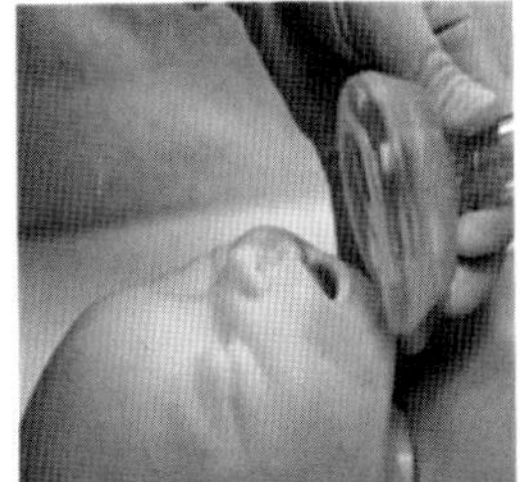
A
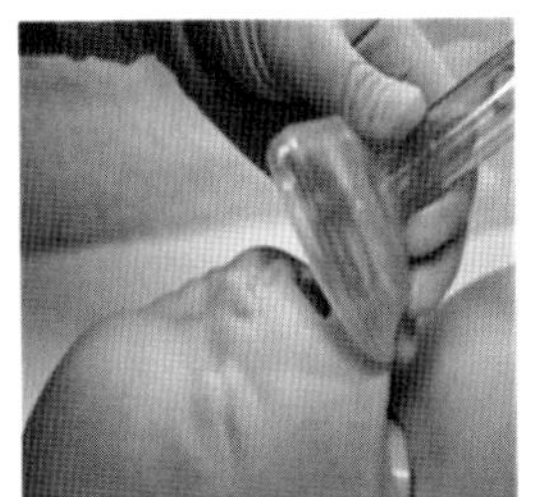
B
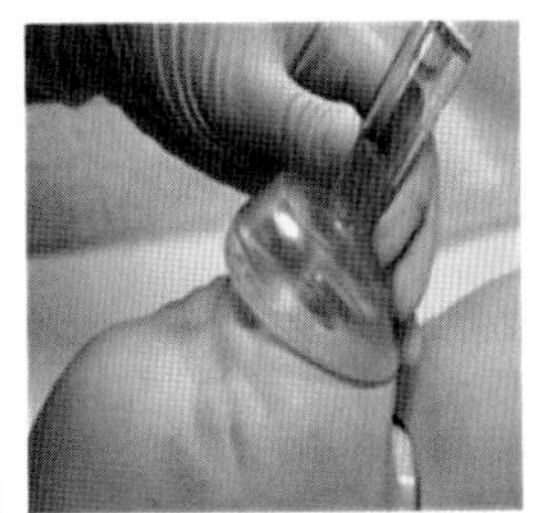
C
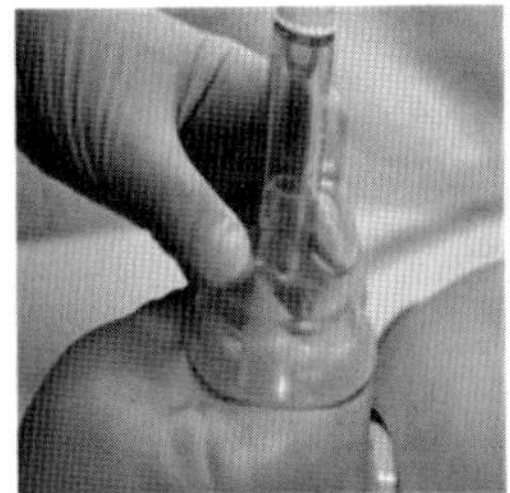
D

Fig. 11.1.4 Technique for using face mask in neonatal resuscitation. (From Schilleman K, Witlox RS, Lopriore E et al 2010 Leak and obstruction with mask ventilation during simulated neonatal resuscitation. Arch Dis Child Fetal Neonatal Ed 2010;95:F398–F402, with permission.)

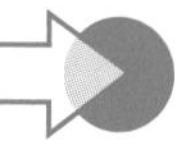

**Practical points**

**Umbilical vein cannulation**

- When urgent venous access is required, placement of an umbilical vein catheter is easy to achieve.
- Place a cord tie around the cord and control any bleeding by tying tight.
- Cut the cord 1 cm from the skin.
- The vein is oval and flush with the cord; the two arteries usually project slightly from the surface.
- Have ready a sterile umbilical catheter, or other sterile catheter, filled with 0.9% saline and attached to a syringe.
- This is inserted 3–5 cm into the vein; there should be no obstruction.

### Meconium exposure

Up to 10–20% of deliveries are accompanied by meconium-stained liquor.

- With delivery of the head it is possible to suction the oropharynx if the meconium is thick and particulate, but a well designed study found no benefit from this practice.
- Following birth, if the infant is vigorous and crying, no suctioning is required.
- If the infant is floppy and has no or inadequate respirations, it is reasonable to aspirate the upper airway under direct vision using a laryngoscope.

### Caesarean sections

The Royal Australasian College of Physicians (RACP) recommends that paediatricians (or the designated person for neonatal resuscitation, such as a trained nurse practitioner) do not need to attend elective caesarean sections under regional anaesthesia, although, as for all births, there must be a person present whose role it is to care for the infant.

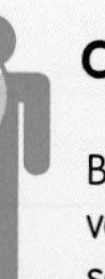

**Clinical example**

Baby Aloisi was born at term following a ventouse-assisted delivery because of a delayed second stage. He cried briefly at birth but at 30 seconds there was noted to be clear fluid coming from both his nose and mouth, which was vigorously suctioned. The heart rate was then noted to fall to 80 bpm and he was apnoeic. The senior midwife immediately positioned the baby on his back with his head in a neutral position and pushed the jaw forward to make sure his airway was open. Baby Aloisi cried, his heart rate rose to 120 bpm and he became fully pink. He was placed on his mother's chest and covered to keep him warm.

## Newborn examination

It takes time to get to know the range of normality and to feel comfortable when examining newborn babies. New parents spend many hours looking at (examining) their offspring and may have concerns that are easily put to rest by a compassionate professional.

### Purpose of newborn examination

- To check successful perinatal transition achieved and that the infant is healthy
- To screen for significant anomalies
- To establish baseline for further assessments (weight, length, head circumference)
- To address any parental concerns and provide reassurance
- To continue provision of health advice (e.g. supine sleeping, breastfeeding, etc.).

Excellent comprehensive guidelines are to be found in textbooks of neonatology.

As in all medicine, the newborn examination must be seen in the context of medical history and family background. Some knowledge of family history, pre-pregnancy maternal history, obstetric history, details of this pregnancy (for instance, any antenatal scans) and birth must be elicited either from the notes and/or the mother. Patient-held obstetric notes greatly facilitate this process.

### Who should do the examination?

Anyone with appropriate training can do the examination: midwife, nurse practitioner, general practitioner, paediatrician or junior doctor as part of the paediatric team. Training will consist of some or all of: tutorials, visual aids that can be reviewed repeatedly, observation of an experienced practitioner and fully observed examination by the student. It will still take some time to become completely familiar with the wide range of normality, and people should not be shy of seeking another opinion *and* telling the parents that this is being done and why.

### When should it be done?

The traditional and still the ideal, if possible, is a three-tiered approach:

- a fairly quick examination at birth to establish the sex, identify major anomalies and to check that the infant is well and kept warm. Most newborns are alert and responsive for some time after birth and this is often a special time for new parents and their infant to get to know each other
- a full and thorough examination in the next 48 hours, in the presence of one or both parents
- a repeat examination sometime later in the first week, particularly to check on feeding, weight gain or loss, jaundice and other aspects of the original examination.

This approach, however, is clearly tempered by early discharge policies and will depend to some extent on the place of birth and the domiciliary facilities, and will often mean there is one main examination in the first 24 hours.

### Frequency of anomalies

Several series suggest as many as 10–20% of newborn infants will have some anomaly, although the great majority are of no importance; 1–1.5% of all infants have a more significant congenital anomaly. The difference between a normal phenotypic variation (common in the population and often familial, for example partial syndactyly of the second and third toes) and an anomaly occurring in less than 4% of the population may be a matter of definition. The presence of three or more minor anomalies greatly increases the risk of there also being a major malformation.

Whether born by vaginal delivery or caesarean section, around 3% may have some form of birth trauma, such as bruising or a transient nerve palsy. Mostly, this resolves quickly.

### Outline of general examination

Ideally, the examination should be when the infant is quietly alert and the parents are present. Clarify that the parents think their child is well or whether they have concerns. Usually a review of feeding and passage of urine and bowel motions, plus enquiry into mother's health, can establish rapport. The room should be warm and the lighting good.

Check that the infant has been weighed and the length and head circumference measured, and these values plotted on an appropriate centile chart.

**Clinical example**

Baby Jane was born at term following a spontaneous vaginal delivery in a community hospital. Baby Jane's mother was 26 years old and had been well in this first pregnancy, but smoked 10 cigarettes a day. A 19-week ultrasound scan agreed with her dates and showed normal growth and anatomy. The birth weight was 2780 g, length 48.5 cm and head circumference 30.2 cm. The birth weight plotted on the third centile on appropriate growth charts and the length on the 10th centile, but the head circumference was not plotted. Baby Jane was thought to be well after birth with normoglycaemia, and went home on day 3. On day 7, she was seen at home when the domiciliary midwife plotted the head circumference and found it to be 4 cm below the third centile. Baby Jane was immediately referred for a paediatric opinion and MRI a few days later showed significant intracranial anomalies.

Well infants have a minor objection to being undressed, but settle easily. Unwell infants are often either unduly irritable or lethargic. Most infants have somewhat flexed limbs and spontaneous movements of all four limbs.

Check that the baby is not unduly pale. The hands and feet are sometimes rather blue but the tongue and mucous membranes should be pink. If there are any doubts as to cyanosis, check with a saturation monitor: healthy term infants should normally have an arterial oxygen saturation ($S_aO_2$) of 95% or more.

Most examiners then generally prefer to carry out a top to toe method of review but take the opportunity to examine out of sequence as it arises. For example, if the infant cries then look in the mouth. Various reflexes can be elicited as the examination proceeds. The Moro, or startle, reflex is when the infant's head is lifted a few centimetres off the bed and then allowed to fall back suddenly on to the examiner's hand. In a normal Moro reflex the infant cries, the arms extend and then abduct across the chest. The Moro adds little to the rest of the examination, is upsetting for the infant, and can usually be left out.

#### Look for the presence of any skin lesions or rashes

A majority of infants will have faint pink lesions over the eyelids, temples, upper lip, nape of the neck, or elsewhere on the face. These *capillary naevi*, also called salmon patches or stork marks, are benign and those on the front of the face nearly always fade completely.

Many infants also have tiny white spots on the forehead, nose or cheeks. These are inclusion cysts in the epidermis called *milia*, and are of no consequence. Similar are small white to yellow papules from *sebaceous hyperplasia* on the nose and face.

#### Head and scalp

- *Caput* is oedema over the presenting part of the scalp and will resolve in a day or two (Fig. 11.1.5).
- A *cephalhaematoma* is a haemorrhage under the periosteum of a skull bone, most commonly the parietal, and so will not cross the suture lines. As this large bruise will organize from the margins, it may feel firm at the edges with a soft, fluctuant centre before fully resolving.
- A *subgaleal haemorrhage*, bleeding into the scalp in the subaponeurotic space, is much rarer and more serious because significant hypovolaemia and anaemia can result. All of the scalp feels boggy and loose.
- There is often considerable *moulding* of the skull (i.e. movement of skull bones to allow passage through the birth canal), and sutures may be overriding but should move separately.

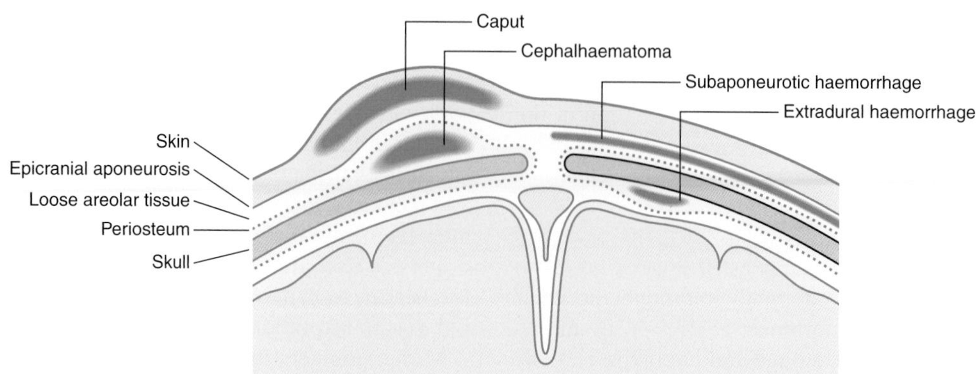


Fig. 11.1.5 Sites of extracranial and extradural haemorrhage in the newborn.

- A clear ridge over the suture, most commonly of the metopic (anterior part of the sagittal) suture, may indicate *craniosynostosis* or premature fusion and will need neurosurgical referral.
- The *anterior fontanelle* may vary hugely in size but should move with respirations and not be tense when the infant is quiet.

### Face

Many syndromes have several minor anomalies affecting the facies (e.g. Down syndrome, fetal alcohol syndrome) (see Chapter 10.3).

- *Facial asymmetry* when the infant cries is most commonly a temporary facial palsy affecting eye closure caused by pressure on the facial nerve during delivery. There is lack of creasing by the nose and side of the mouth, and lack of mouth movement on the side affected with crying. Function usually recovers within a few days but in a few cases the defect is more protracted. There may also be a congenital nerve palsy as opposed to trauma, or isolated congenital hypoplasia of the depressor anguli oris muscle.
- Elicit a *rooting reflex* by stroking the infant's cheek. The infant's suck can be assessed by letting him or her suck on a clean finger, and the roof of the mouth can then be palpated for a submucous cleft.
- *Cleft lips and palate* may be isolated or syndromic.
- *Pierre Robin* sequence comprises micrognathia and cleft palate, and requires careful assessment that the infant can protect the airway.
- *Mucus retention cysts* of the gums are common and benign.
- Occasionally an infant will be born with a (natal) tooth present. These are loose and easily dislodged, so should be removed.

Many infants open their eyes when sucking or may do so spontaneously. It should be easy to see that the infant focuses on the examiner's face (about 50 cm away) and can follow movement visually.

- *Subconjunctival haemorrhages* are common and resolve without problems.
- Elicit a normal red reflex with a small torch.
- An ophthalmoscope is needed to look for *cataracts* (most cannot be seen with the naked eye). Hold the ophthalmoscope about a foot away from the infant.
- If there are *sticky eyes* and the conjunctiva are red and swollen, urgent Gram stain and culture are required to look for gonococcal ophthalmitis. Unilateral sticky eyes are more likely to be a bacterial infection, or blocked tear duct if no redness or swelling is present. Bilateral mildly sticky eyes with no redness is often a chlamydial infection and requires special swabs and a course of oral erythromycin.
- *Pre-auricular skin tags and pits* are common and, together with more major aural defects, such as microtia, should mean the infant has a formal hearing test (see below).

### Chest and heart

- The *respiratory rate* is normally 40–60 breaths per minute and frequently somewhat irregular, faster and slower with brief pauses. Infants with respiratory distress have rapid and often regular breathing, and may have subcostal recession and an expiratory grunt (see Chapter 11.3).
- *Inspiratory stridor*, more obvious when the infant is crying, is common and self-limiting and should be distinguished from inspiratory or expiratory stridor at rest or in the presence of other symptoms.
- The *heart rate* varies from 90 to 160 bpm or more with crying. Sinus arrhythmia and occasional ectopic beats are common.
- Feel the brachial and femoral pulses.
- With coarctation of the aorta there may be absent femoral pulses – not always an easy thing to be sure about. If there are any doubts, check the blood pressure in the arm and leg, a difference of 20 mmHg being significant for possible coarctation.

- Listen for *heart murmurs* when the infant is quiet. The chance of detecting a murmur will depend upon the timing of this exam, up to 50% of infants having a precordial murmur within 6 hours of birth from ductal or other flow. Later in the first week the incidence of murmurs is closer to 1–2%. Although there are reported features that increase the probability that a murmur is innocent in the newborn (soft, grade 1–2/6 systolic murmur at left sternal edge, normal pulses and no other abnormalities), it is recognized that significant heart disease can occur with no or seemingly innocent murmurs. If the murmur persists at a second examination within 24 hours, our policy, in common with others, is to perform echocardiography; this is almost certainly cost-effective and greatly reassuring for parents.

**Clinical example**

Baby Jackie had her first full neonatal examination at 48 hours of age. The only unusual finding was a loud systolic murmur at the left sternal edge, which had not been noted at birth. There was no family history of congenital heart disease. Although there had been an antenatal anatomy scan at 21 weeks' gestation, views of the heart had not been ideal. The resident doctor requested an echocardiogram, which was carried out 2 hours later and showed a small, mid-septal, muscular ventricular septal defect (VSD) with no other problems. Baby Jackie's family were able to be reassured this would cause no problems and that the defect was likely to close spontaneously by 1–2 years of age.

## Abdomen and genitalia

- There is often *divarication of the rectus abdominis*, leading to a soft midline bulge above the umbilicus; this is normal.
- Check the *umbilicus*. The cord separates by a process of low-grade inflammation over several days. In the past, various regimens, including anointing the stump every 4 hours with antiseptic or alcohol, have been used to try to minimize bacterial colonization. It is doubtful whether such practices are useful or necessary, and they may delay cord separation.
- Feel for any *masses*. The liver edge is usually palpable 1–2 cm below the right costal margin. A spleen tip may be felt in normal babies and the lower pole of both kidneys felt on deep bimanual palpation. A distended bladder, such as with posterior valves, can be felt up to the umbilicus.
- *Bile-stained vomitus* is always abnormal and urgent investigations and possible surgical referral are required (see Chapter 11.5).
- *Ambiguous genitalia* should have been detected in the labour ward. There are many causes, and urgent investigations are required. The parents should be clearly told that it is not possible to tell whether their infant is a boy or a girl just now, and a phrase such as 'because the genitalia are immaturely formed' may be useful.
- *Hypospadias* can be subtle and it may be necessary to see the infant micturate to detect the urethral opening.
- *Hydroceles*, demonstrated by transillumination, are common and need no action. Other scrotal swellings and undescended or maldescended testes require surgical referral (see Chapter 11.5).
- The *foreskin* is not retractile in the newborn. Tiny *epithelial pearls*, white papules, are common here.
- There is no medical indication for *circumcision* of the healthy male newborn.
- Checking for *anal agenesis* requires parting the buttocks and fully examining the perineum. It is not uncommon to be fooled by observing some meconium on the perineum or the nappy if there is an associated fistula connected to the bowel.
- *Vaginal mucoid discharges* are common, as is a small *vaginal bleed* in the first few days of life, which needs no treatment (but check that vitamin K has been given – see below). *Vaginal mucosa skin tags* are also common and benign.

## Limbs

- *Extra digits* may be parts of syndromes or isolated and sometimes familial.
- Is there a *grasp reflex* on placing a finger in the open palm? A similar plantar reflex can be found by placing a finger on the sole of the foot.
- *Erb's palsy* occurs in 1–2 per 1000 births, being more common following shoulder dystocia or instrumental deliveries. It is the most common brachial plexus injury and the arm is flaccid by the side or in a 'waiter's tip' position. Most are very transient with improvement over a few days; otherwise physiotherapy is indicated. Sometimes there is also a *fractured clavicle*, usually detected by crepitus over the bone, but no specific treatment is required.
- Infants who have been in a *breech presentation* with extended legs may sometimes still prefer to lie in this position after birth for a few days. For examination for congenital dislocation of the hip see Chapter 8.1.
- *Talipes calcaneovalgus*, with the dorsum of the foot pressed against the front of the shin, is nearly always positional and the ankle can be moved through a full range of movements. *Talipes equinovarus*, with the foot inverted, is more likely to have restricted ankle movements and requires orthopaedic referral (see Chapter 8.1.). There may be associated or isolated *metatarsus varus* in which the forefoot is twisted relative to the heel.

### Other

- Check the infant's *tone*. Placed prone, the infant will lie with flexed limbs and can just move the head at least to the midline. On pulling the infant up by the arms from supine there will be some flexion of the elbows and resistance and tone in the shoulders, but quite marked head lag. On holding the infant in ventral suspension, the hips and shoulders and head will raise up a little in contrast to the 'rag doll' feel if there is significant hypotonia.
- Check *limb reflexes*. One or two beats of clonus at the ankle on sudden dorsiflexion of the foot is normal.
- The *walking reflex* consists of walking movements of the legs stimulated by the soles of the feet touching a surface when the baby is held vertical. It is not necessary to elicit this reflex if the baby otherwise appears normal, but it is often of great interest to parents.
- *Gestational age scoring* – a time-honoured occupation of paediatricians has been estimation of gestational age, but one that is now rarely indicated (such as a concealed pregnancy):
  - Many more pregnancies have early ultrasound examinations that can confirm mother's dates.
  - The time of conception is not a fixed time from the first day of the last menstrual period, so two infants of the same gestation may not have the same physiological maturity.
  - At best, a Dubowitz or Ballard score will estimate the gestational age ±2 weeks.
  - There is little point in the exercise, fun though it is!

## Common minor anomalies and debated importance

More recent series have confirmed earlier evidence that *simple sacral dimples or pits* are not markers for occult spinal dysraphism (such as a tethered cord or dermal sinus). Simple sacral dimples are defined as less than 5 mm and less than 2.5 cm from the anus in the gluteal fold. Lesions outside these limits, or when there are two or more cutaneous markers, should be investigated by ultrasonography (up to 2–3 months of age).

A *single umbilical artery* (SUA), detected antenatally or at the time of birth, occurs in about 1 in 200 infants and 1 in 5 of these have an associated malformation, which is often multiple and chromosomal. Recent reviews suggests that, if the SUA occurs without obvious associated anomalies, there will be only a very small yield from further investigation of the urinary tract, with the majority of findings being self-limiting conditions such as minor degrees of vesicoureteric reflux. Despite this, other authors do recommend a renal ultrasound scan if a SUA is detected.

*Tongue tie* (ankyloglossia) describes a short frenulum with relative tethering of the tongue, After many years of leaving such infants alone unless they have significant feeding difficulties or later speech problems, both uncommon, there has been a recent increase in recommendations that the tongue should be 'released'. The change seems to stem from lactation consultants believing that the short frenulum may affect breastfeeding and lead to maternal pain from poor latching, views that have been supported by several small studies of variable quality. If frenectomy is being considered, it must be performed by a properly trained health professional and preferably with adequate analgesia. Side-effects, including haemorrhage, are rare but have been reported.

## Later examination

- If there is a later examination at around 1 week or beyond, the focus is a little different. It will include a history of feeding and bowel movements, and measurement of weight gain. The five 'Hs' are:
- *Head* – congenital hydrocephalus may now present with a full fontanelle, widened sutures and abnormally increasing head circumference
- *Heart* – some murmurs may now be apparent, or signs of heart failure (tachypnoea, hepatomegaly)
- *Hepar* – jaundice may need assessment (see Chapter 11.2).
- *Hips* – another opportunity to examine for congenital dislocation of the hips (see Chapter 8.1.)
- *Hearing* – does the baby hear, shown by a sudden quieting to his/her mother's voice or a rattle shaken out of view?

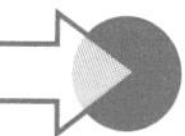

**Practice points**

**Neonatal examination**

- All infants must have a thorough examination within 48 hours of birth.
- Clear and accurate records must be kept of all examinations.
- The findings will to some extent depend upon the timing of the examination.
- Weight, length and head circumference must be accurately recorded on an appropriate centile chart.

## Other issues

### Analgesia

Newborn infants may be subjected to a number of painful procedures, such as heel pricks, and have a right to effective analgesia. The RACP has issued comprehensive guidelines on this topic.

Use of a pacifier with 0.5–1.0 mL 24% sucrose in 0.25-mL aliquots 2 min prior to venepuncture or heel pricks reduces discomfort from these. Some mothers may prefer to breastfeed and swaddle the baby during the procedure.

### Vitamin K

Vitamin K deficiency bleeding is an uncommon but potentially fatal disorder which presents with spontaneous bruising or internal, including intracranial, haemorrhage. There are three recognized forms:

- *Early:* This is very rare, occurs on the first day of life, and is usually associated with maternal medication such as anticonvulsants.
- *Classical:* Bleeding occurs from day 2–6 of life. Without vitamin K prophylaxis it may occur in 1 in 400 exclusively breastfed infants.
- *Late:* Between 1 week and 6 months of age, almost always in breastfed infants and often in association with unrecognized liver disease or malabsorption syndrome.

In both Australia and New Zealand a mixed micelle form of vitamin K is used (Konakion MM). The guidelines state that:

- the recommendations about vitamin K should be discussed with parents before the infant's birth
- the preferred route is intramuscular, 1 mg, following birth
- should parents not agree to an intramuscular injection (and most do), three oral doses of Konakion can be given over several weeks, although this may be a less effective prevention.

### Hearing screening

In the past, referrals for hearing tests have been based on a number of factors conferring increased risk, including congenital deafness in a close relative, malformations of face or ear, very low birth weight, high serum bilirubin level (>340 µmol/L), hypoxic–ischaemic encephalopathy, bacterial meningitis, congenital infection with rubella or cytomegalovirus, or exposure to aminoglycosides. However, such criteria detect only a minority of affected infants and many countries, including Australia and New Zealand, are implementing universal neonatal screening, with either oto-acoustic emissions or automated auditory brainstem responses, or a combination of these tests.

### Immunization

There is a high risk of vertical transmission of hepatitis B during delivery for mothers who are hepatitis B carriers (HBsAg-positive). The risk of the infant acquiring the virus remains high during the first 5 years of life. Infection in early life is associated with a high risk of chronic hepatitis (see Chapter 20.5). In Australia, it is recommended that all term infants receive hepatitis B vaccine at birth.

Infants born to mothers who are hepatitis B carriers should be given:

1. an early bath with 1% chlorhexidine obstetric cream to remove maternal blood and fluids.

Within 12 hours of birth and as early as possible:

2. hepatitis B immunoglobulin 100 IU i.m.
3. hepatitis B vaccine i.m. (opposite thigh).

### Metabolic screening

Following informed parental consent, all infants should have a heel prick performed at 48 hours of age for metabolic screening (commonly called the Guthrie card). Different diseases are screened for in the various states of Australia and in New Zealand, but they usually include phenylketonuria, hypothyroidism and cystic fibrosis. The introduction of tandem mass spectrophotometry has meant that a number of amino acid and fatty acid oxidation disorders are also screened for (see Chapter 10.5).

## Normal infant matters

### Weight

Normal infants lose up to 8% of their birth weight in the first 3–5 days and regain birth weight by 7–10 days.

### Micturition

Normal infants often pass urine soon after birth, then infrequently for the next 24 hours. As feeding is established, urine is passed more often, usually every 3–4 hours. Normal newborn urine is clear and colourless, although in the nappy there may be a pink colour from the presence of urates exposed to the air.

### Bowel actions

Some 20% of infants pass meconium before delivery or during the first 4 hours afterwards, 96% pass meconium by 24 hours and 99.9% by 48 hours. Failure to pass meconium by 48 hours is almost always abnormal and may indicate Hirschsprung disease, meconium plug syndrome or other bowel obstruction.

### Vomiting

Small-volume (<5 mL) occasional vomits are common, as all infants have some degree of gastro-oesophageal reflux in the first week of life. 'Possets' are tiny 1–2-mL vomits. Larger, more frequent, vomits may be a normal variation but also may be the first signs of illness, for example a bacterial infection. Vomits containing bile (which is green, not yellow) are almost always abnormal, strongly suggesting bowel obstruction, and should always be investigated even if other indicators of bowel obstruction (distension and constipation) are absent.

### Waking, sleeping, crying

Normal infants are usually awake and active for 30 minutes or so after birth. Thereafter patterns of sleep, wakefulness and crying are extremely variable. On average, infants sleep for at least 18 hours a day in the first week, with sleep evenly distributed throughout the 24 hours. By 6 weeks of age most infants are sleeping more at night than during the day, and by 12 weeks of age much more sleep occurs at night. Acquisition of this circadian rhythm is clearly affected by various care practices as well as endogenous hormone production. Newborn infants also may cry for an average of 4 hours or more per 24 hours.

Newborns infants will look at objects within a focal distance of 20–45 cm and preferentially focus on the edges of objects, lines and shapes. They can distinguish the human face from other objects. They can hear and distinguish their mother's voice from other sounds. They have a sense of smell and can distinguish their mother's smell from that of others. They distinguish between several tastes. They move in characteristic ways to different rhythms of speech and they mimic adult facial movements, including tongue protrusion.

We attribute many human experiences, emotions and moods to newborn infants, and rightly so, but no one really knows what it is like to be a newborn. Health workers should strive to make this episode in life as rewarding as possible for infants and their parents. The rewards for health workers who achieve these goals are also great.

### List of (normal) newborn topics in other chapters


- Breastfeeding and nutrition – Chapter 3.3
- General resuscitation – paediatric emergencies, Chapter 5.2
- Congenital dislocation of the hip – Chapter 8.1
- Surgical issues (e.g. hydrocele) – Chapters 11.5 and 20.1
- Birth defects – Chapter 10.1
- Dysmorphic child – Chapter 10.3
- Newborn (metabolic) screening – Chapter 10.5
- Jaundice – Chapter 11.2
- Group B streptococcus and other infections – Chapter 11.4
- Antenatal pelvicalyceal dilatation – Chapter 18.1
- Skin disorders – Chapter 21.1
- Hearing screening – Chapter 22.1

# 11.2

# Low birth weight, prematurity and jaundice in infancy

Jane Harding, Jane Alsweiler, Mariam Buksh

## Principles of care

Care of the sick newborn is often complex, and requires specialized training and equipment. However, remembering the basic principles will allow you to provide emergency care for the sick newborn, regardless of diagnosis, until specialized help is available:

- *Keep the baby pink*. Initial resuscitation should follow the usual ABC guidelines (see Chapters 5.1, 5.2 and 11.1). After that, many babies will maintain breathing with supplemental oxygen until more sophisticated respiratory support is available. If an oxygen saturation monitor is available, give only enough oxygen to keep a preterm baby's oxygen saturations between 86% and 94%, and a term baby's saturations above 95%.
- *Keep the baby warm*. Cooling increases the baby's oxygen and glucose requirements and is associated with increased mortality. Dry the baby and put a hat on to reduce heat loss while you are assessing other problems. Use a radiant heater, electric blanket or incubator if available.
- *Keep the baby fed.* Sick babies are at risk of hypoglycaemia, which can cause brain damage. If milk feeds are not possible, give intravenous 10% dextrose 60 mL/kg daily (2.5 mL/kg hourly).
- *Consider infection.* Almost any signs and symptoms of illness in the newborn can be caused by infection, and untreated septicaemia can cause death within hours. If specialized care is likely to be delayed by more than an hour or two, take blood cultures if possible and give intravenous or intramuscular antibiotics.

## Definitions

Babies are commonly classified into groups associated with different disease patterns and different outcomes (Fig. 11.2.1). These include:

- Gestation
  - term: ≥37 completed weeks' gestation
  - preterm: <37 completed weeks' gestation
  - post-term: >42 completed weeks' gestation
- Birth weight
  - low birth weight (LBW): <2500 g
  - very low birth weight (VLBW): <1500 g
  - extremely low birth weight (ELBW): <1000 g
- Weight for gestational age
  - appropriate for gestation (AGA): birth weight between 10th and 90th centiles for gestation
  - small for gestational age (SGA): birth weight <10th centile for gestation
  - large for gestational age (LGA): birth weight >90th centile for gestation.

## The premature infant

### Causes of preterm birth

Although there are many risk factors for preterm birth (Box 11.2.1), approximately half of preterm births occur in the absence of recognized risk factors. Survival rates increase and the incidence and severity of complications all decrease with increasing gestational age and birth weight (Figs 11.2.2, 11.2.3, Table 11.2.1).

**Clinical example**

George is a 900-g (extremely low birth weight) baby born to a 16-year-old mother who received no prenatal care. His mother was admitted after the membranes ruptured and she began to have contractions. She did not remember the date of her last menstrual period and had not had any antenatal ultrasound scans. She smoked a pack of cigarettes per day during the pregnancy. At delivery, George had poor respiratory effort and marked retractions so he was intubated in the delivery room and brought to the neonatal intensive care unit. He required moderate ventilator settings and 50% oxygen. Chest X-ray showed a diffuse ground-glass appearance with air bronchograms consistent with respiratory distress syndrome. A dose of surfactant was given through the endotracheal tube. Gestational age was estimated at approximately 27 weeks based on the Ballard examination, which assesses physical and neuromuscular development. Based on this estimated gestation, the infant's weight, length and head circumference were all at the 25th centile, and were appropriate for his gestational age.

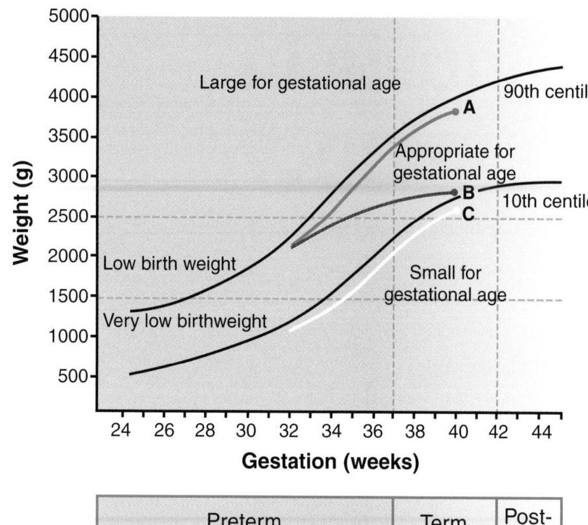


Fig. 11.2.1 Common definitions of size at birth, illustrating the difference between intrauterine growth restriction (IUGR) and small for gestational age (SGA). Baby A is an appropriately grown term baby. Baby B is also born with an appropriate size for gestational age (AGA), but has suffered reduced intrauterine growth compared with baby A and thus has IUGR. Baby C has had normal intrauterine growth, but is born SGA.

**Box 11.2.1 Risk factors associated with preterm birth**

**Maternal**

- Previous preterm birth
- Extremes of maternal age
- Low pre-pregnant weight
- Acute illness (e.g. pyelonephritis)
- Uterine anomalies
- Cervical incompetence
- Pre-eclampsia/eclampsia
- Previous miscarriage or termination of pregnancy
- History of infertility
- *In vitro* fertilization (IVF)

**Fetal**

- Multiple gestation
- Fetal anomalies
- Polyhydramnios
- Fetal demise
- First trimester threatened abortion

**Placenta and membranes**

- Placenta praevia
- Abruptio placentae
- Premature rupture of membranes
- Chorioamnionitis

**Social**

- Low socioeconomic status
- Smoking
- Alcohol abuse
- Illicit drug abuse
- Heavy physical work
- Psychological stress

## Short-term complications of prematurity

### Respiratory

See also Chapter 11.3.

*Respiratory distress syndrome*

Respiratory distress syndrome is also called surfactant deficiency syndrome. Immaturity of the respiratory system with surfactant deficiency results in respiratory distress. This is managed with oxygen, nasal continuous positive airway pressure (NCPAP) or, when more severe, surfactant administration and mechanical ventilation. Corticosteroids given to the mother before preterm birth reduce the incidence and severity of respiratory distress syndrome.

*Periodic breathing, apnoea of prematurity*

Premature babies commonly experience periodic breathing due to immaturity of the respiratory centres of the brain. Cessation of breathing persisting for more than 20 seconds, or less than 20 seconds if there is associated bradycardia or desaturation, is termed apnoea. Premature babies require cardiorespiratory and pulse oximetry monitoring to detect apnoea and associated bradycardia or desaturation. Apnoea of prematurity occurs in almost all extremely premature babies and usually improves around 34–36 weeks' postmenstrual age. Pharmacological treatment includes methylxanthines such as caffeine or theophylline, which improve diaphragmatic contraction and stimulate the respiratory centres. NCPAP is also helpful, partly by reducing any obstructive component to the apnoea and reducing the work of breathing. If apnoea is severe, the baby may have to be ventilated mechanically. Apnoea can also be caused by many other complications of prematurity, such as infection, neurological problems, anaemia, hypoxia, patent ductus arteriosus and upper airway obstruction, so these need to be considered in babies experiencing apnoea.

### Cardiac

*Patent ductus arteriosus*

Before birth, the ductus arteriosus diverts blood from the right ventricle away from the lungs to the aorta. After birth it normally closes functionally within a few days. In premature babies, closure may be delayed, leading to left-to-right shunting of blood from the aorta through the ductus to the lungs. This results in pulmonary congestion, worsening lung disease and decreased blood flow to the gastrointestinal tract and brain. These changes have been implicated in the pathogenesis of necrotizing enterocolitis and intraventricular haemorrhage. A significant patent ductus arteriosus (PDA) is often clinically

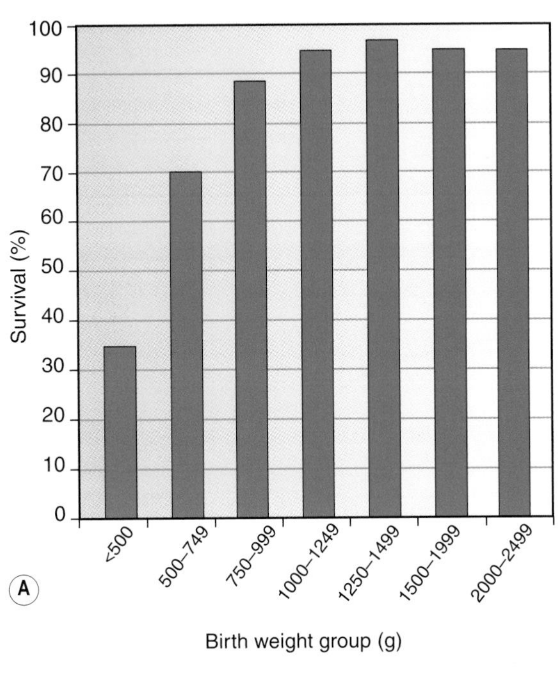


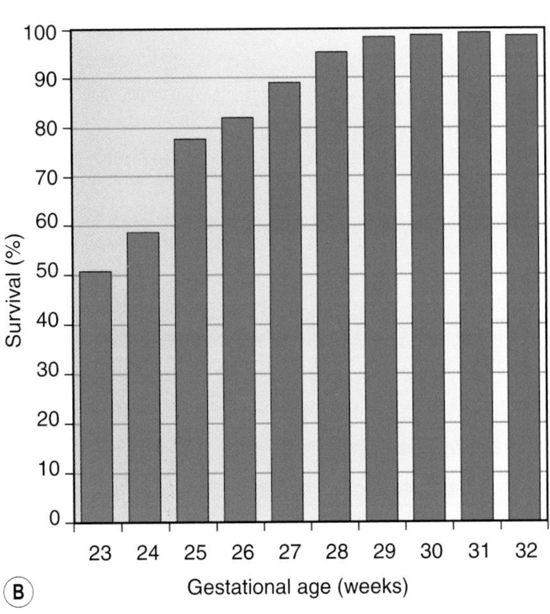


**Fig. 11.2.2** Survival of preterm infants admitted to neonatal units according to (A) birth weight and (B) gestational age. (Source of data: Australian and New Zealand Neonatal Network (ANZNN) 2009 Report of the Australian and New Zealand Neonatal Network 2006. ANZNN, Sydney.)

silent, or there may be a continuous heart murmur, hyperdynamic precordium, bounding pulses and widened pulse pressure. Diagnosis is made by echocardiography. A significant PDA may be treated by giving prostaglandin inhibitors (indometacin or ibuprofen). If these are unsuccessful, surgical ligation may be necessary.

## Neurological

*Intraventricular haemorrhage*

This is due to bleeding from the immature capillary bed of the germinal matrix lining the ventricles, often within the first 48 hours after birth. Risk factors include asphyxia and changes in cerebral blood flow due to hypotension or rapid intravenous fluid

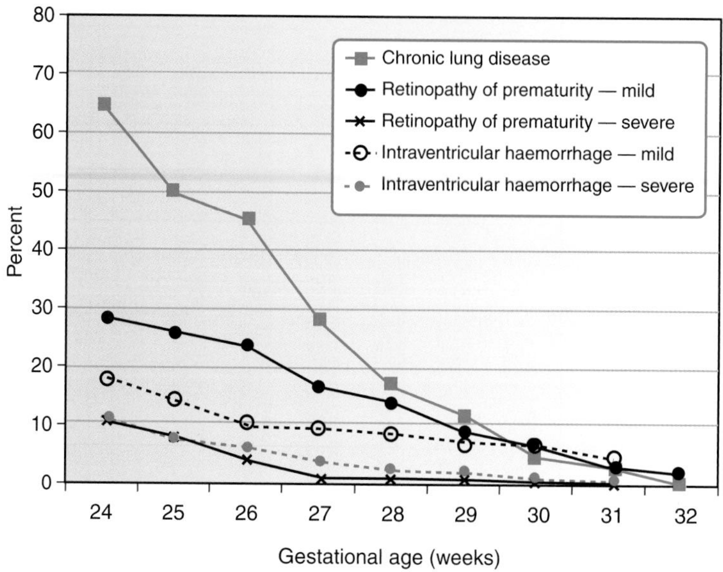


Fig. 11.2.3 Frequency of complications of prematurity in babies admitted to neonatal units according to gestational age. (Source of data: Australian and New Zealand Neonatal Network (ANZNN) 2009 Report of the Australian and New Zealand Neonatal Network 2006. ANZNN, Sydney.)

**Table 11.2.1 Complications of preterm birth**

| | Common | Rare except in very low birth weight |
|---|---|---|
| **Early** | | |
| Respiratory | Respiratory distress syndrome<br>Apnoea | |
| Cardiac | | Patent ductus arteriosus |
| Neurological | | Periventricular haemorrhage<br>Periventricular leukomalacia |
| Hepatic | Hypoglycaemia<br>Hyperbilirubinaemia | Hyperglycaemia |
| Renal | Hyponatraemia | Hyperkalaemia<br>Metabolic acidosis |
| Gastrointestinal | Feeding problems | Necrotizing enterocolitis |
| Other | Anaemia<br>Infection<br>Poor thermoregulation | |
| **Late** | Delayed growth | Retinopathy of prematurity<br>Chronic lung disease<br>Neurodevelopmental delay |

infusion. Intraventricular haemorrhage is diagnosed by cranial ultrasonography and varies in severity from grade I intraventricular haemorrhage (germinal matrix haemorrhage) to grade IV (intraparenchymal haemorrhage). Although lower grades have a good prognosis, grades III and IV intraventricular haemorrhage are often associated with later hydrocephalus and neurological abnormalities such as cerebral palsy.

*Periventricular leukomalacia*

This is an uncommon problem, characterized by ischaemic necrosis of the white matter surrounding the lateral ventricles. Periventricular leukomalacia is diagnosed on head ultrasonography, usually at 4–6 weeks of age. It often results in cerebral palsy.

**Clinical example**

George improved significantly after the administration of surfactant. He was extubated and was placed on nasal continuous positive airway pressure (NCPAP) by age 36 hours. Caffeine was given before extubation in anticipation of apnoea of prematurity. Small feedings of expressed breast milk were started on day 1. Electrolytes were monitored closely because of the potential of large insensible water losses.

On day 4, George began to deteriorate with increasing apnoeas and respiratory distress. A continuous murmur was noted along the left sternal border. The pulses were bounding and the precordium was very active. Echocardiography confirmed the presence of a large patent ductus arteriosus and a course of indometacin was commenced.

George did well during the next week. At 2 weeks of age, he again developed worsening apnoea with feed intolerance and temperature instability. A full blood count revealed anaemia and an increase in immature white cells. Blood cultures, a lumbar puncture, chest X-ray and bladder tap were performed. George was treated with a blood transfusion and antibiotics, with gradual improvement during the next 2 days.

### Hepatic

*Hypoglycaemia* is common because of decreased glycogen stores and increased glucose requirements in premature babies.

*Hyperglycaemia* can also occur in VLBW babies because of high glucose infusion rates, reduced insulin secretion and impaired insulin sensitivity.

*Hyperbilirubinaemia* is common and due to hepatic immaturity coupled with a shorter half-life of red blood cells. Premature babies require treatment at lower bilirubin levels than term babies because their low albumin levels and immaturity of the blood–brain barrier place them at greater risk of bilirubin encephalopathy.

### Renal

Immaturity of the kidneys results in a poor ability to concentrate or dilute the urine. This may be aggravated by immature skin leading to high insensible water losses, contributing to:

- *dehydration*
- *hypernatraemia* and *hyponatraemia*
- *hyperkalaemia*
- *metabolic acidosis* due to inability to conserve bicarbonate.

### Gastrointestinal

*Necrotizing enterocolitis*

This is an uncommon inflammatory process in the bowel wall that can lead to necrosis. Fluctuating gut blood flow, hypotension, hypoxia, infection and feeding practices have all been implicated, but their exact contribution remains unclear. Exclusive breast milk feeding is partially protective against necrotizing enterocolitis. Presentation of necrotizing enterocolitis can be non-specific, including apnoea, bradycardia and temperature instability, then with more focal abdominal signs such as distension, tenderness, feed intolerance, bloody stools and bilious gastric aspirates. Occasionally there may be rapid progression to sepsis, shock and death. Classical X-ray findings are air in the bowel wall (pneumatosis intestinalis) and perforation of the gut. Treatment is by withholding of feeds, antibiotics and, if necessary, surgery. There is emerging evidence that probiotics in the milk feeds may decrease the risk of developing necrotizing enterocolitis.

*Feeding problems*

Premature babies have weak and uncoordinated suck and swallow reflexes, delayed gastric emptying and immature gut motility. Feed intolerance and gastro-oesophageal reflux are common. Parenteral nutrition is usually required initially in extremely premature babies, with gradually increasing volumes of milk, preferably expressed breast milk, given by tube. Supplemental vitamins, minerals, protein and calories may also be required to allow adequate growth. Sucking feeds are usually established at 34–36 weeks' postmenstrual age.

### Haematological

*Anaemia*

Anaemia of prematurity is almost universal, as a result of low iron stores and red cell mass at birth, rapid growth, reduced erythropoiesis and decreased survival of red blood cells, aggravated by repeated blood sampling. Treatment is supportive with transfusion in the early period and iron supplementation.

### Immunological

*Infection*

Premature babies have increased susceptibility to infection due to impaired cell-mediated immunity and reduced concentrations of complement and immunoglobulins, together with exposure to invasive procedures and monitoring. Signs of sepsis are extremely non-specific, including lethargy, temperature instability, apnoea, tachypnoea, feed intolerance and jaundice. Investigation usually requires a full blood count, blood culture, chest X-ray, bladder tap urine and lumbar puncture. Because deterioration can be rapid, early treatment with antibiotics is essential pending culture results.

### Thermoregulation

This is a significant problem in the premature baby due to a relatively large body surface area, thin skin and subcutaneous tissues, and lack of a keratinized epidermal barrier. Nursing preterm infants in an incubator, with humidification if necessary, maintains a stable temperature.

**Clinical example**

George did well throughout the remainder of his hospitalization. He began to suck some feeds by 34 weeks' corrected age, and by 37 weeks he was fully breastfed. His eyes were examined for retinopathy of prematurity (ROP) at 6 weeks of age and were found to be immature but with no evidence of ROP. He would be followed every 2–3 weeks until his retinas were fully mature. His head ultrasound scans were normal at 5 and 28 days of age. He continued to have occasional episodes of desaturation until 36 weeks' corrected age and required oxygen 100 mL/min by nasal cannula to maintain adequate oxygenation. He received his first vaccinations before discharge. He was discharged at 38 weeks' postmenstrual age with an appointment to be seen in the high-risk follow-up clinic 6 weeks later. He was also followed by home health nurses while on oxygen.

## Late-onset complications of prematurity

### Retinopathy of prematurity

ROP results from disruption of the normal process of vascularization of the retina, with new vessel formation and fibrous scarring. Although ROP can result from excessive oxygen exposure, most cases occur in extremely premature babies with multiple other problems even when oxygen monitoring has been meticulous. Severity is classified on the basis of the location and extent of ROP, from grade 1 (mild changes) to grade 4 (retinal detachment). Most mild ROP regresses spontaneously; however, regular eye examinations are required to detect progressive ROP requiring laser therapy to reduce the chances of myopia and blindness.

### Chronic lung disease

This is usually defined as the need for supplemental oxygen at 36 weeks' postmenstrual age. It results from a combination of lung immaturity, oxygen toxicity, ventilator-induced lung injury, inflammatory and free radical-mediated lung injury. Babies with chronic lung disease may require supplemental oxygen for months or even years, and are at increased risk of respiratory infections in the first year and adverse developmental outcome.

### Growth

Because premature babies often do not grow for 2–3 weeks after birth, most are still below birth centiles at discharge; however, steady catch-up growth is usual during the first 2 years of life. Permanent growth failure is more likely in premature babies who were also small for gestational age.

### Neurodevelopmental impairments

Severe impairments (cerebral palsy, mental retardation, blindness, deafness) occur in 10–15% of VLBW babies. More subtle delays in language, attention deficits and social/behavioural difficulties are common. Regular developmental assessment is recommended for all VLBW babies.

### Growth and developmental expectations

Growth according to centiles and developmental achievements are usually corrected for prematurity up until the end of the second year of life.

### Immunizations

Immunizations should be administered according to the baby's chronological age and the timing should not be adjusted for prematurity.

## The late preterm baby

Babies born at 34–36 weeks' gestational age make up the largest proportion of preterm births. These babies are often managed in a similar fashion to term babies owing to their relatively large size and functional maturity. However, late preterm babies have an increased incidence of neonatal mortality and morbidity, and in later life have a higher rate of behavioural and developmental problems compared with term babies.

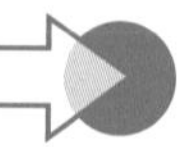

**Practical points**

**Low birth weight**

- May be due to a number of underlying causes.
- Consider whether appropriately grown preterm infant or small-for-gestational-age (SGA) infant.
- Monitor for hypoglycaemia and hypothermia.
- Prognosis will depend on the underlying cause.

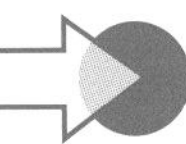

### Practical points

**Prematurity**

- Antenatal corticosteroids given to a mother at risk of preterm delivery decrease mortality and morbidity in preterm babies.
- Keep a preterm baby pink, warm and fed until specialized help is available.
- The more preterm the baby, the greater the likelihood of complications of prematurity and decreasing survival.
- Complications of prematurity can affect every organ system and can have lifelong effects.

## Small for gestational age

### Clinical example

Rachel was born at 36 weeks' gestation to a 30-year-old mother in her first pregnancy. Labour was induced because of poor growth and maternal pregnancy-induced hypertension. Delivery was by emergency caesarean section for fetal distress. Rachel was vigorous at birth with a birth weight of 1800 g, which was less than the 3rd centile. Her length was 45 cm, on the 10th centile, and her head circumference was 33 cm, on the 50th centile. Apart from her small size, no abnormalities were detected on initial examination. In particular, there were no dysmorphic features or signs of congenital infection. She was initially nursed in an incubator because of poor temperature maintenance in a cot. Blood glucose concentrations were monitored because of her small size. Despite early milk feeds, Rachel required an intravenous glucose infusion for the first 24 hours to maintain adequate blood glucose concentrations. She also became jaundiced and required phototherapy for days 3–6 after birth.

### Terminology

Smallness for gestational age (SGA) is usually defined as birth weight below 10th centile for gestation. The distinction between SGA babies and those with intrauterine growth restriction (IUGR) would be useful but is difficult to make clinically (see Fig. 11.2.1). SGA is measured by birth weight because this is easy and accurate, but babies with IUGR suffer a variety of complications even when birth weight is in the normal range. Similarly, some SGA babies are small normal babies, for example the small infant of a small mother in some ethnic groups. This problem is reduced by the use of centile charts specific for the relevant population.

**Box 11.2.2 Causes of being small for gestational age**

**Intrinsic: altered growth potential**

- Chromosomal
- Congenital anomalies
- Dysmorphic syndromes
- Congenital infections

**Extrinsic: reduced fetal nutrient supply**

- Reduced substrates in maternal blood (e.g. severe maternal undernutrition, eating disorders, chronic illness)
- Reduced uterine blood flow (e.g. hypertension, renovascular disease, vigorous exercise)
- Reduced placental transfer of substrates to the fetus (e.g. placental infarcts, abruption)
- Factors acting at all of these points (e.g. drugs, smoking, alcohol)

### Causes and complications

It is useful to think of the causes and complications of SGA in two main groups (Box 11.2.2):

- *Intrinsic fetal problems*: altered fetal potential for growth, such as chromosomal anomalies, intrauterine infection and congenital anomalies. Management and outcome in this group depend on the underlying cause.
- *Extrinsic problems in fetal supply*: the baby is undernourished *in utero* as a result of factors limiting nutrient supply at one or more places along the fetal supply line. Complications and outcome can be thought of as those of intrauterine starvation (Table 11.2.2).

However, in a large proportion of cases (perhaps 30%), no cause is identified.

### Treatment

No specific treatments have been shown to improve growth before or after birth. Treatment is directed to preventing and managing complications (see Table 11.2.1).

### Clinical example

Clinically Rachel did well. She fed vigorously, lost little weight after birth, and by 12 days she was weaned from the incubator to the cot. Her weight at that time was 1900 g. She was discharged home at 2 weeks of age. On follow-up at age 2 years, all of her measurements were at the 10th percentile and she had normal developmental milestones.

### Prognosis

- *General.* Prognosis depends on the cause of growth restriction. For the intrinsic group, outcome is that of the underlying problem. For the extrinsic group,

**Table 11.2.2 Pathophysiology of intrauterine growth restriction**

| Fetal nutrient limitation | Consequences for the fetus | Possible clinical consequences for the newborn | Long-term consequences |
|---|---|---|---|
| Reduced supply of glucose | Reduced body fat<br>Reduced glycogen stores | Hypothermia<br>Hypoglycaemia | Increased mortality<br>Neurological damage |
| Reduced supply of oxygen | Stillbirth<br>Asphyxia<br>Increased haematopoiesis<br><br><br>Redistributed cardiac output<br>Cardiac failure | Meconium aspiration<br>Hypoxic ischaemic encephalopathy<br>Coagulopathy<br>Polycythaemia<br>Jaundice<br>Relatively big head (head-sparing)<br>Pulmonary haemorrhage | Neurological damage |
| Reduced supply of amino acids | Impaired immune function<br>Delayed bone maturation<br>Reduced muscle mass | Infection<br>Hypocalcaemia<br>Insulin resistance | Poor growth |

outcome depends on severity and time of onset of the growth restriction. In general, the earlier the onset in gestation and the more severe the growth restriction, the greater the likelihood of permanent growth and developmental problems.

- *Growth.* Most SGA babies catch up in the first 6 months after birth. However, babies born short tend to remain short, and account for approximately 20% of short adults.
- *Neurodevelopment.* If growth restriction is of late onset and head size is normal, outcome may be good. However, many of the complications of growth restriction impair developmental outcome, and on average performance is reduced (see Table 11.2.1).
- *Adult disease.* Babies born small are at increased risk of a number of chronic diseases in adulthood, particularly coronary heart disease, stroke, hypertension and non-insulin-dependent diabetes. This is thought to be because fetal adaptations to undernutrition *in utero* result in both small size at birth and permanent resetting of homeostatic mechanisms (programming) that increase risk of later disease (the developmental origins of health and disease or Barker hypothesis).

## Jaundice

See also Chapter 20.5.

Jaundice is the visible yellow coloration of the skin due to raised bilirubin levels. It is extremely common, affecting approximately 50% of all newborns. In most babies jaundice is physiological. However, it should always be taken seriously, as it is a common sign of illness, and at high levels bilirubin can cause permanent brain damage (kernicterus).

### Bilirubin synthesis

Bilirubin is derived from haemoglobin, and to a lesser degree from myoglobin and the cytochromes. These haem proteins are oxidized in the reticuloendothelial system to form biliverdin and then *unconjugated bilirubin*. Because unconjugated bilirubin is not water-soluble, most of it circulates bound to albumin. Circulating bilirubin is taken up by the liver, and conjugated in the endoplasmic reticulum by the enzyme glucuronyl transferase to form bilirubin monoglucuronides and diglucuronides. *Conjugated bilirubin* is excreted via the biliary tree into the gastrointestinal tract and then into the faeces. However, some of the conjugated bilirubin is converted back to unconjugated bilirubin and is reabsorbed into the circulation by a process known as *enterohepatic circulation.*

### Evaluation of jaundice

Jaundice usually becomes visible at serum bilirubin levels of 85–120 μmol/L; however, the depth of jaundice is an extremely unreliable guide to the bilirubin level. Jaundice progresses in a cephalocaudal fashion and is more likely to be significant if it affects the arms or lower legs. Unconjugated hyperbilirubinaemia is the most common type and can be physiological or pathological. Conjugated hyperbilirubinaemia, defined as a serum conjugated bilirubin above 35 μmol/L, always requires urgent evaluation (see Chapter 20.5).

The extent of evaluation required in a jaundiced baby depends on the wellness of the baby and the pattern of jaundice (Fig. 11.2.4). As a minimum, all jaundiced babies should have a history taken, physical examination and measurement of the serum bilirubin level.

### History

- *Family history*: previous sibling, other family members with jaundice (hereditary causes?)

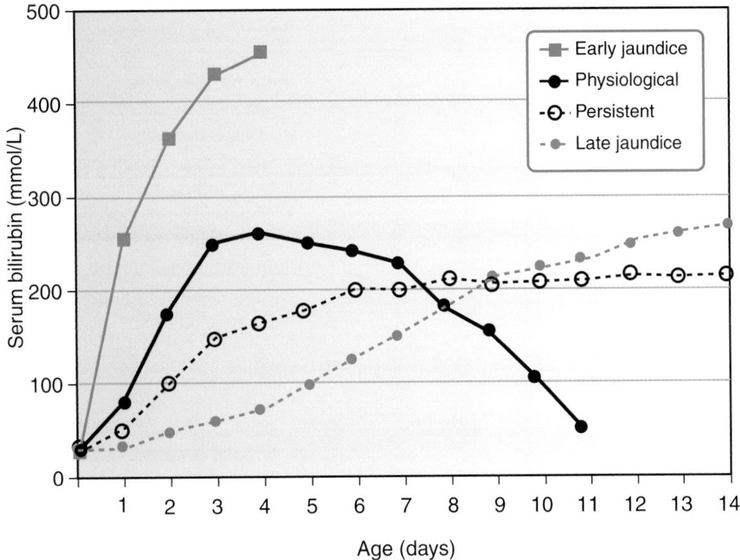


Fig. 11.2.4 Trends in serum bilirubin levels in common types of jaundice: early-onset haemolytic jaundice, physiological jaundice, prolonged jaundice and late-onset jaundice.

- *Maternal history*: history of splenectomy, haemolytic anaemia, gallstones, blood type
- *Pregnancy history*: gestational diabetes, illnesses (polycythaemia, infections?)
- *Delivery history*: type of delivery (forceps, vacuum extraction, trauma?), medications, length of rupture of membranes (sepsis?), delay in cord clamping (polycythaemia?), Apgar score (asphyxia?)
- *Newborn history*: feeding history (dehydration, starvation?), stool pattern (Hirschsprung disease?), vomiting (intestinal obstruction, pyloric stenosis?).

### Physical examination

- *Measurements*: small for gestational age or infant of a diabetic mother (polycythaemia?)
- *Colour*: plethora (polycythaemia?), pallor (anaemia?)
- *Wellness*: activity, tone, cry (sepsis?)
- *Presence of bruising*, petechiae, cephalhaematoma
- *Umbilical cord*: infection or umbilical hernia (hypothyroidism?)
- *Hepatosplenomegaly* (haemolysis, intrauterine infection?)
- *Neurological examination*: evidence of bilirubin encephalopathy.

### Laboratory evaluation

#### Early jaundice (<24 hours of age)

Always pathological.

- Evaluate for haemolysis and sepsis:
  - serum bilirubin
  - full blood count
  - maternal and infant blood type
  - Coombs test
  - assess risk for hereditary haemolytic diseases
  - consider cultures for infection.

#### Jaundice at more than 24 hours of age

Is it physiological? (Normal history and examination, normal pattern of jaundice)

- Monitor, no further investigations.

Not definitely physiological?

- Assess for haemolysis and sepsis as above.
- Assess feeding and weight gain/loss.
- Assess for gastrointestinal obstruction.
- Urinalysis for reducing substances (galactosaemia).

#### Persistent or late jaundice (>2 weeks in term baby, >3 weeks in preterm baby)

- Total and conjugated bilirubin (conjugated requires immediate investigation)
- Breast milk jaundice?
- Full blood count
- Thyroid function tests
- Liver function tests.

### Physiological jaundice

Physiological jaundice begins after 24 hours of age, peaks on approximately day 3 and resolves around the end of the first week (see Fig. 11.2.4). It is unconjugated and caused by a number of factors, including increased bilirubin load and impaired excretion (Box 11.2.3). The infant is healthy with a relatively slow rise in serum bilirubin (<85 µmol/L daily), which does not generally

**Box 11.2.3 Causes of physiological jaundice**

**Increased bilirubin load**
- Increased red blood cell volume
- Decreased red blood cell survival
- Increased enterohepatic circulation

**Defective hepatic uptake**
- Relative hepatic uptake deficiency

**Defective bilirubin conjugation**
- Decreased synthesis and activity of glucuronyl transferase

**Defective bilirubin excretion**
- Higher concentration of β-glucuronidase in intestinal mucosa increasing bilirubin breakdown
- More alkaline pH in proximal small intestine causing breakdown of conjugated bilirubin
- Lack of intestinal flora

**Box 11.2.4 Causes of haemolytic jaundice**

**Immune-mediated**
- ABO incompatibility
- Rhesus disease
- Minor blood group incompatibilities
- Drug-induced
- Maternal autoimmune haemolysis

**Acquired, non-immune**
- Congenital intrauterine infection
- Bacterial sepsis

**Hereditary**
- Membrane defects: hereditary spherocytosis, elliptocytosis, and others
- Enzyme abnormalities: glucose-6-phosphate dehydrogenase (G6PD) deficiency, pyruvate kinase deficiency

**Haemoglobinopathies**

exceed 250 μmol/L. In the premature baby, the bilirubin peaks towards the end of the first week and resolves in the second week.

Physiological jaundice is a diagnosis of exclusion. In a well baby whose jaundice is following the predicted course, no further investigation or treatment is required; however, any signs of illness in the baby or alterations in the pattern of jaundice require immediate investigation.

### Breast milk jaundice

Breast milk jaundice is a prolonged unconjugated hyperbilirubinaemia common in breastfed babies. The jaundice peaks in the second week but resolves only very slowly and may last up to 3 months (see Fig. 11.2.4). The infant is healthy and thriving. Breast milk jaundice is thought to be due to factors in breast milk that cause increased enteric absorption of bilirubin.

Diagnosis is based on the pattern of jaundice and wellness of the baby. As for any prolonged jaundice, conjugated hyperbilirubinaemia must be excluded. The diagnosis can be confirmed by improvement of the jaundice on temporary interruption of breastfeeding, but this is rarely required.

### Pathological unconjugated jaundice

#### Haemolysis

The onset of jaundice before 24 hours of life is always pathological and usually caused by haemolysis (Box 11.2.4). Haemolytic jaundice is most commonly immune-mediated and due to blood group incompatibilities, such as ABO and rhesus incompatibility. If investigations for immune-mediated haemolysis are negative, further investigations are necessary to determine whether haemolysis is due to other causes such as glucose-6-phosphate dehydrogenase (G6PD) deficiency, an X-linked disorder seen in Mediterranean and Asian ethnic groups, or hereditary spherocytosis, an autosomal dominant disorder affecting the cell membrane.

#### Non-haemolytic jaundice

Unconjugated hyperbilirubinaemia can be caused by increased production or decreased clearance of bilirubin, or sometimes by a combination of these factors (Box 11.2.5).

### Complications of jaundice

Unconjugated bilirubin is lipid-soluble, so can cross cell membranes and is toxic to cells, especially the brain. *Kernicterus* is a term used to describe the yellow

**Clinical example**

**Jaundice**

David is a term male infant born to a 33-year-old G2P1 blood group O+ serology-negative mother by normal vaginal delivery. Jaundice was noted at 18 hours of life, with an unconjugated bilirubin of 220 mmol/L.

A full blood count showed a normal haemoglobin level. The peripheral smear showed occasional spherocytes and some fragmented red blood cells, and the reticulocyte count was significantly raised. The baby was found to be blood type A+ with a positive direct Coombs test. A diagnosis for ABO incompatibility jaundice was made. Phototherapy was started and the serum bilirubin was monitored. The bilirubin rose to near exchange transfusion levels on day 2 before stabilizing. On day 7 a full blood count showed a slightly low haemoglobin level due to haemolysis. Phototherapy was stopped on day 14. Blood counts were monitored after discharge to look for worsening anaemia.

**Box 11.2.5 Other causes of unconjugated hyperbilirubinaemia**

**Increased haem load**
- Haemorrhage
  - Haematoma (especially cephalhaematoma), pulmonary haemorrhage, cerebral haemorrhage, birth trauma, occult
- Polycythaemia
- Swallowed blood

**Increased enterohepatic circulation**
- Bowel obstruction or ileus
- Pyloric stenosis

**Impaired hepatic uptake and conjugation**
- Inborn errors of bilirubin metabolism
  - Non-haemolytic inherited disorders: type I, type II, Gilbert disease
  - Metabolic disease: galactosaemia, tyrosinosis, hypermethionaemia
- Endocrine
  - Hypothyroidism, hypopituitarism, drugs
- Inhibitors
  - Lucey–Driscoll syndrome, breast milk

**Mixed**
- Asphyxia
- Prematurity
- Sepsis
- Infants of diabetic mothers

staining of the brain and the associated neuronal death seen on histology. The cerebellum, basal ganglia and cranial nerve nuclei tend to be most severely affected. *Bilirubin encephalopathy* refers to the clinical manifestations of bilirubin injury to the central nervous system. These can include abnormalities of muscle tone, lethargy, seizures, opisthotonus (arching of back), cerebral palsy and deafness. The risk of brain damage can be increased by:
- high serum unconjugated bilirubin concentration
- reduced binding of bilirubin to albumin, due to prematurity with low serum albumin concentrations, acidosis and displacement of bilirubin by fatty acids (e.g. intralipid) or certain drugs
- impairment of the blood–brain barrier due to prematurity, asphyxia, meningitis.

## Treatment of jaundice

The aim of treatment is to prevent encephalopathy by reducing bilirubin levels.
- *General.* Ensure adequate calorie and fluid intake and adequate stool production to reduce enterohepatic circulation. Treat with antibiotics if sepsis is suspected.
- *Phototherapy.* The baby is nursed under blue light at wavelengths of 450–460 nm. This transforms bilirubin near the skin into a water-soluble form through photo-isomerization. Bilirubin can then be excreted in the bile and urine. This is a safe, simple treatment, designed to avoid exchange transfusion.
- *Exchange transfusion.* The baby's blood is replaced with donor blood in order to decrease the bilirubin level rapidly. The procedure carries a small risk of morbidity and mortality, and is now rarely undertaken.

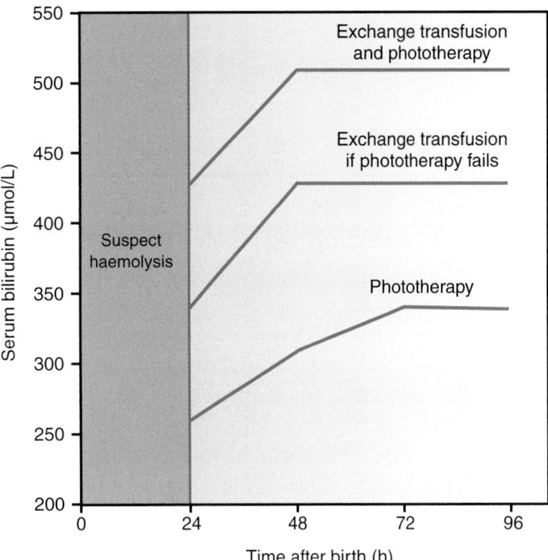


Fig. 11.2.5 Example of a nomogram for the treatment of jaundice in healthy term infants.

The levels at which phototherapy and exchange transfusion are performed are usually determined using standard hospital nomograms. An example is illustrated in Figure 11.2.5. The threshold for treatment is lower if the infant is premature, asphyxiated, ill or haemolysing.

*Intravenous immunoglobulin* may be helpful in the treatment of immune-mediated haemolytic disease, probably by blocking the Fc receptors on the red blood cells and thereby inhibiting haemolysis.

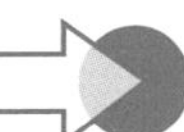

**Practical points**

**Jaundice**
- History and physical examination – is the baby well and feeding?
- Jaundice on day 1 is not physiological – think haemolysis, sepsis.
- Jaundice in the first week– baby well? Pattern of jaundice appropriate? – think physiological jaundice.
- Late jaundice – conjugated or unconjugated? Conjugated always requires investigation.

# 11.3 Breathing problems in the newborn

Luke Jardine, Mark Davies

## Introduction

The establishment and maintenance of breathing is vital for the newborn infant. Problems with breathing are common and dealing with them forms the bulk of neonatal care. The establishment of lung function is dealt with in Chapter 11.1. Respiratory problems beyond the immediate post-birth period include respiratory distress (from a myriad of causes), airway obstruction and hypoventilation (including apnoea and various neuromuscular problems).

## Respiratory distress

Respiratory distress is a broad term that refers to a constellation of signs seen in the neonate who has difficulty breathing and has increased respiratory effort. The signs that the infant with respiratory distress exhibits include the following:

- *Tachypnoea* – is defined as a respiratory rate of more than 60 breaths per minute. In order to clear more carbon dioxide, the infant increases the respiratory rate and therefore the minute ventilation.
- *Expiratory grunt* – this sound is produced by the exhalation of gas from the lungs through a partially closed glottis; this helps with the maintenance of the functional residual capacity. It can be misinterpreted by the inexperienced observer as the baby crying or moaning.
- *Recession* – with increased inspiratory effort the baby generates more negative intrapleural pressure. This increases the gradient between the atmosphere and the intrapleural space. This gradient occurs across the chest wall, and the softer or more compliant parts of the chest wall are sucked in during inspiration – usually the intercostal spaces and the sternum (the lower part is especially mobile and can be sucked in considerably during inspiration). There is also indrawing of the lower costal margin during inspiration, but this occurs owing to a different mechanism, namely contraction of the diaphragm, and is sometimes erroneously called subcostal recession.
- *Nasal flare* – the alae nasi flare during inspiration and this decreases airway resistance.
- *Central cyanosis* – almost invariably some alveoli that are not ventilated remain perfused. The resultant ventilation/perfusion mismatch leads to cyanosis. It is important to remember that babies who are relatively polycythaemic will have cyanosis at relatively high oxygen saturation, and babies with low haemoglobin will not appear cyanosed until their saturation is extremely low.

Not all babies with respiratory distress have all of the signs listed above. For example, an infant may have significant respiratory distress and yet have a respiratory rate of 40 breaths per minute. Often, the somewhat more subjective impression that the baby has increased respiratory effort or is 'working hard' is just as important.

## General principles of management of respiratory distress

The general principles of management apply no matter what the diagnosis or gestational age. The causes of respiratory distress are many, and some are immediately life-threatening. As always, you must attend to any need for resuscitation and ensure that the infant is physiologically stable.

- *Put the baby somewhere you can watch it.* This is best achieved by admission to a neonatal nursery with the baby nursed in an incubator, unclothed initially (this allows frequent observation and the status of the baby's breathing and colour can be assessed instantly upon looking in the incubator). The incubator should also keep the baby warm.
- *Monitor the vital signs* including heart rate, respiratory rate and pre-ductal oxygen saturations (put the oximeter probe on the right hand). These should be noted frequently so that any changes over time can be determined with a glance at the observation record.
- *Assume the baby is infected* until the results of investigations confirm or exclude this. Take cultures: a blood culture is best, with or without surface swabs and a gastric aspirate. Then start antibiotics.

- *Start intravenous fluids.* If you are struggling to breathe you do not need a stomach full of milk. If a peripheral venous cannula cannot be readily inserted then insert an umbilical venous line. Infusing 10% dextrose at 60 mL/kg daily is more than adequate in the first couple of days of life.
- *Get a chest X-ray.* There are some conditions that require an immediate change in management, such as a pneumothorax, congenital diaphragmatic hernia or intrapleural fluid. Although many conditions have characteristic appearances on chest X-ray, none of the findings is definitive. You can never exclude infection by looking at a chest X-ray.
- *Get advice.* If you are not in a neonatal unit that has a paediatrician or neonatologist then you should ring your local neonatal unit. Do this after attending to any requirements for resuscitation and after you have started antibiotics.

The baby may require respiratory support for the respiratory failure that accompanies the respiratory distress. This may include oxygen therapy, continuous positive airway pressure (CPAP) or intubation and mechanical ventilation. Some specific lung diseases will also require exogenous surfactant treatment.

- *Oxygen treatment.* Remember that oxygen is a toxic substance, so use only the minimum amount necessary. If pre-ductal oxygen saturations are below 90%, it is reasonable to increase the fraction of inspired oxygen ($FiO_2$). In infants who do not require any other form of respiratory support this is best achieved by running oxygen into the incubator. Start with a flow of 2 L/min and increase or decrease to keep the pre-ductal oxygen saturations in the low 90s.
- *Blood gas monitoring.* Usually, if an infant requires an $FiO_2$ of more than about 0.4 on CPAP or is intubated and ventilated, they should have an arterial line. This is best achieved by inserting an umbilical arterial catheter, but this should be done by someone who is experienced in doing it. Get advice.
- *Continuous positive airway pressure (CPAP).* This is usually delivered with some form of nasal or nasopharyngeal tube. The aim is to provide a continuous positive background pressure to the infant's airway to help keep the airway open, maintain good lung volume and treat any atelectasis. Usually, a pressure of around 7 $cmH_2O$ is used. This will help to minimize any ventilation/perfusion mismatch.
- *Intubation and mechanical ventilation.* The decision to ventilate a baby with respiratory distress needs to be taken in discussion with the relevant paediatrician or neonatologist. A baby with respiratory distress is at least breathing and achieving some gas exchange – you don't want to convert that situation into something worse with multiple unsuccessful attempts at intubation.
  - Generally accepted criteria for the need for ventilation are unresponsive, severe or frequent apnoea; acidosis (arterial pH $<7.25$ with an arterial partial pressure of carbon dioxide ($PaCO_2$) $>60$ mmHg or pH $<7.25$ with base excess below $-10$ not corrected by bicarbonate or volume loading), requiring a $FiO_2 > 50\%$ to maintain oxygen saturation above 88%.
- *Exogenous surfactant* is usually given via an endotracheal tube to any intubated baby with hyaline membrane disease. Natural, animal-derived surfactants are usually used, including Survanta (a calf lung extract), Curosurf (a porcine product) and BLES (bovine lipid extract surfactant). It is also used before the diagnosis is made in infants of less than 26 weeks' gestational age, as soon as they are intubated.

Once any necessary resuscitation has been attended to, the management principles above applied and any respiratory support given, you can think about working out a cause for the respiratory distress.

- *Take a history.* Get details of the pregnancy, labour and delivery: results of antenatal screening including ultrasound findings, poly- or oligohydramnios, gestational age, risk factors for infection, meconium-stained liquor, need for resuscitation after birth.
- *Examine the baby:* be gentle. Look for any obvious congenital abnormalities.
- *Get a chest X-ray* if you haven't already done so. Take blood for a full blood count and film examination. A blood culture should already have been taken. Send a gastric aspirate and surface swabs (include groin and ear) for bacterial culture.
- If an airway problem is suspected, make sure the nares and oesophagus are patent. The successful passing of a nasogastric tube should confirm this.

## Causes of respiratory distress

A wide variety of congenital and acquired disorders can present in the newborn period as respiratory distress (Box 11.3.1). A systematic approach, which includes taking a thorough history, performing a complete physical examination and undertaking ancillary investigations, will readily determine most of these. The most common causes are explained in greater detail below.

**Box 11.3.1 Causes of respiratory distress**

- Infection (e.g. congenital infection, acquired infection)
- Retained fetal lung fluid, also known as transient tachypnoea of the newborn or 'wet lung'
- Infant respiratory distress syndrome, also known as hyaline membrane disease
- Pulmonary air leak (e.g. pneumothorax, pneumomediastinum, pneumopericardium, pulmonary interstitial emphysema)
- Aspiration (including meconium aspiration syndrome, blood, liquor amnii and milk)
- Surgical conditions (congenital diaphragmatic hernia, cystic hygroma, haemangioma, congenital lobar emphysema, congenital cystic adenomatoid malformation, sequestration of lung, lung cysts)
- Pulmonary hypoplasia (e.g. oligohydramnios from prolonged premature rupture of membranes or decreased fetal urine output, space-occupying thoracic lesions, fetal dyskinesia)
- Chronic neonatal lung disease
- Airway obstruction (e.g. choanal atresia, oesophageal atresia with tracheo-oesophageal fistula, micrognathia, laryngomalacia, tracheomalacia, vascular ring, subglottic stenosis)
- Cardiac disease (e.g. pulmonary hypertension, transposition of the great arteries with intact septum, total anomalous pulmonary venous return, patent ductus arteriosus, large ventriculoseptal defect, atrioventricular canal)
- Other respiratory causes (pulmonary haemorrhage, pulmonary lymphangiectasia, pleural/chylous effusions, hydrops fetalis, eventration of the diaphragm)
- Abdominal distension (e.g. bowel obstruction, necrotizing enterocolitis, massive ascites)
- Other – severe anaemia, polycythaemia, ischaemia, metabolic disease, increased metabolic demand such as hyperthermia, acidaemia, decreased chest wall compliance (e.g. severe oedema or skeletal dysplasia)

It is important to remember that not all cases of respiratory distress are caused by respiratory disease. One of the most common non-respiratory causes is metabolic acidosis (as seen in hypoxic ischaemic encephalopathy); the baby compensates for the acidosis by increasing the respiratory effort in order to clear more carbon dioxide. Some of the other non-respiratory causes of respiratory distress are listed in (Box 11.3.1.)

## Respiratory causes of respiratory distress

Regardless of the lung disease that causes the respiratory distress, the single most important aspect of its pathophysiology is atelectasis. Almost all of the conditions listed below will have an element of lung atelectasis. Atelectasis decreases respiratory compliance and therefore increased pressure is required to achieve adequate tidal volumes. Atelectasis also leads to ventilation/perfusion mismatch and cyanosis. These features in turn lead to a need for increased ventilation and therefore respiratory distress.

### Infection

It can be impossible to differentiate infection from other causes of respiratory distress such as respiratory distress syndrome, retained fetal lung fluid or meconium aspiration syndrome. Therefore, in all babies with respiratory distress, there should be a high index of suspicion for infection and a low threshold for septic workup and commencement of antibiotic therapy. Infection may be contracted *in utero* (congenital) and present at birth or soon afterwards (usually during the first 48 hours of life), or acquired and present later (this is often nosocomial). Maternal risk factors for congenital infection include known colonization with a pathogenic organism (e.g. group B streptococcus); previous infant with early-onset neonatal septicaemia; prolonged rupture of membranes (≥18 hours); multiple vaginal examinations; intrapartum or postpartum temperature ≥38°C; and preterm labour (<37 completed weeks of gestation).

Signs of infection in the baby are non-specific and include respiratory distress, an unexpected need for resuscitation, lethargy, apnoea, hypoglycaemia, hyperglycaemia, bradycardia, poor perfusion, hypotension, increased respiratory tract secretions, temperature instability (especially hypothermia) and feed intolerance. Infection may be found in any normally sterile or non-sterile site, but is most commonly seen in the blood (septicaemia), respiratory tract, urinary tract or cerebrospinal fluid. A large number of organisms including bacteria, viruses and fungi have been reported to cause congenital and nosocomial infection in neonates.

Unless you are absolutely certain that the baby does not have a bacterial infection (and this is rarely the case in a baby with respiratory distress), you should start antibiotics. Antibiotic regimens vary according to local patterns of disease, the age of the baby and previous organisms isolated (from mother or baby). Generally speaking, initial antibiotic choices should be broad-spectrum and then tailored once an organism and its antibiotic sensitivities have been identified. For early infection, a penicillin and aminoglycoside are usually used. Antibiotic choice for late infection is very much driven by the type of bacteria prevalent in the neonatal unit at the time and known colonizing bacteria.

### Clinical example

Baby Caleb was born via vaginal delivery at 41 weeks and 5 days' gestation. His 30-year-old primigravida mother had undergone induction for being post dates and had received two doses of dinoprostone (Prostin). An artificial rupture of membranes was performed 19 hours prior to delivery and no intrapartum antibiotics had been administered. Caleb was unexpectedly flat at delivery but responded well to 60 seconds of intermittent positive-pressure ventilation via bag and mask for resuscitation. His birth weight was 3200 g and the Apgar score was 4 and 8 at 1 and 5 minutes respectively. At 60 minutes of age he was noted to have grunting respirations, poor perfusion and seemed lethargic. Caleb was admitted to the nursery, had a full blood count and blood culture collected, and was commenced on intravenous antibiotics and a 10% dextrose infusion at a rate of 8 mL/h. He proceeded to have major apnoea, which required intubation and mechanical ventilation. Umbilical venous and arterial catheters were placed. Caleb continued to deteriorate with increasing oxygen requirements, hypotension and hypoglycaemia. At 14 hours of age the laboratory called to inform that the blood culture was positive and growing Gram-positive cocci. Despite intravenous antibiotics, inotropic support and mechanical ventilation, Caleb died at 20 hours of age. The culture subsequently revealed group B streptococcus, which was sensitive to penicillin.

## Retained fetal lung fluid or transient tachypnoea of the newborn

Retained fetal lung fluid (RFLF), also commonly known as transient tachypnoea of the newborn (TTN) or 'wet lung', occurs when either there is an excess of lung fluid or clearance mechanisms are inefficient. It is generally a benign, self-limiting disorder and occurs in 1–2% of term newborn infants. Risk factors include caesarean section without labour, breech delivery, male sex, birth asphyxia and heavy maternal analgesia. Babies present with respiratory distress and are sometimes described as 'mucusy' owing to the increased nasal and oral secretions. Infection should always be considered as a possible cause. A chest X-ray should be performed to rule out other causes of respiratory distress (e.g. pneumothorax, congenital diaphragmatic hernia). The lung fields on a chest X-ray show coarse streaking with fluid in fissures, giving a 'wet lung' appearance (Fig. 11.3.1). Most babies will settle with minimal handling in 24–48 hours and cot oxygen, but occasionally require respiratory support (e.g. CPAP, rarely ventilation).

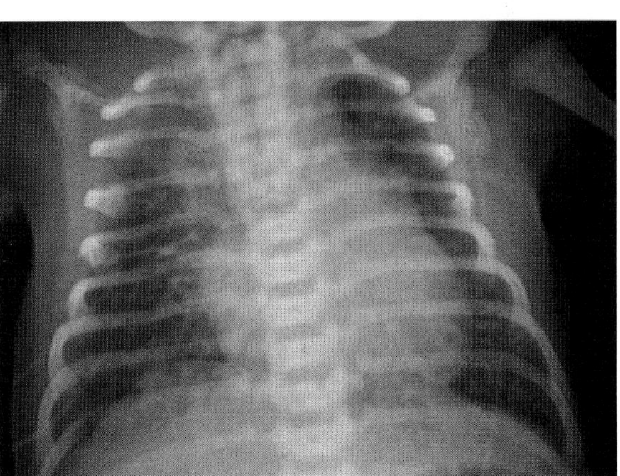

Fig. 11.3.1 Chest X-ray of retained fetal lung fluid.

## Respiratory distress syndrome or hyaline membrane disease

Respiratory distress syndrome (RDS), also known as hyaline membrane disease (HMD), is a specific entity in preterm infants; it is caused by surfactant deficiency in the alveoli. Surfactant is produced by the type 2 pneumocytes and is a surface tension lowering agent that allows alveoli to expand more easily and helps to prevent their collapse. The incidence is directly related to gestational age (Fig. 11.3.2) and can be prevented by administering antenatal corticosteroids or treated with surfactant replacement therapy (either prophylactic or rescue). The natural history of RDS is that it presents at or shortly after birth, increases in severity for 24–72 hours, the baby then starts to diurese and recovery subsequently occurs over the next 48–72 hours. This is often abbreviated by the administration of exogenous surfactant but can be prolonged in the extremely preterm infant. Treatment of RDS with exogenous surfactant decreases mortality and the incidence of pulmonary air leak.

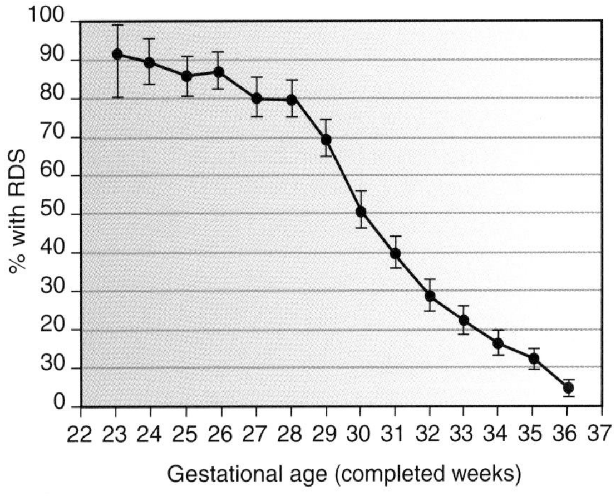


Fig. 11.3.2 Incidence of respiratory distress syndrome (RDS) with gestational age.

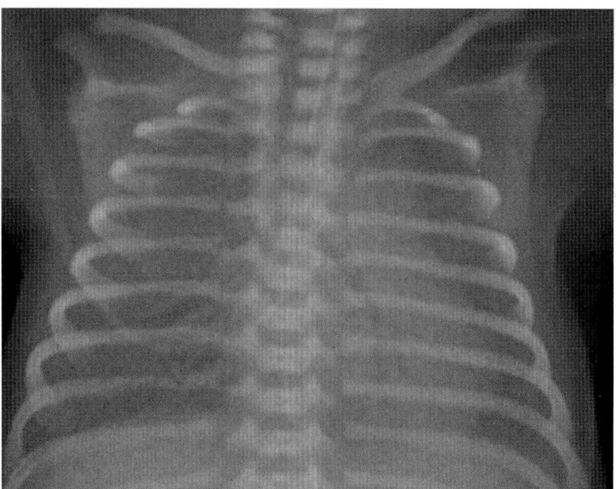

Fig. 11.3.3 Chest X-ray of respiratory distress syndrome.

RDS has a characteristic clinical picture and chest X-ray shows hypoaeration, a diffuse granuloreticular pattern (ground-glass appearance), air bronchograms and, in its most severe form, a diffuse 'white out' (Fig. 11.3.3).

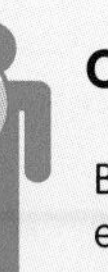

### Clinical example

Baby Kate was born at 29 weeks' gestation via emergency caesarean section to a 31-year-old G2P1 mother who presented with a blood pressure of 150/100 mmHg, abnormal liver function test results and hyperreflexia, presumably secondary to pregnancy-induced hypertension. Her mother was given one dose of betamethasone only 1 hour prior to delivery. Kate weighed 1100 g and had Apgar scores of 3 and 6 at 1 and 5 minutes of age. She was commenced on nasal CPAP shortly after birth, but over the next 4 hours had increasing work of breathing and oxygen requirements, which increased to 35%. Umbilical and venous catheters were inserted. After a premedication she was intubated with a 3.0-mm endotracheal tube, given a dose of exogenous surfactant and ventilated with synchronous intermittent positive-pressure ventilation. Her ventilatory requirements weaned rapidly and she was subsequently extubated to CPAP 12 hours later. She remained CPAP dependent for a further 16 days.

## Pulmonary air leaks

Pulmonary air leaks are more common in the neonatal period than at any other time of life. There are several types:

- pneumothorax: air in the pleural cavity
- pneumomediastinum: air in the mediastinum
- pneumopericardium: air in the pericardial space
- pulmonary interstitial emphysema (PIE): air in the interstitial lung spaces
- pneumoperitoneum: air in the peritoneal cavity (although this is more often secondary to a perforated abdominal viscus).

The pathophysiology of these conditions is similar, in that the alveoli become hyperinflated and rupture. Air escapes into the lung interstitium (PIE) or tracks along the perivascular spaces and ruptures into the mediastinum (pneumomediastinum), through the visceral pleura (pneumothorax) or rarely into the pericardial space (pneumopericardium).

Predisposing factors include the administration of positive-pressure breaths (including during active resuscitation at birth) and lung disease (especially hypoplastic lungs, meconium aspiration syndrome, RDS and RFLF). Spontaneous pneumothorax occurs in 1% of vaginal and 1.5% of caesarean section deliveries, but is usually asymptomatic.

Signs of a pulmonary air leak are non-specific and include respiratory distress, chest asymmetry, decreased air entry on auscultation on the affected side, trachea deviated away from the affected side, increased transillumination on the affected side, increasing ventilatory or oxygen requirements, and sudden deterioration with cardiorespiratory collapse. If the baby is stable, pulmonary air leak can be confirmed by chest X-ray. If the baby with a pneumothorax is unstable, emergency 'needle' aspiration and then drainage with an intercostal catheter may be required. A pneumomediastinum rarely needs to be drained.

### Clinical example

Baby Isabelle was born via elective lower-segment caesarean section at 38 weeks' gestation to a 27-year-old primigravida mother. Her birth weight was 3000 g and her Apgar score was 9 and 9 at 1 and 5 minutes respectively. She developed early respiratory distress with a respiratory rate of 70 breaths per minute, expiratory grunting, intercostal recession and cyanosis. She was found to have oxygen saturations in the low 80s, which improved with oxygen. She was commenced on nasal CPAP and seemed to settle until 4 hours of age when her oxygen requirement and work of breathing suddenly increased and she became bradycardic. Clinical examination revealed decreased air entry on the right, the trachea deviated to the left, an asymmetrical chest wall with the right side appearing full compared with the left, and the right chest bright on transillumination. A tension pneumothorax was suspected and an emergency needle aspiration was performed. Some 80 mL air was removed, with an immediate improvement in her condition. An intercostal catheter was placed on the right side and she was commenced on a morphine infusion for analgesia.

## Aspiration

Any liquid or solid that enters into the respiratory tract can lead to obstruction, atelectasis and an inflammatory response. In newborn babies, the most commonly aspirated agents are meconium, liquor amnii, blood, milk and gastric contents.

Meconium staining of liquor occurs in 10–20% of births, especially breech, post-term and where there is fetal distress. Staining of the amniotic fluid may range from thin green/brown-stained fluid to thick particulate matter. Meconium aspiration syndrome (MAS) occurs in only about 5% of infants born through meconium-stained amniotic fluid. Aspiration probably occurs *in utero* as the fetus starts to gasp with hypoxia. Suction of the airway under direct vision at birth of an infant with meconium-stained liquor is recommended only if the infant is non-vigorous and has not yet established respiration. A vigorous baby is one that has strong breathing efforts, a heart rate greater than 100 beats per min and good tone.

## Meconium aspiration syndrome

MAS has a constellation of features, which usually include the following:

- birth asphyxia requiring resuscitation
- infant covered in meconium with staining of cord, skin and nails
- meconium in the airway
- early-onset respiratory distress that may increase in severity as inflammatory response develops
- pulmonary hypertension
- surfactant dysfunction
- secondary bacterial infection (occurs late but always consider congenital infection as a potential cause).

Chest X-ray can show widespread, coarse, pulmonary infiltrate and atelectasis, areas of hyperinflation, and often both (Fig. 11.3.4).

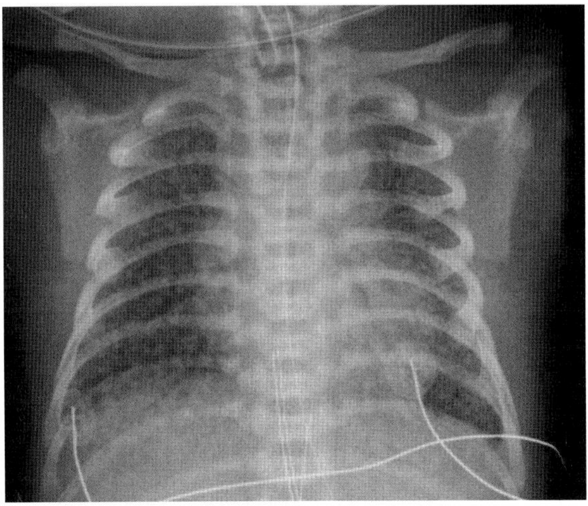

Fig. 11.3.4 Chest X-ray of meconium aspiration.

### Management

Morbidity and mortality from MAS can be prevented or minimized by optimal perinatal management. Treatment for established MAS is as for respiratory distress, with emphasis on humidification of inspired gases, postural drainage and airway suction, and antibiotics. Other management strategies include mechanical ventilation optimizing lung expansion, surfactant, inhaled nitric oxide, high-frequency oscillator ventilation and, possibly, extracorporeal membrane oxygenation.

## Congenital diaphragmatic hernia

See also Chapter 11.5.

Abdominal contents herniate through a muscular defect in the diaphragm into the chest. The incidence is 1 in 3800 births, with 60% isolated and 40% associated with other anomalies or chromosomal defects. The hernia is usually a posterolateral (Bochdalek) type, with 85% occurring on the left side. The defect in the diaphragm permits bowel or liver to herniate into the thorax with lung compression and pulmonary hypoplasia (worse on the side of the hernia but also present on the opposite side). Most cases are diagnosed by routine obstetric ultrasonography at 17–19 weeks' gestation or following investigation for polyhydramnios. If not diagnosed in the antenatal period, an infant may present immediately after birth with respiratory distress, dextrocardia (if a left-sided hernia) and a scaphoid abdomen. Diagnosis is confirmed by demonstration of abdominal contents (especially bowel loops) in the thorax on chest X-ray.

### Management

Management involves gastric decompression and cardiorespiratory support. Surgical repair is typically delayed for 3–7 days to enable maximum stabilization. Prognosis depends on age at presentation, coexisting problems, degree of pulmonary hypoplasia, presence of polyhydramnios and the severity of pulmonary hypertension. Overall only 30–60% of children with an isolated lesion survive.

## Pulmonary hypoplasia

Normal fetal lung development requires adequate amniotic fluid volume and fetal breathing movements. Although unilateral lung hypoplasia may be an isolated developmental anomaly, bilateral hypoplasia is secondary to other factors, such as:

- oligohydramnios (e.g. prolonged membrane rupture and liquor leak, or severe renal disease with little fetal urine output). The baby with renal agenesis may exhibit additional features of Potter deformation sequence with facial dysmorphism, joint contractures and amnion nodosum of the placenta
- a space-occupying lesion in the thorax (e.g. diaphragmatic hernia, pleural effusion, cystic adenomatoid malformation of the lung)
- chest wall deformities (e.g. skeletal dysplasia)
- fetal dyskinesia causing a decrease in fetal breathing patterns.

Infants with pulmonary hypoplasia present with progressive respiratory failure from birth, with marked hypoxia, hypercarbia and metabolic acidosis. Pneumothorax is common, due to the increased ventilatory pressures used to try to achieve adequate gas exchange. Death, ventilator dependence or bronchopulmonary dysplasia may result.

### Pulmonary haemorrhage

Pulmonary haemorrhage most commonly presents in very preterm infants with haemorrhagic pulmonary oedema (with blood welling up the endotracheal tube), which will compromise ventilation and lead to cardiovascular collapse. It may be seen in a large patent ductus arteriosus, severe perinatal asphyxia, coagulation disturbances, severe intrauterine growth restriction, hypothermia or congenital heart disease, and occasionally following exogenous surfactant therapy for RDS. Treatment consists of positive-pressure ventilation with high positive end-expiratory pressure to keep the lungs open and management of any coexisting shock, coagulation disturbance or patent ductus arteriosus.

### Congenital lobar emphysema

This is a rare anomaly due to cartilaginous deficiency in lobar bronchus (left upper lobe 50%, right middle lobe 24%, right upper lobe 18%). It may present as an insidious onset of respiratory distress over 2–3 weeks. It is associated with congenital heart disease in 30% of cases. On chest X-ray there is a hyperinflated lobe with surrounding pulmonary collapse and mediastinal displacement. Surgical lobectomy is usually curative.

### Cystic adenomatoid malformation

This is often diagnosed on antenatal ultrasonography. Polyhydramnios, hydrops fetalis, prematurity or stillbirth may result. There are three types:

- type 1 (70%) – single or multiple large cysts in one lobe
- type 2 (18%) – multiple medium-sized cysts
- type 3 (10%) – large cysts containing smaller cysts.

Differential diagnosis is from lobar emphysema, sequestration of lung and pulmonary lymphangiectasia. Surgical resection is usually curative.

### Neonatal chronic lung disease

Neonatal chronic lung disease (CLD) usually follows acute lung disease (most often RDS) in babies at high risk – the extremely preterm and those requiring mechanical ventilation with high pressures and large tidal volumes. The lung disease is characterized by chronic inflammation of the alveoli and airways with small airway narrowing, areas of atelectasis and hyper-expansion, increased airway secretions and, in the extremely preterm, altered lung architecture with decreased numbers of distorted alveoli. For research and audit purposes, neonatal CLD in ex-preterm infants is best defined as infants who require respiratory support or oxygen beyond 36 weeks' postmenstrual age. CLD may also complicate other lung diseases, such as meconium aspiration or pulmonary hypoplasia.

Infants with neonatal CLD have persistent chest recession, increased work of breathing, episodes of cyanosis and crackles/wheeze on auscultation of the chest. They are prone to lung infections, gastro-oesophageal reflux, aspiration, systemic hypertension, bronchospasm, progressive pulmonary hypertension with or without cor pulmonale, poor growth, developmental delay and sensorineural disability.

### Other lung diseases

Other disorders presenting in the newborn include sequestration of lung, pulmonary lymphangiectasia, lung cysts (especially bronchogenic), pleural/chylous effusions and eventration of the diaphragm.

## Airway obstruction

Any form of obstruction to the upper airway or lower airway can cause respiratory distress. The normal anatomy of the upper airway is shown in Figure 11.3.5. Babies with severe airway obstruction from birth usually present with respiratory distress immediately after birth with rapid onset of cyanosis, bradycardia and eventually apnoea.

#### Nasal obstruction

As newborn infants are obligatory nose-breathers, choanal atresia (caused by a bony obstruction of the nasopharyngeal meatus) can present with

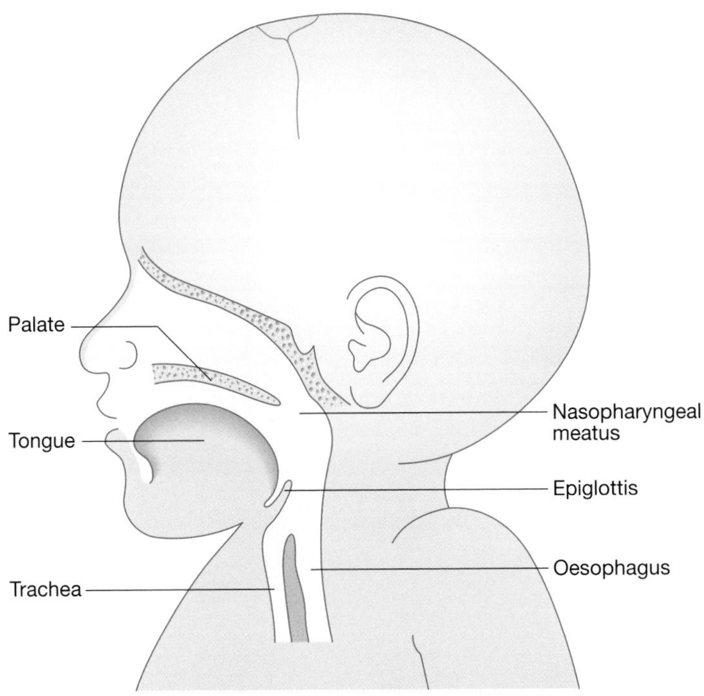


Fig. 11.3.5 Normal upper airway anatomy.

obstructed breathing and apnoea. The atresia can be confirmed by failure to pass a nasogastric tube through either nare. This can be managed temporarily by the insertion of an oropharyngeal airway (Fig. 11.3.6).

## Pharyngeal obstruction

Micrognathia (as seen in the Pierre Robin sequence) causes a backward displacement of the tongue which obstructs the pharynx. This can be managed temporarily by insertion of a nasopharyngeal airway

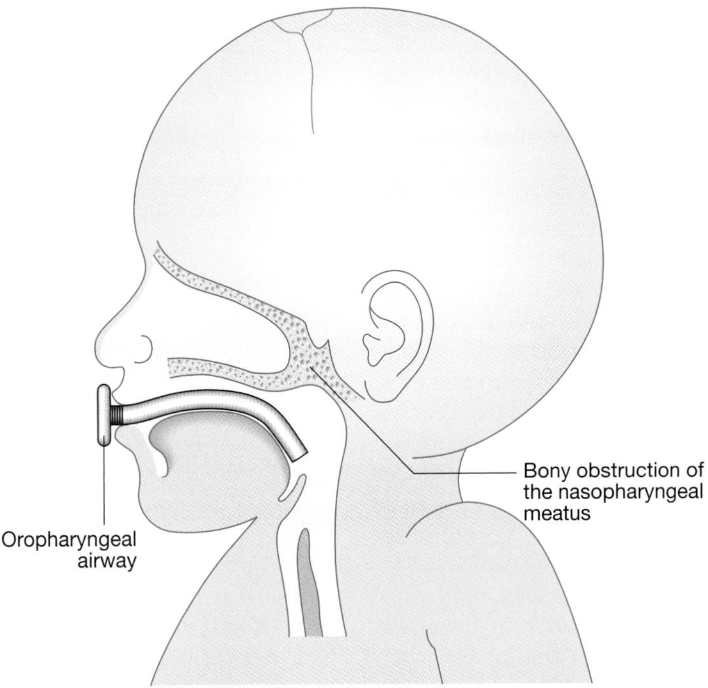


Fig. 11.3.6 Choanal atresia and oropharyngeal airway.

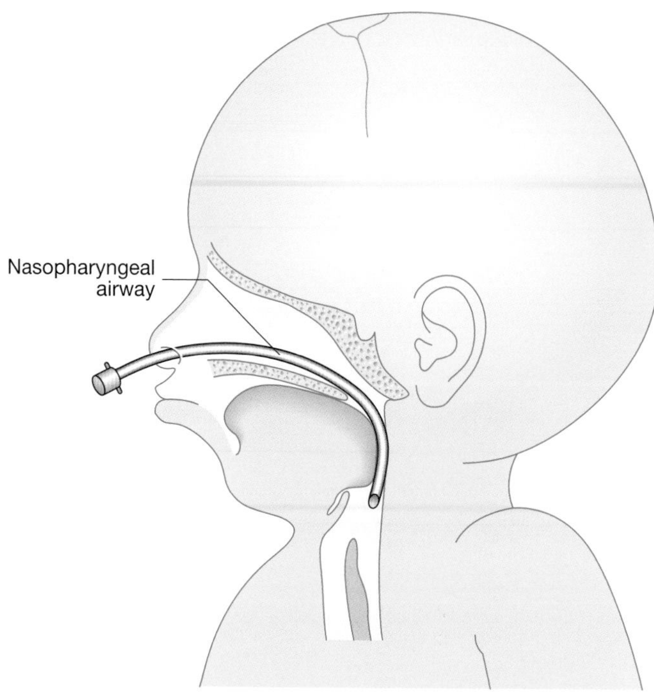


Fig. 11.3.7 Micrognathia and nasopharyngeal airway.

(Fig. 11.3.7). Severe macroglossia (as seen in trisomy 21 and Beckwith–Weidemann syndrome) can be managed in a similar fashion. Rare causes of upper airway obstruction include tumours and cysts of the tongue or floor of the mouth, as well as cystic hygromas.

### Laryngeal and/or tracheal obstruction

Laryngomalacia, due to a large floppy larynx (secondary to decreased cartilage) that narrows on inspiration, may rarely present in the newborn period as respiratory distress (most commonly as inspiratory stridor when crying). Most cases are benign. However, if severe, consult with an ENT surgeon as surgical laser excision of the aryepiglottic folds may be curative. Other causes of upper airway obstruction include subglottic stenosis (often due to repeated or traumatic intubations), laryngeal webs, laryngeal oedema/inflammation (due to prolonged/traumatic intubation) or haemangiomas. Unilateral vocal cord paralysis will partially obstruct the larynx; bilateral paralysis causes complete obstruction. Other causes of obstruction in the lower airway include tumours, haemangiomas of the airway (can be in the lumen, in the wall of the larynx or trachea, or compressing from outside the airway), vascular rings, broncho/tracheomalacia, and tracheal stenosis or webs. Examination of the airway under direct vision (laryngoscopy and/or bronchoscopy) is often required to define the cause and extent of the airway obstruction.

## Hypoventilation

The physiology of breathing requires more than a pair of lungs with a functional gas-exchanging surface and matching circulation. It also requires an intact mechanism to enable the mechanics of breathing (i.e. moving a bulk volume of air in and out of the lungs with each breath). A clear airway is essential, as is an intact pathway from the respiratory signals in the brainstem to the muscles of breathing. Any malfunction of the neuromuscular pathway (Fig. 11.3.8), from brain to respiratory muscles, can lead to hypoventilation and inadequate gas exchange, especially carbon dioxide clearance.

### Apnoea

The ultimate form of hypoventilation is apnoea. Apnoea is defined as a cessation or absence of air flow in and out of the lungs. In a practical sense, neonates are said to have had an apnoea when either there is: (1) no air flow for 20 seconds or more, or (2) no air flow for 10 seconds or more if it is accompanied by bradycardia or desaturation.

Apnoea does not necessarily mean there is no respiratory effort. Complete airway obstruction will not allow any airflow, but, at least initially, there will be respiratory effort – this is the case with obstructive apnoea.

The most common cause of apnoea in neonates is apnoea of prematurity. The immature respiratory centres in the brainstem regulate breathing poorly until around

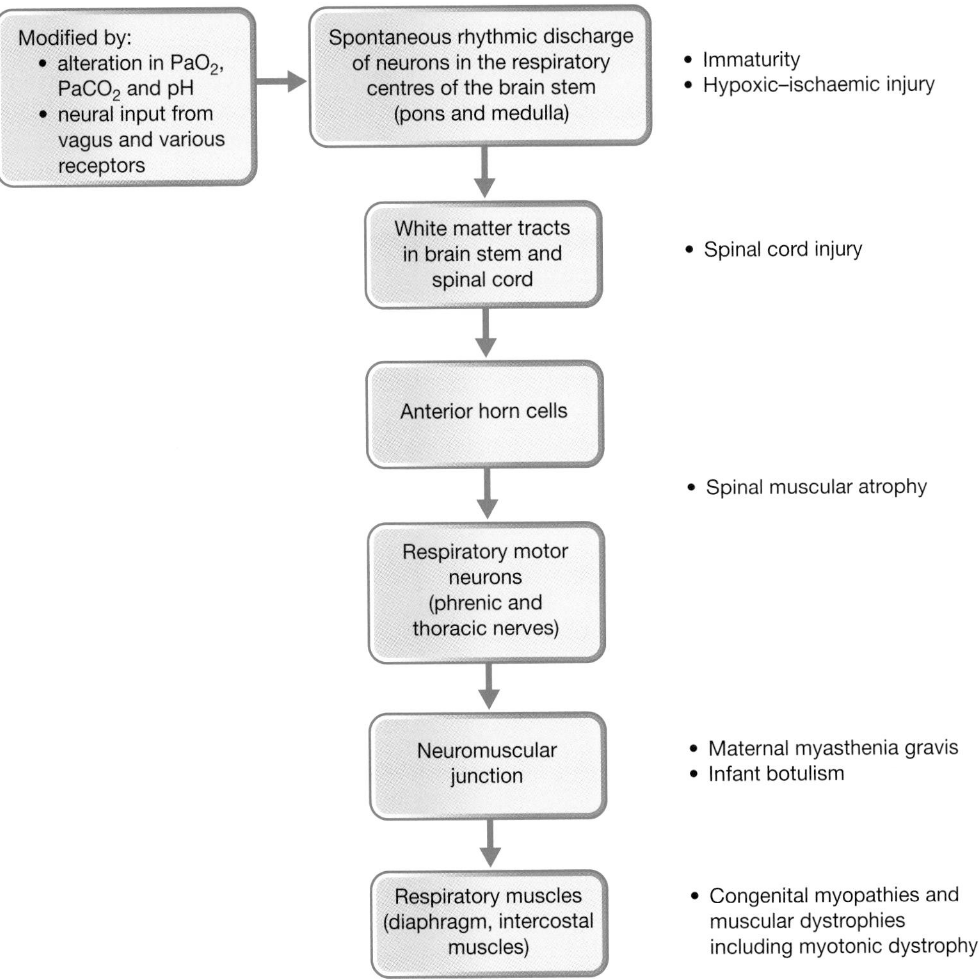


**Fig. 11.3.8** Flow diagram showing control of respiration.

34 weeks' gestational age. Breathing patterns will vary from regular, irregular and periodic; all may be accompanied by apnoea in a well preterm infant. Periodic respirations refer to a cyclical pattern of changes in the size of the infant's breaths – usually alternating periods of normal breathing with hypoventilation.

Apnoeas commonly occur in otherwise well preterm infants. They often resolve spontaneously or gentle stimulation is required to restart breathing.

Because of preterm infants' immature respiratory centres, they are prone to developing apnoea (or more severe or more frequent apnoea) from a variety of causes. These include:

- lung disease
- hypoxia
- acidaemia
- drugs (e.g. narcotics (including those given to the mother), dinoprostone, magnesium sulphate)
- metabolic disturbance (e.g. hypoglycaemia, hypocalcaemia, hypomagnesaemia, hypermagnesaemia)
- infection – generalized or focal; bacterial or viral
- intracranial haemorrhage
- polycythaemia with hyperviscosity
- necrotizing enterocolitis
- patent ductus arteriosus
- seizures
- temperature instability (e.g. incubator temperature too high, hypothermia, too rapid warming or cooling).

Any previously well preterm infant who develops apnoea or has an increase in the frequency or severity of their apnoea warrants investigation for a cause. This must include a blood culture (with or without cerebrospinal fluid culture), a full blood count and blood film examination, and then commencement of antibiotics.

Apnoea in a term infant is *always* abnormal and a cause must be sought. Cover with antibiotics until bacterial infection is ruled out. Consider covering for treatable viral infections such as herpes.

It is sometimes useful to classify apnoea as central, obstructive, mixed or reflex:

- *Central apnoea* – apnoea secondary to factors affecting the respiratory centres in the brainstem. It is characterized by an absence of respiratory effort.
- *Obstructive apnoea* – complete obstruction of the central airways will cause obstructive apnoea. Nasal obstruction can also cause obstructive apnoea because newborn infants are obligatory nose-breathers. Causes of airway obstruction have been discussed above. Transient causes include milk and mucus, or foreign bodies lodged in the airway. Obstructive apnoea is characterized initially by increased respiratory efforts.
- *Mixed apnoea* – a mixture of central and obstructive types; seen especially in the preterm infant where an obstruction can trigger central apnoea. This is difficult to diagnose clinically.
- *Reflex apnoea* – reflex or vagally mediated apnoea can occur after suction of the pharynx, larynx or stomach, secondary to passage of a nasogastric tube, or even in response to defaecation. Apnoea associated with gastro-oesophageal reflux may be reflex and/or obstructive.

### Neuromuscular causes

Sometimes hypoventilation presents without overt apnoea. Any interruption of the pathway shown in Figure 11.3.8 can decrease ventilation; this usually causes carbon dioxide retention initially, with or without hypoxia. Often babies with neuromuscular causes for their hypoventilation will have a high $PaCO_2$ in the absence of any increased respiration. If the respiratory neuromuscular pathway is intact, a high $PaCO_2$ will usually cause dramatically increased respiratory efforts.

Hypoxic–ischaemic encephalopathy can interfere with respiratory centre function secondary to direct neuronal injury. Any accompanying seizures are more likely to cause apnoea. Spinal cord injury is a rare complication of traumatic delivery (e.g. following rotational forceps delivery). In congenital spinal muscular atrophy the anterior horn cells of the motor neurons degenerate, leading to generalized muscle weakness that includes the respiratory muscles. Blockage of the neuromuscular junction can occur with infant botulism (rare in the developed world but not infrequent in the developing world) or maternal myasthenia gravis (maternal anti-acetylcholine receptor antibodies block the neuromuscular junction). Any weakness of the respiratory muscles from congenital myopathies and muscular dystrophies (including myotonic dystrophy) will also lead to hypoventilation.

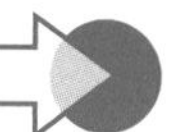

#### Practical points

- The signs of respiratory distress may include any of the following: tachypnoea, expiratory grunt, recession, nasal flare and central cyanosis.
- A baby with respiratory distress should be monitored closely for signs of respiratory failure.
- Infection should always be considered as a possible cause of respiratory distress. Unless you are absolutely certain that the baby does not have a bacterial infection (and this is rarely the case in a baby with respiratory distress), you should collect a blood culture and start intravenous antibiotics.
- A chest X-ray is useful to exclude causes of respiratory distress such as pulmonary air leak and congenital diaphragmatic hernia.

# Congenital and perinatal infections 11.4

Mike Starr

## Introduction

Infections in the fetus and newborn (perinatal infections) may be acquired *in utero* (congenital infection), around the time of delivery or in the neonatal period.

### Modes of acquisition of infection

- *In utero*
  - haematogenous – placental infection and/or transplacental transmission
  - ascent from the maternal genital tract – across intact membranes, or after the membranes rupture
- During delivery
  - from maternal genital secretions
  - from maternal blood
- After birth
  - from breast milk
  - by conventional (horizontal) routes from mother or other contacts.

The route by which the fetus or newborn acquires the infection has important implications for management during pregnancy and the neonatal period, and for the development of appropriate intervention strategies to prevent mother-to-child transmission.

The outcome of perinatal infection may include particular constellations of congenital abnormalities, spontaneous abortion or stillbirth, or acute neonatal infection. Common clinical manifestations include:

- growth retardation
- prematurity
- hepatitis, thrombocytopenia
- meningoencephalitis
- microcephaly
- intracerebral calcifications
- rash
- chorioretinitis
- deafness
- neurological defects.

For some congenital infections, there may be no symptoms or signs in the neonatal period and it may be weeks, months or even years before the effects first become evident.

Many organisms can cause infection in the fetus and newborn. Box 11.4.1 lists some of the more common or clinically significant.

### Risk assessment

The risk of fetal damage can be estimated, based on:

- the likelihood of maternal exposure and infection
- the likelihood of transmission to the fetus
- the stage in gestation at which infection occurs – this influences the risk of vertical transmission and/or the fetal or perinatal consequences.

Only a small number of exposed infants are infected and, of these, a minority will have adverse effects. Many infections that can damage the fetus are mild or asymptomatic in the mother, and diagnosis may depend on routine antenatal screening. Whether this is appropriate depends on the frequency and severity of fetal or neonatal disease and the availability of a suitable screening test and effective intervention.

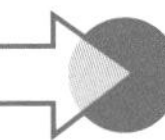

**Practical points**

**Congenital infections**

- Some common viral infections (e.g. cytomegalovirus, parvovirus, rubella, varicella-zoster virus) can cause fetal infection with severe consequences if acquired during pregnancy by a non-immune woman.
- Ensuring that a woman has antenatal testing and is immunized with all recommended vaccines is an important part of care during pregnancy.
- Management of a pregnant woman exposed to relevant viral infections depends on a careful risk assessment, which includes knowledge of the woman's immune status, history of the exposure, stage in the pregnancy, and clinical presentation in the woman.

## Organisms associated with perinatal infection

### Cytomegalovirus

Primary cytomegalovirus (CMV) infection is usually asymptomatic or causes a non-specific illness with fever, atypical lymphocytosis and mild hepatitis. The

**Box 11.4.1 Organisms commonly associated with perinatal infection**

**Associated with congenital abnormalities**
- Cytomegalovirus
- Parvovirus B19
- Rubella
- *Toxoplasma gondii*
- *Treponema pallidum* (syphilis)
- Varicella zoster virus

**Associated with acute neonatal infection**
- *Chlamydia trachomatis*
- *Escherichia coli*
- Enterovirus
- Herpes simplex virus
- *Listeria monocytogenes*
- Group B streptococcus

**Associated with chronic infection**
- Hepatitis B virus
- Hepatitis C virus
- Human immunodeficiency virus

virus remains in a latent state with periodic asymptomatic reactivation and excretion in urine, saliva or genital secretions. Primary maternal infection or reactivation can result in fetal CMV infection, although fetal damage is more likely to be associated with primary infection. CMV can infect the fetus transplacentally to cause congenital infection.

Cytomegalovirus can also be transmitted during or after delivery when the neonate comes in contact with maternal genital secretions or with breast milk. However, it appears that there are no hearing or neurodevelopmental sequelae.

Congenital CMV affects approximately 3–12 per 1000 births and causes 10–30% of childhood sensorineural hearing loss (SNHL). Infants with asymptomatic congenital CMV have a risk of developing hearing loss or intellectual disability. Early intervention can minimize the impact of SNHL on language development. Moreover, antiviral treatment may improve outcome.

The best evidence for primary maternal infection is seroconversion but this may not be demonstrable if investigation is delayed. Specific immunoglobulin (Ig) M may indicate recent infection but is unreliable: it may be detectable for months, can rise after reactivation, and false-positive results are not uncommon.

### Primary infection

- 50% of young women are seronegative (susceptible). In developing countries and lower socioeconomic groups, primary infection occurs at a younger age and fewer women are susceptible.
- 1% of women seroconvert during pregnancy.
- 30% of fetuses of women with primary infection are infected.
- The risk of congenital CMV infection after primary maternal CMV infection remains increased for up to 4 years after seroconversion, with the highest risk being in the first 2 years.
- Infection is transplacental; severe fetal damage is more likely early in gestation.
- 10% of infants infected during primary maternal infection are symptomatic at birth: of these, 90% have significant long-term handicap.
- 90% of infants infected during primary maternal infection are asymptomatic at birth: of these, 10% go on to develop deafness or intellectual handicap.
- The overall incidence of congenital infection due to primary maternal infection is 1 in 1000.

### Reactivation

- 20–30% of seropositive women reactivate latent infection during pregnancy.
- 2–5% of their infants are infected *in utero* but significant CMV disease is rare; mild sequelae (unilateral deafness) occur infrequently (<10%).
- The overall incidence of congenital infection is 1–2% – the majority are unaffected.

### Clinical features

The clinical features of severe intrauterine CMV infection include:
- intrauterine growth restriction
- hepatosplenomegaly, hepatitis
- anaemia, thrombocytopenia
- pneumonitis
- microcephaly, encephalitis, cerebral calcification and chorioretinitis
- SNHL in congenital CMV affects 50% of symptomatic infants and 10% of asymptomatic infants. It is the most common long-term consequence. It ranges from mild unilateral to profound bilateral hearing loss. In asymptomatic infants it may be underdiagnosed because the SNHL is detected too late to prove congenital infection
- cerebral palsy, intellectual disability, epilepsy and visual impairment.

### Diagnosis

If primary maternal infection is suspected or cannot be excluded, fetal infection can be diagnosed by culture and/or polymerase chain reaction (PCR) analysis of amniotic fluid at 18 weeks' gestation.

Depending on when maternal infection occurred, the risk of fetal damage may justify termination of pregnancy.

Congenital CMV infection is diagnosed by a positive culture of urine or saliva collected in the first 3 weeks of life; after that it is difficult to distinguish congenital from postnatal infection. Testing for CMV IgM in the infant's serum is less sensitive and specific. Congenital infection may be confirmed by PCR analysis of dried blood spots (e.g. Guthrie card).

### Treatment

Antiviral drugs active against CMV are contraindicated during pregnancy but have been used with limited success in congenitally infected infants. Intravenous ganciclovir and oral valganciclovir have been shown to reduce hearing deterioration in infants with symptomatic congenital CMV and central nervous system involvement. However, use of these medications is limited by their side-effects. There is currently no indication for systemic antiviral therapy for infants with asymptomatic infection at birth.

**Clinical example**

A 32-year-old woman delivered a small-for-gestational-age baby boy weighing 2400 g at 38 weeks' gestation. His head circumference was smaller than expected for his weight and he had hepatosplenomegaly. He also had thrombocytopenia.

Rubella, CMV, *Toxoplasma* and syphilis serology were performed on the baby and compared with the mother's antenatal serological results. The baby had urine collected for viral culture. The baby had CMV IgG and IgM present, and CMV was cultured from the urine, confirming congenital CMV infection.

The potential side-effects of 6 weeks of intravenous ganciclovir therapy in this child must be weighed against a possible small benefit in terms of reduction of hearing deterioration. Affected neonates should have baseline audiology testing, and this should be repeated in the first 6 months of life. They should also be monitored for developmental delay.

## Parvovirus B19

Most cases of parvovirus B19 infection are asymptomatic. The most common clinical presentation of infection is erythema infectiosum, or 'slapped cheek disease' in children.

Parvovirus B19 can also cause:

- asymptomatic infection
- mild respiratory tract illness without rash
- petechial or purpuric rash
- arthritis in adults
- chronic bone marrow failure in immunodeficient patients
- transient aplastic crisis in patients with haemolytic anaemia (e.g. sickle cell disease).

Approximately 60% of adult women are immune. The risk of infection in seronegative women is greatest in women exposed to an infected child at home (approximately 50%). The risk for childcare and primary school teachers exposed is 20–30%, and the risk overall depends on exposure to children but is approximately 10–20%.

### Fetal risks following maternal infection

In 50% of cases of maternal infection, the fetus is unaffected. Fetal damage occurs only if maternal infection occurs before 20 weeks' gestation. The complications include:

- fetal loss in the first 20 weeks of pregnancy (15% compared with 5% in controls, i.e. 10% excess fetal loss)
- congenital abnormalities: <1% (anecdotal reports only)
- hydrops fetalis: following maternal infections at 9–20 weeks' gestation (incidence is approximately 3%); may result in:
  - spontaneous resolution (one-third of cases)
  - fetal death (usually without intrauterine transfusion; occasionally despite it)
  - resolution after intrauterine transfusion (most cases in which it is attempted)
  - long-term sequelae: chronic congenital anaemia after intrauterine transfusion is rare.

See also Table 11.4.1.

There are no specific congenital abnormalities associated with maternal parvovirus infection.

**Table 11.4.1 Risk assessment – parvovirus B19**

| | Any pregnant woman exposed to parvovirus (%) | Pregnant woman with proven recent infection (%) |
|---|---|---|
| Excess fetal loss in first 20 weeks | 0.4–1 (1 in 100–250) | 5 (1 in 20) |
| Death from hydrops or its treatment | 0.05–0.1 (1 in 850–2000) | 0.6 (1 in 170) |

### Diagnosis

Diagnosis in children is mainly clinical. In potentially infected women, serology and PCR can be performed. IgM is detectable within 1–3 weeks of exposure and usually remains detectable for 2–3 months. Specific IgG may rise 2–3 weeks following infection. Parvovirus DNA can be detected in serum for up to 9 months after the acute viraemic phase in some patients, so it does not necessarily indicate acute infection.

### Management

Pregnant school teachers or childcare workers do not need to be excluded from work, even during an epidemic (nor do infected children). It is certainly not practicable to prevent exposure at home. Pregnant women who have been exposed to parvovirus, and those with an illness consistent with parvovirus, should be tested serologically. If maternal infection is confirmed, the pregnancy should be monitored with serial ultrasonography.

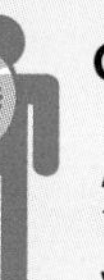

**Clinical example**

A 24-year-old primary school teacher is 12 weeks' pregnant. She has a 3-year-old who is well at the moment. She is concerned because there is a boy in her class with 'slapped cheek disease'. What advice should be given to her?

The likelihood is that she is immune – 60% of women of child-bearing age are seropositive. She should have her serology done to check. Even if she is not immune, there is no point in her staying away from school. The boy with slapped cheek disease is probably no longer infectious – once the rash is apparent children are not infectious, and there may well have been others in the class with asymptomatic infection. If there have been many cases of parvovirus infection around, her 3-year-old may have had it too, and the greatest risk of infection for a pregnant mother is from her own children.

If the woman is seronegative when checked, she should be offered repeat serology in 2 weeks. If the serology is negative at this time, nothing further needs to be done. If she has evidence of seroconversion, there is a 50% chance that the fetus will be infected and a very small risk that she will lose the pregnancy or that the fetus will develop hydrops. She should have ultrasonography at 1–2-week intervals for the next 8 weeks, checking for the development of fetal hydrops. Even if this develops, at least 60% of fetuses will have a good outcome.

## Rubella

The teratogenic effects of rubella were first noted in 1941 by an Australian ophthalmologist, who recognized several cases of congenital cataract following a large outbreak of rubella. Maternal rubella is now rare in many industrialized countries with rubella vaccination programmes. However, in many developing countries, congenital rubella syndrome remains a major cause of developmental anomalies, particularly blindness and deafness.

### Clinical features

The risk of fetal infection and damage is greatest during the first 8 weeks of pregnancy and damage is rare after 16 weeks. Congenital rubella syndrome (Fig. 11.4.1) may include a number of clinical features, some of which may not present until adolescence or adulthood:

- intrauterine growth restriction
- neonatal purpuric rash and hepatosplenomegaly
- microcephaly and developmental delay
- cardiac: pulmonary artery hypoplasia, patent ductus arteriosus
- eye: cataract, retinopathy; microphthalmia
- deafness – develops later
- diabetes mellitus – develops later.

### Diagnosis

Congenital rubella is confirmed by:

- isolation of rubella virus from saliva, tears, urine, cerebrospinal fluid (CSF) or tissue during the first 3 months of life
- demonstration of specific IgM antibody or persistence of IgG antibody beyond 6 months of age.

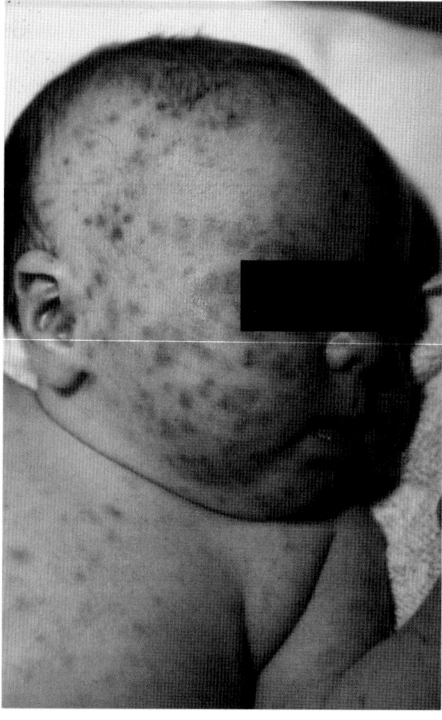

Fig. 11.4.1 Characteristic purpuric ('blueberry muffin') rash of congenital rubella.

### Prevention

Congenital rubella is preventable by immunization in childhood (see Chapter 3.5). Routine antenatal screening and postpartum immunization of susceptible women provides additional protection. If rubella infection or contact is suspected during pregnancy, investigation to detect or exclude infection (specific IgM or IgG seroconversion) should be done, even in women with known past immunity, as re-infection occasionally occurs. Termination of pregnancy may be recommended after proven infection during the first trimester.

## *Toxoplasma gondii*

*Toxoplasma gondii* is a protozoan parasite that infects up to a third of the world's population. Infection is acquired mainly by ingestion of food or water that is contaminated with oocysts shed by cats or by eating undercooked or raw meat containing tissue cysts. Primary infection is usually subclinical but may cause lymphadenopathy or ocular disease. Infection acquired during pregnancy may cause severe damage to the fetus. The risk of fetal infection increases, but that of fetal damage decreases with advancing gestation (Table 11.4.2). There is geographical variation in the incidence of congenital infection; in Australia it is estimated to be less than 1 in 1000 births.

### Clinical features

- Most congenitally infected infants are asymptomatic at birth.
- Many later develop signs and sometimes symptoms of chorioretinitis (up to 80%, with some visual impairment in about half).
- Some 10% develop neurological sequelae and/or hearing deficit.
- Signs of severe symptomatic congenital toxoplasmosis include:
  - anaemia, hepatosplenomegaly, jaundice, lymphadenopathy
  - thrombocytopenia, petechial rash

**Table 11.4.2 Risk assessment – *Toxoplasma gondii***

| | Fetal infection (%) | Fetal damage (%) |
|---|---|---|
| First trimester | 5–15 | 60–80 |
| Second trimester | 25–40 | 15–25 |
| Third trimester | 30–75 | 2–10 |

  - central nervous system damage – intracranial calcification, hydrocephalus and microcephaly
  - neurological and/or visual impairment in most survivors.

### Diagnosis and management

Toxoplasmosis during pregnancy is ideally diagnosed by demonstrating seroconversion. More commonly, it is suspected because specific IgM is detected in serum by antenatal screening. IgM can remain detectable for many months and, in the absence of symptoms, further testing is needed. Tests for the avidity of IgG antibodies can discriminate between recently acquired and previous infection. If recent infection is confirmed or cannot be excluded, treatment of the mother with spiramycin can reduce the risk of vertical transmission.

Appropriate management depends on diagnosis of intrauterine infection by amniotic fluid PCR at about 18 weeks' gestation. If fetal infection occurs during the first trimester, termination of pregnancy is often recommended. If infection occurs during the second or third trimester, treatment of the mother with a combination of pyrimethamine and a sulphonamide is likely to reduce sequelae of the disease in the newborn.

Specific IgM in the infant's serum or persistence of IgG beyond the first few months of life is evidence of congenital toxoplasmosis. *T. gondii* may be detected in tissue by histological examination or PCR, or in CSF by PCR. Treatment of a congenitally infected infant with spiramycin, pyrimethamine and a sulphonamide can reduce progressive damage after birth.

## *Treponema pallidum* (syphilis)

Syphilis is a sexually transmitted infection caused by *Treponema pallidum*. Congenital syphilis is now a rare disease in most countries but it remains a severe adverse outcome of pregnancy in many less developed countries. Untreated syphilis in pregnancy can cause stillbirth, preterm labour and intrauterine growth restriction. Later in life, a range of neurological disorders can occur, including paretic neurosyphilis; all of these manifestations respond poorly to treatment.

Fetal infection is a result of haematogenous spread from an infected mother, although transmission at the time of delivery can occur from direct contact with infectious genital lesions. Transmission from mother to fetus can occur at any stage of pregnancy, particularly during early (primary, secondary or early latent) syphilis. Maternal syphilis is often asymptomatic and recognized only because of a positive routine antenatal serological test. Early antenatal screening and treatment of maternal syphilis can prevent most cases of congenital infection.

The fetal outcome of untreated maternal syphilis depends on the stage of the disease:

- primary or secondary: premature delivery or perinatal death, 50%; congenital syphilis, 50% (few normal infants)
- early latent syphilis (or indeterminate): at least 50% normal, 20–40% congenital syphilis; increased risk of perinatal death and preterm birth.

### Clinical features

At least 50% of infants with congenital syphilis are asymptomatic, so diagnosis may rely on serology. Clinical features typical of congenital syphilis include:

- an abnormally bulky placenta – histological examination should be done
- hydrops fetalis due to severe anaemia and/or severe liver disease
- lymphadenopathy, hepatosplenomegaly, jaundice
- osteochondritis with typical radiological changes; arthropathy or pseudoparalysis
- rhinitis ('snuffles')
- vesiculobullous rash on back, legs, palms and soles, followed by desquamation
- condylomata lata – fleshy lesions in moist areas of skin.

The diagnosis is confirmed by serological tests on the mother and infant: neonatal IgG antibody titres that are significantly higher than the mother's and/or the presence of specific IgM in the infant. A lumbar puncture should be performed on the infant. Neurosyphilis is suggested by CSF pleocytosis, raised protein level and positive CSF serology.

### Treatment

Congenital syphilis is treated with parenteral penicillin. Serological and clinical follow-up is needed to confirm successful treatment and exclude neurological or ophthalmological abnormality or deafness.

Congenital syphilis may present in a variety of ways. It is important to screen for maternal syphilis following stillbirth or if an unusual lesion or condition consistent with syphilis is present in the newborn infant. Routine antenatal screening for syphilis is cost-effective and still recommended, although the prevalence in Australia is low. Adequate treatment of an infected mother during pregnancy will prevent fetal damage.

**Clinical example**

A 19-year-old intravenous drug user has a past history of a stillbirth at 36 weeks' gestation, for which no cause was found. She is known to be hepatitis C positive, but her human immunodeficiency virus (HIV) status is unknown. She is now pregnant and presents at term, having had no antenatal care. She delivers a baby boy who is noted to have hepatosplenomegaly. What tests should be done?

With no antenatal care and a baby with hepatosplenomegaly, the concern is that the baby may have a congenital infection. Given the history that she was an intravenous drug user and hepatitis C positive, particular concerns would include syphilis, hepatitis C, hepatitis B and HIV.

Mother and baby should have serological tests for syphilis: rapid plasma reagin test (RPR) and *Treponema pallidum* haemagglutination test (TPHA). If the neonatal antibody titres are significantly higher than the mother's, the baby's IgM should be tested. A lumbar puncture should also be performed on the baby. Neurosyphilis is suggested by CSF pleocytosis, raised protein level and positive CSF serology.

The mother should have other serological testing: HIV antibodies, hepatitis B surface antigen and hepatitis C antibody, and viral load. The baby should have hepatitis C antibody testing no earlier than 12 months, and preferably at 18 months of age. If performed earlier, a positive result may simply reflect the mother's antibody.

## Varicella-zoster virus

At least 90% of adults are immune to varicella, but exposure during pregnancy is common. Fetal outcomes following maternal infection early in pregnancy include:

- uncomplicated self-limiting infection (10%)
- herpes zoster (shingles) in the first year of life (2–3%)
- fetal varicella syndrome (2–3% of cases), manifestations of which include:
  - growth restriction
  - skin scarring over a dermatomal distribution (Fig. 11.4.2)
  - ipsilateral limb or other skeletal hypoplasia
  - encephalopathy and abnormalities of various organs.

The risk of fetal varicella syndrome in children exposed to varicella-zoster virus (VZV) *in utero* is around 0.5% after maternal infection at 2–12 weeks of pregnancy, 1.4% after infection at 12–28 weeks, and does not occur after infection from 28 weeks onwards. It occurs in around 1.6 per 100 000 births in the population. Shingles in the mother does not carry a risk of fetal varicella syndrome.

VZV infection of the newborn results from transmission from a mother with chickenpox to her infant

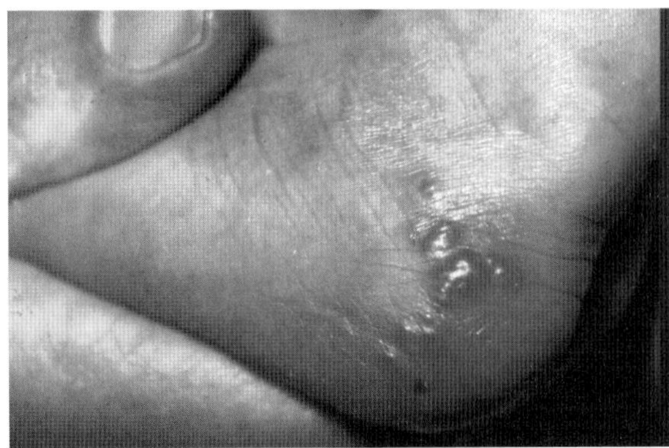

Fig. 11.4.2 Skin scarring from congenital varicella-zoster virus infection.

around the time of delivery, where the infant lacks the protection of maternal antibodies. The likelihood of infection depends on the timing of delivery in relation to when the mother develops the chickenpox rash. If the rash develops more than 7 days before delivery, this generally allows time for the development and transfer of protective maternal antibodies. However, as transfer of antibodies from the mother to the infant is limited before 26–28 weeks of gestation, maternal immunity to VZV does not usually protect preterm infants delivered before 28 weeks' gestational age.

If maternal VZV infection occurs during the week from 5 days before delivery until 2 days afterwards, infection of the infant may be complicated by pneumonia, hepatitis or encephalitis, and high mortality. When maternal infection occurs more than 5 days before delivery, infection in the infant is usually mild. Infants exposed to varicella after the first few days of life also usually have mild disease, although this is variable and depends, amongst other factors, on the mother's immune status.

### Prophylaxis and treatment

Zoster immune globulin (ZIG) can prevent or modify varicella if given within 4 days (preferably 48 hours) of exposure to:

- pregnant women with no past history of chickenpox who are seronegative or whose immune status is unknown
- newborn infants of women who develop varicella within 5 days before to 2 days after delivery.

Severe varicella in mother or infant should be treated with intravenous aciclovir.

Varicella vaccine is now a component of the routine immunization schedule (see Chapter 3.5). Immunization of susceptible women of child-bearing age will protect the fetus from the risk of congenital varicella.

> **Clinical example**
>
> A 30-year-old mother of two has just had her third baby. The day after delivery, her 2-year-old developed chickenpox. She had cuddled and kissed her mother and the new baby. The 4-year-old has not had chickenpox and the mother is not sure whether she has had it herself. The father had chickenpox as a child. What should be done for this family?
>
> The mother should have her VZV serology checked immediately. If she is seronegative, the baby should be given ZIG within 96 hours of exposure. ZIG may not abrogate the risk of fetal infection, so the baby should be watched for development of vesicles, and aciclovir should be given if he develops chickenpox.
>
> The mother and 4-year-old should be offered VZV vaccine, as post-exposure administration of the vaccine within 5 days of exposure can prevent or limit severity of disease.
>
> If the mother is found to be seropositive, nothing needs to be done for her or the baby.

## Neonatal sepsis

Neonatal sepsis is generally divided into early and late-onset sepsis (EOS and LOS). The cut-off for these definitions is variable throughout the literature. EOS is often defined as sepsis occurring within the first 7 days after birth, and LOS after 7 days. EOS is associated with maternal risk factors and acquisition of pathogens from the birth canal, whereas LOS is associated with infection by pathogens acquired at delivery but invading later, acquired at home or in hospital.

The bacterial pathogens that classically cause EOS are:

- *Streptococcus agalactiae* (group B streptococcus, GBS) – the most common in industrialized countries
- *Escherichia coli*
- *Listeria monocytogenes* – uncommon but often occurring in clusters.

Numerous bacteria can cause LOS, including coagulase-negative staphylococci, Gram-negative bacilli, streptococci, anaerobes, *Staphylococcus aureus*, *Chlamydia trachomatis* and genital mycoplasmas.

Neonatal infection with herpes simplex virus and enterovirus may mimic bacterial sepsis.

Risk factors for neonatal sepsis include premature rupture of the membranes, chorioamnionitis and maternal fever.

### Clinical features

Intrauterine infection can cause premature labour or fetal distress with or without maternal fever. The clinical manifestations of neonatal sepsis are non-specific:

- respiratory distress, tachypnoea, apnoea

- temperature instability, irritability
- feeding difficulty, vomiting, diarrhoea and jaundice
- haematological changes – neutrophilia or neutropenia, increased proportion of immature neutrophils, thrombocytopenia and coagulopathy.

Focal disease such as pneumonia, meningitis, or urinary tract, bone, soft tissue or middle ear infections may complicate disseminated sepsis or occur alone, often with only non-specific systemic symptoms.

### Diagnosis

Investigations for suspected neonatal sepsis may include:

- full blood examination and acute phase reactants such as C-reactive protein
- culture of blood, CSF or urine (preferably collected by suprapubic bladder aspiration)
- CSF examination (if indicated): typical findings in bacterial meningitis are pleocytosis, with a predominance of polymorphonuclear leukocytes, a raised protein and decreased glucose level; in viral meningoencephalitis the cell counts are usually lower, mononuclear cells usually predominate and glucose levels are normal
- chest X-ray.

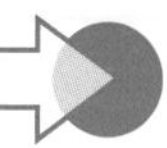

**Practical points**

**Neonatal sepsis**

- Newborn infants can develop bacterial sepsis from the same postnatally acquired infections as older infants (e.g. *Streptococcus pneumoniae, Staphylococcus aureus, Haemophilus influenzae*), but in addition, are at risk of infection from perinatally acquired organisms.
- These organisms include group B streptococcus, *Escherichia coli* and *Listeria monocytogenes*.
- Herpes simplex virus and enterovirus infection in the newborn can mimic bacterial sepsis.
- Investigations and empiric antibiotic treatment for sepsis in the neonatal period must take account of these organisms.

## Organisms associated with acute neonatal infection

### *Chlamydia trachomatis*

*Chlamydia trachomatis* is a sexually transmitted organism that causes cervicitis, pregnancy complications and secondary infertility in women, and can be transmitted vertically during delivery. Neonatal chlamydial infection, which manifests principally as ophthalmia neonatorum or pneumonia, is a significant cause of neonatal morbidity. *C. trachomatis* is the most common infectious cause of ophthalmia neonatorum in industrialized countries and is a significant cause of neonatal conjunctivitis in developing countries.

The incidence of chlamydial infection varies widely according to geography and socioeconomic group. The incidence is relatively high in young, single women with multiple sexual partners, in socially disadvantaged groups and in developing countries. Additional risk factors include presence of another sexually transmitted infection or a partner with urethritis.

Most infants of infected women are normal at delivery, but about 60% of those exposed are infected and, of these, about half develop symptoms: 18–50% develop conjunctivitis, 15–20% nasopharyngeal colonization and 5–20% pneumonia.

#### Clinical features

- Conjunctivitis:
  - may develop a few days to several weeks postpartum, typically between 5 and 14 days after delivery
  - severity ranges from mild conjunctival injection to severe conjunctivitis with purulent discharge
  - usually begins in one eye with progressive involvement of the other eye after 2–7 days
  - symptoms are often persistent but are eventually self-limiting.
- Pneumonia:
  - usually occurs between 2 and 19 weeks postpartum, typically around 6 weeks of age
  - is associated with conjunctivitis in only half of all cases
  - subacute onset and insidious course
  - paroxysmal cough, vomiting and weight loss; often misdiagnosed as pertussis
  - systemic symptoms are minimal and fever absent
  - prolonged but eventually self-limiting course.

#### Diagnosis

Diagnosis involves culture, immunofluorescence or PCR analysis of conjunctival scrapings or nasopharyngeal aspirate.

#### Treatment

Infection in an infant is a marker of maternal infection; if untreated, a woman may develop postpartum salpingitis with a risk of secondary infertility. Thus, it is important for both mother and infant that a specific diagnosis be made, even if mild conjunctivitis is the only symptom. The mother and her sexual partner(s) should be treated. Treatment of chlamydial pneumonia should reduce the duration of illness.

Conjunctivitis or pneumonia should be treated with azithromycin. Topical therapy does not eradicate *C. trachomatis* from the nasopharynx or prevent pneumonia.

## *Escherichia coli*

*Escherichia coli* causes bacteraemia, urinary tract infection and meningitis in the first week of life. However, there is a continued risk up to 2 months of age. Premature infants are more commonly affected.

Treatment is with intravenous antibiotics for 3 weeks.

## Enterovirus

Enteroviruses, which include Coxsackie A, B and echoviruses, cause hand, foot and mouth disease, gastroenteritis and meningitis. Neonatal infection may be acquired from maternal infection in the 2 weeks prior to delivery or postnatal exposure. In newborn infants, enteroviral disease may be particularly severe and is associated with high morbidity and mortality. During summer and autumn, neonatal enteroviral disease may be more common than diseases caused by GBS or herpes simplex virus. Despite this, it is frequently unrecognized as a cause of neonatal sepsis.

### Clinical features

- Meningoencephalitis
- Thrombocytopenia
- Disseminated intravascular coagulopathy
- Cardiomyopathy
- Hepatitis.

### Diagnosis

Viral culture or PCR analysis of CSF, stool or throat swab.

### Treatment

There are no readily available antiviral agents for treating enteroviral infection. Intravenous immunoglobulin has been used to treat neonatal disease, but there is limited evidence.

## Herpes simplex virus

Perinatal herpes simplex virus (HSV) infection can be acquired in one of three ways:

- *in utero* – maternal viraemia during primary infection (HSV-1 or HSV-2) – 5%
- peripartum – maternal genital tract during delivery (HSV-1 or HSV-2) – 85%
- postpartum (postnatal) – contact after birth with cold sores, infected saliva or hands (usually HSV-1) – 10%.

Primary maternal HSV infection can cause fever, systemic symptoms and severe mucocutaneous lesions, but is often asymptomatic (and diagnosed by seroconversion). Transplacental infection is rare, but spontaneous abortion or preterm labour can occur.

### Risk factors for vertical transmission

- Type of maternal infection – recurrent genital herpes infections are the most common form of genital HSV during pregnancy. However, women with primary genital HSV infections who are shedding HSV at delivery are 10–30 times more likely to transmit the virus to their babies than women with a recurrent infection. The difficulty is that approximately 66% of women who acquire genital herpes during pregnancy remain asymptomatic.
- Maternal (and neonatal) antibody status – transplacental passage of anti-HSV-neutralizing antibodies reduces the risk of transmission and of disseminated disease.
- Prolonged rupture of membranes.
- Poor integrity of mucocutaneous barriers (e.g. use of fetal scalp electrodes).
- Mode of delivery – caesarean section reduces risk of HSV transmission in women shedding HSV at the time of birth, particularly in women with first-time infections who are HSV type-specific antibody-negative.

### Clinical features

Perinatal HSV infections can be classified as:

- Disseminated disease
  - involving multiple visceral organs, including lung, liver, adrenal glands, skin, eye and the brain
  - 25% of perinatal HSV disease (with early treatment)
  - usually presents at 10–12 days of life
  - fever, disseminated intravascular coagulation, shock, hepatitis, pneumonia, encephalitis
  - 80% mortality rate untreated
  - high incidence of sequelae in survivors.
- CNS disease
  - meningoencephalitis
  - one-third of perinatal HSV disease
  - usually presents at 16–19 days of life
  - 60% have skin lesions at some point

  - seizures, lethargy, irritability, poor feeding
  - presentation may be indistinguishable from neonatal sepsis.
- Skin, eye, mouth (SEM) disease
  - disease limited to the skin, eyes and/or mouth
  - 45% of perinatal HSV disease (with early treatment)
  - usually presents at 10–12 days of life
  - infants with apparently localized mucocutaneous HSV infection may have neurological sequelae from unrecognized encephalitis.

See Figure 11.4.3.

### Diagnosis

Neonatal HSV infection is diagnosed by isolation or detection of HSV by immunofluorescence or PCR in skin lesions, blood, CSF, saliva, urine or tissue biopsy.

### Treatment

Early treatment with high-dose intravenous aciclovir reduces mortality and morbidity, and should be given for suspected neonatal HSV infection. Treatment must be continued for 3 weeks if HSV is proved (or cannot be excluded).

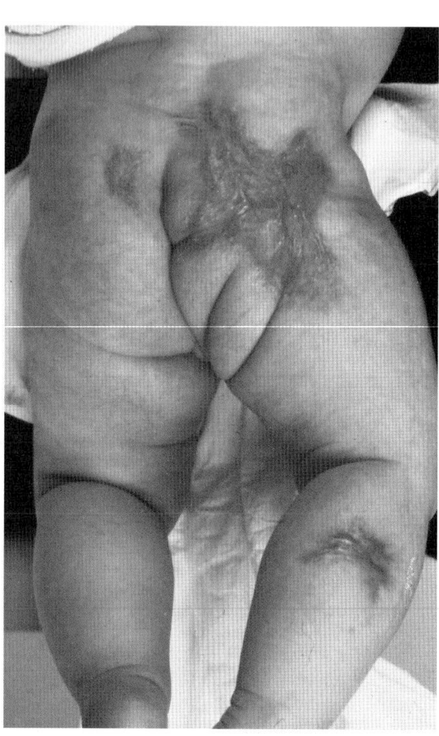

Fig. 11.4.3 Localized herpes simplex virus skin lesions.

### Prevention

- Caesarean delivery in a woman with active genital lesions can reduce the risk of perinatal HSV infection.
- Prophylactic aciclovir beginning at 36 weeks' gestation reduces the risk of clinical HSV recurrence at delivery, caesarean delivery for recurrent genital herpes and the risk of HSV viral shedding at delivery. However, it is not clear whether there is a reduction in perinatal disease.
- There may be a role for the use of condoms and oral antivirals in a seronegative woman with a seropositive sexual partner.

## *Listeria monocytogenes*

- Listeriosis is usually acquired from contaminated food such as dairy products and processed meats.
- Pregnant women, neonates, the elderly and the immunocompromised are most at risk.
- Maternal infection is often asymptomatic or mild.
- Spontaneous abortion, stillbirth or premature delivery, and neonatal sepsis or meningitis can occur.

### Diagnosis

Culture of blood and CSF.

### Treatment

High-dose intravenous benzylpenicillin.

## Group B streptococcus

The burden of EOS due to *Streptococcus agalactiae* or GBS has declined substantially over the past 20 years as a result of widespread use of intrapartum antibiotic prophylaxis. However, it remains the most common cause of neonatal sepsis overall. GBS is carried in the vaginal flora of 25% of healthy women. Less than 1% of the infants of carriers are infected. The overall incidence of neonatal GBS sepsis in Australia is 0.4 per 1000 live births.

### Clinical features

- GBS can cause neonatal sepsis, pneumonia, meningitis and, less frequently, focal infections such as osteomyelitis, septic arthritis or cellulitis.
- Early-onset disease occurs within the first week of life; most occur on the day of birth or within 72 hours.
- Late-onset disease occurs after the first week, and cases are relatively evenly distributed over the first 3 months of life.

- Some 50% of infections begin *in utero*; associated with preterm labour, prolonged rupture of membranes and chorioamnionitis.
- The mortality rate varies with gestational age at infection:
  - 2% after 37 weeks
  - 10% for neonates aged 34–36 weeks
  - 30% for neonates aged less than 33 weeks.

#### Risk factors for early-onset disease

- Maternal GBS colonization
- Prolonged rupture of membranes
- Preterm delivery
- GBS bacteriuria during pregnancy
- Previous GBS-infected baby
- Maternal chorioamnionitis
- Young maternal age
- Low levels of serotype-specific IgG antibody against GBS.

These factors often coexist, but maternal age and gestational age have been shown to be independent predictors of early-onset disease risk.

#### Risk factors for late-onset disease

- Preterm gestation
- Young maternal age
- Maternal GBS colonization.

#### Intrapartum antibiotic prophylaxis

Intrapartum penicillin given to carrier mothers has been shown to decrease early-onset neonatal GBS sepsis. Two strategies have been used to identify which women should receive intrapartum chemoprophylaxis; routine antenatal screening for vaginal GBS carriage and identification of clinical risk factors during labour. Recent data suggest that screening programmes for the detection of GBS carriage may be more effective than risk-based strategies to prevent early-onset neonatal GBS sepsis. Combined vaginal and rectal swabs, collected between 35 and 37 weeks' gestation, either by a health-care worker or by the patient herself, and inoculated on to selective media after enrichment, provide the optimum conditions to detect carriage. Increasingly, erythromycin and clindamycin resistance is being described overseas; this may influence the choice of antibiotics used in those allergic to penicillin. Widespread antibiotic use, particularly with broad-spectrum agents, may lead to increasing neonatal sepsis with ampicillin-resistant organisms. Although rates of non-GBS neonatal sepsis are generally stable, there is evidence suggesting that *E. coli* sepsis in premature infants is increasing.

#### Diagnosis

Culture of blood and CSF, plus chest X-ray if indicated.

#### Treatment

High-dose intravenous Benzylpenicillin plus synergistic gentamicin.

## Organisms associated with chronic infection

### Hepatitis B virus

Women who are chronic carriers of hepatitis B virus (HBV) (i.e. have persistently detectable hepatitis B surface antigen (HBsAg) in serum), or who have acute hepatitis B late in pregnancy, often transmit the virus to their infants. The three main modes of transmission from the mother to the infant are:

- *in utero* infection – unusual except in the setting of acute hepatitis B infection during the third trimester
- direct inoculation during delivery – most common mode of transmission. As the fetus passes through the vaginal canal, maternal blood may be swallowed by the fetus. Up to 95% of infants born to mothers who are HbsAg-positive have the antigen in their gastric fluid
- postnatal (horizontal) transmission.

The risk and the outcome depend on the amount of live virus in maternal serum. A relatively high level of infectivity is indicated by the presence in serum of the hepatitis B e antigen (HBeAg) or DNA polymerase, both of which are associated with active viral replication. About 90% of infants of HbeAg-positive carriers are infected during delivery and will become chronic carriers; they are at risk from chronic liver disease, cirrhosis and hepatocellular carcinoma, which does not usually occur before early adulthood. Children who are HBsAg carriers are a potential source of horizontal transmission of HBV to other young children.

The risk of becoming a carrier is much lower (approximately 10%) for infants of HBsAg carriers with antibody to HBeAg (indicating lower infectivity), but these infants may develop acute HBV infection.

The risk of chronic infection and subsequent liver disease is inversely proportional to age at the time of infection:

- 90–95% of HBV infections under 1 year of age result in chronic liver disease
- 25–50% of HBV infections in 1–5-year-olds result in chronic liver disease
- 6–10% of HBV infections in adults result in chronic liver disease.

### Prevention

Universal HBV immunization is the most effective means of preventing HBV transmission (see Chapter 3.5). Routine antenatal screening and immunization of infants of HBsAg carriers can prevent neonatal HBV infection. The infant should be given hepatitis B immune globulin (HBIG) as soon as possible after birth (no later than 48 hours) and a course of HBV vaccine starting in the first week. Three further doses should be given at 2, 4, and 6 or 12 months (the timing depends on the combination vaccine used). This prevents HBV infection in more than 95% of infants at risk.

Lamivudine has been used to prevent the transmission of HBV to neonates in mothers with high viral load.

## Hepatitis C virus

Approximately 1% of pregnant women are infected with hepatitis C virus (HCV). Perinatal transmission has been shown to be the leading cause of HCV infection among infants and children. However, the risk of vertical transmission is low (approximately 5%). There is an increased risk with high maternal viral load and maternal co-infection with HIV.

Perinatally-acquired HCV infection has a slower, more indolent course than infection in older children and adults. Approximately 20% of children appear to clear the infection, 50% develop chronic asymptomatic infection and 30% develop chronic active infection.

The general recommendation for testing a well child with perinatal HCV exposure is to test for HCV antibodies at ≥18 months of age, as passively transferred maternal HCV antibodies will have cleared by then. When follow-up cannot be guaranteed, however, testing by HCV RNA PCR should be performed earlier, but not before 1 month of age, as the sensitivity of the test is low (22%). A positive PCR result should always be confirmed on a separate occasion.

There is no evidence that HCV transmission occurs during breastfeeding, nor that caesarean delivery reduces the risk of transmission.

## Human immunodeficiency virus

The rate of mother-to-child transmission of HIV around the world varies according to availability of antenatal care, antiretroviral drugs and background prevalence rates. In the absence of antiviral and obstetric interventions, the risk overall of mother-to-child transmission is reported as 20–40%.

There are three routes of vertical transmission of HIV:

- *in utero*
- during labour and delivery – 70%
- breastfeeding – transmission risk is highest in the first few months of life.

Perinatal transmission risk can be reduced to less than 1% with measures including:

- antiretroviral therapy (for the mother during pregnancy and labour) and to the infant for the first 6 weeks of life
- elective caesarean section (it is generally thought that interventions to minimize infant contact with maternal vaginal secretions and infected blood during passage through the birth canal is important to reduce the risk of vertical transmission)
- avoidance of invasive obstetric procedures
- avoidance of breastfeeding.

The Royal Australian and New Zealand College of Obstetricians and Gynaecologists recommends that all pregnant women should be assessed for risk of HIV infection and should be offered HIV antibody testing following appropriate counselling.

# 11.5 Surgical conditions in the newborn

Sebastian K. King, Spencer W. Beasley

The majority of the conditions discussed in this chapter will present initially to the paediatrician, general practitioner or obstetrician as emergencies. Delay in diagnosis may seriously compromise recovery and will almost certainly increase morbidity. Disorders that are obvious at birth but do not require urgent surgical referral have not been included in this chapter. For information on these, the reader is referred to paediatric surgical texts.

## Oesophageal atresia

Any newborn infant who appears to salivate excessively (drooling) at birth should be suspected of having oesophageal atresia. This is a congenital abnormality where the mid-portion of the oesophagus is missing. In most there is an abnormal communication between the trachea and the lower oesophageal segment, called a distal tracheo-oesophageal fistula.

The diagnosis is confirmed by passing a large, firm catheter, for example a 10-French gauge orogastric tube, through the mouth and finding that it cannot be passed more than about 10 cm from the gums. The child must not be fed; otherwise, aspiration of feeds into the lungs is likely to occur. A plain X-ray of the torso will show gas in the bowel, confirming the presence of a distal tracheo-oesophageal fistula. About 50% of these infants have other congenital abnormalities, most of which form part of the VACTERL association (vertebral, anorectal, cardiac, renal and limb abnormalities; see Chapter 10.3). Major chromosomal abnormalities are seen in 5%, of which trisomy 18 and trisomy 21 are the most frequent. Many are premature and a history of maternal polyhydramnios is common.

Initial management involves regular suctioning of the upper oesophageal pouch to prevent aspiration until the tracheo-oesophageal fistula has been divided. The oesophageal ends are anastomosed at the time of surgery to close the fistula.

## Duodenal obstruction

Bile-stained vomiting starts soon after birth. The obstruction may be:

- intrinsic (e.g. duodenal atresia, duodenal web)
- extrinsic (e.g. malrotation with volvulus).

In duodenal atresia there may be other abnormalities, such as Down syndrome and imperforate anus (see Chapter 10.3). In the absence of birth asphyxia these infants are usually alert and feed well, but they vomit bile-stained material almost immediately. There may be epigastric distension. The diagnosis of duodenal atresia is made on plain X-ray of the abdomen, which reveals a characteristic 'double bubble' due to gas in the stomach and proximal duodenum (Fig. 11.5.1). Little or no gas will be visible distal to the obstruction. Duodenoduodenostomy is performed after resuscitation and correction of any fluid or electrolyte disturbance.

Bile-stained vomiting may also be an indication of malrotation complicated by volvulus. The small bowel mesentery has a narrow attachment to the posterior abdominal wall, the so-called 'universal mesentery', which allows the midgut to twist around the superior mesenteric vessels. This is a true surgical emergency as the blood supply to the midgut may be cut off as the midgut twists around this axis. The diagnosis can be confirmed with an urgent barium meal or by ultrasonography. If signs of peritonitis with abdominal distension and guarding are already present, the infant should be taken immediately to theatre.

## Distal bowel obstruction

In more distal bowel obstructions, vomiting remains a major feature but tends to occur later and is associated with abdominal distension. The more distal the obstruction, the later the vomiting and the more pronounced the distension (Fig. 11.5.2). The vomitus may become faeculent. An erect film of the abdomen will show distended loops of bowel and fluid levels (Fig. 11.5.3). The number of loops is dependent on the level of obstruction. The radiological appearances of Hirschsprung disease, meconium ileus and ileal atresia may be similar, and a contrast study, rectal biopsy or laparotomy may be required to make the definitive diagnosis.

### Hirschsprung disease

Hirschsprung disease (congenital megacolon) is the most common cause of neonatal bowel obstruction. There is an absence of ganglion cells for a variable distance proximal to the anus. Peristalsis is abnormal

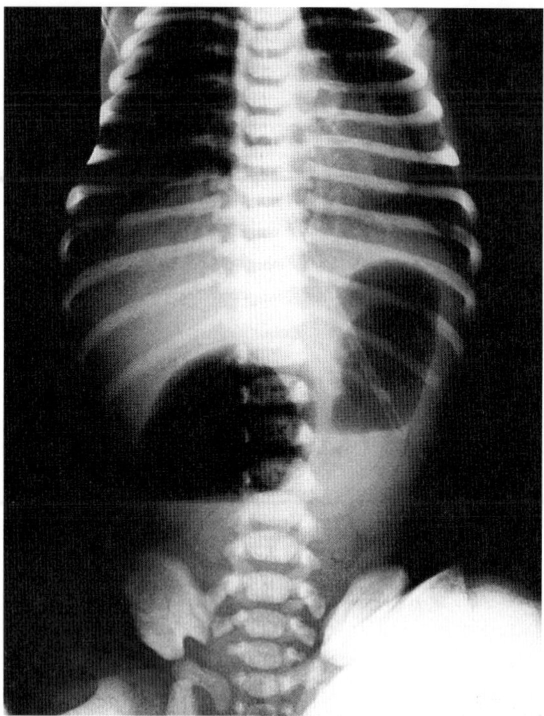

Fig. 11.5.1 X-ray of the abdomen in a neonate demonstrating the 'double bubble' sign. Note the absence of gas in the bowel distal to the second bubble. This child had duodenal atresia.

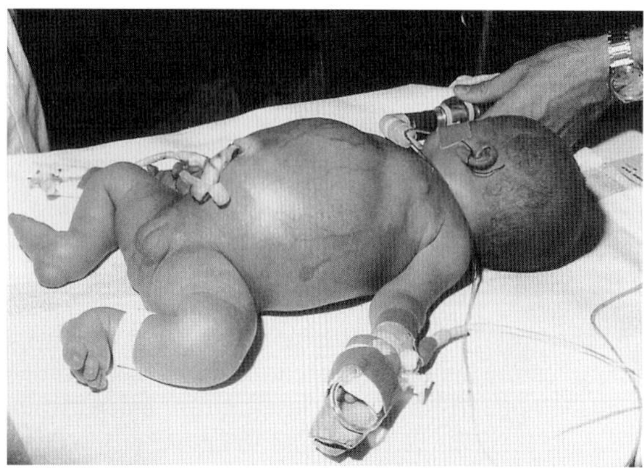

Fig. 11.5.2 Distal bowel obstruction in a neonate. Gross abdominal distension was evident and associated with vomiting of faeculent material.

in the aganglionic segment and results in an incomplete lower intestinal obstruction with severe constipation. The bowel proximal to the aganglionic segment becomes dilated and hypertrophied. The diagnosis is confirmed on suction rectal biopsy. Most of these infants present at 3 or 4 days of age with increasing abdominal distension and delay in the passage of meconium. Surgical correction involves:

- excision of the aganglionic segment
- anastomosing ganglionated bowel to the anus.

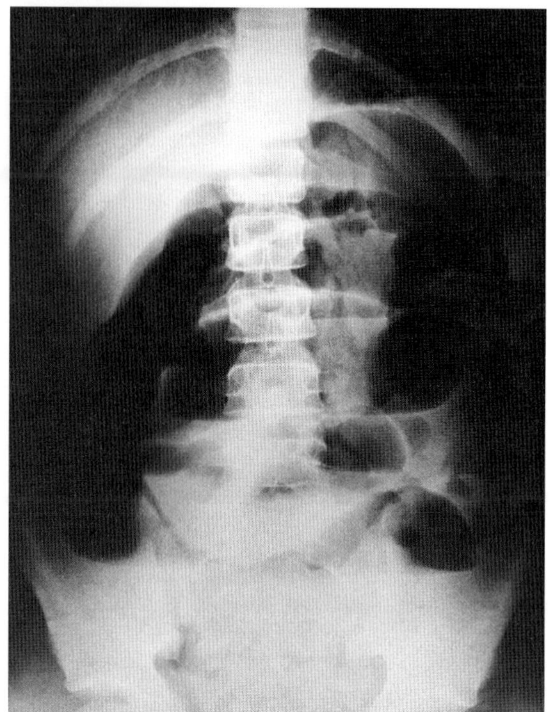

Fig. 11.5.3 Erect X-ray of the abdomen, showing marked dilatation of multiple loops of bowel and several fluid levels. The most likely diagnoses include Hirschsprung disease, meconium ileus and ileal atresia.

It is often performed as a single-stage procedure at diagnosis in the neonate, but in certain circumstances requires a staged approach.

## Meconium ileus

Meconium ileus occurs in infants with cystic fibrosis. In this condition meconium becomes excessively thick and tenacious, causing obstruction, and the distal ileum is jammed with hard pellets of inspissated meconium. The colon is empty and no meconium is passed after birth. The infant has a distended abdomen and commences vomiting shortly after birth. A contrast enema will demonstrate a microcolon.

Sometimes the impacted pellets can be dislodged with a Gastrografin enema, but usually surgery is required. A temporary ileostomy allows the bowel to be irrigated to clear the inspissated meconium. The diagnosis of cystic fibrosis is confirmed subsequently (see Chapter 14.6).

## Small bowel atresias

Atresias of the jejunum are often multiple (Fig. 11.5.4). There is gross distension of the proximal jejunum proximal to the first atresia, followed by multiple short segments of jejunum and collapsed normal bowel distally. Ileal atresia tends to be an isolated lesion. Colonic atresia is extremely rare.

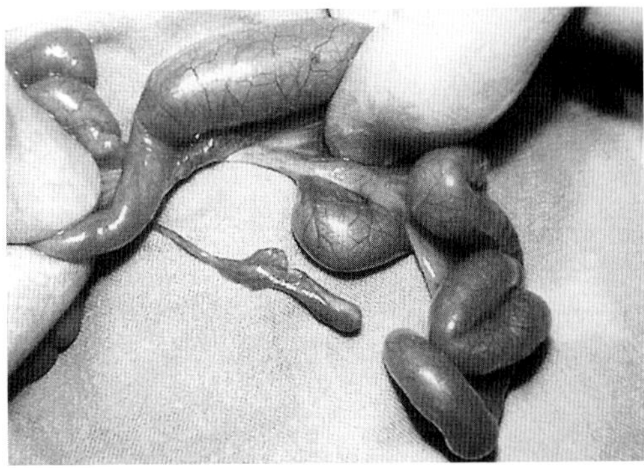

Fig. 11.5.4 Intraoperative photograph showing multiple areas of jejunal atresia in a neonate who presented with vomiting after the first two feeds after birth.

## Neonatal necrotizing enterocolitis

Neonatal necrotizing enterocolitis (NEC) is an acquired condition that predominantly afflicts the premature neonate who has undergone severe perinatal stress (see Chapter 11.2). The neonate becomes lethargic and unwell, usually between 2 days and 2 weeks after birth. There is bile-stained vomiting and the abdomen becomes distended. Loose stools are passed, which may contain blood. As the disease progresses, signs of peritonitis develop: there is redness and oedema of the abdominal wall and increasing abdominal tenderness. Both small and large bowel may be involved. Plain X-rays of the abdomen show:

- dilated loops of bowel
- intramural gas (pneumotosis intestinalis) – this is a pathognomic sign on radiology
- portal venous gas – this is a sign of severe disease and poor prognosis in which surgery is usually required
- pneumoperitoneum – results from full-thickness perforation and surgery is almost always required.

Initial management involves cessation of all enteral feeds, decompression of the gastrointestinal tract by nasogastric aspiration, fluid resuscitation and antibiotics. Where there is continued clinical deterioration despite appropriate resuscitation, or there is evidence of full-thickness bowel necrosis (e.g. free intraperitoneal gas on X-ray), surgery is indicated. Necrotic bowel is excised and a defunctioning stoma may be required. Malabsorption, short gut syndrome and colonic strictures may complicate the condition.

## Anorectal malformations

These include a spectrum of abnormalities that affect the anorectum, loosely called 'imperforate anus' (Fig. 11.5.5). They fall into two main groups:

- low lesions – the rectum continues beyond the pelvic levator ani musculature
- high lesions – the rectum stops at or above the pelvic levator ani musculature (Fig. 11.5.5A).

Low lesions usually have a fistulous communication with the skin as an anocutaneous fistula, for which a cutback anoplasty is performed as a neonate (Fig. 11.5.5B). High lesions tend to be more complicated and are more likely to be associated with other congenital abnormalities, particularly of the urinary tract. In the male with a high lesion there is either no opening at all or the rectum communicates with the urinary tract via a rectourethral or rectovesical fistula (Fig. 11.5.5C). In the female with a high lesion the rectum usually communicates with the vestibule or vagina as a rectovestibular or rectovaginal fistula respectively (Fig. 11.5.5D). High lesions require an anorectoplasty – a considerably more complicated procedure, performed either at birth or as a staged procedure later. In addition, a rare and even more severe group of abnormalities may occur in the female; in these cloacal malformations there is only one opening for the rectum, vagina and urinary tract.

### Clinical example

Thomas was born normally after an uneventful pregnancy and labour. Meconium was first passed at 36 hours. At the age of 4 days he was noted to be feeding poorly and his abdomen was becoming increasingly distended but no mass was palpable. He vomited twice. On rectal examination a 'squirt' of meconium was passed. A plain upright film of the abdomen revealed several fluid levels suggestive of intestinal obstruction. A provisional diagnosis of Hirschsprung disease was made. This was confirmed on suction rectal biopsy, which demonstrated the absence of ganglion cells in the submucosa. A primary pull-through procedure via the perineum was performed, with the transition zone being determined by intraoperative frozen sections.

# Abdominal wall defects

The two main major abdominal wall defects are:

- exomphalos (omphalocele)
- gastroschisis.

Frequently, a diagnosis of exomphalos or gastroschisis is made on antenatal ultrasonography. This may influence the location and timing of delivery, but does not influence the mode of delivery. It also provides an opportunity for antenatal counselling.

### Exomphalos

This is a large defect at the umbilicus with herniation of bowel and liver into a sac covered by fused amniotic membrane and peritoneum (Fig. 11.5.6). The sac

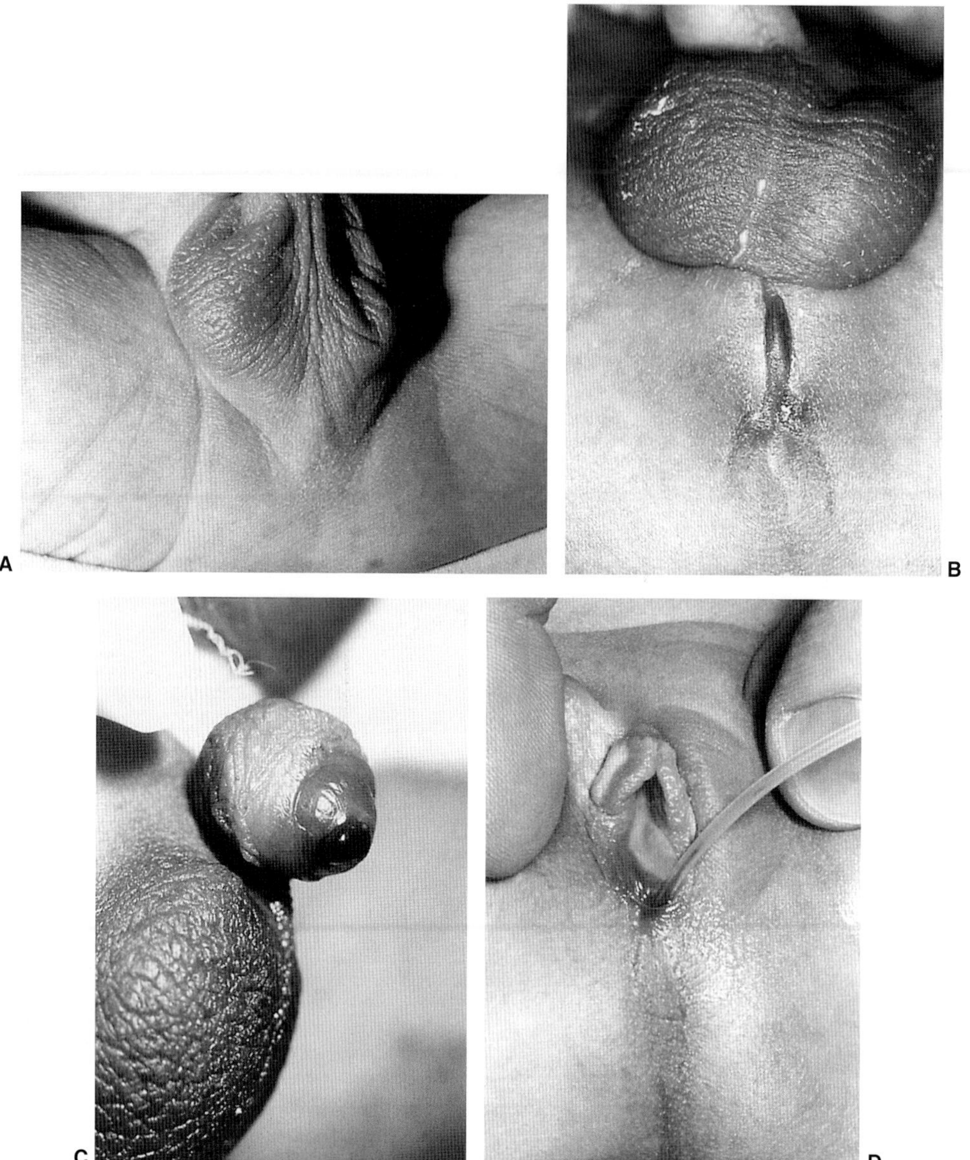

Fig. 11.5.5 Anorectal anomalies presenting as imperforate anus in the neonatal period. **(A)** High imperforate anus, the lesion being above the levator ani musculature. **(B)** Imperforate anus due to a low lesion. Meconium is visible behind the distended skin of the median raphe. **(C)** Passage of meconium from the urethra. This has occurred in a neonate with a high imperforate anus and an associated rectourethral fistula. **(D)** Anorectal anomaly in a newborn girl. The catheter has been passed into the rectum.

is translucent at birth but quickly becomes opaque as it desiccates. Coexisting abnormalities are common and usually involve the heart and kidneys. Beckwith–Wiedemann syndrome may also be present and must be recognized as it is associated with severe hypoglycaemia that requires immediate correction at birth (see Chapter 10.3).

The early management of exomphalos involves placing the neonate in a warm Humidicrib incubator and wrapping the entire torso, including the exposed viscera, in clear plastic wrap to prevent evaporative heat loss. A nasogastric tube keeps the stomach empty, aiding subsequent closure of the defect. The defect can usually be repaired at birth but the largest defects, particularly those that contain liver, may require a period of external compression or staged procedures.

## Gastroschisis

In gastroschisis there is a small defect immediately to the right of the umbilicus through which bowel (and sometimes the gonads) herniate (Fig. 11.5.7). There is

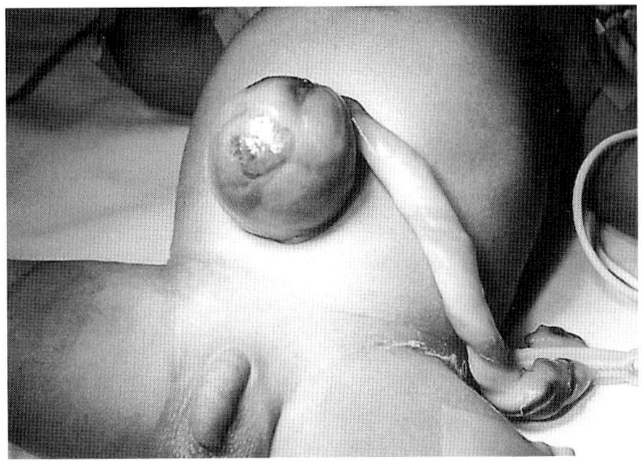

Fig. 11.5.6 Exomphalos, showing the site of the defect at the umbilicus. In some affected neonates the lesion is much larger and may contain most of the bowel and liver.

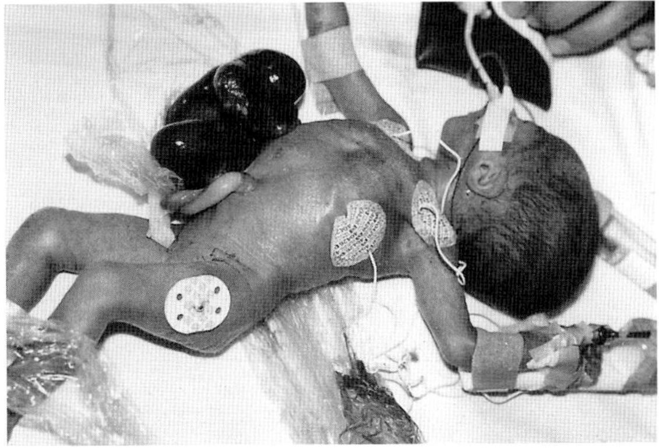

Fig. 11.5.7 Gastroschisis, with herniation of abdominal contents through an abdominal wall defect lateral to the umbilicus.

no covering sac, and the eviscerated small and large bowel is thickened and densely matted with exudate as a result of amniotic peritonitis before birth. These infants have a significant risk of hypothermia, and exposed viscera should be wrapped in clear plastic wrap to prevent evaporative heat loss. Surgery is directed at returning the bowel to the peritoneal cavity and repairing the defect. Where the peritoneal cavity is too small to accommodate the bowel, it may be necessary to create a temporary prosthetic silo that contains the remaining bowel. After surgical repair the bowel may take many weeks to function normally. Coexisting abnormalities are normally confined to the gastrointestinal tract.

## Diaphragmatic hernia

In the most common type of congenital diaphragmatic hernia (Bochdalek hernia) there is a defect of the left posterolateral part of the diaphragm that allows the contents of the abdomen to herniate into the left thoracic cavity. This limits the space available for the lungs to develop *in utero*. The resulting pulmonary hypoplasia results in severe respiratory distress within minutes of birth and in some neonates is not compatible with long-term survival. The more severe the lung hypoplasia, the earlier the neonate becomes symptomatic and the poorer the prognosis. Diagnosis of the condition may be made antenatally on routine ultrasonography.

The diagnosis is confirmed after birth by a chest X-ray, which shows loops of bowel in the left thoracic cavity. The heart is displaced to the contralateral side and there is little room available for the lungs. Right-sided diaphragmatic hernias account for only 15% of such lesions. Early treatment involves aggressive cardiorespiratory support and decompression of the bowel with a nasogastric tube. When the child is stable, operative repair of the diaphragm is undertaken.

## Sacrococcygeal teratoma

This is a rare tumour that is usually evident at birth; the baby is born with a large mass protruding from the lower back and arising from the tip of the coccyx or sacrum. In other infants it may expand predominantly into the pelvis. It may be extremely large and cause obstetric difficulties. The tumour is removed soon after birth. Malignant change is possible and is more likely if surgery is delayed or where the tumour is uniformly solid and devoid of cysts.

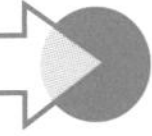

**Practical points**

- Oesophageal atresia is often associated with other congenital anomalies (e.g. VACTERL association) and presents with excessive salivation at birth.
- Bile-stained vomiting may have a serious underlying cause, such as malrotation with volvulus, which must be excluded with an upper gastrointestinal contrast study.
- The most common cause of neonatal bowel obstruction is Hirschsprung disease.
- Necrotizing enterocolitis most commonly affects premature neonates who have suffered perinatal stress.
- Exomphalos is a midline defect where bowel and liver protrude from beneath the umbilicus, whereas the defect in gastroschisis is typically to the right of the umbilicus and the bowel has no covering sac.

PART 12

# INFECTIONS

# 12.1 Infectious diseases

David Burgner, David Isaacs

## Infectious diseases presenting with fever and rash

Infectious diseases of childhood are a significant cause of illness in children, especially in the first years of life. Globally, infection is responsible for the majority of the more than 10 million childhood deaths that occur each year. Many of these infections are preventable by immunization and the high mortality rate is compounded by malnutrition and low birth weight (see Chapter 11.2). In resource-rich countries such as Australia, infectious diseases are the commonest cause of admission to hospital and amongst the commonest reasons for a child to consult a general practitioner. The burden of infectious diseases falls mainly on infants and the preschool child and disproportionately on Indigenous children.

Many infections and related conditions manifest as fever and rash, and a timely and accurate diagnosis is important. This chapter discusses some of the more important and common of these conditions, highlighting the epidemiological and clinical features that may point to a specific diagnosis, as well as the complications, treatment and prevention. Other causes of fever and rash include drug reactions, toxins and autoimmune diseases and these are discussed in related chapters (see Chapters 13 and 21).

The child with rash and fever needs careful assessment. The most important aspect is identifying potentially life-threatening conditions, of which meningococcal septicaemia (also known as meningococcaemia; see Chapter 12.3) is the most common and important. Meningococcal septicaemia may occur in isolation or together with meningococcal meningitis. It progresses rapidly, has a high mortality, and requires prompt identification and aggressive treatment. Meningococcal disease should be considered in any febrile child with signs of shock even if there is no rash. Other indicators of severe illness include pallor, meningism, abnormal cry, lack of eye contact and failure to respond to normal social clues. Early in the illness, the typical non-blanching rash may be absent in up to a third of cases, may be difficult to find (so undress the child fully and remember to look at the conjunctivae and palate), or initially may be maculopapular with subtle petechial elements. The meningococcus replicates rapidly in the bloodstream and the rash may evolve very quickly. A non-blanching petechial rash is not specific for meningococcal infection; only about 10% of children with a petechial rash have meningococcal disease and the remainder have viral infections, other bacterial infections, or have suffered minor trauma. Early treatment is potentially life-saving; intravenous or intramuscular antibiotics should be given immediately if the diagnosis is suspected and prior to urgent transfer to hospital (Fig. 12.1.1).

The terminology used to describe infections causing fever and rash can be confusing and some terms are largely of historical interest. An exanthem (from the Greek *exanthema*, 'a breaking out') usually refers to a widespread rash, often of viral origin. An enanthem refers to small spots on the mucous membranes, such as Koplik's spots seen in measles. In the early 20th century, prior to immunization, six common exanthems of childhood were categorized. Historically these were known as 'the six diseases of childhood' (Table 12.1.1). This numerical terminology is still used occasionally, although the existence of the 'fourth disease' is questionable.

## Measles (rubeola, morbilli)

Measles is a leading cause of childhood mortality, and in 2008 caused an estimated 164 000 deaths globally, or nearly 18 deaths per hour. Malnourished and vitamin A-deficient children are at increased risk. More than 95% of measles deaths occur in low-income countries and there are over 20 million measles cases per year. There is a highly effective vaccine and increased measles immunization coverage has resulted in a decline by over 75% in total deaths between 2000 and 2008. Most deaths result from bacterial complications. Even in resource-rich countries, measles has a significant mortality rate, approaching 1 in 25 000. From 1978 to 1992, about 10 Australian children died from measles each year, as a result of acute encephalitis or pneumonia. With increasing immunization coverage, the number of deaths fell to 1–2 per year from 1992, and there have been no deaths since 1995, when a second preschool dose of measles vaccine was introduced.

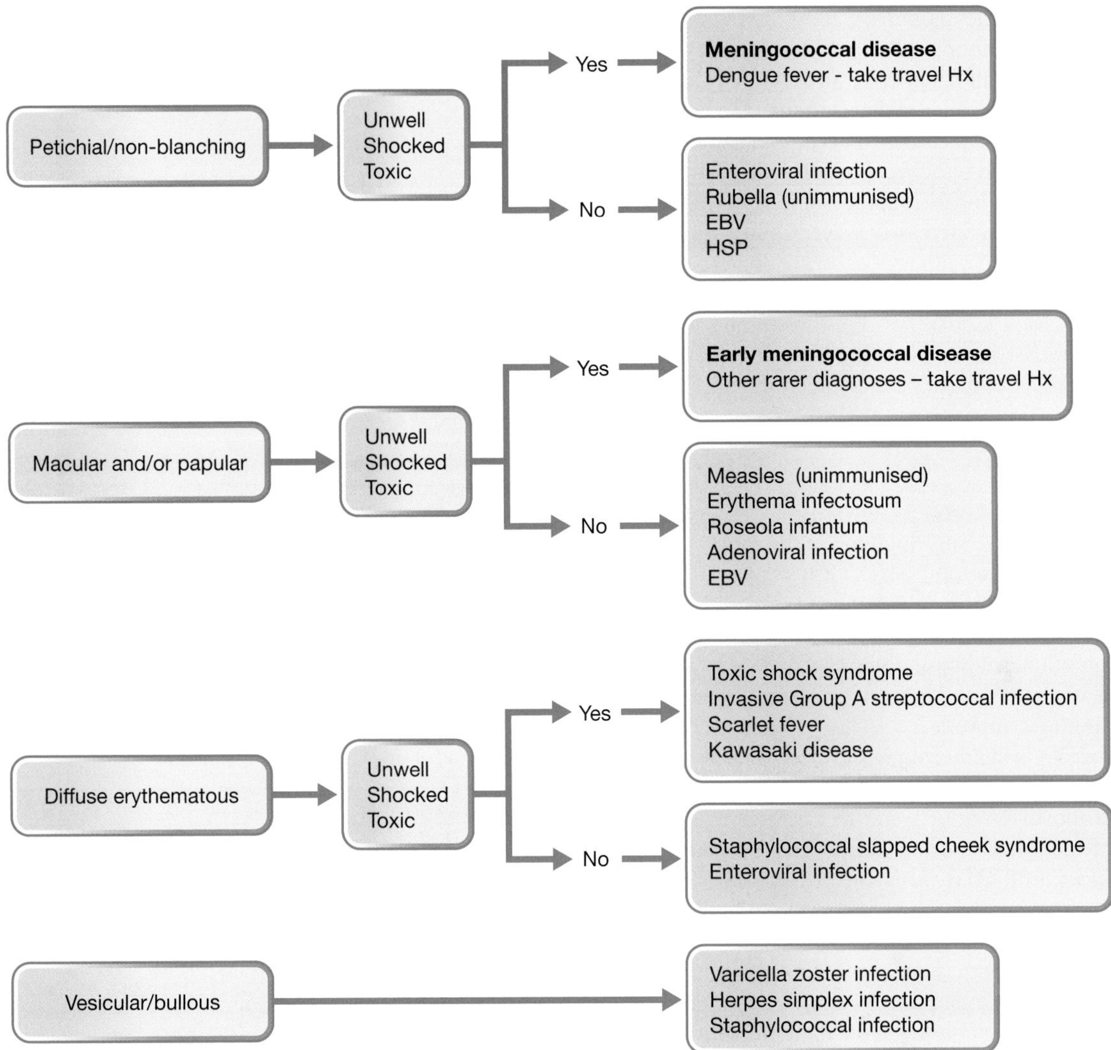


Fig. 12.1.1 An approach to the patient with rash and fever.

**Table 12.1.1 The 'six diseases' or 'six exanthems' of childhood**

| Historical name | Name | Synonym(s) | Aetiological agent |
|---|---|---|---|
| First disease | Measles | Rubeola, morbilli | Measles virus (= morbillivirus) |
| Second disease | Scarlet fever | Scarlatina (milder form) | *Streptococcus pyogenes* (= Lancefield group A streptococcus) |
| Third disease | Rubella | German measles | Rubella virus (= rubivirus) |
| *Fourth disease* | *Filatow–Dukes' disease* | *The existence of Fourth disease as a separate entity is controversial – term not widely used* | |
| Fifth disease | Erythema infectiosum | Slapped cheek disease | Parvovirus B19 |
| Sixth disease | Roseola infantum | Exanthem subitum | Human herpesvirus 6 (HHV-6) and less commonly HHV-7 |

In resource-rich countries, most cases are imported or occur in unimmunized children. Measles is caused by measles or morbillivirus, an RNA virus with high infectivity and virulence that is thought to have evolved from the virus that causes rinderpest in cattle. However, humans are the only hosts of measles virus. Infection results in significant suppression of T-cell immune responses, with increased susceptibility to diarrhoea and respiratory illness, and an increased overall infection-related mortality for up to a year following measles. Measles can be a life-threatening infection in the immunocompromised (e.g. oncology patients) and suspected cases require strict infection control.

## Epidemiology

- Humans are the only known host.
- Infants and young children are the most susceptible to severe infection.
- Respiratory droplet or airborne spread, highly infectious, causing outbreaks every 2 years in unimmunized populations.
- Incubation period is 8–14 days from the exposure to onset of symptoms.
- Measles is highly contagious and over 98% of adults in unimmunized communities are seropositive.
- Infected individuals are infectious for 4 days before until 4 days after the rash appears (but immunocompromised patients are infectious for the duration of the illness).
- Measles virus may survive in air and on inanimate surfaces for some hours.
- In developing countries, the high mortality rate is due mainly to pneumonia, often with bacterial (staphylococcal or pneumococcal) superinfection.

## Clinical features (Figs 12.1.2, 12.1.3)

- Prodromal period (symptoms before rash) 3–5 days, with sudden onset of high fever, irritability, brassy or hacking cough, exudative conjunctivitis, rhinorrhoea, otitis media, and a characteristic enanthem on buccal mucosa (Koplik's spots).
- Rash starts behind ears and spreads caudally. It is a blotchy, raised rash, confluent in places. The more confluent the rash, the more severe the illness.
- Child is miserable and febrile when rash is present but fever resolves rapidly after a few days; persistent fever suggests bacterial superinfection.
- Immunocompromised patients may have minimal rash (showing that T cells are important in the aetiology of measles rash) and may develop fulminant giant cell pneumonia.

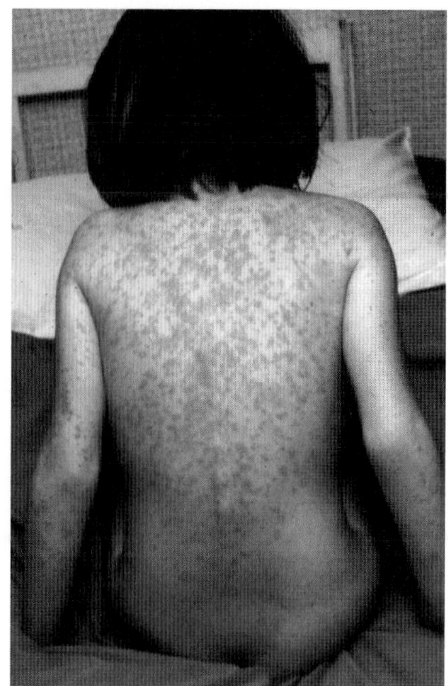

Fig. 12.1.2 Measles: blotchy, raised rash.

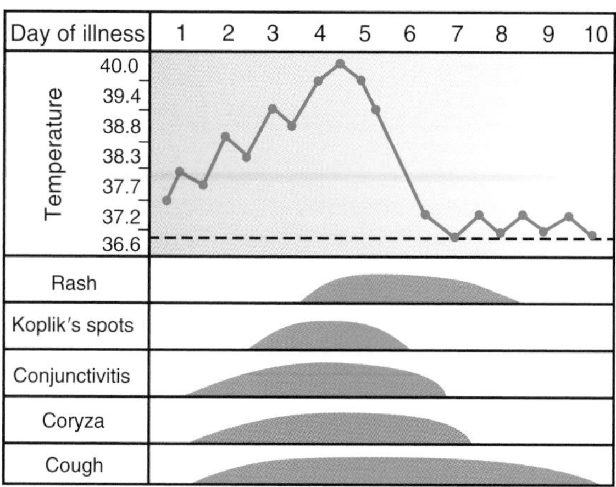


Fig. 12.1.3 The development of measles.

## Complications

- Acute complications reflect the intense inflammatory response to measles infection, possibly with associated immune suppression.
- Otitis media is the commonest acute complication, followed by lower respiratory tract infection.
- Encephalitis is a rarer but more serious complication, possibly related to the host immune response. It may be fatal (15%) or result in neurological sequelae (25%).

- In resource-poor countries, mastoiditis and diarrhoea are common and life-threatening complications.
- Subacute sclerosing panencephalitis (SSPE) is a rare (1 in 100000), devastating, invariably fatal, neurological condition that occurs about 7–8 years after wild-type measles infection (but not vaccination), especially in children infected in infancy. It is characterized by developmental regression with deteriorating intellectual function, seizures, coma and death.

### Differential diagnosis

- In roseola infantum (see below) the rash may be identical to measles but appears as the fever subsides, and the child looks well when the rash appears, in contrast to children with measles who are unwell with the rash.
- Other viruses causing morbilliform (measles-like) rash on occasions: enteroviruses, Epstein–Barr virus (EBV), adenoviruses, influenza and parainfluenza viruses.
- Antibiotics, especially amoxicillin or ampicillin, may cause a rash, particularly if given to a child with EBV infection.
- Kawasaki disease.
- Scarlet fever.

### Laboratory diagnosis

- Rapid antigen detection: immunofluorescent or PCR staining of nasopharyngeal secretions.
- Serology: measles-specific immunoglobulin (Ig) M or 4-fold rise or greater in IgG titre – less helpful in making a rapid diagnosis.

### Treatment

- Mainly symptomatic in industrialized countries.
- Vitamin A therapy recommended for severe cases and malnourished children more than 6 months of age, as reduces severity and mortality.
- Antibiotics for bacterial complications, particularly pneumonia.

### Prevention

- Measles is a *vaccine-preventable disease*; it should be possible to eradicate measles from the world by immunization, because humans are the only host.
- Measles vaccine is a live, attenuated vaccine, that can be given alone (monovalent) or in combination with mumps and rubella (MMR) and also varicella vaccines (MMRV). It is not immunogenic if significant maternal measles IgG antibodies are present or if children have received recent intravenous immunoglobulin.
- In Australia, measles–mumps–rubella (MMR) vaccine is given at 1 year of age and a second dose at 4–5 years of age (note that maternal antibody is generally protective before 1 year and interferes with immunogenicity if vaccine is given earlier).
- Live vaccines are generally contraindicated in those with significant immunodeficiency. If exposed to measles, intramuscular or intravenous immunoglobulin gives 'passive' protection.

**Clinical example**

Harriet, 3 years old, was in preschool with a friend who, 10 days earlier (1), had a cough and fever (2) and later came out in a rash. Neither had been immunized against measles (3). Harriet developed a high fever, runny nose and cough (4) and was irritable. Her eyes became red and weepy (5) and her ears were sore (6). After 3 days (2) her doctor found bilateral otitis media (6) and white spots on a red background on her buccal mucosa (7). Next day she remained miserable and hot, and developed a rash behind her ears, which spread over the next 2 days to her face, trunk and limbs, and was pink to red and blotchy (8). In some areas the rash joined up and was raised (8). She had scattered wheezes bilaterally (4). She remained febrile and unwell for 3 days, when the rash faded leaving brown discoloration of the skin with desquamation of the fingers and toes (9).

The following are features typical of measles infection:

- Incubation period 8–14 days (1)
- Infectious during the prodromal period, which lasts 3–5 days (2)
- Immunization over 95% protective (3)
- Bronchitis (4), exudative conjunctivitis (5) and otitis media (6) are almost invariable features
- Enanthem called Koplik's spots (7)
- Rash is classically descending, blotchy to confluent (8), may be papular (raised) and may desquamate, often more marked in children from developing countries (9).

## Roseola infantum (exanthem subitum, sixth disease)

### Epidemiology

- Caused by infection with human herpesvirus 6 (HHV-6) and occasionally HHV-7, both DNA viruses.
- Many HHV-6 and HHV-7 infections are asymptomatic or have non-specific symptoms (e.g. fever).
- Mainly affects infants aged 3–18 months.

- Infants usually infected by asymptomatic shedding of virus from family member.
- Incubation for HHV-6 is about 10 days; unknown for HHV-7.

### Clinical features and complications

- High fever, irritability, lymphadenopathy, upper respiratory tract signs with inflamed tympanic membranes and diarrhoea are common but non-specific features.
- Morbilliform (measles-like) rash appears as high fever subsides in classical roseola infantum, although pattern is less predictable in many HHV infections.
- Bulging fontanelle and febrile convulsions in acute phase are more common than with other viral infections.
- Virus persists in host (herpesvirus latency) and may reactivate, especially if immunocompromised.

### Prevention and treatment

There is no vaccine and no specific antiviral treatment for HHV-6 and HHV-7 infections (aciclovir is ineffective).

#### Clinical example

Mark, a previously well 9-month-old baby, developed a runny nose, fever and irritability (1) and went off his feeds. After 2 days of fever, he had a generalized tonic–clonic seizure (2), which stopped after 2 minutes. He was admitted to hospital, where he was found to have a fever of 40 °C and cervical lymphadenopathy (3) but no rash or enanthem (4). A lumbar puncture was normal. After 24 hours' observation in hospital his fever subsided but he developed a diffuse maculopapular rash on his trunk, thought at first to be measles (5). He was well and was discharged home. Serology for HHV-6 revealed positive specific IgM.

The following are features typical of classical roseola infantum:

- Usual presenting features, lasting 2–3 days (1), (3)
- Febrile convulsion (2) is a recognized complication
- No enanthem (4)
- Rash often misdiagnosed as measles but, unlike measles, the child with roseola becomes afebrile as the rash appears and looks well (5).

## Rubella (German measles, third disease)

Rubella is a rare infection in resource-rich countries where vaccination is widespread. Its main importance is congenital infection, which can cause miscarriage, fetal death or a constellation of teratogenic effects on the fetus, called 'congenital rubella syndrome'.

### Epidemiology

- RNA virus; humans are the only host.
- Respiratory droplet spread; patients are infectious for about 5 days before and after development of the rash.
- Incubation period is 2–3 weeks.
- Spring and summer epidemics in non-immunized populations.
- Mainly affects children aged 5–10 years, but also non-immune pregnant women.
- Less infectious than measles: 15–20% of adults in unimmunized populations are non-immune.

### Clinical features (Figs 12.1.4, 12.1.5)

- Rubella is usually a mild or subclinical disease in children.
- Rash much fainter and less florid than measles, not raised.

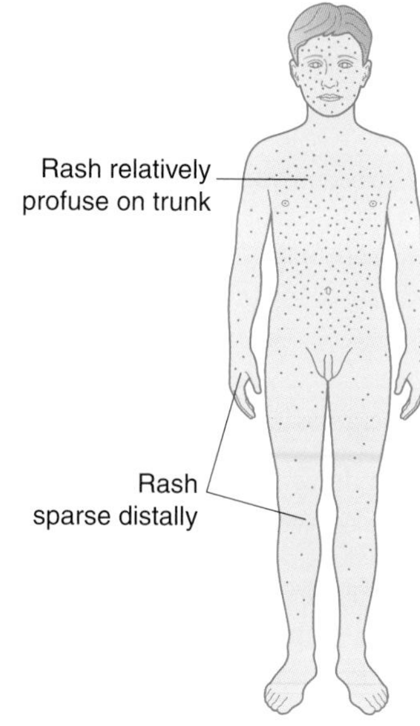


Fig. 12.1.4 The distribution of rash in rubella.

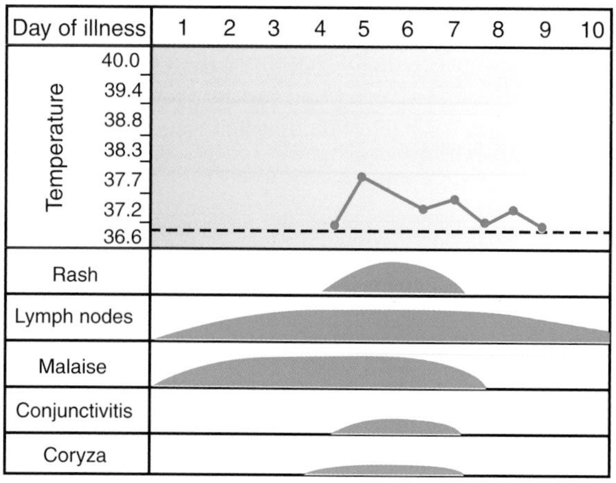

Day of illness 1 2 3 4 5 6 7 8 9 10
Temperature 40.0 39.4 38.8 38.3 37.7 37.2 36.6
Rash
Lymph nodes
Malaise
Conjunctivitis
Coryza

Fig. 12.1.5 The development of rubella.

- Rash often starts on face in young children, spreads to neck, trunk and extremities.
- Lymphadenopathy common, particularly suboccipital, postauricular and cervical.
- Adolescents and adults often have constitutional symptoms: conjunctivitis, arthralgia or arthritis, malaise and fever.
- Encephalitis and purpura are rare complications.
- Congenital rubella syndrome results from first-trimester rubella infection (see Chapter 11.4).
- There is no specific therapy.

### Diagnosis

In non-immune pregnant woman exposed to possible rubella, send serum for rubella-specific IgM and repeat 2–4 weeks later for rising IgG titre. If baby or cord blood has positive rubella IgM (which does not cross placenta), this indicates recent or congenital infection.

### Differential diagnosis

- Many other viruses cause rubelliform rashes.
- Clinical diagnosis of rubella is notoriously unreliable.
- Rubella is very rare in infancy: other viruses (e.g. enteroviruses, HHV-6) are much more likely to cause infantile rashes.

### Prevention

- Live attenuated rubella vaccine is usually given universally as MMR in resource-rich countries.
- Congenital rubella syndrome is rare in industrialized countries such as Australia, but more common in developing countries.

## Erythema infectiosum (slapped cheek disease, fifth disease)

- Caused by human parvovirus B19 (*parvo* = small), a DNA virus.
- Spread by respiratory route or vertical transmission from mother to fetus.
- Incubation period 4–14 days.
- May cause epidemics in school-aged children and household contacts.
- Initial presentation is mild, with fever in only 15–30%, cervical lymphadenopathy and an intensely red, 'slapped cheek' rash often with circumoral pallor (viraemic phase).
- Subsequently develop lacy, reticular rash on limbs and trunk, sometimes with arthralgia or arthritis (immune complex-mediated) (Figs 12.1.6, 12.1.7).
- The virus infects red cell precursors in the bone marrow, usually with mild, non-significant

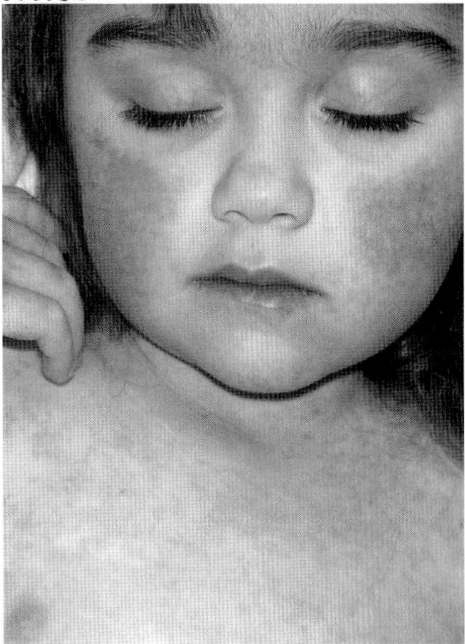

Fig. 12.1.6 Fifth disease: slapped cheeks and lacy rash (with permission of Bernard Cohen, DermAtlas: http://www.dermatlas.org).

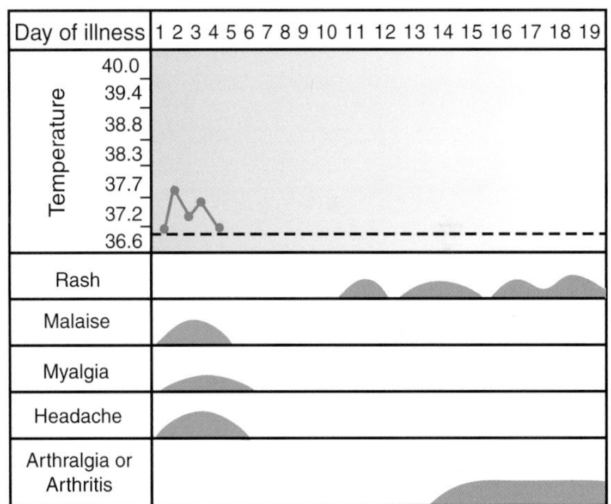


Fig. 12.1.7 The development of erythema infectiosum (fifth disease).

anaemia but with severe anaemia in those with shortened red cell survival (e.g. children with haemoglobinopathies or fetuses).

- In sickle cell disease and other hereditary anaemias, infection may cause a severe but transient aplastic crisis due to red cell aplasia.
- Infection during the second trimester of pregnancy may result in fetal hydrops due to fetal anaemia, with a mortality rate of about 5%.
- There is no specific treatment. Aplastic crises may require transfusion and severe fetal hydrops may necessitate intrauterine transfusion.

## Varicella (chickenpox)

Chickenpox (Figs 12.1.8, 12.1.9) is a highly infectious disease causing a bullous (pox-like) rash. The DNA virus responsible, varicella-zoster virus (VZV), is a herpesvirus and has the ability to remain dormant in the dorsal root ganglia and reactivate as herpes zoster (shingles, discussed below).

### Epidemiology

- Occurs worldwide, although spreads less readily in tropical countries.
- Highly infectious, spread by respiratory route, due to infectious particles from burst vesicles and from respiratory tract.
- Incubation period 10–21 days, short prodromal period of 1–2 days, which is the most infectious period.
- Infectivity persists until the last skin lesion has crusted.
- Peak age incidence is 2–8 years.

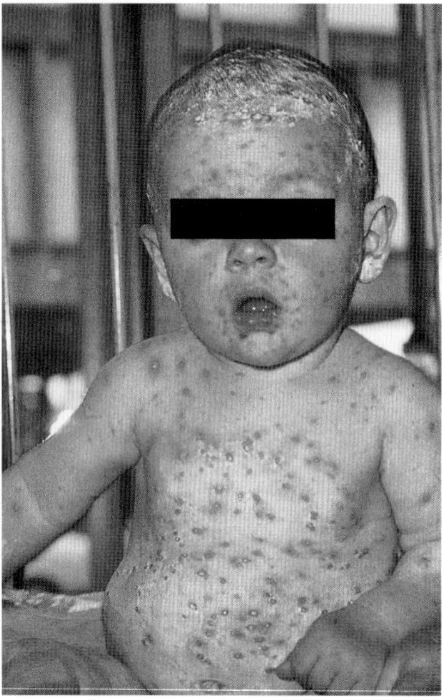

Fig. 12.1.8 Chickenpox: vesicles and pustules on trunk and scalp.

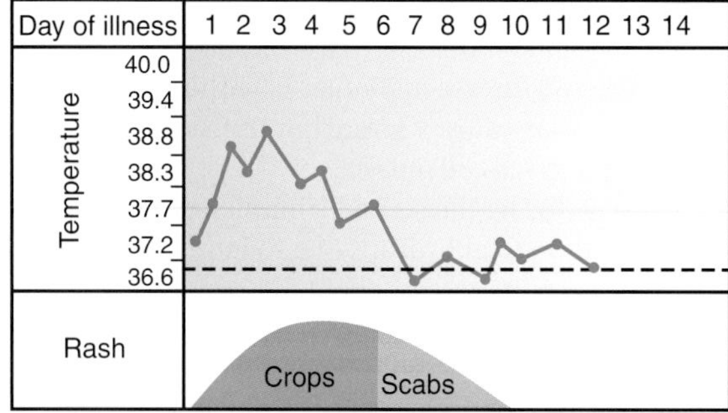


Fig. 12.1.9 The development of chickenpox.

- Humans are only host.
- Effective live attenuated vaccine available.

### Clinical features

- Typically causes 250 to 500 intensely pruritic skin/palatal lesions that are initially vesicular or bullous and then crust.
- Skin lesions may scar.
- Illness is more severe in adolescents and adults.
- May result in severe congenital syndrome if maternal infection occurs at less than 20 weeks' gestation.
- If infection occurs just before delivery, transplacental transfer of virus before protective antiviral antibodies can cross the placenta may result in severe and potentially fatal infection in the newborn (neonatal varicella).

### Complications

- Bacterial superinfection of skin.
- Pneumonia/pneumonitis:
  - varicella pneumonitis particularly affects immunocompromised children, but also pregnant women and normal adults
  - bacterial pneumonia (pneumococcal or staphylococcal) can rarely complicate varicella pneumonitis.
- Encephalitis:
  - incidence about 1 in 1000 cases
  - most common form is pure cerebellar ataxia, with complete recovery over days to weeks
  - severe form is acute disseminated encephalomyelitis (ADEM), a post-infectious demyelinating illness.
- Haemorrhagic chickenpox – severe illness in those with cellular immune deficiency (e.g. oncology patients), indicating importance of T cells in recovery from VZV infection.
- Streptococcal toxic shock syndrome, due to *Streptococcus pyogenes* superinfection.

### Diagnosis

- Usually clinical.
- PCR of virus from blister fluid in tissue culture or detect antigen by PCR or immunofluorescence on vesicle fluid.
- Can use serology (IgM).

### Prevention

- Live attenuated VZV vaccines are highly protective, but contraindicated in pregnancy and in those with impaired immunity.
- Given early, vaccines are effective in preventing infection following exposure.
- Varicella-zoster immune globulin (ZIG or VZIG) is an immunoglobulin preparation with a high titre of anti-VZV IgG antibodies. It is used for passive

prophylaxis of immunocompromised patients (e.g. oncology patients, neonates) exposed to VZV.

### Treatment

Aciclovir is used to treat children with, or at risk of, severe varicella. It is not indicated in uncomplicated primary varicella in an immunocompetent child.

**Clinical example**

Charles, aged 6, had been in contact with a school friend who was off school 2 weeks ago with chickenpox (1). Charles had a sore throat and fever of 38 °C but no spots. Next day, a few small red spots like mosquito stings appeared on his trunk and limbs (2) and on his scalp under the hair (3). These became raised, then developed into small, fluid-filled blisters surrounded by a small area of erythema (4). They were intensely itchy and when scratched readily became superinfected and left a scar (5). These spots crusted over within hours, but fresh crops of vesicles kept appearing on Charles' face, trunk and limbs (6). He had difficulty swallowing and his eyes were red and sore. He was miserable but not unwell and was troubled by the intense pruritus. On the fifth day he became febrile again and a lesion on his leg developed surrounding erythema, diagnosed as cellulitis (7). He recovered after a course of intravenous antibiotics in hospital.

The following are features typical of varicella:

- Incubation period 10–21 days (1)
- Short 1–2-day prodrome during which infectious (not infectious during the incubation period) (2)
- Spots under hairline characteristic and distinguish varicella from insect bites (3)
- Start as macules, then progress to papules, vesicles or pustules (4)
- If scratched they may become infected, the commonest complication, and leave a scar or pockmark (5)
- They come in crops, and can infect the pharynx, palate and conjunctivae of the lids. The child is infectious until the last spot crusts (6)
- Children are usually febrile only during the initial viraemic phase. Prolonged or recurrence of fever suggests bacterial superinfection or other complications (7).

## Zoster (herpes zoster, shingles)

- VZV remains dormant in the dorsal root ganglia of sensory nerves after primary infection and can reactivate many years later as zoster. Zoster follows a dermatomal distribution that does not cross the midline. Historically the distribution of the sensory nerves was mapped by areas affected by zoster infection, which may occur on the trunk and limbs or follow cranial nerves.
- Zoster infection in a previously well child is almost always benign and not suggestive of underlying immune deficiency.
- About 10% of children whose mothers developed chickenpox during pregnancy will develop zoster in early childhood; if a young child gets zoster, ask about chickenpox in pregnancy.
- Immunocompromised children are at increased risk of zoster, which may disseminate.
- Neuralgia before, during and after zoster is very uncommon in children, in contrast to adults.
- Most childhood zoster does not need specific treatment but intravenous aciclovir is indicated for ophthalmic zoster (to prevent eye damage; Fig. 12.1.10) or if the child is immunocompromised (to prevent life-threatening disseminated infection).

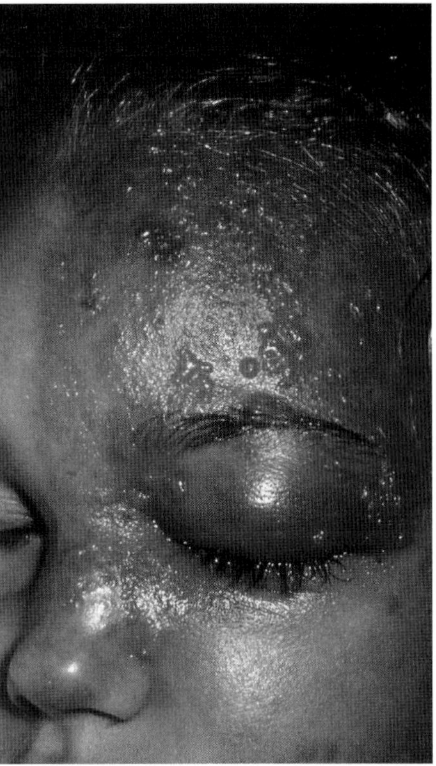

Fig. 12.1.10 Ophthalmic zoster: zoster affecting the ophthalmic division of the Vth nerve. Needs urgent admission and treatment as potentially sight-threatening.

## Scarlet fever and scarlatina

- Group A streptococcus causes a range of infections, most commonly pharyngitis and scarlet fever, but also toxic shock and necrotizing fasciitis (see Chapter 21).
- Post-infectious complications include acute rheumatic fever (see Chapter 12.2) and glomerulonephritis (see Chapter 18.2).
- Scarlet fever (Fig. 12.1.11) is a toxin-mediated disease caused by exotoxins from group A streptococcus (*S. pyogenes*).
- It is commonest at age 5–10 years.
- Toxins act as 'superantigens', causing widespread T-cell activation by bypassing the usually highly specific human leukocyte antigen (HLA)

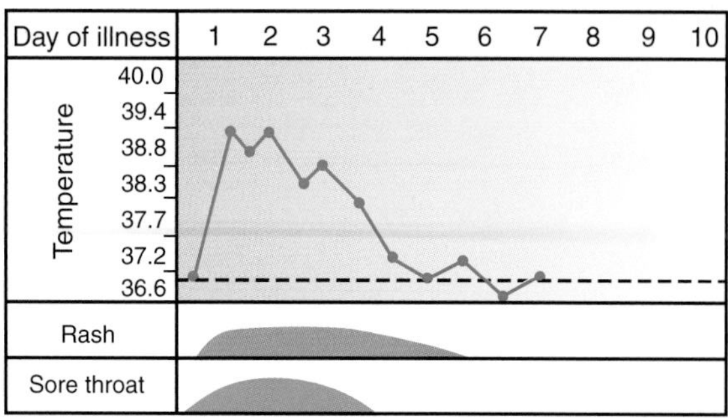


Fig. 12.1.11 The development of scarlet fever.

presentation of antigens to T cells. Analogous superantigen-mediated diseases include toxic shock syndrome and possibly Kawasaki disease.

- The primary site of group A streptococcal infection is the throat, causing exudative tonsillitis and/or pharyngitis.
- *Scarlatina* is a mild form of scarlet fever, usually affecting preschool-aged children.

### Clinical features

- Usually occurs in association with pharyngitis, rarely with pyoderma or wound infection.
- Confluent sandpaper-like rash, which may be pruritic.
- Strawberry tongue and circumoral pallor may occur.
- Treatment is with oral penicillin.

### Diagnosis

Positive throat swab (although asymptomatic carriage of *S. pyogenes* is common in school-aged children) or positive serology: high or rising titre to streptolysin O (anti-streptolysin O titre; ASOT) or deoxyribonuclease B (anti-DNAase B). ASOT and anti-DNAase B are generally higher in Australian Aboriginal children.

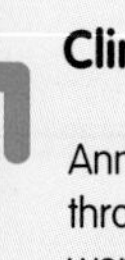

**Clinical example**

Anna, 7 years old, presented with fever and sore throat for 2 days, followed by a rash. Her tonsils were red and covered in spots of white exudate. Her tongue had prominent red papillae. Her face looked red but was white around the mouth, like a clown's. The rash was red, patchy and rough to the touch, and covered her whole body. In the axillae and groins there were lines of petechiae. Her cervical lymph nodes were enlarged and tender. She was treated with penicillin and rapidly improved. Two weeks later she had extensive peeling of her hands and feet.

The following are features typical of scarlet fever: exudative tonsillitis; strawberry tongue; circumoral pallor; sandpaper rash; Pastia's lines; tender cervical lymphadenitis; peripheral desquamation.

## Infectious mononucleosis (glandular fever)

### Epidemiology

- Infectious mononucleosis is caused by Epstein–Barr virus (EBV), a DNA herpesvirus; humans are the only host.
- Typically a disease of adolescence.
- Transmission from infected saliva by the oral route (known as the 'kissing disease').
- Asymptomatic secretion of the virus is common.
- A similar clinical syndrome may be caused by infection with cytomegalovirus (CMV) and *Toxoplasma gondii* (toxoplasmosis).

### Clinical features

- Fever, exudative pharyngitis, lymphadenopathy and splenomegaly.
- Palatal petechiae may be present.
- Rash may be subtle but typically becomes more florid if amoxicillin is given.
- Infections in younger children may be subclinical or cause severe enlargement of the tonsils.
- Severe disseminated infection may occur in the immunocompromised.

### Diagnosis

- Specific IgM or rising IgG titre to EBV. The Paul–Bunnell test and monospot test detect non-specific (heterophil) antibodies produced because of the polyclonal B cell proliferation caused by EBV. They have low sensitivity in preschool children. False-positive EBV serology may occur in other febrile illnesses.
- The blood film is often suggestive, showing many atypical mononuclear cells. PCR of blood may be helpful in immunocompromised patients.

### Treatment

- Contact sports should be avoided until the spleen is no longer palpable, as there is a risk of rupture.
- Corticosteroids may be considered if airway obstruction is developing due to tonsillar hypertrophy.

**Clinical example**

Beth, 6 years old, presented with fever, sore throat and malaise. She was treated with amoxicillin for exudative tonsillitis. Two days later, she developed a florid rash. When reviewed, she had marked tonsillar enlargement and large matted nodes in the neck, which were moderately tender.

She had petechiae on the soft palate. Her eyelids were puffy and her spleen was palpable 2 cm below the costal margin. Pulse oximetry, performed overnight to exclude significant upper airway obstruction, was normal, so dexamethasone was withheld and Beth was sent home.

'Purulent' exudative tonsillitis may be due to group A streptococcus or EBV at this age. Ampicillin or amoxicillin causes a dramatic rash in EBV infection. Tender lymphadenitis occurs in both infections, but palatal petechiae, puffy eyelids and splenomegaly are typical features of EBV infection. There is no specific treatment, although steroids are sometimes used to reduce upper airway obstruction.

## Herpes simplex virus

### Epidemiology and clinical features

- Herpes simplex virus (HSV) is a DNA herpesvirus, with two serotypes, HSV-1 and HSV-2.
- HSV-1 is primarily oropharyngeal, whereas HSV-2 is primarily genital.
- Neonates may acquire HSV around delivery, usually (about 90%) HSV-2.
- HSV infection can disseminate in the skin of children with eczema (eczema herpeticum, Kaposi varicelliform eruption) if not treated promptly with aciclovir.
- Neonatal HSV infection may be localized to skin, eye (conjunctivitis) and/or mouth, may cause isolated encephalitis or isolated pneumonitis or, if not treated with aciclovir, will usually disseminate to cause hepatitis, disseminated intravascular coagulation, encephalitis and death.
- Neonatal HSV encephalitis (see Chapter 11.4) is usually due to primary maternal genital infection and more rarely following reactivation of maternal genital herpes.
- Most post-neonatal infections are symptomatic.
- The commonest primary HSV infection in childhood is gingivostomatitis; it causes nasty ulceration of the gums (gingivae), buccal mucosa (*stoma* = mouth) and pharynx.
- In primary infection, HSV is shed for about 1 week; in recurrent infection for 3–4 days.
- Incubation period beyond the neonatal period is from 2 days to 2 weeks.
- Herpes encephalitis can occur at any age, may be primary or secondary, due to HSV-1 or HSV-2, and has a poor prognosis, even if treated with aciclovir.
- As a herpesvirus, local recurrences of HSV are common, often at the mucocutaneous junction of the lip ('cold sores'), but can be on the finger ('whitlow') or on the skin elsewhere. They may be exacerbated by sunlight exposure.
- Try to avoid the child inoculating virus into the genital area.

### Diagnosis

Rapid diagnosis by immunofluorescence of blister fluid or polymerase chain reaction (PCR) of blister fluid and/or cerebrospinal fluid is preferred to culture or serology (IgM).

### Treatment

Aciclovir is effective against HSV and may be given topically (e.g. for keratitis), orally (for mild disease) or intravenously (for severe or neonatal infection).

## Enteroviruses

- The enteroviruses, as the name suggests, are gut viruses, usually transmitted faecal–orally, although respiratory spread can occur.
- Commonly spread in swimming pools.
- Faecal shedding may continue for months, often asymptomatically; respiratory shedding is for less than 1 week.
- Spring and summer peaks.
- They are picornaviruses (from *pico* = small + RNA).
- They can affect the central nervous system, causing a variety of syndromes.
- The major groups of enteroviruses are:
  - coxsackieviruses
  - echoviruses
  - enterovirus types (somewhat confusingly).
- Polioviruses are usually considered separately from non-polio enteroviruses.

### Clinical features

Enteroviral infection may result in a broad range of clinical infections.

- *Fever*: common cause of isolated fever in infancy.
- *Rashes*:
  - hand, foot and mouth disease – blistering rash on palms, soles and palate caused by coxsackievirus A16 and other enteroviruses, including enterovirus (EV) 71
  - various non-specific rashes – macular, papular, papulo-urticarial, vesicular, morbilliform, rubelliform, etc.
- *Enanthem*: herpangina (= ulcerative pharyngitis) due to coxsackievirus A.
- *Neurological*:
  - paralytic – poliomyelitis due to infection of anterior horn cells by poliovirus, but similar syndrome can be caused by other enteroviruses
  - monoplegia – EV 71, other enteroviruses
  - 'aseptic' meningitis and encephalitis – coxsackieviruses, echoviruses, EV 71.
- *Cardiac*: myocarditis – mainly coxsackievirus B.
- *Liver*: hepatitis – mainly echoviruses.

- *Eyes*: epidemic haemorrhagic conjunctivitis – EV 71.
- *Gastrointestinal*: vomiting, diarrhoea, abdominal pain and hepatitis.
- *Musculoskeletal*: Bornholm disease (epidemic pleurodynia) due to coxsackie virus B.

### Diagnosis

PCR or PCR from throat and rectal swabs, stool and CSF. Serology is not possible.

### Treatment

The antiviral drug pleconaril has activity against enteroviruses, but is not widely available.

### Prevention

Immunization against polio with oral polio vaccine (live, attenuated) or inactivated polio vaccine (injected, killed).

## Adenoviruses

- Multiple serotypes.
- In infancy, adenoviruses are an important cause of exudative tonsillitis with high fever (at this age, group A streptococcal infection is rare).
- Can cause epidemics of conjunctivitis, often with red throat (pharyngoconjunctival fever).
- Can cause disseminated infection with pneumonia, hepatitis and encephalitis (particularly adenovirus 7 and 21); rare, but may be fatal.
- Enteric adenoviruses can cause gastroenteritis.

### Diagnosis

Viral culture or immunofluorescence on throat swab.

## Kawasaki disease (mucocutaneous lymph node syndrome)

- Kawasaki disease is an important but poorly understood cause of prolonged fever, rash and other features.
- Results in coronary artery damage in 25% of untreated and 5% of treated children.
- The cause is unknown; probably an abnormal immune response to an infectious trigger.
- Predominantly affecting those between 6 months and 4 years, but can occur at any age. Commoner in boys.
- Much more common in north-eastern Asians (Japanese, Koreans) but seen in all ethnic groups.
- Diagnosis is made clinically with fever of at least 5 days and classically at least four other diagnostic criteria:
  - polymorphous rash (petechiae and vesicles do not occur)
  - changes to mucous membranes (red lips, strawberry tongue, red pharynx, no exudates)
  - changes to the extremities (swollen erythematous hands and feet, desquamation especially around nail-beds in subacute phase)
  - non-purulent bilateral conjunctival injection
  - lymphadenopathy (unilateral, >1 cm, largely in older children).
- Clinical features appear sequentially and are rarely present at same time.
- Children are usually very irritable and often have white cells (but no pathogens) in CSF and urine.
- C-reactive protein (CRP) and neutrophil count usually high acutely; platelets rise in subacute phase.
- Coronary artery damage may occur in those with fewer than four features ('incomplete Kawasaki disease'); consider the diagnosis in any child with prolonged unexplained fever unresponsive to antibiotics.
- Treatment with intravenous immunoglobulin given before day 10 reduces coronary artery damage. Usually given with low-dose aspirin.

### Clinical example

Josh, an 18-month-old child of Japanese and Australian parents, presents with a 4-day history of fever, unresponsive to antipyretics and oral amoxicillin, given by his general practitioner for a red throat. Josh has had red eyes, which have largely resolved, and an erythematous rash with target lesions. His mother noticed very red lips ('as though he had put on my lipstick'), swollen feet and a reluctance to walk. He was extremely irritable.

Following admission to hospital, examination of blood, urine and CSF showed inflammatory changes, but cultures were sterile and there was no response to intravenous broad-spectrum antibiotics. The diagnosis of Kawasaki disease was made on day 7, and Josh defervesced following intravenous immunoglobulin. An echocardiogram at diagnosis showed mild coronary artery dilatation, which was found to have resolved after 6 weeks, when low-dose aspirin therapy was ceased.

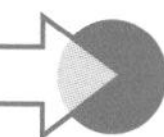

### Practical points

- Measles is a severe vaccine-preventable childhood infection.
- Children with measles are sick when the rash appears; children with roseola infantum are sick until the rash appears.
- Rubella is usually mild but can cross the placenta in the first trimester to cause congenital rubella syndrome.
- Chickenpox and measles can be devastating in children with impaired cell-mediated (T cell) immunity.
- Scarlet fever is a toxin-mediated disease caused by an exotoxin produced by group A streptococci.
- Consider Kawasaki disease in a child with fever persisting for more than 5 days and no clear diagnosis.

# Bone and joint infections 12.2

Jonathan Carapetis, Andrew Steer

## Introduction

Infections of bones (osteomyelitis) and joints (septic arthritis) can occur at any age but are much more common in children than adults. They are often difficult to diagnose, can be difficult to treat and, if not diagnosed and treated promptly, can lead to permanent disability. Many children and adults have shortened or deformed limbs, fused joints or even amputations because osteomyelitis or septic arthritis was diagnosed too late or treated inadequately. Almost all these poor outcomes need not have happened; with careful history-taking and examination, prudent use of investigations – particularly imaging – and close observation, virtually all bone and joint infections can be diagnosed and treated before permanent damage ensues.

## Pathogenesis

The area around the growth plates of children's bones is particularly prone to infection. Although the metaphysis has a plentiful blood supply from nutrient arteries, blood flow through capillary loops and sinusoidal veins at the metaphyseal–epiphyseal junction is slow, which allows bloodborne bacteria to deposit in this region (Fig. 12.2.1). This area also has poor penetration of white blood cells and other immune mediators, so deposited bacteria are relatively protected. As the infection progresses, pus accumulates under pressure, further limiting the blood supply to the region. Increased stasis and activity of cytokines encourages clots to form in blood vessels, leading to ischaemic bone necrosis. Infection then spreads to the cortex through the Volkmann canals and haversian system, and subsequently into the subperiosteal space.

If the infection remains untreated, bone necrosis may lead to development of a sequestrum – an area of dead cortical bone separated from normal bone. Sometimes the infection becomes walled off by granulation tissue that forms a fibrous capsule, the so-called Brodie abscess, usually located in the metaphysis and presenting subacutely with pain and tenderness, but rarely fever.

Chronic osteomyelitis is usually the result of untreated or inadequately treated acute osteomyelitis. Sequestra and Brodie abscesses are sometimes found in chronic osteomyelitis. Most cases of chronic osteomyelitis, like acute osteomyelitis, are caused by *Staphylococcus aureus*, but chronic presentations increase the likelihood of unusual organisms, including *Mycobacterium tuberculosis*, fungi and *Kingella kingae*.

Septic arthritis may occur *de novo*, as a result of deposition of bacteria in the joint. Alternatively there may be extension from adjacent osteomyelitis, which is more common in children than adults, possibly because of transport of bacteria through blood vessels that cross the epiphyseal plate. In some joints, the metaphysis is intra-articular, which means that osteomyelitis can transform directly into septic arthritis. These joints are:

- proximal femur → hip joint
- proximal humerus → shoulder joint
- proximal radius → elbow joint
- distal lateral tibia → ankle joint.

Synovial joints are poor at clearing infection and the connective tissue may be damaged by enzymes released by bacteria. Initially, the inflammation results in a joint effusion, which may be purulent; if left untreated, the articular and growth cartilage can be destroyed. Longer-term complications may include dislocation, avascular necrosis of intra-articular epiphyses and joint destruction.

## Microbiology

Although occasionally caused by fungi, and rarely by parasites or viruses, osteomyelitis and septic arthritis are predominantly bacterial infections, most often caused by *S. aureus*. The major bacterial pathogens are:

- *Staphylococcus aureus* (80–90% of culture positive cases) – usually methicillin-susceptible but community-acquired methicillin-resistant *S. aureus* (CA-MRSA) is on the rise in many places.
- *Kingella kingae* – recent studies using polymerase chain reaction (PCR) diagnosis suggest that this organism is a common cause of osteomyelitis and septic arthritis in young children (usually under 2 years), but is often not identified using standard laboratory cultures.

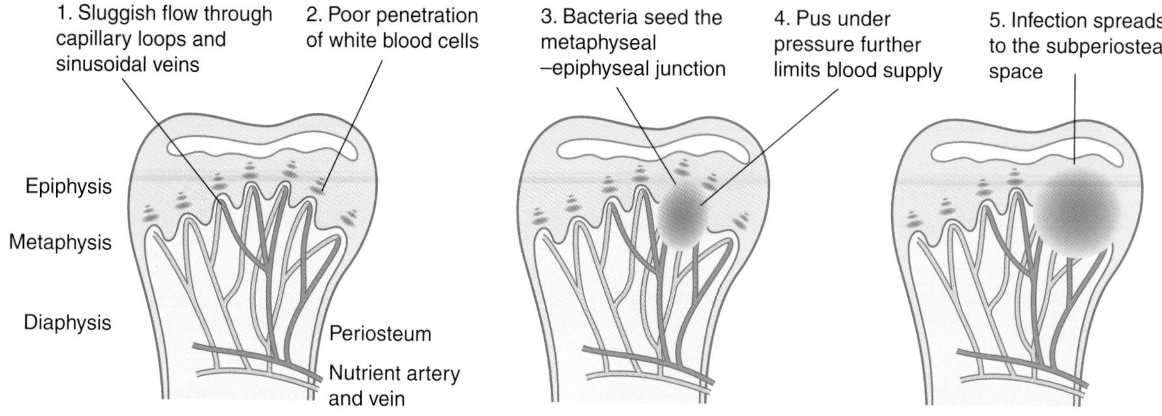
1. Sluggish flow through capillary loops and sinusoidal veins
2. Poor penetration of white blood cells
3. Bacteria seed the metaphyseal –epiphyseal junction
4. Pus under pressure further limits blood supply
5. Infection spreads to the subperiosteal space
Epiphysis
Metaphysis
Diaphysis
Periosteum
Nutrient artery and vein

Fig. 12.2.1 Anatomical evolution of osteomyelitis. (Adapted with permission from Krogstad P, Smith AL 2004 Osteomyelitis and septic arthritis. In: Feigin RD, Cherry JD, Demmler GJ, Kaplan SL (eds) Textbook of pediatric infectious diseases, 5th edn. WB Saunders, Philadelphia, PA, pp 683–703.)

- *Streptococcus pyogenes* (group A streptococcus) – sometimes associated with varicella infection.
- *Streptococcus pneumoniae* – mainly in children aged less than 2 years.
- *Pseudomonas aeruginosa* – immunocompromised patients or traumatic (classical cause is a nail through a tennis shoe causing calcaneal osteomyelitis).
- Group B streptococcus or *Escherichia coli* – especially in neonates.
- *Haemophilus influenzae* type b – in unimmunized populations (mainly in developing countries).
- *Mycobacterium tuberculosis* – mainly in children from developing countries or immigrant populations; 50% of cases affect the spine. Often subacute presentation.
- *Salmonella* spp – particularly in people with sickle cell anaemia.
- *Neisseria gonorrhoeae* – mainly in developing countries; may cause multifocal septic arthritis in neonates or sexually active adolescents.

## Clinical presentation

Although osteomyelitis and septic arthritis are usually considered distinct entities, in paediatric practice they are sometimes difficult to distinguish and may occur together. Children with septic arthritis are more likely than adults to have osteomyelitis in the adjacent bone. In neonates and infants, osteomyelitis and septic arthritis coexist so commonly that the preferred term is 'osteoarticular infection'.

The typical child with osteomyelitis or septic arthritis is aged less than 5 years: approximately 50% of cases occur under the age of 5 years and of these 25% are under the age of 1 year. Usually the symptoms have been present for 2–3 days prior to presentation. Early in the illness, when bacteraemia is present, the child may be unwell with fever and malaise. Later, as the infection establishes itself, the symptoms relate to the main site of infection. Both diseases usually present with fever and limb pain; in younger children this will most often manifest as a limp, or disuse of a limb or other body part. Septic arthritis is more likely than osteomyelitis to have obvious localized clinical signs.

### Osteomyelitis

In osteomyelitis, there is pain, which may be poorly localized, especially in young children. Neonates may present with a generalized febrile illness, without any localizing features. The precise location of the infection can often be elicited with careful physical examination, looking particularly for metaphyseal tenderness. Erythema and swelling are signs of abscess formation, which occurs late in the illness. In one-third of cases there is a history of mild preceding trauma to the affected area so such a history should increase rather than reduce the suspicion of osteomyelitis.

Osteomyelitis most commonly affects, in order:

1. femur
2. tibia
3. humerus
4. calcaneus.

The pelvis and vertebrae are less commonly affected but more likely to present with advanced disease because of delayed presentation (in vertebral osteomyelitis) or delayed diagnosis (in pelvic osteomyelitis). The diagnosis of osteomyelitis in long bones may also be delayed – and hence become subacute or chronic – because of formation of a Brodie abscess or the presence of low-grade infection, sometimes due to unusual organisms. In these cases, diffuse pain or tenderness is prominent and fever may be absent.

### Septic arthritis

Differentiating septic arthritis from osteomyelitis can be difficult. Children with osteomyelitis may not want to move the adjacent joint because of either pain or muscle spasm. In addition to fever and limb pain, the hallmark of septic arthritis is a warm, tender joint with a dramatically restricted range of movement and an effusion. However, these signs are not always present. Septic arthritis of the shoulder or hip is very difficult to diagnose early, because of the lack of visible joint swelling in the early stages.

The following features should raise suspicion that there is coexistent osteomyelitis and septic arthritis:

- osteomyelitis in a bone with an intra-articular metaphysis (proximal femur, proximal humerus, proximal radius, distal lateral fibula)
- slow clinical response to therapy
- slow response of inflammatory markers (e.g. C-reactive protein) to therapy
- age less than 18 months
- delayed presentation
- previous antibiotic therapy.

## Differential diagnosis

The most important diagnosis to exclude in possible osteomyelitis is malignancy. Bone tumours can cause local bone destruction, and leukaemia may present with fever and bone pain. Cellulitis may mimic the focal tenderness and erythema of late-presenting osteomyelitis. Patients with sickle cell disease may develop bone infarction, which can be difficult to differentiate from osteomyelitis.

Chronic recurrent multifocal osteomyelitis (CRMO) is a rare, non-infectious, inflammatory syndrome of unknown pathogenesis that affects children and young adults and is most common in girls. Affected children have prolonged symptoms of pain and swelling that relapse and recur. The clavicle is a classical site of involvement. Treatment with antibiotics does not alter the course of the disease but steroids and anti-inflammatory medication may provide symptomatic relief. CRMO usually resolves, although it may relapse and recur over a prolonged period (up to 15 years), and there is a danger of premature epiphyseal closure.

Septic arthritis of the hip can present similarly to transient synovitis ('irritable hip'), which usually occurs following minor injury or a viral illness. Children with transient synovitis are usually not unwell and their joint signs are not as severe as those in children with septic arthritis, but in the early stages of either illness the diagnoses can be confused. Sometimes the only way to be sure of the diagnosis is to aspirate the joint and observe the child. It is important not to treat empirically with antibiotics without first obtaining a diagnostic specimen.

Acute joint swelling may be caused by inflammatory arthritis (e.g. juvenile chronic arthritis, inflammatory bowel disease, other connective tissue diseases), reactive arthritis (which may occur in association with a wide range of pathogens including *Mycoplasma*, cytomegalovirus, Epstein–Barr virus, parvovirus, hepatitis, rubella, *Yersinia*, *Salmonella* and *Shigella* species), rheumatic fever and Henoch–Schönlein purpura.

Rarely, osteomyelitis or septic arthritis may affect multiple bones or joints at the same time. This should raise the suspicion of a distant source of persistent bacteraemia such as endocarditis or occult abscess, and should lead to a thorough investigation for other sites of infection (e.g. heart, liver, spleen, brain, eyes). It should also raise suspicion of unusual organisms (e.g. *N. gonorrhoeae*) as a cause of multifocal septic arthritis or an alternative diagnosis if an organism cannot be identified (e.g. CRMO, inflammatory or reactive arthritis, or rheumatic fever).

## Confirming the diagnosis

As a minimum, all patients with suspected bone or joint infections should have a blood culture, blood count and film, C-reactive protein (CRP) measurement and plain radiography. Other investigations are tailored to the likelihood of bone or joint infection (Fig. 12.2.2).

### Osteomyelitis

Diagnosis depends upon the presence of two of the following:

- clinical signs (fever, localized tenderness, erythema, oedema)
- pus aspirated from bone
- positive blood or bone culture
- evidence of osteomyelitis on plain radiography, bone scan or magnetic resonance imaging (MRI).

Other laboratory tests can provide supportive evidence for the diagnosis:

- The peripheral white cell count (WCC) is normal in half or more of osteomyelitis cases. However, WCC and blood film examination should be performed to exclude leukaemia.
- Erythrocyte sedimentation rate (ESR) and CRP are raised at presentation in more than 90% of cases. CRP is preferred to ESR to monitor response to therapy because it rises faster (within 6 hours, compared with 24 hours for ESR) and responds more quickly to treatment (returning to normal in 2 weeks, compared with 3–4 weeks for ESR in typical cases).

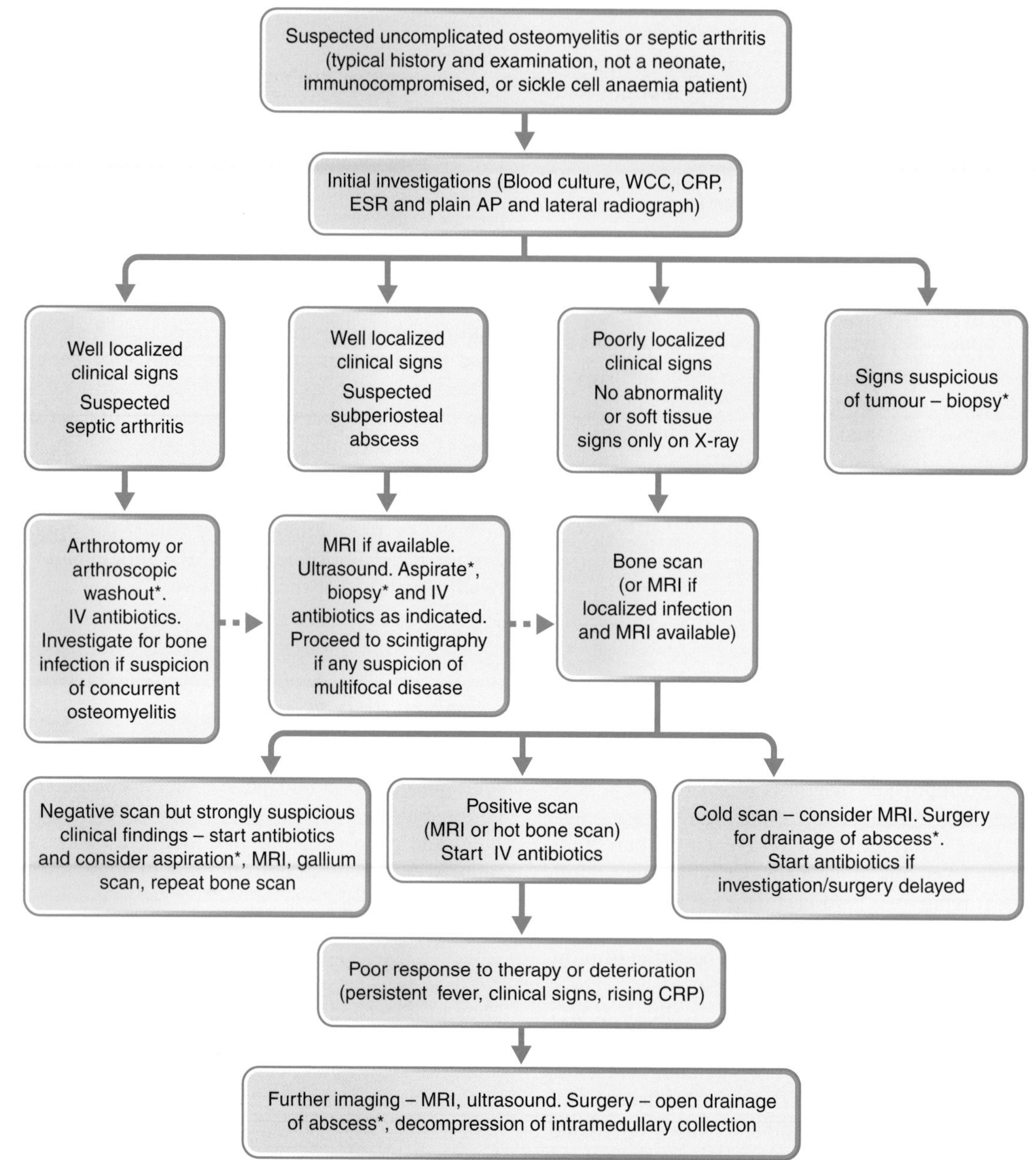


**Fig. 12.2.2** Approach to the management of osteomyelitis and septic arthritis in children. AP, anteroposterior; CRP, C-reactive protein; ESR, erythrocyte sedimentation rate; IV, intravenous; MRI, magnetic resonance imaging; WCC, white cell count. (Adapted with permission from Steer AC, Carapetis JR 2004 Acute hematogenous osteomyelitis in children: recognition and management. Pediatric Drugs 6:333–346.)

## Pus aspirated from bone

Although some advocate diagnostic bone aspiration or biopsy as a routine, the majority of children do not need these invasive tests. A diagnostic specimen should be obtained in any of the following situations:

- delayed presentation
- a child with any predisposing condition (e.g. immune compromise, sickle cell disease, other haemoglobinopathies)
- unusual radiographic findings (e.g. lucency on plain radiography at presentation)

- geographical region where there is a high likelihood of CA-MRSA
- reason to suspect a complication such as an abscess
- reason to suspect an alternative diagnosis such as malignancy
- delayed response to antibiotics.

## Positive blood or bone culture

Cultures from bone aspiration or biopsy are positive at admission in 50–70% of osteomyelitis cases, and culture-negative cases may have a positive Gram stain or typical histological features of acute osteomyelitis. However, as stated above, this procedure is usually not needed. Blood cultures are positive in 30–50% of cases.

## Imaging

*Plain radiography*

Plain radiography should be performed routinely to exclude a fracture or malignancy. There are no changes of osteomyelitis in the first 3 days. From days 3–10 there may be non-specific, deep, soft tissue swelling followed by poor distinction of muscular planes. From days 10–21 periosteal elevation or lytic lesions may be seen (Fig. 12.2.3). Because these changes indicate longer-standing disease, if they are seen on radiography at presentation the child should not be treated as having acute, uncomplicated osteomyelitis (i.e. the child requires more prolonged courses of antibiotics, initially intravenous and subsequently oral).

*Bone scan*

The typical bone scan uses technetium-99 m-labelled phosphates or phosphonates, which bind to hydroxyapatite crystal as they flow through bone. Uptake is increased with increased blood flow, inflammation and increased osteoblastic activity. The sensitivity of bone scans in the diagnosis of osteomyelitis is more than 90%, but a negative bone scan does not exclude the diagnosis. False-negative bone scans in osteomyelitis can be caused by focal ischaemia due to compression from abscess formation, leading to a 'cold' rather than the typical 'hot' scan. There is a 5–30% false-positive rate of bone scans, usually due to difficulty in differentiating infection in surrounding soft tissue or joints from bone. Bone scans are considered the investigation of choice by many people for osteomyelitis because they are sensitive, cheap, usually positive within 48 hours of onset of symptoms, rarely require sedation and allow for the detection of multifocal disease (because the whole skeleton is visualized). However, bone scans give a relatively high radiation dose (equivalent to 100 chest X-rays, or half that for computed tomography (CT) of the chest) and do not give detailed anatomical information, particularly relating to collections of pus.

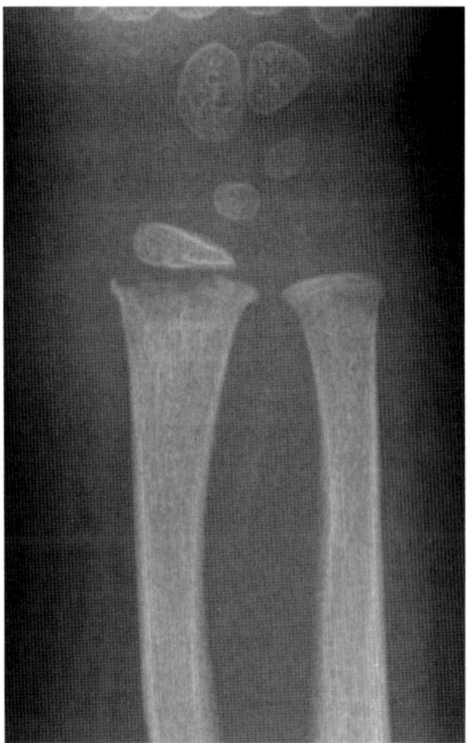

Fig. 12.2.3 Osteomyelitis in a 3-year-old girl who presented with pseudoparalysis. Radiographs at presentation were normal. This radiograph, taken 2 weeks after presentation, shows early abscess formation in the distal radius with erosion of the radial metaphysis and loss of fat plane definition. (Courtesy of Professor Kerr Graham; reproduced with permission from Steer AC, Carapetis JR 2004 Acute hematogenous osteomyelitis in children: recognition and management. Pediatric Drugs 6:333–346.)

**Clinical example**

Michael, aged 15 months, was noted by his parents to be reluctant to bear weight on his right leg and had a low-grade fever. He was seen by his general practitioner and referred immediately to the emergency department, from where he was admitted with 'possible osteomyelitis' of the right distal femur because of mild metaphyseal tenderness and refusal to bear weight. Osteomyelitis was confirmed by positive blood culture (*S. aureus*) and a positive bone scan. Plain radiographs were normal. Michael was managed with intravenous flucloxacillin for 3 days, followed by oral flucloxacillin for 3 weeks. He was followed for 6 months and had no long-term sequelae.

*Ultrasonography*

Ultrasonography is used mainly to guide aspiration of subperiosteal fluid collections. There may be other changes that suggest osteomyelitis (e.g. cortical breaches and soft tissue swelling), but ultrasonography is rarely used by itself for diagnosing osteomyelitis. It may also detect fluid collections in adjacent joints suggestive of septic arthritis.

*Magnetic resonance imaging*

MRI is the best test for osteomyelitis in cases where symptoms and signs are localized (Fig. 12.2.4). A finding of dark bone marrow intensity on T1-weighted images has almost 100% sensitivity. The specificity is not quite so high, although the use of fat-suppressed contrast-enhanced imaging improves specificity. The other advantages of MRI are that it will show abscesses and sinus tracts, and is particularly useful in planning surgery in complex cases. MRI is often used in vertebral osteomyelitis because of the risk of epidural abscess, and in the pelvis, where there is a higher risk of abscess formation. However, it is often difficult to obtain an MRI scan at short notice, scans are expensive and younger children may need to be anaesthetized for a scan. MRI may also be useful in cases where there is high clinical suspicion of localized osteomyelitis but a negative (and therefore possibly false-negative) bone scan.

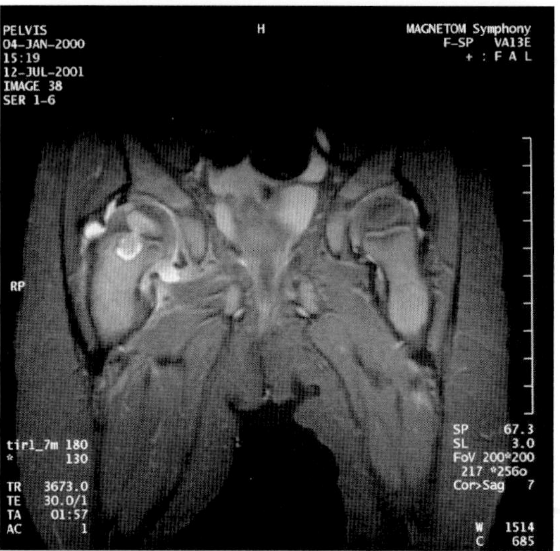


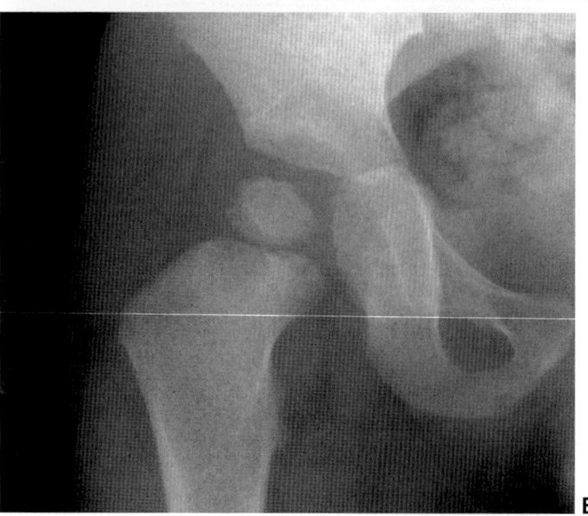


**Fig. 12.2.4** An 18-month-old child who presented with fever and limp. **(A)** Magnetic resonance image shows an abscess that originates in the metaphysis of the right proximal femur crossing the physeal cartilage to the epiphysis. **(B)** Plain radiograph shows an abscess in the proximal femur. (Courtesy of Professor Kerr Graham; reproduced with permission from Steer AC, Carapetis JR 2004 Acute hematogenous osteomyelitis in children: recognition and management. Pediatric Drugs 6:333–346.)

## Septic arthritis

Septic arthritis can usually be diagnosed more easily than osteomyelitis because the signs are more obvious and a diagnostic specimen is obtained more easily. Traditional teaching is that any child with a possibly infected joint requires urgent surgical intervention, usually a formal arthroscopic washout or arthrotomy in the operating theatre under general anaesthesia. In general, joint aspiration should be performed to obtain a specimen only when the diagnosis is in doubt – with the intention of proceeding to the operating theatre if the diagnosis is confirmed – or if there is an unavoidable delay before getting the child to the operating theatre. However, recent published experience from Finland suggests that diagnostic joint aspiration may be the procedure of choice; more research is needed in this area before firm recommendations can be made.

Joint fluid should be sent immediately to the laboratory for Gram staining and culture. The Gram stain is not a reliable method of microbiological diagnosis, so Gram staining results should not be used as a reason to cease anti-staphylococcal antibiotics in favour of other antimicrobials. Instead, Gram staining suggesting other organisms (e.g. Gram-negative bacilli) is an indication to add broader-spectrum cover to the anti-staphylococcal antibiotic. The antimicrobial treatment can be rationalized when definitive culture and susceptibility results are known.

Occasionally, pus from an obviously infected joint may not grow organisms on culture, even if a child has not received prior antibiotics. This is probably because of the high levels of natural cytokines and other antibacterial agents in the effusion, although sometimes it may be because the infection is caused by an organism, such as *K. kingae*, that is not easily identified using standard culture techniques. Microbiological yield from joint fluid can be increased by inoculating the fluid directly into a blood culture. Most culture-negative cases can be managed as *S. aureus* infections, but sometimes the negative culture result is because the joint is not actually infected. A number of patients with juvenile chronic arthritis and rheumatic fever present initially with culture-negative 'septic arthritis'. Therefore, a negative culture of synovial fluid should lead to a thorough re-evaluation of the patient and exclusion of other diagnoses.

## Treatment

The choice of empirical antimicrobial therapy is similar for septic arthritis and osteomyelitis. The duration of treatment is identical for uncomplicated cases. Osteomyelitis is more likely than septic arthritis to be complicated and then to require longer courses of initial parenteral and subsequent oral therapy. Surgery is always required for septic arthritis, but only occasionally required for osteomyelitis.

### Antibiotic choice

*S. aureus* is the most common cause of bone and joint infections in all age groups, and in most parts of Australia CA-MRSA rates are low (< 10% of all community-acquired *S. aureus* infections). In these regions, empirical antibiotic therapy should always contain an anti-staphylococcal antibiotic such as a β-lactamase-resistant penicillin (e.g. flucloxacillin) or first-generation cephalosporin (e.g. cephalothin or cefazolin). Where rates of CA-MRSA infection are high, either clindamycin or vancomycin should be used empirically (in some regions, clindamycin resistance is also rising, in which case vancomycin is the best choice) until microbiological diagnosis is confirmed and antibiotics can be tailored according to susceptibility testing. Note that *K. kingae* is usually susceptible to most antibiotics used empirically, including penicillins and cephalosporins, but is commonly resistant to clindamycin and vancomycin.

The following patients should have other antibiotics added to (not substituted for) the anti-staphylococcal antibiotic regimen:

- *neonates*: add gentamicin or a third-generation cephalosporin (e.g. cefotaxime, ceftriaxone)
- *sickle cell anaemia*: add a third-generation cephalosporin (e.g. cefotaxime, ceftriaxone)
- *puncture wounds to the feet*: add an anti-pseudomonal antibiotic (e.g. ceftazidime, piperacillin, ticarcillin)
- *immunocompromise*: add an anti-pseudomonal antibiotic, as above. If there is no response, consider also adding an antifungal (e.g. amphotericin or voriconazole)
- children aged less than 5 years and not immunized against *H. influenzae* type b (Hib): add a third-generation cephalosporin (e.g. cefotaxime, ceftriaxone).

Following identification of the organism, antibiotic choice is dictated by susceptibility testing. If unable to obtain cultures or if cultures are negative, the initial empirical choice should be continued provided the clinical response is adequate.

### Duration of antibiotic therapy

Adult patients are usually treated for osteomyelitis or septic arthritis with 4–6 weeks of intravenous antibiotics. By contrast, children can often be treated for a shorter time and most of the treatment course can be given orally. The typical child with acute, uncomplicated osteomyelitis or septic arthritis who responds quickly to initial therapy can be treated with 3 days of intravenous antibiotics followed by 3 weeks of oral antibiotics. However, this regimen should be used only in otherwise healthy children with classical acute presentations, no evidence of chronicity on initial radiography and a rapid response to treatment. Children with atypical presentations, underlying illness, evidence of chronicity, complications or delayed response to treatment should all be treated with longer initial courses of intravenous antibiotics and longer total duration of therapy. When the switch is made from parenteral to oral antibiotics, they should be used at two to three times higher doses than normally given to achieve adequate serum and bone concentrations. Children usually tolerate this well, with few side-effects. Recent evidence suggests that even shorter courses may be possible – a total of 10 days (including an initial 3-day intravenous course) for septic arthritis, or a total of 20 days (with an initial 4-day intravenous course) for acute haematogenous osteomyelitis with or without adjacent septic arthritis. However, such abbreviated courses should be considered only in uncomplicated cases that show a rapid and sustained response of signs, symptoms and CRP to intravenous treatment, in whom close follow-up is assured, and when the carers appreciate the possibility that the treatment failure rate may be greater than after more prolonged treatment courses.

### Surgical management

As mentioned above, the current recommendation is that all children with septic arthritis require a formal arthroscopic washout or arthrotomy as a diagnostic and therapeutic procedure. Recent data suggesting that diagnostic aspiration alone may be preferable require confirmation before a change to routine management can be recommended. Splinting an infected joint may be useful to reduce pain in the first few days, but joint mobility should be encouraged once the acute signs have settled. An infected hip may require abduction bracing to prevent or treat septic dislocation in the younger child.

The main place for surgery in osteomyelitis is to confirm the diagnosis or manage complications such as abscesses, chronic osteomyelitis, sequestra, pseudarthroses or growth defects. In chronic osteomyelitis, both long-term antibiotics and surgical debridement are needed. Deformities that result from chronic osteomyelitis or growth plate damage may require limb reconstruction techniques. Destruction to articular cartilage causes lifelong problems that are not correctable by surgery.

### Adjunctive treatment

A recent placebo-controlled randomized controlled trial found that 4 days of intravenous dexamethasone in addition to antibiotic and surgical management led to a significant reduction in residual dysfunction, from 26% in the control group to 2% in the treatment group, 12 months later. However, because the baseline rate of dysfunction in that study was much higher than would be normal in Australia, adjunctive corticosteroids cannot be routinely recommended until further evidence of their efficacy is available.

### Monitoring therapy and follow-up

The child should be followed clinically to ensure that pain, tenderness, mobility and systemic symptoms all respond quickly and do not relapse on or after antibiotic treatment. Inflammatory markers are usually also followed. The CRP is the best marker in bone and joint infections – it is almost always raised initially, unlike the WCC, and responds more quickly to treatment than the ESR. It is not necessary to wait for the ESR to normalize before ceasing antibiotic treatment, provided the child has fully responded clinically and the CRP has normalized or dramatically improved. A rise in CRP after antibiotics have been started may indicate the presence of complications or septic arthritis in addition to osteomyelitis.

If there is persistent fever or local symptoms and/or the CRP has not begun to fall 2–3 days after commencing intravenous antibiotics, there may be a complication such as an abscess, coexistent septic arthritis or a sequestrum. In these cases, re-imaging is usually needed with MRI or ultrasonography. Any collection should be drained and, if no collection is present, aspiration at the site of infection should be undertaken for histology and culture/Gram staining.

Typical cases that respond well to initial treatment and can be switched to oral treatment in the first week can be discharged from hospital shortly after commencing oral antibiotics. They should be assessed clinically and with CRP measurement for 3 weeks and reviewed occasionally (e.g. every 6 months) for the next 2 years to monitor for relapse.

## Prognosis

In affluent countries, children almost never die from osteomyelitis but some children develop recurrent infection (which may occur many months or even years later) or chronic osteomyelitis. Other rare complications include pathological fractures and bone deformities, including growth arrest, and leg-length discrepancy. The outcome of septic arthritis is also usually good but delayed or inadequate treatment can lead to joint damage or destruction, with long-term problems of poor function and osteoarthritis. All of these complications are more common in children whose diagnosis is not made sufficiently early or who receive inadequate initial treatment.

> **Clinical example**
>
> Jennifer, aged 6 months, was admitted to hospital with a diagnosis of 'pyrexia of unknown origin'. She was investigated extensively. Eventually she was treated with oral antibiotics for a 'possible urinary tract infection'. This made her afebrile, but the fever returned within 2 days of completing the antibiotic course. Septic arthritis of the right hip and proximal femoral osteomyelitis was diagnosed 3 weeks after the onset of fever. Jennifer progressed to develop septic dislocation of the right hip, avascular necrosis of the femoral capital epiphysis and growth arrest. She required more than 20 hospital admissions for orthopaedic operations throughout childhood. At the age of 15 years, she is a very troubled teenager with a painful hip, short leg and severe limp.

## Discitis and vertebral osteomyelitis

Musculoskeletal infection of the spine is uncommon but does occur in children. There are two distinct entities of spinal infection: vertebral osteomyelitis and discitis (or diskitis). In their initial phases, both present with poorly localized back pain and absent or only low-grade fever.

Children with vertebral osteomyelitis are usually older (>8 years) and eventually become febrile and toxic, developing localized back pain that may affect any part of the spine. The cause is usually *S. aureus* infection and, because of delayed presentation, complications such as paraspinal abscesses are often found. These children require prolonged antibiotics and frequently also surgical drainage of abscesses to prevent spinal cord or nerve compression.

Discitis tends to occur in the lower lumbar spine and in younger children (<5 years) who present with non-specific symptoms such as a limp or refusal to bear weight. The ESR is usually raised and by 4 weeks, plain radiography of the spine reveals narrowing of one or more disc spaces. MRI may provide further detailed anatomical information. In many cases of discitis no clear evidence of infection can be found, and surgery is usually not recommended when the diagnosis is clear from history, examination and imaging. It is generally accepted that the treatment is prolonged anti-staphylococcal antibiotics such as flucloxacillin.

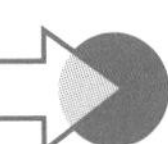

## Practical points

**Osteomyelitis**

- Fever and limb pain is a common presentation of osteomyelitis in older children, with the femur and the tibia being the most commonly affected bones.
- Osteomyelitis in neonates and infants presents non-specifically with fever – neonates are more likely to have multifocal disease and Gram-negative organisms.
- Bone malignancy is an important differential diagnosis and must be excluded (usually by X-ray at presentation).
- A bone scan or MRI is indicated in the investigation of suspected osteomyelitis – MRI is the best test where symptoms are clearly localized, because of the detailed information it provides.
- Treatment of simple, uncomplicated cases is with an anti-staphylococcal antibiotic (tailored according to local rates of CA-MRSA) given intravenously for 3–5 days followed by a high-dose oral anti-staphylococcal antibiotic for 3 weeks, or even as little as 20 days' total treatment for simple and very responsive cases.
- In cases that are not simple or have a delayed response to treatment, further investigation, obtaining a surgical specimen, and longer and broader-spectrum antibiotic therapy are indicated.

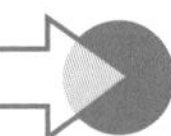

## Practical points

**Septic arthritis**

- Most cases of uncomplicated acute septic arthritis are due to *Staphylococcus aureus*.
- Gram stain result of aspirated fluid that suggests organisms other than *S. aureus* is an indication to add broader-spectrum antibiotic therapy.
- Septic arthritis is more likely to coexist with osteomyelitis when the joint involved has a metaphysis that is intra-articular (hip, shoulder, elbow and ankle), when there has been slow response to therapy, in infants, and when there is delayed presentation.
- Every child with septic arthritis requires urgent surgical intervention – this means a washout of the joint.
- Treatment of uncomplicated cases following joint washout is with an anti-staphylococcal antibiotic (tailored according to local rates of CA-MRSA) given intravenously for 3 days followed by a high-dose oral anti-staphylococcal antibiotic for 3 weeks, although simple cases that respond very quickly may be treated with courses for as little as 10 days.
- In cases that are not simple or have a delayed response to treatment, prolonged antibiotic therapy and possibly surgical intervention may be indicated.

# 12.3 Meningitis and encephalitis

Robert Booy, Cheryl Jones

Meningitis and encephalitis are both life-threatening infections that require rapid recognition and treatment for a child to survive without sequelae. They are on the differential diagnosis for all febrile ill children, particularly those with altered consciousness.

## Bacterial meningitis

The improving control of leading causes of bacterial meningitis has reduced both mortality and morbidity; both vaccination and improved quality of life have contributed to dramatic declines in the incidence of the big three causes: *Haemophilus influenzae* type b, *Neisseria meningitidis* and *Streptococcus pneumoniae*. Consequently, the reduced familiarity of doctors with disease must be balanced by better training in the early recognition and treatment of these deadly infections.

Knowledge of local epidemiology should direct antibiotic use. Appropriate adjustments in antibiotics rely heavily on culture and sensitivity results. Improved supportive and resuscitative measures in recent decades have reduced the range of case fatality rates from 5–25% (pneumococcal meningitis and meningococcal sepsis being the most deadly) to 2%–8%. What has made the difference, at least in developed countries, includes paying close attention to:

- fluid resuscitation for circulatory compromise
- elective intubation before respiratory failure
- management of convulsions
- control of cerebral oedema
- electrolyte and glucose balance.

### Epidemiology

The annual incidence of bacterial meningitis is about 10–20 cases per 100 000 children aged 0–5 years, highest in infants. In Australia, the pneumococcus bacteria is now the commonest cause, and Hib immunization means that there are only a few sporadic Hib cases. Pneumococcal and meningococcal cases are sporadic too, except for occasional outbreaks of meningococcal disease. As with other serious infections, the risk of disease and its severity are determined by factors to do with the environment, the microbe and the host.

### The environment

The incidence of bacterial meningitis is higher in the Indigenous and the poor, the two all too often occurring together. Prior viral respiratory infection and crowding (including school and daycare attendance) increase risk and perhaps explain why disease peaks during late winter and spring. Exposure to smokers and close personal contact is also important.

### Microbe: polysaccharide capsule

A key virulence determinant is the microbe's polysaccharide capsule. Specific human antibody to each capsule is protective.

### Human genetic factors

Human genetic factors predisposing to disease are increasingly recognized, although so far they account for only a small proportion of cases. Our understanding in this area is growing rapidly.

- Defects in the various complement pathways predispose to meningococcal disease. First recognized were mutations of terminal complement components, then properdin.
- More recently, variants in mannose-binding protein and factor H binding protein have been identified as increasing the risk of meningococcal infection.
- For Hib, genetic variation in Toll-like receptor-4 and associated pathways are linked to increased risk.
- The risk of pneumococcal disease is increased by an inherited defect in interleukin-1 receptor-associated kinase-4 (IRAK-4), leading to a failure to make cytokines following stimulation with Toll-like receptor agonists such as interleukin-1β.
- Congenital absence of the spleen may have a genetic basis and predisposes to infection with encapsulated organisms.
- Immunoglobulin deficiencies (X-linked or recessive) predispose to meningitis generally, whereas recurrent meningococcal disease may be associated with immunoglobulin (Ig) M deficiency.

## Other factors that increase the risk of meningitis:

- Acquired impaired immunity (e.g. human immunodeficiency virus infection) and splenectomy
- Congenital or acquired neuroanatomical defects (e.g. base of skull fracture)
- Penetrating head injuries, neurosurgical procedures
- Cerebrospinal fluid (CSF) leak
- Congenital dural defect (dermal sinus or myelomeningocele)
- Cochlear implants.

## Aetiology

The most common pathogens in each age group are:

- Neonates and infants aged under 3 months:
  - *Escherichia coli*
  - *Streptococcus agalactiae*
  - *Listeria monocytogenes*
- Infants and children:
  - *Streptococcus pneumoniae* (pneumococcus)
  - *Neisseria meningitidis* (meningococcus)
  - *Haemophilus influenzae* type b (Hib)
- Children older than 5 years:
  - *N. meningitidis*
  - *S. pneumoniae.*

## Pathogenesis

The development of bacterial meningitis usually follows: (1) colonization of the nasopharynx by encapsulated bacteria; (2) invasion of the host causing bacteraemia and then invasion of the meninges; (3) bacterial multiplication and induction of inflammation within the subarachnoid space; and (4) neuronal injury (Fig. 12.3.1).

## Clinical presentations

### Infants

Many symptoms and signs within this age group are non-specific:

- poor feeding, vomiting
- fever, irritability, drowsiness.

Neck stiffness or a bulging fontanelle are more specific but may be absent, especially early in the illness.

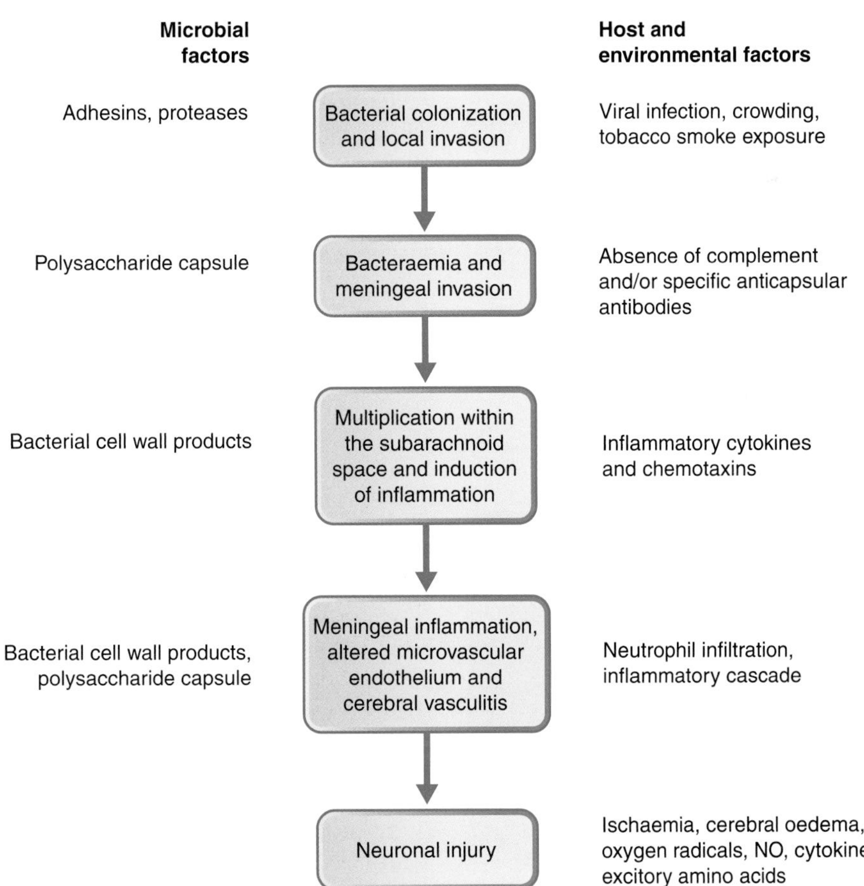


**Fig. 12.3.1** The pathophysiological cascade of meningitis.

### Children aged at least 3 years

Symptoms and signs are more obvious:

- severe headache, vomiting, photophobia
- fever, neck stiffness, delirium or deteriorating consciousness.

Convulsions are a presenting feature in 20–30% of infants and children with bacterial meningitis. Those with meningococcal meningitis or septicaemia may have a petechial and/or purpuric rash over the trunk, limbs and, in extremis, the face. Initially the rash may be blanching, but within hours become non-blanching purpuric lesions that may progress through dermal vascular necrosis to peripheral gangrene (Fig. 12.3.2).

## Diagnosis

*Lumbar puncture* (LP) helps to establish and localize the infection through obtaining a sample for microscopy, culture, biochemistry and molecular diagnostic testing. Unless the child is already treated with antibiotics, LP has a very high sensitivity. *Molecular diagnostic testing* using polymerase chain reaction (PCR) on blood or CSF can identify the cause of meningitis in patients pretreated with antibiotics.

Owing to concern over the dangers of cerebral herniation, circulatory compromise or disseminated intravascular coagulation, in recent years LP has often been postponed; immediate collection of *peripheral blood* samples for diagnosis (*culture, PCR*) is helpful but diagnostic sensitivity may be reduced by up to 50%. The suspicion of bacterial meningitis should prompt rapid commencement of antibiotics; this is ultimately a clinical decision.

Paired serology is helpful, but only in retrospect.

- *Needle aspirate from skin lesions* for Gram stain and culture is useful for diagnosis in meningococcal disease.
- *Suprapubic aspirate* or catheter urine specimen, if less than 6 months old, may reveal dual sites of infection.

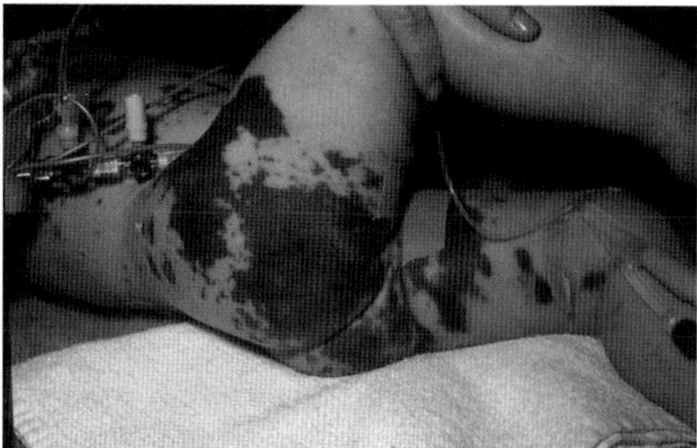

Fig. 12.3.2 Meningococcal infection with purpura and ecchymoses.

- *Full blood count*, including white blood cell differential, C-reactive protein or procalcitonin may all point to the seriousness of infection.
- *Serum electrolytes, glucose and creatinine* should be monitored and managed.

*Lumbar puncture is delayed* for patients with any of the following:

- absent or non-purposeful responses to pain
- focal neurological signs (or a false localizing sixth nerve palsy)
- abnormal pupil size or reaction
- decerebrate or decorticate posturing
- irregular breathing, rising blood pressure and falling pulse (despite peripheral vasoconstriction)
- papilloedema
- continuous fitting.

Such patients require intensive care management, including measures to reduce intracranial pressure. LP should still be performed, but only when the child is stable, usually within 2–3 days. Cerebral herniation occurs in about 5% of cases, with or without LP, and may account for 30% of the deaths.

The typical CSF changes in bacterial meningitis are outlined in Table 12.3.1. Organisms are often seen on Gram stain of the CSF, making a presumptive diagnosis possible.

CSF examination may be difficult to interpret, especially when prior antibiotics have been given.

Parameningeal foci, such as brain abscess or subdural empyema, and tuberculous meningitis can have a similar CSF profile to partially treated bacterial meningitis, so should be in the differential diagnosis.

Cerebral imaging, by either computed tomography (CT) or magnetic resonance imaging (MRI), is not recommended routinely and is not useful for determining whether there is raised intracranial pressure. It has a role when there is concern that conditions that may mimic meningitis are present, such as intracranial mass lesions, and LP is contraindicated.

## Antibiotic treatment

The antibiotics selected should cover the commonly encountered causative bacteria. As strains of *S. pneumoniae* resistant to penicillin and cephalosporin are relatively common in many settings, vancomycin may be used with a third-generation cephalosporin as initial empirical therapy, except in infants aged less than 3 months for whom amoxicillin should be given in addition to cover *Listeria*.

Subsequent adjustments depend on culture and sensitivity results.

Dosage and duration of antibiotic treatment are outlined in Table 12.3.2.

**Table 12.3.1 Cerebrospinal fluid: normal values and typical changes in some pathological conditions**

| | Total WCC ($\times 10^6$/L)* | Predominant cell type | Glucose (mmol/L) | Protein (g/L) |
|---|---|---|---|---|
| Normal | <5 | Lymphocytes | 2.5 | <0.4 |
| Normal neonate | <20 (<3 neutrophils) | Lymphocytes | Normal | Mildly increased |
| Bacterial meningitis | 1000s | Neutrophils | Reduced or undetectable | Moderately raised |
| Partially treated bacterial meningitis† | 100–1000s | Neutrophils | Reduced or undetectable | Moderately raised |
| Tuberculous meningitis | 50–100s | Neutrophils/mononuclear cells | Reduced or undetectable | Moderately to markedly increased |
| Viral meningitis | <10–100s | Lymphocytes‡ | Usually normal | Normal to <1 |
| Encephalitis | <10–100s | Lymphocytes | Usually normal | Mildly to moderately raised |
| Brain abscess and other mass lesions§ | Normal to mild increase | Variable neutrophils | Normal | Normal to mildly raised |

*A traumatic tap is the commonest cause of blood-stained cerebrospinal fluid; for every $1000 \times 10^6$/L red blood cells, add $2 \times 10^6$/L white blood cells and 0.01 g/L protein to normal values, but can also be seen in HSV encephalitis.
†Partially treated meningitis is seen when children receive oral antibiotics before the diagnosis of meningitis has been made.
‡Neutrophil predominance may be present in enterovirus meningitis.
§Lumbar puncture is not done if a mass lesion is suspected. CSF changes depend on the site of the lesion; for example, if near the cerebral surface pleocytosis occurs.
WCC, white cell count.

**Table 12.3.2 Antibiotic therapy for bacterial meningitis**

| Pathogen | Antibiotic | Dose (mg/kg) | Duration (days) |
|---|---|---|---|
| *Streptococcus pneumoniae* | | | |
| Penicillin susceptible | Penicillin G | 60 IV 4-hourly | 7–10 |
| Penicillin non-susceptible | Cefotaxime* | 50 IV 6-hourly | 7–10 |
| Penicillin + third-generation cephalosporin non-susceptible | Vancomycin + Cefotaxime* | 15 IV 6-hourly<br>75 IV 6-hourly | 10–14 |
| *Neisseria meningitidis* | Penicillin G | 60 IV 4-hourly | 4–7 |
| *Haemophilus influenzae* b and non-b species | | | |
| Non-β-lactamase-producing | Amoxicillin | 50 IV 4-hourly | 7 |
| β-Lactamase-producing | Cefotaxime* | 50 IV 6-hourly | 7 |
| Unknown pathogen | Cefotaxime* ±<br>Vancomycin | 50 IV 6-hourly<br>15 IV 6-hourly | 7 |

Maximum doses: penicillin G, 2.4 g; amoxicillin, 2 g; cefotaxime, 3 g; ceftriaxone, 2 g; vancomycin, 500 mg.
*Ceftriaxone 50 mg/kg 12-hourly can be substituted for cefotaxime.

### Supportive treatment

#### Clinical observations

Keeping a regular record of heart and respiratory rates, blood pressure, temperature and conscious state can detect important trends such as falling heart rate and rising blood pressure with rising intracranial pressure. The head circumference in infants should be measured daily.

#### Fluid therapy

Intravenous fluids are administered initially to restore circulating blood volume, to correct glucose or electrolyte disturbance, and to minimize the need to swallow, with its attendant risk of aspiration.

In contradiction to past recommendations, recent studies have shown that fluid restriction is not helpful for children with bacterial meningitis and, indeed, the use of maintenance fluid is associated with fewer neurological complications. Fluid administration should be adjusted according to vital signs and adequacy of circulation. The low serum sodium levels and reduced urine output that may occur in bacterial meningitis are due to fluid depletion rather than inappropriate antidiuretic hormone secretion.

#### Corticosteroids

Dexamethasone for treating bacterial meningitis is controversial and depends on the cause. Children with Hib meningitis have a reduced risk of deafness if dexamethasone is given prior to antibiotics. Benefit, or detriment, in children with either pneumococcal or meningococcal meningitis remains unproven; however, a recent Cochrane review showed a lower case-fatality rate and fewer long-term sequelae in a combined adult/child group of bacterial meningitis cases. A reasonable approach for bacterial meningitis of, as yet, uncertain aetiology might be to give dexamethasone 0.15 mg/kg just before the first dose of empirical antibiotics and to continue 6 hourly for 4 days, but to cease if *N. meningitidis* becomes the principal diagnosis.

### Acute complications

During meningitis, complications from central nervous system infection or systemic effects of infection are common. Children with recurrent or protracted convulsions, circulatory instability or signs of cerebral oedema should be managed in an intensive care unit.

#### Convulsions

About 30% of children with bacterial meningitis have convulsions, more commonly with pneumococcal or Hib meningitis than meningococcal meningitis. Benzodiazepines such as diazepam or midazolam will control most convulsions, but if these recur or are prolonged they may raise intracranial pressure and worsen the cerebral ischaemic injury. Administration of phenytoin or phenobarbital, and mechanical ventilation may be necessary. Consider aberrations in sodium, calcium or glucose levels.

#### Cerebral oedema

Careful observation for signs of increased intracranial pressure (IIP) is essential. These are listed above under reasons for delaying a LP. Refer also above to section on fluid therapy. The child with suspected raised IIP should be nursed head-up and in midline, be sedated, intubated and ventilated, and given boluses of hypertonic saline or mannitol to reduce pressure. Regular oral glycerol (with or without dexamethasone) may reduce both mortality and neurological sequelae, especially in cases caused by Hib.

#### Circulatory shock

Approximately 5–10% of children with bacterial meningitis present in shock and initially require large-volume fluid resuscitation in 10–20-mL/kg boluses. If a second bolus is required, strong consideration should be given to elective intubation and ventilation, but in a third-world setting without ventilator support research suggests fluids be given more slowly (i.e. not by bolus).

Inotropic agents may be needed to help support the circulation.

#### Neurological lesions

Hard neurological deficits (central, cranial and/or peripheral) are present in 10–20% of children during the acute illness, although some may be reversible. Long-term follow-up studies suggest an average IQ diminution of 5 points and significantly more psychological, social and educational impediments.

#### Subdural effusion

This is a fluid accumulation in the subdural space that is usually sterile but needs to be differentiated from subdural empyema (see below). An effusion is quite a common complication of bacterial meningitis, usually asymptomatic and occasionally associated with:

- persistent or recurring high fever
- focal or generalized convulsions
- persistent vomiting
- increasing head circumference or fontanelle tension
- development of a focal neurological deficit.

Most resolve spontaneously. Subdural empyema is uncommon but should be suspected when the above features are accompanied by ongoing irritability and raised erythrocyte sedimentation rate (ESR)/C-reactive protein levels. Cerebral CT (Fig. 12.3.3) or MRI establishes the diagnosis of subdural effusion or empyema.

### Persistent (>7 days) or secondary fever

Differential diagnosis:

- viral nosocomial infection
- subdural effusion
- thrombophlebitis
- other suppurative lesions
- immune-mediated disease – reactive arthritis or pericarditis.

Uncommonly, fever may also result from:

- inadequately treated meningitis
- a parameningeal focus (e.g. abscess or subdural empyema)
- drugs (e.g. penicillin, co-trimoxazole)
- Munchausen by proxy syndrome (parent infecting child deliberately).

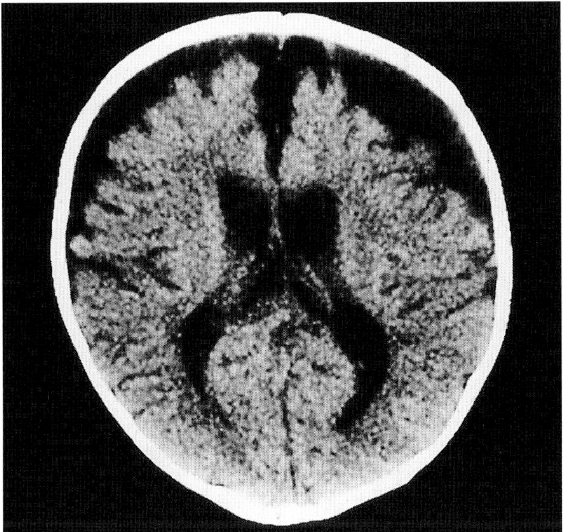

Fig. 12.3.3 Cranial computed tomogram of a 5-month-old boy with pneumococcal meningitis who developed secondary fever and generalized convulsions on his seventh day in hospital. It shows subdural effusions over both frontal lobes. He received anticonvulsant therapy and the effusion resolved spontaneously.

## Cerebral imaging

Cranial CT or MRI is useful in identifying:

- subdural collections
- brain abscess
- cerebral vascular thrombosis
- hydrocephalus.

These investigations are considered for patients with:

- prolonged coma
- sustained irritability or convulsions
- persistent focal neurological deficits
- enlarging head circumference
- recurrent disease.

## Outcome

- Mortality rate 2–8% (industrialized countries), lowest in meningococcal and highest in pneumococcal meningitis.
- Intellectual disability, spasticity, convulsions, hydrocephalus, deafness 5–15%.
- Later learning and behaviour disorders 25–40% (may be subtle).

Independent risk factors for severe neurological or intellectual disability are meningitis in infancy, delayed diagnosis, persistent or late-onset convulsions and focal neurological signs.

All children should have their hearing tested following meningitis, by brainstem (auditory) evoked potentials or formal audiometry. Regular review should be continued in children, particularly for those with persisting auditory and neurological abnormalities. Even in first-world settings, up to 50% of children and adolescents discharged after bacterial meningitis are not assessed routinely in outpatients.

## Primary prevention

Antibodies directed against the capsular components of Hib, *S. pneumoniae* and *N. meningitidis* are especially important for protection. Polysaccharide–protein conjugate vaccines are commercially available against:

- Hib
- *S. pneumoniae*
- *N. meningitidis* A, C, Y and W135.

Cases of Hib, pneumococcal and meningococcal serogroup C meningitis have substantially decreased in countries where routine implementation has occurred, but following use of the 7-valent pneumococcal conjugate vaccine there has been evidence of replacement disease with non-vaccine serotypes (e.g. 19A) in some countries (see Chapter 3.5).

### Clinical example

Mousaka, a 7-month-old female infant, presented after a 15-minute right-sided focal convulsion. She had been unwell for 12 hours with poor feeding. Her past medical history, growth and development were normal. Her primary immunizations were up to date for age. There was no family history of convulsions. Her temperature was 39.3°C. She was pale and very irritable when handled. There was no neck stiffness, bulging fontanelle or rash. No focal neurological signs were present.

A lumbar puncture revealed turbid CSF. Numerous Gram-negative coccobacilli were seen in the CSF, and non-typeable *H. influenzae* was isolated. Mousaka's clinical course was complicated by a secondary fever, a tense fontanelle with increasing head circumference, recurrent focal convulsions, right hemiplegia, and persistently raised peripheral white blood cell counts and C-reactive protein concentrations. Subdural pus was surgically drained after MRI demonstrated a left-sided subdural empyema. This was followed by rapid clinical improvement. Subsequent testing found no signs of underlying immunodeficiency.

Less than 1% of children with febrile convulsions have meningitis. Infants and those with complex febrile convulsions are more likely to have bacterial meningitis. It is important that, following a febrile convulsion, children are evaluated carefully for signs of meningitis. The impact of conjugate vaccines means that rarer causes of bacterial meningitis are relatively more important. Although the incidence of non-typeable *H. influenzae* meningitis has hardly changed, in fully immunized children it has become a more common cause of meningitis than Hib. Such children often have an underlying medical condition and, compared with Hib infection, they have a more severe illness with greater mortality.

The monovalent C meningococcal conjugate vaccine has dramatically reduced the incidence of C disease in children and adolescents. The newer quadrivalent conjugate, which also incorporates protection against serogroups A, Y and W135, is offered routinely in the USA and soon, perhaps, in other countries. It provides especial benefits when travelling to meningitis-prone areas such as the sub-Saharan region. The success of conjugate vaccines rests not only on inducing immunity in young children and establishing immunological memory but also on engendering herd immunity. Challenges remain over the cost and delivery of these vaccines to children in developing nations where they are most needed. The poorly immunogenic meningococcal B capsular polysaccharide has necessitated a different approach; various outer membrane proteins have been incorporated in new candidate meningococcal B vaccines based on 'reverse vaccinology' techniques.

## Chemoprophylaxis

Transmission of Hib and the meningococcus bacteria is by oral and respiratory secretions. Those at increased risk of infection are:

- household members
- childcare contacts
- persons intimately exposed to oral secretions.

At-risk contacts of a case of meningococcal meningitis should immediately receive oral rifampicin, 10mg/kg (neonates 5mg/kg) to a maximum of 600mg, twice daily for 2 days. Alternatively a single dose of intramuscular ceftriaxone (125mg for children under 12 years of age, 250mg for older children and adults) is given, or adults may receive 500mg oral ciprofloxacin. The index case does not require further prophylaxis if treatment has included a third-generation cephalosporin. Parents must be warned that if they, or their children, are unwell immediate medical attention should be sought.

Because of the increased risk of Hib infection in young contacts, rifampicin 20mg/kg (maximum 600mg) as a single daily dose for 4 days is prescribed for the index case of Hib meningitis and all household contacts, if the child is aged less than 2 years or the household contacts include unimmunized children aged younger than 4 years of age. Unlike *N. meningitidis*, single doses of ceftriaxone do not eradicate Hib from the nasopharynx. Chemoprophylaxis is not required in cases of pneumococcal meningitis.

## Special circumstances

### Neonatal meningitis

Neonates, particularly if premature, are at increased risk of meningitis. The responsible pathogens are mainly:

- *S. agalactiae* (group B streptococcus)
- *Escherichia coli* and other Gram-negative bacilli
- *L. monocytogenes.*

As in infants, the symptoms and signs of meningitis are often non-specific. Approximately 5–15% of septic neonates have concomitant meningitis. Initial therapy is with amoxicillin and cefotaxime until culture and antibiotic sensitivities are available. Antibiotic treatment should be for at least 2 weeks for Gram-positive meningitis, and 3 weeks for Gram-negative bacillary cases.

### Infants aged 1–3 months and the immunocompromised

These patients may have meningitis from pathogens common to both neonates and older children. Empirical therapy (usually with amoxicillin and cefotaxime) must cover a wide range of pathogens. When the clinical circumstances (e.g. asplenia), CSF Gram stain and/or PCR testing suggest that *S. pneumoniae* is the causative agent, vancomycin should replace amoxicillin.

### Meningococcaemia

Although *N. meningitidis* serogroup A is associated with epidemics in sub-Saharan Africa, in industrialized countries serogroups B, C and Y (at least in the USA) are endemic, but serogroup B causes most sporadic meningococcal disease. Large increases in disease caused by meningococcal clones have been observed over recent decades.

The majority of invasive meningococcal disease is acute meningococcaemia, which is almost always septicaemic. Although about two-thirds have concomitant meningitis, signs of sepsis dominate the clinical presentation and the necessary management. Half of cases occur in children aged less than 5 years in whom serogroup B strains predominate. Cases may deteriorate rapidly within a few hours, initially with:

- fevers, rigors
- severe pain in the limbs, abdomen or back
- vomiting, plus or minus headache
- mottled or pale skin, with cool extremities.

Additional non-specific signs in infants include:

- fever, irritability or drowsiness
- grunting or moaning respirations.

A rash is present, or develops during illness, in most cases irrespective of age. Initially it may be a blanching macular or maculopapular rash before evolving into the characteristic petechial or purpuric rash of meningococcaemia (Fig. 12.3.2). The clinical course can be rapidly progressive, with the time from onset of fever until death as short as 12 hours. The overall mortality rate for invasive meningococcal disease is 10%, but the case fatality rate reaches 20% for fulminant forms of the disease.

Many of the clinical features of meningococcaemia are provoked by antibiotics causing the release of cell wall products which, in turn, activate proinflammatory cytokines and complement; this leads to endothelial injury with capillary leak and loss of vasomotor tone. The major cause of death in meningococcaemia is circulatory collapse from capillary leak, intravascular volume depletion, vasodilatation and myocardial failure. Haemodynamic collapse in combination with disseminated intravascular coagulation (DIC) leads to multiorgan dysfunction.

Treatment is urgent and is commenced immediately (preferably by the intravenous (IV) route, but intramuscular acceptable) the diagnosis is suspected, and ideally after taking blood cultures. Penicillin G is the drug of choice, the recommended dose being 60 mg/kg IV given 4-hourly. The patient is managed in respiratory isolation during the first 24 hours of treatment. Management of those with signs of septic shock should be in an intensive care unit (preferably paediatric) and includes aggressive fluid resuscitation to restore the circulating blood volume, cardiac and respiratory support, and careful management of blood electrolyte and glucose levels. Short-term corticosteroids may benefit those in septic shock. The use of other adjunctive therapies, such as recombinant human activated protein C and monoclonal antibody to endotoxin, is not supported by results of clinical trials. Although prehospital treatment with penicillin has reduced the proportion of culture-confirmed cases, the use of PCR to detect meningococcal DNA in normally sterile fluids has improved the sensitivity of diagnosis without materially affecting the specificity.

### Tuberculous meningitis

This is most common in children younger than 5 years. The onset is gradual, with headache, malaise, fever and irritability, progressing over 1–2 weeks to drowsiness, neck stiffness, convulsions, cranial nerve palsies and coma. Typical CSF changes are listed in Table 12.3.1. There may be no history of infectious contact. Tuberculin skin testing (Mantoux) is often negative and a chest X-ray abnormality is present in only half of cases. Gastric aspirates, urine and CSF should be sent for culture and PCR, and some experts also recommend that a sample of sputum be induced with hypertonic saline, usually performed by a physiotherapist wearing mask, gown and gloves. Cranial CT or MRI may detect hydrocephalus and basilar meningeal inflammation; basal ganglia infarction is a late radiographic sign. Initial treatment is with isoniazid, rifampicin and pyrazinamide. A fourth drug is added if there are concerns over potential drug resistance. High-dose steroids are also used during the first weeks of therapy.

#### Clinical example

Tom, aged 14 years, had developed chills on the day of presentation and complained of pain in his head, neck and limbs. He rapidly became confused, agitated and started to vomit. When seen by his family doctor, Tom was pale and a faint red macular rash had appeared over his buttocks and legs. A diagnosis of possible meningococcaemia was made and Tom received 1.2 g penicillin intramuscularly before immediate transfer to hospital. On arrival he was pale and shocked, was difficult to arouse, and had an evolving purpuric rash. He received cefotaxime, aggressive fluid resuscitation, inotropes and assisted ventilation. He gradually improved and a lumbar puncture 2 days later showed 150 white blood cells $\times 10^6$/ L only. Although cultures were sterile, PCR testing of whole blood collected upon arrival at hospital confirmed meningococcal infection and Tom completed a 5-day course of intravenous penicillin G.

### Recurrent meningitis

This is uncommon and an underlying cause should be sought:

- immunodeficiency (see Chapter 13.2)
- neuroanatomical defects: intracranial or lumbosacral.

Consider neuroanatomical defects when enteric bacteria or *Staphylococcus aureus* are cultured from the CSF. Cranial and spinal MRI, or high-resolution CT of the temporal and frontal bones, may be indicated.

## Aseptic and viral meningitis, and infectious encephalitis

'Aseptic' meningitis is inflammation of the meninges, as shown by leukocytes in the CSF, in the absence of bacteria. Viruses are the commonest cause of aseptic meningitis. Encephalitis is inflammation of the brain with associated neurological symptoms. It is usually due to infection, most commonly viruses, although an aetiological agent is not identified in many cases. Immune-mediated encephalitides are also being recognized increasingly in children. Box 12.3.1 lists common causes of infectious encephalitis and viral meningitis.

### Viral meningitis

The absence of an altered sensorium and focal neurological findings generally helps to distinguish viral meningitis from encephalitis. Non-polio enteroviruses cause 80–90% of identifiable cases. The onset is often acute with:

- fever
- headache
- vomiting
- neck or spine stiffness.

Abdominal pain and diarrhoea are common and occasionally a macular rash appears, suggesting an enterovirus as the causative agent. The illness may be biphasic, with return of fever and neurological manifestations after an interlude. Signs of meningism indicate the need for LP. Typically, there is a CSF pleocytosis with normal to mildly raised protein and normal glucose levels (see Table 12.3.1).

PCR testing of CSF specimens for enterovirus or herpes simplex virus DNA have become important diagnostic tools. Other disorders that may present in a similar fashion include:

- partially treated bacterial meningitis
- tuberculous meningitis
- cryptococcal meningitis
- *Mycoplasma* meningitis
- cerebral abscess
- cerebral tumour.

A repeat LP or cerebral imaging may also be required to clarify the diagnosis.

Viral meningitis is usually a benign disease, and requires symptomatic treatment only. Complete recovery without sequelae is expected within a few days to weeks.

### Infectious encephalitis and myelitis

Infectious agents may cause encephalitis directly, by invading the central nervous system, or indirectly, by inducing proinflammatory responses or vasculitis

**Box 12.3.1 Viruses and non-bacterial infecting agents that may commonly cause meningitis and encephalitis**

**Para- or post-infectious encephalitis without direct invasion of the CNS**

- Measles, influenza, *Mycoplasma pneumoniae*, RSV, parainfluenza viruses, *Rickettsia*, rubella, varicella, EBV, mumps, post-immunization

**Meningitis and/or encephalitis with direct CNS infection**

- Enteroviruses – ECHO, Coxsackie, enteroviruses and polio viruses. These usually cause meningitis but can occasionally cause encephalitis. EV71 is associated with demyelinating disease
- HSV type 1 can cause focal (usually temporoparietal) encephalitis (HSV-1 or -2 can cause encephalitis in neonates)
- Mumps – usually meningitis, less often meningoencephalitis
- Other herpes group viruses – human herpesvirus 6/7, EBV, varicella, cytomegalovirus (neonates, immunocompromised)
- Other viruses – adenoviruses, measles, rubella, rotaviruses, rabies viruses, lyssavirus
- Arbovirus (arthropod-borne virus) – e.g. flaviviruses and alphaviruses, such as Japanese encephalitis, West Nile encephalitis, Murray Valley encephalitis, Dengue virus, Nipah virus
- Bacteria – *Haemophilus influenzae, Streptococcus pneumomiae, Neisseria meningitidis, Listeria monocytogenes*
- Other agents – *Toxoplasmosis gondii, Coxiella burnetii*

**Progressive encephalitis**

- For example, subacute sclerosing panencephalitis due to measles virus infection, HIV, or human prion disease

CNS, central nervous system; EBV, Epstein–Barr virus; ECHO, Enteric Cytopathic Human Orphan; EV, enterovirus; HIV, human immunodeficiency virus; HSV, herpes simplex virus; RSV, respiratory syncytial virus.

in the brain during or after infection at other sites. Viruses are the major known cause of infectious encephalitis, although a confirmed aetiology is not identified in many cases. Worldwide, vector-borne viruses are becoming an important cause of infectious encephalitis. Acute disseminated encephalomyelitis (ADEM) is a neurological syndrome associated with white matter demyelination that is thought to be immune-mediated after a variety of viral and bacterial infections, or rarely immunization (see Box 12.3.1). It is subacute in onset and usually presents without fever after a non-specific respiratory or gastrointestinal illness.

Infectious encephalitis presents with an array of neurological signs:

- altered conscious state
- confusion and disorientation
- behaviour, personality or speech disturbance
- generalized or focal convulsions
- ataxia or other movement disorders
- headache, vomiting
- focal neurological deficits
- fever, or history of fever.

Meningism is frequently absent. The involvement of the spinal cord (transverse myelitis) may develop in isolation and can lead to flaccid paralysis, loss of tendon reflexes, neurogenic bladder and a definable sensory level. When it occurs, acute cord compression from a spinal epidural abscess or some other cause must also be considered and excluded urgently by MRI or CT myelography.

Causes of acute encephalitis may be suggested by:

- the season
- recent travel history
- prior personal or family illness
- animal exposures or insect bites
- drug and immunization history
- presence of lymphadenopathy, parotitis, rash or pneumonia.

Investigations to identify the aetiological agent include:

- PCR of CSF, blood, respiratory secretions
- viral culture of CSF, blood, respiratory secretions, faeces and urine
- serology.

The CSF profile of encephalitis is outlined in Table 12.3.1, although patients may have normal CSF parameters. PCR analysis provides a rapid and accurate diagnosis for a wide range of pathogens. Electroencephalographic (EEG) abnormalities are seldom specific but may be helpful in herpes simplex virus (HSV) encephalitis. MRI is more sensitive than cranial CT and helps differentiate encephalitis from ADEM (Fig. 12.3.4). MRI T2-weighted images in viral encephalitis demonstrate one or more diffuse areas of hyperintensity involving the grey matter of the cerebral cortex and the underlying white matter, with involvement of the basal ganglia, brainstem and cerebellum to a lesser extent. In contrast, ADEM is characterized by multiple asymmetrical areas of increased focal signal in the white matter of both hemispheres, basal ganglia, cerebellum and, on occasions, the spinal cord. Other treatable causes of acute encephalopathy should also be sought.

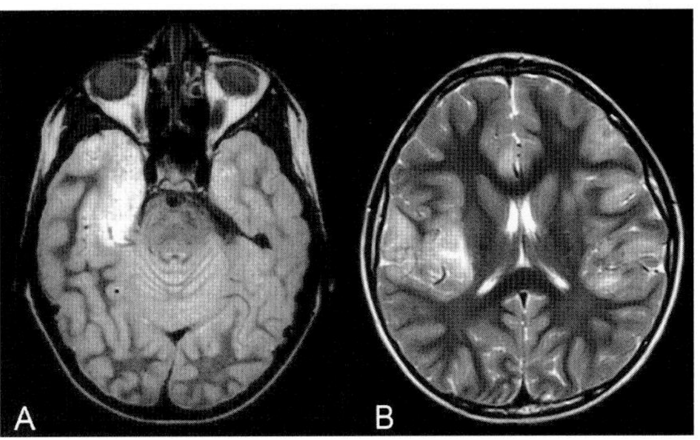


**Fig. 12.3.4** T2-weighted axial magnetic resonance images. **(A)** A 6-year-old girl with HSV encephalitis (see text for clinical details), which shows an increased signal in the right temporal lobe. **(B)** A 4-year-old boy with focal convulsions and dysphasia following a respiratory illness. The bilateral and asymmetrical multifocal increased signal in the white–grey junction and subcortical white matter is characteristic of acute disseminated encephalomyelitis.

Initially, aciclovir is given in all cases of suspected encephalitis until a diagnosis of HSV encephalitis can be excluded on clinical, radiological and PCR criteria. Early initiation of appropriate antiviral therapy (e.g. oseltamivir) should be also considered if influenza is suspected. Treatment of viral encephalitis and ADEM is otherwise supportive, involving:

- careful fluid and electrolyte management
- control of convulsions
- monitoring for signs of raised intracranial pressure
- circulatory support to maintain cerebral perfusion
- assisted ventilation for respiratory failure
- maintenance of nutrition.

Corticosteroids should be considered when MRI shows striking enhancement of multifocal white matter lesions consistent with ADEM.

Almost 10% of children with encephalitis die, and long-term studies suggest that nearly half of the survivors have neurological or educational disabilities. Young age, coma, delayed presentation, high CSF protein and infection with HSV or *Mycoplasma pneumoniae* are associated with a poor prognosis. However, patients can also make an excellent recovery, even after prolonged coma.

## Herpes simplex encephalitis

Herpes simplex virus causes a severe, sporadic focal encephalitis. Outside the newborn period, individuals with defects in innate immunity such as a deficiency of signalling protein Unc-93B, are at increased risk of HSV encephalitis. Treatment with the antiviral agent aciclovir reduces the mortality rate to below 20%. However, most survivors still have severe neurological or behavioural sequelae. Neonatal herpes simplex encephalitis can be due to either HSV-1 or HSV-2, whereas cases outside the neonatal period are almost exclusively caused by HSV-1. One-third of cases in older infants and children result from a primary infection.

CSF PCR for HSV DNA is the diagnostic test of choice. Although frontal and temporal lobe localization is characteristic, PCR and MRI have shown that the disease can be diffuse in neonates and young children. The course described in the clinical example is typical of HSV encephalitis.

**Clinical example**

Rachael, aged 6 years, was hospitalized with a 3-day history of fever, headache, intermittent confusion and progressive lethargy. On presentation she had several left-sided focal convulsions. Her temperature was 40.1°C; she was drowsy with mild neck stiffness and left hemiparesis.

Her CSF had $100 \times 10^6$/L lymphocytes. The protein content of the CSF was mildly raised and the glucose concentration was normal. HSV encephalitis was suspected and aciclovir (500 mg/m$^2$ IV 8-hourly) was started. Phenytoin controlled Rachael's convulsions. An EEG demonstrated periodic discharges localized to the right temporal lobe, and MRI showed increased signal in T2-weighted images of this region (see Fig. 12.3.4A). PCR of the CSF was positive for HSV-1 DNA.

Rachael gradually improved over several days, but was still febrile after 2 weeks of treatment. A repeat lumbar puncture at 3 weeks revealed persisting HSV-1 DNA. Aciclovir was continued for a total of 4 weeks. Her fever settled, but the hemiparesis remained and she was left with major behaviour and learning disabilities.

### Arthropod-borne encephalitis viruses

Viruses transmitted to humans by biting arthropods (mainly mosquitoes and ticks) are a major cause of encephalitis. Flaviviruses are the most common and include Japanese encephalitis (Asia), West Nile encephalitis (Africa, Middle East, North America) and Australian encephalitis (Australia). West Nile encephalitis has recently become established in North America following its introduction into New York in 1999, and Japanese encephalitis has expanded throughout Asia and into Australia.

Most infections are mild or subclinical, with less than 1% developing neurological symptoms. However, when symptomatic, the disease is often severe with fever, headache, vomiting, altered consciousness, convulsions, tremor and dystonia. Both Japanese encephalitis and West Nile encephalitis may present with acute flaccid paralysis. The mortality rate for Japanese and Australian encephalitis is 20–30%, with 50% of survivors experiencing severe neurological and intellectual sequelae. Vector control programmes and personal protection are important preventative measures, and there is a vaccine for Japanese encephalitis.

### Slow virus infection

Some viruses can cause a subacute or chronic neurodegenerative disorder. The major example in childhood is subacute sclerosing panencephalitis, a rare late complication of measles, especially if measles occurs early in life. Rubella is a less common cause. The disorder is manifest by:

- deterioration of behaviour, personality and intellect
- myoclonic convulsions
- motor disturbance.

The onset is usually several years after measles. As the disease progresses, spastic paresis, tremors, athetosis and ataxia develop. The disease runs a variable but progressive course and is usually fatal within 2 years. Initially, the EEG shows a typical 'suppression-burst pattern'. The typical clinical picture and high-titre CSF measles antibody establish the diagnosis.

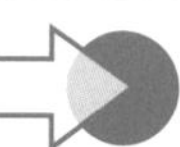

**Practical points**

- Meningitis and encephalitis should always be considered in ill-appearing infants and children but impaired conscious state or altered behaviour especially suggests encephalitis.
- Unless contraindicated by signs of raised intracranial pressure, haemodynamic instability or DIC, lumbar puncture should be performed as part of the diagnostic work-up to establish the diagnosis and to help identify the causative organism.
- Control of infection, shock, electrolyte imbalance and convulsions are the immediate treatment goals for bacterial meningitis. Steroids at disease onset are often indicated.
- Bacterial meningitis that is recurrent, caused by an unusual pathogen or the consequence of vaccine failure in a fully vaccinated child raises the possibility of an underlying disorder, including immunodeficiency or a neuroanatomical defect.
- The absence of an altered sensorium and focal neurological findings helps distinguish viral meningitis from acute encephalitis.
- Antiviral therapy with aciclovir should be commenced if there are clinical signs of encephalitis until herpes simplex virus can be excluded.

# Infections in tropical and developing countries

# 12.4

Stephen Graham, David Brewster

Most of the world's population lives in the tropics and subtropics in developing countries where health outcomes are much poorer than in developed countries such as Australia or New Zealand. Infections are a major cause of childhood disease in these settings and an important contributor to overall child mortality. Rather than geography and climate, however, it is socioeconomic factors that have most influence on susceptibility to infections, leading to high mortality. These factors are highlighted in Chapter 1.2: Child health in a global context. They include low levels of female literacy, lack of access to clean water, poor sanitation and hygiene, nutritional insecurity, and inadequate health-care resources, including human resources. The main causes of morbidity and mortality are not exotic tropical diseases but common conditions such as pneumonia, malaria, diarrhoea, sepsis and human immunodeficiency virus (HIV) infection caused by common pathogens.

The main seasonal influences in the tropics are the rainy season, when there is increased exposure to pathogens (e.g. malaria and diarrhoea), and the hungry season, when there is food insecurity. These seasons tend to coincide resulting in a strong seasonal influence on the prevalence of childhood malnutrition. Poor nutrition is an important contributor to the high childhood mortality rate from infectious diseases in the developing world, including intrauterine growth retardation resulting in low birth weight. Over half of child deaths are due to the potentiating effect of malnutrition on infections. Malnutrition can also be a consequence of recurrent or chronic infections.

The purpose of this chapter is to give an overview of common infections in tropical regions, including Australia, and developing countries. It is not possible to discuss in detail the many disorders endemic to these areas. The focus of the chapter is on the common infectious causes of childhood disease, with an emphasis on public health and prevention.

## An overview

### Prevention and disease control

Three of the seven Millennium Development Goals (MDGs) set in 2000 for 2015 have direct relevance to childhood infections:

- MDG 4: Reduce by two-thirds the mortality rate among children under 5 years of age
- MDG 6: Halt and begin to reverse the spread of HIV/AIDS and the incidence of malaria and other diseases
- MDG 7: Reduce by half the proportion of people without sustainable access to safe drinking water and basic sanitation.

Although these MDGs are unlikely to be achieved in many high-mortality settings, they have provided an important focus and substantial progress has been made in the last decade. Important child health programmes that reduce the burden of infectious disease include the Expanded Programme on Immunization (EPI), breastfeeding promotion and infectious disease control programmes. Immunization against measles and polio, for example, has been highly effective and highly cost-effective. EPI continues to be expanded with the addition of *Haemophilus influenzae* type b (Hib) conjugate vaccine and hepatitis B vaccine to the schedules of many low-income countries in recent years. Vaccines against *Streptococcus pneumoniae* (pneumococcus) and rotavirus are the likely next candidates for wider implementation in low-income countries.

Gains are also being made by disease control programmes using a combination of reducing transmission of infections and more effective treatment. Three infections that have received particular attention and funding support to national control programmes are HIV, tuberculosis (TB) and malaria. HIV has had a profound impact on child morbidity and mortality in high HIV-endemic countries. Strategies that lead to a reduction in antenatal HIV prevalence and prevent mother-to-child transmission of HIV will reduce HIV-related child mortality as well as reduce the burden on child health-care services. Antiretroviral treatment of the mother during and after pregnancy can reduce the risk of HIV transmission to the newborn to less than 1%, and make breastfeeding a feasible option. The HIV epidemic has also increased the prevalence of TB, including drug-resistant infection. In malaria-endemic settings, children and pregnant women are particularly susceptible to severe disease. Malaria control is being improved with increased usage of insecticide-treated bed-nets and more effective first-line therapy.

### Integrating and improving clinical case management

The usual clinical presentations of infections in tropical and developing countries are as one or more of typical clinical scenarios (e.g. respiratory distress, diarrhoea with dehydration, sepsis, anaemia or febrile seizures). There is clinical overlap between disease groups, a range of possible causes including the possibility of co-infections with more than one pathogen, and the need for health workers to assess and promptly treat the most likely infectious causes, often empirically on the basis of clinical assessment alone. Further, these challenges are particularly common in those at greatest risk of death, such as the young infant, the malnourished or the HIV-infected.

The World Health Organization (WHO) has developed treatment protocols for the common diseases, based upon simple clinical indicators, that can be assessed by health workers with minimal training. The Integrated Management of Childhood Illness (IMCI) initiative aims to reduce child morbidity and mortality in developing countries by improved management of common illnesses (Box 12.4.1). This integrated horizontal approach aims to avoid the limitations of a vertical single-disease approach. This will hopefully provide improved patient care as well as recognition of the importance of integration between national disease control programmes. Evaluation studies of the quality of care at hospitals and health centres in the developing world consistently report major deficiencies in triage, emergency care, monitoring, drug availability, staffing levels and the use of protocols for clinical care. On the other hand, implementation studies show what can be achieved when such deficiencies are addressed, even with limited resources. In 2005, WHO published a pocketbook of guidelines for the management of common illnesses in health facilities with limited resources.

**Box 12.4.1 Diagnostic classifications and clinical signs for referral to hospital**

**Young infants (0–2 months)**

1. Possible serious bacterial infection – seizures, tachypnoea (≥60 breaths/min), severe chest indrawing, nasal flaring, grunting, bulging fontanel, perforated eardrum, omphalitis, fever or hypothermia (≥38°C or <30°C), many or severe skin pustules, difficult to wake up or cannot be calmed within 1 hour
2. Diarrhoea with severe dehydration – lethargic or unconscious, sunken eyes and skin pinch goes back very slowly
3. Severe persistent diarrhoea (≥14 days)
4. Not able to feed

**Children (2 months to 5 years)**

1. General danger signs – not able to drink or breastfeed, vomits everything, convulsions, or lethargic or unconscious
2. Severe febrile disease – fever (rectal temperature ≥38°C) and any general danger sign, or stiff neck
3. Severe pneumonia – cough or difficult breathing and any general danger sign, chest indrawing, or stridor when calm
4. Diarrhoea with severe dehydration – abnormally sleepy or difficult to wake up, sunken eyes, not able to drink or drinking poorly, skin pinch goes back very slowly
5. Severe persistent diarrhoea (≥14 days) with dehydration – restless/irritable, sunken eyes and skin pinch goes back slowly
6. Severe malnutrition or severe anaemia – visible severe wasting, oedema of both feet, or severe palmar pallor

Adapted from World Health Organization Integrated Management of Childhood Illness.

### Travel bug

The ease of air travel and the frequency of people of all ages visiting the tropics have made it essential for the student and practising doctor to have an appreciation of tropical medicine. Migration, including for humanitarian reasons (refugees), makes it almost certain that some will carry disease undetected by the medical screening process. The majority of children with TB infection or disease identified in Australia have recently immigrated from or spent time in TB-endemic countries. It is of the greatest importance that a history of overseas travel is sought in any unusual disease presentation, particularly a febrile illness.

## Invasive bacterial disease

Serious bacterial infections are much more common in children in tropical and developing countries than in temperate and developed countries, and 25% or more of children dying in hospital have bacteraemia. Studies from tropical Africa in infants and children hospitalized with a wide range of presentations, including severe malaria, have documented that invasive bacterial infections are common and associated with a high case-fatality rate.

Common clinical presentations include:

- pneumonia
- septicaemia with or without focus
- meningitis
- bone and joint sepsis
- soft tissue sepsis (e.g. abscess, cellulitis, pyomyositis).

Important risk factors for disease incidence and/or poor outcome include:

- Age: particularly common in infants and young children. Neonatal sepsis is a major contributor to the high neonatal mortality in developing countries.

- Co-morbidities: such as malnutrition, HIV infection, measles or sickle cell disease.
- Late presentation to health services: common in resource-limited settings.

*Pneumococcus* and Hib have been the commonest causes of invasive bacterial disease in children beyond the neonatal age group. The increasing uptake of Hib conjugate vaccine into EPI schedules has resulted in a dramatic reduction in the burden of invasive disease due to Hib, including meningitis. Pneumococcus is the commonest cause of bacterial pneumonia and meningitis in developing countries. Uptake of the pneumococcal conjugate vaccine has been limited in low- and middle-income countries due to cost constraints. However, wider implementation of a vaccine that covers the majority of the serotypes causing disease is high on the global public health agenda, such as the GAVI Alliance.

Other causes of invasive bacterial disease include the Gram-negative enteric pathogens (e.g. *Salmonella* spp, *Escherichia coli*, *Klebsiella pneumoniae*) and *Staphylococcus aureus*. They are important causes in the young including neonates, the malnourished and HIV-infected. Resistance of Gram-negative bacilli to multiple antibiotics is common. *S. aureus* is an important cause of bone, joint and soft tissue sepsis, as well as of pneumonia in association with measles and HIV infection.

*Salmonella* infections occur worldwide but are particularly important in tropical and developing countries. Enteric or typhoid fever is due to *Salmonella typhi* and *S. paratyphi*. Typhoid fever is confined to humans, and occurs where standards of hygiene, water supply and sanitation are poor. The typical presentation is fever, malaise, headache, abdominal discomfort, and sometimes vomiting and diarrhoea. In severe disease, toxaemia is profound and complications such as small bowel perforation can occur in older children. This typical presentation of typhoid fever is mainly in children of school age. In younger children, *S. typhi* often presents with a non-specific febrile illness. Invasive disease due to *S. typhi* is particularly common in Asia and some Pacific Islands.

There are over 2000 serotypes of non-typhoidal salmonellae. In developed countries, the usual presentation is acute gastroenteritis due to food poisoning. In malaria-endemic regions of Africa, non-typhoidal salmonellae commonly cause severe invasive disease in children, including meningitis in infants, especially during the rainy season, presenting as a non-specific febrile illness with a high case-fatality rate of 20–25%. Consistent clinical associations include young age, malaria, anaemia, malnutrition and HIV infection.

Antibiotic resistance to ampicillin, co-trimoxazole and chloramphenicol (multidrug resistance) is now common for *S. typhi* in Asia and for non-typhoidal *Salmonella* in Africa. This poses a management challenge in settings where availability and choice of antibiotics is limited. Third-generation cephalosporins (e.g. ceftriaxone) or quinolones (e.g. ciprofloxacin) are usually effective alternatives, although quinolone resistance is increasing in Asia.

Group A streptococcus is also important in developing countries, not as a major cause of invasive disease in children, but more as a cause of pharyngitis and skin sepsis in communities where rheumatic heart disease and acute glomerulonephritis are common and cause significant morbidity.

## Viruses

Finally, it is important to recognize that viruses are a common cause of lower respiratory tract infection and diarrhoea in developing countries. The causes are similar to those in developed countries, but with less marked seasonal variation in the tropics. With improved socioeconomic conditions in communities in the Asia–Pacific region, viruses are responsible for a larger proportion of disease than bacteria, and virus-induced airway disease (e.g. acute bronchiolitis, asthma) is increasingly common. This has important implications for clinical management guidelines such as IMCI protocols, and appropriate use of antibiotics.

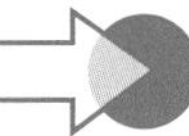

### Practical points

**Bacterial infections**

- Serious bacterial infections are common in children in developing countries and associated with a high case-fatality rate.
- Important causes include pneumococcus, *Haemophilus influenzae* type b, multiresistant Enterobacteriaceae (e.g. *Salmonella, E. coli*) and *Staphylococcus aureus*.
- IMCI guidelines aim to help primary care health workers to identify children needing antibiotic treatment.

## Tuberculosis

It is estimated that a third of the world's population is infected with *Mycobacterium tuberculosis* and almost all live in developing countries. Most of these people have latent TB infection and will not develop TB disease. However, many do develop disease, most commonly pulmonary tuberculosis (PTB), and infection is readily transmitted through coughing. Children are usually infected by contact with an adult or older child with sputum smear-positive PTB. Generally, children under 8–10 years of age do not develop pulmonary cavities; thus they have pauci-bacillary disease which is not considered contagious, and do not require isolation.

If a child is infected, the risk of developing symptomatic TB disease depends on:

- Age: infants and children aged less than 3 years have a much higher risk of disease than older children, and a high risk of severe disseminated forms of disease such as TB meningitis.
- HIV co-infection: HIV-infected children are at increased risk of exposure/infection because they live in families with TB/HIV, and at much higher risk of disease than HIV-uninfected. Antiretroviral therapy (ART) reduces the risk of developing disease following infection in HIV-infected children.
- Other co-morbidities: severe malnutrition, recent measles or other conditions associated with immunosuppression.
- Bacille Calmette–Guérin (BCG) vaccination: given to newborns in TB-endemic countries, this provides some protection against severe forms of TB in young children, such as TB meningitis and miliary TB. It is recommended that BCG is not given to HIV-infected infants because of the risk of disseminated BCG infection.

The commonest form of TB in children is PTB (about 75% of cases) and most cases present in young children, as do TB meningitis and miliary TB. Other forms of extrapulmonary TB that tend to present in older children include TB adenitis (cervical TB is commonest), TB pleural effusion, TB ascites or spinal TB.

Common clinical features associated with a diagnosis of TB include a persistent cough not responding to broad-spectrum antibiotics, weight loss or failure to thrive, persistent fever, and fatigue or reduced playfulness. A history of contact with an infectious case should be carefully sought, and is often positive in young children. The diagnosis of PTB is usually based on clinical and radiological features because young children have pauci-bacillary disease and have difficulty in providing sputum for microscopy. Sputum smear-positive disease is not unusual in older children and adolescents, but the yield from gastric aspirates or induced sputum in young children is very low. Thus, TB diagnosis in young children remains one of the most challenging issues in paediatric practice in tropical and developing countries with HIV and malnutrition, and diagnostic algorithms perform poorly.

An HIV test should be routine in assessment of children with suspected TB. This is because HIV infection increases risk of TB disease and is associated with a poorer outcome. Further, the diagnosis of TB in children with chronic respiratory symptoms can be more challenging in HIV-infected children because there are other forms of HIV-related lung disease to consider such as lymphoid interstitial pneumonitis and bronchiectasis.

Children with TB receive similar regimens to adults depending on the type of disease, but at higher dosages in milligrams per kilogram (mg/kg). Children tolerate anti-TB therapy very well and serious adverse events are rare. HIV-infected children with TB require co-trimoxazole preventative therapy and antiretroviral therapy (ART) in addition to anti-TB therapy. ART improves outcome in HIV-infected children treated for TB disease, and is generally commenced as soon as TB treatment is tolerated. Although there is a risk of immune reconstitution inflammatory syndrome (IRIS) in the severely immunosuppressed child, early HIV treatment appears not to increase mortality.

Children who are close household contacts of source cases with TB, especially those with sputum smear-positive disease, should be screened. Those with symptoms suggestive of TB disease should be assessed and investigated as appropriate for possible TB disease. Asymptomatic children at risk of developing disease after exposure: any child contact aged less than 5 years, or an HIV-infected child of any age, should be given preventative therapy following exclusion of active disease.

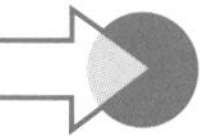

**Practical points**

**Tuberculosis**

- Childhood TB is common in countries with a high incidence of sputum smear-positive TB in the community.
- Diagnosis is usually clinical, and important features in children include persistence of symptoms, history of contact with a source case, age and nutritional status of the child, and HIV infection status.

## Malaria

Malaria is a major global health problem, with an estimated 50% of the world's population in 88 countries in 2010 exposed to various degrees of risk, almost exclusively in tropical regions. In holo-endemic settings, children are the most vulnerable group for severe disease and death due to malaria. Immunity to severe disease is acquired with age. Pregnant women are also vulnerable in the third trimester of pregnancy and malaria in pregnancy is an important cause of low birth weight babies.

Severe malaria in children:

- is caused mainly by *Plasmodium falciparum* infection
- is most common during the rainy season
- presents mainly as cerebral malaria or severe anaemia, or as a combination of both.

Thick blood film microscopy remains the 'gold standard' for malaria diagnosis. However, parasitaemia is not necessarily synonymous with disease. In 1000 children bitten by an infected mosquito there might be 400 asymptomatic infections, 200 cases of clinical malaria (febrile illness), 12 cases of severe malaria and 1 death. Rapid diagnostic tests that detect *Plasmodium*-specific antigens are now available, but are expensive and not species specific.

Cerebral malaria is characterized by acute encephalopathy with coma (Table 12.4.1) and often with seizures, and presents in older children (mean age 3–4 years) in areas with seasonal and moderate transmission. In Africa, cerebral malaria has a mortality of around 10% and significant neurological sequelae can occur in survivors. The main features of severe disease with poor outcome are prolonged unresponsive coma, deep breathing, decerebrate posturing and hypoglycaemia.

Severe malarial anaemia is most frequent in younger children (mean 1–2 years) in regions with high malarial transmission. Severe malarial anaemia presents to hospital with severe pallor and often respiratory distress due to lactic acidosis and/or heart failure from an abrupt drop in haemoglobin levels.

Treatment for malaria depends on severity and may include:

- Anti-malarial therapy:
  - non-severe disease: the most widely recommended treatment is currently artemether combination therapy (ACT), because resistance to chloroquine and sulfadoxine–pyrimethamine has emerged in many parts of the world
  - severe disease: parenteral quinine or artesunate (in south-east Asia where there is quinine resistance).
- Exclude other diagnoses: for example, meningitis, because there is overlap with the clinical diagnosis of cerebral malaria.

**Table 12.4.1 Modified Blantyre Coma Score as used for cerebral malaria**

| Score | Responses to painful fingernail and sternal pressure |
|---|---|
| 0 | No response or decerebrate/decorticate or opisthotonic postures |
| 1 | Non-specific response (e.g. moans or moves) |
| 2 | Withdraws the limb |
| 3 | Localizes the painful stimulus |
| 4 | Responds and cries momentarily but relapses into coma |
| 5 | Normal or fully conscious |

- Supportive care: management of hypoglycaemia and seizures.
- Blood transfusion: the decision to transfuse is based on severity of anaemia, evidence of cardiac failure and degree of parasitaemia.
- Antibiotics should be considered in severe cases as bacteraemia is common and associated with a worse outcome. Severe malarial anaemia is associated with invasive disease due to non-typhoidal *Salmonella*.

The most effective malaria control measures available to clinicians are insecticide-treated bed-nets (ITNs) (e.g. permethrin), personal protection with mosquito repellents (e.g. DEET – *N*,*N*-diethyl-meta-toluamide) and effective malaria treatment. In systematic reviews, the protective efficacy of ITNs and indoor-residual spraying on reducing the malaria-attributable mortality rate in children aged under 5 years in *P. falciparum* settings is 55% (range of 49–61%). WHO has formulated a global strategic plan (2005–2015) called Roll Back Malaria. Its priorities include:

- locally appropriate vector control methods (e.g. ITNs)
- prompt diagnosis and treatment with effective anti-malarial medicines (e.g. ACT)
- pregnant women receive intermittent preventative treatment.

Although there have been major international efforts to develop malaria vaccines, an effective, affordable vaccine is at least a decade away from implementation.

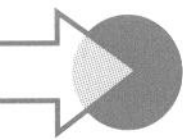

**Practical points**

**Malaria**

- Malaria affects 50% of the world's population in 88 countries.
- Important malaria control activities include the use of insecticide-treated bed-nets and effective first-line treatment.
- Clinical algorithms for malaria diagnosis perform poorly, so thick blood film or rapid diagnostic tests are important diagnostic tools.
- Cerebral malaria and malarial anaemia are the two forms of severe *falciparum* malaria in children.
- Parenteral artesunate or quinine is the drug of choice for severe malaria.

## Dengue virus infection

A number of viruses are capable of producing haemorrhagic disease in humans. They are mainly arthropod-borne, the most common vectors being ticks and mosquitoes. Dengue is the most widespread, vector-borne, viral infection in humans, with 50–100 million cases annually, being particularly common in tropical countries where the mosquito vector *Aedes aegypti* is present. Dengue is a leading cause of childhood mortality in Asia and South America, and is the most rapidly spreading and important arboviral disease in the world with a geographical distribution of more than 100 countries. Most dengue cases are sporadic, but dengue is endemic in south-east Asia and recent epidemics have occurred in the Asia-Pacific region (e.g. East Timor, Fiji, New Caledonia). The incubation period is 2–7 days and asymptomatic infections are common.

The clinical features are abrupt onset of high fever with generalized aches and pains, and a macular skin eruption. The influenza-like illness lasts 2–6 days and then may relapse a day or two later with fever and rash, followed by fatigue for several weeks. Severe dengue is characterized by the two syndromes:

- *Dengue haemorrhagic fever (DHF):* a petechial rash appears on about the third day, with bleeding from the gums, nose, gastrointestinal tract and venepuncture sites. After the initial phase as fever begins to subside, signs of circulatory failure appear, with restlessness, pallor, diaphoresis and cool peripheries. T-cell activation with a rapid increase in cytokines and chemical mediators leads to malfunction of vascular endothelial and haemocoagulation systems. Typical laboratory findings include thrombocytopenia, raised haematocrit, increased liver enzymes and abnormal coagulation test results.
- *Dengue shock syndrome (DSS):* shock results from marked plasma leakage due to a diffuse vasculitis often with features of disseminated intravascular coagulation (DIC). It usually progresses from haemorrhagic fever, but some develop signs of shock earlier in the illness.

The management of dengue fever is symptomatic and supportive:

- circulatory support – adequate fluid intake, the use of plasma expanders
- replacement of coagulation factors
- careful clinical monitoring.

Most children will recover and proper management of severe disease is crucial for reducing case-fatality rates, but a mortality rate of 2% persists, even in sophisticated centres.

It is still not clear why some children with dengue progress to shock or haemorrhagic syndromes, but the key immunopathological mechanisms are viral strain virulence and host immune responses, which augment the severity of infection. A notable risk factor for DHF is the existence of heterotypic dengue virus antibodies, present because the host has previously been infected with a different strain of dengue virus. These antibodies are associated with increased viraemia in second infections, indicating the importance of the immune response in the pathogenesis of severe disease and complicating vaccine development. Epidemics can be contained only by vector control until a vaccine is available, hopefully in the near future.

## Diarrhoeal disease

Diarrhoea is a major cause of morbidity and mortality in children in developing countries. Important environmental, socioeconomic and host risk factors for infection and severe disease are well known, and have already been mentioned in the introduction. Similar to child pneumonia, there is a wide range of possible aetiological agents that include bacteria, viruses and protozoa, and the relative importance of each of these varies between regions and populations. The principles of management are similar to those outlined in Chapter 20.2. This chapter will briefly highlight a few issues that are particularly relevant to management of children with diarrhoea in developing countries.

Diarrhoea is generally divided into three categories for clinical management purposes:

- *Acute watery:* the commonest form, often seasonal. Cholera and enterotoxigenic *E. coli* are important causes of severe dehydrating diarrhoea in some regions. Viruses also important worldwide, especially rotavirus. Effective fluid management of dehydration and maintenance is critical. The widespread use of pre-packaged oral rehydration solution has had a major impact in reducing diarrhoea-related mortality in children, particularly from dehydration and hypokalaemia.
- *Acute bloody (or dysentery):* usually due to invasive bacterial pathogens such as *Shigella dysenteriae*. Antibiotics are indicated in the acute phase, in addition to fluid management.
- *Persistent diarrhoea:* may follow the presentation of either of the above. More common in malnourished or HIV-infected children – and may lead to malnutrition by persistent malabsorption. Nutritional support is very important to promote catch-up growth.

Nutrition is important for recovery from acute diarrhoea. Children with diarrhoea should continue to feed with normal diet to facilitate recovery. Zinc supplementation for 10–14 days significantly reduces the duration of diarrhoea and time to recovery.

No particular pathogen is associated with persistent diarrhoea in children under 5 years in low- and middle-income countries, although enteropathogenic *E. coli* is the only organism found in over 10% of cases. Pathogens detected in children with persistent diarrhoea may not necessarily be the cause of the illness, as up to 43% of non-diarrhoeal controls have at least one organism isolated from stool. There is therefore no evidence to justify routine antimicrobial use for children with persistent diarrhoea of unknown cause. Dietary management of carbohydrate intolerance is important, particularly in poor hygiene settings and with HIV-infected infants.

In terms of diarrhoeal disease control, the key interventions of proven effectiveness are handwashing with soap and water, improved water quality and access, and breastfeeding promotion. Children living in poor hygiene circumstances or with HIV infection are likely to be affected by tropical or environmental enteropathy with partial villous atrophy of the small intestinal mucosa, mucosal T-cell activation and crypt hyperplasia. Indigenous Australians living in remote communities have particularly high rates of enteropathy, and a superimposed enteric infection with *E. coli*, rotavirus, *Cryptosporidium* or *Strongyloides* results in complete villous atrophy with lactose intolerance, hypokalaemia, acidosis and dehydration. Tropical enteropathy also appears to contribute significantly to growth failure in young children unresponsive to dietary interventions, and may also contribute to iron deficiency anaemia.

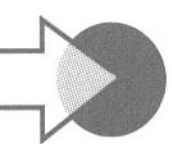

**Practical points**

**Diarrhoea**

- Acute diarrhoea is very common and, due to a wide range of pathogens, variable between regions.
- Effective management of dehydration is extremely important to avoid deaths, irrespective of the cause.
- Acute bloody diarrhoea or dysentery is usually due to invasive bacteria and antibiotics are indicated.
- Continued feeding and zinc supplementation improves recovery from acute diarrhoea.
- The management of persistent diarrhoea can be complicated and nutritional support is important in recovery.

## Parasitic infections

Human parasites are classified into five major divisions:

- Protozoa (e.g. amoebae, sporozoans)
- Platyhelminths (cestodes, trematodes)
- Acanthocephala (thorny-headed worms)
- Nematodes (roundworms)
- Arthropods (spiders, ticks).

Geohelminths are a subgroup of soil-transmitted intestinal nematodes such as *Strongyloides*, hookworm, *Ascaris* and *Trichuris* (Table 12.4.2). The WHO estimates that some 3.5 billion people are infected by intestinal parasitic and protozoan infections, and that 450 million have disease, the majority being children. In China, for example, a nationwide survey, including stool microscopy on 1.5 million people, found a prevalence of 63%, of whom 43% had multiple parasites. The five most common parasites were *Ascaris lumbricoides* (47%), *Enterobius vermicularis* (26%), *Trichuris trichiura* (19%), *Giardia lamblia* (2.5%) and *Entamoeba histolytica* (0.9%). This compares to prevalence estimates in sub-Saharan African schoolchildren of 32% for hookworms, 30% for *Ascaris* and *Trichuris*, and 14% for *Schistosoma mansoni.*

### Giardiasis

*G. lamblia* is one of the most common parasitic infections in humans, with a prevalence of 20–30% in many developing countries, although it is also common in developed countries. The clinical manifestations of *Giardia* vary from asymptomatic passage of cysts to chronic diarrhoea with malabsorption and weight loss. The usual clinical syndrome is characterized by watery diarrhoea, foul-smelling stools, bloating and abdominal cramps. Only about half of patients develop symptoms following ingestion of cysts. The course is frequently prolonged and some go on to develop syndromes of chronic diarrhoea or frequent relapses. Children in the developing world with chronic diarrhoea and malnutrition often have giardiasis but are also co-infected with other enteric pathogens. The diagnosis relies upon stool microscopy finding trophozoites or cysts. Presumptive treatment with tinidazole or metronidazole for children with persistent diarrhoea is common practice. *Giardia* is waterborne and cysts are highly resistant to chlorine and ozone, so filtration provides the best protection against transmission.

### Amoebiasis

Although this organism is commonly found in stools in children in the tropics, recent molecular and immunological techniques have demonstrated two distinct species of *Entamoeba* that are morphologically identical. *E. histolytica* is pathogenic, causing symptomatic disease in 10% of infections, whereas *E. dispar* causes only asymptomatic colonization. Abdominal discomfort may be the only symptom of amoebiasis, but an acute attack may provoke severe diarrhoea, cramps, tenesmus and toxaemia, with stools containing blood and mucus but little pus. Amoebic liver abscess, a well-known complication in adults, is rare in childhood. Risk factors for invasive disease are interaction with bacterial flora, host genetic susceptibility, malnutrition, male sex, young age and immunodeficiency.

### Schistosomiasis (bilharzia)

There are seven human species of this trematode, including *Schistosoma haematobium*, which affects the renal tract, and *S. mansoni*, which affects the

Table 12.4.2 Common intestinal parasites

| Infection | Other name | Symptoms | Transmission | Treatment of choice | Alternative treatments |
|---|---|---|---|---|---|
| **1. Protozoa** | | | | | |
| *Entamoeba histolytica* | Amoebiasis | Dysentery | Faecal–oral | Metronidazole | |
| *Entamoeba dispar* | – | Asymptomatic | Faecal–oral | Nil | |
| *Giardia lamblia* | Giardiasis | Chronic diarrhoea, or malabsorption | Faecal–oral | Tinidazole | Metronidazole or nitazoxanide |
| *Cryptosporidium parvum* | Cryptosporidiosis | Persistent diarrhoea | Faecal–oral | Nitazoxanide* | |
| *Cyclospora cayetanensis* | Cyclosporiasis | Diarrhoea | Faecal–oral | Co-trimoxazole | |
| *Isospora belli* | Isosporiasis | Diarrhoea with AIDS | Faecal–oral | Co-trimoxazole | |
| **2. Nematodes** | | | | | |
| *Ascaris lumbricoides* | Roundworm | Intestinal obstruction | Faecal–oral | Albendazole† | Levamisole, pyrantel |
| *Enterobius vermicularis* | Pinworm/threadworm | Nocturnal anal pruritus | Faecal–oral | Albendazole | Levamisole, pyrantel |
| *Ancylostoma duodenale* | Hookworm | Iron deficiency anaemia | Percutaneous | Albendazole | Levamisole, pyrantel |
| *Necator americanus* | Hookworm | Iron deficiency anaemia | Percutaneous | Albendazole | Levamisole, pyrantel |
| *Strongyloides stercoralis* | Strongyloidiasis | Diarrhoea | Percutaneous | Ivermectin | Albendazole |
| *Trichuris trichiura* | Whipworm/trichuriasis | Dysentery, rectal prolapse | Faecal–oral | Albendazole | Levamisole, pyrantel |
| **3. Cestodes** | | | | | |
| *Hymenolepis nana* | Dwarf tapeworm | Asymptomatic | Faecal–oral | Nitazoxanide* | Praziquantel |
| **4. Trematodes** | | | | | |
| *Schistosoma mansoni* | Bilharzia | Melaena/portal hypertension | Percutaneous | Praziquantel | Oxamniquine |
| *Fasciolopsis buski* | Giant intestinal fluke | | Percutaneous | Praziquantel | |

*Where treatment is indicated. Note that nitazoxanide has not been found to be effective in human immunodeficieny virus (HIV)-infected children with cryptosporidiosis.
†Or mebendazole.

gastrointestinal tract. It has been estimated that 220 million people are infected by schistosomiasis in 74 countries and that 20 million have severe disease. Eggs of *S. mansoni* or *S. haematobium* are passed in the faeces or urine respectively. They hatch in warm water and the ciliated larvae penetrate freshwater snails, producing thousands of tiny cercariae. These penetrate human skin in water, enter peripheral lymphatics or veins, and are carried via the lung to mature in portal or vesical vessels. Adult worms may survive 5 years or longer, producing eggs that cause granuloma formation in bowel, liver or bladder. Most infections are light and asymptomatic. However, the host's inflammatory reaction to eggs carried to the liver can lead to portal hypertension. Severe disease with hepatosplenomegaly affects about 10% of *S. mansoni* cases in endemic areas, taking 5–15 years to develop. Normally the condition presents with blood in stools, abdominal discomfort, tiredness and weight loss in children The key early feature of *S. haematobium* infection is terminal haematuria which, untreated, may progress over years of heavy exposure to obstructive uropathy, hydronephrosis and pyelonephritis.

Diagnosis is based on finding eggs in the faeces, but stool concentration methods and numerous immunological techniques (e.g. enzyzme-linked immunosorbent assay; ELISA) are more sensitive for milder infections. Treatment is with praziquantel 40 mg/kg as a single dose. Prevention involves avoidance of water sources containing cercariae and promotion of latrine use. Control programmes for schistosomiasis involve mass chemotherapy, destruction of snails, environmental sanitation, prevention of water contact and health education.

## Ascariasis

Ascariasis is one of the most prevalent infections in the world, affecting approximately 1400 million people (23% of the world's population), with 59 million, mostly children, at risk of morbidity. The highest prevalence is in countries where sanitation is deficient. Curiously, ascariasis was never common in tropical Australia, unlike other intestinal parasites. Morbidity is directly related to worm load. Geophagy (eating soil) is a significant risk factor for ascariasis and trichuriasis. *Ascaris* infection is not associated with mucosal damage, and 85% of infected individuals have light infections that remain asymptomatic. Heavy infection may induce a pneumonitis from migrating pulmonary larvae, with cough, wheeze, eosinophilia and transient patchy infiltrates, which may be difficult to differentiate from pneumonia, asthma or bronchitis. This syndrome of tropical pulmonary eosinophilia (Loeffler), common in adults, is rarely recognized clinically in children with *Ascaris* or hookworm.

The most common clinical feature of ascariasis is intestinal obstruction from a bolus of worms, which occurs in 0.2% of infections in children but accounts for 72% of all complications of *Ascaris* infection. Surgical management can invariably be avoided with experience with this syndrome, using daily nasogastric administration of anthelminthics with supportive therapy until the bolus is passed. Worms are often vomited or passed in stools on presentation of sick children. The diagnosis is based upon identification of the characteristic eggs on microscopy of stool or identification of the adult worm passed spontaneously or after treatment. Eggs are plentiful in faeces, as each female produces a mean of 200 000 eggs daily. A lack of latrines and soap for handwashing are risk factors for infection.

## Hookworm

The two major species of hookworm are *Ancylostoma duodenale* and *Necator americanus*, which have similar life cycles and disease. The gravid female hookworm produces about 5000–30 000 eggs per day in faeces. The eggs hatch into rhabditiform larvae that grow into infective larvae and enter the host, usually by boring through bare feet, and reach venules or lymphatics. The larvae then migrate into the lungs, ascend the respiratory tract and descend to the small intestine, where they attach and mature in the jejunum.

Hookworms are probably the second most prevalent intestinal parasite after ascariasis, with 1200 million people infected worldwide (two-thirds by *Necator*), including 90–130 million with morbidity. *Necator* predominates in Central and South America, and *Ancylostoma* in India, China, North Africa and tropical Australia, but mixed infections occur in many regions. Unlike *Ascaris* and *Trichuris*, hookworm transmission is associated with rural rather than urban settings. There are several other species of dog and cat helminth (e.g. *Toxocara* spp) that can cause eosinophilic enteritis, cutaneous larva migrans or viscera larva migrans in humans.

Hookworm larvae entering the skin can result in a papulovesicular rash at the site of entry, or cutaneous larvae migrans for animal hookworms. Although eosinophilia accompanies the larval migration phase, pneumonitis is mild and is rarely recognized in children. The main morbidity from hookworm is iron deficiency anaemia, particularly with heavy infections. The diagnosis of hookworm is based upon identifying hookworm eggs on microscopy of faeces. Eosinophilic enteritis due to animal hookworm may require endoscopy for definitive diagnosis, as stool microscopy will be negative. Charcot–Leyden crystals in the stools reflect breakdown of eosinophils, which is a non-specific feature of early infection.

Measures to prevent hookworm include ceasing the use of human faeces as fertilizer, use of toilets, wearing shoes and generally improving living standards. In high-prevalence areas of hookworm and schistosomiasis, regular mass de-worming campaigns using albendazole or praziquantel are effective in reducing anaemia rates.

### Whipworm

A mature *Trichuris trichiura* female worm produces up to 20 000 eggs/day, which are not infectious over 2–4 weeks. Once ingested, larvae penetrate the epithelium of the mucosal crypt in the caecum, where they moult and the hairlike worm remains attached while the broader distal end extends into the lumen. The adult worm is 4 cm long and survives 1–2 years in the host. Trichuriasis is a very common infestation with an estimated 1049 million cases worldwide, including 114 million preschool- and 233 million school-aged children. Most infections in children are light (<20 adult worms) and asymptomatic, with symptoms developing in less than 10% of infected children. Light infections incite a local inflammatory response involving eosinophils and neutrophils in the colon. With heavy infestations, frequent watery or mucous stools occur, sometimes with frank blood. Rectal prolapse can occur with heavy infestations, and occasionally heavily infected children develop a dysentery syndrome characterized by chronic dysentery, stunting, anaemia and finger clubbing.

The diagnosis is based on finding eggs on stool microscopy. The use of proper latrines, good hygiene with handwashing, and washing vegetables will interrupt the life cycle. Overcrowded urban slums with limited water supply and heavily faecally contaminated soil for growing vegetables place children at particular risk. Mass chemotherapy is highly effective but re-infection occurs rapidly in high-exposure settings.

### Cryptosporidiosis

The protozoa *Cryptosporidium parvum*, *Isospora belli*, *Cyclospora cayetanensis* and *Sarcocystis hominis* all belong to the group of intestinal coccidial infections, which cause diarrhoea. They have come into prominence in recent years through causing severe and protracted diarrhoea in people with acquired immune deficiency syndrome (AIDS) and infecting piped water supplies as a result of the chlorine resistance of oocysts. However, *Cryptosporidium* can also cause persistent diarrhoea and proximal small intestinal enteropathy in children with normal immune function.

Transmission is from person to person and from animals to people by ingestion of faecally contaminated food or water. Cryptosporidial infection causes watery diarrhoea with low-grade fever, vomiting and often cramps, severe dehydration and hypokalaemia. Among Aboriginal children in Darwin, *Cryptosporidium* was found in the stool of 7.4% of admissions with diarrhoeal disease, with a mean age of 12 months and mean admission serum potassium of 2.7 mmol/L. It was associated with severe and prolonged mucosal damage and inflammation.

Cryptosporidiosis is diagnosed by finding oocysts in stool using an acid-fast stain, which is sensitive only in diarrhoeal cases. Immunofluorescent and ELISA techniques are more sensitive, and polymerase chain reaction (PCR) may be even more sensitive for detecting low numbers of oocysts in stool specimens. The high infectivity and ubiquitous oocysts in the environment make prevention by water, hygiene and sanitation programmes very difficult – indeed impossible in the developing world, where up to 95% of children in some areas have positive serology by the age of 2 years. Precautions for travellers include handwashing, boiling water, avoiding animals, proper cooking of food, peeling fruit and avoiding uncooked food in contact with unboiled water (e.g. salads).

### Strongyloidiasis

Although not a major cause of morbidity worldwide, the nematode *Strongyloides stercoralis* is unique in its ability to persist indefinitely within the host through autoinfection and to cause disseminated disease associated with prolonged use of corticosteroids or other causes of immunosuppression.

*S. stercoralis* is present in tropical and subtropical regions, but estimates of worldwide prevalence vary widely (3–100 million), with the best estimate that of 30 million people in 70 countries. Strongyloidiasis accounts for about 8% of acute diarrhoeal admissions in Australian Aboriginal children in Darwin, with a mean age of 23 months, this group being significantly older than for other children with diarrhoeal admissions. Prevalence rates vary with climate, geographical region, soil characteristics and socioeconomic status, such as quality of housing, hygiene standards and crowded population density.

Malabsorption and small-bowel bacterial overgrowth occur with strongyloidiasis, and symptoms of abdominal pain, diarrhoea and weight loss. As with hookworm, larval migration may affect the lungs (eosinophilic pneumonitis) or skin ('ground itch' on the foot or 'larva currens' on the buttocks) but these are not usually recognized in children. The commonest manifestation of *S. stercoralis* infection in children is an acute diarrhoeal illness with foul stools with a typical musty odour. Severe dehydration is uncommon, but hypokalaemia and malabsorption occur commonly. Eosinophilia (5–15% of total white blood cell count) is a common but not universal finding. A syndrome of partial intestinal obstruction with strongyloidiasis has been described in Aboriginal children in the Northern Territory. *Strongyloides fulleborni* is a more virulent infection affecting young children in Papua New Guinea, which may be transmitted via breast milk, and is characterized by abdominal swelling, ascites, pleural effusions and a high mortality rate.

Disseminated strongyloidiasis (hyperinfection) occurs with impaired cell-mediated immunity, such as children treated with prolonged courses of steroids or children with malignancy (e.g. lymphoma, leukaemia) on immunosuppressive drugs. Eradication of *Strongyloides* is essential before immunosuppressive therapy is commenced. Disseminated infection is always a serious complication with high mortality, usually affecting bowel, lungs and central nervous system, and often accompanied by sepsis.

The diagnosis is established by identification of larvae on stool microscopy, which is very reliable in acute diarrhoea but less reliable in chronic or asymptomatic infection because larvae excretion is irregular and the parasite load is often low, so a single stool examination may detect larvae in only 30% of cases of latent infection. The stool culture technique is more sensitive. Various serological tests are also available. Disposal of human excreta, wearing shoes, treatment of cases and improved hygiene reduce the risk of transmission of strongyloidiasis in communities. Regular mass chemotherapy programmes have a modest impact on strongyloidiasis.

### Drug treatments for parasitic diseases

The benzimidazoles albendazole and mebendazole have broad-spectrum activity against roundworm, whipworm, hookworm, pinworm and wireworm species. Pyrantel pamoate is active against *Ascaris* and *Enterobius*. Levamisole is an immune stimulant that is effective against intestinal infection caused by *Ascaris* and hookworm. Ivermectin has broad-spectrum activity against helminths and filariasis but is the drug of choice against strongyloidiasis. Metronidazole and tinidazole are used for giardiasis and amoebiasis. Nitazoxanide is a new broad-spectrum antimicrobial agent with activity against nematodes, trematodes, anaerobic bacteria and protozoal parasites such as *Cryptosporidium*. However, it does not appear to be effective in HIV-infected children with cryptosporidiosis.

The results of systematic reviews of preventative programmes show the public health benefits of combining health interventions such as integrated school health packages, which may include deworming, iron supplementation, school feeding and malaria control. The impact of anthelmintic treatment is greatest when albendazole is co-administered with praziquantel. Although there are strong theoretical reasons to be concerned about the effect of iron on predisposing to infection, including malaria, prevention of iron deficiency is clearly beneficial, so the benefits outweigh the risks even in sub-Saharan Africa.

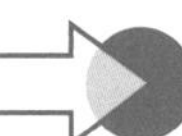

**Practical points**

**Intestinal parasites**

- Intestinal parasitic and protozoan infections are highly prevalent, with 3.5 billion people infected and 450 million having disease.
- Roundworms, whipworms and protozoa are transmitted faecally–orally (poor hygiene), hookworms and *Strongyloides* percutaneously (walking barefoot), and schistosomiasis from water (bathing, wading).
- Amoebic organisms in stool are most likely to be *Entamoeba dispar*, which is not pathogenic.
- Only *Cryptosporidium* and *Strongyloides* are significantly associated with diarrhoea; *Giardia* can cause chronic diarrhoea but is found more commonly in stools of children without diarrhoea.
- Control of intestinal parasites in high-prevalence communities is best achieved through integrated health interventions including periodic anthelminthic administration and improved water and sanitation.

## Specific infections of the Australian tropics

Box 12.4.2 lists the common infections in hospitalized children in the Top End of Australia. Murray Valley encephalitis is endemic in north-west Australia, with significant rates of exposure but a low clinical attack rate of about 0.1% of those infected. However, those with clinical illness develop devastating encephalitis with fever, coma, seizures and neurological signs of cerebellar, spinal cord and brainstem involvement, with a mortality rate of 20% and neurological sequelae in up to 40% of survivors. Although more common in the tropical north of Australia, Ross River and Barmah Forest viruses can cause outbreaks throughout Australia. Infection in children is usually asymptomatic and it is likely that infection in childhood accounts for the very low incidence of clinical disease in Aboriginal communities in northern Australia despite high rates of seropositivity.

Melioidosis is caused by the bacterium *Burkholderia pseudomallei*, which is ubiquitous in soil and water in northern Australia and is even more common in Thailand. Disease in children is relatively uncommon compared with adults (only 4% of cases at Royal Darwin Hospital are in children), who often have predisposing chronic disease risk factors, such as diabetes and alcoholism. Although pneumonia is the commonest presentation of melioidosis, there is a wide spectrum of manifestations, from mild cutaneous lesions to fulminant disease with multiple visceral abscesses. Prolonged treatment is required, usually with the antibiotics ceftazidime or imipenem and co-trimoxazole.

**Box 12.4.2 Common infections in Aboriginal community children in tropical Australia**

**Respiratory infections**
- Otitis media – especially chronic suppurative otitis media (CSOM)
- Airway disease – acute bronchiolitis, chronic mucopurulent bronchitis progressing to *bronchiectasis
- Bacterial pneumonia (N.B. pneumococcal and Hib infections now uncommon because of the use of conjugate vaccines)

**Infectious diarrhoea**
- *Enteropathogenic *Escherichia coli* (EPEC) and enteroaggregative *E. coli* (EAEC)
- Rotavirus (*complicated by metabolic acidosis and secondary lactose intolerance)
- **Strongyloides stercoralis*
- **Cryptosporidium parvum*
- *Salmonella* (N.B. clinical dysentery uncommon)

**Intestinal nematodes**
- *Whipworm – *Trichuris trichiura* (N.B. *Ascaris* or roundworm is very rare)
- **Strongyloides*, which causes diarrhoea and occasionally disseminated infection
- *Hookworm – *Ancylostoma duodenale* (less common now because of widespread use of albendazole)

**Skin infections**
- Impetigo and cellulitis – usually *Streptococcus pyogenes*
- Boils and abscesses – usually *Staphylococcus aureus*
- *Scabies, often with pyoderma
- Tinea corporis – usually *Trichophyton rubrum*

**Bone, joint and muscle infections**
- Septic arthritis, osteomyelitis and *pyomyositis, usually *S. aureus*

**Other**
- *Rheumatic fever (group A streptococcus)
- *Acute post-streptococcal glomerulonephritis (group A)
- *Epidemic gonococcal conjunctivitis (occasionally)
- *Trachoma (*Chlamydia trachomatis*)
- Hepatitis A (usually anicteric)

*Occurs predominantly in Aboriginal children.

PART 13

# ALLERGY, IMMUNITY AND INFLAMMATION

# 13.1 Atopy

Mike Gold

## General principles

### Definition, prevalence and burden of disease

Atopy is defined as the ability of an individual to form specific immunoglobulin (Ig) E antibodies to one or more common inhaled aeroallergens such as animal dander, pollen, mould or house dust mite. An allergen is defined as an antigen (usually a protein) that is recognized by the immune system, is usually harmless, and induces an allergic inflammatory response. The atopic or allergic diseases include eczema, asthma and allergic rhinoconjunctivitis. These are complex inflammatory conditions that are associated with immune dysregulation. Not all atopic individuals express clinical disease, but the majority of children who have these diseases are atopic. For example, 30–40% of individuals in developed countries can be shown to be atopic (have detectable allergen-specific IgE antibodies), yet only 5–20% may manifest an atopic disease. The reasons for this variable disease expression are not known.

There is a marked variation in the global and regional prevalence of the atopic diseases, with the highest disease burden in industrialized countries and urbanized communities. In these countries, atopic diseases are now the commonest ailments of childhood, and Australian and New Zealand children have the fifth highest global rates of atopic disease (Table 13.1.1). Since the industrial revolution, the prevalence of atopic diseases has been increasing in most communities, for reasons that are not yet apparent. Environmental factors are thought to account for the variable and increasing prevalence of atopic disease. A commonly cited hypothesis, the 'hygiene hypothesis', proposes that the lack of early childhood exposure to infections and/or other environmental factors (such as bacterial endotoxin) may predispose to atopic disease in genetically susceptible individuals. Such a hypothesis can be supported by epidemiological and possibly immunological evidence.

Because atopic diseases are common, often chronic and usually begin in early childhood, the burden to the community, family and individual is considerable. The cost of allergic disease to the Australian community is estimated to be $7 billion per annum. Importantly, the impact of severe atopic disease such as atopic dermatitis on a family may exceed that of other chronic childhood disorders such as diabetes mellitus or juvenile rheumatoid arthritis.



### Pathogenesis

Although atopy is defined by an excessive production of IgE, this is only one of many immunological changes that characterize the allergic diseases, as these are also associated with a complex dysregulation of the humoral and cellular immune systems (Fig. 13.1.1). For this process to occur, both a genetic predisposition and early life environmental exposure are important. During early life, naive T-helper lymphocytes respond in a particular way to environmental allergen exposure as well as a host of other non-allergen immunomodulatory factors (such as endotoxin). T-regulatory cell function and the pattern of cytokine secretion are central to the factors that result in the production of antibodies, including IgE.

## Approach to diagnosis, investigation and management

### History and examination

The history and examination should cover the following aspects:

- Specific symptoms
  - nature, timing (seasonal, perennial, episodic), situational (specific site or circumstance)
- Severity of symptoms and degree of disability
  - medication required to control symptoms, medical visits and hospitalization, school absenteeism, interference with sleep, sport or play
- Use of medication
  - current and past medications, efficacy, compliance, technique of use and side-effects
- Environmental history – identification of triggers
  - exposure to common allergens (Box 13.1.1) and non-allergen (e.g. cigarette smoke) triggers should be considered
  - a trigger may be identified easily if the onset of symptoms is acute and occurs soon after exposure, if symptoms occur in a specific geographical location, are seasonal, or occur repeatedly following similar exposures
  - a trigger may be difficult to identify when continuous exposure results in chronic symptoms
  - identification of possible triggers requires knowledge of the likely circumstances of allergen exposure.

| Table 13.1.1 Prevalence of atopic disorders among Australian children | | |
|---|---|---|
| Disorder | 6–7-year-olds (%) | 13–14-year-olds (%) |
| Eczema ever | 23 (11) | 16 (10) |
| Asthma ever | 27 (25) | 28 (29) |
| Hayfever ever | 18 (12) | 43 (20) |

Values in parentheses show the percentage that currently have the condition. Data obtained from the International Study of Asthma and Allergy in Childhood questionnaire-based survey of 10 914 children in Melbourne, Sydney, Adelaide and Perth.

On examination, atopic children may have a typical appearance (Table 13.1.2).

## Assessment

Once the history and examination are completed, there is seldom difficulty in diagnosing the presenting atopic disease. However, as many children manifest more than one atopic disease, it is important to consider whether any other atopic condition is present. A differential diagnosis should be considered, as uncommon disorders may present similarly to an atopic disease (Table 13.1.3).

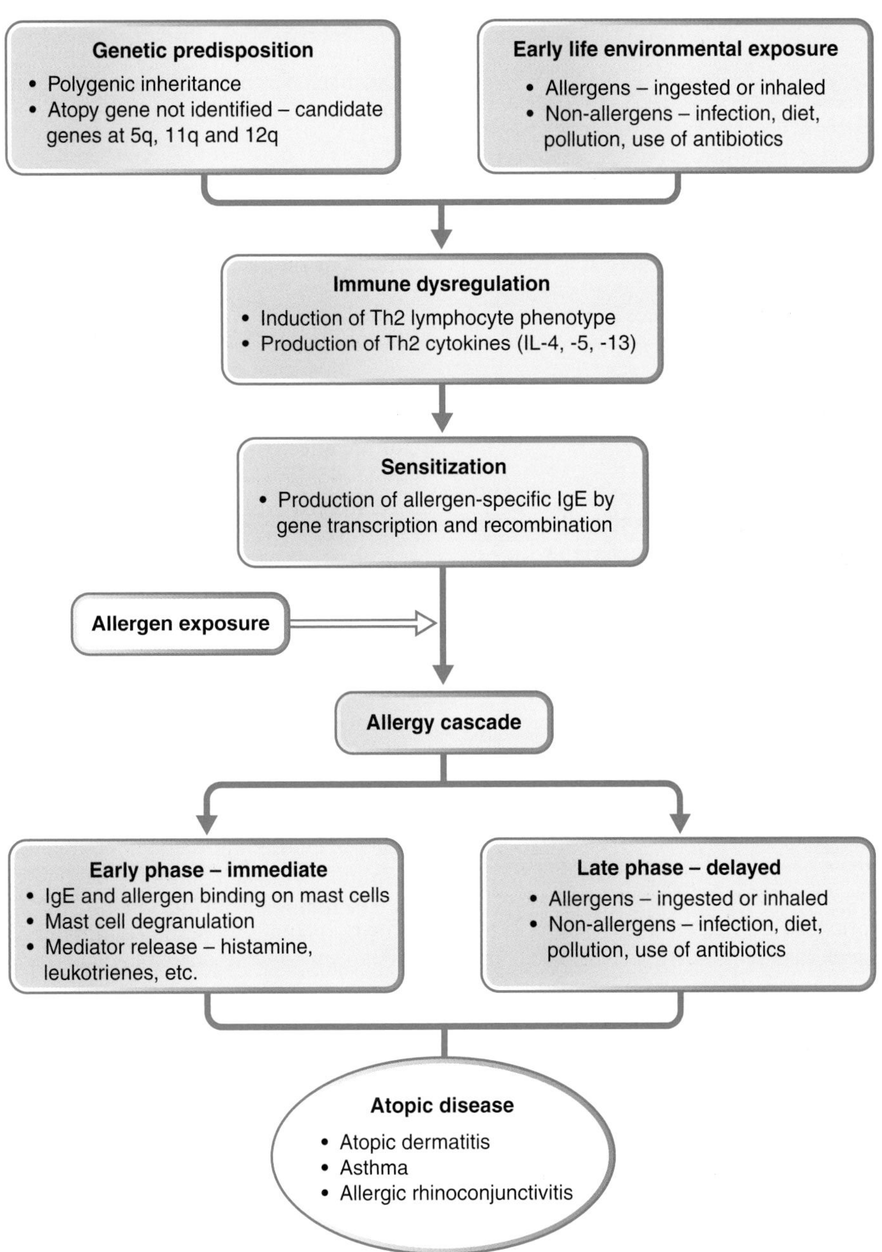


Fig. 13.1.1 Pathogenesis of atopic disease. Ig, immunoglobulin; IL, interleukin; Th2, T-helper type 2.

### Clinical example

Michaela, aged 10 years, had severe, persistent asthma. She presented for follow-up after a recent admission to the intensive care unit for acute respiratory symptoms diagnosed as status asthmaticus. In passing, her mother mentioned that immediately prior to her most recent episode she had inadvertently eaten a chocolate containing peanuts. She did not usually eat peanuts because she said that they made her mouth 'feel funny'. Her mother recalled that as an infant Michaela experienced two episodes of generalized skin rash immediately following peanut ingestion.

The history is suggestive of an IgE-mediated peanut anaphylaxis. Children with asthma are at increased risk of death from anaphylaxis. Additional questions in the history should ascertain whether Michaela had experienced any urticaria, angio-oedema, abdominal pain or vomiting with the most recent episode, as this would suggest the recent presentation was due to anaphylaxis rather than status asthmaticus. An assessment of allergen specific IgE (skin or serological test) to peanut should be obtained. Management of severe peanut allergy should include the complete dietary exclusion of peanut, an anaphylaxis action plan, adrenaline (epinephrine) for first aid use (EpiPen or Anapen) and a MedicAlert bracelet. Michaela's parents and other carers (including those at school) should be trained to use the anaphylaxis action plan. At this age, nut allergy is likely to be lifelong.

## Investigations

Investigations in the atopic child are limited. Total IgE concentration is raised in the majority of children with atopic disease but there is substantial overlap with values in non-atopic children. Measurement of total IgE levels is seldom indicated. Allergen-specific IgE (ASE) is more useful and can be determined using both *in vivo* (skin testing) and *in vitro* (serological) methods (Table 13.1.4). Measurement of ASE may be helpful in identifying a specific allergen trigger. However, interpretation of the skin test or ASE result is critical:

- The presence of specific IgE to an allergen is only one factor in establishing whether the allergen is a clinically significant trigger.
- The result should always be correlated with the history and/or a trial of allergen avoidance with or without subsequent challenge.
- The predictive value of a negative result is higher than the predictive value of a positive result.
- The skin test or ASE result should always be discussed with the parent or caregiver to avoid misinterpretation.
- Failure to discuss often leads to inappropriate avoidance measures such as excluding foods from the diets of children solely on the basis of a positive skin test or ASE result.

**Box 13.1.1 Allergens that may trigger symptoms in atopic children**

**Inhaled allergens**
- Animal dander – cat, dog, horse, rabbit
- Pollen – grass (rye, couch, timothy), weed (plantain), tree (olive, plane)
- Mould – *Alternaria, Aspergillus, Cladosporium, Penicillium* spp
- House dust mite – *Dermatophagoides pteronyssinus, Dermatophagoides farinae*
- Cockroach

**Ingested allergens**
- Food – cow's milk, egg, nuts, fish, shellfish, soy, wheat, fruit
- Medication – antibiotics (penicillin) and non-antibiotic medication

**Miscellaneous**
- Latex contained in balloons and surgical gloves

## Management

The aims of management in atopic disease may vary depending on the clinical context.

### Primary prevention of atopic disease

The most useful predictor for the development of an atopic disease is the family history. If one or both parents are affected, the risk to an infant of developing an atopic disease is 40–60%. With no positive family history, the risk of developing an atopic disease is 10%. General primary prevention advice should be to avoid exposure to tobacco smoke and promotion of breastfeeding, although the evidence concerning the protective effects of breastfeeding for allergy prevention remains variable. Maternal allergen avoidance during pregnancy is not thought to be effective. Still under current investigation is maternal intake of omega-3 fish oils and probiotics during pregnancy. There is evidence that use of a partially hydrolysed cow's milk formula (if breastfeeding is not possible) may be of benefit in high-risk infants, and also under investigation is the use of infant formulae containing prebiotics and probiotics. The timing of the introduction of 'allergenic foods' (e.g. cow's milk, egg and nuts) and the association with the development of food allergy is under investigation. However, there is currently no evidence to support prolonged empirical avoidance of allergenic foods beyond 6 months of age, even in high-risk infants.

### Management of symptomatic atopic disease

Once the child has developed symptomatic atopic disease, management involves allergen identification and avoidance, and symptomatic treatment. Immunotherapy may be appropriate for selected children.

**Table 13.1.2 Examination of the atopic child**

| System | Clinical findings |
|---|---|
| Growth | Weight<br>Height |
| Facies | Facial pallor<br>Allergic shiners – infraorbital dark circles due to venous congestion<br>Dennie–Morgan lines – wrinkles under both eyes<br>Mouth breathing<br>Dental malocclusion – from long-standing upper airway obstruction<br>Sinus tenderness |
| Skin | Atopic dermatitis<br>White dermatographism – white discoloration of skin after scratching<br>Xerosis – dry skin<br>Urticaria and/or angio-oedema |
| Nose | Horizontal nasal crease<br>Inferior nasal turbinates – pale and swollen<br>Clear nasal discharge |
| Respiratory | Chest deformity – Harrison sulcus, increase in anteroposterior diameter<br>Respiratory distress<br>Wheeze and/or stridor |
| Eyes | Conjunctivitis<br>Subcapsular cataracts associated with conjunctivitis |
| Ears | Tympanic membrane dull and retracted |
| Throat | Tonsillar enlargement<br>Postpharyngeal secretions and cobblestoning of mucosa |
| Cardiovascular | Blood pressure |

**Table 13.1.3 Differential diagnosis of atopic disease**

| Atopic disease | Differential diagnosis |
|---|---|
| Atopic dermatitis | Seborrheic dermatitis<br>Psoriasis<br>Wiskott–Aldrich syndrome*<br>Hyper-IgE syndrome* |
| Asthma | Infection – viral, bacterial, mycobacterial<br>Congenital anomaly (e.g. vascular ring)<br>Cystic fibrosis<br>Immunodeficiency disease<br>Aspiration syndrome secondary to gastro-oesophageal reflux, incoordinate swallowing or tracheo-oesophageal fistula<br>Inhaled foreign body<br>Cardiac failure |
| Allergic rhinitis | Infective rhinitis<br>Non-allergic rhinitis<br>Vasomotor rhinitis<br>Rhinitis medicamentosa<br>Sinusitis<br>Adenoidal hyperatrophy<br>Nasal polyps<br>Nasal foreign body<br>Choanal atresia (unilateral, bilateral) |

*These immunodeficiency diseases may have atopic dermatitis as a component.

**Table 13.1.4 Determination of allergen-specific IgE**

| | Skin testing | Serology |
|---|---|---|
| Method | Skin puncture test | UniCAP |
| Availability | Limited | Widely |
| Expense | Cheap | Expensive |
| Results | Immediate | Delayed |
| Risk of anaphylaxis | Rare | Nil |
| Interference | Antihistamines<br>Extensive atopic dermatitis<br>Dermatographism | High total IgE |
| Sensitivity | ++++ | ++ |
| Specific | ++++ | ++ |

Ig, immunoglobulin; UniCAP, radioallergosorbent test.

*Allergen identification and avoidance*
When possible, this remains an important component of management. Avoidance measures may involve considerable parental education, effort and expense. Note that:

- with ingested allergens identification and avoidance are particularly important when atopic disease is associated with a food allergy, as this is the only means of therapy
- with inhalant allergens, methods have been evaluated to reduce exposure to indoor allergens, most importantly house dust mite (Box 13.1.2). A number of studies in sensitized individuals have demonstrated improvements in atopic dermatitis and allergic rhinitis following house dust mite reduction measures. The benefit of house dust mite avoidance in asthma is much more controversial

**Box 13.1.2 Methods to reduce house dust mite exposure**

**Definitely useful**
- Encase bedding in impermeable covers (dust mite covers): most important measure, because the bed is the major source
- Hot water washing of bedding and clothes (>56°C): will destroy house dust mite and remove allergens

**Probably useful**
- Replacement of fitted carpets with smooth flooring
- Hard-surface cleaning with a damp cloth, at least once a week

**Possibly useful**
- Air filtration, ionizers and air conditioning

**Unlikely to be useful**
- Acaricides (dust mite sprays) for the carpet and mattress

- other indoor allergens (cat, cockroach, mould) and outdoor allergens are less easily avoided and alternative forms of therapy may be required.

*Symptomatic treatment*
When allergen avoidance is difficult, the response is partial or the allergen cannot be identified, symptomatic treatment is indicated. A number of medications are available, including antihistamines, sympathomimetics, mast cell stabilizers, corticosteroids and leukotriene antagonists (Table 13.1.5).

*Induction of tolerance: immunotherapy*
Allergen immunotherapy was first used for grass pollen-induced allergic rhinitis almost 100 years ago and is effective only for IgE-mediated inhalant or venom (bee, wasp, jumper ant) allergic disease. Although the exact mechanism is not known, the induced state of tolerance to an allergen is associated with the production of blocking antibodies, downregulation of T-helper type 2 (Th2) lymphocytes and a decrease in ASE.

Immunotherapy should be initiated and supervised by an experienced allergist. Pollen-induced allergic rhinoconjunctivitis remains the main indication for immunotherapy and should be considered in children who have intractable and disabling symptoms that have failed to respond to allergen avoidance and to symptomatic treatment. Immunotherapy for children who present primarily with asthma is controversial. Not only is the risk of an adverse reaction higher in these children, but they are often sensitized to both seasonal and perennial allergens. No form of immunotherapy is currently available for atopic dermatitis.

## Specific atopic disorders

The majority of children who develop atopic dermatitis (eczema) or asthma present by 6 years of age, with most individuals manifesting symptoms of allergic rhinoconjunctivitis by age 20 years. However, there is a predictable pattern of disease expression, which is called the 'allergic march':

- Expression of atopy usually starts with atopic dermatitis, which presents in the first 6 months of life and often improves in the second year of life.
- Approximately 50% of children with atopic dermatitis will then develop asthma in early childhood.
- With resolution of asthma in late childhood some children then develop allergic rhinitis, which may be lifelong.
- Importantly, in a number of children all forms of atopic disease may be expressed concurrently. For this reason, although one atopic disease may be predominant at a particular age, it is always important to consider which other atopic conditions may be present.

| Table 13.1.5 Medications for the symptomatic treatment of allergic disease | | |
|---|---|---|
| | Important mechanisms of action in allergic disease | Examples |
| Antihistamines | | |
| First and second generation | $H_1$-receptor antagonism | Diphenhydramine<br>Promethazine<br>Hydroxyzine |
| Second generation | Above plus antiallergic effects<br>Decrease mediator release<br>Decreased migration and activation of inflammatory cells<br>Reduced adhesion molecule expression | Cetirizine<br>Loratadine<br>Terfenadine |
| Sympathomimetics | | |
| β-agonists | Bronchial smooth muscle relaxation<br>Reduce mast cell secretion | Salbutamol<br>Albuterol<br>Terbutaline |
| α- and β-agonists | Bronchial smooth muscle relaxation<br>Vasoconstriction – skin and gut<br>Inotropic and chronotropic effects<br>Reduce mast cell secretions<br>Glycogenolysis | Adrenaline (epinephrine) |
| Cromolyn | Mast cell stabilizer<br>Inhibits chemotaxis of eosinophils<br>Inhibits pulmonary neuronal reflexes | Cromolyn sodium<br>Nedocromil sodium |
| Corticosteroids | Reduce T-cell cytokine production<br>Reduce eosinophil adhesion, chemotaxis<br>Reduce mast cell proliferation<br>Reduce vascular permeability<br>Reverse adrenoreceptor downregulation | Hydrocortisone<br>Beclomethasone<br>Budesonide<br>Fluticasone/flunisolide<br>Triamcinolone acetonide |
| Leukotriene antagonists | 5-Lipo-oxygenase enzyme inhibition, or LTD4 receptor antagonist | Montelukast |

LT, leukotriene.

## Atopic dermatitis

See also Chapter 21.1.

### Definition and clinical presentation

Atopic dermatitis is a chronic inflammatory skin disorder that is associated with overproduction of IgE and eosinophils due to a systemic Th2 cytokine response. Histamine, neuropeptides, proinflammatory cytokines, mast cells, eosinophils and antigen-presenting cells are all increased in skin affected by atopic dermatitis. The cardinal features of atopic dermatitis include:

- intense pruritus
- a relapsing course
- a typical distribution of skin rash
- a personal or family history of an atopic disease
- additional features that may be present:
  - dry skin (xerosis), skin infection, white dermatographism
  - other atopic diseases and atopic facies (see Table 13.1.4)
  - food allergy and intolerance.

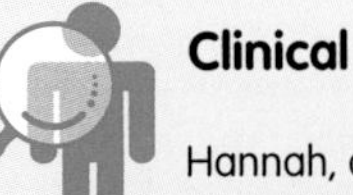

**Clinical example**

Hannah, aged 8 months, had severe atopic dermatitis. Her skin was permanently excoriated and erythematous. She had been breastfed and was on solids, which included rice, vegetables and wheat. A dietary history revealed that she also had food that contained small amounts of egg and cow's milk protein. A UniCAP performed by her general practitioner showed specific IgE antibodies to egg of more than 100 U/L (very high) and to cow's milk of 30 U/L (moderate). No specific IgE had been detected to wheat and rice.

The treatment of atopic dermatitis involves avoidance of skin irritants, use of skin moisturization, topical anti-inflammatories and the identification and avoidance of triggers. Approximately 50% of infants with atopic dermatitis have IgE sensitization to one or more of the common food proteins. Some of these infants may have an IgE-mediated food allergy, and in some ingestion of these food proteins may trigger atopic dermatitis. This infant should have dietary exclusion of egg and cow's milk protein, and the effect on her atopic dermatitis should be assessed. It is important not to continue a prolonged exclusion diet unless there is a significant clinical improvement in the eczema as a result. Therefore, if possible, this should occur under the supervision of a dietitian and alternative sources of protein and calcium should be included in the diet. Egg and cow's milk allergy usually resolve by 5 years of age, so regular review of the diet and other management is mandatory.

The main symptom of atopic dermatitis is intense pruritus, which when severe may be associated with disruption of sleep, school and social interactions, and can profoundly affect the quality of life. In older children and adolescents, disfigurement and teasing may be important. The appearance of the skin in atopic dermatitis may be variable:

- In infants with an acute presentation the lesions are erythematous, papulovesicular and occur mostly on the face, scalp, extensor surfaces of the limbs and trunk.
- With increasing age the lesions localize to the hands, feet, and the antecubital and popliteal flexures.
- Chronic changes include lichenification of the skin, which is a skin thickening resulting from persistent rubbing and scratching.
- The skin is almost invariably dry and its appearance may be altered by intense excoriation and secondary bacterial infection.

### Investigations

Determination of specific IgE to inhaled or ingested allergens by skin test or UniCAP should be considered if the atopic dermatitis is extensive and has not responded to measures of general skin care and symptomatic treatment.

Most affected children above 2 years of age have a raised total IgE concentration and have measurable specific IgE to common inhaled and ingested allergens. This is a marker of atopic status rather than indicating that a specific allergen may be a trigger for atopic dermatitis. Response to withdrawal of the allergen is currently the only way to determine the significance of these results.

### Management

A number of triggers may exacerbate atopic dermatitis, including:

- skin irritants (e.g. soap, heat)
- viral infection
- food allergens
- allergens such as house dust mite, animal dander, mould and pollen
- bacterial (*Staphylococcus aureus*) or viral (herpes simplex virus) skin infection
- stress.

The aim of management is to reduce as many of these triggers as possible and to provide symptomatic relief until the disorder improves, which fortunately occurs in most children.

The majority of children respond to general measures of skin care, which include:

- avoidance of skin irritants – soaps, shampoo, woollen clothing, hot baths
- frequent use of topical moisturizers (at least twice daily)
- antiseptic measures – antiseptic bath oil, topical antiseptic cream (intermittent)
- wet wraps – wet dressings (bandages) applied to the affected skin.

If symptoms persist despite these general measures then medication should be considered:

- Topical corticosteroids are used commonly:
  - The least potent steroid should always be used for maintenance therapy.
  - If possible, steroids should be used intermittently.
  - Potent steroids must be avoided on the face.
- Antihistamines may be useful for skin itch. Non-sedating antihistamines may be useful during the day and sedating antihistamines may be used intermittently, particularly for night-time itch in children older than 2 years of age.
- Antibiotics may also be useful for secondary bacterial infection of the skin.

If symptoms persist and are severe despite general measures of skin care and topical steroids, an allergy review would be appropriate; the aim would be to identify allergens that could be significant triggers. Allergen avoidance is particularly important in infants and children who have associated food allergies and those who have been sensitized to house dust mite.

Unfortunately, a small number of children have severe and disabling atopic dermatitis despite all of these measures and may require intermittent hospitalization for intensive topical therapy, phototherapy and immunosuppressive medication.

## Asthma

See also Chapter 14.3.

### Definition and clinical presentation

Asthma is defined as a chronic inflammatory lung disorder usually associated with bronchial hyperactivity, and presents as a symptom complex of cough, wheeze and shortness of breath. As asthma is discussed elsewhere (see Chapter 14.3), this section will review asthma in the context of the atopic child.

Although the exact cause of asthma is not known, the two most significant risk factors are a family history and atopy. Specifically, 60–80% of asthmatic children are atopic. Furthermore, sensitization to indoor allergens (house dust mite and cockroach) combined with exposure to high levels of these allergens is an important risk factor associated with symptomatic asthma. The implication is that exposure to indoor allergens may contribute to the development of asthma and that ongoing exposure or intermittent exposure may be a trigger factor for asthma.

*Allergen triggers and asthma*

Asthma has multiple triggers, the most important of these being viral infections and physical factors such as cold air and exercise. However, in individuals who have become sensitized to inhaled allergens, further allergen exposure may act as a trigger for asthma:

- Bronchial challenge studies show that acute bronchospasm can be induced in atopic asthmatics by inhalation of aeroallergens.
- Epidemics of asthma have been documented in association with airborne allergens.
- The level of exposure to indoor allergens has been correlated with the extent of asthma severity.
- In controlled settings asthmatic symptoms, peak expiratory flow rate and bronchial hyperresponsiveness improve when individuals avoid allergens to which they are allergic.

### Investigations

Demonstration of ASE (positive skin tests or UniCAP) may be useful in children who:

- present with the symptom complex of cough and/or wheeze and in whom the diagnosis of asthma may not be clear, because atopy is commonly associated with asthma
- have persistent asthma in association with allergic rhinitis. Determination of ASE to inhaled allergens could be considered part of routine asthma management in children with persistent asthma. Identification of those individuals sensitized to animal dander and house dust mite may be useful because allergen avoidance would be important for control of allergic rhinitis. Treatment of allergic rhinitis usually results in improvement of asthma.

Determination of ASE is not indicated in episodic asthma because viral infection is the most frequent trigger. However, if a specific inhaled allergen trigger is suspected from the history, ASE may be helpful.

### Management

The management of asthma depends on the frequency and severity of the condition. Episodic asthma may require intermittent treatment, whereas persistent asthma may require continuous treatment (see Chapter 14.3). Asthma education is critical and includes an explanation of the disease, education about techniques of using the inhalers and spacers, home monitoring, an explanation of the side-effects of medications, an action plan for home treatment, and education about allergen avoidance.

### Allergen identification and avoidance in asthma

Studies of house dust mite reduction in atopic asthmatics with persistent asthma have had variable results. It is clear that studies that have markedly reduced the exposure of asthmatics to house dust mite (e.g. by hospitalization) have shown an improvement in asthma. However, clinical trials that have aimed to reduce dust mite exposure in patients' homes have had more variable results, which probably correlate with the effectiveness of dust mite reduction methods. Although effective methods have been evaluated to reduce house dust mite levels, these are expensive and time-consuming and often not adhered to by patients (see Box 13.1.2). Removal of pets from the homes of sensitized asthmatics should be recommended, but occurs uncommonly.

Ingested allergens rarely trigger asthma as a sole manifestation. Other features of ingested allergens in relation to asthma are:

- acute bronchospasm – may be part of anaphylaxis in asthmatic children, but usually occurs with other manifestations of anaphylaxis, such as skin rash or vomiting
- a history from parents that cow's milk appears to cause respiratory tract symptoms, including asthma; however, empirical removal of cow's milk from the diet of children with asthma without such a history is not justified
- in some asthmatics, ingestion of metabisulphite can result in immediate bronchospasm. This is because of a pharmacological intolerance to metabisulphite, possibly as a result of direct irritation of the airway. Metabisulphite is a commonly used preservative in a number of food substances including meat, dried fruit, fruit juices and hot chips.

## Allergic rhinoconjunctivitis

See also Chapter 22.1.

### Definition and clinical presentation

Allergic rhinoconjunctivitis is rare in infants under 6 months old. Perennial allergic rhinoconjunctivitis may occur at any age in childhood, and seasonal allergic rhinoconjunctivitis often develops in older children.

The primary functions of the nose are olfaction and air filtration and humidification. This is achieved by the nasal structure, which ensures that inhaled air is in contact with an extensive and highly vascular mucosal membrane. In sensitized individuals, mucosal contact with inhaled allergens in the nose and conjunctiva elicits IgE-mediated mast cell degranulation and a chronic inflammatory response.

The history should determine the specific symptoms, as the presentation is quite variable, with either rhinitis or conjunctival symptoms predominating:

- The symptoms of allergic rhinitis are nasal obstruction, itch, sneezing and clear rhinorrhoea.
- Conjunctival symptoms include itching and an increase in tear fluid.

The timing of symptoms provides important information concerning possible triggers. Symptoms may be seasonal, perennial, a combination of perennial and seasonal, or episodic:

- Symptoms during spring, summer or autumn indicate seasonal allergic rhinoconjunctivitis, which may be triggered by pollen (grass, weed or tree) or mould.
- Perennial symptoms may be due to indoor allergens (house dust mite, animal dander, cockroach).
- Episodic symptoms are most often due to exposure to animal dander but may occur in response to other allergens.

Examination of the nose and eyes is important (see Table 13.1.4):

- The inferior nasal turbinates can be visualized with a light source (using an otoscope), with the diagnostic features being pallor and swelling. When severe, the swollen nasal turbinates may extend to the nasal septum and may be mistaken for nasal polyps, which are uncommon in children. Typical findings may not be present.
- Conjunctival injection and oedema affect both the bulbar and tarsal conjunctiva, and appear as redness and swelling.

Rhinitis symptoms may occur without evidence of an allergic cause (see Table 13.1.4). If nasal obstruction is the main symptom, it is important to exclude an anatomical cause. If symptoms such as sneezing, mucoid rhinorrhoea and/or obstruction are predominant, alternative diagnoses such as vasomotor or infective rhinitis need to be considered.

### Investigations

Determination of ASE is not indicated in seasonal allergic rhinitis unless symptoms are intractable and immunotherapy is being contemplated. ASE is indicated in perennial allergic rhinitis if symptoms are troublesome because, if specific IgE to an indoor allergen(s) can be demonstrated, a trial of allergen avoidance measures would be justified.

### Management

In children sensitized to indoor allergens a trial of avoidance measures should be instituted. The choice of symptomatic treatment depends on the nature, severity and timing of symptoms. Intermittent and infrequent symptoms can be treated with antihistamines. Prolonged symptoms are best treated with topical steroids combined with antihistamines if control is inadequate. For seasonal allergic rhinoconjunctivitis, treatment should be commenced before the onset of spring:

- Topical nasal corticosteroids are most effective for nasal obstructive symptoms but also reduce rhinorrhoea, sneezing and conjunctival symptoms. Steroids may take up to a week to work and may require prior use of a decongestant to allow adequate nasal delivery. In general, nasal steroids have been shown to be safe in children but epistaxis may be a problem in some children. This can be reduced by directing the nasal spray away from the nasal septum.
- Antihistamines (oral or topical) are useful for symptoms of rhinorrhoea, nasal or eye itch, and watery eyes, but are not effective for nasal obstruction. When given orally, non-sedating and long-acting antihistamines are preferred but often are more expensive.
- Use of nasal decongestants (vasoconstrictors), either topical or oral, for longer than 5 days should be discouraged.
- Conjunctival symptoms can be controlled with mast cell stabilizers or, if severe, short-term topical ocular steroid drops.

Immunotherapy should be considered in children with aero-allergen-induced seasonal allergic rhinoconjunctivitis who have failed to respond to symptomatic treatment, provided the selection criteria have been fulfilled.

## Complications of atopic disease and important associated conditions

A number of important conditions occur more commonly in children with atopic disease. The exceptions are medication and insect venom allergy, which are not more common in atopic children.

### Food allergy and intolerances

Adverse reactions to food are often reported in children with atopic disease. The important reactions to consider are food allergies and intolerances, particularly in infants and young children with atopic dermatitis (Table 13.1.6).

**Table 13.1.6 Food allergy versus food intolerance**

| | Food allergy | Food intolerance |
|---|---|---|
| **Mechanism** | Immune-mediated:<br>• IgE-mediated<br>• Non-IgE-mediated – cell-mediated | Non-immune-mediated:<br>• Pharmacological |
| **Food triggers** | **Food proteins**<br>• Cow's milk<br>• Egg<br>• Nuts<br>• Fish and shellfish<br>• Soy<br>• Wheat<br>• Fruits | **Food chemicals**<br>Food additives:<br>• Preservatives<br>• Food colourings<br>• Monosodium glutamate<br>Natural constituents:<br>• Salicylates<br>• Amines<br>• Monosodium glutamate |

Conversely, food is an uncommon trigger for asthma and allergic rhinitis. Food allergy and intolerance may occur in children without any atopic disease.

## Food allergy

*IgE-mediated food allergy*

It is important to recognize IgE-mediated food allergy in children with atopic disease:

- The condition is more common in infants and children with atopic dermatitis. In some studies of children presenting with atopic dermatitis up to one third may have an IgE-mediated food allergy.
- Those children who have asthma and IgE-mediated food allergy are at greater risk of experiencing more severe reactions, and rarely death from anaphylaxis may occur in this group of children.

*Diagnosis.* The diagnostic hallmark of IgE-mediated food allergy is that symptoms usually occur immediately (minutes to hours) after ingestion of the food. Although the most severe manifestation of IgE-mediated food allergy is anaphylaxis, a generalized or facial skin rash may be the sole manifestation. Anaphylaxis is a multisystem disorder characterized by respiratory and/or cardiac involvement, usually in combination with involvement of another system, most often the skin. The following symptoms and/or signs may occur with a generalized allergic reaction, including anaphylaxis:

- skin – generalized skin erythema, urticaria or angio-oedema
- respiratory system – rhinorrhoea, sneezing, cough, wheeze, stridor, respiratory distress
- gastrointestinal system – abdominal pain, vomiting, diarrhoea
- cardiovascular system – hypotension (if severe, collapse with loss of consciousness).

Up to 60% of children who have an IgE-mediated allergy to one food protein are allergic to another food, mainly cow's milk, egg, nuts, soy, fish and wheat. Hence, if an infant presents with a reaction to one food, it is always important to exclude others.

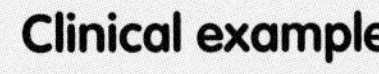

**Clinical example**

John, aged 12 years, had asthma. While swimming he was stung by a bee on his hand. Within 5 minutes he developed generalized urticaria, facial angio-oedema, cough, wheeze and difficulty breathing. An ambulance was called and intramuscular adrenaline (epinephrine) was administered, with resolution of John's symptoms.

Anaphylaxis is defined as a multisystem and generalized allergic reaction with involvement of the cardiorespiratory system. The emergency treatment is adrenaline, which initially is easily administered by the intramuscular route. The incidence of bee venom anaphylaxis is not increased in asthmatics. However, asthma is a risk factor for more severe episodes of anaphylaxis in anyone with a food, medication or insect venom allergy. For this reason, in someone who has asthma and anaphylaxis, first aid measures should be in place, including access to an adrenaline auto-injector device, which should be prescribed together with an anaphylaxis action plan. Immunotherapy is recommended for the long-term treatment of bee venom anaphylaxis.

*Non-IgE-mediated food allergies*

Non-IgE-mediated food allergies are thought to be mediated by cellular mechanisms, probably involving T lymphocytes. Cow or soy milk protein is the usual trigger, but other food proteins may be involved:

- Exacerbation of underlying atopic dermatitis, which usually presents as a delayed reaction hours after exposure to the offending food

- A number of gastrointestinal manifestations of non-IgE-mediated food allergy may occur:
  - cow's milk protein-induced colitis presents as a well infant with fresh blood in the stools, which resolves once cow's milk is excluded from the infant's diet or from the diet of the mother if breastfeeding
  - food protein-induced enterocolitis may present as sudden vomiting, dehydration and collapse, which may be mistaken for a gastroenteritis or bowel obstruction and occurs within hours of exposure to the food trigger
  - other manifestations include an enteropathy, which may present as failure to thrive, irritability, chronic diarrhoea and anaemia, or eosinophilic eosophagitis, which presents with abdominal pain, recurrent vomiting and dysphagia and may be mistaken for gastro-oesophageal reflux.

### Food intolerances

Food intolerances are thought to be pharmacological in nature. Important food intolerances in atopic children include:

- metabisulphite, a common food preservative, which may trigger acute wheeze in a small minority of children with asthma
- facial skin rashes, due to contact irritation from foods such as tomato and citrus, common in children with atopic dermatitis
- generalized exacerbations of eczema due to food intolerance have been proposed in children with atopic dermatitis, but the evidence is poor and this remains a controversial area.

### Investigation of food allergy and intolerance

The investigation of food allergy and intolerance is limited:

- If an adverse food reaction is thought to be IgE-mediated, determination of ASE is indicated. However, foods should not be excluded from the diet solely on the basis of a skin test or UniCAP.
- There are no validated tests for non-IgE-mediated food allergy or food intolerances. The only investigation is to demonstrate an improvement of symptoms following withdrawal of the food trigger and recurrence of symptoms with rechallenge. Double-blind and placebo-controlled challenges are preferable but are seldom available except in specialized facilities. An open and non-blind challenge is more practical but is less accurate.
- Empirical use of a diet that eliminates a number of naturally occurring food substances should never be instituted for more than 4 weeks and should be used as a diagnostic trial. If the child responds, this should be followed by appropriate challenges to identify specific food triggers.
- Unsubstantiated tests (e.g. Vega or cytotoxic tests) should never be used to diagnose food allergy or intolerance.

### Management

The only management available for food allergy or intolerance is exclusion of these foods from the child's diet. Additionally:

- education of the parents and other carers, particularly when young children attend childcare and kindergarten, is essential and may require the advice of a dietitian
- in breastfed infants with atopic dermatitis and food allergy, exclusion of food triggers from the maternal diet may also be tried, although this is best done with the support of a dietitian and may not be beneficial in all infants
- with any exclusion diet it is important to ensure that the diet is nutritionally adequate. This is particularly important as regards calcium intake when milk products are excluded.
- In atopic children who have had food anaphylaxis the following points are important:
  - anaphylaxis is a medical emergency and requires prompt recognition and treatment (Box 13.1.3)
  - all children should undergo subsequent specialist review
  - appropriate dietary advice is essential to avoid recurrent episodes
  - adrenaline (epinephrine) for first aid use by parents and other carers should be considered. This is prescribed most conveniently in the form of an auto-injector device. Appropriate training and documentation in the form of an anaphylaxis action plan is essential.

**Box 13.1.3 Emergency management of anaphylaxis**

1. Remove the trigger.
2. Administer adrenaline (epinephrine) by deep intramuscular injection: 0.01 mL/kg 1:1000 adrenaline (maximum dose 0.5 mL).
3. Establish an airway if required and administer oxygen.
4. Assess circulation. If hypotensive: administer IV fluids, normal saline 10–20 mL/kg as a bolus.
5. Repeat doses of intramuscular adrenaline can be administered every 5 min until clinical improvement occurs. Consider intravenous adrenaline if hypotension and poor response to IV fluids and intramuscular adrenaline.
6. Antihistamines and steroids are not administered for the initial management but should be given as second-line therapy.

## Clinical example

Justine was 12 months old and was known to have atopic dermatitis. She had been otherwise well and her weight was 10 kg. She was breastfed and, because her mother was about to return to work, Justine was offered her first bottle-feed containing a cow's milk protein formula. Immediately after drinking a small amount she became irritable, vomited and then developed generalized urticaria, a persistent cough, difficulty breathing and stridor.

Justine had experienced an anaphylactic reaction to cow's milk protein. Although this was the first apparent exposure, she was likely to have been exposed to cow's milk protein in maternal breast milk.

Adrenaline (epinephrine) is required for the emergency management and is most easily administered by deep intramuscular injection (0.01 mL/kg of 1 : 1000 (i.e. 0.1 mL at Justine's weight of 10.0 kg). The response is usually rapid but the dose can be repeated until a clinical response is obtained.

It was important to ensure that the family was educated regarding subsequent exclusion of cows' milk from Justine's diet. Tolerance to cow's milk develops by school age in the majority of children. Approximately 60% of children with a cow's milk allergy may have an allergy to other foods – most commonly egg and nuts. Therefore, a careful history should be taken to ensure that these foods have been ingested and tolerated. If there has been no ingestion (for example of nuts), the options of determining IgE to these foods (by a skin prick test or UniCAP) or a graded home introduction can be discussed with the family.

### Prognosis

The natural history of food allergy and intolerances is to improve with increasing age. Therefore, carefully supervised challenge with the implicated food at 12-month intervals is recommended. Determination of ASE may predict when it is appropriate to consider a challenge. IgE-mediated nut, fish and shellfish allergies may require a challenge less frequently because these allergies may be lifelong, although tolerance may develop in up to 10% of children.

## Recurrent or chronic sinusitis in allergic rhinitis

Allergic rhinitis should be considered as a possible predisposing factor in children who:

- have recurrent or chronic sinusitis. The orifices of the frontal, ethmoid and maxillary sinuses are located in close proximity to the nasal turbinates, and rhinitis may predispose to ostial obstruction. Symptoms of sinusitis in older children and adults are typical, and include facial pain, toothache, headache and fever (see Chapter 22.1). However, young children may present with rhinorrhoea, cough, post-nasal discharge, periorbital swelling and otitis media
- have secretory otitis media, in whom the incidence of atopy is increased. However, it remains unclear whether allergic rhinitis is a significant underlying factor because of eustachian tube obstruction. If indicated, allergic rhinitis should be treated in such children, but this may not improve the secretory otitis media.

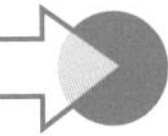

## Practical points

- The atopic diseases of childhood are eczema, asthma and allergic rhinitis. The majority of children who have these conditions will be atopic – have allergen-specific IgE (ASE) to one or more common allergens.
- The presence of ASE does not always indicate an allergen trigger, and should be interpreted together with the history and/or a trial of allergen avoidance with or without subsequent challenges.
- The management of atopic disease includes identification and avoidance of allergens (if possible), symptomatic treatment and immunotherapy for selected children.
- Anaphylaxis is a generalized multisystem allergic reaction, which includes cardiorespiratory involvement.
- The emergency treatment of anaphylaxis is adrenaline (epinephrine), which, unless hypotension is present, can be administered via the intramuscular route.
- All children with anaphylaxis should undergo a specialist review so that the trigger can be identified, avoidance strategies implemented and first aid measures established, including use of injectable adrenaline.

## Obstructive sleep apnoea in allergic rhinitis

Nasopharyngeal obstruction in children may present with snoring and, if severe, obstructive sleep apnoea (OSA). OSA may present in children with early morning headache, daytime sleepiness and poor concentration. Children who present with allergic rhinitis should be questioned about these symptoms, and those children presenting with upper airway obstruction should be evaluated and, if needed, treated for allergic rhinitis.

## Skin infection in atopic dermatitis

Bacterial, viral and fungal skin infection is an important complication of atopic dermatitis:

- *Staphylococcus aureus* is detected almost universally in atopic dermatitis. The organism produces exotoxins, which may potentiate the inflammatory process. Topical antiseptic measures are important but oral antibiotics may be required.
- Herpes simplex virus (HSV) type I may infect lesions and present as vesicular lesions, which soon ulcerate. Generalized HSV skin infection may be severe and would be an indication for hospitalization and parenteral aciclovir.
- Dermatophyte infections may occur in atopic dermatitis and should be considered in resistant lesions.

### Spasmodic croup

Spasmodic croup is a condition of recurrent sudden upper airway obstruction that presents as stridor and cough, usually in the early hours of the morning (see Chapter 14.2). Typically, the condition is short-lived and there are no features to suggest an infective laryngotracheobronchitis such as fever or coryza. Approximately 50% of these children have an atopic disease. The condition is managed symptomatically and there is no evidence to suggest that measures such as allergen avoidance or symptomatic treatment with antihistamines are useful.

# 13.2 Immunodeficiency and its investigation

Melanie Wong

Recurrent infections, especially in the small child, are common. It can be challenging, but important, to determine which children warrant investigation to exclude an underlying immunodeficiency, and which tests are most appropriate. Primary immunodeficiencies (PID) are rare, but with increasing physician and community awareness and rapid technological advances, the number of recognized genetic defects predisposing to infection risk is increasing exponentially. Some defects are essential to diagnose early, with appropriate treatment influencing morbidity and mortality. Others contribute to our understanding of the complexity of the immune response, allow tailoring of treatment and provide an explanation to concerned families.

Susceptibility to infection varies, influenced by age, genetic and environmental factors, including atopy, siblings, daycare, exposure to cigarette smoke, drug therapies and anatomical variations, all secondary factors that may be the sole cause of increased manifestations of infection, or contribute to the severity of an underlying primary immune defect. Despite the emphasis on primary disease, the clinical significance of secondary immunodeficiencies cannot be underestimated.

The aim of this chapter is to provide an approach for differentiating primary immunodeficiency from other factors predisposing to a real or apparent increased risk of infection, based on history, examination and appropriate initial investigation. A selection of PIDs will be highlighted but it is beyond the scope of this chapter to discuss in depth the pathophysiology and specialized treatment of these disorders, or specifically to cover all potential PIDs. A list of recent references is provided for further reading.

## Host factors and resistance to infection

Immune defence is provided by multiple well-orchestrated components, which can be categorized into two main groups:

1. Innate, non-antigen-specific responses are initiated early. There are an increasing number of recognized components, including:
   - barriers: epithelial surfaces, mucosal barriers
   - secretions: saliva, respiratory secretions, tears, urine
   - normal microbial flora: gastrointestinal, genital tract
   - phagocytic cells: neutrophils, macrophages
   - natural killer cells
   - proteins: complement, mannose-binding lectin, antimicrobial peptides
   - pattern recognition receptors: toll-like receptors and the associated transcription pathways.
2. Adaptive, antigen-specific immune responses are the basis of immunological memory and are essential for maturation of protective immune responses and efficacy of vaccination. The components are:
   - T cells: cellular immunity
   - B cells and antibody: humoral immunity.

Deficiencies or disruption of any of these components can predispose to infection. These defects may be the result of immaturity, primary or acquired deficiency, influencing age and severity of presentation as well as management and prognosis. Some disorders will result in localized disease, whereas others predispose to infection with specific microorganisms, as shown in Figure 13.2.1.

### The influence of atopy

When recurrent respiratory infections are the sole infectious manifestation, allergy must be considered. Features that suggest an allergic or atopic condition may be responsible include absence of fever, clear non-purulent discharge, personal and/or family history of atopic conditions such as eczema, food allergies, asthma and allergic rhinitis, seasonal or exposure-related pattern, variable response to antibiotics, and good response to antihistamines, bronchodilators and/or topical steroids. In addition, atopic tendencies can prolong and adversely modify the severity of otherwise minor, often viral, infections for which antibiotics may be prescribed, contributing to the perception of frequent severe infection.

### Acquisition of immunological memory

The adaptive immune response develops with recurrent exposure to infection. Primary exposure often resulting in clinical infection occurs most frequently in infancy and early childhood. Secondary exposure in the presence of an intact adaptive immune system, results in a more rapid and efficient response, and avoidance of subsequent infection in older children and adults. In association with increasing exposure,

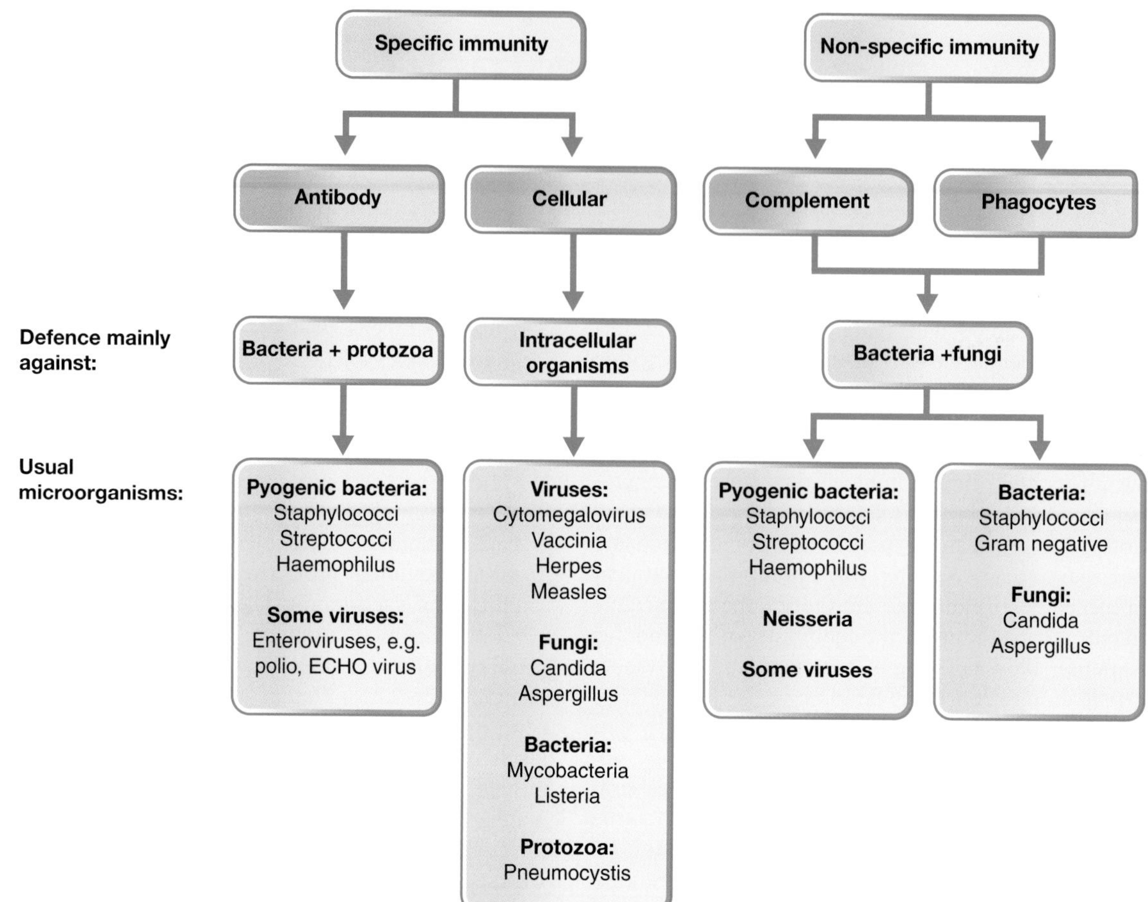


Fig. 13.2.1 Common infections associated with immunodeficiency.

this results in the peak number of infections between the ages of 2 and 4 years, with an average of six infections a year. Existence of siblings, daycare attendance and exposure to cigarette smoke further increase this number. Children attending daycare or preschool can experience 10 to 12 upper respiratory tract infections and 1 to 2 gastrointestinal tract infections per year.

The induction of immunological memory is the principle underlying vaccination. Not only does vaccination enable protection from and/or attenuation of the severity of targeted infections, measurement of specific antibody levels after vaccination provides a means by which the function of the immune system can be assessed.

### Age of presentation, infective complications and diagnosis

Deficiencies of humoral immunity typically present after the age of 4–5 months, when maternally-derived antibody has waned. Significant deficiencies of T-cell function present earlier, within the first months. The type of infection(s) as well as associated clinical features may provide clues to the deficient immune component (see Fig. 13.2.1, Table 13.2.1). In children presenting with recurrent fever without obvious and/or identifiable infection, the possibility of an autoinflammatory syndrome should be considered. Many primary immunodeficiencies present in infancy with dermatological manifestations such as severe or atypical eczema, thrombocytopenic purpura, recalcitrant candidiasis and abscesses. Some are diagnosed in association with other conditions such as cardiac, endocrine and neurological anomalies (e.g. DiGeorge syndrome, ataxia telangiectasia). Conditions such as common variable immunodeficiency, natural killer cell and complement deficiencies can present at a range of ages, from late infancy to young adulthood.

## Defects associated with prematurity and delays in immunological development

In the absence of intrauterine infection, the fetus exists in a sterile environment until birth, at which time specific immune responses begin to develop. Active transplacental transport of immunoglobulin (Ig) G (but not IgA, IgM or IgE) occurs during the third trimester, providing humoral protection to the newborn.

**Table 13.2.1 Clinical features suggestive of some immune defects**

| Clinical feature | Immunodeficiency |
|---|---|
| Recurrent sinopulmonary infections/chronic diarrhoea and failure to thrive (and, less commonly, cytopenias, arthritis, hepatitis, coeliac disease, inflammatory bowel disease, granuloma formation, malignancy) | Humoral |
| Recurrent fungal, opportunistic infections/chronic diarrhoea, failure to thrive, neonatal hypocalcaemia | Cellular |
| Recurrent periodontal disease, gingivitis, skin and deep abscesses, fungal pneumonia, osteomyelitis | Phagocytic |
| Recurrent or severe meningococcal or pneumococcal infection | Complement |

Physiological hypogammaglobulinaemia of infancy occurs between 3 and 6 months of life at the nadir of waning maternal IgG balanced by increasing infant production of IgG (Fig. 13.2.2). This can be accentuated and prolonged in premature infants by a reduced store of maternally derived IgG, or alternatively by delay in IgG production, the latter termed transient hypogammaglobulinaemia of infancy.

In most cases, these measurable abnormalities are asymptomatic and resolve completely, usually by 9–15 months of age, but in some cases low levels of IgG, and sometimes also IgA and IgM, may persist for longer. With more sophisticated follow-up, spontaneous resolution has been documented up to the end of the first decade. Immunoglobulin replacement therapy may rarely be required in affected infants experiencing significant infections despite prophylactic antibiotics, such as co-trimoxazole. If commenced, a trial of cessation of intravenous immunoglobulin (IVIG) should be undertaken after a period free of significant infection. A small number of these children continue to have immune abnormalities and require ongoing IVIG, the diagnosis evolving to common variable immunodeficiency (CVID). This diagnosis cannot be made definitively before the age of 2 years.

T cell-independent antibody responses, for example to polysaccharide antigens, which are important for humoral protection from encapsulated microorganisms such as pneumococcus, *Haemophilus* and meningococcus, are poor in infants aged less than 2 years. Protein-conjugated vaccines induce T cell-dependent antibody production in younger infants, enabling vaccination from 2 months of age.

Neonates have relatively low levels of complement and impairment of neutrophil chemotaxis, both of

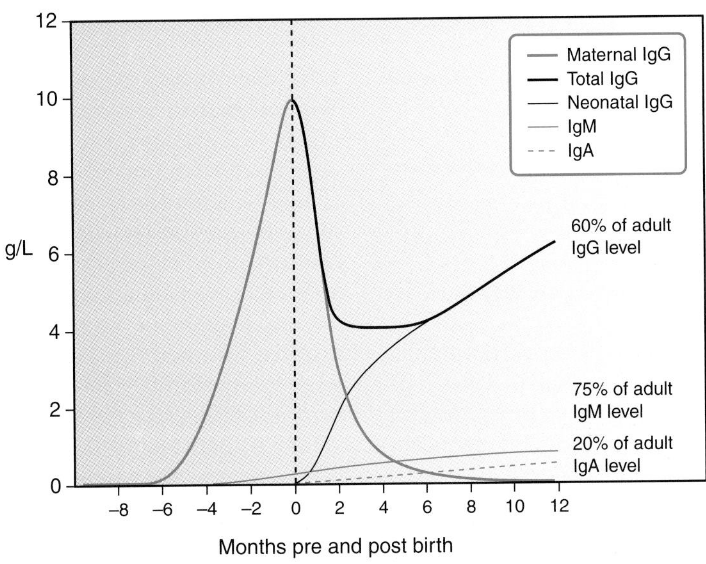


Fig. 13.2.2 Evolution of serum immunoglobulin (Ig)G, IgA and IgM levels *in utero* and during the first year after birth, illustrating the contribution of maternal and neonatal IgG. Levels of IgM reach adult equivalents by approximately 3 years of age, IgG by 5–6 years and IgA by 9–12 years.

which mature rapidly during early infancy. T-cell proliferative responses are reasonable but cytokine production, particularly of proinflammatory (T-helper type 1, Th1) cytokines such as interferon (IFN)-γ, is immature, which may compromise T-cell help. This immaturity may persist in some infants with an atopic tendency, potentially contributing to infection risk.

**Clinical example**

Thomas presented at 12 months of age with a history of six episodes of otitis media associated with green nasal discharge since the age of 6 months. Each responded to antibiotics with recurrence soon after cessation. There was discharge from the left ear on two occasions from which *Streptococcus pneumoniae* and non-typeable *Haemophilus influenzae* were isolated. Thomas was thriving and had no other symptoms. He was an only child, his immunizations were up to date, and he did not attend daycare. There was no significant family history.

Examination revealed a perforated left tympanic membrane. Tonsillar tissue was present. Full blood count was unremarkable. Serum IgG (2.5 g/L, normal range 3.4–11.6 g/L) and IgA (0.1 g/L, normal range 0.2–1.2 g/L) were moderately reduced but IgM level was normal for age. Both IgG1 and IgG2 levels were slightly below the normal range. T-and B-cell numbers were normal. Levels of antibodies to vaccine antigens (tetanus, diphtheria, and conjugated *Haemophilus influenzae* B and pneumococcal vaccines) were acceptable.

A provisional diagnosis of transient hypogammaglobulinaemia of infancy was made. A trial of prophylactic, daily, low-dose co-trimoxazole successfully prevented further recurrences of ear infection, until an attempt to cease therapy after a year. Antibiotic prophylaxis was ceased uneventfully at 3 years of age. Serum IgG and IgA levels rose gradually into the lower end of the normal range by the age of 2 and 5 years respectively.

## Primary and secondary immunodeficiencies

More than 150 primary immunodeficiencies (PID) have been identified and characterized, and the number is growing constantly. An expert international committee of the International Union of Immunological Societies (IUIS) meets regularly to update continually the known primary immunodeficiencies and, where identified, the underlying genetic cause. The publication by Notarangelo and co-workers, summarizing the most recent meeting in 2009, contains detailed tables summarizing clinical features, laboratory findings, genetics and relative frequency of known PIDs. Although, individually, most are rare or extremely rare, many affect similar pathways or categories of immune function and thus collectively are not uncommon. Table 13.2.2 lists these conditions as categorized by IUIS and, where known, the mode of inheritance.

An underlying PID may be suggested by the frequency, severity and type of infection, the response or lack of response to antimicrobial therapy, associated failure to thrive and existence of significant family history (Box 13.2.1).

Secondary immunodeficiency, usually as a result of suppression, reduced production or loss of components of the immune system, is much more common. Important causes, listed in Box 13.2.2, include prematurity, metabolic diseases, infiltrative diseases and their treatment, malnutrition, infection, trauma, immunosuppressive therapy and ageing.

### Investigations

The proportion of PIDs in each of the categories listed in Table 13.2.2 has been calculated from data derived from four major international PID registries: European Society for Immunodeficiencies (ESID), Latin American Group for Primary Immunodeficiencies (LAGID), Australia and New Zealand, and Iranian registries. Predominantly antibody deficiencies accounted for 56%, combined antibody and cellular deficiencies for 8.4%, other well defined immunodeficiencies 18.3%, diseases of immune dysregulation 2.7%, disorders of phagocytic cells 11.2%, defects of innate immunity 0.4%, and complement defects for 2.5% of all reported cases. As most of the first three categories affect humoral immune responses, screening of antibody levels will detect a large proportion of cases. Blood count and film will identify patients with asplenia, neutropenia, neutrophil granule abnormalities and thrombocytopenia associated with small platelet size, the latter features pathognomic of Wiskott–Aldrich syndrome. Second-tier investigations (Table 13.2.3), some of which are available only from specialized laboratories, will depend on clinical suspicion of either humoral, cellular, phagocytic or complement abnormalities. Genetic testing may be available to confirm some PIDs and/or used for genetic counselling and future prenatal testing.

Consideration of age-related reference ranges are essential for interpretation of serum immunoglobulin levels (particularly the IgG subclass), lymphocyte numbers and subset analyses. However, there is significant variability in the rate of rise in levels as well as biological fluctuations over time. The division of age groups for each reference range is arbitrary, such that children at the boundaries of age groups may be erroneously affected. This may not be obvious to the requesting clinician because reference ranges are usually reported without information regarding the actual age range or the reference range of adjacent age groups. Thus normal

**Table 13.2.2 International Union of Immunological Societies (IUIS) classification of primary immunodeficiencies**

| Disease | Inheritance |
|---|---|
| **Combined T- and B-cell immunodeficiency** | |
| $T^-$ $B^+$ SCID | |
| γc deficiency | XL |
| JAK3 deficiency | AR |
| IL-7 receptor α deficiency | AR |
| CD45 deficiency | AR |
| CD3δ/CD3ε/CD3ζ deficiency | AR |
| Coronin-1A deficiency | AR |
| $T^-$ $B^-$ SCID | |
| RAG1/RAG2 deficiency | AR |
| DCLREIC (Artemis) deficiency | AR |
| DNA $PK_{cs}$ deficiency | AR |
| Adenosine deaminase (ADA) deficiency | AR |
| Reticular dysgenesis | AR |
| Omenn syndrome | AR (most) |
| DNA ligase IV deficiency | AR |
| Cernunnos deficiency | AR |
| CD40 ligand deficiency | XL |
| CD40 deficiency | AR |
| Purine nucleoside phosphorylase deficiency | AR |
| CD3γ deficiency | AR |
| CD8 deficiency | AR |
| ZAP-70 deficiency | AR |
| $Ca^{2+}$ channel deficiency | AR |
| MHC class I deficiency | AR |
| MHC class II deficiency | AR |
| Winged helix deficiency (nude) | AR |
| CD25 deficiency | AR |
| STAT5b deficiency | AR |
| Itk deficiency | AR |
| DOCK8 deficiency | AR |
| **Predominantly antibody deficiencies** | |
| Severe reduction in all serum Ig isotypes with profoundly decreased or absent B cells | |
| Btk deficiency | XL |
| μ heavy chain deficiency | AR |
| λ5 deficiency | AR |
| Igα deficiency | AR |
| Igβ deficiency | AR |
| BLNK deficiency | AR |
| Thymoma with immunodeficiency | None |
| Severe reduction in at least 2 serum Ig isotypes with normal or low numbers of B cells | |
| Common variable immunodeficiency disorders | Variable |
| ICOS deficiency | AR |
| CD19 deficiency | AR |
| TACI deficiency | AD or AR |
| BAFF receptor deficiency | AR |
| Severe reduction in serum IgG and IgA with normal/raised IgM and normal B-cell numbers | |
| CD40L deficiency | XL |
| CD40 deficiency | AR |
| AID deficiency | AR |
| UNG deficiency | AR |
| Isotype or light chain deficiencies with normal numbers of B cells | |
| Ig heavy chain mutations or deletions | AR |
| κ chain deficiency | AR |
| Isolated IgG subclass deficiency | Variable |
| IgA with IgG subclass deficiency | Variable |
| Selective IgA deficiency | Variable |
| Specific antibody deficiency with normal Ig concentrations and normal B cell numbers | Variable |
| Transient hypogammaglobulinaemia of infancy with normal B-cell numbers | Variable |
| **Other well-defined immunodeficiency syndromes** | |
| Wiskott-Aldrich syndrome | XL |
| DNA repair defects | |
| Ataxia telangectasia | AR |
| Ataxia telangectasia-like disease | AR |
| Nijmegen breakage syndrome | AR |
| Bloom syndrome | AR |
| Immunodeficiency with centromeric instability and facial anomalies (ICF) | AR |
| PMS2 deficiency | AR |
| Thymic defects | |
| DiGeorge anomaly | *De novo*/AD |
| Immune osseous dysplasias | |
| Cartilage hair hypoplasia | AR |
| Schimke syndrome | AR |
| Comel–Netherton syndrome | AR |
| Hyper-IgE syndromes (HIES) | |
| AD-HIES | AD |
| AR-HIES | AR |
| Chronic mucocutaneous candidiasis | AD/AR/sporadic |
| Hepatic veno-occlusive disease with immunodeficiency | AR |
| XL dyskeratosis congenita | XL |
| **Diseases of immune dysregulation** | |
| Immunodeficiency with hypopigmentation | |
| Chediak–Higashi syndrome | AR |
| Griscelli syndrome, type 2 | AR |
| Hermansky–Pudlak syndrome, type 2 | AR |
| Familial haemophagocytic lymphohistiocytosis | |
| Perforin deficiency | AR |
| UNC13-D deficiency | AR |
| Syntaxin 11 deficiency | AR |
| Lymphoproliferative syndromes | |
| XLP1, SH2D1A deficiency | XL |
| XLP2, XIAP deficiency | XL |
| Itk deficiency | AR |
| Syndromes with autoimmunity | |
| Autoimmune lymphoproliferative syndrome (ALPS) | |
| CD95 (Fas) defects, ALPS type 1a | AD |
| CD95L (Fas ligand) defects, ALPS type 1b | AR |
| Caspase 10 deficiency, ALPS type 2a | AR |
| Caspase 8 deficiency, ALPS type 2b | AR |
| Activating N-ras, N-ras-dependent ALPS | AD |
| APECED (autoimmune polyendocrinopathy with candidiasis and ectodermal dystrophy) | AR |
| IPEX (immune dysregulation, polyendocrinopathy, enteropathy, X-linked) | XL |
| CD25 deficiency | AR |

(Continued)

**Table 13.2.2 International Union of Immunological Societies (IUIS) classification of primary immunodeficiencies—cont'd**

| Disease | Inheritance |
|---|---|
| **Congenital defects of phagocyte number, function or both** | |
| Severe congenital neutropenias | AD |
| Kostman disease | AR |
| Neutropenia with cardiac and urogenital malformations | AR |
| Glycogen storage disease type 1b | AR |
| Cyclic neutropenia | AD |
| X-linked neutropenia/myelodysplasia | XL |
| P14 deficiency | AR |
| Leukocyte adhesion deficiency type 1 | AR |
| Leukocyte adhesion deficiency type 2 | AR |
| Leukocyte adhesion deficiency type 3 | AR |
| Rac2 deficiency | AD |
| β-Actin deficiency | AD |
| Localized juvenile periodontitis | AR |
| Papillon–Lefèvre syndrome | AR |
| Specific granule deficiency | AR |
| Schwachman–Diamond syndrome | AR |
| X-linked chronic granulomatous disease | XL |
| Autosomal chronic granulomatous diseases | AR |
| IL-12 and IL-23 receptor β1-chain deficiency | AR |
| IL-12p40 deficiency | AR |
| IFN-γ receptor 1 deficiency | AR, AD |
| IFN-γ receptor 2 deficiency | AR |
| STAT1 deficiency | AR |
| AR hyper-IgE syndrome | AR |
| AD hyper-IgE syndrome | AD |
| Pulmonary alveolar proteinosis | Bi-allelic |
| **Defects in innate immunity** | |
| Anhidrotic ectodermal dysplasia with immunodeficiency (EDA-ID) | XL |
| AD EDA-ID | AD |
| IL-1 receptor-associated kinase 4 (IRAK4) | AR |
| deficiency | AR |
| MyD88 deficiency | AD |
| WHIM (warts, hypogammaglobulinaemia, infections, myelokathexis syndrome) | |
| Epidermodysplasia verruciformis | AR |
| Herpes simplex encephalitis (HSE) – UNC93B1 | AR |
| HSE – TLR3 | AD |
| Chronic mucocutaneous candidiasis – CARD9 | AR |
| Trypanosomiasis | AD |

| Disease | Inheritance |
|---|---|
| **Autoinflammatory disorders** | |
| Familial Mediterranean fever | AR |
| TNF receptor-associated periodic fever syndrome (TRAPS) | AD |
| Hyper-IgD syndrome | AR |
| Muckle–Wells syndrome | AD |
| Familial cold autoinflammatory syndrome | AD |
| NOMID/CINCA | AD |
| Pyogenic sterile arthritis, pyoderma gangrenosum, acne (PAPA) syndrome | AD |
| Blau syndrome | AD |
| Chronic recurrent multifocal osteomyelitis and congenital dyserythropoietic anaemia (Majeed) | AR |
| DIRA (deficiency of IL-1 receptor antagonist) | AR |
| **Complement deficiencies** | |
| C1q deficiency | AR |
| C1r deficiency | AR |
| C1s deficiency | AR |
| C4 deficiency | AR |
| C2 deficiency | AR |
| C3 deficiency | AR |
| C5 deficiency | AR |
| C6 deficiency | AR |
| C7 deficiency | AR |
| C8 deficiency | AR |
| C9 deficiency | AR |
| C1 inhibitor deficiency | AD |
| Factor I deficiency | AR |
| Factor H deficiency | AR |
| Factor D deficiency | AR |
| Properdin deficiency | AR |
| Mannose-binding lectin deficiency | AR |
| MASP2 deficiency | AR |
| Complement receptor 3 (CR3) deficiency | AR |
| Membrane cofactor protein (CD46) deficiency | AD |
| Membrane attack complex inhibitor (CD59) deficiency | AR |
| Paroxysmal nocturnal haemoglobinuria | Acquired |
| Immunodeficiency associated with ficolin-3 deficiency | AR |

AD, autosomal dominant; AR, autosomal recessive; IFN, interferon; Ig, immunoglobulin; IL, interleukin; XL, X-linked.
Modified from: Notarangelo LD, Fischer A, Geha RS et al 2009 Primary immunodeficiencies: 2009 update. *Journal of Allergy and Clinical Immunology* 124:1161–1178.

screening tests, particularly at the lower end of the reference range, in the presence of a suspicious clinical picture, should not prevent specialist referral.

Many primary immunodeficiencies are associated with an increased risk of malignancy. Thus, where possible, exposure to excess radiation should be avoided. The indication for each chest X-ray and computed tomography scan, especially repeated high-resolution scans to assess the presence of bronchiectasis, should be considered carefully.

**Box 13.2.1 Warning signs of primary immunodeficiency**

Patients are advised to seek medical review if affected by 2 or more of the following 10 warning signs of primary immunodeficiency (Jeffrey Modell Foundation, New York):

1. Eight or more new ear infections within 1 year
2. Two or more serious sinus infections within 1 year
3. Two or more months on antibiotics with little effect
4. Two or more pneumonias within 1 year
5. Failure of an infant to gain weight or grow normally
6. Recurrent, deep skin or organ abscesses
7. Persistent thrush in the mouth or on the skin, after age 1 year
8. Need for intravenous antibiotics to clear infections
9. Two or more deep-seated infections such as meningitis, osteomyelitis, cellulitis or sepsis
10. A family history of primary immunodeficiency

### Treatment

Management will depend on the diagnosis but may include:

- awareness of types of infection most likely for that PID
- early, appropriate antibiotic treatment
- prophylactic therapy – for example, co-trimoxazole for chronic granulomatous disease (CGD) and severe combined immunodeficiency (SCID), antifungals for CGD and mucocutaneous candidiasis (MCC), IFN-$\gamma$ for CGD
- awareness and management of autoimmune and atopic disease complications, for example in common variable immunodeficiency (CVID) and Wiskott–Aldrich syndrome (WAS)
- immunoglobulin replacement therapy, mostly as a monthly intravenous infusion in hospital, but increasingly via subcutaneous infusion at home
- avoidance of live vaccinations where a T-cell defect is suspected and live polio vaccination in hypogammaglobulinaemia. Routine immunization is unnecessary when receiving immunoglobulin replacement therapy and any potential response may be inhibited. However, influenza vaccination may be of benefit in some patients, such as those with CVID
- bone marrow transplantation, for example in SCID or WAS
- gene therapy for some rare PIDs – gene therapy for X-linked SCID has been the most successful to date, but remains experimental in view of ongoing safety and technical concerns.

## Specific primary immunodeficiency disorders

Examples of some important primary immunodeficiency disorders are discussed.

### Predominantly antibody deficiencies

#### X-linked agammaglobulinaemia/Btk deficiency

Affected boys have a defect in *BTK* (Bruton tyrosine kinase) gene on the X chromosome. The gene product, Btk, has a major role in activated B-cell receptor

**Box 13.2.2 Secondary immunodeficiency**

**Premature and newborn**

**Hereditary and metabolic diseases**
- Chromosomal abnormalities (e.g. Down syndrome)
- Uraemia
- Diabetes mellitus
- Malnutrition
- Vitamin and mineral deficiencies
- Protein-losing enteropathies
- Nephrotic dystrophy
- Myotonic dystrophy
- Sickle cell disease

**Immunosuppressive agents**
- Radiation
- Immunosuppressive drugs
- Corticosteroids
- Anti-lymphocyte or anti-thymocyte globulin
- Anti-T- or B-cell monoclonal antibodies

**Surgery and trauma**
- Burns
- Splenectomy
- Anaesthesia
- Head injury

**Infectious diseases**
- Congenital rubella
- Viral exanthema – measles, varicella
- HIV infection, AIDS
- Cytomegalovirus
- Infectious mononucleosis
- Bacterial infections
- Mycobacterial, fungal or parasitic diseases

**Infiltrative and haematological diseases**
- Histiocytosis
- Sarcoidosis
- Hodgkin's disease and lymphoma
- Leukaemia
- Myeloma
- Agranulocytosis and aplastic anaemia
- Lymphoma in immunocompromised transplant recipients

**Miscellaneous**
- Lupus erythematosus
- Chronic active hepatitis
- Alcoholic cirrhosis
- Ageing

**Table 13.2.3 Investigations for immunodeficiency**

| Test | Suspected deficiency |
|---|---|
| **Screening** | |
| Blood count and film | |
| Immunoglobulin G, A and M levels | |
| **Second tier dependent on clinical suspicions** | |
| Immunoglobulin G subclass titres (IgG 1, 2, 3, 4) | H, Com |
| Immunoglobulin E | H, Com, N |
| Isohaemagglutinins | H, Com |
| Specific antibody titres | H, Com |
| • After routine vaccinations – tetanus, diphtheria, Hib, pneumococcal | |
| • After pneumococcal polysaccharide vaccine – non-conjugate vaccine serotypes | |
| Lymphocyte subsets (T, B and NK cell) | H, C, Com |
| Check chest X-ray for thymus (neonates and young infants) | C, Com |
| Lymphocyte proliferation to mitogens (e.g. PHA, ConA) (non-specific) | C, Com |
| Lymphocyte proliferation to specific antigens (e.g. *Candida*) | C, Com |
| Adenosine deaminase and purine nucleotide phosphorylase measurements | C, Com |
| Neutrophil function testing | N |
| • Nitroblue tetrozolium (NBT)/equivalent dihydrorhodamine (DHR)-based assay | |
| • More extensive testing of chemiluminescence, chemotaxis | |
| • Surface expression of CD11 and CD18 | |
| NK cell cytotoxicity | NK |
| Complement testing | Complement |
| C3, C4, CH50 (AH50, specific complement components) | |
| C1 esterase inhibitor and function | C1-INH |
| HIV testing | C, Com |
| Genetic studies | |

C, cellular; Com, combined humoral and cellular; ConA, concanavalin A; H, humoral; HIV, human immunodeficiency virus; INH, inhibitor; N, neutrophil/phagocyte; NK, natural killer cell; PHA, phytohaemagglutinin.

signalling and is required for normal B-cell development. In X-linked agammaglobulinaemia (XLA), precursor cells in the marrow fail to develop into mature circulating B cells. Absence of peripheral mature B cells is also a feature of several rarer autosomal recessive forms of early-onset hypogammaglobulinaemia with clinical features similar to XLA, but also affecting girls (see Table 13.2.2).

Most boys with XLA are asymptomatic for the first 4–6 months of life. Nearly all develop symptoms by 18 months of age, and the diagnosis is usually made within the first 3 years of life. The commonest manifestations are recurrent mucopurulent otitis media, upper and lower respiratory tract infections with common respiratory tract organisms, in particular *Streptococcus pneumoniae* and *Haemophilus influenzae* type b, despite vaccination, as well as *Staphylococcus aureus* infections. Resolution is often slow and incomplete, eventually leading to bronchiectasis in the absence of intervention. Meningitis, septicaemia, diarrhoea, aseptic mono- or oligo-articular arthritis, septic arthritis, osteomyelitis, chronic or recurrent conjunctivitis, and chronic or disseminated enteroviral infection occur more frequently.

The most useful clinical feature is absent or markedly hypoplastic tonsils. Serum IgG levels are markedly reduced with undetectable IgA and IgM. There is an absence of circulating B cells and no functional/specific antibody response to common antigens such as tetanus and diphtheria vaccination. Absent Btk expression can be demonstrated on flow cytometry and *BTK* mutations on genetic testing, both of which detect female carrier status. If prenatal diagnosis is not undertaken, newborn males with a family history can be screened non-invasively for absent cord blood B cells. Early diagnosis allows institution of therapy before the development of infective complications.

Early commencement of lifelong immunoglobulin replacement therapy will minimize complications, significantly reducing the incidence of chronic lung disease and prolonging life expectancy. However, as these infusions replace only IgG, recurrent conjunctivitis and diarrhoea may not be eliminated because secretory IgA function is not restored. The usual dose is 400 mg/kg intravenously every 4 weeks, but varies to maintain adequate trough IgG levels and to prevention infection. This 4-week interval between infusions is based on a half-life of IgG in normal individuals of 21–28 days, but some individuals require more frequent infusions. Alternatively immunoglobulin replacement can be given by subcutaneous infusions once to three times a week, facilitating administration at home. Specific infections are treated with appropriate antibiotics.

### Hyper-IgM syndrome

Most cases of hyper-IgM syndrome are X-linked, and are secondary to mutations in the CD40 ligand gene. Hyper-IgM syndrome is characterized by defective B-cell switching from IgM to IgG and IgA production, as well as abnormalities of T-cell function. An autosomal recessive form secondary to mutations in the CD40 gene has similar clinical features, whereas there is no T-cell dysfunction in the other known recessive forms, AID and UNG deficiency. Raised IgM levels can also be found in other immunodeficiencies such as CVID and anhidrotic ectodermal dysplasia with immunodeficiency (NEMO deficiency).

The spectrum of respiratory infections is similar to that observed in XLA, but *Pneumocystis* pneumonia is a frequent presentation. Intermittent or persistent neutropenia commonly causes oral and upper gastrointestinal tract ulceration. Haemolytic anaemia, thrombocytopenia, nephritis and arthritis also occur. Infection with *Cryptosporidium* is common and may lead to sclerosing cholangitis.

Serum IgA and IgG levels are low with a normal or raised IgM concentration. B- and T-cell numbers are normal. However, there is an absence of switched memory B cells. Primary and secondary antibody responses are reduced and limited to IgM. Hyper-IgM syndrome must be considered when there is a history of proven *Pneumocystis* pneumonia and a normal mitogen-induced T-cell proliferative response, making SCID unlikely. X-linked hyper-IgM syndrome can be confirmed by absent CD40 ligand expression on activated T cells or identification of mutations in the CD40 ligand gene. CD40 deficiency can be identified by absence of CD40 expression on B cells.

Treatment consists of intravenous immunoglobulin replacement therapy, appropriate antibiotic treatment of specific infections, and prophylaxis for *Pneumocystis* infection. Granulocyte–macrophage colony-stimulating factor (GM-CSF) may be required if neutropenia is severe. Measures to avoid *Cryptosporidium* infection may prevent liver disease.

### Common variable immunodeficiency

CVID is a heterogeneous group of disorders due to either an intrinsic B-cell defect or a B-cell dysfunction secondary to abnormal T cell–B cell interaction. Underlying genetic defects are being identified increasingly, some shared by other well-defined immunodeficiencies such as mutations in genes for Btk in XLA, CD40 ligand in hyper-IgM syndrome, and SLAM-associated protein (SAP) in X-linked lymphoproliferative disease. In recent years, mutations in a number of novel genes have been identified, including BAFF-receptor, TACI, CD20, CD81, Toll-like receptors and CD21, which all result in a failure to produce an adequate humoral immune response. Despite these advances, however, many of the defects underlying CVID are not yet known. The majority of individuals with CVID have no family history of CVID. However, 10–20% may have a relative with selective IgA deficiency.

CVID is an acquired hypogammaglobulinaemia, with onset usually in the second and third decades but sometimes in childhood. The spectrum of respiratory infections is similar to that observed in XLA, but onset of the symptoms may be more insidious. Uncommonly pneumonia has been associated with *Pseudomonas aeruginosa* or *Pneumocystis jiroveci* (previously *P. carinii*). Occasionally, lymphoid interstitial pneumonitis develops, presenting with cough, dyspnoea, weight loss and an interstitial infiltrate, causing a restrictive lung disease pattern. Diarrhoea due to *Campylobacter jejuni* or *Giardia lamblia* is common. Other manifestations include hepatosplenomegaly, autoimmune haemolytic anaemia, thrombocytopenia, neutropenia, non-caseating granulomas of lungs, spleen, skin and liver, and atypical lymphoid hyperplasia. There is an increased incidence of lymphoma.

The diagnosis of CVID depends on exclusion of other well-defined syndromes on the background of significantly reduced serum IgG levels (usually not as low as in XLA) and reduced IgA and/or IgM with defective specific antibody responses. T- and B-cell numbers are variable, as are T-cell proliferative responses. A diagnosis of CVID cannot be made in children less than 2 years of age, although a small number of children with presumed transient hypogammaglobulinaemia, selective antibody, IgA or IgG subclass deficiency may subsequently develop definitive features of CVID. Measurement of switched memory B cells may prove helpful in determination of diagnosis, prognosis and therapeutic decisions. The subset of children and adults with CVID who have low numbers of switched memory B cells tends to have more infections, as well as autoimmune, granulomatous and lymphoproliferative complications.

Treatment consists of intravenous immunoglobulin replacement therapy and appropriate antibiotic treatment of specific infections. Autoimmune phenomena may need corticosteroid and immunomodulatory therapy, and those considered at risk of *Pneumocystis* infection should receive co-trimoxazole prophylaxis.

### Selective IgA deficiency

Selective IgA deficiency is defined as a serum IgA level of less than 0.05–0.07 g/L (the lower limit of detection of most commercial assays) with normal IgG and IgM levels, probably secondary to impaired switching from IgM to IgA production. No underlying genetic defect has been identified and there is usually no family history. It is the commonest primary immunodeficiency, with reported prevalence ranging from 1 in 200 to 1 in 1000 of the normal population. Most are asymptomatic but there is an increased incidence of recurrent infections, particularly bronchitis and otitis media. More severe suppurative sinopulmonary disease is less common and is often associated with reduced IgG2 subclass levels and specific antibody deficiency. Secretory IgM is thought to compensate for IgA deficiency in asymptomatic individuals.

Serum IgA levels are low in normal infants, reaching adult equivalents by 9–12 years of age. IgA deficiency may be transient, reflecting a maturational delay. The detection of salivary IgA may help distinguish this group, as salivary IgA levels reach normal adult levels by 6 months of age. However, this test is not routinely available. The clinical significance of detectable serum IgA but at a level below the normal reference limit is uncertain, but in most children IgA levels are likely eventually to increase to the normal range. Transient IgA deficiency in infants and young children is unlikely to predispose to increased frequency or severity of infections.

IgA deficiency is associated with an increased incidence of autoimmune diseases, allergic disorders and malignancy. Acute reactions, including anaphylaxis, to residual IgA in blood transfusions and intravenous immunoglobulin can occur due to the development of anti-IgA antibodies.

### IgG subclass deficiency and specific antibody deficiency

There are four subclasses of IgG. IgG1 accounts for 65% of total serum IgG, IgG2 for 25%, IgG3 for 7% and IgG4 for less than 5%. Antibody responses to peptides are predominantly IgG1 and IgG3, whereas responses to polysaccharides are predominantly IgG2 and, to a lesser extent, IgG1. Deficiency may occur in one or more subclasses. However, the diagnosis is hampered by the significant individual variation in IgG subclass levels with age, and the logistic difficulties in establishment of age-related normal ranges.

There is poor correlation between the diagnosis of IgG subclass deficiency and susceptibility to infection, resulting in controversy regarding whether IgG subclass deficiency is a true immunodeficiency. Coexistence of a functional antibody deficit is of more relevance, particularly specific antibody responses to polysaccharide antigens, such as unconjugated pneumococcal vaccine, in children older than 2 years.

Maturational delay of T cell-independent antibody responses may prolong susceptibility to infections (particularly sinopulmonary infections) with encapsulated bacteria in children over the age of 2 years, even in the presence of quantitatively 'normal' levels of IgG, IgA and IgM. Defective antibody responses associated with quantitatively normal IgG and IgG subclass levels is referred to as specific antibody deficiency (SAD). Many children with SAD also do not respond to conjugated pneumococcal vaccination. However, conjugated vaccine will benefit those children who do respond.

Clinical features of SAD and IgG subclass deficiency with defective antibody responses include chronic otitis media with discharge, bronchitis, sinusitis and pneumonia. Affected individuals usually present in the first 7 years of life. The range and severity of infections may be similar to those in other antibody deficiencies such as XLA and CVID.

Management of symptomatic children with defective antibody responses with or without IgG subclass deficiency includes ready access to antibiotic therapy, a trial of antibiotic prophylaxis and, in a small subset, intravenous immunoglobulin therapy with periodic reassessment of ongoing requirement. In many, the defect will resolve with age, but in a smaller proportion the defect is permanent or evolves into CVID.

## Combined T- and B-cell immunodeficiency

### Severe combined immunodeficiency

SCID encompasses a heterogeneous group of conditions associated with a profound deficiency of both T- and B-cell function, the genetic basis of which is being increasingly identified (see Table 13.2.2). X-linked SCID, secondary to a mutation in the common γ chain of the interleukin (IL)-2 receptor, accounts for over half of all cases. Autosomal recessive forms include defects of recombinase activating genes (RAG-1 and RAG-2), IL-7 receptor, signalling components after T-cell receptor activation such as ZAP-70 and Jak3, enzymes essential for lymphocyte metabolism such as adenosine deaminase (ADA) and purine nucleoside phosphorylase (PNP), and DNA repair mechanisms such as Artemis.

SCID usually presents within the first 6 months of life. There is often a history of diarrhoea, lower respiratory tract infections, failure to thrive, candidiasis and rash. *Pneumocystis* pneumonia is common and its occurrence should always prompt investigation to exclude SCID. It is often insidious in onset with cough and pulmonary infiltrates that progress over several weeks (Fig. 13.2.3). Children

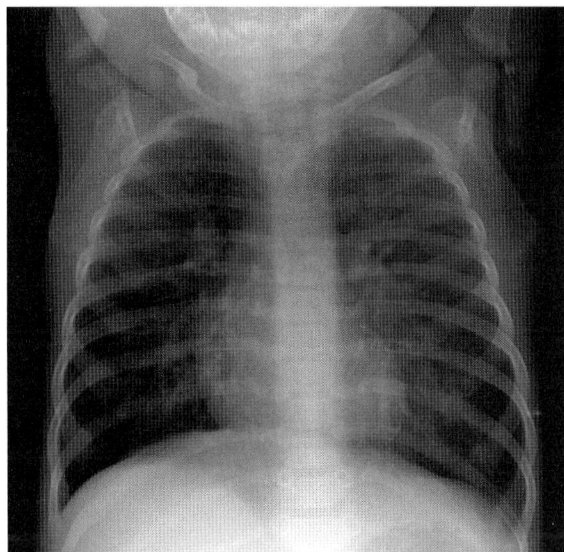

Fig. 13.2.3 Chest X-ray of a 6-month-old child with *Pneumocystis* pneumonia associated with severe combined immunodeficiency. The mediastinum is narrowed by absence of the thymic shadow. The lungs are hyperinflated and there is bilateral diffuse pulmonary infiltrate.

with SCID are extremely susceptible to bacterial, viral and fungal infection. Without bone marrow transplantation, death usually occurs within the first 2 years of life.

Immune abnormalities vary but usually include lymphopenia with markedly reduced T-cell numbers and reduced serum IgG, IgA and IgM levels. The presence or absence of normal B-cell numbers may help to identify the underlying genetic defect (see Table 13.2.2). T-cell proliferative response to mitogens is abnormal, and specific antibody responses, including isohaemagglutinins, are absent. Molecular diagnosis should be undertaken where available to aid genetic counselling and future prenatal diagnosis.

Supportive treatment involves protective isolation, specific antimicrobial therapy, intravenous immunoglobulin replacement and prophylaxis against *Pneumocystis*. Live virus vaccines should be avoided and blood products must be irradiated to prevent graft-versus-host disease from transferred T cells. Definitive therapy is bone marrow transplantation. Early transplantation from a human leukocyte antigen (HLA)-identical sibling has a success rate of over 90%, but is lower with matched unrelated donors. ADA deficiency can be treated with ADA replacement. Patients with X-SCID and ADA deficiency have been treated successfully with gene therapy, but this remains experimental owing to technical and safety concerns.

**Clinical example**

Daniel presented to the emergency department of his local hospital at 4 months of age with a 2-week history of increasing cough and respiratory distress. He also had persistent oral and napkin-area thrush associated with chronic loose stools, irritability and poor weight gain over the preceding couple of months. He had received his routine vaccinations at 2 months of age. There was no known family history of immunodeficiency.

On physical examination, he had evidence of failure to thrive, with reduced subcutaneous fat and his weight was significantly below the third percentile for age. Lymph nodes were not palpable and no tonsils were seen. He was tachypnoeic and had generally reduced air entry. Chest X-ray revealed hyperinflated lungs with a diffuse interstitial infiltrate. There was no thymic shadow.

Daniel was found to be lymphopenic ($0.2 \times 10^9$/L) on full blood count. Serum IgG was very low (0.4 g/L, normal range 1.6–7.8 g/L) and IgA undetectable, whereas IgM was mildly reduced (0.26 g/L, normal range 0.33–1.05 g/L). Isohaemagglutinins were not detected. Lymphocyte subsets demonstrated absence of T and natural killer (NK) cells, but the presence of some B cells. There were no detectable antibodies to his routine vaccinations and no T-cell proliferative response to the mitogen, phytohaemagglutinin (PHA). Stool culture detected vaccine associated poliovirus. *Pneumocystis jiroveci* was isolated from bronchoalveolar lavage (BAL) sampling.

The diagnosis of X-linked severe combined immunodeficiency was made. Daniel commenced treatment for *Pneumocystis* pneumonia with high-dose intravenous co-trimoxazole and corticosteroids, and started replacement with monthly intravenous immunoglobulin (IVIG). On recovery from his respiratory illness, the co-trimoxazole was reduced to a prophylactic dose to prevent recurrence of *Pneumocystis* infection. Daniel underwent a successful HLA-matched unrelated bone marrow transplant from cord blood 3 months later, having no suitable HLA-matched relatives. Daniel is now well with no detectable immune abnormality.

Genetic testing confirmed the diagnosis of X-SCID and Daniel's mother's carrier status. This enabled prenatal diagnosis in subsequent pregnancies.

## Other well-defined immunodeficiency syndromes

### Wiskott–Aldrich syndrome

Wiskott–Aldrich syndrome is an X-linked condition that usually presents with refractory atopic dermatitis and thrombocytopenic purpura. Otitis media and pneumonia are common and associated with defective antibody response to polysaccharide antigens. There is a variable T-cell defect and children with WAS are at risk of *Pneumocystis* infection. Serum IgA and IgE levels are usually high, with low or normal IgG and IgM levels. There is a variable reduction in T-cell number and function, which deteriorates with age. Platelets are typically small. Definitive diagnosis can be made by demonstrating a mutation in the *WASP* gene.

Treatment consists of IVIG for demonstrated antibody deficiency, appropriate antibiotic treatment of specific infections, and prophylaxis for *Pneumocystis* infection. Life expectancy is reduced by infection, haemorrhage and a high incidence of malignancy, often B-cell lymphoma, in early adult life. Splenectomy can reduce the risk of life-threatening haemorrhage but increases the risk of serious infection with encapsulated organisms. Definitive treatment is bone marrow transplantation, although the preliminary results of gene therapy in children with WAS appear promising.

### Ataxia telangectasia

Ataxia telangectasia (AT) is an autosomal recessive chromosomal breakage syndrome, resulting from a defect in DNA repair. Most patients present with ataxia in infancy or early childhood, then develop telangiectasia of the skin and bulbar conjunctivae associated with hyperpigmented and depigmented cutaneous patches.

The degree of immune dysfunction is variable. Suppurative sinopulmonary infections occur in half of the patients. Aspiration may contribute, the severity of respiratory tract disease usually correlating with the severity of neurological impairment. Pneumonia is a major cause of death. There is a high incidence of lymphoreticular malignancy.

IgA deficiency, often with associated IgG2 subclass deficiency, is common. IgE is often absent. Defects in T-cell function and number are variable. Serum α-fetoprotein levels are raised in virtually all cases. Defects in DNA repair lead to an increased incidence of chromosome breaks in cytogenetic studies.

Infections should be treated early with appropriate antibiotics, whereas IVIG may be indicated if a significant antibody defect is demonstrated.

### DiGeorge syndrome (velocardiofacial syndrome, Sprintzen syndrome)

DiGeorge syndrome is the result of interrupted embryonic development of the third and fourth pharyngeal pouches. Deletions of chromosome 22q11.2, detectable by fluorescence *in situ* hybridization (FISH), are found in over 85% of cases, whereas deletions of chromosome 10p13-14 are found in a smaller number.

There is a significant phenotypic variability, but the syndrome is characterized by conotruncal cardiac defects (e.g. interrupted aortic arch or truncus arteriosus), symptomatic neonatal hypocalcaemia secondary to parathyroid hypoplasia, characteristic facies with palatal dysfunction leading to feeding difficulties, speech delay and aspiration, behavioural and developmental problems, and thymic absence or hypoplasia resulting in T cell-mediated immunodeficiency.

Complete absence of the thymus resulting in a SCID phenotype is rare. Most patients have mild immune impairment. Susceptibility to otitis media and sinusitis is usually more a result of anatomical and functional airway compromise than of systemic immunodeficiency. The commonest finding is a mild reduction in total T-cell numbers (CD3), particularly of the CD4 subset, which is usually of no clinical significance. Occasionally there is an associated specific antibody deficiency that requires immunoglobulin replacement therapy. Live vaccines should not be given until the degree of immune impairment has been determined.

### Chronic mucocutaneous candidiasis

Chronic mucocutaneous candidiasis (CMC) is characterized by persistent or recurrent *Candida* infections of the skin, mucous membranes and nails. In most, isolated defects in cell-mediated immunity to *Candida* can be demonstrated by delayed hypersensitivity skin tests or *in vitro* techniques.

There are several distinct clinical syndromes. The classical autosomal recessive form, secondary to mutations in the *AIRE* gene, is associated with autoimmune polyendocrinopathies (APECED). An autosomal dominant form is associated with thyroid disease. Although candidiasis usually manifests before the age of 5 years, endocrine dysfunction may present at any age. Deficiencies of CARD-9 and Dectin-1 have been identified in CMC without endocrinopathy. CMC is also a prominent feature of hyper-IgE syndrome. Defects in the Th17/IL-17 pathway, involving either Th17 cell numbers, ligand binding, signalling pathways, IL-17 and/or IL-22 production or neutralizing antibodies to these cytokines, appear to be the unifying aetiology of CMC in these diverse conditions.

Long-term oral antifungal therapy is usually required to prevent recurrence.

### Hyper-IgE syndrome

Hyper-IgE syndrome is characterized by recurrent infections and eczematous or vesicular rash from infancy. There is progressive development of coarse facial features, osteopenia, retained primary dentition and skeletal abnormalities. Subcutaneous cold abscesses and suppurative lower respiratory tract disease caused by staphylococcus, *Haemophilus influenzae,* pneumococcus, *Candida* and *Pseudomonas* are common. Persistent pneumatoceles (Fig. 13.2.4) following infection occur in most patients.

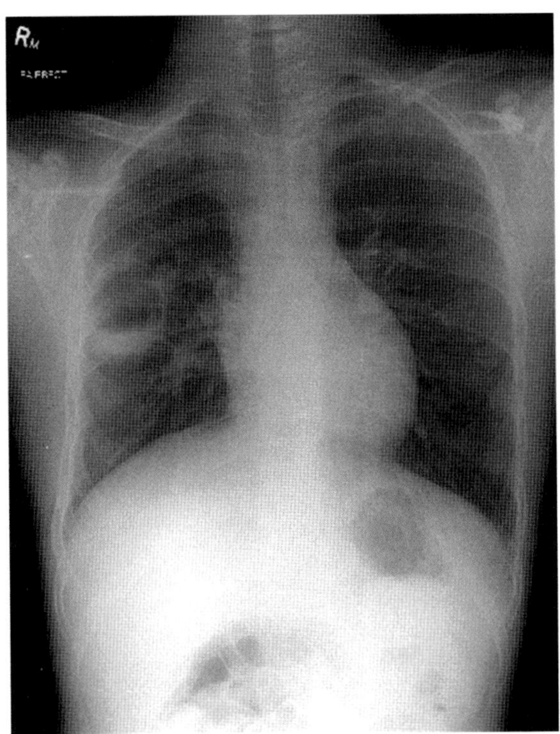

Fig. 13.2.4 Staphylococcal pneumonia with pneumatocele in hyper-IgE syndrome.

Serum IgE levels are usually markedly raised, but may be near normal in infancy. Extremely high IgE levels can also be detected in infants with severe atopic dermatitis, but this can be differentiated from hyper-IgE syndrome by the localization of infection to superficial skin and by the distribution and characteristics of the rash. Levels IgG, IgA and IgM are also typically increased. There are variable defects in neutrophil chemotaxis. Some subjects have a defective functional antibody response to polysaccharide antigens.

Most cases of hyper-IgE syndrome are autosomal dominant or sporadic. These are secondary to mutations in the *STAT3* gene which causes deficiency of Th17 cells and, as a consequence, of cytokines such as IL-17 and IL-22, which have important roles in humoral immune responses and defence against mucocutaneous candidiasis. The mechanism by which *STAT3* mutations cause the musculoskeletal associations is yet to be fully elucidated. Mutations in *Tyk2* and *DOCK-8* are causes of autosomal recessive hyper-IgE syndrome. Patients with autosomal recessive hyper-IgE syndrome typically do not develop the musculoskeletal abnormalities, and have a higher incidence of viral infections and malignancy than those with autosomal dominant disease.

Management consists of long-term anti-staphylococcal antibiotic prophylaxis and treatment of acute infections.

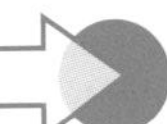

**Practical points**

- Recurrent infections are common in early childhood.
- Resistance to infection is provided by non-specific mechanisms and through the adaptive immune response.
- A small number of children with recurrent infections will have a primary immunodeficiency disorder.
- Some components of the immune response are immature at birth.
- A blood count, blood film and measurement of serum immunoglobulin concentrations can be a useful screen for primary immunodeficiency disorders.

Surgical intervention may be required and IVIG may reduce the incidence of infection if a functional antibody deficiency is demonstrated.

## Phagocytic cell disorders

### Chronic granulomatous disease

CGD is caused by a defect of one of the four subunits of phagocyte NADPH oxidase (phox), required to produce the respiratory burst that generates reactive oxygen intermediates, such as superoxide and hydrogen peroxide, which are used to kill phagocytosed pathogens. The majority (60–70%) of cases are due to an X-linked mutation of the $gp91^{phox}$ gene; the remainder are due to autosomal recessive mutations of $p22^{phox}$, $p47^{phox}$ or $p67^{phox}$.

Failure to thrive, bacterial adenitis, abscesses or osteomyelitis may occur within the first year of life. Pneumonia and lymphadenitis due to catalase-positive organisms such as *Staphylococcus* and *Serratia*, or fungi such as *Candida* and *Aspergillus* are the most common infections. Intestinal or urinary tract obstruction can be caused by granuloma formation. Gingivitis (Fig. 13.2.5), inflammatory

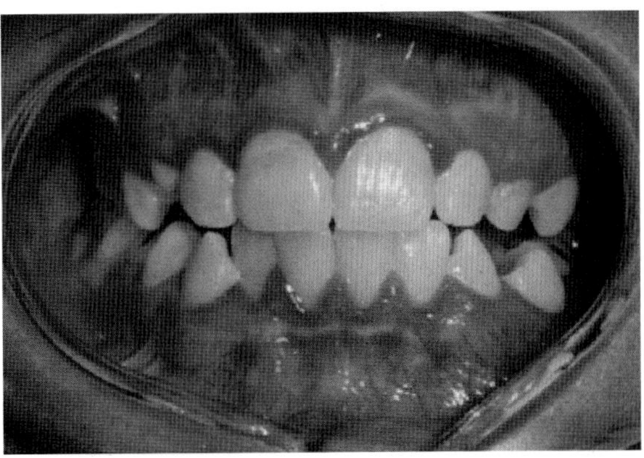

Fig. 13.2.5 Gingival inflammation secondary to infection in an individual with cyclic neutropenia. Symptoms included halitosis and bleeding gums with minor trauma.

bowel disease, hepatosplenomegaly and lymphadenopathy are other features.

The diagnosis is made by demonstrating absence of an oxidative burst in activated neutrophils on nitroblue tetrazolium (NBT) testing or an equivalent flow cytometric assay. These tests can detect female carriers of X-linked CGD, but not autosomal recessive carriers. CGD can be confirmed on formal neutrophil function testing and/or by molecular testing.

Early diagnosis and co-trimoxazole prophylaxis has dramatically reduced the incidence of infections and improved survival. Additional antifungal and/or IFN-γ prophylaxis is also beneficial. Development of invasive fungal infections is associated with poorer prognosis. Bone marrow transplantation is generally limited to patients with more severe disease, preferably where there is a related HLA-matched donor, and is associated with significant mortality. Promising results had been reported in preliminary trials of gene therapy, but the response proved short-lived owing to lack of a selective advantage in gene-modified cells.

### Leukocyte adhesion deficiency

These rare conditions are secondary to abnormalities of cell surface expression of proteins responsible for the adhesion, activation and movement of phagocytes out of blood vessels into areas of inflammation. The most common defect, leukocyte adhesin deficiency (LAD) type I, is due to an autosomal recessive deficiency of β-integrins (CD18).

Affected children suffer from recurrent severe infections and usually die in the first few years of life without bone marrow transplantation. Severe gingivitis and periodontitis, and impaired healing of traumatic or surgical wounds are major features among all patients who survive infancy.

The characteristic features are delayed separation of the umbilical cord, a significantly raised peripheral blood neutrophil count, and paucity of neutrophils in areas of infection. Diagnosis is confirmed by flow cytometry showing absence of CD18 and associated molecules (CD11a, CD11b and CD11c) on stimulated neutrophils.

### Defects of the interleukin-12/interferon-γ axis

A number of gene defects affecting the IL-12/IFN-γ axis have been identified (see Table 13.2.2) that predispose affected individuals to atypical mycobacterial and salmonella infections.

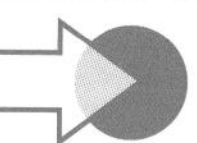

**Practical points**

- Primary immunodeficiency disorders may present with severe or unusual infections.
- Many of the primary immunodeficiency disorders are associated with specific gene mutations.
- Treatment of a primary immunodeficiency disorder depends on a specific diagnosis, treatment and prevention of a variety of infections, and therapies such as intravenous immunoglobulin and bone marrow transplantation.
- Demonstration of a specific genetic defect is important information for genetic counselling.

## Complement disorders

Deficiencies of early classical complement components are associated with an increased incidence of immune complex-mediated autoimmune disease, particularly systemic lupus erythematosus (SLE). Patients with deficiency of terminal complement components are at increased risk of recurrent neisserial infections, whereas deficiency of some components of the alternative pathway (e.g. properdin) predispose to overwhelming/fatal neisserial and pneumococcal infection. C3 deficiency predisposes to severe recurrent bacterial infection and is associated with a high mortality rate.

Integrity of the classical and alternate complement pathways is tested by the classical (CH50) and alternate (AH50) haemolytic complement assays, respectively. Although CH50 and the complement components C3 and C4 are readily available, AH50 and assays of other individual components are often available only from specialized laboratories.

# 13.3 Arthritis and connective tissue disorders

Kevin Murray, Navid Adib

Chronic inflammatory arthritis and connective tissue disorders are associated with immune dysregulation and may affect many systems, involving joints, skin and internal organs. Although the exact aetiology of most of these disorders remains unknown, it is believed that they may be the result of interaction between genetic and environmental factors.

Box 13.3.1 lists some of the important forms of chronic arthritis and connective tissue disorders of childhood.

## Frequency

The chronic arthritis and connective tissue disorders in childhood are generally uncommon. The most common type of chronic arthritis is juvenile idiopathic arthritis (JIA). The prevalence is estimated to be 1 in 1000, although the condition may be even more common. Other causes of arthralgia or musculoskeletal pains are seen far more often, such as pain related to mechanical disorders, ligamentous laxity or joint hypermobility.

## Arthritis in children

Arthritis is inflammation of, or related to, a joint and symptoms of arthritis may include:

- pain
- heat
- swelling
- deformity or loss of range of motion
- stiffness, particularly early morning
- loss of function
- occasionally erythema.

In the evaluation of the acute onset of joint inflammation, infection or trauma must be considered. Infection may occur as primary septic arthritis or extension of infection from a nearby focus of osteomyelitis into the joint space (see Chapter 12.2). Meningococcal septicaemia and *Haemophilus influenzae* type b meningitis may be complicated by septic arthritis, or by sterile reactive arthritis. Where trauma is suspected with joint swelling, both accidental and non-accidental injury must always be considered. Inflammation in a joint may also result from bleeding into the joint in haemophilia (see Chapter 16.2), from chloroma associated with neoplastic disease, or rarely from foreign-body penetration.

## Juvenile idiopathic arthritis

Persistent or chronic arthritis in the absence of any other associated diagnosis or disorder, in a young person under 16 years of age, is diagnosed as JIA. The term 'juvenile' refers to the onset of this disorder, and arthritis commonly persists into adulthood.

In 1996, efforts to harmonize research and clinical care in juvenile forms of chronic arthritis resulted in the development of an international classification system, which is now widely recognized. The most recent revision of this classification is detailed in Box 13.3.1. The three main broad clinical presentations are:

- oligoarthritis
- polyarthritis
- systemic arthritis.

### Oligoarthritis

Oligoarthritis, defined as four or fewer joints involved during the first 6 months after onset of symptoms, is the commonest form of JIA, accounting for over 60% of cases. Most children present between 1 and 4 years of age, girls twice as frequently as boys. Knees are affected most commonly, followed by ankle (and subtalar) joints, wrists and elbows. Hip disease is rare, and a child presenting with isolated hip involvement must be investigated carefully for disorders such as septic arthritis or osteomyelitis and, in the appropriate age groups, avascular necrosis of the femoral head (Perthes disease) and slipped femoral capital epiphysis (see Chapter 8.1).

There is usually no systemic disturbance in oligoarthritis. Radiographs may show soft tissue swelling, effusions and widening of the joint space, but erosions are rare. Where treatment has been delayed, epiphyseal overgrowth and lengthening of the involved limb is common. Untreated children ultimately develop erosive disease, whereas growth plate involvement may result in arrest of linear growth and limb deformity

**Box 13.3.1 Chronic inflammatory arthritis and connective tissue disorders of childhood, including the new International League of Associations for Rheumatology (ILAR) classification system for juvenile idiopathic arthritis**

- Juvenile idiopathic arthritis
  1. Systemic arthritis
  2. Oligoarthritis
     a) persistent oligoarthritis
     b) extended oligoarthritis
  3. Rheumatoid factor-negative polyarthritis
  4. Rheumatoid factor-positive polyarthritis
  5. Psoriatic arthritis
  6. Enthesitis-related arthritis
  7. Undifferentiated arthritis
- Systemic lupus erythematosus
- Juvenile dermatomyositis
- Scleroderma
- Overlap syndromes
- Primary vasculitic disorders

(Fig. 13.3.1A,B). More than 70% have a positive serological test for antinuclear antibody (ANA), and rheumatoid factor is usually negative. Oligoarthritis onset has the greatest association with anterior uveitis (see below), which if untreated can cause blindness. Approximately 25% of patients with oligoarthritis will develop progressive polyarthritis after the first 6 months, and are classified as having extended oligoarthritis.

## Clinical example

Tianna, 2 years old, had an 8-week history of a painful left knee that was stiff in the mornings and became progressively more swollen. The orthopaedic team performed arthroscopic drainage of the knee joint and gave antibiotics with little improvement in her knee. The synovial fluid showed more than 20 000 white blood cells but was negative on culture. The histopathology report of a synovial biopsy showed synovial hypertrophy with 'non-specific' inflammation.

Rheumatology review noted a knee effusion, synovial thickening and 15° flexion deformity with significant quadriceps wasting. Tianna also had mild (asymptomatic) swelling of her left ankle that had gone unnoticed. Investigations revealed an erythrocyte sedimentation rate (ESR) of 41 mm/h and a positive ANA titre of 1:160. Ophthalmological review revealed evidence of cells and flare in the anterior chamber of Tianna's left eye, consistent with chronic iridocyclitis. The diagnosis was juvenile idiopathic arthritis of the oligoarthritis type with uveitis.

Tianna was treated with a non-steroidal anti-inflammatory drug (NSAID), aspiration of involved joints, with intra-articular injection of long-acting corticosteroid (triamcinolone) and regular physiotherapy. Within 3 weeks all signs of her arthritis had resolved and her range of motion was near normal. Her eye disease responded rapidly to topical steroids and mydriatics, although it recurred several times over the next 2 years. The arthritis recurred twice in the following few years, requiring further corticosteroid injections with further excellent response. By 10 years of age, Tianna's arthritis and uveitis had been in remission off all treatment for over 2 years.

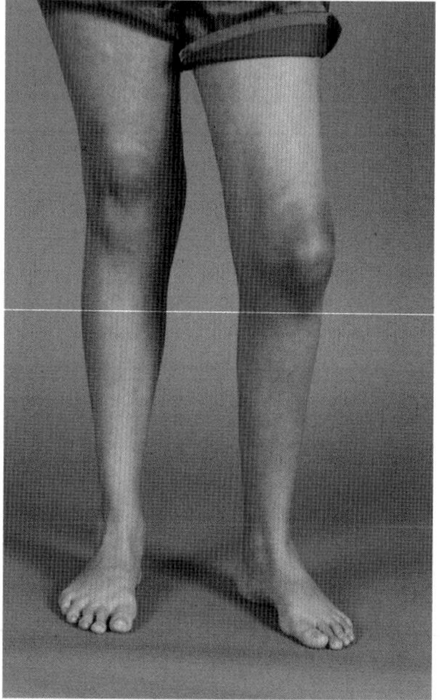

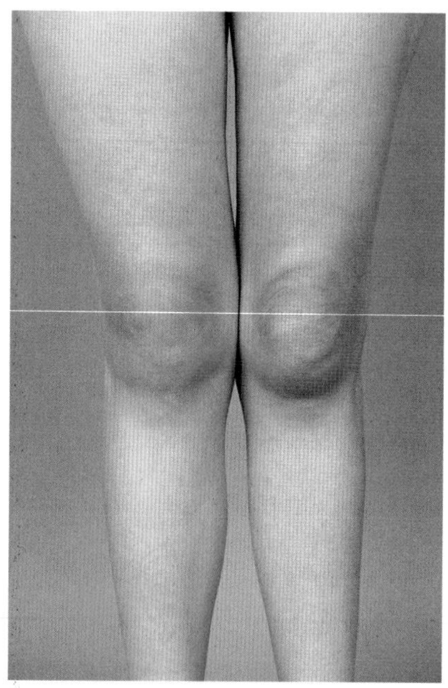

Fig. 13.3.1 A 15-year-old girl with oligoarthritis-onset form of juvenile idiopathic arthritis from age 5 years, largely untreated. (**A**) Marked flexion deformity and overgrowth of the left leg. (**B**) Response to multiple joint injections, methotrexate and intensive physiotherapy for 12 months.

## Polyarthritis

Polyarthritis, defined as involvement of five or more joints in the first 6 months of disease, accounts for about 25% of JIA cases. Girls are affected twice as often as boys. Onset is most common between the ages of 2 and 4 years, but can be at any age.

Asymmetrical large and small joint involvement is usual. Hip disease may occur, particularly later. Untreated polyarthritis may cause severe disability, joint deformities, asymmetrical overgrowth (particularly knees) and undergrowth (temporomandibular joint and mandible; Fig. 13.3.2), destruction, ankylosis (especially the wrist and cervical spine) and considerable muscle wasting.

Only a small subgroup is rheumatoid factor-positive, usually adolescent females with a symmetrical small and large joint arthritis (see below). Tests for ANA are positive in 30–40%, and uveitis may also occur, mandating screening, although not as commonly as with oligoarthritis. Radiographs are similar to those in oligoarthritis, but radiological progression is more frequent.

## Systemic arthritis

Systemic arthritis (formerly called Still's disease) may present at any age in childhood, although rarely in the first year. Adults may rarely develop a similar 'adult-onset Still's disease'. Presentation is classically with systemic symptoms and extra-articular manifestations, and affected children may not develop joint disease for many months, making diagnosis difficult.

Systemic arthritis affects both sexes equally and accounts for about 10% of cases of JIA. The initial presentation is often with daily or twice-daily spiking fevers, usually above 39 °C, returning to normal between spikes. Affected children are very irritable and movement appears painful, although joints may not appear inflamed. A classical evanescent rash, usually salmon-pink macules, may occur on the upper trunk, arms and thighs associated with fever, a warm bath or scratching the skin (Koebner phenomenon) (Fig. 13.3.3). Notably, in some individuals, particularly darker-skinned children, the rash may be more urticarial and papular.

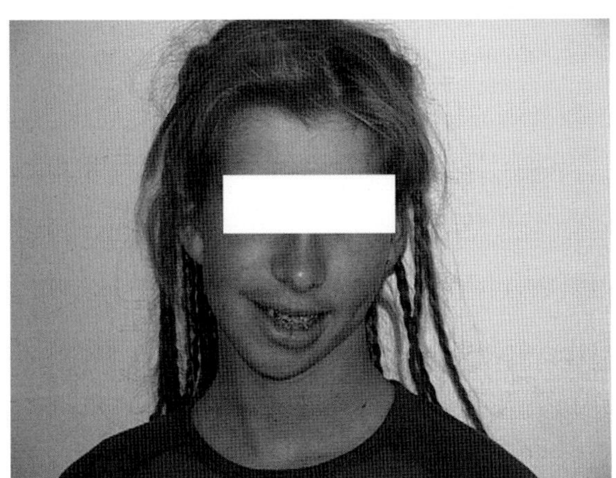

Fig. 13.3.2 A 14-year-old girl with severe mandibular deformity due to asymmetrical right-sided temporomandibular joint involvement causing failure of growth of the right ramus.

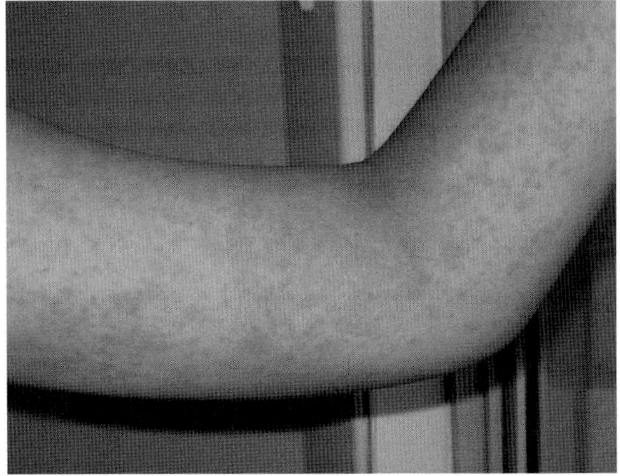

Fig. 13.3.3 Typical salmon-pink macular rash of systemic onset form of juvenile idiopathic arthritis in a 10-year-old boy.

Other features include generalized lymphadenopathy, hepatosplenomegaly, serositis causing abdominal pain (peritonitis), pleuritis and pericarditis. Pericardial effusions may result in cardiogenic shock in young children.

Early systemic arthritis mimics infection and malignancy, and diagnosis may be difficult, especially when there is no joint involvement. Haematological features include anaemia, leukocytosis, thrombocytosis, and markedly raised acute-phase reactants.

Both large and small joint involvement occurs. About half of children with arthritis respond relatively well to treatment and eventually remit within a few years. In others, the course is of relentless polyarthritis, often initially with persistent fever and rash. Occasionally children die from infections or macrophage activation syndrome. In the era before methotrexate and other cytotoxics, systemic amyloidosis could cause fatal multisystem failure. In recent years, biological agents that inhibit interleukin (IL)-1, IL-6 or tumour necrosis factor (TNF)-α have been used increasingly in severe disease.

### Clinical example

Andrew, aged 3 years, had been unwell for 4 weeks with a daily high-spiking fever and a widespread rash that was worse with fever or if he scratched himself. He had not responded to several courses of antibiotics. He presented to the emergency department with chest pain and difficulty breathing. He was unwell, dyspnoeic, febrile to 39.5 °C and had a widespread, erythematous, macular rash. He had generalized lymphadenopathy and mild hepatosplenomegaly. His heart sounds were muffled and his peripheral pulses weak.

Andrew's haemoglobin was 89 g/L, white cell count 29 000/mm$^3$, platelets 829 000/mm$^3$ and ESR 131 mm/h. Tests for ANA and rheumatoid factor were negative, as were multiple blood cultures. He had cardiomegaly on chest X-ray and a moderate pericardial effusion on echocardiography.

A diagnosis was made of JIA of the systemic arthritis type. Andrew had minimal response to NSAIDs and developed a widespread polyarthritis of both small and large joints. He was given intravenous pulse (high-dose) methylprednisolone for 3 days followed by oral steroids, with a dramatic improvement in his fever, rash and joint swelling. His pericarditis resolved within a week. He was commenced on low-dose methotrexate (15 mg/m$^2$) as a 'steroid-sparing agent', but relapsed whenever steroids were tapered.

Six months later Andrew's polyarthritis deteriorated, with only a transient response to methylprednisolone. He was started on the biological agent etanercept (anti-TNF) subcutaneously twice weekly, with a moderate improvement over 6 months. The etanercept therapy was switched to anakinra (an IL-1 receptor antagonist), used for several years with methotrexate. He improved markedly and was eventually weaned successfully off all medication.

## Other forms of juvenile idiopathic arthritis

### Rheumatoid factor-positive polyarthritis

Rheumatoid factor-positive polyarthritis usually presents in later childhood or adolescence with a symmetrical arthritis involving predominantly small joints initially, but in time large joints equally. Erosions occur early in untreated disease, and the course is often severe and deforming. Early, aggressive treatment with disease-modifying antirheumatic drugs and newer biological agents is usually needed. This disorder resembles adult-onset rheumatoid arthritis, although complications of vasculitis, Felty syndrome and cardiopulmonary disease are not common.

### Psoriatic arthritis (PsA)

Some children with oligoarthritis or polyarthritis have nail dystrophy and skin rash consistent with psoriasis, although the rash may not appear for many years. Dactylitis (sausage-like swelling of one or more fingers or toes) and distal interphalangeal (DIP) arthritis are features. Skin involvement may be subtle, for instance umbilical, scalp, external auditory meatus, or behind the ears. The severe form, arthritis mutilans, is very rare in childhood. A family history of psoriasis is typical. Treatment is as for other forms of JIA. Skin disease may also respond to methotrexate and anti-TNF therapy.

### Enthesitis-related arthritis (ERA)

Enthesitis refers to inflammation of tendons, ligaments or fascia at their points of insertion into the bone, particularly the Achilles tendon, patellar tendon and plantar fascia insertions. ERA was previously called juvenile spondyloarthropathy or HLA-B27-associated arthritis. HLA-B27 antigen is present in about 60–90% of affected patients. Boys aged 6 years or older typically present with lower-limb asymmetrical arthritis (similar to the oligoarthritis pattern) with a predilection for the tarsus and great toe. Unlike oligoarthritis, hips may be the first (or only) joints involved. In later adolescence, sacroiliac and lumbar spine inflammation is typical, although peripheral joints are usually involved also. In some (<10%) the arthritis persists into adulthood, resembling ankylosing spondylitis. Early-onset cases often remit later, although if HLA-B27-positive may develop acute anterior uveitis or inflammatory bowel disease.

### Arthritis in association with other connective tissue diseases or conditions associated with immune dysregulation

Chronic or episodic arthritis may be seen in other connective tissue disorders such as systemic lupus erythematosus (SLE), juvenile dermatomyositis, sarcoidosis, vasculitides (e.g. polyarteritis nodosa), and scleroderma (both localized and systemic). Furthermore, velocardiofacial and Down syndrome, as well as some specific immune deficiency disorders, may feature chronic inflammatory arthritis. Cystic fibrosis and other suppurative lung diseases may develop inflammatory arthropathy, possibly due to immune complex deposition. Hypertrophic pulmonary osteoarthropathy (HPOA) associated with congenital cyanotic heart disease or severe cystic fibrosis involves large joints symmetrically, closely resembling inflammatory arthritis.

## Eye disease in juvenile arthritis

Inflammatory disease of the uveal tract (uveitis or iridocyclitis) can complicate most forms of JIA, and is an important cause of acquired paediatric eye disease and blindness in developed countries. Young girls with oligoarthritis who are ANA-positive are at highest risk, whereas young boys may be more refractory to treatment (Fig. 13.3.4).

Acute anterior uveitis presents as unilateral painful red eye with photophobia and reduced vision. Chronic anterior uveitis, however, is painless and usually goes unnoticed, so slit-lamp examination by an ophthalmologist at diagnosis and in follow-up is essential. Treatment is with mydriatics and topical steroid preparations. Untreated eye disease may lead to severe impairment of vision due to band keratopathy and adhesions of the iris (synechiae). Glaucoma and cataracts may also occur due to persistent inflammation.

A granulomatous pan-uveitis or posterior uveitis may occur in paediatric sarcoidosis, which is rare.

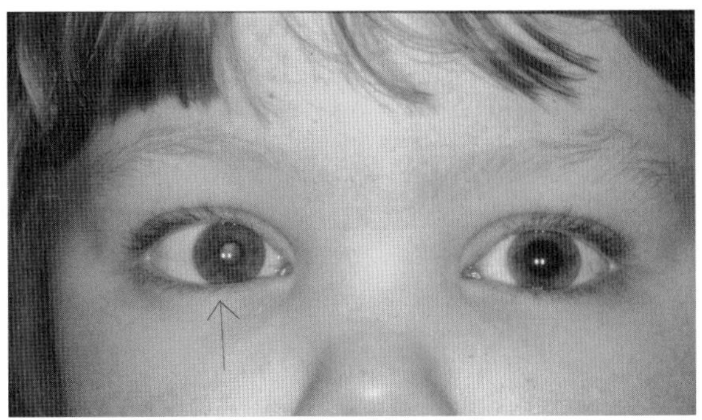

Fig. 13.3.4 Abnormal right eye of a 5-year-old boy with juvenile idiopathic arthritis and chronic silent anterior uveitis, showing an irregular fixed pupil and early cataract formation.

## Investigation of chronic arthritis in childhood

### Pathology and laboratory findings

Useful initial investigations are listed in Box 13.3.2. Common findings on investigation in a child with one of the arthritis or connective tissue disorders are:

- hypochromic microcytic anaemia
- raised erythrocyte sedimentation rate (ESR) and C-reactive protein (CRP) level
- autoantibodies, for example antinuclear antibody (ANA) and, less commonly, rheumatoid factor (RF+ polyarthritis) or anti-cyclic citrullinated peptide (anti-CCP) antibodies
- HLA-B27 antigen in ERA
- inflammatory synovial fluid (white cell count > $2000/mm^3$, and protein)
- histological evidence of chronic inflammation in synovium.

### Radiology

Plain radiographs are often normal in early arthritis, or show only periarticular osteopenia or soft tissue changes, but can rule out other diagnoses (e.g. bone dysplasia, bone or synovial tumours, unsuspected fractures and radio-opaque foreign bodies) and serve as baseline measurements. Later changes include loss of joint space, bone overgrowth (e.g. fusion of spinous processes in cervical spine), joint damage and ultimately joint ankylosis, (usually cervical spine or wrist), or subluxation. Erosive disease occurs in aggressive disease, such as rheumatoid factor-positive enthesitis-related and psoriatic arthritis. Magnetic resonance imaging (MRI) is used increasingly for difficult diagnoses, to assess deep joints such as the hip, for enthesitis, and with gadolinium to show the presence and extent of synovitis. High-frequency ultrasound imaging shows promise in assessing synovial pathology, although is operator-dependent and requires patient cooperation.

**Box 13.3.2 Initial investigations in suspected juvenile arthritis**

- Full blood count (FBC) and film
- Erythrocyte sedimentation rate and/or C-reactive protein
- Rheumatoid factor
- Antinuclear antibody
- HLA-B27 (children aged ≥6 years, especially males)
- Liver function, coagulation profile, iron studies and renal function tests in those who are systemically unwell
- Radiography of major involved joints (may X-ray contralateral joints for comparison)

## Management of idiopathic arthritis

Management of JIA has been revolutionized in the last few decades with vastly improved drug regimens and the evolvement of multidisciplinary centres with allied health professionals. The overall aim of such therapy is to normalize major outcomes such as health-related quality of life (HRQOL) and prevent structural damage. A concerted and integrated approach will ensure that the psychosocial wellbeing of the young person, in relation to their environment (family, friends, school), has been optimally promoted.

### Relief of pain

Persisting pain in the involved joints is a major burden for children and their families. Pain in any joint can lead to poor sleeping, irritability and depressed mood, as well as decreased appetite. Inability to do simple activities because of pain has a marked effect on the child and family. Pain in the joints of the lower limbs interferes with walking and mobility, and children with painful wrists and fingers may no longer be able to dress or feed themselves. Splinting may reduce pain, but prolonged disuse may accelerate osteopenia and irreversible loss of range of movements. Heat application may relieve stiff joints, whereas the hot inflamed joint may be more comfortable with cold packs. Simple analgesics such as paracetamol and non-steroidal anti-inflammatory agents (NSAIDs) can help with pain control and inflammation. Early intervention with intensive medical therapy, including intra-articular corticosteroids and disease-modifying antirheumatic drugs (DMARDs), has improved pain control in JIA.

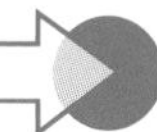

**Practical points**

- In an acutely swollen joint with marked pain, limitation of motion or associated fever, septic arthritis should be considered, and should be ruled out by aspiration and culture.
- Swelling of a joint or joints, lasting longer than 6 weeks, and with other causes excluded, is highly likely to be juvenile idiopathic arthritis (JIA).
- All children diagnosed or suspected as having JIA should be seen by an ophthalmologist to screen for uveitis. The risk is highest in young females with oligoarthritis and a positive antinuclear antibody (ANA) test result.
- Chronic arthritis in the lower limbs in an older boy who is HLA-B27-positive, associated with painful/ swollen entheses, is likely to be enthesitis-related arthritis (ERA).
- For any joint with persistent chronic synovitis unresponsive to NSAIDs, injection with a long-acting steroid is usually very efficacious
- For any polyarthritis unresponsive to simple therapies, use of a disease-modifying drug such as methotrexate is mandated.
- Most forms of JIA are treatable, with an excellent outcome expected for most, although some require treatment into their adult years.

### Maintenance of joint function and prevention of disability

Physiotherapy limited by pain is ineffective, so medical treatment to relieve pain is needed first. As inflammation improves, an active exercise programme can be introduced to improve the range of joint movement and to strengthen muscles around the involved joint. Joint function is maintained by active and passive physiotherapy and occupational therapy, and attention to overall fitness and stamina facilitates other aspects of treatment. Occasionally night-time or functional splinting may be required to restore range of movement, but regular physiotherapy is needed to prevent osteopenia and loss of movement in other joints. Hydrotherapy in a heated pool is especially helpful for lower limb joints. Home exercise programmes and guidance with sporting activities are essential. Appropriate ergonomic seating at home and at school, encouragement and assistance with activities of daily living, and information for schoolteachers and peers are all important.

Surgical intervention is rarely needed in JIA, unless joints have become severely deformed, causing functional impairment, or cause severe pain. Severe long-standing hip disease may benefit from muscle/tendon release or joint replacement, for example. Adults whose disease 'burned out' in childhood may require surgery for accelerated degenerative disease.

Children with severe disease with significant disability or pain need ongoing psychological support. Many children, particularly adolescents, who face challenges of altered body image and threats to their independence, benefit from appropriate counselling. Parents often require supportive therapy, particularly soon after diagnosis. Social work involvement is often required for children with severe arthritis. For example, disabled parking access, health-care cards and disability support allowances are an important part of assistance for parents to provide the extra care needed. Patient travel allowances and specific pharmaceutical benefits for children with chronic diseases and high drug costs are also available. Parent and patient support groups (such as the Arthritis Foundation) are valued greatly by families with affected children.

## Management of associated abnormalities

The management of uveitis has been described above. Growth may be impaired in any chronic inflammatory state, and nutritional assessment and advice is important. Growth hormone has been used in selected patients to help restore growth velocity, particularly during less active phases of disease. Osteoporosis is a well-recognized complication of severe JIA through persistent inflammation and reduced activities, and is exacerbated by steroid use. Attention to calcium and vitamin D intake is important. Bone densitometry is indicated in severe cases and with long-term corticosteroid use. For children at risk of pathological fractures, bisphosphonates (e.g. pamidronate) may be necessary.

## Outcomes of juvenile arthritis

There has been rapid progress in management. Long-term outcome studies relate to patients treated in the previous 20–30 years and are biased towards more severe cases, but suggest that most children with significant joint involvement are still affected by disability and pain in adulthood. Milder cases and those with oligoarthritis undoubtedly fare better, although eye complications are usually more severe in the latter. Long-term disability is most frequent with severe polyarticular-onset disease and with systemic disease that progresses rapidly to widespread polyarticular involvement. The biological therapies have improved outcomes, but treatment may be needed long into adulthood. Physical function, level of education and employment prospects may be impaired even with moderate disease if multidisciplinary input was not provided.

## Other disorders associated with arthritis in childhood

Arthritis due to viral infections may be due to viral invasion of the synovium or immune complex deposition. The viruses most commonly associated with arthritis or arthralgia are rubella, parvovirus B19, Epstein–Barr virus, hepatitis B virus and, in Australia, Ross River virus. Post-infectious inflammatory arthritis is usually of less than 6 weeks' duration. Transient synovitis of the hip or 'irritable hip' is probably post-viral, typically occurs in early childhood and is self-limiting.

Bacteria can also cause inflammation. Rheumatic fever (see Chapter 15.2) is well known. Post-streptococcal arthritis and post-*Mycoplasma* arthritis are increasingly recognized clinical entities, and arthritis is common with gastrointestinal bacteria such as *Shigella*, *Salmonella*, *Yersinia* and *Campylobacter*. Treatment with NSAIDs is usually effective, but occasionally a short course of steroids is beneficial.

Some bacterial infections may cause a persistent arthritis; tuberculosis is still an important cause of chronic joint infection in some countries and may also be associated with a reactive arthritis (Poncet disease).

Lyme disease does not occur in Australia unless contracted overseas, but is a very important cause of arthritis in some parts of the world. Infection with tickborne *Borrelia* species leads to a rash known as erythema chronicum migrans, neurological signs and a relapsing arthritis, usually of one or more large joints.

Henoch–Schönlein purpura (see Chapters 16.2, 18.2) is associated with transient arthritis. Haemophilia (see Chapter 16.2) with recurrent intra-articular joint bleeding leads to chronic synovitis and destructive changes in joints often indistinguishable from inflammatory arthritis, particularly in the knee and the ankle. Polyarthritis due to chloromatous involvement of joints in leukaemia may be difficult to distinguish from JIA; severe night pain and complete refusal to mobilization and a low platelet count are suggestive.

## Other disorders that may present as joint pain or dysfunction in childhood

Other conditions that may present with joint pain or dysfunction are listed in Box 13.3.3.

**Box 13.3.3 Miscellaneous conditions that may be associated with joint pain or dysfunction in childhood**

- Legg–Calvé–Perthes disease
- Slipped upper femoral epiphysis
- Transient synovitis (e.g. irritable hip)
- Chronic recurrent multifocal osteomyelitis
- Foreign-body synovitis (e.g. plant-thorn synovitis)
- Chondromalacia patellae and anterior knee pain syndromes
- Unrecognized trauma
- Metabolic and inherited disorders and syndromes
- Malignancy, including acute lymphoblastic leukaemia
- Dysplastic bone/cartilage disorders
- Conditions with joint hypermobility as clinical feature
- Overuse conditions, especially in elite child athletes and gymnasts
- Reflex sympathetic dystrophy (complex regional pain syndrome II)
- Chronic pain and fatigue syndromes ('fibromyalgia')
- Conversion symptoms and hysterical gait abnormalities

## Systemic lupus erythematosus

SLE is a chronic multisystem disorder. Polyclonal activation of B cells is associated with excessive antibody formation, and disease results from immune complex deposition. Autoantibodies are seen in serum and tissue biopsy samples, but their specific role in the manifestations of disease remains speculative.

SLE is uncommon in childhood, but 10–20% of all cases of SLE have onset at less than 18 years of age, although rarely under age 5 years. Disease in children may be severe. Females are more commonly affected. SLE is seen both with higher frequency and severity in some populations (e.g. South-East Asia or Africa, including after migration). In Australia, SLE is up to four times more common in Indigenous than non-Indigenous children.

SLE often presents with non-specific symptoms of lethargy, low-grade fever, loss of appetite and oral ulceration. Raynaud's phenomenon may be present, and patchy alopecia or scalp ulceration may occur. The typical lupus rash, a photosensitive vasculitis rash with clear demarcation and associated scaling and erythema over the malar area of the face, is present in 70% of cases. Vasculitic lesions may be present on the pulp of the digits, extensor surfaces of the arms and legs, and the palate. Purpura or ecchymoses may result from thrombocytopenia or associated coagulopathy.

There may be arthralgia or symmetrical painful arthritis with some swelling (Jaccoud's arthropathy). Joint symptoms often resolve rapidly when treatment is commenced. Myositis may contribute to weakness. Renal involvement can cause microscopic or frank haematuria, proteinuria may be mild or in the nephrotic range, and children may present with a mixed nephritic–nephrotic picture with oliguria and hypertension. Rarer manifestations are autoimmune hepatitis and pancreatitis.

Neurological manifestations from cerebral lupus include severe headache, mood disorder and cognitive dysfunction. Seizures, psychosis, chorea, polyneuropathy or transverse myelitis are less common, but are associated with poorer disease outcome. Lung and cardiac abnormalities may also occur.

### Laboratory findings

Common laboratory findings are:

- Coombs-positive haemolytic anaemia or anaemia of chronic disease
- raised ESR but normal CRP levels
- leukopenia (specifically lymphopenia)
- thrombocytopenia
- low C3 and/or C4 levels
- microscopic haematuria, proteinuria, cellular casts and altered renal function
- ANA-positive (often homogeneous pattern) in almost all cases, with anti-double-stranded DNA present in only 30% of cases initially.

Important diagnostic immunological findings in SLE are the presence of autoantibodies. ANA is present universally, often in very high titre. The ANA may be directed against specific identifiable extractable nuclear antigens (ENA) such as anti-Sm (Smith), which is diagnostic for SLE, anti-Ro (SSA) and anti-La (SSB). Antibody to double-stranded (native) DNA in high concentrations is almost specific for SLE, and is associated with more severe renal disease and central nervous system disease. Anti-cardiolipin antibody may be present and may be associated with lupus anticoagulant. The associated risk of thrombosis with such antibodies seems to be rarer in children than in adults, but may be a severe complication.

Biopsy of involved tissues such as skin and kidney shows evidence of characteristic inflammation, and immunoglobulin and complement deposition in blood vessels and tissues. The staging of renal disease by biopsy is important for guiding therapy and determining outcomes. Diffuse proliferative glomerulonephritis (grade IV), the most severe form, is the commonest finding in children with kidney disease.

### Management

Treatment of SLE requires careful and expert supervision, often by multiple specialists. Steroids are the mainstay of initial management of SLE, and administration of high doses by oral or intravenous route is often required. Prednisolone (2mg/kg daily) may be needed, and in very severe disease pulsed intravenous methylprednisolone. High-dose steroids may lead to significant side-effects, such as weight gain, osteoporosis and an increased risk of infections. Because SLE itself increases susceptibility to infection and immunosuppressives may mask symptoms, a high index of suspicion regarding infections is critical.

To minimize the long-term and undesirable side-effects of systemic steroids, steroid-sparing or disease-modifying immunosuppressive agents should be used in most patients. Methotrexate or azathioprine are often the first agents used. Hydroxychloroquine has long-term cardiovascular protective effects and may help severe skin rash. Cyclophosphamide is usually used for severe nephritis, cerebral vasculitis, or severe pulmonary interstitial disease. Mycophenolate mofetil may be used, but evidence less emphatic. Plasmaphaeresis is sometimes used in refractory cases. Autologous stem cell transplantation has induced remission in some severe, treatment-resistant cases. Rituximab, an anti-B-cell (CD20) monoclonal antibody, may be effective, especially in patients with severe haematological manifestations, although because of its anti-B cell properties there is a risk of life-threatening infections.

Multidisciplinary involvement of medical specialists, dietitians, psychologists and physiotherapists is often needed. Most children with SLE will require steroid use for some or all of their disease, and many will develop significant dyslipidaemia with risk of atherosclerotic complications in adult life, which thus needs to be monitored and treated.

The outcome for children with SLE has improved markedly in recent decades with earlier intensive and successful therapies. With careful therapy, renal function is usually maintained. Side-effects of steroid therapy and persistently active disease, including avascular necrosis of the femoral heads, decreased spinal mineralization and growth suppression, remain difficult areas of management. For many children, however, the aim should be a near normal life expectancy and preservation of fertility, with minimal disease and minimal treatment morbidity.

### Neonatal lupus syndrome

Some infants born to mothers with serological evidence of SLE-type antibodies will have transient manifestations of SLE. The mothers rarely have a diagnosed rheumatic disorder (such as SLE or Sjögren disease) but may go on to do so in later life. The neonatal manifestations are due to transplacental passage of maternal IgG autoantibody, particularly anti-Ro and anti-La antibodies. The most common abnormality is a discoid lupus-like skin rash (Fig. 13.3.5), mild thrombocytopenia and transaminitis, which gradually improve as maternally-acquired antibody titres decrease. Usually no treatment is required. The most important complication is isolated congenital heart block, which may be diagnosed antenatally, can cause fetal or neonatal death, and may require cardiac pacemaker for its treatment.

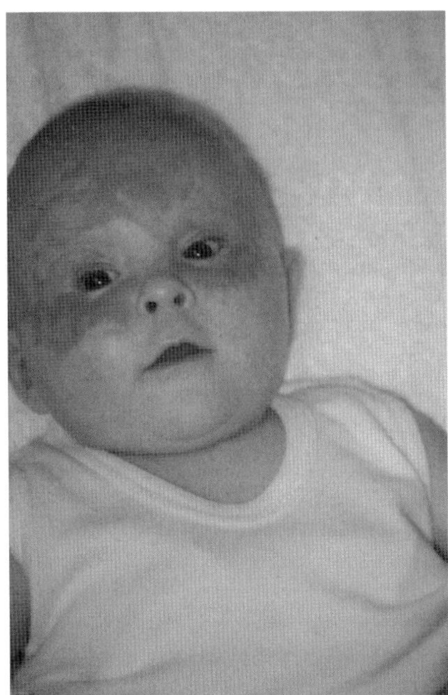

Fig. 13.3.5 A 6-week-old boy with neonatal lupus erythematosus showing facial rash ('racoon facies'); his mother was well but had passed 52-kDa anti-Ro antibodies transplacentally. The baby was well, had mild transaminitis, and all features resolved without treatment in 3 months.

## Sjögren disease

Primary Sjögren syndrome is very rare in childhood, presenting with constitutional symptoms, rash, recurrent or chronic parotitis and conjunctivitis. Xerostomia and the sicca complex are rarely seen in isolation, although more commonly in association with mixed connective tissue disease (MCTD) or overlap syndromes. Serological markers may be similar to those of SLE, with a prominence of anti-Ro and anti-La antibodies.

## Juvenile dermatomyositis

Dermatomyositis in children is seen most commonly between the ages of 4 and 10 years. Weakness and pain in the proximal muscle groups of the limbs are universal. Gait abnormality or difficulty walking are common presenting features. Weakness of muscles may progress to involve the trunk and respiratory muscles, and pharyngeal muscle weakness may increase the risk for aspiration. In some children, onset may be rapid and life-threatening, whereas in others progression may be insidious.

The typical rash of dermatomyositis is a heliotrope (purplish) discoloration around the eyes and involving the eyelids. There is commonly an associated erythematous facial rash without clear demarcation as seen with SLE, and oedema is common. Extreme oedema (anasarca), as well as ulcerative skin disease around the face and ears, may predict a severe disease course. A scaly erythematous rash over the dorsum of the small joints of the hands (Gottron's papules) and elbows and knees is common. Occasionally other patterns such as a 'shawl' or 'V' neck photosensitive distribution may be seen. Extensive subcutaneous calcification may be seen, usually associated with severe treatment-resistant disease. Muscle enzyme levels in serum are usually raised (creatine kinase, lactate dehydrogenase, transaminases). Diagnostic imaging using MRI is useful. Electromyography shows myopathic features with muscle irritability, short duration and low-amplitude potentials. Muscle biopsy is useful for atypical or severe cases when treatment with immunosuppressive regimens (e.g. cyclophosphamide) is contemplated early.

Treatment is initially with high-dose corticosteroids (oral or intravenous), reduced gradually. Early cytotoxic treatment with methotrexate or ciclosporin has a steroid-sparing effect, although some children require steroids for many years. Few children are able to have treatment withdrawn in less than 2 years.

**Clinical example**

Joshua, aged 6 years, developed a scaly, erythematous rash over his face after sun exposure that persisted for several months despite topical allergy treatments. He became very fatigued, often sleeping on return from school for several hours. He stopped playing sport and riding his bike, and complained of painful legs. Over several weeks his rash worsened and spread to his elbows, knees and the back of his hands. He had lost 2 kg in weight, and had difficulty getting up on to the family doctor's examination couch.

Examination revealed a thin boy with a scaly, red rash over the small joints of his hands, knees and elbows. He had a macular erythematous rash on his face, and his eyelids had a violaceous hue. He had marked weakness in his proximal leg muscles, shoulders and trunk, was unable to get up from lying unaided, and was unable to raise his arms above his head for more than a few seconds.

Joshua had a normal blood count, ESR of 25 mm/h, normal renal function, an aspartate transaminase level of 145 IU/L (normal < 50) and alanine transaminase 109 IU/L (normal < 50) with normal bilirubin and albumin levels. His creatine kinase concentration was 2988 IU/L (normal < 200) and lactate dehydrogenase 1468 IU/L (normal < 200). He was diagnosed with an inflammatory myositis. MRI of his thighs showed typical widespread but patchy signal changes in the muscle and fascial tissues of the gluteal region and thighs. A biopsy of the lateral thigh confirmed the inflammatory nature of the myositis. His specific diagnosis was juvenile dermatomyositis based on the clinical picture (facial rash, Gottron's papules and muscle weakness) and investigations (raised muscle enzymes, MRI and histological findings). By this stage, Joshua was having difficulty walking any distance and getting up out of a chair, and had considerable muscle pain.

Treatment was commenced with pulse intravenous methylprednisolone for 3 days followed by 1 mg/kg oral steroids and oral methotrexate 20 mg/m². Joshua started a graduated physiotherapy programme in the hydrotherapy pool. During the first week he gradually improved, and after a second course of intravenous methylprednisolone was discharged with marked improvement in his skin rash and muscle strength. He could walk and started to use stairs. Over the subsequent 3 months his steroids were slowly weaned, he had progressive improvement in his muscle strength and was able to start junior soccer training. His parents had noticed several small lumps on Joshua's knees and inner thighs, which proved to be calcinosis on X-ray. These gradually reduced in size and disappeared over the next 12 months. Joshua was kept on methotrexate for 2 years and, never having experienced a major relapse, was weaned off this medication and discharged after another year in long-term remission.

Some children have persistent chronic disease activity or multiple relapses despite intensive therapy for many years. Other treatments used or added in these situations are azathioprine, ciclosporin and cyclophosphamide (particularly in ulcerative disease). Intravenous immunoglobulin (IVIG) may be useful early in the disease course. Complications include muscle wasting, joint contractures, a form of progressive chronic arthritis, calcinosis of areas of skin and subcutaneous tissue with ulceration of the overlying skin, and, rarely, a lipodystrophy syndrome. However, many children have a very good outcome after a number of years with appropriate intensive multidisciplinary treatment.

## Scleroderma

The major feature of scleroderma is induration or sclerosis of skin and subcutaneous tissue with subsequent atrophy of sweat and sebaceous glands and of underlying muscle and bone. This may occur in several forms. Systemic sclerosis occurs in a diffuse or limited form (the latter being known formerly as CREST syndrome). It is very rare in childhood, but occasionally seen in adolescents. A typical widespread, symmetrical, waxy, tightened, indurated skin with atrophy of muscles is seen, and is associated with anti-PM/Scl antibody in some. The associated vasculopathy causes serious renal and cardiopulmonary disease, and major gut involvement with reflux and malabsorption is seen. Oesophageal dysmotility may cause dysphagia and decreased oral intake with severe weight loss. Contrast studies or upper gastrointestinal endoscopy may reveal achalasia. Intestinal transit time is often increased, with moderate to severe constipation. Treatment remains difficult, with methotrexate and cyclophosphamide offering some benefit. Symptomatic treatment with antihypertensives (e.g. angiotensin-converting enzyme (ACE) inhibitors) and pulmonary vasodilators contribute to management and a reduction in the early mortality rate. Autologous stem cell transplantation has also been used successfully in a number of patients.

Localized scleroderma, although uncommon, is seen 10–20 times more frequently than systemic sclerosis in childhood. It occurs as either morphea (isolated patches) or linear scleroderma, or as combinations of the two lesions, and may be very widespread. The involved skin becomes shiny and thickened, deeply tethered, and has patches of depigmentation, which may evolve into areas of excess pigmentation. The involved areas with active disease feel warmer than the surrounding skin. Major joint contractures occur when it crosses joints, and linear growth in the limb may be arrested. A form occurring on the head (known as *en coup de sabre*) may be severe enough to cause hemifacial atrophy (Parry–Romberg syndrome), occasionally with uveitis and central nervous system involvement (Fig. 13.3.6). There are usually no associated systemic features, although inflammatory polyarthritis may be coexistent.

Evidence now indicates that early treatment with steroids and maintenance with methotrexate for more severe lesions over a number of years may benefit many patients. Such treatment may reverse the severe

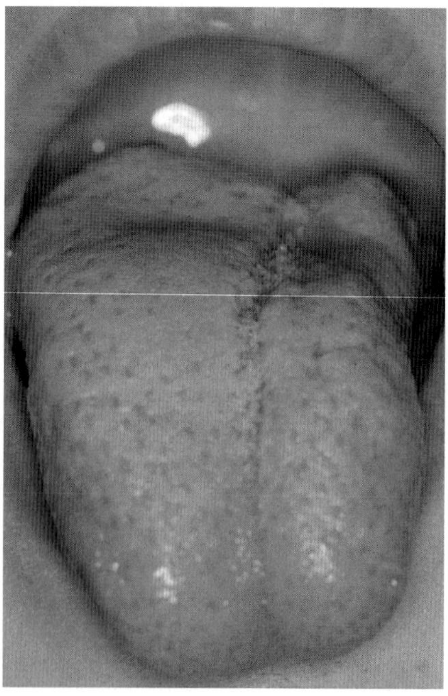

Fig. 13.3.6 A 12-year-old girl with left facial localized scleroderma and associated atrophy of the tongue.

and disfiguring fibrosis if commenced in the inflammatory stage of the disease. Topical treatments have been largely unsuccessful, and cosmetic and corrective surgery may be required.

## Overlap syndromes

Some children appear to have features of several of the disorders described above, or some features without having any complete disorder. One specific type of 'overlap syndrome' disorder is called mixed connective tissue disease (MCTD), in which there is Raynaud's phenomenon, skin nodules, arthralgia or arthritis, sclerodactyly and sometimes myositis. Patients with MCTD characteristically have a speckled-pattern high-titre ANA with specificity for U1RNP. Some children with MCTD later develop major manifestations of SLE or scleroderma. Other children may present with what is termed *undifferentiated connective tissue disease*, where they may have a positive ANA and phenomena such as Raynaud's and mild, small vessel vasculitis. They may rarely develop connective tissue disorder in later life.

**Box 13.3.4 Primary vasculitic disorders in childhood based on predominant size of vessel involved**

**Classification of childhood vasculitis (International Consensus Conference, Vienna, 2005)**

I. Predominantly large vessel vasculitis
- Takayasu arteritis

II. Predominantly medium-sized vessel vasculitis
- Childhood polyarteritis nodosa
- Cutaneous polyarteritis
- Kawasaki disease

III. Predominantly small-vessel vasculitis

A) Granulomatous
- Wegener's granulomatosis
- Churg–Strauss syndrome

B) Non-granulomatous
- Microscopic polyangiitis
- Henoch–Schönlein purpura
- Isolated cutaneous leukocytoclastic vasculitis
- Hypocomplementaemic urticarial vasculitis

IV. Other vasculitides
- Behçet's disease
- Vasculitis secondary to infection (including hepatitis B-associated PAN), malignancy and drugs including hypersensitivity vasculitis
- Isolated vasculitis of the central nervous system
- Cogan syndrome
- Unclassified

## Vasculitis syndromes

Box 13.3.4 provides a classification of primary vasculitic disorders occurring in childhood according to the predominant vessels involved. The commonest are Henoch–Schönlein purpura (see Chapter 16.2, 18.2) and Kawasaki disease (see Chapter 12.1). Acute secondary vasculitis of the skin may be associated with acute infectious syndromes such as with streptoccocal or *Mycoplasma* infection (Fig. 13.3.7) and rarely meningoccocal and gonococcal infection. The other vasculitic disorders are rare in childhood, often presenting with constitutional symptoms, fever, weight loss and rash. They may evolve later into more organ-specific features, such as nephritis and hypertension in polyarteritis nodosa, or respiratory symptoms in Wegener granulomatosis. Biopsy of affected tissues or angiography is usually required to establish the diagnosis. Therapy usually involves corticosteroids and immunosuppressive or cytotoxic medications for long periods, with significant risk of morbidity and mortality.

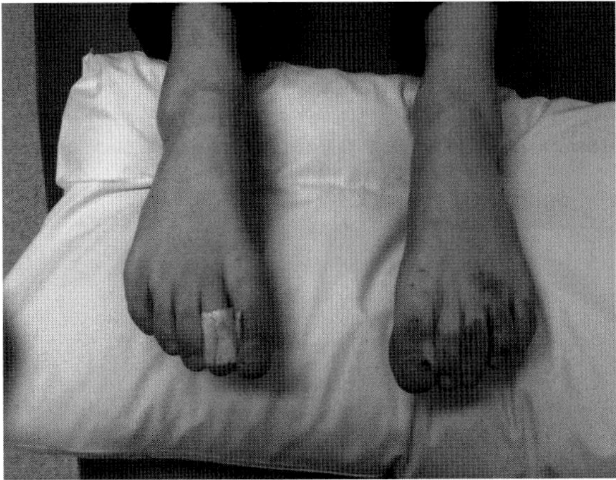

Fig. 13.3.7 An 11-year-old girl with peripheral vasculitis secondary to *Mycoplasma* infection and cold agglutinins which resolved in 4 weeks.

### Kawasaki disease

Kawasaki disease is a systemic vasculitis that occurs worldwide but is more common in children of Japanese descent. It is most common under 4 years of age. The aetiology is unknown. The major complication is aneurysms of major arteries, particularly the coronary arteries, which can be prevented in most cases by early treatment with IVIG (see Chapter 12.1). Criteria were developed for diagnostic and epidemiological purposes, but some children will be considered atypical or have an incomplete version of the disorder, and the diagnosis should still be a clinical one.

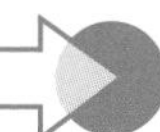

**Practical points**

- When more than one system appears to be involved in an inflammatory disorder, suspect a connective tissue disorder or vasculitis.
- Autoantibodies such as ANA may be useful in a child suspected of a connective tissue disorder and are more specific if found in high titre or with specific antibodies such as double-stranded DNA or extractable nuclear antigens such as anti-Ro, anti-La and anti-Sm.
- In children with an acute illness comprising high fever, rash, lymphadenopathy and oral mucosal changes, Kawasaki disease should be considered, and echocardiography and IVIG treatment considered.
- When steroid therapy is required, the minimal effective dose should be used and steroid-sparing agents should be introduced as soon as practical if prolonged use is expected.
- All children who require any prolonged steroid therapy should have calcium and vitamin D supplementation and bone mineral density studies to help treat and prevent osteoporosis.

## Chronic recurrent multifocal osteomyelitis

Chronic recurrent multifocal osteomyelitis (CRMO) is a chronic inflammatory condition that usually presents in older children and mimics pyogenic osteomyelitis. The disease causes inflammatory, painful, bony swelling and arthritis if near a joint, or occasionally atypical pain in a limb or in the back. Radiology reveals characteristic lesions with bone lysis and new bone formation, and nuclear bone scans may reveal (usually) multiple areas of increased uptake. The most common site is the medial third of the clavicle (Fig. 13.3.8A,B), distal tibia or femur, vertebrae or mandible. Multiple lesions may be associated with some constitutional symptoms and increased inflammatory markers. Some children have features of psoriasis or a family history of psoriatic arthritis, or features of the same arthritis themselves such as dactylitis (Fig. 13.3.9).

The constellation of synovitis, acne, pustulosis, hyperostosis and osteitis (so-called SAPHO syndrome) is rare in childhood. Biopsy reveals non-specific chronic inflammatory changes and is always negative on culture. Affected children often received recurrent antibiotics without benefit. Treatment is with NSAIDs, or even with steroids or DMARDs (e.g. methotrexate) for severe cases.

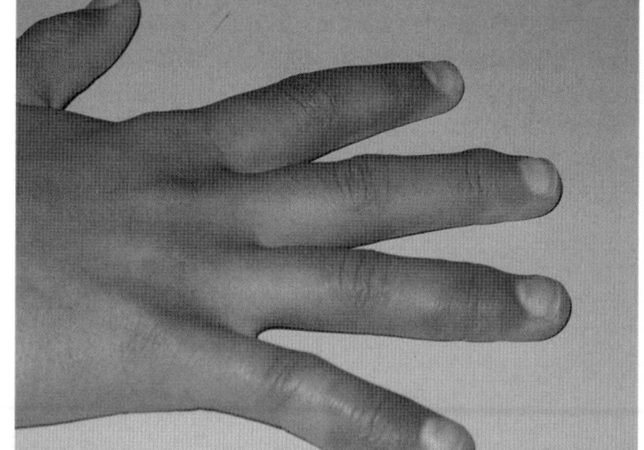

Fig. 13.3.9 A 10-year-old boy with a history of pustulosis and bony osteolysis with acute dactylitis of the hand. Prominent distal interphalangeal (DIP) joint involvement is seen with overlying erythema as part of his SAPHO syndrome.

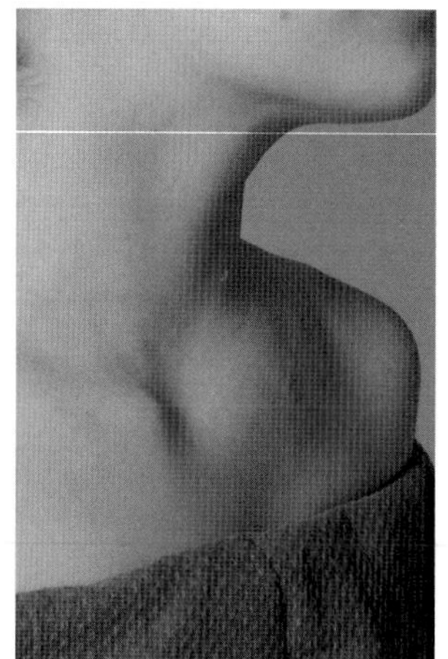

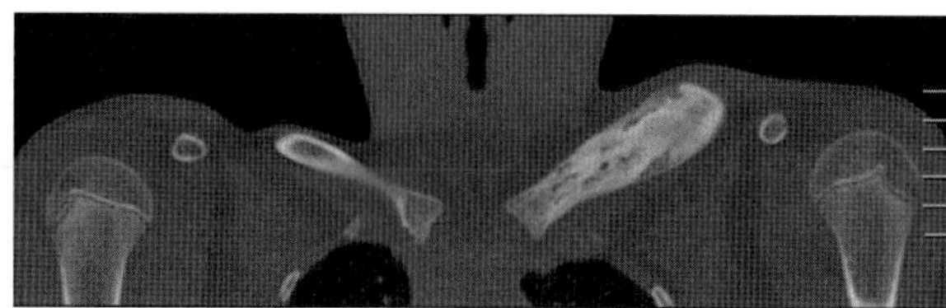

Fig. 13.3.8 (**A**) A 12-year-old girl with left clavicular enlargement as part of chronic recurrent multifocal osteomyelitis (CRMO). (**B**) Computed tomogram of the same girl with bony lysis and new bone formation typical of CRMO.

## Non-inflammatory musculoskeletal disorders

General practitioners and paediatricians see many children with joint symptoms, the majority of whom will not have an inflammatory arthritis or connective tissue disorder. The history for these children is often shorter or more episodic, and usually the joint discomfort is associated with activities and relieved by rest. These symptoms are mechanical in origin and are related to underlying factors such as ligamentous laxity (hypermobility), overuse, poor fitness or specific inherited physiques (such as pes planus or genu valgus).

### Hypermobility disorders

Marked ligamentous (and soft tissue) laxity is often seen in specific genetic disorders such as Ehlers–Danlos and Marfan syndromes, but also occurs in Down syndrome and Stickler disease. Far commoner is so called benign joint hypermobility, where inherited ligamentous laxity is associated with musculoskeletal symptoms such as 'growing pains', recurrent lower-limb arthralgia, painful flat feet, anterior knee pain syndrome and adolescent mechanical back pain. Bursitis and tendonitis can also be seen, particularly in older children. Mechanical spinal pain disorders in adolescence are becoming more common and appear to be associated with increasing sedentary lifestyle and obesity. It is possible that these may predispose to premature degenerative spinal disease and osteoarthritis in later life.

### Chronic pain disorders

In some children, musculoskeletal symptoms develop in the absence of any definable cuastive organic pathology. Fibromyalgia or chronic widespread pain disorder is a symptom complex of chronic muscle and joint pain, marked sleep disturbance, and the presence of typical tender or trigger points in the musculature. Another form of chronic pain disorder is often localized to an extremity and is known as reflex sympathetic dystrophy or complex regional pain syndrome. This takes the form of a limb or joint that becomes painful after minor injury and is immobilized to control the pain. Subsequent sensory and vasomotor disturbance may follow with discoloration, altered sweating and eventually atrophy of tissue if untreated (Fig. 13.3.10). Patients are typically pre-adolescent or early-adolescent females who are often highly disabled by their symptoms, with cessation of their physical activities and frequent school absenteeism.

These disorders are considered by most practitioners to have a major psychogenic component, although physical deconditioning and tissue changes may become established. Hence, physical treatment is an important part of rehabilitation. Psychological treatment of the young person and their family, and counselling, are usually required to ensure a timely and complete recovery.

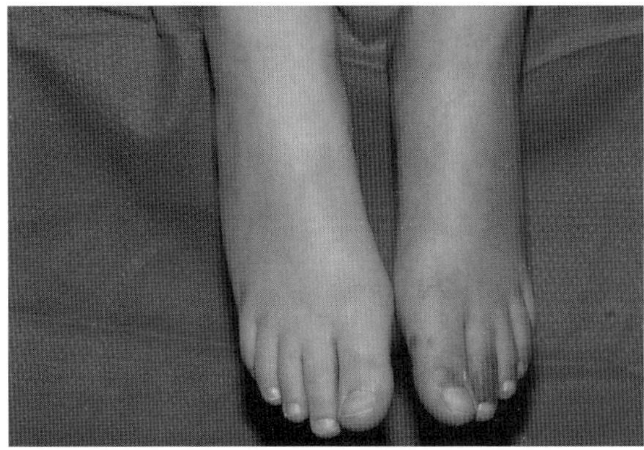

Fig 13.3.10 A 13-year-old girl with a swollen left foot after cold immersion and mild chilblains with associated hypersensitivity to touch and prolonged immobilization typical of reflex sympathetic dystrophy.

PART 14

# RESPIRATORY DISORDERS

# 14.1 Acute upper respiratory infections

Craig Mellis

Because of their frequency, upper respiratory tract infections (URTIs) are a major burden for young children and their parents. Although the common cold is the most common ailment in humans, it is particularly frequent in preschool-aged children, who average six to eight episodes per year. The timing and frequency of these infections depends on the level of exposure, occurring earlier and more often in those with older siblings, and those who attend daycare (Fig. 14.1.1). The vast majority of URTIs are viral in origin, mild, and of short duration (5–7 days), and usually described as a 'common cold'. Numerous different viruses are responsible, and the age of the child and the specific respiratory virus are the major predictors of the symptoms, severity and extent of respiratory tract involvement (Tables 14.1.1, 14.1.2).

## Respiratory complications

The importance of these recurring infections of early childhood should not be underestimated. A significant percentage of children will suffer from local complications of viral URTIs, especially acute otitis media and acute sinusitis (Fig. 14.1.2). Moreover, progression of the infection into the lower respiratory tract is a risk, particularly in the very young. This is especially likely with the more potent respiratory viruses, such as respiratory syncytial virus (RSV – the usual cause of acute viral bronchiolitis), parainfluenza (the usual cause of viral 'croup'), influenza virus (A and B) and the recently recognized human metapneumovirus (HMP – a close relative of RSV). Some children are particularly vulnerable to these lower respiratory tract complications, suggesting additional important host and environmental factors (Fig. 14.1.3).

## Systemic complications

As well as their direct respiratory morbidity, viral URTIs can cause serious indirect or systemic complications. For example, respiratory viruses are by far the most common trigger of severe acute exacerbations of wheeze and asthma in young children, resulting in high rates of attendance at emergency departments and hospitalization. Viral URTIs can also trigger vascular syndromes, such as Henoch–Schönlein purpura. Further, it is difficult clinically to differentiate viral pharyngitis (very common – and relatively harmless) from streptococcal pharyngitis (uncommon – but can result in serious complications such as acute glomerulonephritis or rheumatic fever).

## Incubation period of viral respiratory infections

Knowledge of the incubation period of these respiratory viruses is useful when considering the likely timing of infection, the source and quarantine decisions. A systematic review of over 400 publications described the median incubation period (and 95% confidence intervals) for the respiratory viruses of public health importance; these are listed in Table 14.1.2. Most have a short incubation period, with symptoms generally developing within 2–3 days of exposure.

## Identifiable URTI syndromes

Arbitrary definitions are used to describe the many 'URTI syndromes', such as rhinitis, rhinosinusitis, stomatitis, pharyngitis (tonsillitis) and otitis media. These descriptive terms signify the site of predominant symptoms – nose, sinuses, mouth, throat and ear (earache) respectively. Clearly there is substantial overlap with these syndromes, as viral infections ignore anatomical boundaries. Indeed, as a general rule, viral inflammation of the respiratory tract is usually diffuse rather than focal, whereas bacterial infections of the respiratory tract (such as streptococcal tonsillitis) are often more localized anatomically.

The two most common forms of URTI are the 'common cold' (with predominant symptoms being nasal) and pharyngitis (predominant symptom being sore throat), which are discussed in detail below.

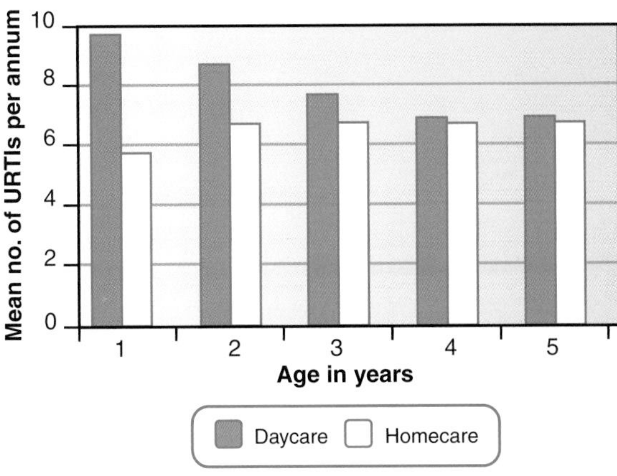


Fig. 14.1.1 Number of respiratory tract infections per year in infants and preschoolers (daycare versus homecare). (From data in Isaacs D, Moxon ER 1996.)

**Table 14.1.2 Incubation period of viral respiratory infections**

| Virus | Median incubation period (95% confidence interval) |
|---|---|
| Influenza A | 0.6 (0.5 to 0.6) days |
| Rhinovirus | 1.9 (1.4 to 2.4) days |
| Parainfluenza | 2.6 (2.6 to 3.1) days |
| Adenovirus | 3.2 (2.8 to 3.7) days |
| Respiratory syncytial virus | 4.4 (3.9 to 4.9) days |
| Influenza B | 12.5 (11.8 to 13.3) days |

## Common cold (uncomplicated viral URTI or 'head cold')

This is defined as an acute illness where the major symptoms are:

- nasal (snuffliness, sneezing and rhinorrhoea)
- mild sore throat
- conjunctival irritation (red, watery eyes).

The symptoms are mild, fever is often minimal or absent, and all symptoms resolve between 5 and 7 days. The usual pathogen responsible for an uncomplicated viral URTI is rhinovirus, which has over 100 types. However, there are many other respiratory viruses that can produce this syndrome (see Table 14.1.2). These viruses are highly infectious and spread via both droplets (particularly by sneezing) and nasal secretions on hands and fomites (clothing, handkerchiefs, toys, cot sides). Viral shedding is maximal in the 7 days after inoculation and most have a short incubation period (2–3 days). Therefore, close proximity such as household contacts with older school-aged siblings, daycare attendance, overcrowding, lower socioeconomic status and poor personal hygiene are all associated with higher rates of URTI (see Fig. 14.1.3).

Local ENT complications of the common cold include otitis media and acute rhinosinusitis (see Fig. 14.1.2), and a small proportion progress to involve the lower respiratory tract.

**Table 14.1.1 Age of child and type of respiratory tract infection**

| Age | Type of infection |
|---|---|
| Newborn | Risk of acute, generalized systemic illness with respiratory syncytial virus (looks 'septic') |
| Infant | High risk of lower respiratory tract involvement with respiratory viruses (particularly acute viral bronchiolitis from respiratory syncytial virus) |
| Toddler/preschooler | Very frequent viral respiratory tract infections, mostly confined to upper respiratory tract<br>High risk of viral laryngotracheobronchitis ('croup') from parainfluenza viruses |
| School age (5–15 years) | Lower rates of viral respiratory tract infection<br>Suspect:<br>• bacterial (streptococcal) tonsillitis<br>• Epstein–Barr viral pharyngitis/tonsillitis<br>• *Mycoplasma pneumoniae* if lower respiratory tract involvement (bronchitis and bronchopneumonia) |

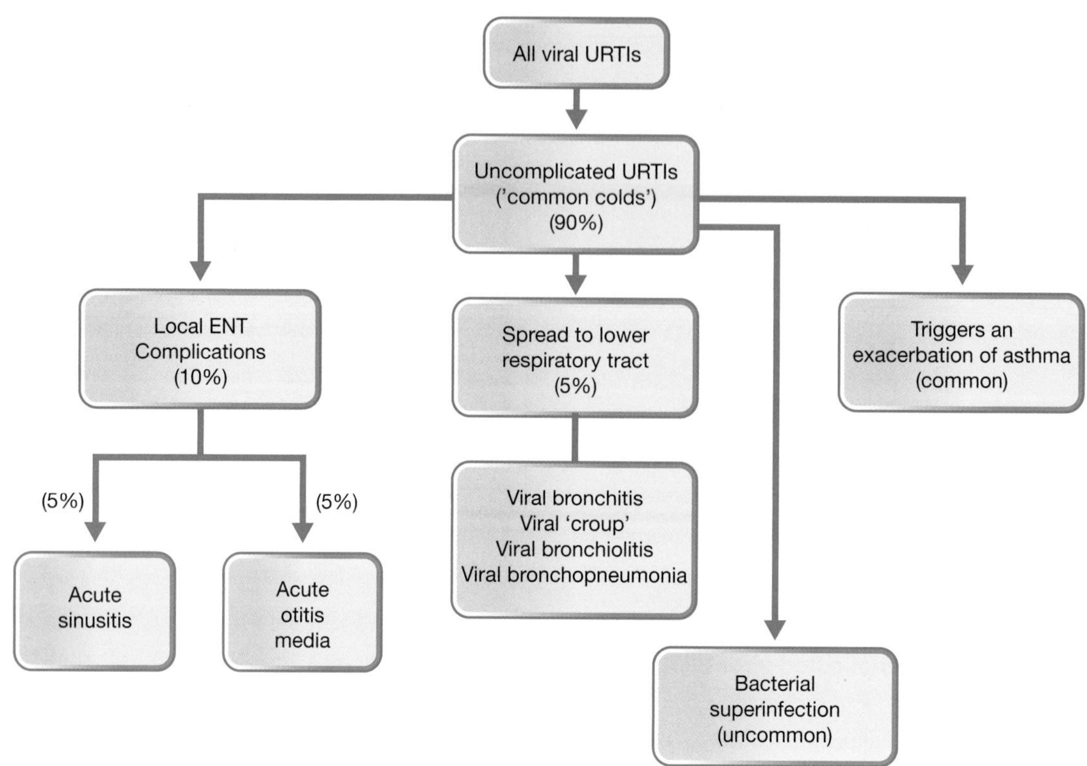


Fig. 14.1.2 Complications of viral upper respiratory tract infections (URTIs).

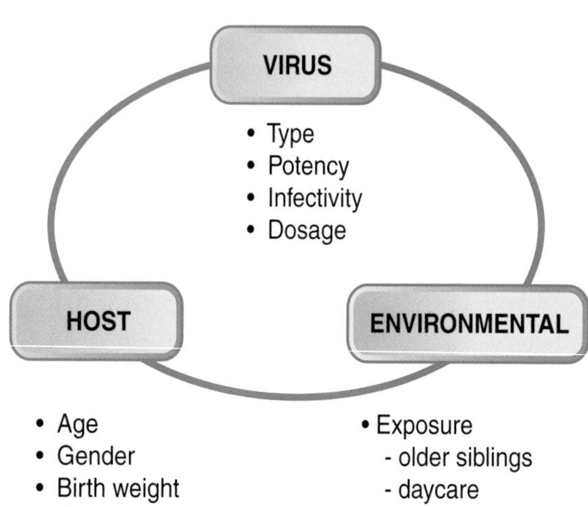


Fig. 14.1.3 The frequency and severity of viral upper respiratory tract infections depend on a complex interaction between virus, host and environment. ATSI, Aboriginal or Torres Strait Islander; ETS, environmental tobacco smoke.

## Pharyngitis (oropharyngitis/tonsillitis)

Pharyngitis is a clinical syndrome in which the major complaint is acute sore throat and/or discomfort on swallowing (dysphagia). The illness is common, generally mild and self-limiting, with three-quarters of patients free of pain within 2–3 days of onset, whether due to a respiratory virus or to β-haemolytic streptococcus. Many respiratory viral infections begin with a sore throat, before the development of the more obvious symptoms and signs such as rhinorrhoea/sneezing. However, there are a number of specific, recognizable syndromes of oropharyngitis/tonsillitis, which are described briefly below.

### Ulcerative pharyngotonsillitis

This is usually due to an adenovirus infection and typically occurs in infants and toddlers. It produces an isolated exudative tonsillitis resembling streptococcal tonsillitis or Epstein–Barr virus pharyngitis. Adenoviruses (types 3, 4, 7, 14 and 21) also produce the very specific 'pharyngoconjunctival fever'. The enteroviruses (Coxsackie virus and echovirus) and herpes simplex virus can also produce ulcerative pharyngotonsillitis. Other respiratory viruses (including RSV and parainfluenza) usually cause a more diffuse nasopharyngitis rather than this focal tonsillar inflammation.

### Epstein–Barr virus pharyngitis/tonsillitis

Although this typically occurs in older, school-aged children, it can also cause an exudative tonsillitis in the very young. The tonsillitis is associated with a membrane and marked cervical lymphadenopathy. Generalized symptoms, including fever, lethargy, anorexia and headache, can also occur, especially in older children and adolescents, and the condition is usually referred to as infectious mononucleosis, or 'glandular fever'.

### Primary herpes simplex virus stomatitis

Primary infection with herpes simplex virus (HSV), usually HSV type 1, typically causes multiple discrete ulcers on the anterior regions of the oropharynx – tongue, gums and palate (gingivostomatitis), most commonly in children aged 1–3 years. Other characteristic features are vesicles on the lips or circumoral region, significant fever and lymphadenopathy (especially submental and anterior cervical lymph glands). The ulcers persist for 5–7 days and can cause considerable pain, feeding difficulty and irritability. Asymptomatic oral shedding of HSV henceforth is common and can transmit the virus. Infection may be widespread in children with eczema and severe in the immunocompromised.

The usual treatment is analgesics, such as paracetamol. Local anaesthetic gels are commonly tried but are often poorly tolerated because they sting and the child already has a painful mouth. There have also been adverse effects reported, including aspiration from pharyngeal numbness and seizures from excessive absorption. Aciclovir is generally reserved for immunocompromised children. A study has shown benefit from aciclovir in HSV stomatitis in normal hosts, but it is effective only when given within 72 hours of onset, which is often before presentation to medical care.

**Clinical example**

At the age of 18 months, Jennifer developed a high fever and irritability. She cried loudly when given cordial to drink and spat it out. She could not swallow her saliva and was dribbling constantly. Her mouth looked red and inflamed, and her mother took her immediately to see her family doctor.

Jennifer was difficult to examine, but had submental and cervical lymphadenopathy. With gentle persuasion, she was encouraged to open her mouth. The gingivae and anterior oropharynx were bright red, and there were many small ulcers on her gums, tongue and hard palate.

Jennifer had acute gingivostomatitis, almost certainly due to herpes simplex virus. She was given small frequent sips of water and milk to maintain her hydration. She could not take paracetamol because she had difficulty swallowing in the first 24 hours, and it was difficult to apply a topical analgesic gel because of pain. The first night, a paracetamol suppository was used to provide some analgesia. The ulcers healed after 4 days and did not leave any scars.

The virus may result in persistent dormant infection in the oral region, with recrudescent orolabial infections ('cold sores'). These episodes may be triggered by intercurrent viral infections, stress, menstruation, and exposure to cold or ultraviolet radiation.

### Herpangina

Herpangina typically occurs in preschool-aged children, due to enteroviruses (Coxsackievirus A or B, or echoviruses). It results in a number of discrete mouth ulcers, localized to the back of the oropharynx: tonsillar pillars, pharyngeal wall, uvula and palate. This distribution contrasts with the anterior ulcers due to HSV.

### Hand, foot and mouth disease

Hand, foot and mouth disease affects young children and is also due to enteroviruses (mainly Coxsackie A and enterovirus 71), causing oral ulcers similar to those of HSV. The usual symptoms are sore throat and refusal to eat and drink. There is often an associated vesicular or papular rash on the hands, feet, buttocks or trunk. The mouth ulcers are generally around the mouth (circumoral), tongue, palate and buccal mucosa. The illness classically occurs in mini-epidemics, is moderately contagious, has an incubation period of 3–7 days, and clinical recognition is relatively simple.

### Acute bacterial tonsillitis ('streptococcal pharyngitis')

Group A β-haemolytic streptococcus is the usual bacterial cause of acute pharyngitis (Box 14.1.1) and is more common in school-aged children. Although it is important to distinguish viral pharyngitis from streptococcal pharyngitis, unfortunately this is not easy on clinical grounds. However, if three or more of the

**Box 14.1.1 Clinical features of group A β-haemolytic streptococcal tonsillitis**

**History**
- Age 3–15 years
- Abrupt onset
- Severe sore throat (pain and difficulty swallowing)
- Systemic symptoms
  - headache
  - abdominal pain/nausea/vomiting
- No cough or coryzal/nasal symptoms

**Examination**
- Tonsillar exudates, purulent and patchy (rather than a membrane); marked inflammation of throat and tonsils
- Enlarged, tender bilateral anterior cervical lymph nodes
- No nasal discharge

following characteristics are present then it is more likely that the child has a streptococcal infection:
- age 3–14 years
- high fever
- tonsillar exudate
- tender, enlarged anterior cervical lymph nodes
- absence of cough and/or coryzal symptoms.

Although this clinical dilemma can be overcome by use of rapid laboratory (antigen detection) tests, a throat culture remains the 'gold standard' for confirming the presence of streptococcal pharyngitis and rational use of antibiotics.

It would appear logical to give antibiotics in the presence of streptococcal pharyngitis, but current evidence casts doubts on efficacy. A Cochrane review of randomized controlled trials concluded that antibiotics confer little benefit (in terms of pain relief) in the treatment of sore throat, irrespective of whether the infection is due to a virus or to streptococcus. However, in children known to be at high risk of complications of streptococcal infection (post-streptococcal glomerulonephritis and/or rheumatic fever), the threshold for giving antibiotics should be considerably lower. Populations at particular risk include Aboriginal and Torres Strait Islanders, Maori and Pacific Islander children.

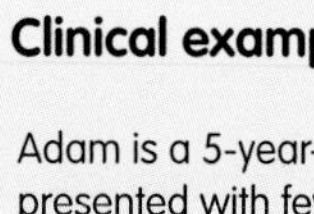

**Clinical example**

Adam is a 5-year-old Caucasian child who presented with fever, sore throat and difficulty swallowing over the previous 24 hours. When first seen he had an axillary temperature of 38.2 °C and both tonsils were swollen and inflamed, with a visible yellow exudate scattered over both tonsils. There was bilateral enlargement of the lymph nodes in the anterior cervical chain. A clinical diagnosis of acute streptococcal tonsillitis was made, and a throat swab was taken for culture. Oral penicillin was considered, but not prescribed at this time as Adam was considered to be at low risk of suppurative or rheumatic complications of streptococcal infection. He re-presented several days later because of ongoing fever and the development of a clear nasal discharge and watery eyes. He had a mild dry cough but was now drinking well and not complaining of a sore throat. His throat culture was sterile. The illness was almost certainly due to a respiratory virus (probably an adenovirus). Several days later Adam's mother rang to say that he was now virtually back to his normal self. This case clearly demonstrates the major clinical difficulty in distinguishing a bacterial from a viral tonsillitis/pharyngitis.

## Mumps (epidemic parotitis)

Mumps is primarily a disease of childhood; 90% of cases occur before adolescence. It is preventable by immunization with live attenuated virus vaccine (usually given with measles and rubella vaccines as MMR vaccine). Mumps classically causes swelling, pain and tenderness of the parotid glands. It can rarely be unilateral, but unilateral neck swelling is more suggestive of alternative diagnoses (e.g. lymphadenopathy, Kawasaki disease, recurrent benign parotitis of childhood). Other salivary glands, sublingual and submandibular, may be involved in mumps. Complications include viral meningitis (symptomatic in 10% of children with mumps, asymptomatic in over 50%), encephalitis, orchitis, oophoritis, pancreatitis, thyroiditis, deafness and rarely ophthalmitis, arthritis, myocarditis and nephritis.

## Acute sinusitis (rhinosinusitis)

Bacterial infection of the paranasal sinuses occurs as a complication of approximately 5–10% of viral URTIs and generally involves the maxillary sinuses. The usual manifestation is a profuse, mucopurulent nasal discharge with nasal obstruction. Uncomplicated acute viral rhinosinusitis normally resolves without specific treatment in 7–10 days. Thus, if the child has a purulent nasal discharge continuing beyond 10 days, the possibility of secondary bacterial sinusitis needs to be considered.

A Cochrane review of randomized controlled trials concluded that antibiotics have a small beneficial effect in uncomplicated acute sinusitis, which needs to be weighed against the potential for adverse effects due to the antibiotics. However, as complications of acute bacterial sinusitis can be serious, the sicker the child (high fever, toxic or constitutionally ill), or the more prolonged the symptoms (more than 10–14 days), the more prudent it is to prescribe antibiotics. The usual organisms responsible for acute bacterial sinusitis are *Streptococcus pneumoniae*, non-typeable *Haemophilus influenzae* and *Moraxella catarrhalis*. Amoxicillin plus clavulanic acid is, therefore, generally considered the antibiotic of choice.

## Acute otitis media

See also Chapter 22.1.

Acute otitis media is characterized by earache, fever, reduced hearing, and non-specific discomfort and irritability in the very young child. Examination shows a red tympanic membrane, loss of the normal anatomical landmarks on the tympanic membrane, the presence of a middle ear fluid, and the eardrum may be visibly bulging. However, because not all of these signs may be observed easily, the diagnosis of acute otitis media is often made with a degree of uncertainty, particularly in infants and very young children.

Acute otitis media is the most frequent complication of viral URTI, particularly in the very young (from 6 months to 2 years of age). Virtually all children will have at least one episode of otitis media and some are particularly prone to this complication. Viral inflammation of the nasopharynx disrupts the function of the eustachian tubes, impairing ventilation, thus rendering the middle ear liable to infection. The microbiology of otitis media has been well documented. In a Finnish study, middle ear fluid was obtained (by myringotomy) in over 90% of 2500 episodes of clinical acute otitis media during the first 2 years of life, and a bacterial pathogen, particularly *S. pneumoniae, M. catarrhalis* and *H. influenzae*, was cultured from over 80%.

Although this suggests that young children with acute otitis media should be treated with an antibiotic, the evidence is unimpressive. A Cochrane review found no reduction in earache at 24 hours between antibiotics and placebo, and only a small (6%) absolute reduction in pain at 2–7 days. Approximately 80% of all children with acute otitis media, irrespective of treatment, will be pain-free by 2–7 days. This small benefit of antibiotics is possibly outweighed by the 5% risk of adverse effects (rash, diarrhoea and/or vomiting). The duration of antibiotic administration has also been addressed in a Cochrane review, which concluded that 5 days of antibiotics is adequate for uncomplicated ear infections in children.

Consequently, simple oral or topical analgesics (anaesthetic ear-drops) are the mainstay of therapy. However, as with streptococcal pharyngitis, in patients considered at increased risk of complications of otitis media (particularly Aboriginals, Torres Strait Islanders, Maoris and Pacific Islanders) the threshold for prescribing antibiotics should be substantially lower.

*S. pneumoniae* is the most common reported bacterial cause of acute otitis media (between one-third and one-half of all cases) and initial trials of multivalent conjugate vaccines against the serotypes responsible for otitis media have been shown to be effective. An updated summary of the primary care management of otitis media in Australia was published in the *Medical Journal of Australia* in 2009, and includes the management of otitis media with effusion (glue ear) and chronic suppurative otitis media.

# Approach to management of respiratory tract infections

## Prevention and treatment

Provided they are uncomplicated, URTIs are self-limiting and require no specific pharmacological intervention. An extraordinary number of therapeutic agents has been studied in an attempt either to prevent or to treat the common cold, an indicator that there is probably nothing that makes any real difference. Indeed, there are currently 16 Cochrane systematic reviews of various interventions, most of which conclude either 'no difference from placebo', or that the studies are of such poor quality that 'no firm recommendation can be made'. Interventions studied include garlic, *Echinacea*, vitamin C, Chinese medicinal herbs, zinc and antibiotics. Although NSAIDs improve symptoms of pain (e.g. earache, headache, joint pain), they have no impact on respiratory symptoms. However, the transmission of respiratory viruses can be largely prevented by hygienic measures such as simple handwashing, face masks and isolation (Box 14.1.2).

**Box 14.1.2 Prevention of upper respiratory tract infections (URTIs)**

**Reduction of exposure in daycare**
- Cohorting (both by age and if symptomatic of respiratory tract infection)
- Reducing overcrowding
- Improving ventilation
- Individual use of personal items (e.g. toothbrushes and facecloths)
- Strict handwashing by both staff and children

**Education of parents about spread of respiratory viruses and appropriate care**
- Similar issues to those outlined above for daycare
- Education concerning no antibiotics for URTIs
- Symptomatic treatment should be minimal (e.g. oral analgesics)

**Reduced exposure to environmental tobacco smoke, especially in homes and cars**

**Vaccination**
- Influenza vaccine
  - to prevent serious influenza A and B infections in young children
  - to reduce the pool of infection to protect the elderly community
- Pneumococcal conjugate vaccine (to reduce rates of acute otitis media)

### Reduced exposure to environmental tobacco smoke

Although the evidence concerning respiratory infections and passive smoking relates predominantly to lower respiratory tract infections, there is also evidence that URTIs in young children are increased in those exposed to environmental tobacco smoke.

### Immunization

Immunization with pneumococcal conjugate vaccines reduces the incidence of pneumococcal otitis media due to serotypes in the vaccine, but there is often replacement by non-vaccine serotypes, so that the overall incidence of otitis media is only slightly lower. New pneumococcal conjugate vaccines incorporating increasing numbers of serotypes are being introduced.

Although often recommended, the use of influenza vaccine in infants and young children remains controversial. During years when influenza viruses predominate, the rates of hospitalization with acute respiratory disease in children under 2 years of age (without specific risk factors) can be as high as 2% per annum. Studies have also found that routine immunization of schoolchildren results in a reduction in mortality from influenza in the elderly. This confirms that children are the major disseminators of influenza, and routine annual influenza immunization for children should be considered in all young children.

In children over the age of 1 year, it is possible to use neuraminidase inhibitors, which are potent, safe agents effective against both influenza A and B viruses. A Cochrane review concluded that both inhaled zanamivir and oral oseltamivir were effective in shortening illness duration (by 1.0–1.5 days) and hastening return to normal activity in previously healthy children with influenza. Efficacy in 'at risk' children remains to be proved. Emergence of drug-resistant strains of viruses is a potential problem.

## Summary

The vast majority of respiratory tract infections in young children are uncomplicated 'common colds' that require no specific treatment. Although local ENT complications are not uncommon, antibiotic treatment for acute otitis media and acute sinusitis offers limited benefit and can cause adverse effects (particularly rashes and gastrointestinal symptoms). A very small proportion of URTIs are bacterial. Streptococcal tonsillitis resolves quickly without complication in the majority of children without antibiotics. When treating populations known to be at high risk of suppurative complications, and/or high rates of post-streptococcal glomerulonephritis or rheumatic fever, there must be a substantially lower threshold for antibiotic treatment.

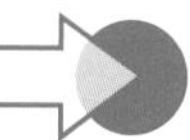

### Practical points

- Young children experience six to eight viral URTIs per year. The vast majority are mild, self-limiting 'common colds', that require no treatment.
- Local ENT complications of viral URTIs (e.g. acute sinusitis, acute otitis media) occur in approximately 10% of URTIs. Although these may benefit from symptomatic therapy (such as analgesics), antibiotics are not generally necessary.
- A very small proportion of URTIs are bacterial (and may benefit slightly from antibiotics). The most common is streptococcal pharyngitis ('tonsillitis'), especially in school-aged children.
- Spread of the viral infection into the lower respiratory tract and secondary bacterial infection are both uncommon complications.
- The age of the child, the specific infective agent, and other host and environmental factors have a major bearing on the nature of the respiratory infections, including the timing, frequency, severity and likelihood of either local or distant complications.
- A number of recognizable viral oropharyngeal syndromes occur in young children, including herpes gingivostomatitis and the enteroviral syndromes – herpangina, and hand, foot and mouth disease.

# Stridor 14.2

Sadasivam Suresh, Peter Sly

Stridor is a symptom of airway obstruction that predominantly involves the upper and larger airway. Croup is the commonest cause of stridor in children.

## Stridor

### Physiological principles

Stridor is defined in *Dorland's Illustrated Medical Dictionary* (28th edition) as 'a harsh, high-pitched respiratory sound such as the inspiratory sound often heard in acute laryngeal obstruction'. Although this definition is strictly correct, it is not all that helpful and gives no information about how and why stridor comes about. Stridor is a harsh, high-pitched noise heard predominantly during inspiration. Consideration of the physiological principles underlying this fact gives some clue as to the site of the lesion causing the stridor. The presence of an added respiratory sound implies an obstruction to the free flow of gas through the airway tree. This obstruction is usually known as flow limitation. Flow limitation in a compliant tube, such as the airways, is accompanied by fluttering of the walls, which occurs to conserve energy when driving pressure exceeds the pressure required to produce the maximal flow. The fluttering of the walls produces a respiratory noise. When this phenomenon occurs during inspiration the resultant noise is known as stridor, and when it occurs during expiration the noise is known as wheeze.

During breathing, there are pressure gradients between the airway opening and the alveoli. Inspiration occurs when alveolar pressure is lowered below atmospheric pressure and air flows in to equalize the pressures. At the onset of expiration, alveolar pressure exceeds atmospheric pressure and air flows out. There are also pressure gradients across the airway wall and these tend to alter airway calibre. The pressure around the extrathoracic airways, that is, those above the thoracic inlet, is atmospheric, whereas the pressure around the intrathoracic airways essentially is equal to the pleural pressure. As illustrated in Figure 14.2.1, the pressure gradients across the airway wall during inspiration means that there is a net force tending to narrow the extrathoracic airways and to dilate the intrathoracic airways (Fig. 14.2.1A). During expiration, the direction of the forces is opposite, resulting in a tendency to narrow intrathoracic airways and dilate extrathoracic airways (Fig. 14.2.1B).

As stridor is an inspiratory noise, the predominant site of obstruction (the site responsible for the flow limitation) is generally in the extrathoracic airways. Stridor with an expiratory component, that is, where the noise can also be heard at the beginning of expiration, can result either from a severe obstruction producing flow limitation during expiration as well, or from a lesion that extends into the intrathoracic airways.

### Differential diagnosis

When considering the differential diagnosis, several factors need to be taken into consideration. These include:

- *Age of onset.* A stridor present from the first few days of life suggests a congenital or structural cause.
- *Speed of onset of symptoms.* Infective causes such as croup tend to come on quickly; however, most cases of congenital or structural stridor commonly first present following a viral upper respiratory illness.
- *Progression of stridor.* Stridor increasing in severity over weeks to months suggests a progressive lesion, such as subglottic haemangioma.
- *Effect of body position.* Stridor that is worse when lying supine is seen commonly with laryngomalacia.
- *Presence of an expiratory component.* This suggests a more severe obstruction that limits flow during expiration as well as during inspiration.
- *Quality of voice.* Although the voice is frequently normal, a hoarse voice would suggest a vocal cord lesion.
- *Other medical conditions that could contribute to the pathogenesis or presentation:* febrile illness, ex-premature infant, gastro-oesophageal reflux, cutaneous haemangiomas, Möbius syndrome (a very rare syndrome characterized

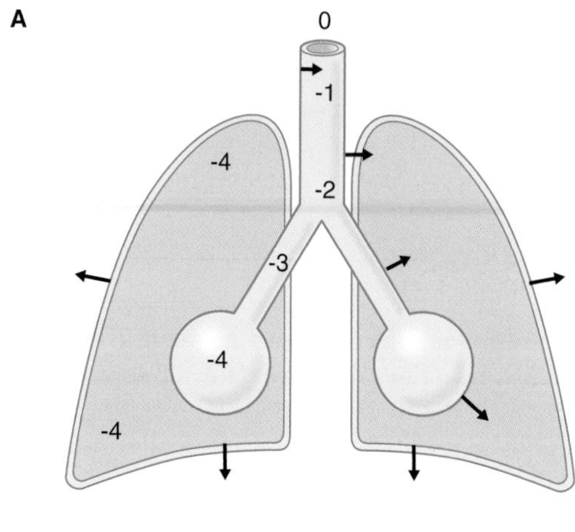


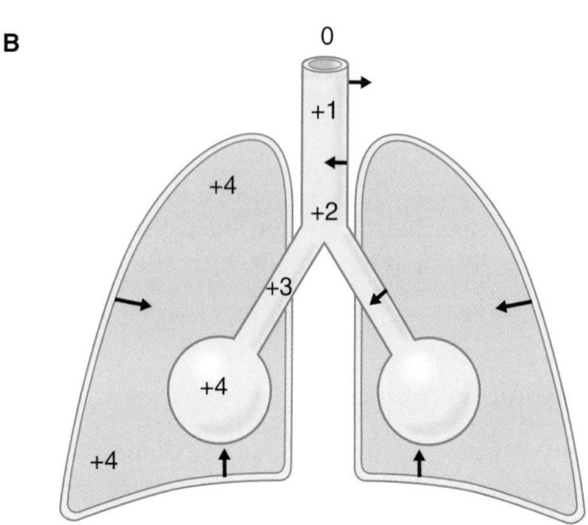


Fig. 14.2.1 The distribution of pressures throughout the respiratory system during (**A**) inspiration and (**B**) expiration. Atmospheric pressure is shown as zero. During inspiration, the expansion of the thorax results in pleural pressure falling below atmospheric. This relatively negative pressure is transmitted to the alveoli and a pressure gradient is established between the airway opening and the alveoli. Gas flows into the lungs along this pressure gradient. The pressure outside the airways is essentially pleural pressure, and results in net forces that tend to expand intrathoracic airways and to collapse the extrathoracic trachea. As shown in **B**, the pressure gradients are opposite during expiration.

by congenital palsy of the external rectus and facial muscles, usually bilateral, associated with paralysis of the sixth and seventh nerves).

## Classification

### 1. Acute stridor

a. Common causes:
- laryngotracheobronchitis (croup)

b. Rare causes (in developed countries):
- laryngeal trauma
- acute angioneurotic oedema
- retropharyngeal abscess
- peritonsillar abscess (quinsy)
- acute epiglottitis (typically a low-pitched rumbling noise coming from the supraglottic area)
- diphtheria.

### 2. Persistent stridor

a. Common causes:
- laryngomalacia (infantile larynx)
- congenital subglottic stenosis
- acquired subglottic stenosis in a premature infant who required intubation

b. Uncommon causes:
- subglottic haemangioma
- vocal cord palsy (unilateral or bilateral)
- laryngeal webs
- cysts of the posterior tongue or aryepiglottic folds
- subglottic mucus retention cysts in a premature infant who required intubation
- vascular ring (note that this usually presents with a predominantly expiratory noise)

c. Rare causes:
- laryngocele
- laryngeal cleft
- tracheal stenosis (note that this usually presents with a predominantly expiratory noise).

## Characteristics of the more important causes of stridor

### Laryngomalacia

Laryngomalacia, which is sometimes known as infantile larynx, is the most common cause of persistent stridor. The supraglottic tissues appear as if they are too large for the size of the glottis and narrow the glottic aperture during inspiration instead of the more normal widening during inspiration. This can occur in a number of ways, the most common being:
- a long, curled (sometimes called omega-shaped) epiglottis collapsing during inspiration so that the lateral walls touch, restricting the free passage of air (Fig. 14.2.2A)
- floppy arytenoid processes prolapsing into the glottic aperture during inspiration (Fig. 14.2.2B)
- a long epiglottis collapsing against the posterior pharyngeal wall during inspiration.

In more severe cases, combinations of these mechanisms may be responsible for the inspiratory obstruction.

Laryngomalacia classically produces a cog-wheel stridor, with no expiratory component. The cog-wheel nature to the stridor is likely to come from vibrations of the supraglottic tissues as the degree of obstruction varies during the inspiratory effort. The stridor

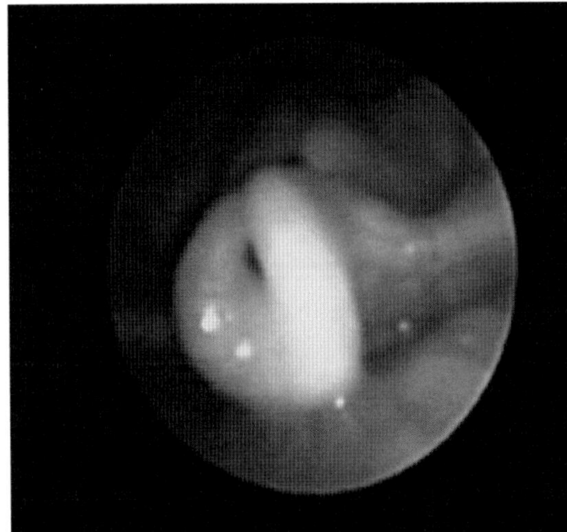

A

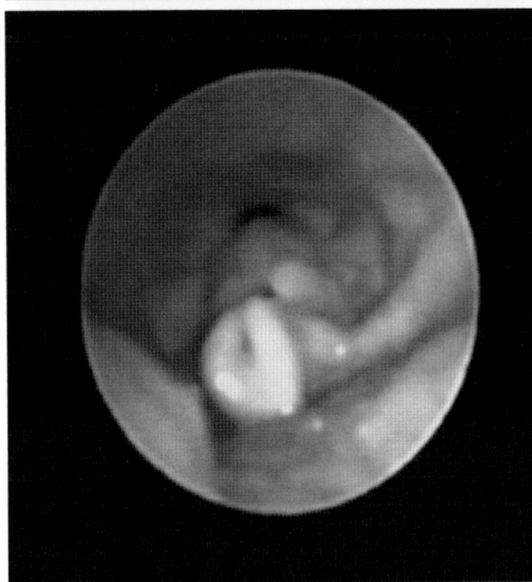

B

Fig. 14.2.2 Flexible bronchoscopy images showing (**A**) omega-shaped epiglottis and (**B**) prolapse of the arytenoids into the glottic aperture.

may be worse when the infant is lying supine, although this feature is not always seen. More severe obstruction may be associated with suprasternal and sternal retraction during inspiration.

Laryngomalacia is usually a benign condition that does not require any treatment, except to reassure the parents that this is the case. Severe laryngomalacia may be associated with failure to thrive and gastro-oesophageal reflux. The importance of parental reassurance should not be underestimated, as the stridor is likely to last for 2–3 years. Frequently, parents find the most distressing part of having a child with laryngomalacia are the looks from people when they take the child out in public and the well-intentioned advice received from relatives.

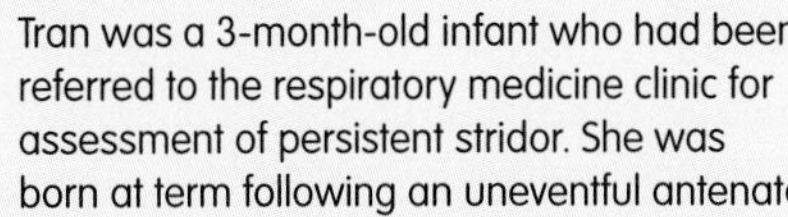

**Clinical example**

Tran was a 3-month-old infant who had been referred to the respiratory medicine clinic for assessment of persistent stridor. She was born at term following an uneventful antenatal course and normal vaginal delivery. The stridor was not present at birth and was noticed for the first time at the age of 2 months when she caught a cold from her older brother. Her mother was extremely concerned that something was seriously wrong with her baby as several relatives had told her it is not normal for a baby to make this type of noise.

Since that time the stridor had been present on most days but was heard less commonly when Tran was sleeping. Her mother was concerned that the stridor was becoming louder and, on questioning, reported that sometimes an expiratory component could be heard. The stridor was typically worse when Tran was crying or when lying supine for nappy changes.

Examination revealed a female infant who looked scrawny. Her height was on the 50% percentile but her weight was just below the 10% percentile. She had two typical strawberry naevi on her trunk. While being held in her mother's arms, a cog-wheel stridor with no expiratory component could be heard clearly. When she was lying supine, the stridor was associated with a soft but definite expiratory component and mild suprasternal retraction.

**Discussion points**

- What is the most likely diagnosis?
- What investigations are warranted?

A flexible bronchoscopy was performed under general anaesthesia and revealed laryngomalacia, with a tightly coiled epiglottis and prolapsing arytenoid processes. The subglottic area and lower airways were normal.

**Discussion points**

- Is any treatment warranted?
- Is the fact that Tran's weight percentile is lower than her height percentile of concern?
- Is the laryngomalacia likely to be responsible for her relative failure to thrive (lower weight percentile than height percentile)?
- How could this come about?

The bronchoscopic findings are diagnostic of laryngomalacia and one can be confident that the symptoms will resolve spontaneously with time. The relative failure to thrive may be related to the increased work of breathing required to overcome the obstruction. However, a dietary assessment is warranted before attributing the failure to thrive to this mechanism. As the obstruction decreases with time, Tran's work of breathing will also decrease and the failure to thrive should resolve.

## Subglottic stenosis

Subglottic stenosis refers to a narrowing in the upper part of the trachea, immediately below the glottis. This narrowing may be congenital or acquired. Congenital subglottic stenosis occurs typically at the level of, and involves, the cricoid cartilage. The tracheal epithelium typically appears normal but the cross-sectional area of the lumen is reduced and typically does not vary with respiration. Acquired subglottic stenosis usually results from trauma and is most commonly seen in premature infants who required intubation. Older infants and children who require prolonged intubation are also at risk. Here the tracheal epithelium is more likely to be replaced by scar tissue.

Subglottic stenosis may present soon after birth or the presentation may be delayed. The stenosis, either congenital or acquired, is usually not progressive but the degree of obstruction may increase, for example as the child's activity levels increase or at times of respiratory infection. The typical presentation is with stridor, particularly at times of respiratory infection. If the obstruction is severe enough, the stridor may have an expiratory component and be associated with suprasternal and sternal retractions.

Many cases of subglottic stenosis do not require treatment and most will improve with growth. Laser and dilatation treatments are generally disappointing. More severe obstruction may require surgery, usually involving a procedure in which the cricoid cartilage is split and reconstructed.

### Subglottic haemangioma

The subglottic area can also be narrowed by a haemangioma occurring in this area. These are typical haemangiomas occurring in the submucosal layer of the tracheal wall (Fig. 14.2.3). As with other haemangiomas, they enlarge during the first year of life and typically present with increasing stridor and inspiratory obstruction. The stridor is rarely present at birth and most come to attention around 4–6 months of age. As the obstruction becomes worse, the stridor develops an expiratory component and is associated with sternal and suprasternal retractions. Approximately 50% of subglottic haemangiomas are associated with cutaneous haemangiomas, although the converse association is much less frequent.

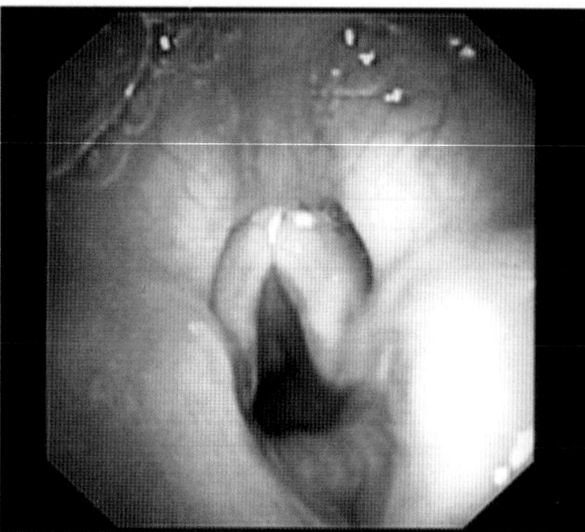

Fig. 14.2.3 Flexible bronchoscopic image showing subglottic haemangioma at the 5–7 o'clock position.

The earlier a subglottic haemangioma presents, the more likely that surgical treatment will be necessary. Tracheostomy remains the definitive treatment if airway obstruction is marked. Medical management is also shown to be of benefit in a subgroup of patients. Commonly used agents are propranolol, corticosteroids or interferon. The milder forms of haemangioma regress, not needing further intervention.

## Investigations

The most important investigations in elucidating the cause of a stridor are a thorough history and physical examination. As discussed above, the characteristics of the stridor, the time of onset, the progression, and whether or not an expiratory component is present will clarify the cause of the stridor on many occasions.

The definitive investigation for stridor is bronchoscopy, preferably performed with a flexible, fibreoptic bronchoscope. Laryngoscopy is not sufficient as the subglottic area and lower trachea cannot be assessed safely and adequately. Frequently the trachea can be visualized on penetrated radiography of the chest and lateral neck; however, these X-rays rarely replace the need for bronchoscopy.

### Clinical example

Jane was a 4-year-old girl who was brought to the emergency department by her mother, who reported increased wheezing over the past day, associated with a cold. Jane had a history of troublesome episodes of asthma for the past 3 years. She was reasonably well between episodes but, since starting preschool, her mother had noticed that Jane wheezed when running and appeared to tire more easily. Jane's mother reported that the wheeze was not really helped by bronchodilators and that inhaled steroids did not help prevent the attacks. On examination, Jane had an expiratory wheeze but had a prominent inspiratory component to her wheeze. She was not particularly distressed and her oxygen saturation was normal.

**Discussion points**

- What is the most likely diagnosis?
- What investigations are warranted?

A chest X-ray showed an odd appearance to the upper mediastinum but was otherwise normal. A barium swallow was performed which demonstrated a well-defined indentation at the upper half of the oesophagus (Fig. 14.2.4). This confirmed the clinical diagnosis made by the emergency department consultant that the stridor was due to a vascular ring.

**Discussion points**

A vascular ring causes an obstruction to the intrathoracic portion of the trachea. Using the distribution of pressures throughout the respiratory system shown in Figure 14.2.1, explain the physical signs Jane presented with.

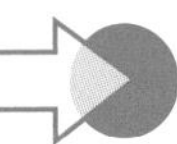

**Practical points**

- A careful history of the age of onset, features of preceding viral infection, nature and respiratory timing of the stridor are important for diagnosis.
- Many children with stridor need no investigations.
- Persistent stridor with an expiratory component always warrants further investigation.

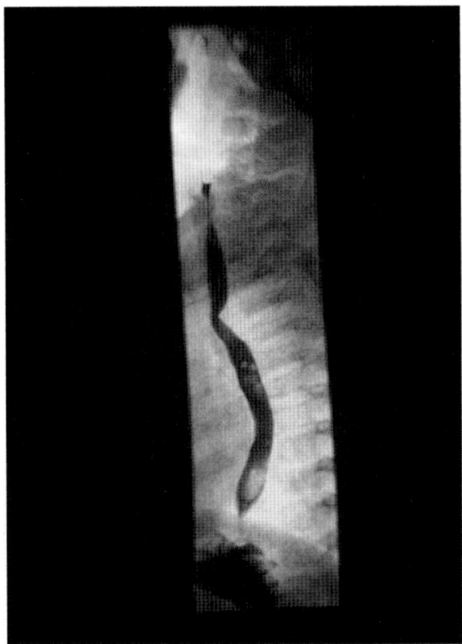

Fig. 14.2.4 Barium swallow demonstrating extrinsic compression of the oesophagus by the vascular ring.

## Croup (laryngotracheobronchitis)

Croup is usually considered to exist in two forms:

- acute viral croup
- recurrent (or spasmodic) croup.

Although these two conditions have a number of similarities, they are likely to be distinct entities. They have in common that they involve the larynx, trachea and bronchi, and present with a typically barking cough. The cough is so typical it is usually referred to as a 'croupy' cough.

### Acute viral croup

Acute viral croup is typically a disease of toddlers, being rare in the first 6 months of life and reaching a peak incidence of 5 cases per 100 children per year during the second year of life. Boys are affected more commonly than girls. Most children who get acute viral croup will only ever have one or two episodes. These episodes typically begin with the symptoms of an upper respiratory infection and progress to typical croup over 1–2 days. The most common viruses isolated from children with croup are parainfluenza virus type 1 (up to 50% in some series), parainfluenza virus type 3 (up to 20%) and respiratory syncytial virus (approximately 10%).

#### Clinical manifestations

As mentioned above, croup usually begins with signs and symptoms of an upper respiratory infection, including fever and rhinitis. A cough may be present. The typical barking, croupy cough usually begins during the night or the early hours of the morning. As the disease progresses, stridor may be heard on exertion initially. If the subglottic obstruction progresses further, stridor may be heard at rest and an expiratory component may be heard. The typical cough continues to be heard.

If the degree of obstruction continues to worsen, the stridor may become more difficult to hear and the child may become distressed and restless. Cough may be absent at this stage. The lack of stridor comes about because the amount of air moving through the obstructed airway is not sufficient to generate the noise (see above). The distress and restlessness are most likely to be due to hypoxia and signal impending complete respiratory obstruction.

The viral illness generally lasts 7–10 days, but the typical croupy cough usually only occurs on the first 2–3 nights.

#### Investigations

Most children with croup do not warrant any investigations. Viral diagnosis on nasal secretions, usually obtained by per nasal aspiration, can be helpful from an epidemiological point of view but will not alter management. Chest X-rays are not helpful for children with typical croup.

Children less than 6 months old who present with croup or those whose croup runs an atypical course warrant investigation. The most useful investigations are likely to be a lateral neck X-ray and flexible bronchoscopy.

#### Management

The majority of children with croup do not require any treatment. Symptomatic treatment for fever and cold symptoms may be warranted. Children with a croupy cough and stridor on exertion (but not at rest) can usually be managed with supportive treatment only. There is a widespread belief that exposing these children to steam, especially by steaming up the home bathroom, helps relieve stridor. There is no evidence to support this treatment. The only benefit that is likely to come from sitting with the child in a steamy bathroom is from sitting quietly with the child and not from the steam.

Children with stridor at rest warrant medical assessment. The most useful treatment for croup that has reached this severity is corticosteroids. These can be giving orally in syrup form or inhaled (nebulizer or metered-dose inhaler and spacer). The mechanism of action is not known but is likely to be via a topical action. A single dose of steroids decreases the risk of hospitalization dramatically.

More severe obstruction can be relieved by nebulized adrenaline (epinephrine). Traditionally this has been given as a 50:50 mix of the L- and D-isoforms (known as racemic adrenaline), but the L-isoform (as found in standard ampoules of intravenous adrenaline) is as effective and is now commonly used. This relieves obstruction by causing a topical vasoconstriction, which wears off in 1–4 hours, depending on the severity of the underlying obstruction.

Severe obstruction may require intubation or even tracheostomy, although the need for these types of treatment has become much less with the widespread use of oral corticosteroids in the emergency departments of paediatric hospitals in Australia.

A management flowchart from a recent review article summarizes acute outpatient management of croup (Fig. 14.2.5).

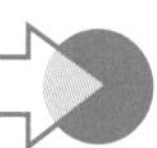

**Practical points**

- Use of corticosteroids can favourably modify the course of acute viral croup.
- Severe croup can lead to complete airway obstruction and death.

## Recurrent (spasmodic) croup

Some children suffer recurrent episodes of croup, frequently without the preceding viral prodrome usually seen in acute viral croup. Typically these children are well when they go to bed and wake in the early hours of the morning with a barking cough and stridor. Fever is unusual in this form of croup. The same viruses as found in acute viral croup may be found in the upper airways of children with spasmodic croup, although the relationship between the viruses and the symptoms is less clear. Frequently children with recurrent croup have a family history of atopy and asthma, or have asthma themselves. This, together with the uncertain relationship between the clinical symptoms and the presence of a virus, have led to the concept that spasmodic croup may be a manifestation of upper airway hyperresponsiveness. There are no direct data to support or refute this hypothesis. The viral isolates from these patients are similar to those found in children with acute croup. There is some literature supporting the association between gastro-oesophageal reflux disease and episodes of recurrent croup.

Spasmodic croup may be severe enough to require treatment with oral corticosteroids, nebulized adrenaline or even intubation; however, the episodes are frequently short-lived and often settle by the time the child presents to the emergency department.

Although controlled trials have not been carried out, there is a substantial body of anecdotal evidence that frequent bouts of recurrent croup can be prevented by maintenance therapy with inhaled corticosteroids via a spacer.

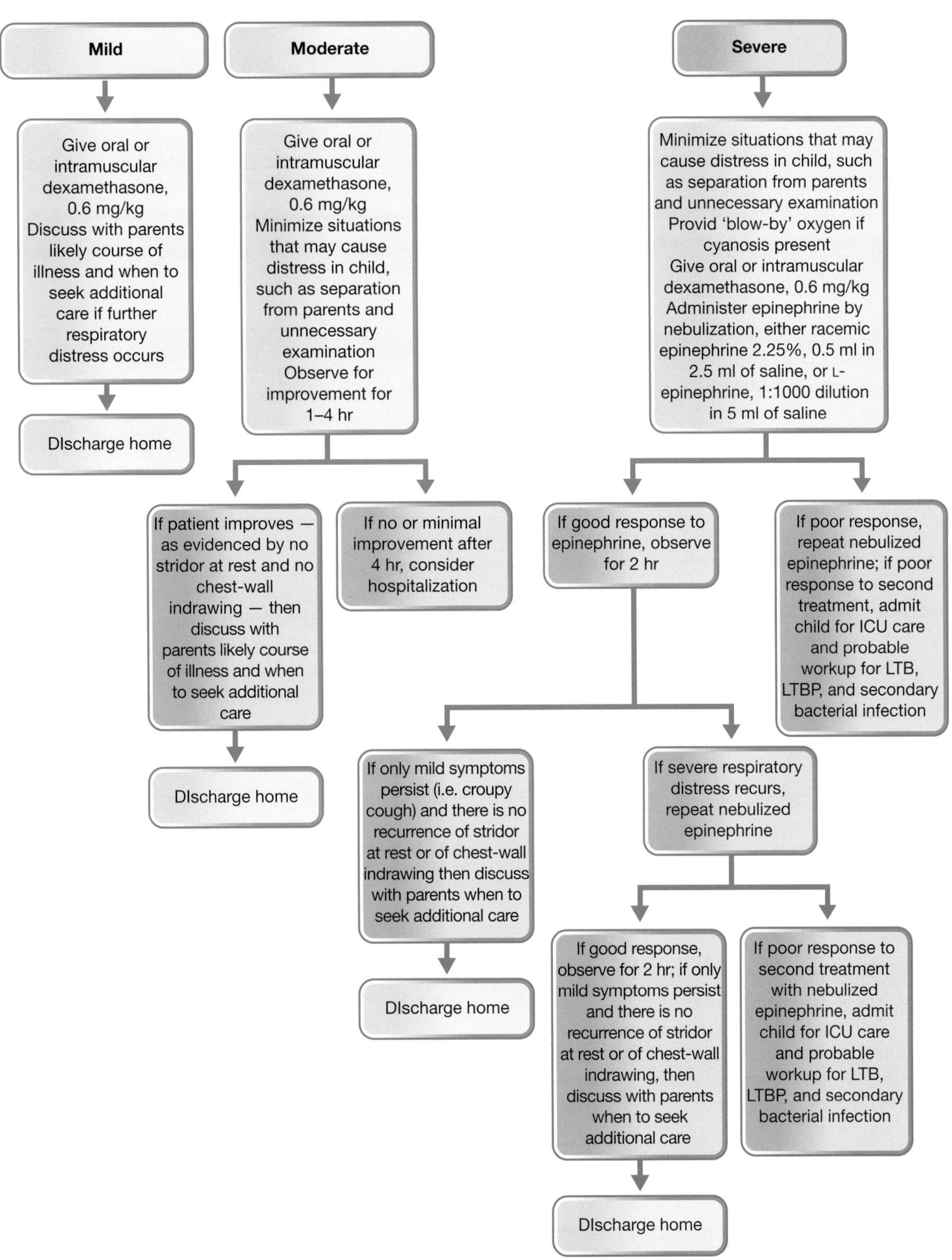


Fig. 14.2.5 Outpatient management flow chart. ICU, intensive care unit; LTB, laryngotracheobronchitis; LTBP, laryngotracheobronchopneumonitis. (Source: Cherry JD 2008 Clinical practice. Croup. N Engl J Med 358:384–389.)

# 14.3 Asthma

Adam Jaffé

## Definition

The word 'asthma' is a derivative of the Greek verb *aazein* , meaning 'to pant'. In an attempt to describe it more precisely, the Global Initiative for Asthma (GINA) has defined asthma as 'a chronic inflammatory disorder of the airways in which many cells and cellular elements play a role. The chronic inflammation is associated with airway hyper-responsiveness that leads to recurrent episodes of wheezing, breathlessness, chest tightness, and coughing, particularly at night or in the early morning. These episodes are usually associated with widespread, but variable, airflow obstruction within the lung that is often reversible either spontaneously or with treatment'. Although this is a complex definition and is of limited practical value in making the diagnosis in an individual, it highlights the interplay between inflammation, airway hyper-responsiveness, obstruction and clinical symptoms.

## Burden of asthma

Asthma is estimated to affect 300 million people worldwide. Although the burden of asthma continues to increase in some countries, its prevalence is stabilizing and even declining in others. In the UK the prevalence of asthma is 1 in 11, and in Australia it is 1 in 9 children. The International Study of Asthma and Allergies in Childhood (ISAAC) has identified Australia, along with the UK, New Zealand and the Republic of Ireland, as having a relatively high prevalence of asthma in children compared with other countries. It is one of the commonest presentations to the primary physician and emergency department. In most developed countries the mortality rate remains low, but death still occurs in childhood. Like many respiratory diseases, the prevalence of asthma is higher in Indigenous children.

The return to school after the summer holidays is associated with a peak in hospital admissions; this occurs in February in the southern hemisphere, and in October in countries in the northern hemisphere, and is likely to be caused by the spread of viruses such as rhinovirus in the classroom.

## Age of onset

The onset of asthma can occur at any age, including within the first few years of life; children under 4 years of age are more likely to be hospitalized or to seek medical attention. However, the diagnosis of asthma is particularly difficult in the preschool child as there are many different wheezing phenotypes in this age group (see Chapter 14.4). It is often difficult to distinguish young children who wheeze with upper respiratory tract viral infections from those with intermittent asthma. The importance of this distinction is that those with virus-induced wheeze will usually get better by 6 years of age.

The Asthma Predictive Index is a helpful guide in the clinical setting for predicting whether children under 3 years of age with recurrent wheeze will develop asthma when older. Children are at a high risk of developing asthma if they have either:

one of:

- parental history of asthma (particularly maternal)
- eczema
- sensitization to aeroallergens

or two of:

- allergic rhinitis
- >4% eosinophilia
- food allergies
- wheezing in circumstances not related to upper respiratory tract infections.

## Pathogenesis

### Genes

The cause of asthma is multifactorial and complicated, and involves an interaction between genetic determinants and environmental stimuli (Table 14.3.1). Although asthma has been known to run in families, the inheritance pattern remains unclear. Asthma is polygenic and, although many potential candidate

**Table 14.3.1 Factors involved in the pathogenesis of asthma**

| Host | Environment |
|---|---|
| Innate immunity<br>• Hygiene hypothesis<br><br>Genetic candidates<br>• $\beta_2$-adrenoreceptor<br>• Tumour necrosis factor $\alpha$<br>• Interleukin-4<br>• Interleukin-4 receptor<br>• Clara cell protein<br>• CD14<br>• $\beta$-chain of IgE receptor<br>• RANTES (a chemokine) promoter polymorphism<br>• ADAM33 (a disintegrin and matrix metalloproteinase domain-containing protein 33)<br><br>Sex<br>• More prevalent in boys<br>• From puberty, more prevalent in females | Allergens<br>• Aeroallergens (house dust mite, cockroaches, *Alternaria)*<br><br>Respiratory infections<br>• Viruses (e.g. RSV) (association but causation not yet proven)<br><br>Environmental tobacco smoke<br>• *In utero* causes smaller airways and increased wheeze in early life<br>• Continued exposure associated with increased asthma severity<br><br>Air pollution (association but causation not fully proven)<br><br>Low intake of antioxidants (association but causation not yet proven)<br><br>Low intake of omega-3 fatty acids (association but causation not yet proven)<br><br>Obesity (via inflammatory mediators)<br><br>Chlorinated swimming pools in infancy (association but causation not yet proven)<br><br>Paracetamol (controversial – association *in utero* and first 12 months of life but causation not proven) |

Ig, immunoglobulin; RANTES, regulated upon activation, normal T cell expressed and secreted; RSV, respiratory syncytial virus

genes have been discovered, no single gene accounts for more than 10% of the susceptibility of an individual for developing asthma. Boys generally have smaller airways than girls and tend to suffer more from asthma. However, after adolescence the prevalence is higher in females.

## Allergy

The role of allergy in asthma is very important and more than 80% of people with asthma have an allergy. Sensitization and chronic exposure to aeroallergens such as house dust mite, cockroach and animal dander are implicated in the development of asthma; however, this research area remains confusing as there is evidence that early exposure to animals such as dogs may be protective.

## Hygiene hypothesis

This is another explanation for why children develop asthma. At birth, there is an overexpression of the T-helper cell type 2 (Th2) pathway. Th2 cells produce cytokines (interleukin (IL)-4, -5, -6, -9 and -13) that mediate allergic inflammation, and this pathway is associated with the development of atopy and asthma. Factors that favour the Th2 phenotype include antibiotic use, diet, urban environment and lifestyle, and sensitization to allergens. Exposure to environmental stimuli such as lipopolysaccharide stimulates the immune system to develop along the Th1 pathway with expression of IL-2 and interferon-γ. Having older siblings or living in a rural environment also favours the expression of the Th1 phenotype; these children generally do not develop an allergic phenotype.

## Viruses

Although viruses such as human rhinovirus C cause asthma exacerbations, it is increasingly recognized that exposure to viruses may lead to the development of asthma. Some researchers have demonstrated that babies exposed to winter viruses are more likely to develop asthma later in life. The role of respiratory syncytial virus (RSV) is important but controversial. Infection with RSV is certainly associated with the development of asthma, but whether it causes asthma directly or is simply a marker for those likely to develop asthma remains to be elucidated.

Most children with asthma have an underlying immunoglobulin (Ig) E-mediated eosinophilic response, but it is increasingly being recognized that there are other phenotypes such as neutrophilic asthma. This has potential implications with regard to therapy, as children with neutrophilic asthma may benefit from medications such as macrolides. Future research will help to define better the different phenotypes and causes of asthma in children.

## Clinical features

The diagnosis of asthma is likely in children with the following symptoms, particularly if they occur at night or early in the morning or have identified triggers:

- Wheeze – the main symptom is wheeze which is a musical note caused by turbulent air flow and is usually, but not always, present in children with asthma. Parents often mistake wheeze for other sounds such as stertor or rattle, so it is important to ensure that parents understand what is meant by the term 'wheeze' (see Chapter 14.4)
- Cough
- Difficulty breathing
- Chest tightness.

The likelihood of asthma is increased if there is a personal history of atopy or a family history of atopy or asthma. A clinical or lung function bronchodilator response to β-agonists further supports the diagnosis of asthma. It is a myth that asthma cannot be diagnosed under 2 years of age, although it is often difficult to do so in the absence of confirmatory lung function testing.

### Clinical example

John was a 12-year-old boy who presented with a history of breathlessness and chest pain that occurred towards the end of an 800-metre run. Neither cough nor wheeze was present. He had received bronchodilators and sodium cromoglycate before exercise, without benefit. A trial of inhaled corticosteroids for 6 weeks followed by a leukotriene receptor antagonist had also been ineffective. His parents were both keen athletes and hoped that John would become a champion athlete.

Physical examination was normal. $FEV_1$ was normal and a mannitol challenge test was negative, with no evidence of airway hyper-responsiveness. John was non-atopic on allergen skin testing. After an explanation to John and his parents that he did not have asthma, John indicated that he was not interested in competitive athletics. He was discharged on no treatment. One year later he was completely well. He could play regular sport with no difficulties. The tests used were helpful in confirming that John did not have asthma.

## History

The key points to concentrate on are:

- antenatal history: smoking (causes smaller airways)
- birth history: prematurity, need for ventilator support (premature babies may wheeze for other reasons such as bronchomalacia)
- atopy: development of food intolerance, eczema, hay fever
- triggers: viruses, exercise, allergen exposure, cold air, emotions such as laughter, thunderstorms
- symptom pattern: this helps classify the type and severity of asthma
- family history: asthma, eczema, hay fever, atopy (particularly parental)
- social history: exposure to environmental tobacco smoke (parental smoking outside still results in exposure to the child), pets, mould, cockroaches, house dust mite.

## Examination

The key signs on examination in both acute and chronic asthma are summarized in Figure 14.3.1.

An alternative diagnosis should be sought in children who are clubbed, have a history of a moist cough, have cough as their only symptom, have normal clinical signs and spirometry when symptomatic, and do not respond to asthma treatment.

## Classification

A useful way to classify asthma is according to symptom pattern, which helps to determine the need for a controller medication (Table 14.3.2). Infrequent intermittent asthma occurs in 70–75% of all childhood asthmatics. Frequent intermittent asthma occurs in 20% of asthmatic children, and only 5% of children have persistent asthma.

Questions that are particularly helpful in clarifying the pattern of asthma include:

- Are there nocturnal symptoms?
- Are there symptoms on waking in the morning?
- Is there normal exercise tolerance?
- How much school is missed because of asthma?
- How frequent is the use of bronchodilator medication?
- How frequent are asthma symptoms?

### Clinical example

Jane presented with her first episode of wheeze at 8 months of age. She responded well to a bronchodilator. She did not have eczema and there was no history of asthma or hay fever in the family. She continued to become wheezy when she caught a viral upper respiratory tract infection. The episodes occurred approximately every 3 months and she was treated with inhaled salbutamol via a spacer only. When she started school, her symptoms disappeared. Her case is typical of those children with infrequent intermittent asthma where a preventer is not necessary; most children grow out of it by 6 years of age.

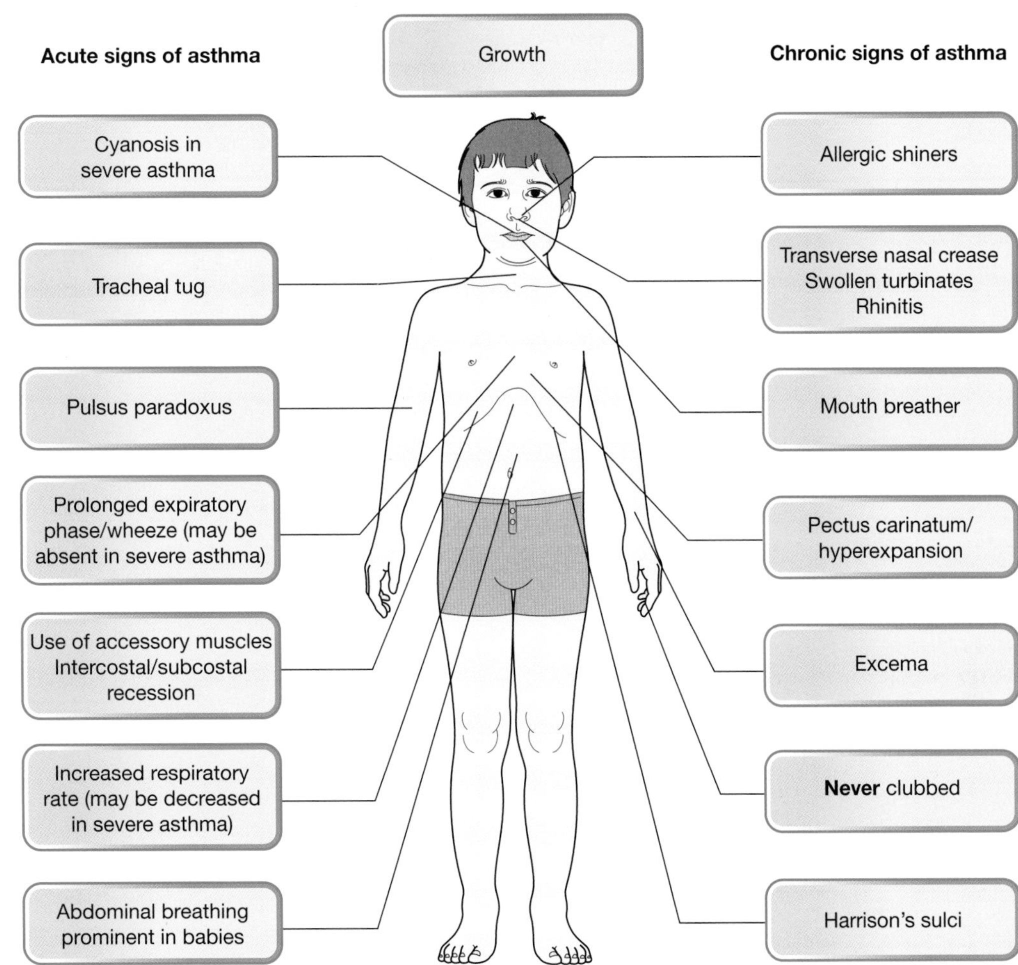


Fig. 14.3.1 Key examination findings in acute and chronic asthma.

## Investigations

- Chest X-ray: there is no role for a routine chest X-ray. This should be done only if the diagnosis is uncertain.
- Skin prick tests to common aeroallergens in children of all ages are usually helpful but may change over time in the very young child whose immune system is developing.
- Spirometry: typically children from age 5 years onward can perform reproducible spirometry, although children from 3½ years may be able to do this with incentive software on lung function testing equipment. Typically the flow volume loop will show an obstructive picture with classical 'scooping' of the expiratory flow volume loop (Fig. 14.3.2) with a reduced forced expiratory volume in 1 second ($FEV_1$) to forced vital capacity (FVC) ratio of less than 0.70.
- Bronchodilator response: an increase in $FEV_1$ or FVC of ≥12% or ≥200 mL 10–15 minutes following the administration of a β-agonist indicates a significant positive bronchodilator response and supports the diagnosis of asthma.
- Bronchial provocation tests help in assessing whether the child has bronchial hyper-responsiveness. There are different techniques available but they all rely on the principle of inhaling increasing doses of a stimulus that causes bronchoconstriction and measuring the fall in $FEV_1$:
  - *Direct challenge* of bronchial smooth muscle cells: methacholine; histamine. Although responsiveness correlates well with asthma severity, a response is not necessarily specific to asthma diagnosis.
  - *Indirect challenge* by the action of inflammatory mediators released from intermediary cells such as mast cells in response to a stimulus to: adenosine; hypertonic saline; cold air; eucapnic voluntary hyperpnoea (hyperventilating with a dry gas); exercise; mannitol (useful for the diagnosis of exercise-induced asthma).

**Table 14.3.2 Classification of asthma by symptom pattern in children**

| | Intermittent | | Persistent | | |
|---|---|---|---|---|---|
| | Infrequent | Frequent | Mild | Moderate | Severe |
| Symptoms | None | None | >1 per week but <1 per day | Daily | Continual |
| Exacerbations | Brief, mild, occur <4–6 weeks | >2 per month | May affect activity and sleep | ≥2 per week<br>Affects activity and sleep | Frequent<br>Restricts activity |
| Nocturnal symptoms | None | None | >2 per month | >1 per week | Frequent |
| $FEV_1$ or PEF (in children over 5 years of age) | >80% predicted | >80% predicted | >80% predicted | 60–80% | ≤60% |
| Variability of $FEV_1$ and PEF (in children over 5 years of age) | <20% | <20% | 20–30% | 30% | >30% |

$FEV_1$, forced expiratory volume in 1 second; PEF, peak expiratory flow.
Adapted with permission from: Global Initiative for Asthma (GINA) 2008 Global strategy for asthma management and prevention, Bethesda, and National Asthma Council Australia 2006 Asthma management handbook 2006, South Melbourne.

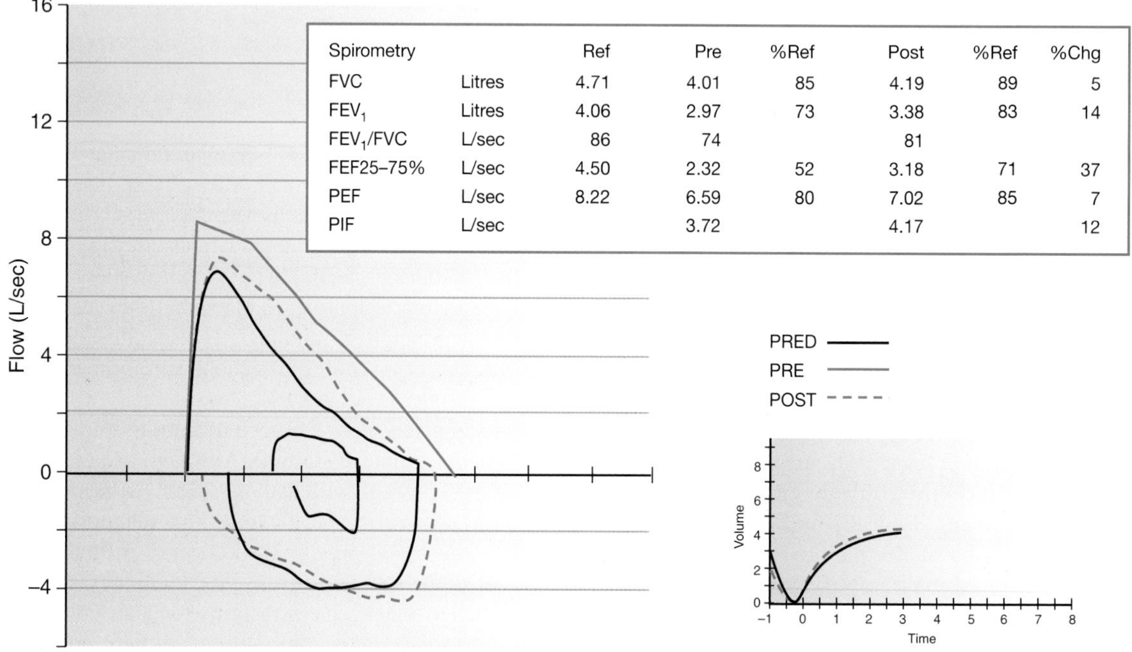

| Spirometry | | Ref | Pre | %Ref | Post | %Ref | %Chg |
|---|---|---|---|---|---|---|---|
| FVC | Litres | 4.71 | 4.01 | 85 | 4.19 | 89 | 5 |
| $FEV_1$ | Litres | 4.06 | 2.97 | 73 | 3.38 | 83 | 14 |
| $FEV_1$/FVC | L/sec | 86 | 74 | | 81 | | |
| FEF25–75% | L/sec | 4.50 | 2.32 | 52 | 3.18 | 71 | 37 |
| PEF | L/sec | 8.22 | 6.59 | 80 | 7.02 | 85 | 7 |
| PIF | L/sec | | 3.72 | | 4.17 | | 12 |



Fig. 14.3.2 Spirometry demonstrating a scooped flow volume loop seen in obstructive disease in asthma. Following bronchodilator use (PRED, predicted) there is a positive bronchodilator response of >12% in forced expiratory volume in 1 second ($FEV_1$). FEF, forced expiratory flow rate; FVC, forced vital capacity; PEF, peak expiratory flow rate; PIF, peak inspiratory flow rate.

- Exhaled nitric oxide is a marker of lower airway eosinophilic inflammation and may have a role in helping make the diagnosis of asthma and assessing the impact of therapy. It is often raised in children with allergies.

## Management

### Acute asthma

The focus of management of acute attacks is the assessment of severity of the episode and treatment to restore to normal baseline lung function. The initial assessment identifies children whose asthma is mild and may be managed at home and those who require admission to hospital and may require management in an intensive care unit. The key signs on examination in acute asthma are displayed in Figure 14.3.1. The assessment of a child with acute asthma is outlined in Table 14.3.3.

Initial management consists of oxygen and repeated doses of an inhaled $\beta_2$-agonist, preferably by a spacer device. A nebulizer driven by oxygen may be required in severe asthma. Ipratropium may be considered in moderate to severe cases for its additive effect. Systemic steroids should be given either by the oral route or intravenously in severe cases. In deteriorating cases, salbutamol may be given intravenously with regular monitoring of potassium. Intravenous aminophylline may also be used in severe asthma, although its popularity in various paediatric departments fluctuates. A loading dose should be avoided in those taking oral theophylline owing to its potentially cardiotoxic nature. In deteriorating severe cases, intravenous magnesium sulphate may avoid intubation. Any child requiring 3-hourly or more frequent $\beta_2$-agonists should be admitted to hospital.

The resolution of an acute attack of asthma is not the end of treatment and should be used as an opportunity to consider the background control and educate the child and parents in the ongoing management.

### Chronic asthma

All children should have an asthma action plan reviewed at least 6-monthly. The school should be aware of the child's medical condition and have a copy of the plan.

- Preventative strategies:
  - environmental tobacco smoke avoidance
  - aeroallergen avoidance (such as pets)
- Pharmacological management. There are two principal classes of medication used in the chronic management of asthma:
  - *Relievers* – short-acting bronchodilators have a rapid onset and are used as required. Rapidly acting inhaled $\beta_2$-agonists are generally more effective than ipratropium bromide. Children with infrequent intermittent asthma require treatment only during exacerbations and do not need controller medications. Those who have more regular symptoms require a controller medication.

**Table 14.3.3 Assessment of a child with acute asthma**

| Symptoms | Mild | Moderate | Severe and life-threatening |
|---|---|---|---|
| Saturations in air | >94% | 90–94%* | <90%* |
| Central cyanosis | None | None | Present |
| Heart rate | Normal range for age | Mild–moderate tachycardia for age | Marked tachycardia for age (bradycardia suggests imminent arrest) |
| Ability to talk | Sentences/long cry | Phrases/shortened cry | Words/weak cry/unable to vocalize |
| Use of accessory muscles | None | Mild to moderate | Moderate to severe |
| Presence of wheeze | Variable | Moderate to loud | Quiet/absent |
| Consciousness | Alert | Easily engaged | Agitated, drowsy, confused |

*Inhaled β-agonists can cause an increase in ventilation perfusion mismatch and a decrease in oxygen saturations. A low reading should be interpreted in the context of other clinical symptoms.

Adapted with permission from: National Asthma Council Australia 2006 Asthma management handbook 2006, South Melbourne.

- *Controllers* – inhaled steroids; leukotriene receptor antagonists; cromones; combination therapy of inhaled steroid and long-acting $\beta_2$-agonist; theophylline.

Children with frequent intermittent asthma may benefit from a controller, particularly over the winter months. Controller medications are required in those with persistent asthma. Although there are subtle differences in the stepwise management in various guidelines worldwide (Figs 14.3.3 & 14.3.4), the principal aim is to start at the most appropriate level and step up or down depending on the level of control (Table 14.3.4).

> **Clinical example**
>
> Craig was an 8-year-old boy who had eczema and rubbed his nose. He coughed most nights and when tickled. He wheezed with exercise. His mother had severe asthma and smoked. There were two cats at home. Craig demonstrated a bronchodilator response of 21% $FEV_1$. Skin-prick testing was positive to house dust mite, cat and grasses. Think about how you would classify his pattern of asthma and develop an asthma management plan. Remember to address environmental factors, treat the nose, assess the level of control and choose an appropriate step to commence a controller medication.

## Unified airway hypothesis

The nose is that part of the airway accessible to the finger. Nasal inflammation is likely to exert effects on the lower airway through a, yet to be proven, 'naso-bronchial reflex'. It is essential that allergic rhinitis is treated appropriately as this can improve asthma control and lung function with a reduction in lower airway inflammation. The most effective treatment is with topical steroids, but leukotriene receptor antagonists, inhaled cromones and antihistamines (oral or inhaled) are alternative strategies.

## Drug side-effects

### Steroids

The growth of children on long-term inhaled steroids may be affected. Although final adult height is attained, it may be delayed. Use of high-dose inhaled steroids (>500 μg fluticasone, >800 μg beclomethasone diproprionate, >800 μg budesonide per day) is associated with adrenal suppression and has resulted in death due to adrenal crisis. These overall potential risks are well balanced by their benefits. Children on inhaled corticosteroids at these doses should have their adrenal function tested; they may require steroid replacement in times of stress if they have adrenal insufficiency.

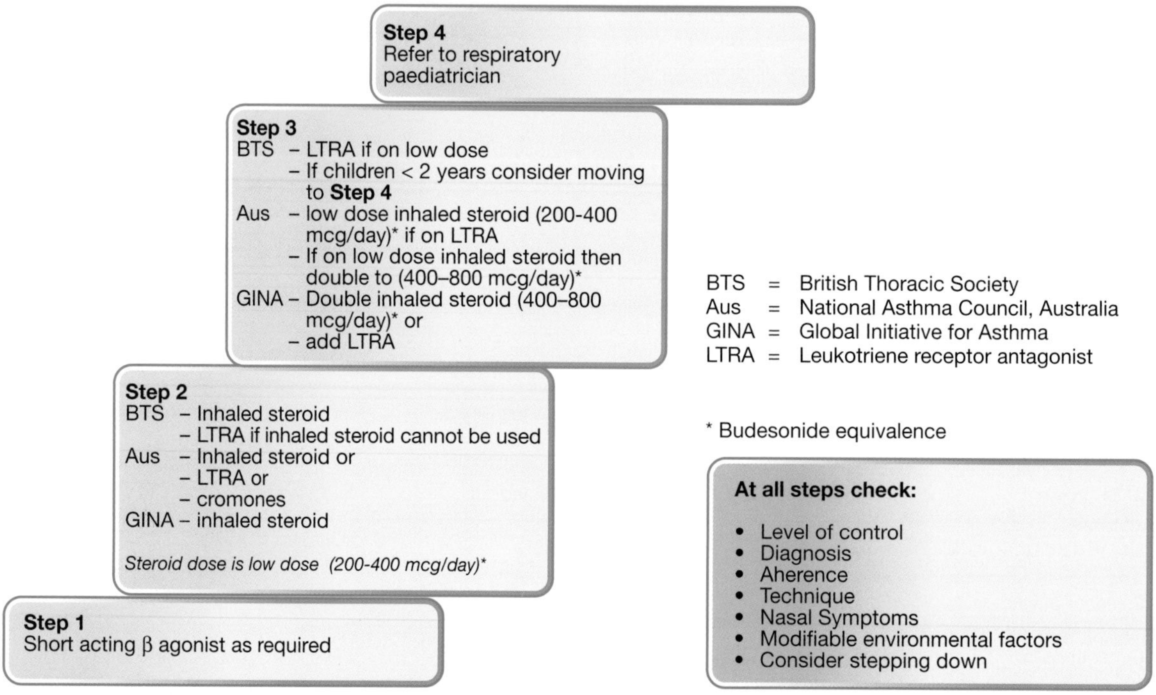

**Step 4**
Refer to respiratory paediatrician

**Step 3**
BTS – LTRA if on low dose
– If children < 2 years consider moving to **Step 4**
Aus – low dose inhaled steroid (200-400 mcg/day)* if on LTRA
– If on low dose inhaled steroid then double to (400–800 mcg/day)*
GINA – Double inhaled steroid (400–800 mcg/day)* or
– add LTRA

**Step 2**
BTS – Inhaled steroid
– LTRA if inhaled steroid cannot be used
Aus – Inhaled steroid or
– LTRA or
– cromones
GINA – inhaled steroid

*Steroid dose is low dose (200-400 mcg/day)**

**Step 1**
Short acting β agonist as required

BTS = British Thoracic Society
Aus = National Asthma Council, Australia
GINA = Global Initiative for Asthma
LTRA = Leukotriene receptor antagonist

* Budesonide equivalence

**At all steps check:**

- Level of control
- Diagnosis
- Aherence
- Technique
- Nasal Symptoms
- Modifiable environmental factors
- Consider stepping down

Fig. 14.3.3 Stepwise pharmacological management of asthma in children aged 5 years and younger, incorporating Australian National Asthma Council (Aus), British Thoracic Society (BTS) and Global Initiative for Asthma (GINA) guidelines. *Budesonide equivalence. LTRA, leukotriene receptor antagonist. LABA, long acting β agonist.

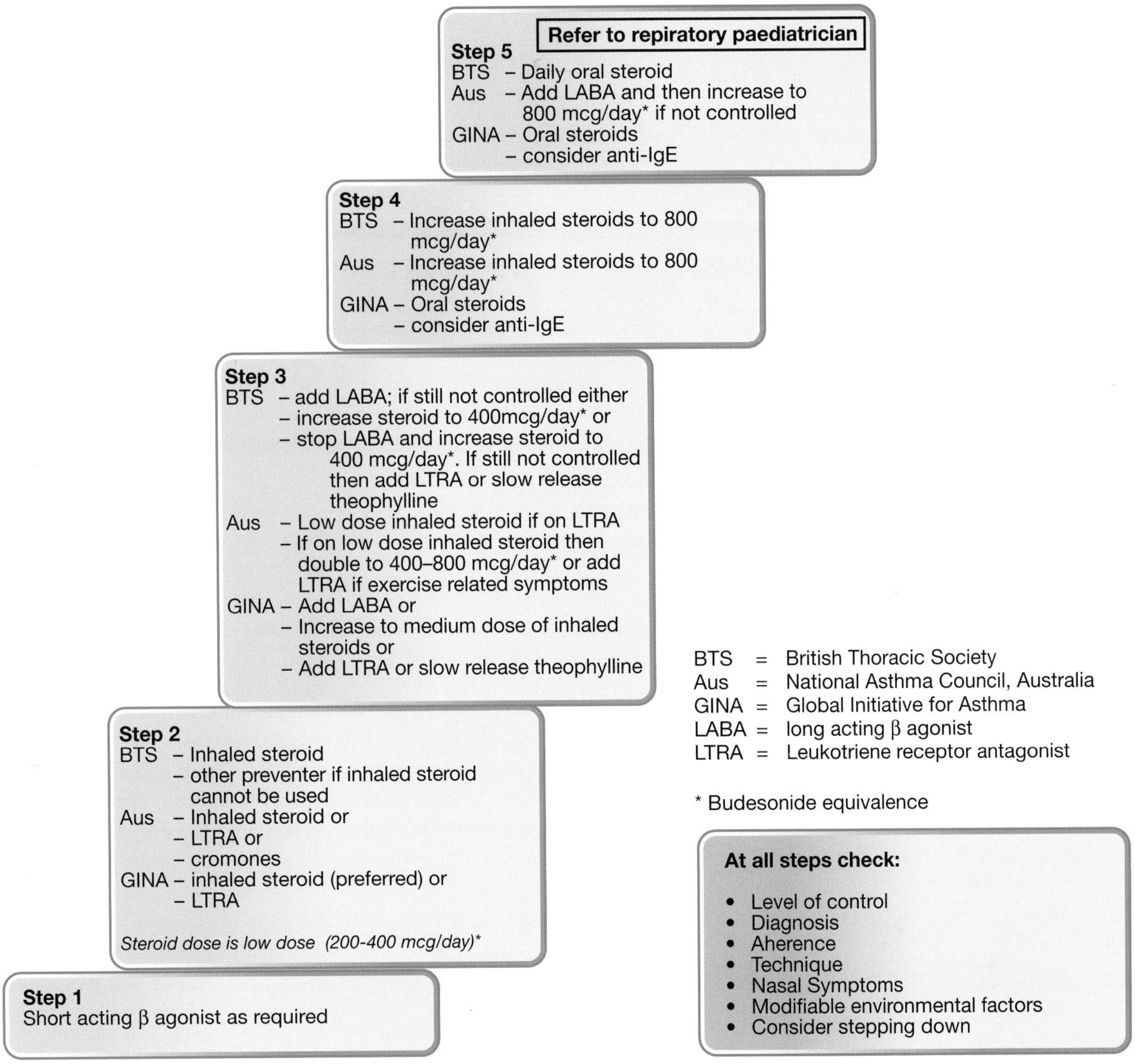

**Step 5** **Refer to repiratory paediatrician**
BTS – Daily oral steroid
Aus – Add LABA and then increase to 800 mcg/day* if not controlled
GINA – Oral steroids
– consider anti-IgE

**Step 4**
BTS – Increase inhaled steroids to 800 mcg/day*
Aus – Increase inhaled steroids to 800 mcg/day*
GINA – Oral steroids
– consider anti-IgE

**Step 3**
BTS – add LABA; if still not controlled either
– increase steroid to 400mcg/day* or
– stop LABA and increase steroid to 400 mcg/day*. If still not controlled then add LTRA or slow release theophylline
Aus – Low dose inhaled steroid if on LTRA
– If on low dose inhaled steroid then double to 400–800 mcg/day* or add LTRA if exercise related symptoms
GINA – Add LABA or
– Increase to medium dose of inhaled steroids or
– Add LTRA or slow release theophylline

**Step 2**
BTS – Inhaled steroid
– other preventer if inhaled steroid cannot be used
Aus – Inhaled steroid or
– LTRA or
– cromones
GINA – inhaled steroid (preferred) or
– LTRA

*Steroid dose is low dose (200-400 mcg/day)**

**Step 1**
Short acting β agonist as required

BTS = British Thoracic Society
Aus = National Asthma Council, Australia
GINA = Global Initiative for Asthma
LABA = long acting β agonist
LTRA = Leukotriene receptor antagonist

* Budesonide equivalence

**At all steps check:**

- Level of control
- Diagnosis
- Aherence
- Technique
- Nasal Symptoms
- Modifiable environmental factors
- Consider stepping down

Fig. 14.3.4 Stepwise pharmacological management of asthma in children aged over 5 years, incorporating Australian National Asthma Council (Aus), British Thoracic Society (BTS) and Global Initiative for Asthma (GINA) guidelines. *Budesonide equivalence. Ig, immunoglobulin; LABA, long-acting β-agonist; LTRA, leukotriene receptor antagonist.

## Long-acting β-agonists

The use of long-acting β-agonists (LABAs) alone has been associated with an increase in death in adults and should never be used without an inhaled steroid in combination. Some children with the *Arg/Arg* mutation at position 16 of the $\beta_2$-adrenoreceptor gene treated with LABAs may develop tachyphylaxis/tolerance to β-agonists, resulting in worsening of asthma control and poor response to short-acting β-agonists. Given these potential problems, LABAs should be used only in children with severe uncontrolled persistent asthma (approximately 5% of all children with asthma).

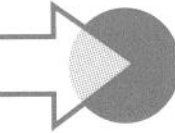

### Practical points

- The severity pattern of asthma indicates whether a controller medication should be used.
- All children should have an asthma action plan that is reviewed regularly.
- Aeroallergens and exposure to environmental tobacco smoke should be avoided.
- Treatment is aimed at controlling symptoms.
- Regularly check the level of control, diagnosis, inhaler technique, response to treatment and adherence.
- Allergic rhinitis should be treated.

**Table 14.3.4 Assessment of asthma control in children of all ages**

| Characteristic | Controlled (all of the below) | Partly controlled (any measure in a week) | Uncontrolled (3 or more features of partly controlled in any week) |
|---|---|---|---|
| Daytime symptoms | None (≤2 per week) | >2 per week | >2 per week |
| Limitations of activities | None (≤2 per week) | Any | Any |
| Nocturnal symptoms | None | Any | Any |
| Need for reliever | None (≤2 per week) | >2 per week | Any |
| Exacerbations | None | ≥1 per year | 1 in any week |
| Lung function (over 5 years only) | Normal | <80% predicted or best | <80% predicted or best |

Adapted with permission from: Global Initiative for Asthma (GINA) 2008 Global strategy for asthma management and prevention, Bethesda, and GINA 2009 Global strategy for the diagnosis of management of asthma in children 5 years and younger, Bethesda.

## Inhaler devices

The most effective way for delivering an inhaled medication at any age is by a metered-dose inhaler and valved spacer device. Children should use a spacer with mask until 3 years of age, and after that use a spacer with mouthpiece. One actuation at a time should be used to ensure optimal delivery. Owing to the impracticality of carrying around a spacer device, particularly for short-acting β–agonists, a dry-powder device may be used in older children. Irrespective of which device the child uses, it is essential that it is age-appropriate and that inhaler technique is assessed regularly.

## Prognosis

Most children who have wheezed in childhood will grow out of it by adulthood. The rates vary from 58% (Melbourne study) to approximately 75% (UK and Tasmanian studies). The discrepancies may be due to the classification of asthma in these studies. The long-term prognosis depends on the pattern of asthma in childhood. Some 60% of those with intermittent (previously called episodic) asthma will have grown out of it, but as many as 90% of those children with severe persistent asthma will continue to have symptoms in adulthood and have reduced lung function. However, with appropriate therapies, asthma should be well controlled, ensuring a normal quality of life.

# 14.4 Wheezing disorders other than asthma

Hiran Selvadurai

The previous chapter discussed the diagnosis and management of asthma. An important feature of asthma is wheeze. Although asthma is the most common cause of recurrent wheeze in childhood, there are several other causes of wheezing that need to be considered. The non-asthmatic causes of wheeze in childhood are frequently seen by general practitioners and may provide a diagnostic conundrum. The purpose of this chapter is to present some of the more common causes of wheezing that are not due to asthma. Although space precludes an exhaustive and detailed list of non-asthmatic causes of wheeze, it is hoped that when the typical signs and symptoms of asthma do not 'fit', the clinician is prepared to consider other causes of wheeze.

## Definition and pathophysiology

It is important to have a clear definition of a wheeze in order to obtain an accurate history from the child's parent. A 'wheeze' can be defined as a high-pitched whistling noise that occurs during the respiratory cycle. The high-pitched whistle is caused by air flowing rapidly through compressed or partially obstructed airways. Although a wheeze can occur in either the inspiratory or the expiratory phases of the respiratory cycle, the latter is significantly more common in childhood. The reason is that, owing to the small size, partially obstructed flow most commonly occurs in the bronchioles. The bronchioles lay in the intrathoracic section of the respiratory system. During inspiration, the highly negative intrapleural pressures relative to the intraluminal pressures keep the bronchioles patent. However, during expiration, the intrapleural pressures relative to intraluminal pressure are positive. Hence, the lumen of the bronchioles and other intrathoracic structures may be compromised. Consequently, partial obstruction of the bronchioles tends to occur during the expiratory phase of the respiratory cycle.

Although it is correct that partial obstruction can occur in the larger airways and turbulent flow can cause a wheeze to occur, this is less common as plates of cartilage that are present in the trachea serve to keep it firm and less likely to be compressed. If there is partial obstruction in the larger airways that lay in the extrathoracic compartment, wheezing may be heard in the inspiratory phase of the respiratory cycle. Other sounds such as stridor, snoring and nasopharyngeal congestion may all be erroneously reported to the clinician as a 'wheeze'. Unlike a typical wheeze, these sounds tend to be low-pitched and guttural in nature.

The aetiology of non-asthmatic wheeze can be categorized according to the age of presentation. As such, non-asthmatic wheeze in infants and preschool children will be presented separately to non-asthmatic wheeze in school-aged children.

## Causes of non-asthmatic wheeze in infancy and preschool children

### Transient infantile wheeze

Transient infantile wheeze is typified by wheeze that is associated with an intercurrent respiratory tract illness within the first 3 years of life. Unlike in children with asthma, children with transient infantile wheeze are non-atopic and generally do not have a family history of asthma. There is no hypoxia or significant morbidity with this condition. The children are generally thriving. After the age of 3 years, children with transient infantile wheeze become less symptomatic and generally are symptom-free by the age of 6 years. The pathophysiology of this condition is thought to be congenitally small, poorly developed, airways. Although the aetiology is uncertain, there is an association with maternal smoking. Bronchodilators are not usually effective in treating the wheeze in children with transient infantile wheeze.

### Infections

The common viruses that can infect the respiratory tract of infants and preschool children are respiratory syncytial virus (RSV), metapneumovirus, influenza, parainfluenza and rhinovirus. Children with acute bronchiolitis may present with a short history of coryza, cough and wheeze, together with tachypnoea and a mild fever. On auscultation, coarse crackles are a more common finding than wheeze. See Chapter 14.5 for a detailed review of this topic.

Most children with *Mycobacterium tuberculosis* infection do not develop clinical disease. Uncommonly, young children with tuberculosis may present with cough, fever, weight loss and wheeze as the constellation of symptoms. These symptoms are more typical of adulthood. Tuberculosis in the young child differs to that in adolescence or adulthood in that it is unlikely to be infective to contacts. The diagnosis can be made with a tuberculin skin test (Mantoux test). Three-quarters of children with a positive tuberculin test have a normal chest radiograph.

## Bronchopulmonary dysplasia

Children who are born prematurely with a history of hyaline membrane disease are at risk of developing bronchopulmonary dysplasia (BPD). BPD is defined by the need for supplemental oxygen therapy beyond 28 days of life and is associated with chronic radiological changes. The radiological changes associated with BPD are characterized by areas of fibrotic, thickened markings with cystic changes. Children with BPD may present with an acute viral infection that precipitates a respiratory decompensation. On examination, they may demonstrate signs of increased work of breathing (such as tachypnoea, nasal flare, intercostal muscle recessions and use of accessory muscles of respiration). On auscultation, widespread expiratory wheeze may be present. The long-term prognosis for children with BPD is good in terms of lung function but there is growing evidence of ongoing exercise limitation into adulthood.

## Cystic fibrosis

Cystic fibrosis (CF) is a cause of chronic suppurative lung disease with an estimated carrier rate of 1 in 20 in the Caucasian population and an incidence of 1 in 2500 live births. More than 1700 genes are associated with CF. Although newborn screening is now widely performed, a small proportion of infants may fail to be diagnosed if they have uncommon mutations. If symptoms of failure to thrive, recurrent chest infections, cough and wheeze are noted, the clinician should consider CF as a diagnosis. If the child has associated pancreatic insufficiency, steatorrhoea may be present. Chest radiographs may be normal or demonstrate upper lobe bronchiectasis (Fig. 14.4.1). A sweat test may aid in making the diagnosis and should be performed after consultation with a paediatrician.

## Non-cystic fibrosis suppurative lung disease

Recurrent wheeze can be a presenting feature in children with other non-CF causes of suppurative lung disease. Causes of generalized wheeze and crackles would include underlying immune deficiency such as

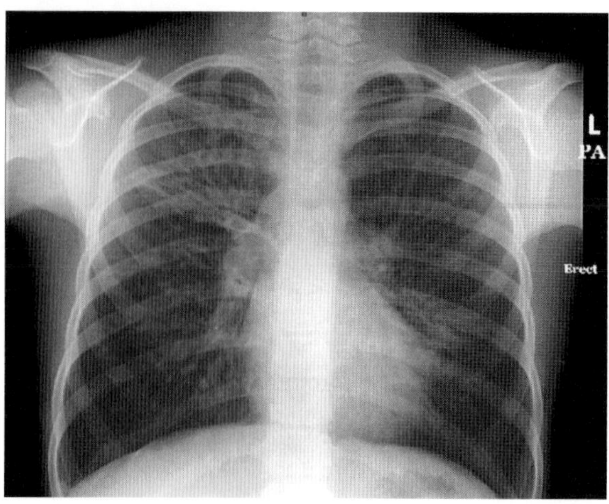


Fig. 14.4.1 Child with cystic fibrosis demonstrating classical upper lobe bronchiectasis.

X-linked hypogammaglobulinaemia and immotile cilia syndrome. The latter, also called primary ciliary dyskinesia, is due to absent or abnormally functioning cilia that line the respiratory tract. Children with this condition typically have other upper airway manifestations such as recurrent middle ear infections and sinusitis. In approximately half the children with primary ciliary dyskinesia, there is associated dextrocardia. This constellation is referred to as Kartagener syndrome (Fig. 14.4.2). Management is aimed at achieving good airway clearance with physiotherapy and antibiotics to treat infective exacerbations.

## Aspiration pneumonia

Aspiration pneumonia could occur from below the diaphragm due to gastro-oesophageal reflux of gastric contents. It can also occur if a child has a discoordinate

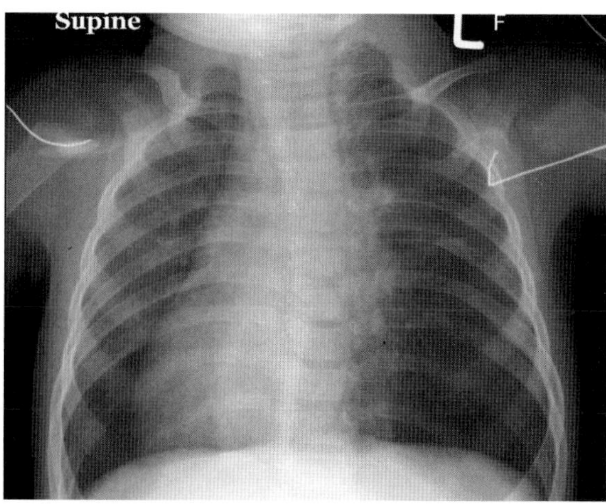


Fig. 14.4.2 Child with primary ciliary dyskinesia with dextrocardia (Kartagener syndrome).

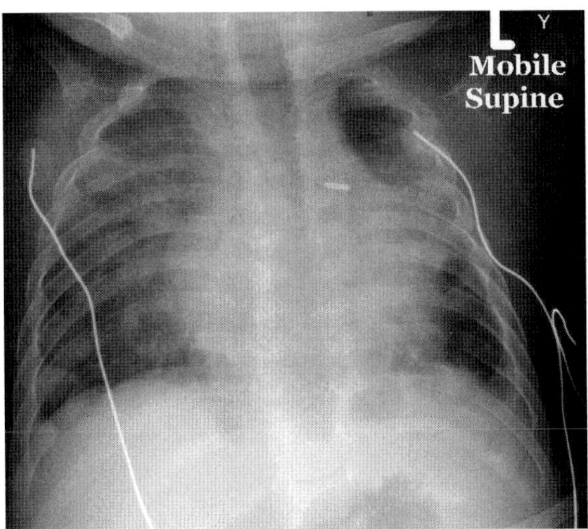


Fig. 14.4.3 Child with neurological impairment and chronic pulmonary aspiration.

oral swallow and aspirates non-particulate matter. The latter presentation is more common in children with neurological impairment. Figure 14.4.3 depicts a child with chronic aspiration who, due to a poor swallowing coordination, had no oral intake and was fed via a gastrostomy button. Underlying anatomical abnormalities such as a tracheo-oesophageal fistula may result in aspiration pneumonia. Clinical presentations may vary, and recurrent wheeze may be a feature. Bronchoscopy, barium studies, pH studies and milk scans may all be needed to confirm this diagnosis, as each of these investigative tools has limitations when used in isolation.

## Bronchiolitis obliterans

Bronchiolitis obliterans is a chronic form of bronchiolitis where the child presents with a waxing and waning history of wheeze, episodes of atelectasis and tachypnoea. Radiographic findings are variable, with areas of atelectasis as well as areas of hyperinflation with peribronchial thickening. High-resolution computed tomography may reveal pruning of the bronchial tree. There may be some evidence of traction bronchiectasis (Fig. 14.4.4).

Bronchiolitis obliterans may be a long-term sequela to significant respiratory tract infection. Long-term follow-up studies demonstrate that the majority of children who are infected with adenovirus types 7 and 21 have pulmonary function and radiological findings that are consistent with a diagnosis of bronchiolitis obliterans. More common viruses such as RSV have been associated with bronchiolitis obliterans if the child has other predisposing factors such as immunodeficiency or if they are immunosuppressed.

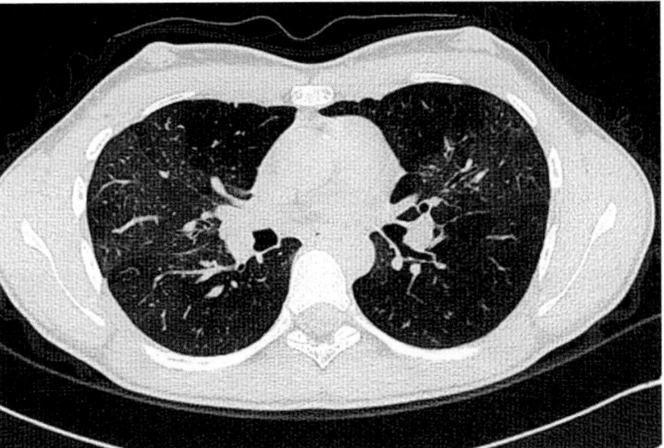

Fig. 14.4.4 High-resolution computed tomogram of a child with bronchiolitis obliterans. Note the areas of hyperlucency, traction bronchiectasis and peripheral bronchial pruning.

Bronchiolitis obliterans has also been reported as a long-term sequela of *Mycoplasma pneumoniae* and influenza virus infection.

Management is based on treating hypoxia and any intercurrent infection. Systemic steroids and macrolide antibiotics have been used to manage this condition, with variable benefit.

## Structural airway abnormalities

A variety of structural abnormalities can present with wheeze as one of the signs. Generally, however, there are other clues to the diagnosis.

### Subglottic haemangiomas

Subglottic haemangiomas may present with stridor in infancy. The stridor is described as biphasic, as it may be heard in both inspiration and expiration. Expiratory wheeze may be another presenting sign. The diagnosis may be considered in children between the ages of 6 weeks and 6 months. Haemangiomas of the skin may occur concurrently, especially along the neck and jaw, but their absence should not dissuade the clinician from considering this diagnosis. Bronchoscopy is usually required to make the diagnosis and, if the obstruction is significant, laser therapy may be considered.

### Airway 'malacia'

Bronchomalacia may present with tachypnoea and cough. On auscultation, a localized wheeze may be heard. Radiological evidence of atelectasis, recurrent localized pneumonia or even gas trapping may be noted. The pathophysiology of bronchomalacia is thought to be due to an absence or deficiency of functioning cartilage. Bronchomalacia may occur in isolation or be associated with congenital pulmonary malformations such as lobar emphysema. One-third of children with congenital lobar emphysema have localized bronchomalacia to the affected lobe.

Children may have a deficiency of effective cartilage in the tracheal wall that will result in tracheomalacia. Children with tracheomalacia have a typical 'brassy' cough. If the condition is severe enough, these children may have episodes of acute respiratory collapse. Airway 'malacia' is best diagnosed using a flexible fibreoptic bronchoscope.

### Airway stenosis

Congenital tracheal stenosis is rare, and the signs and symptoms will depend on the locality and extent of the defect. Stridor is the predominant feature but these children may present with a wheeze.

### Congenital vascular ring

A congenital vascular ring may be formed when the usual attachments of the large vessels to the heart are misplaced. For example, a right-sided aortic arch with a ligamentum arteriosum, or a double aortic arch, or an aberrant right subclavian artery, or an anomalous innominate artery may each entrap the trachea and the oesophagus, and cause compression. Although this may cause a wheeze, the infant will generally have other signs such as failure to thrive and feeding difficulties. The diagnosis may be considered with a barium study that demonstrates a posterior or lateral indentation on the oesophagus (Fig. 14.4.5). Computed tomography with angiography will help make the definitive diagnosis, and surgical treatment is considered.

## Other causes of wheeze in infancy and preschool children (Box 14.4.1)

### Cardiac causes of wheeze

A child with an underlying cardiac defect may present with wheeze and shortness of breath. The large and small airways may be compressed in a variety of cardiac defects. The large airways may be compressed by an enlarged left atrium or large pulmonary vessels. The small airways may be compressed by engorged pulmonary vasculature, which may be due to a large left to right shunt. The wheeze is caused by the turbulent air flow through partially compressed airways.

Children with a history of cardiac surgery (especially the Fontan procedure) may present with an acute severe bronchitis with wheeze. This condition is referred to as 'plastic bronchitis'. Unlike the plastic bronchitis that can occur with asthma, those with prior cardiac disease have bronchial casts that are devoid of eosinophilic inflammation and Curschmann's spirals. Figure 14.4.6 demonstrates a bronchial cast that was

**Box 14.4.1 Causes of non-asthma wheeze in infants and preschool children**

**Obstruction of small airways**
- Transient infantile wheeze
- Acute infection (e.g. bronchiolitis)
- Suppurative lung disease
- Chronic lung disease of prematurity
- Secondary to cardiac causes

**Obstruction of large airways**
- Inhaled foreign body
- Structural abnormalities
- Mediastinal masses

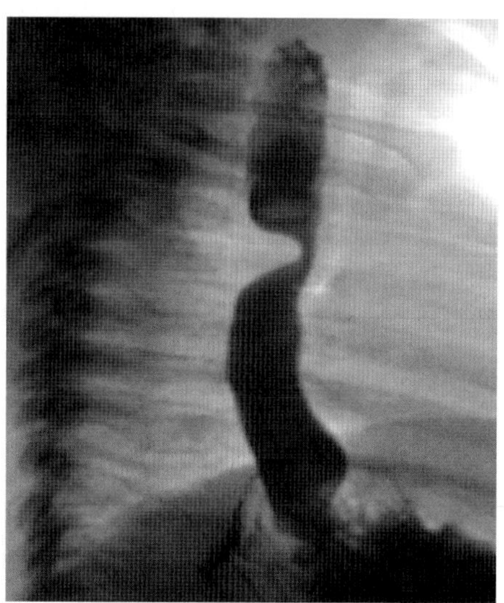

Fig. 14.4.5 Barium study in a child with a vascular ring demonstrating an oesophageal indentation.

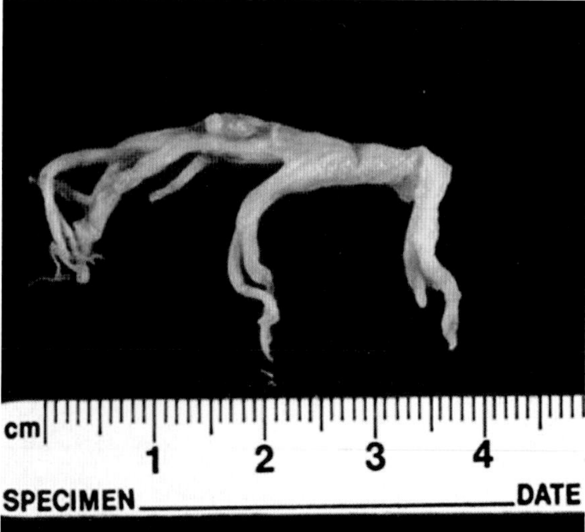


Fig. 14.4.6 Bronchial cast from a 5-year-old boy in acute respiratory distress who had a history of cardiac disease.

removed during emergency bronchoscopy in a child who presented in acute severe respiratory distress with a history of known cardiac disease.

### Inhaled foreign body

An inhaled foreign body may present with localized wheeze, cough and shortness of breath. Clinicians should be aware that the typical history of choking soon after the child was playing with a toy or food is uncommon. Children are capable of inhaling a variety of objects such as nuts, seeds and components of plastic toys. For anatomical reasons, the most common area for the object to get lodged is the right main stem bronchus. On examination, asymmetrical air entry may be noted. Although the inspiratory film of a chest radiograph may be relatively unremarkable, gas trapping may become evident on the expiratory film (Fig. 14.4.7). This is due to the ball-valve effect of the foreign body. If the foreign body has been lodged for a prolonged period of time, atelectasis, rather than gas trapping, will be noted in the affected region. This is due to reabsorption of the trapped gas. If the clinical examination is suggestive, a normal chest radiograph should not dissuade the clinician from requesting a bronchoscopy in search of a foreign body. It is reported that one-third of children with inhaled foreign bodies have unremarkable chest radiographs.

### Mediastinal masses

Posterior mediastinal masses such as neuroblastomas and neuroenteric cysts are less likely to compress the airways and cause wheeze.

Masses in the anterior and middle mediastinum may cause airway compression. Teratomas and dermoid cysts may present with wheeze as one of the constellation of symptoms.

Enlarged hilar lymph nodes may compress the main bronchi and may uncommonly present with cough, dyspnoea and wheeze. This may occur in primary tuberculosis. Endobronchial tuberculosis may also occur by compromising the patency of the airway, resulting in radiographic evidence of atelectasis. A detailed history is important and may reveal other symptoms such as fever, night sweats and weight loss. Sarcoidosis is a rare cause of hilar lymphadenopathy, and may mimic tuberculosis clinically and radiologically.

Lymphomas may present with non-tender swelling of the cervical or supraclavicular region, of short duration. If the anterior mediastinum is affected, the child may present with cough, dyspnoea and wheeze. Case reports of the use of systemic steroids to treat the wheeze resulting in catastrophic acute tumour lysis syndrome are well documented.

Oesophageal duplication cysts may lay in the middle mediastinum and cause airway compression. Figure 14.4.8 demonstrates the barium study of a 4-year-old boy who presented with a provisional diagnosis of difficult-to-treat asthma that was not responsive to asthma medication. A barium study demonstrated that the child had achalasia that caused airway obstruction by the mass effect. When the achalasia was treated with oesophageal myotomy, the child's wheeze and respiratory symptoms also regressed.

## Causes of non-asthmatic wheeze in school-aged children (Box 14.4.2)

### Infection

Many of the infective causes of wheeze that were discussed in the preschool age group may also present in the school-aged group. However, infections such

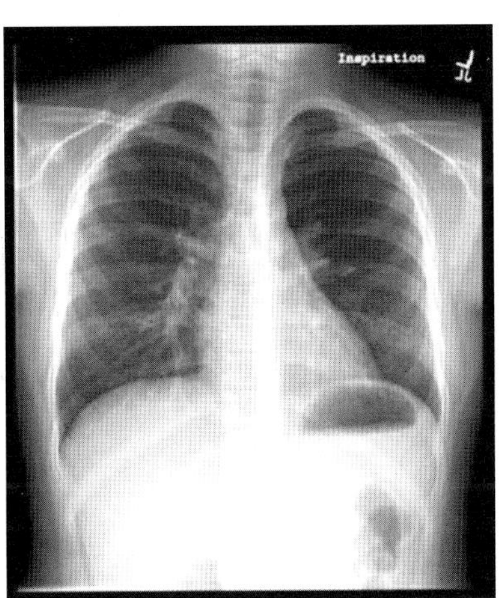


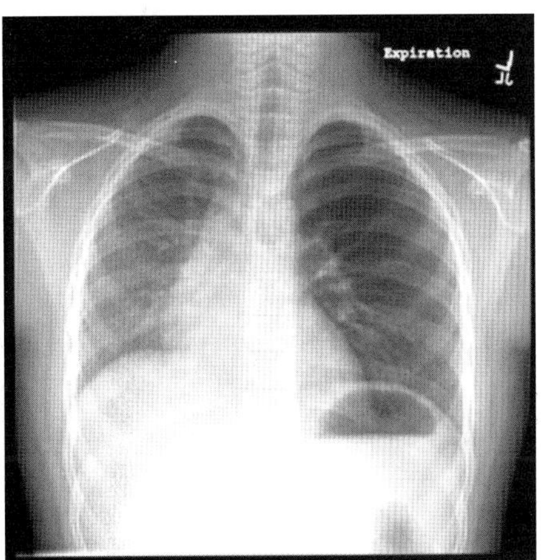


Fig. 14.4.7 The inspiratory film (**A**) appears normal, whereas the expiratory film (**B**) shows gas trapping in left lung. The left lung remains fully inflated while the right lung partially deflates, as is normal in expiration. At bronchoscopy, a small plastic toy building brick was found in the left main bronchus. (Image reprinted with permission of radRounds Radiology Network – http://www.radrounds.com).

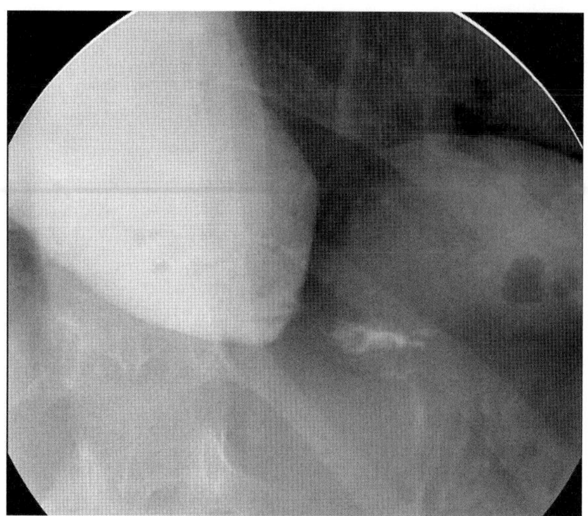

Fig. 14.4.8 Barium study demonstrating oesophageal achalasia.

**Box 14.4.2 Causes of non-asthmatic wheeze in school-aged children**

**Obstruction of small airways**
- Infection (e.g. *Mycoplasma pneumoniae*)
- Suppurative lung disease
- Mixed connective tissue diseases

**Obstruction of large airways**
- Inhaled foreign body
- Mediastinal masses
- Endobronchial lesions (e.g. tuberculosis, bronchial adenomas)

**Vocal cord dysfunction**

as *M. pneumoniae* are more common in school-aged children. Infection with *M. pneumoniae* may present in a variety of ways and should be considered in a child with cough and fever who, on auscultation of the chest, may demonstrate mild crackles or wheeze but on chest radiography has diffuse and extensive parenchymal disease. Infection with *Chlamydia pneumoniae* may cause wheeze, either by the primary infection or by acting as an inflammatory trigger for asthma. The presentation is non-specific and similar to that of *M. pneumonia*. The diagnosis is made by isolation of the organism from nasopharyngeal or throat swabs.

Infections due to tuberculosis should be considered in this age group. The presentation may be with non-specific symptoms of malaise, cough and fever. Wheeze may occur if there is compression of the airways by hilar nodes or endobronchial extravasation.

## Mixed connective tissue disorders

Mixed connective tissue disorders, such as systemic lupus erythematosus and scleroderma, typically have other symptoms and signs, such as rash and arthralgia, suggesting the condition (see Chapter 13.3). Uncommonly, in school-aged children, wheeze may be part of the clinical spectrum either as part of the primary disease process or secondary to evolving bronchiolitis obliterans.

## Mediastinal masses and malignancy

As in the preschool group, school-aged children may develop extrinsic airway compression due to mediastinal masses and present with wheeze. Malignancies such as lymphomas may present with non-specific malaise, weight loss and fever. They may also present more insidiously with a non-specific wheeze that the clinician is tempted to treat as asthma. Endobronchial lesions due to tuberculosis and malignancy, such as bronchial adenomas, may present with a unilateral wheeze and tachypnoea. Occasionally, there may be a history of haemoptysis. Partial ball-valve effect may occur and cause hyperinflation in the manner of an inhaled foreign body.

## Uncommon causes of wheeze in school-aged children

A variety of hypersensitive pneumonitis due to exposure to an array of triggers such as bird droppings, mould and even medications such as paracetamol (acetaminophen) may result in a clinical presentation of tachypnoea and wheeze. The diagnosis is suggested by the rapid improvement in symptoms when the child is removed from the offending environment.

A condition that may mimic the clinical presentation of asthma is Churg–Strauss syndrome. This is a systemic vasculitis that differs from asthma by the concurrent presence of gastrointestinal symptoms such as diarrhoea and abdominal pains.

$\alpha_1$-Antitrypsin deficiency typically presents with gastrointestinal symptoms in childhood. Respiratory symptoms due to restrictive lung disease usually present in adulthood but there are sporadic case reports of children presenting with wheeze, cough and tachypnoea.

## Vocal cord dysfunction

The pathophysiology of vocal cord dysfunction is not clear. Children may present with symptoms suggestive of exercise-induced asthma. Unlike typical exercise-induced asthma, where maximal bronchoconstriction occurs on completion of exertion, children with vocal cord dysfunction may report wheeze early in the course of exercise. On auscultation, the wheeze is heard maximally in the neck and there is no evidence of lung hyperinflation. Figure 14.4.9 shows the exercise flow volume loop of a child with vocal cord dysfunction. The wavering inspiratory loop is typical of vocal cord dysfunction. Counselling and psychological support have been beneficial in children with this condition.

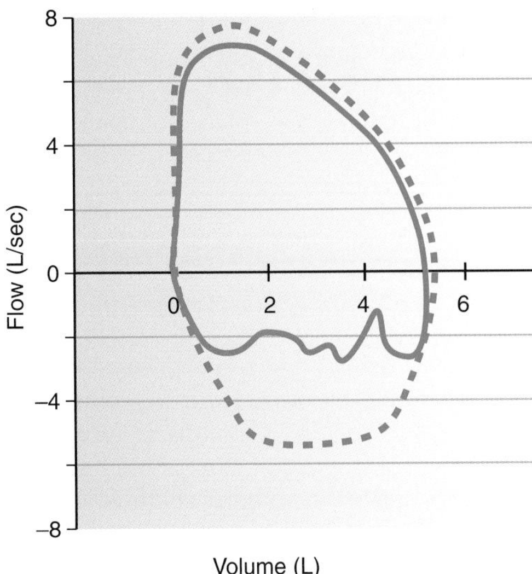


Fig. 14.4.9 Exercise flow volume loop demonstrating variable inspiratory flow obstruction (Dashed lines denote predicted normal flow. Solid lines denote actual measured flow).

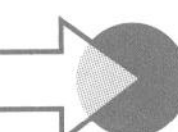

### Practical points

- All infants and children who wheeze do not necessarily have asthma.
- Be prepared to consider other causes of wheeze in children if the history is suggestive.
- The aetiology of non-asthma wheeze differs according to the age group.
- Referral to a paediatrician is needed when the diagnosis or management is not clear.

# 14.5 Lower respiratory tract infections and abnormalities

Peter LeSouëf

## Lower respiratory tract infections

Lower respiratory tract infections (LRTIs) are a major cause of morbidity in developed and developing countries and the greatest cause of mortality in children under 5 years of age in developing countries, with more than 2 million deaths from pneumonia in this age group annually. Respiratory tract infections often involve both the upper and lower respiratory tracts, particularly those due to viruses. For respiratory tract infections that appear to involve mainly the upper airway, involvement of the lower respiratory tract is usually present to some degree. Over the last few years, acute asthma has been shown to be caused mainly by respiratory viral infection of the lower airway, and this is now recognized as the most common form of LRTI. However, this form of LRTI is discussed in the chapter on asthma (see Chapter 14.3).

### Pneumonia

Pneumonia is a common cause of morbidity and mortality in children and is characterized by infection, inflammation and consolidation of the lung. There are many different causes of pneumonia. Viruses are the most common cause. Bacteria cause fewer cases of pneumonia, but the morbidity and mortality is several times higher than for viral pneumonia. Atypical infectious agents cause fewer cases of pneumonia, except in the increasing number of children with human immunodeficiency virus (HIV) infection.

Symptoms of acute infective pneumonia include dyspnoea, fever and malaise. Cough may be dry or moist, but is not always present. Pleuritic chest pain is often present. If the pneumonia involves the apices, neck pain may be present and can be confused with the neck stiffness of meningism. If the diaphragmatic pleural surface is involved, pain can be referred to the abdomen or shoulder tip.

Signs include tachypnoea and respiratory distress, dullness to percussion, and, on auscultation, localized crackles and bronchial breathing. Of these signs, tachypnoea is the most consistent and reliable, and may be the only sign pointing to this diagnosis. Pneumonia should be suspected in any child with an unexplained tachypnoea. Cyanosis is rare, but low levels of oxygen saturation are common. Clinical signs are less reliable in younger children and can be virtually absent in the presence of obvious radiological changes.

However, none of the symptoms or signs is specific for pneumonia, and the clinical diagnosis should be suspected when the history and examination are consistent. Signs of complications of pneumonia include those related to:

- pleural effusion – shifting of mediastinum or trachea, dullness to percussion (stony dullness with large effusions), reduced or absent breath sounds, and bronchial breathing above the effusion
- pneumothorax – uncommon, shifting of mediastinum or trachea, reduced breath sounds.

#### Investigations

*Chest radiography* is the most reliable investigation to confirm the presence of pneumonia. If the chest radiograph is normal, pneumonia can be reasonably excluded at that time, but if the X-ray is taken very early in the disease process this does not preclude radiological changes developing later. In general, patchy or peripheral consolidation may be more in keeping with a viral infection, lobar opacification is suggestive of bacterial pneumonia, and a more central peribronchial infiltrate may indicate *Mycoplasma* infection, but the specificity of these changes is relatively poor. Importantly, all of these radiological features can be found with asthma.

Repeat X-ray to establish resolution of the pneumonia is important to reduce the risk of missing an unrecognized, underlying or unresolved pathology, particularly those related to mechanical obstruction of the airway. Preferably this should be done at least 4–6 weeks after the acute illness has settled down, as the radiological abnormalities of pneumonia can be slow to resolve and may still be present if the repeat X-ray is done too early.

*Blood culture* may be performed if clinically indicated. Bacteraemia is not common in bacterial pneumonia.

*A nasal aspirate* should be taken if the diagnosis is unclear or viral aetiology is suspected. The aspirate should be subjected to polymerase chain reaction (PCR) analysis to detect the presence of causative respiratory viruses, but care is needed in interpreting results as positive results for respiratory viruses are common in asymptomatic children, and the presence of a virus in a nasal aspirate does not exclude the possibility of a bacterial pneumonia. Human rhinovirus detection should be included in the PCR detection panel as increasing recent evidence suggests that this virus is responsible for many LRTIs in hospitalized children. Rhinovirus typing may also be included in the near future, as even more recent evidence has shown that the newly discovered human rhinovirus group C is the most common virus group causing LRTI in hospitalized children, and also causes more pathology than previously known rhinovirus groups, as well as the majority of acute asthma admissions in children.

*Sputum* is often difficult to obtain and of limited usefulness due to contamination by upper airway bacteria.

*Pleural fluid specimen.* In more serious cases where a pleural effusion of sufficient size is present, obtaining pleural fluid should be considered, as it provides a more reliable possibility of obtaining a bacteriological diagnosis. Ultrasonography may be employed to guide the aspiration.

*Bacterial antigen detection* in the peripheral blood is also of limited use.

*Immune function.* In recurrent or atypical pneumonia, consideration should be given to the possibility of immunodeficiency. Initial investigations may include assessment of serum immunoglobulins and tests for HIV.

## Pneumococcal pneumonia

*Streptococcus pneumoniae* is the most common cause of bacterial pneumonia in children at any age. Pneumococcal pneumonia is most common in children under 3 years of age. Risk factors include male sex, Indigenous ethnicity and pre-term delivery.

Pneumococcal pneumonia may be preceded by symptoms suggestive of a mild upper respiratory tract infection, and typical symptoms and signs of pneumonia may then appear. Although these can be non-specific, compared with viral pneumonia, symptoms are likely to include fever, dyspnoea, pleuritic chest pain and cough. Cough can, however, be absent and sputum production is less likely in younger children. Signs are more likely to include tachypnoea, grunting, nasal flaring, reduced movement of the chest wall on the affected side, dullness to percussion, reduced breath sounds and bronchial breathing over the area involved. Dullness to percussion may indicate the presence of an empyema. If the upper lobes are involved, neck stiffness may be present and lead to the misdiagnosis of meningitis.

Chest X-ray findings vary widely, but the most common and classic finding is lobar involvement (Fig. 14.5.1). A well-defined round opacification is not uncommon and patchy changes can occur. Empyema, abscesses and pneumatoceles are less common than in staphylococcal pneumonia. Increases in white cell count and indices of inflammation are commonly found in peripheral blood, and blood culture may be positive.

The diagnosis should be made as early as possible and treatment commenced with penicillin and a third-generation cephalosporin. The response to treatment is usually rapid and complete recovery can be expected.

**Clinical example**

Jack, a 3-year-old boy, presented with a 4-day history of cough and fever. He was noted to be mildly unwell, to have a respiratory rate of 60 breaths per minute and bronchial breathing over the left base posteriorly. A chest X-ray showed opacification confined to the left lower lobe. He was treated with parenteral then oral penicillin, and was afebrile within 8 hours. The bronchial breathing had disappeared the next day and Jack was back to normal health within a week. A repeat X-ray 1 month later was normal.

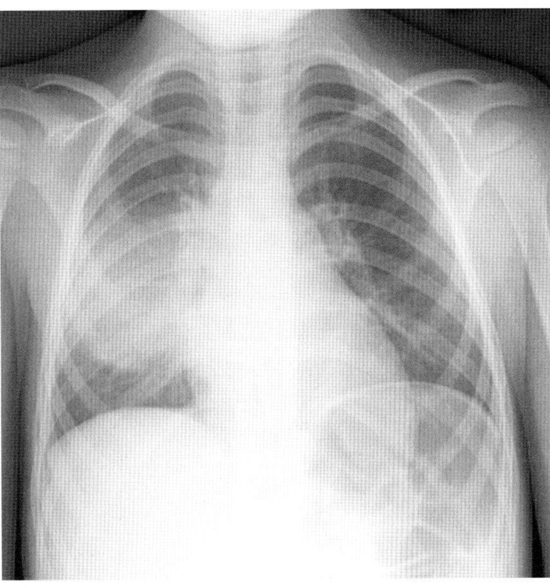

Fig. 14.5.1 Pneumococcal pneumonia in a 5-year-old girl, showing opacification in the midzone of the right lung.

## Staphylococcal pneumonia

Pneumonia due to *Staphylococcus aureus* is important as it is usually more severe than pneumonia due to other infective agents and is more common in younger children, especially those under 1–2 years of age. However, even in this younger age group, pneumococcal pneumonia is more common. Another important risk factor for staphylococcal pneumonia is a socially disadvantaged or Indigenous background.

Compared with other forms of pneumonia, the child with staphylococcal pneumonia is more likely to have a shorter acute history, to appear more unwell, and to have a high fever, marked tachypnoea and significant respiratory distress. The onset is usually acute and the course more rapid. Chest signs are often nonspecific. The chest X-ray may be normal early in the disease, but later is more likely to show severe involvement. The early radiological features may be similar to those of other forms of bacterial pneumonia, including lobar consolidation, patchy shadowing and a small pleural effusion. However, more serious complications are common and these can develop quickly within the first few days; they include:

- widespread opacifications, displaced intrathoracic structures and pleural effusions
- more specific to staphylococcal pneumonia:
  - large or encysted pleural effusions with thick walls
  - empyema
  - abscesses, either single or multiple
  - air leaks are common, occurring in around half of cases and include pneumothorax, pneumomediastinum, pneumopericardium and, in particular, pneumatoceles (Fig. 14.5.2A). Although highly specific to staphylococcal pneumonia, these complications are not pathognomonic of this condition, as air leaks including pneumatoceles can very occasionally be found in bacterial pneumonias caused by pneumococci, *Escherichia coli, Klebsiella, Pseudomonas* and group A streptococci.

High-resolution computed tomography (HRCT) of the chest (Fig. 14.5.2B) is often useful in defining the nature and extent of these complications.

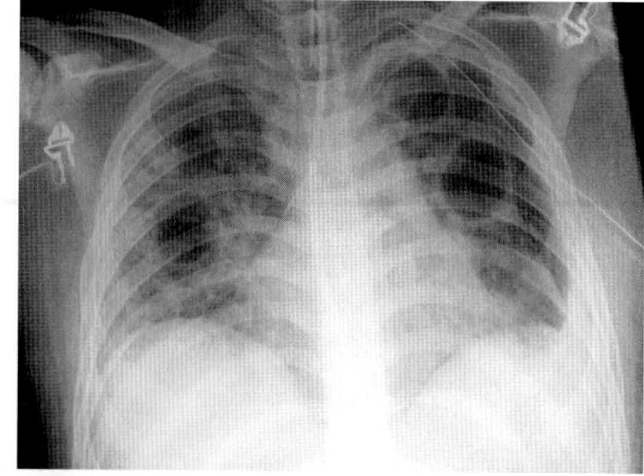
A

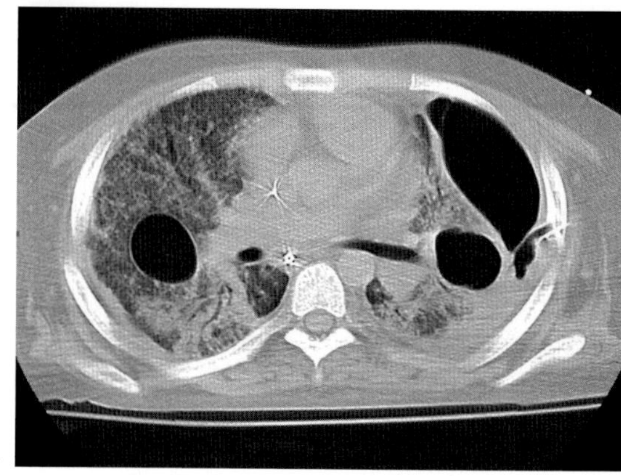
B

Fig. 14.5.2 **(A)** Chest X-ray and **(B)** a single slice from thoracic high-resolution computed tomography in an immunocompromised 15-year-old with staphylococcal pneumonia and bronchopleural fistulae. There is diffuse air space opacification with several pneumatoceles and a left-sided pneumothorax.

*Investigations*

Blood cultures are positive in the acute phase of the illness. Pleural effusions should be aspirated, when large enough, to assist with diagnosis, but the fluid from an empyema may be sterile if sufficient antibiotic treatment has been given.

*Management*

Owing to the increased risks from staphylococcal pneumonia, infants in whom this diagnosis is suspected should be hospitalized to allow adequate observation during the acute phase of the illness. Deterioration can be rapid, and air leaks can occur and require immediate treatment. Broad-spectrum antibiotics should be used until an accurate diagnosis can be made. The combination of a β-lactamase-resistant penicillin such as flucloxacillin and a third-generation cephalosporin, both given intravenously, is useful in this situation, as it combines direct treatment of staphylococci as well as coverage of other common respiratory pathogens. In any child under 2 years of age with clinically significant pneumonia, flucloxacillin should be included in the treatment regimen because of the much higher prevalence of staphylococcal pneumonia in this age group.

Resistance to β-lactamase-resistant penicillins (methicillin-resistant *Staphylococcus aureus* (MRSA)) is now common in staphylococcal pneumonia caused by community-acquired organisms, and multiresistant organisms have become more common in nosocomially acquired cases. Hence, from a therapeutic viewpoint, nosocomial staphylococcal infections are more likely to show multiple drug resistance than community-acquired MRSA infections. Treatment needs to be tailored to the prevailing local situation, but other drugs such as clindamycin should be considered. Given the high risk of relapse, the duration of antibiotic treatment is often extended to around 6 weeks, particularly in more severe cases or those with complications.

*Surgical intervention*

*Staphylococcus* is the more common cause of empyema in Western society, and whether or not to undertake drainage of effusions or empyema depends on their size and the severity of the case. In appropriate cases, drainage may be undertaken early in the course of the illness to assist in diagnosis or to reduce the mechanical effects of large effusions. The use of video-assisted thoracoscopic surgery (VATS) to drain empyemas depends on the availability of an appropriately trained and skilled surgeon. Whether or not drainage reduces the total duration of illness is less clear, but the need to reduce the space-occupying and pressure effects of a large effusion, as well as reducing the recovery time, should be considered.

*Long-term outcome*

Clinical recovery from staphylococcal pneumonia is usually good, with a very high likelihood of a complete return to normality. Radiological recovery is usually also complete, as children examined radiologically some years after recovery generally show no evidence of previous problems, despite extensive, serious abnormalities on chest X-ray at the time of the illness. However, a strong risk factor for more severe staphylococcal pneumonia, necrotizing pneumonia, and a higher morbidity and mortality is the presence of the Panton–Valentine leukocidin (PVL) toxin, which is common in community-acquired staphylococcal pneumonia.

**Clinical example**

Jayda, a 9-month-old girl, was brought to the local doctor by her mother. She had been unwell for 12 hours, with increasing fever, lethargy and difficulty feeding. The doctor noticed that she was pale, listless and tachypnoeic, and scattered coarse inspiratory and expiratory crackles were heard on auscultation of her chest. She was transferred by ambulance to hospital where a chest X-ray showed opacification in the right upper and left lower lobes. Jayda was treated with oxygen and intravenous flucloxacillin and cefotaxime. Blood culture was positive for *Staphylococcus aureus*, and treatment with flucloxacillin was continued for 6 weeks. Jayda slowly improved and she was fully recovered when seen after the antibiotic treatment had been completed.

### *Haemophilus influenzae* type b pneumonia

Pneumonia due to *Haemophilus influenzae* is now uncommon in countries with efficient immunization programmes against this organism. In countries without effective immunization policies, it remains a common and important cause of pneumonia. The organism colonizes the upper respiratory tract of the majority of normal, non-immunized children, but does so less commonly in those who have been immunized. Risks factors for *H. influenzae* infection include age less than 5 years, Indigenous ethnicity, lower socioeconomic group, male sex, and congenital and acquired immunodeficiency.

The signs, symptoms and radiological features of *H. influenzae* pneumonia are not specific or distinguishable from those found in other pneumonias. Other foci of infection including the meninges and the epiglottis are common in children with *Haemophilus* pneumonia. For children in whom *H. influenzae* pneumonia is suspected who are either under 12 months of age or significantly unwell, treatment with a parenteral third-generation cephalosporin is recommended, and for children who are less unwell, oral amoxicillin–clavulanic acid is appropriate. Other children in the family do not require prophylactic treatment if they are adequately immunized.

### *Mycoplasma* pneumonia

*Mycoplasma pneumoniae* is a frequent cause of community-acquired pneumonia in children, particularly those over 5 years of age, as it is most common in young school-aged children. The clinical course is characterized by the gradual development over several days of fever, malaise, upper respiratory symptoms and cough. The cough tends to be non-productive initially and may become productive and troublesome. In children with a tendency to asthma, wheeze is commonly present, but wheeze can occur in children with no prior history of asthma. Signs also often include widespread sparse fine or coarse crackles. Both clinical signs and chest X-ray changes are typically more striking than expected for the degree of clinical illness. The radiological findings themselves are usually non-specific, but can include perihilar opacification, and consolidation of one or more lobes (Fig. 14.5.3). The diagnosis is supported by positive serology.

Treatment with a macrolide is indicated as *M. pneumoniae* is usually susceptible to this group of antibiotics. However, the response to treatment may be restricted to a reduction in general symptoms, as the clinical course of the pneumonia itself may not be affected by treatment unless this is started within the first few days of symptoms. The anti-inflammatory effects of macrolides could also contribute to the modest efficacy of treatment.

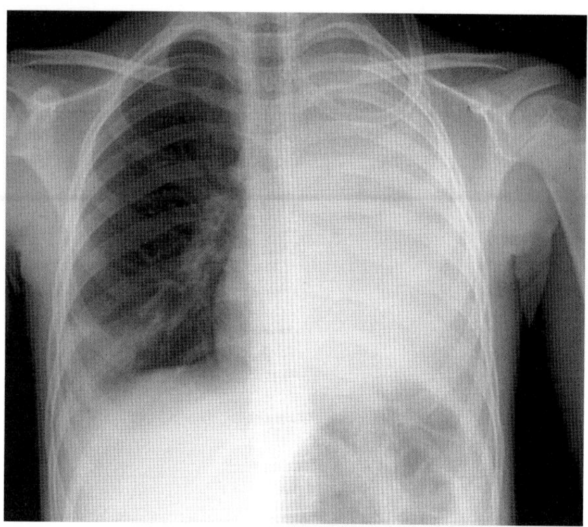

Fig. 14.5.3 *Mycoplasma* pneumonia in a 7-year-old girl presenting with cough and fever. There is extensive consolidation in the left lung with air bronchogram formation and focal consolidation in the lateral basal segment of the right lower lobe.

## Other less frequent causes of bacterial pneumonia

*Group A β-haemolytic streptococci (Streptococcus pyogenes)*

This organism is a common cause of bacterial pharyngitis, but a rare cause of pneumonia. When it does cause pneumonia, it tends to be in children over 5 years of age, and the clinical course is rapid, severe and poorly responsive to antibiotic treatment compared with other causes of bacterial pneumonia. Fever, chest pain and haemoptysis are more common than with other forms of pneumonia, and the necrotizing nature of the infection means that serious complications such as air leaks, large pleural effusions and empyema are more likely to occur. Once the organism has been isolated, treatment is with high-dose intravenous penicillin G.

*Other streptococci*

Group B β-haemolytic streptococci are a common and important cause of neonatal pneumonia, which occurs within hours of birth, has a rapidly progressive course, can mimic respiratory distress of prematurity and has a high mortality rate. After the neonatal period, it rarely causes pneumonia and, when it does, the disease course is usually less acute. Group C streptococci are also a rare cause of pneumonia in children and, as for group A, the clinical picture can be severe and protracted.

*Klebsiella pneumoniae*

This organism typically causes pneumonia in neonates and immunocompromised hosts. *Klebsiella* pneumonia is rare in children, and when *Klebsiella* infection is present bacteraemia is more common than pneumonia. The clinical picture of *Klebsiella* pneumonia initially is not distinguishable from other forms of pneumonia, but the complications of lung abscess and pneumatocele may occur and, without appropriate treatment, the mortality rate is high. Recommended treatment depends on individual resistance patterns, but is likely to include an aminoglycoside and a third-generation cephalosporin.

*Other bacteria*

Other bacterial organisms that are rare causes of pneumonia in immunocompetent children include anthrax, *Bordetella pertussis*, *Brucella*, *Burkholderia cepacia*, *Citrobacter* spp., *Corynebacterium* spp., *Coxiella burnetii*, *E. coli*, *Listeria monocytogenes*, *Mycobacterium* spp., *Neisseria meningitidis*, *Pasteurella* spp., *Proteus* spp., *Pseudomonas aeruginosa*, *Salmonella* spp. and *Yersinia* spp.

## Viral pneumonia

Viruses are the most common cause of lower respiratory illnesses in children, and viral pneumonia is the most common form of pneumonia in childhood. The spectrum of disease varies widely, but viruses are the greatest contributor to the 3–5 million children who die worldwide each year from an acute respiratory illness. Risk factors for viral pneumonia include:

- *Age* – children under 5 years of age are at greatest risk of viral pneumonia, but the risk remains high throughout the first decade of life.
- *Season* – peak incidence is in winter.
- *Passive smoke exposure* – maternal smoking increases the risk, especially in the first year of life. Exposure during pregnancy is a much greater risk factor than exposure thereafter.
- *Poor socioeconomic status* – a risk factor in both developing and developed countries.
- *Pre-existing chronic problems* – the risk is increased with chronic problems such as cystic fibrosis, post-neonatal lung disease, congenital heart disease and immunodeficiency.

The most important causative viruses are parainfluenza virus, influenza virus, respiratory syncytial virus (RSV), human metapneumovirus (HMV), adenovirus and human rhinovirus (HRV). All of these viruses can cause other respiratory illnesses apart from pneumonia, including acute upper respiratory tract infection, acute laryngotracheitis, bronchitis and bronchiolitis. Symptoms of these illnesses can coexist with those of pneumonia. Rhinoviruses, cytomegalovirus and measles virus can also cause pneumonia. In recent years, HRV has been identified as the most common cause of exacerbations of acute asthma in both children and adults, so care is needed to avoid misdiagnosing pneumonia in children with X-ray changes due to HRV-induced asthma. The radiological features of viral pneumonias are non-specific, but patchy, widespread infiltrates are more characteristic

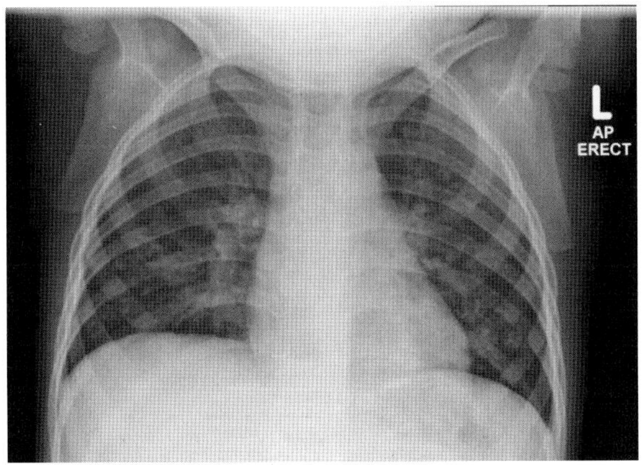


Fig. 14.5.4 Viral pneumonia in a 15-month-old child, with typical non-specific, patchy widespread opacifications in both lung fields.

than lobar involvement (Fig. 14.5.4). Treatment with antiviral agents is of limited efficacy and rarely indicated in normal children, but supportive measures are commonly required.

### Clinical example

Emily, a 4-year-old girl, was brought to her general practitioner with a 3-day history of fever, increasing dry cough and loss of appetite. Her 6-year-old brother had also been unwell with a cough and a fever. On examination, her doctor noted a temperature of 37.8 °C, a respiratory rate of 36 breaths per minute, mild soft tissue recession, and the presence of sparse, coarse crackles bilaterally on auscultation. A chest X-ray showed scattered areas of patchy opacification. She was diagnosed as having viral pneumonia, treated symptomatically and recovered uneventfully over the next few days.

### Fungal pneumonia

Fungal causes of pneumonia or pneumonia-like illnesses occur most commonly in immunocompromised children, and include *Actinomyces, Aspergillus, Candida, Coccidiomycosis, Cryptococcus, Histoplasma* and *Nocardia* spp. Some fungi are endemic in certain areas. For example, *Coccidiomycosis* is endemic in places in the Americas, including the south-west of the USA, and histoplasmosis is endemic in the mid-western USA. Fungal respiratory infections in non-immunocompromised children are usually mild and do not require specific treatment.

### Protozoal pneumonia

Protozoa that cause pneumonia or pneumonia-like illnesses also occur most commonly in immunocompromised children and include *Cryptosporidium* spp., *Pneumocystis jiroveci* (formerly *carinii*) and *Toxoplasma* spp.

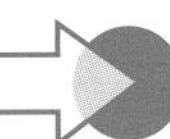

### Practical points

**Pneumonia**

- Tachypnoea is the most useful clinical sign.
- Pneumococcal pneumonia is the most common cause of bacterial pneumonia at all ages, including the first year of life.
- Staphylococcal pneumonia is uncommon, but occurs most commonly in the first year or two of life.
- Follow-up X-rays should be taken to ensure that there is no significant underlying pathology.
- Follow-up X-ray timing: leave for at least 4–6 weeks to allow enough time for complete clearing of the abnormalities.

## Acute viral bronchiolitis

Bronchiolitis is the most common significant LRTI in the first year of life and is also common in the second year. It is the most common cause of hospital admission in the first year and a common cause of mortality globally. Bronchiolitis follows a seasonal pattern with the highest rates occurring during winter in most locations, but in more tropical or subtropical latitudes the highest rates are during the rainy season. The reason for these seasonal patterns is unknown. Maternal smoking is a major risk factor, related mostly to smoking during pregnancy rather than by inhalation during infancy. Other risk factors include pre-term delivery and chronic lung disease of prematurity, allergy, chronic cardiorespiratory diseases (including congenital heart disease and cystic fibrosis) and immunodeficiency.

Classically, acute viral bronchiolitis has been considered to be a disease mainly caused by the respiratory syncytial virus (RSV), as RSV is the most common virus detected in children who are hospitalized with this condition. However, in recent years community studies have shown that milder cases that do not present to hospital are more likely to be due to infection with human rhinovirus (HRV) and that, overall, HRV causes more cases of bronchiolitis than RSV. Dual infection with RSV and HRV is also common. In addition, most other respiratory viruses can cause bronchiolitis, including parainfluenza viruses 1–3, influenza virus A and B, adenovirus and HMV. Bronchiolitis is rarely due to bacteria, and secondary infection with bacteria is also rare.

The clinical course of bronchiolitis tends to be of symptoms gradually increasing over 2–3 days, and consisting of mild or no fever, tachypnoea, a mild dry cough and expiratory wheezing. With increasing severity, dyspnoea becomes more marked and feeding is impaired. Clinical signs typically include soft tissue recession on inspiration, the appearance of increased work of breathing, hyperinflation of the chest, fine inspiratory crackles and wheeze. After 2–3 days the symptoms gradually resolve and the child should have recovered within a week. Slow or prolonged recovery is more common if an underlying predisposing chronic problem is present; if recovery has not been achieved within 2 weeks, further investigations such as a sweat test should be considered.

The main differential diagnosis is early asthma (now more commonly called 'virus-induced wheeze of infancy'). Hyperinflation and fine inspiratory crackles are classical for bronchiolitis, but many infants have a mixture of these signs and those more consistent with asthma, including expiratory wheeze. As the two conditions are caused by the same viruses and overlap so much, in many cases there is no reasonable way to separate these two diagnoses.

Investigations are not needed in mild cases, but in hospitalized children a nasal fluid specimen should be obtained to allow viral detection by PCR and adequate isolation of infectious cases. If a chest X-ray is indicated clinically, the usual findings are of hyperinflation with few other changes in mild cases and more widespread, but non-specific, opacifications in more severe cases. The level of oxygen saturation is a good guide to the severity of the illness, and oxygen should be given accordingly.

Treatment is supportive and consists of ensuring adequate oxygenation and care with fluid intake to avoid aspiration. Particular care needs to be taken with infants who are reluctant to feed, as aspiration can occur if oral fluids are pushed too hard or administration of nasogastric fluids is accompanied by vomiting. In marked respiratory distress where the infant's ability to cough or maintain an airway is impaired, intravenous fluids should be given. No drugs have been proven to be effective in treating bronchiolitis. Despite this, many infants receive bronchodilators even though there is evidence that they increase the need for additional oxygen. Specific treatments targeting the virus have not found their way into routine practice. Anti-RSV immunoglobulins are not indicated for regular use owing to poor efficiency and high expense.

The great majority of cases of bronchiolitis resolve without sequelae, but longitudinal studies have shown that the risk of further wheezing is increased. Whether this is due to pre-existing variations of immune function or to changes induced by the infections that cause bronchiolitis has not been resolved completely. However, the presence of relative deficiencies in innate immunity that predate bronchiolitis in children destined to become atopic and asthmatic suggests that the former is more likely.

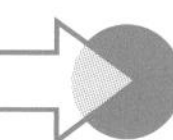

**Practical points**

**Bronchiolitis**

- Bronchiolitis is the most common cause of wheeze in early life.
- Rhinovirus is the most common cause of mild bronchiolitis, RSV is the most common cause of severe bronchiolitis.
- Clinical features include low-grade fever, cough, wheeze, hyperinflation and fine inspiratory crackles.
- Differentiation of some cases of bronchiolitis from early asthma or 'virus-induced wheeze' is often not possible.
- Treatment is supportive only – oxygenation, hydration, nutrition.

## Pertussis (whooping cough)

This serious respiratory illness is caused by the bacterium *Bordetella pertussis*. It can occur at any age but infants, particularly those aged less than 6 months, are at greatest risk of complications, which include apnoea, severe pneumonia, encephalopathy and death.

Immunity from the natural infection is not complete, and reinfection can occur in children and adults. However, the incidence and severity of pertussis is greatly reduced by pertussis vaccine, originally a whole-cell vaccine and now an acellular pertussis vaccine. A major value in immunization is the increased herd immunity that reduces transmission to young babies from older siblings and adults. This is important, as those most at risk from pertussis are those too young to be immunized.

Pertussis is most infectious in the prodromal phase and continues to be infectious for up to 3 weeks.

### Clinical features

The incubation period is usually 7–10 days, and has a prodromal phase with nasal discharge and a mild non-productive cough that lasts for a few days. This precedes the phase when cough becomes pronounced. In most, but not all, cases prolonged paroxysms of coughing are followed by a characteristic 'whoop'. The cough is often accompanied by vomiting and may be so severe that subconjunctival haemorrhages occur. Apnoea is common in very young infants. Less commonly, young infants can develop severe pneumonia or encephalopathy, both of which can be fatal.

### Investigations

A nasopharyngeal specimen is used to detect pertussis using immunofluorescent antibodies or culture. Serology is less reliable.

### Management

Infants less than 6 months of age are more likely to require hospital admission for supportive therapy. Macrolide antibiotics reduce the period of infectivity and can alter the course of the illness, but only if commenced before the paroxysmal phase. Thus, they are indicated in those seen very early in the course of the illness or those with severe symptoms. Household contacts are usually also treated to reduce spread of infection. Infected individuals should avoid contact with other children until they have had at least 5 days of antibiotics or have had the illness for at least 3 weeks.

## Pulmonary tuberculosis

Tuberculosis (TB) is the most common chronic infection in the world and is caused by infection with *Mycobacterium tuberculosis*. Pulmonary TB is an important cause of morbidity and mortality in children worldwide. The tubercle bacillus was discovered by Koch in 1822, and in the 20th century the incidence of the disease was reduced in developed countries by effective public health and therapeutic approaches. In recent years, the TB incidence rates have been stable or falling in many regions, but in other regions the incidence has been slowly increasing. This increase is likely to be due to the presence of large numbers of people with HIV infection who are highly susceptible to TB, and who are responsible for the subsequent increase in the global pool of infective organisms. In developed countries that accept large numbers of refugees from developing countries, high rates have been found in those emigrating, and this has also increased the circulation of the organism.

Children usually acquire the infective agent from an adult or adolescent rather than from other children. TB in children is most common under 5 years of age, with a lower incidence between 5 and 15 years. Other risk factors are low socioeconomic conditions, an Indigenous ethnic background and immunodeficiency. The organism is transmitted mainly by inhalation in the indoor environment, and only a small proportion of those infected will develop disease.

After exposure, signs of pulmonary TB do not appear for weeks, months or years. The initial lesion is often subpleural, occurring with an associated lymph node response that comprises a primary complex. Early symptoms are often absent or few, in which case a dry cough and mild dyspnoea may be noted. The disease does not progress further in most patients but, when it does, effusions may occur, lymph nodes may enlarge and obstruct major airways, and the lung may be damaged by extensive caseation. The disease may then disseminate and produce miliary, meningeal or renal tuberculosis. Hence, later symptoms may include weight loss, malaise, fever, and a dry cough and wheeze if an airway is obstructed.

Diagnosis is established by:

- a positive tuberculin skin test (>15 mm skin induration from 5 tuberculin units (TU) of purified protein derivative (PPD)-S is taken as evidence of disease; 10–15 mm suggests that infection has occurred, but disease may not be present; false-negatives can occur in early or severe disease)
- culture of the organism from early-morning gastric lavage
- radiological findings that include hilar or mediastinal lymphadenopathy, lobar hyperinflation or atelectasis if an airway is obstructed, consolidation, effusions and empyema. Cavitation is uncommon in young children. Miliary TB has a widespread 'snowstorm' appearance. HRCT is often useful if characterizing the anatomy and extent of the findings.
- light microscopic identification of bacilli from sputum, bronchoalveolar lavage fluid or pleural fluid.

Treatment has traditionally been with triple therapy, which consists of 6 months' treatment with rifampicin, isoniazid and pyrazinamide, but World Health Organization recommendations for therapy are frequently updated and the latest of these should be consulted. Patients with a positive skin test without any evidence of pulmonary disease are treated with isoniazid alone for 6–9 months.

## Atypical mycobacterial infection

Atypical mycobacteria (*M. avium, M. intracellulare, M. scrofulaceum*) can, on rare occasions, cause pulmonary disease in immunocompetent children, particularly in Australia. Presentation with symptoms and signs of airway obstruction secondary to pulmonary lymphadenopathy is typical in these cases. Diagnosis is made by specific skin testing and by identification of bacilli from fluid or tissue. Response to treatment is slow, and therapy may need to be continued for 12–24 months, but prognosis for full recovery appears to be excellent.

# Congenital disorders of the lower respiratory tract

## Congenital lung abnormalities

These are rare and may go undetected for life. They often present well into childhood with non-specific symptoms. Most can be detected on chest X-ray.

*Lung cysts* can vary from being simple and solitary to multiple and complex. Cysts can become infected if they communicate with the airway. They can also cause symptoms if they become enlarged and compress surrounding structures.

*Unilateral pulmonary agenesis* may present with neonatal respiratory distress or with non-specific symptoms later in life. Careful radiological investigation including HRCT is needed to confirm the diagnosis.

*Congenital cystic adenomatoid malformation* (CCAM) is caused by either hamartomatous growth of the bronchial tree or a localized arrest in development of the fetal bronchial tree. CCAM generally consists of multiple cysts and abnormal proliferation of lung elements. It can present at birth and, if sufficient lung is involved, cause chronic respiratory insufficiency. Surgery may be needed to remove troublesome cysts. The associated small increase in risk of malignancy requires careful consideration regarding the relative risks of surgery or continued observation.

*Congenital lobar emphysema* is characterized by overinflation of a lung lobe and commonly presents before 6 months of age with respiratory distress or tachypnoea. Surgical intervention may be required if the emphysematous lobe causes significant compression of neighbouring lung.

*Sequestration* of the lung is likely to be the result of a small independent accessory lung bud developing from the foregut. Sequestration is characterized by part of the lung being discontinuous with the rest of the lung, and this can be intrapulmonary or extrapulmonary. The former is much more common, and more likely to become infected and require surgical removal. The latter is most frequently left-sided, with an aberrant systemic blood supply, and is asymptomatic.

## Congenital chest wall abnormalities

*Pectus excavatum* is a common midline concave depression of the lower sternum and is not usually associated with any underlying respiratory abnormality or effect on rib cage or lung function. Cosmetic correction can impair lung function.

*Thoracic dystrophies* are characterized by impaired development of the chest wall and are associated with pulmonary hypoplasia.

*Scoliosis* can cause a restrictive functional defect in chest wall function if the angle of the curve is great enough.

*Congenital eventration of the diaphragm* is a malformation of the diaphragm in which the diaphragmatic muscle is incomplete and replaced by thin fibroelastic tissue that allows the dysfunctional hemidiaphragm to be displaced upwards. It occurs more in males and can be difficult to differentiate from diaphragmatic hernia. More severe cases may present neonatally and require surgery, but minor cases can be found incidentally.

*Congenital diaphragmatic hernia*: see Chapter 11.5.

## Congenital lower airway abnormalities

- Tracheomalacia and bronchomalacia: see Chapter 14.4.
- Oesophageal atresia and tracheo-oesophageal fistula: see Chapter 11.5.
- Bronchogenic cysts: see Chapter 14.4.

# An approach to chronic cough and cystic fibrosis 14.6

Anne Chang, Nitin Kapur

## Introduction

Cough is the most common symptom of respiratory disease for which parents seek medical attention in young children. The presence of cough can indicate the entire spectrum of cardiorespiratory childhood illness, ranging from a symptom of the 'common cold' to a symptom of a severe, life-limiting disorder such as cystic fibrosis (CF). Most cough in children is acute and resolves promptly. Chronic cough is defined as cough lasting longer than 4 weeks. It is abnormal and deserves careful consideration of the cause. In the evaluation of children with chronic cough, determining which children require further investigations and/or treatment is a key management issue.

## Pathophysiology

Cough is generally considered a reflex, but also can be voluntarily generated (or suppressed). Cough is comprised of three phases – inspiratory, compressive and expiratory – and serves as a vital defence mechanism for lung health. The forceful expiration occurs after a build-up of pressure in the thorax (up to 300 mmHg) by contraction of expiratory muscles against a closed glottis. This leads to expulsion of air at high velocity and sweeps material within airways towards the mouth. Inspiration of a variable volume of air occurs when cough is stimulated. Successive coughs may or may not be preceded by inspiration. Cough is an important component of normal respiratory function through two mechanisms. Firstly, mechanical stimulation of the larynx causes immediate expiratory efforts through the expiratory reflex, a primary defence mechanism that is stimulated when foreign objects (such as food or fluid) are inhaled. Secondly, cough enhances mucociliary clearance. The absence of a forceful cough (e.g. generalized muscular weakness) has important clinical repercussions, such as difficulty clearing secretions, atelectasis, lobar collapse and recurrent pneumonia.

Issues to keep in mind when the presenting symptom is cough:

- Cough usually resolves spontaneously (called the period effect), which makes evaluation of therapeutic interventions difficult.
- Many cough treatments are not based on the results of randomized controlled trials.
- As the aetiology and management of cough in childhood are quite different to that in adults, extrapolation of the adult cough literature to children can be harmful.

## Approach to diagnosis and management

Figure 14.6.1 outlines a schematic approach to the diagnosis and management of chronic cough. The key questions are presented in Box 14.6.1. Initial categorization of cough into acute, subacute and chronic cough according to duration is helpful. There is, however, no strict definition of chronic cough. Most acute cough arises from respiratory viruses and settles within 2 weeks. Subacute cough commonly lasts from 2 to 4 weeks, whereas chronic cough can be defined as cough lasting longer than 4 weeks.

### Clinical example

Adrienne, a 13-year-old girl, was referred to a respiratory physician for a chronic cough. She had been managed incorrectly as an asthmatic for more than 10 years. On specific questioning, Adrienne said she had been coughing for as long as she could remember and indicated that her cough was worse in the mornings and that she often expectorated sputum. Her cough had been stable and she had not noticed any exertional dyspnoea. She had no growth failure and did not have digital clubbing. Given that she had some features of bronchiectasis, high-resolution computed tomography of her chest was performed and revealed focal changes in the right basal segment (Fig. 14.6.2). Her serum immunoglobulin levels were normal and she was Mantoux and sweat test negative. On flexible bronchoscopy, a retained foreign body (piece of shell) was visualized and removed from the right medial segment of her right lower lobe. The foreign body had caused prolonged partial bronchial obstruction and was the cause of Adrienne's localized bronchiectasis.

It is important to define the aetiology of any child's chronic cough. This child had features listed in Box 14.6.1 that indicate 'specific cough' and further investigations were indicated. For children, it is best for investigations to be performed in a children's facility.

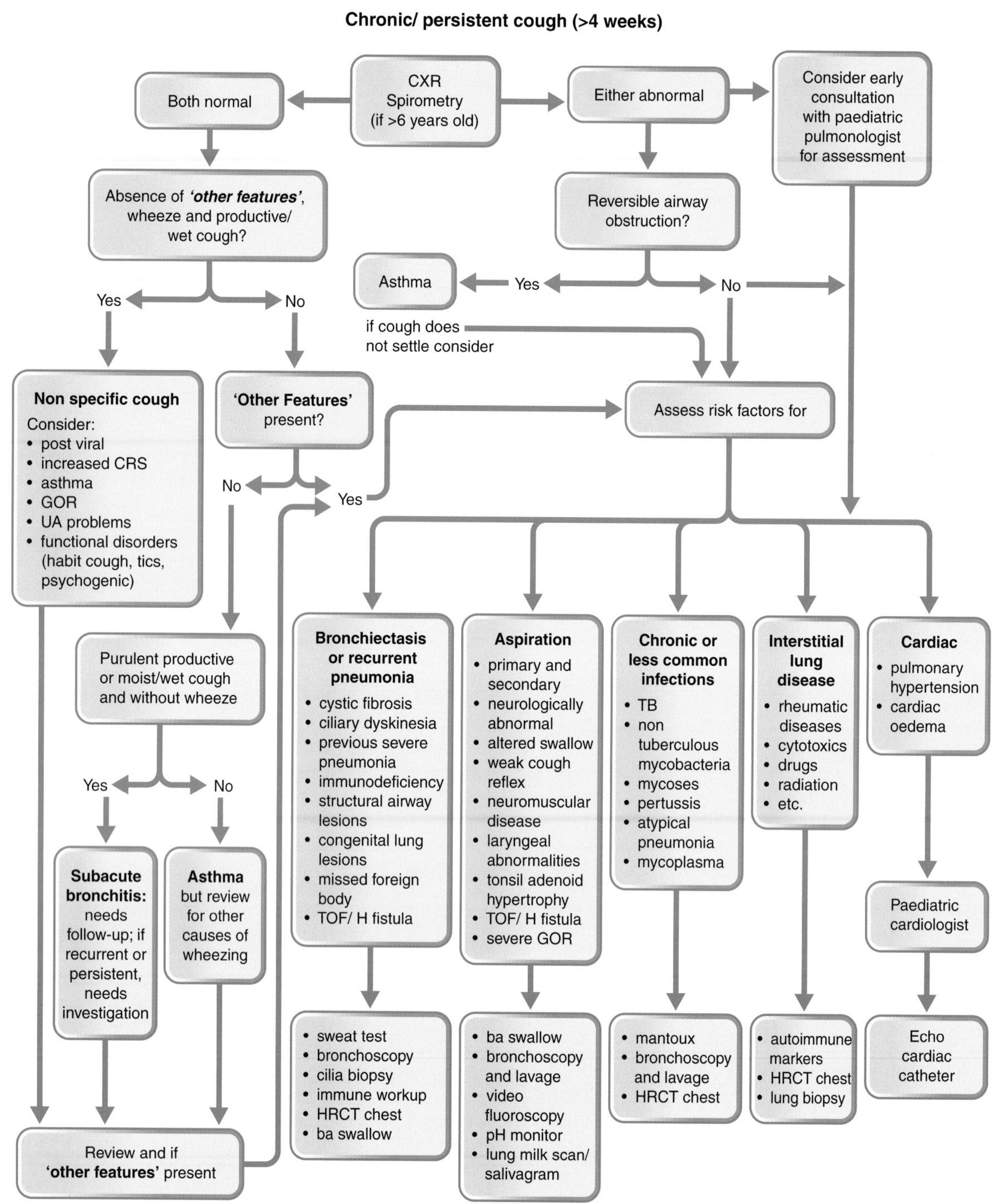


**Fig. 14.6.1** Guide for approaching a child with a persistent cough. Symptoms and signs vary according to age and illness severity. Ba, barium; CRS, cough receptor sensitivity; CXR, chest X-ray; GOR, gastro-oesophageal reflux; HRCT, high-resolution computed tomography; TOF, tracheo-oesophageal fistula, TB, tuberculosis; UA, upper airway.

A key point in the assessment of chronic cough is whether it is specific or non-specific, according to the presence or absence of particular features (Box 14.6.2). Children aged less than 6 years do not generally expectorate sputum. Thus the productive cough of older children and adults manifests as a moist or 'rattly' cough in younger children. The presence of any of these symptoms or signs raises the possibility of an underlying disorder. Certain cough characteristics are associated with particular illness types (see Table 14.6.1).

**Box 14.6.1 Key questions to consider**

- Is the cough representative of an underlying respiratory disorder?
- Are any of the symptoms and signs in Box 14.6.2 present?
- Are exacerbating environmental factors present (passive or active tobacco smoking, other lung toxicants)
- Should the child be referred promptly?

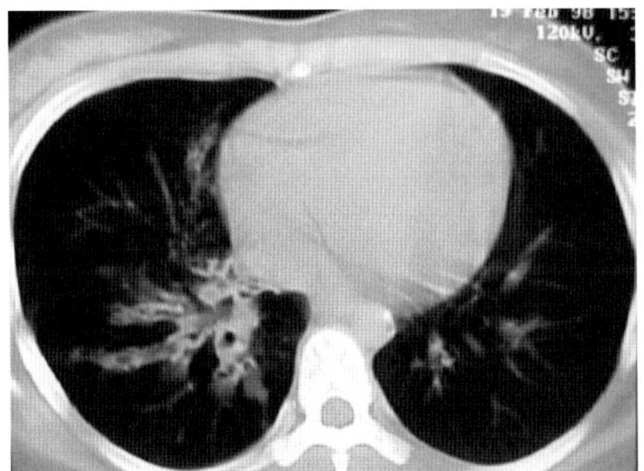

Fig. 14.6.2 High-resolution computed tomogram of Adrienne, as described in Clinical example – a 13-year-old girl with a moist cough for more than 10 years. This child had been incorrectly managed as an asthmatic for 10 years until referred for another opinion. The scan shows focal bronchiectasis of the right basal segment. Flexible bronchoscopy revealed a foreign body (piece of shell) in the right basal medial bronchus.

**Box 14.6.2 Symptoms and signs alerting to the presence of an underlying disorder**

- Auscultatory findings
- Cough characteristics, for example cough with choking, cough quality (see Table 14.6.1), cough starting from birth
- Cardiac abnormalities (including murmurs)
- Chest pain
- Chest wall deformity
- Chronic dyspnoea
- Daily moist or productive cough
- Digital clubbing
- Exertional dyspnoea
- Failure to thrive
- Feeding difficulties
- Haemoptysis
- Immune deficiency
- Neurodevelopmental abnormality
- Sinopulmonary infections

The choice of investigation depends on the clinical findings. Minimum investigation of chronic cough in children is chest radiography and lung spirometry (if aged above 6 years). Diagnoses to be considered include bronchiectasis, asthma, retained foreign body, aspiration lung disease, atypical respiratory infections, cardiac anomalies and interstitial lung disease. If basic investigations are not helpful, referral to a general or respiratory paediatrician is indicated rather than further investigations.

**Table 14.6.1 Classical recognizable cough in children**

| Cough characteristic | Associated illness type |
|---|---|
| Barking or brassy cough | Croup, tracheomalacia, habit cough |
| Honking | Psychogenic |
| Paroxysmal (with/ without whoop) | Pertussis and paratussis |
| Staccato | *Chlamydia* in infants |
| Cough productive of casts | Plastic bronchitis |

## Management of non-specific cough

The majority of children with non-specific cough have post-viral cough and/or increased cough receptor sensitivity. There is no serious underlying cause of non-specific cough and reassurance is a large part of management. Understanding and listening to parental concerns and expectations is important. There is no evidence that 'over the counter' (non-prescription) medications reduce cough in young children.

Identification of exposure to environmental tobacco smoke (ETS) in children and active smoking in adolescents is an important part of respiratory history-taking. ETS exposure can cause non-specific cough and exacerbate a variety of respiratory disorders. If smoking cessation cannot be achieved, aim to reduce smoking in enclosed spaces (e.g. house and car).

Habit cough is a cause of non-specific cough. The age of diagnosis is broad, but is commonly 4–15 years. Severe cases are more common in adolescents than in children. The cough is classically 'honking'. It is generally absent in sleep and worse at times where attention is focused on the cough. Habit cough generally settles promptly once parents are aware that there is no underlying respiratory problem. Mental health expertise is required for those with more severe or prolonged symptoms, especially if there are other features of somatization or concerns of underlying psychopathology.

## Cough, asthma and allergy

There is little doubt that children with asthma can present with cough. However, most children with non-specific chronic cough do not have asthma. Furthermore, although nocturnal cough is a feature of children with asthma, nocturnal cough alone is uncommonly due to asthma. If asthma 'preventer' medication is used, it should be introduced on a trial basis with early review (2–4 weeks) and cessation of medication if the cough does not respond to asthma therapy. Failure to do so will result in escalation of medication dose with the risk of significant side-effects (see Clinical example below).

### Clinical example

Gino was first seen by a paediatric respiratory physician when aged 8 years. He had been receiving 2000 μg/day inhaled corticosteroids for the last 6 years for a chronic dry cough; he had been managed as an 'asthmatic' and his medications were escalated when his cough did not respond to the steroids. When seen, his chest X-ray findings and spirometry were normal, and he was cushingoid (Fig. 14.6.3). Earlier pictures of him showed a normal-sized 3-year-old boy and his 6-year-old brother's body habitus was normal. Gino had been exposed to tobacco smoke and had an element of habitual cough. His asthma medications were subsequently withdrawn and his cough eventually subsided when he was no longer exposed to tobacco smoke and received appropriate counselling.

This example illustrates the importance of obtaining a history of smoke exposure. Also, it is crucial not to 'overdiagnose' asthma based on the presence of isolated cough. In children, when cough is representative of asthma, the cough should subside within 2 weeks of appropriate asthma treatment. If the cough does not subside, the asthma therapy should be withdrawn and not escalated.

A longitudinal population study of cough in infants and children revealed that recurrent cough (rather than chronic cough) presenting in the first year of life resolves over time in the majority of children. The group of children with recurrent cough without wheeze had neither airway hyper-responsiveness nor atopy, and significantly differed from those with classical asthma, with or without cough, in the persistence of symptoms over time. It is believed that infants with recurrent cough without wheeze may have more narrow airways. This group of infants is hard to differentiate clinically from those who continue to have recurrent cough from asthma, making predictions of future illness difficult in infancy.

## Cough, gastro-oesophageal reflux and aspiration lung disease

Gastro-oesophageal reflux (GOR) can be associated with cough. However, although GOR can cause cough, cough can also cause GOR. GOR is neither a specific nor a frequent cause of chronic cough in young children. As cough is very common in children and respiratory symptoms may exacerbate GOR, it is difficult to delineate cause and effect. Infants regularly regurgitate, yet few if any well infants cough with these episodes.

Aspiration lung disease can result from severe GOR or discoordinated swallowing. These children present with chronic cough but usually in the context of developmental or neurological disturbance. The investigatory evidence for aspiration lung disease can be difficult. Ambulatory oesophageal pH studies can

A

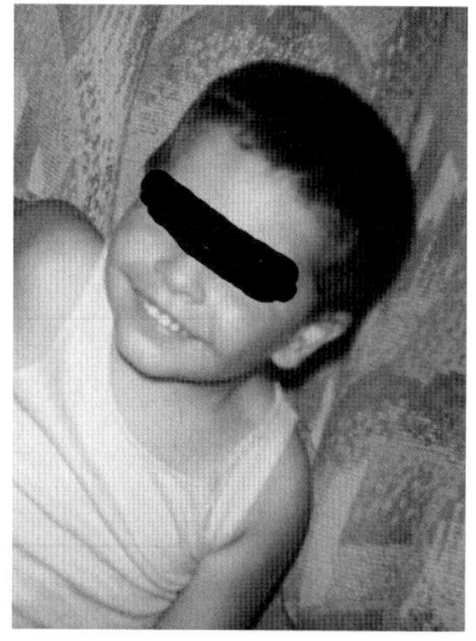

B

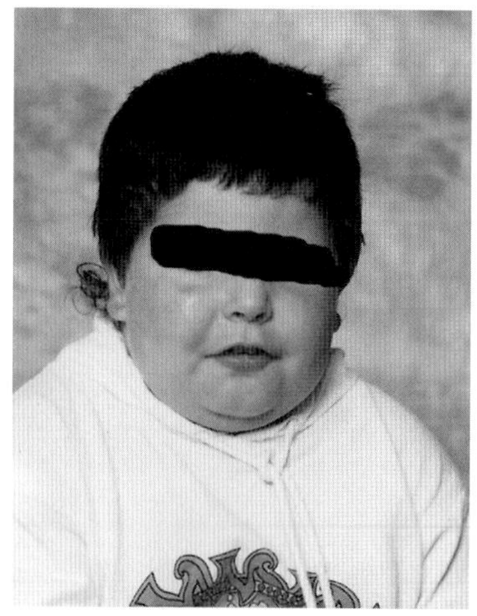

Fig. 14.6.3 **(A)** This previously normal child had a chronic dry cough that had been treated incorrectly with escalating doses of inhaled corticosteroids. **(B)** Two years later, he was cushingoid in appearance without any change in cough. Children with isolated cough should not be treated with increasing doses of asthma therapy.

identify acid GOR, but a positive result does not confirm that aspiration has occurred and a negative result indicates only the absence of reflux related to acid. Similarly primary aspiration (from swallowing discoordination) is also difficult to confirm because current standard tests, such as nuclear medicine milk scan or modified barium swallow, provide only a 'single moment' test that may not be representative of the child's routine feeding pattern.

## Cough, sinusitis and post-nasal drip

Although it is widely stated that sinusitis/post-nasal drip is a common cause of cough, there is little supportive evidence in children. There are no cough receptors in the pharynx or post-nasal space. Although sinusitis is common in childhood, it is not associated with asthma or cough once allergic rhinitis, a common association, has been treated. The relationship between nasal secretions and cough is more likely linked by common aetiology (infection and/or inflammation causing both) or due to throat clearing of secretions reaching the larynx.

## Protracted bacterial bronchitis

The entity of protracted bacterial bronchitis (PBB) was recently described in children where a wet cough resolves completely following antibiotic treatment. PBB, sometimes truncated to protracted bronchitis (PB), is clinically defined as: (a) the presence of isolated chronic (>4 weeks) wet/moist cough, (b) resolution of cough with antibiotic treatment, and (c) absence of pointers suggestive of an alternative specific cause of cough. Many of these children were previously misdiagnosed with asthma, and in some settings they would have been classified as having 'difficult or severe asthma'. PBB is clearly differentiated from acute bronchitis: cough is of shorter duration (≤2 weeks) in paediatric acute bronchitis, and antibiotics are not indicated in acute bronchitis. Some children with PBB go on to have chronic suppurative lung disease or bronchiectasis, and thus should be followed up to ensure the cough resolves.

## Bronchiectasis

Bronchiectasis is now less common compared with its incidence in the mid-20th century. However, in the last decade it has been diagnosed increasingly. Bronchiectasis can be the end result of various disorders, and may be diffuse or focal. Diffuse disease usually develops secondary to an underlying disorder such as cystic fibrosis, immunodeficiency or primary ciliary dyskinesia, although it can be idiopathic. In Indigenous Australians, bronchiectasis is not uncommon and is thought to result from respiratory infections. Focal bronchiectasis more commonly reflects airway narrowing, either congenital (e.g. bronchial stenosis) or acquired (e.g. retained foreign body). Congenital forms of bronchiectasis (e.g. Williams–Campbell syndrome) are rare.

The spectrum of bronchiectasis varies from mild to severe. Symptoms and signs reflect the extent of the disease. Children with bronchiectasis have a chronic moist or productive cough, characteristically worse in the mornings. Physical findings are non-specific: clubbing, chest wall abnormality (hyperinflation or rarely pectus carinatum; Fig. 14.6.4) and inspiratory crepitations. Absence of these signs does not imply absence of disease (see Clinical example below) and most children diagnosed early do not have features associated with more advanced bronchiectasis. Plain radiography may show suggestive features in severe disease (dilated and thickened bronchi may appear as 'tram-tracks'), but are insensitive. Confirmation is by high-resolution computed tomography (CT) of the chest (routine CT provides insufficient detail) with a lower threshold of bronchoarterial ratio used in children.

A child with suspected bronchiectasis should be referred for investigation of a specific cause and specific treatment instituted when indicated (e.g. immunodeficiency). Australian and New Zealand guidelines advocate early diagnosis and appropriate management to improve quality of life and reduce lung function decline. The general approach to managing children with bronchiectasis is similar to (but not exactly the

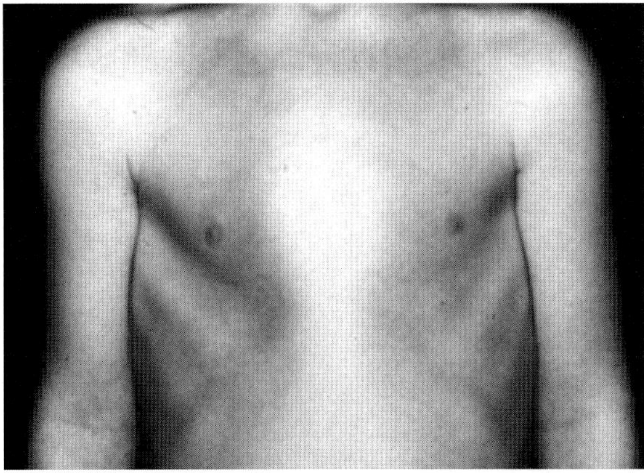

Fig. 14.6.4 Severe pectus carinatum. This can be present in children with any chronic lung disease. Gross pectus carinatum, as shown in this figure, is now rarely seen.

**Clinical example**

Deanna was hospitalized on several occasions for pneumonia, initially at 2 months of age. She was first referred at 2.5 years of age and had a prolonged moist cough. She had a hyperinflated chest wall, early digital clubbing and growth failure. Her weight was below the third percentile and height was at the third percentile. Chest high-resolution CT showed post-infectious bronchiolitis obliterans and bronchiectasis. Other investigations were normal. Deanna's parents were taught home physiotherapy and Deanna was admitted for a prolonged course of intravenous antibiotics. Following discharge she remained on maintenance antibiotics. Her daily moist cough disappeared when her bronchiectasis was treated aggressively with antibiotics and physiotherapy.

same as) that described for CF (see Key elements of respiratory management, below). In addition, children aged above 2 years should receive pneumococcal vaccine. Pooled immunoglobulin replacement is indicated for those with identified immunoglobulin deficiency syndromes. Surgery is very rarely indicated, and only for those with focal disease.

## Primary ciliary dyskinesia

Primary ciliary dyskinesia (PCD) syndromes encompass several congenital disorders, all of which affect the ciliary function of several organs, including the upper and lower respiratory tracts and genitourinary tract. The term includes Kartagener syndrome (situs inversus associated with bronchiectasis), immotile cilia syndrome, ciliary dysmotility and primary orientation defects of ciliary components. PCD has a prevalence of 1 in 20 000, is mostly autosomal recessive in inheritance and probably genetically heterogeneous.

Cilial ultrastructure consists of a 9 + 2 arrangement: the axoneme consists of 9 peripheral microtubular doublets surrounding a central pair of microtubules. Abnormalities in cilial function are due to alteration of its ultrastructure or its function, the ciliary beat frequency. Secondary abnormalities in both ultrastructure and function can also occur as a result of infection, smoking or pollutants. Cilial dysfunction markedly reduces mucociliary clearance and results in recurrent infections of both the upper and lower respiratory tract (middle ear infections, bronchitis, bronchiectasis). In the genitourinary tract, ciliary dysfunction can lead to infertility in males and to ectopic pregnancies in females. Increasingly structural cilial abnormality has been found to be associated with other organ diseases such as the eye (retinitis pigmentosa), the ear (hearing loss) and kidneys (polycystic diseases).

The severity of pulmonary manifestations of PCD varies widely. Presentation can be early in life with neonatal respiratory illness. In infants and older children, the diagnosis should be considered in those with chronic cough, bronchiectasis, recurrent pneumonia, atypical asthma, recurrent rhinosinusitis and chronic secretory otitis media. Specific investigations for PCD include assessment of mucociliary clearance, measurement of ciliary beat frequency, and electronic microscopic identification of cilial ultrastructure.

## Cystic fibrosis

CF is the most common life-threatening autosomal recessive disorder in Australians, affecting approximately 1 in every 2500 births. It is caused by a defect in the CF transmembrane conductance regulator gene (*CFTR*). The *CFTR* gene encodes a protein for a cyclic adenosine monophosphate (cAMP)-regulated chloride channel present on many epithelial cells, including those of the conducting airways, gut and genital tract. The commonest mutation, delta508, accounts for approximately 70% of mutant alleles, and more than 1300 mutations have been described.

### Diagnosis

All infants in Australia are now screened at birth for CF. A two-stage screening procedure is widely used. Initially, immunoreactive trypsin (IRT) is measured in Guthrie blood spot samples. Samples with an IRT level above the 99th percentile are then tested for the common mutation (additional mutations are tested in some states).

Most Australian children with CF are identified by neonatal screening, with the diagnosis confirmed using a sweat test (pilocarpine iontophoresis) at 6–10 weeks. Newborn screening does not detect all children with CF. A sweat test should be arranged if there are phenotypic features suggestive of CF. A raised sweat chloride level (>40 mmol/L) is diagnostic (some centres use a higher cut-off). To minimize the multiple errors that can occur (especially false-negatives), sweat testing should be undertaken in a laboratory that routinely does sweat tests. Very infrequently, patients have been identified with an abnormal CF genotype yet have a normal sweat test result. A borderline sweat test result is more commonly seen in those with retained pancreatic function.

Some 15–20% of Australian infants with CF present before the results of screening with meconium ileus, a form of neonatal intestinal obstruction. Antenatal diagnosis for CF is available when both parents are known carriers of the CF gene owing to the birth of a previous child with CF or a family history.

## Clinical

CF affects multiple organ systems, causing a range of clinical problems of varying severity (Table 14.6.2). It is a severe disorder, although the occasional child has mild disease. Rarely, it is so mild that it is not diagnosed until adult life, following a presentation of *Pseudomonas* pneumonia or male infertility. CF has a major impact on the lungs, where the altered physicochemical properties of the airway epithelium result in abnormally viscid mucus and bacterial colonization of the respiratory tract. The lungs of a child with CF are normal at birth, but over time chronic airway infection develops that causes progressive obstructive lung disease. Clinically, chronic productive cough develops as bronchiectasis progresses and lung function deteriorates. Clubbing is a feature in later stages of the disease (Fig. 14.6.5).

Malabsorption is present in approximately 90% of children with CF, due to failure of the exocrine pancreas.

**Table 14.6.2 Common manifestations of cystic fibrosis disease**

| System | Manifestation |
|---|---|
| Respiratory | Chronic productive or moist cough<br>Features of bronchiectasis<br>Clubbing |
| Ear, nose and throat | Nasal polyps<br>Sinusitis |
| Gastrointestinal | Meconium ileus<br>Features of malabsorption<br>Distal intestinal obstruction syndrome<br>Liver disease<br>Endocrine pancreatic insufficiency (diabetes mellitus) |
| Reproductive | Male infertility |
| General | Growth delay |
| Metabolic | Salt depletion |
| Other | Osteoporosis<br>Urinary incontinence |

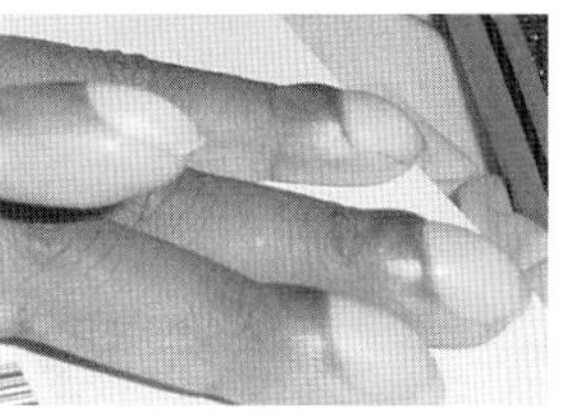

Fig. 14.6.5 Digital clubbing in a boy with bronchiectasis. Digital clubbing is non-specific and may or may not be present in children with suppurative lung disease.

Additionally, there are various degrees of gastric and duodenal hyperacidity, impaired bile salt activity and mucosal dysfunction. Stools are abnormal, being typically frequent and bulky. Growth failure may result from many reasons, including inadequate energy intake, malabsorption and chronic bacterial infection. Long-term retention of pancreatic function is associated with better survival.

As survival of patients with CF improves, a range of CF-related diseases becomes more important. This includes growth and nutrition; diabetes mellitus and liver disease (both seen in approximately 15–20% of adolescents and adults); arthropathy and arthritis; and osteoporosis. Men are generally infertile owing to bilateral absence of the vas deferens. Women are fertile, although pregnancy presents a range of health risks to both the fetus and the mother. Women have increased rates of vaginal yeast infections and stress incontinence.

## Principles of management of a child with cystic fibrosis

The median age of survival has dramatically improved as a range of clinical improvements has developed over time. Four decades ago, median survival was less than 10 years. Current median survival is into the mid-40s, although males survive longer than females. A range of improvements has contributed to these improved health outcomes, including a stronger focus on nutrition and the development of more specific and potent antibiotics. However, a key intervention has been the development of specialized CF centres characterized by a multidisciplinary team of health professionals including respiratory physicians, gastroenterologists, physiotherapists, nutritionists, nurses, surgeons, social workers and mental health therapists. The goal of treatment is to maintain as high a quality of life as possible for as long as possible in order to slow the relentless progression of lung disease that occurs in CF.

The key elements of respiratory management consist of:

- prompt use of antibiotics to reduce bacterial colonization and biofilm formation
- aggressive treatment of recurrent respiratory infections
- promotion of mucociliary clearance by daily physiotherapy
- minimization of other causes of lung damage (e.g. smoking, aspiration)
- additional vaccinations: pneumococcal vaccine and yearly influenza vaccine
- promotion of normal growth through high-energy diet and pancreatic supplementation
- identification and treatment of complications as they arise (asthma-like disease, allergic bronchopulmonary aspergillosis (ABPA), haemoptysis, pneumothorax, etc.).

Respiratory infections should be treated aggressively, because recurrent infection and the accompanying inflammation promotes loss of lung function. The most common respiratory bacteria are *Staphylococcus aureus* and *Haemophilus influenzae* in the early years, followed by *Pseudomonas aeruginosa* and *Burkholderia cepacia*. With increasing use of antibiotics, a plethora of other microorganisms is increasingly isolated, including fungi (*Aspergillus* species, *Scedosporium prolificans*) and other bacteria (*Stenotrophomonas maltophilia*, non-tuberculous mycobacteria, etc.). Most clinic structures currently segregate children to prevent cross-colonization.

Gastroenterological and nutritional management consists of:

- pancreatic enzyme replacement (lipase, protease, amylase) at each meal
- high-energy diet
- vitamin supplementation with vitamins A, D, E and K, and salt tablets
- early identification of liver disease
- early identification of distal intestinal obstruction syndrome.

CF is a life-long chronic condition. As children grow and mature into adolescents and young adults, the psychosocial aspects of the disease take on different dimensions for individuals, siblings and parents. In adolescence, attention to body image issues and feelings of difference due to chronic disease can help maintain young people's adherence with the health-care regimen. Declining health despite good adherence can be especially demoralizing. Lung and liver transplantation are increasingly undertaken to treat end-stage lung and liver disease respectively. Gene therapy is still in the experimental phase.

## Summary

Cough is the commonest manifestation of respiratory problems in children. Although it can be a distressing symptom, its presence is vital for respiratory health. Chest radiography and spirometry are the minimal investigations in a child with a chronic cough (for more than 4 weeks). When cough is associated with other symptoms ('specific cough'), investigations and/or referral

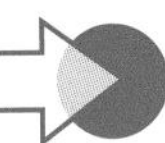

### Practical points

1. Children with chronic cough should:
   - be evaluated carefully for symptoms and signs of an underlying respiratory or systemic disease (termed 'specific cough pointers'; see Box 14.6.2)
   - have a chest X-ray performed and (if age appropriate) spirometry
   - be followed up, because minimal airway secretions may be present in dry cough and hence wet cough may initially present as dry cough
   - be assessed for a history of environmental exposures, particularly tobacco smoke exposure, and intervention initiated if appropriate
   - be reviewed to ensure there is resolution of the cough.
2. Chronic cough can be classified based on the likelihood of an underlying disease or process, specific cough and non-specific cough (an overlap is present).
3. Over-the-counter (OTC) or prescription medications are ineffective for chronic non-specific cough and should not be used for the symptomatic relief of cough.
4. Treatment for chronic cough should be aetiology based. Medications are largely unhelpful for non-specific cough. If medication trials are undertaken, a follow-up review to assess response should be undertaken. Asthma should not be diagnosed based on a single episode in the absence of other symptoms of asthma.
5. Chronic suppurative lung disease or bronchiectasis should be suspected in children with chronic wet cough that does not resolve on oral antibiotics or that recurs frequently. These children should be investigated for an underlying cause such as cystic fibrosis, primary ciliary dyskinesia, immune deficiency and aspirated foreign body.
6. Children with chronic suppurative lung diseases should be managed by a multidisciplinary team. The medical elements include airway clearance techniques, attention to nutrition, and early intervention for pulmonary exacerbations and other complications.

are required to identify the cause. Non-specific cough is largely managed expectantly, trying to explore parent anxieties, minimize investigations and identify environmental triggers such as tobacco smoke. There is little evidence that the common causes of persistent, isolated cough in adults (asthma, GOR, sinusitis and nasal disease) are common causes of chronic cough in children.

## Acknowledgements

The authors thank Professor Susan Sawyer for her contribution to the previous version of this chapter from which this new version has been adapted.

PART 15

# CARDIAC DISORDERS

# 15.1 Suspected heart disease: assessment

Michael Cheung

## Scale of the problem

Cardiac abnormalities or disease affect approximately 1% of children in the developed world and 2–3% in developing countries. This difference is largely due to the higher incidence of rheumatic heart disease in the latter.

The prevalence of congenital heart disease is approximately 8 in 1000 newborn infants. In Australia, heart disease remains one of the major causes of infant mortality.

## Presentation

Significant heart disease in children presents with symptoms and signs of heart failure or cyanosis. These will, of course, vary depending on the age of the patient and severity of disease. Milder forms of heart disease may present by the detection of an asymptomatic murmur.

## Assessment

### History

It is important to determine the onset and type of symptoms. In babies, breathlessness, feeding difficulties, inability to complete feeds and poor weight gain are important to elucidate and may be indicative of a significant heart problem. Cyanosis due to heart disease is usually persistent but may intermittently increase in severity. Intermittent peripheral and circumoral cyanosis are common in normal children, typically occurring when cold (e.g. swimming) or conversely when febrile. Cyanosis may also be associated with breath-holding in children with normal hearts, and in these situations clearly defining the sequence of events leading up to the cyanotic episode is important.

Chest pain in children is rarely due to heart disease. The history of the chest pain is useful in distinguishing cardiac from non-cardiac chest pain; however, this may be difficult to elicit in young children. Pain consistently associated with exertion is more likely to be cardiac in nature, although its location may indicate a musculoskeletal rather than cardiac origin. Oesophageal and gastric pain may be indicated by the history. Brief episodes of chest discomfort may be associated with viral illnesses and myopericarditis.

Palpitations associated with collapse are clearly concerning but the majority of children presenting with palpitations do not lose consciousness with episodes of tachycardia. It is useful to determine the rate, duration, nature of onset and offset of these episodes, in addition to the circumstances surrounding them. Most children may be able to tap out with their hand how fast their heart rate is, or parents can be taught to measure the pulse and keep a diary of events.

### Pulses

Examination of pulses should include both left and right arms and femoral pulses. The upper and lower limb pulses are best compared when palpated simultaneously. Relatively reduced lower-limb pulses suggest coarctation, but femoral pulses may be difficult to feel in the first few days of life. Bounding pulses due to a wide pulse pressure may be associated with patent ductus arteriosus, significant aortic regurgitation, and high cardiac output states. The physiological increase in heart rate in children varies markedly with activity and so it is the resting rate that should be noted (Table 15.1.1).

### Blood pressure

Measurement of blood pressure should be a routine part of examination in children. Use of an appropriate cuff is vital. The balloon/bladder of the cuff should be wide enough to cover two-thirds of the upper arm. In practice, the largest cuff that can be fitted to the upper arm without covering the antecubital fossa is used. Blood pressure should normally be recorded by auscultation of Korotkoff sounds, as in adults, although palpation (of the brachial or radial pulse) may be employed to assess systolic pressure in young children and infants if auscultation proves to be difficult. Significant errors in blood pressure are more likely to result from the use of a cuff that is too small than one that is overlarge. Newer automated devices are able to detect the arterial pulsation and limit the upper pressure of inflation; however, these devices are still relatively slow and may overestimate blood pressure in restless or uncooperative children.

**Table 15.1.1 Approximate normal upper limit for pulse, respiratory rate and systolic blood pressure at rest; resting measurements consistently above these values should arouse suspicion**

| Age group | Pulse rate (beats/min) | Respiratory rate (breaths/min) | Systolic BP (mmHg) |
|---|---|---|---|
| 0–8 weeks | 160 | 50 | 70 |
| Older infant (2–12 months) | 145 | 40 | 85 |
| Toddler (1–3 years) | 130 | 30 | 100 |
| Older child (4–7 years) | 115 | 20 | 115 |

For measurement of leg blood pressure, a cuff may be placed on the thigh. An adult arm cuff may be large enough for young children, but larger children or adolescents will require a 'thigh cuff', which is larger than an adult arm cuff.

Normal blood pressure varies at different ages (see Table 15.1.1).

## Palpation of the cardiac impulse

Location of the apex beat and documentation of any abnormal/forceful impulses/thrill of the precordium is important.

## Auscultatory findings

Splitting of the second heart sound should be noted (Fig. 15.1.1). Splitting is widened during inspiration. Fixed splitting, a feature of atrial septal defect, implies absence of variation between inspiration and expiration (Fig. 15.1.2) and is also typically widely split.

Accentuation of the pulmonary component of the second sound tends to be associated with a loud second sound, which may be palpable, often with no definite splitting, and implies the presence of pulmonary hypertension. However, it should be noted that the normal aortic closure sound may be loud in children with a thin chest wall and is sometimes palpable at the upper left sternal border. The presence of an ejection click (see Fig. 15.1.1) is a useful ancillary auscultatory finding. Such sounds are heard shortly after the first heart sound and tend to be high-frequency and discrete in character. If heard at the apex, it usually implies a bicuspid aortic valve or aortic valve stenosis. When originating from the pulmonary valve, it is heard at the left sternal edge and varies with respiration, being louder on expiration. This finding is characteristic of pulmonary valve stenosis.

Normal heart sounds

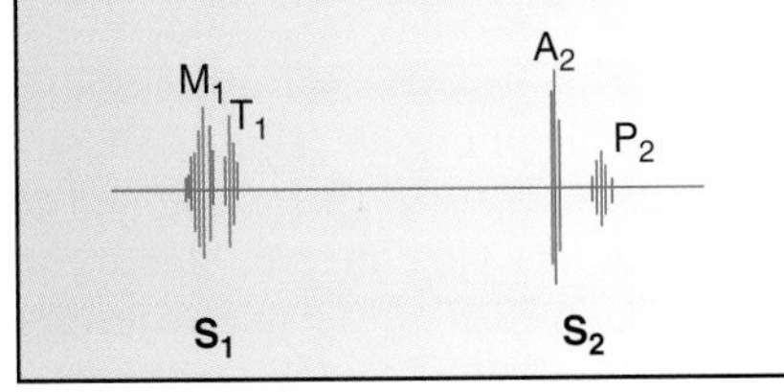


Variation in splitting of the second sound

Inspiration

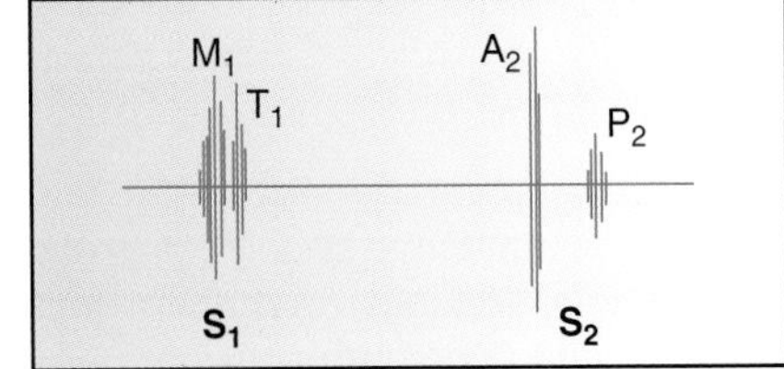


Ejection click

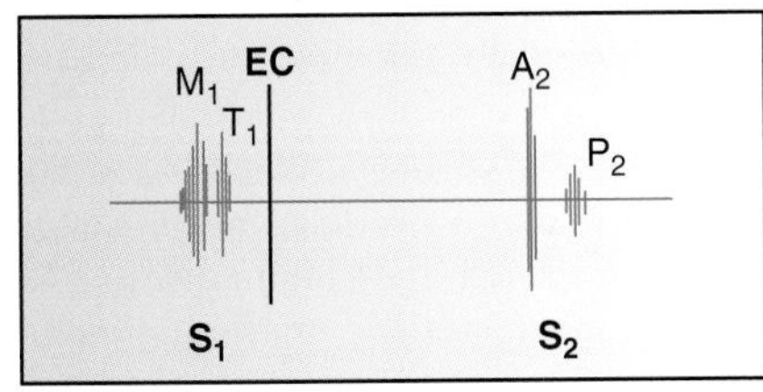


Expiration

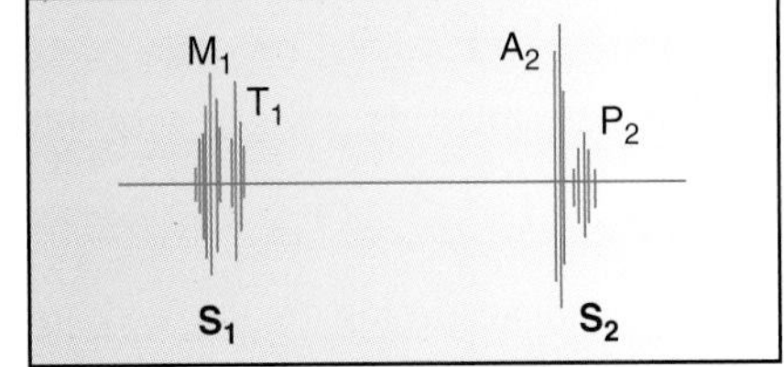


Fig. 15.1.1 Illustration of normal heart sounds, normal splitting of the second sound and ejection click (EC).

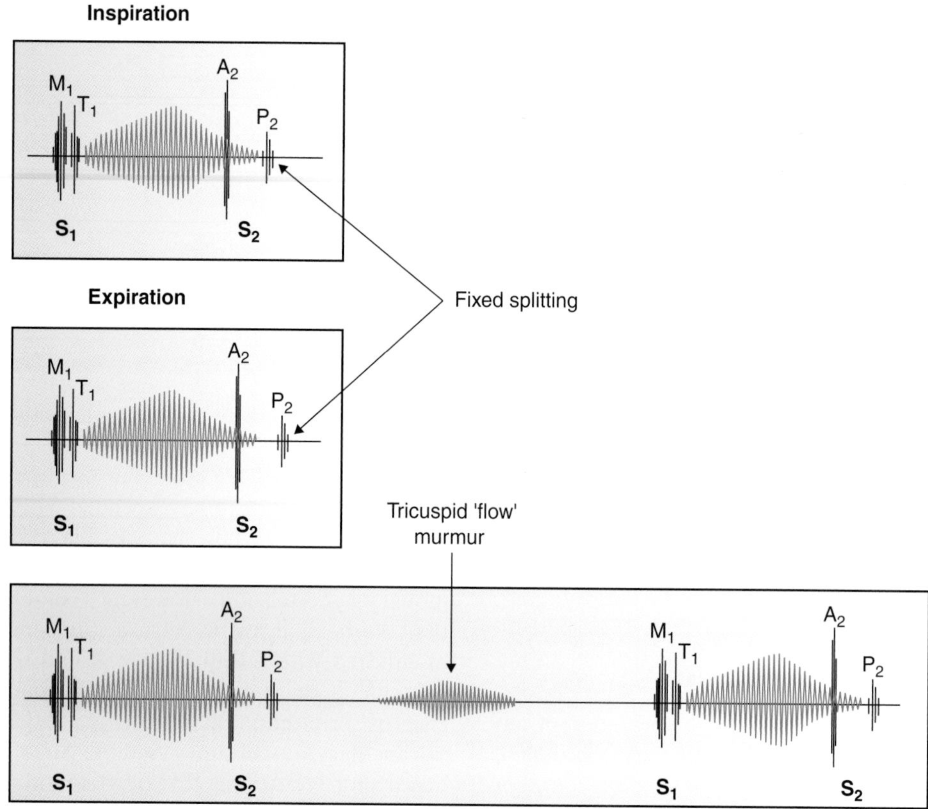


Fig. 15.1.2 Auscultatory signs associated with an atrial septal defect showing ejection systolic murmur, fixed splitting of $S_2$ and tricuspid flow murmur (see Chapter 15.2).

## Murmurs

The following features of the murmur should be determined:

- timing
- location
- amplitude (grading)
- characterization
- radiation.

*Timing*

Murmurs may be systolic (limited to systole), diastolic (limited to diastole) or continuous (extending from systole into diastole). Note that continuous murmurs are not necessarily present throughout the cardiac cycle. Murmurs may be timed by simultaneously palpating a peripheral pulse.

*Location*

The point of maximum intensity of the murmur should be identified.

*Amplitude*

Murmurs may be graded according to the scale in Table 15.1.2. The amplitude of the murmur is affected by the thickness of the chest wall, and the direction, volume and velocity of blood flow relative to the stethoscope position.

*Characterization*

Ejection murmurs (Fig. 15.1.3) are systolic and crescendo–decrescendo in character, starting shortly after the first sound. Good examples are the murmurs of pulmonary or aortic valve stenosis.

Pansystolic murmurs (Fig. 15.1.3) are murmurs that commence at the first sound and continue to the second sound. They may be due to atrioventricular valve incompetence (e.g. mitral incompetence) or a ventricular septal defect (VSD).

Diastolic murmurs may be *early diastolic* (see Fig. 15.1.4) (commencing at the second sound) or *mid-diastolic* (see Fig. 15.1.2). The former reflect either aortic or pulmonary incompetence, whereas mid-diastolic murmurs occur during ventricular filling and reflect either stenosis of or increased blood flow through an atrioventricular valve (e.g. mitral stenosis or secondary to a large left–right shunt due to a VSD).

Other characteristic murmurs include *early* (see Fig. 15.1.4) and *late systolic* murmurs (reflecting a tiny muscular VSD or mitral valve prolapse, respectively),

**Table 15.1.2 Grading of murmurs**

| Grade | Amplitude | Thrill | Comments |
|---|---|---|---|
| 1 | Very soft | Absent | Scarcely audible |
| 2 | Soft | Absent | Easily audible |
| 3 | Loud | Absent | Very easily audible |
| 4 | Loud | Faint/localized | Very easily audible |
| 5 | Very loud | Easily felt/widespread | Very easily audible |
| 6 | Very loud | Easily felt/widespread | Heard with stethoscope off chest wall |

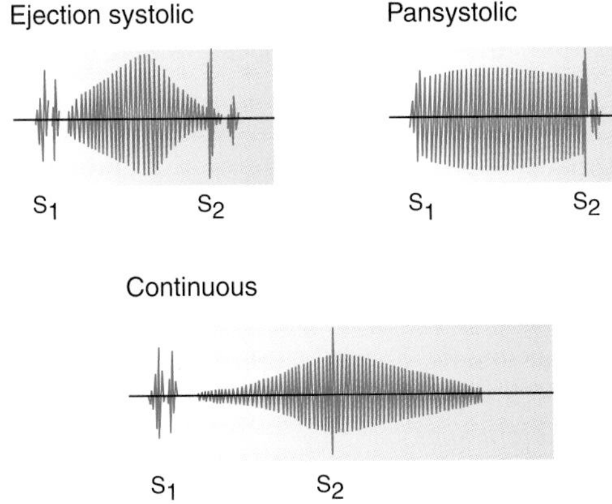


**Fig. 15.1.3** Common murmurs and their relationship to the heart sounds $S_1$ and $S_2$.

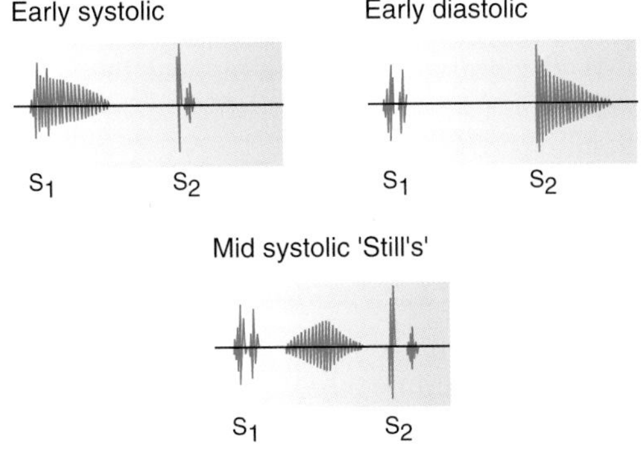


**Fig. 15.1.4** Other murmurs: early systolic, early diastolic and Still's murmur.

and the *late diastolic* murmur associated with atrial contraction in patients with mitral stenosis.

Characterization of murmurs also includes assessment of the pitch of the murmur and its quality, for example 'harsh', 'musical' or 'vibratory'.

*Radiation*

A murmur that is easily audible/loud away from the precordial area (e.g. the neck or axilla) is said to 'radiate' towards the area in question.

## Innocent murmurs

There are four characteristic types of innocent murmur that are, by definition, not associated with cardiac symptoms:

- Still's murmur
- pulmonary flow murmur
- carotid bruit
- venous hum.

*Still's murmur*

This is a short mid-systolic murmur best heard at the left sternal border or between the apex and left sternal edge. This murmur is sometimes referred to as 'Still's' murmur (see Fig. 15.1.4) or a 'vibratory' murmur. The murmur is of medium frequency and has a vibratory or slightly musical quality. It tends to become softer if the patient stands and is louder when the patient is squatting or lying supine.

*Pulmonary flow murmur*

This is a soft, blowing ejection murmur, maximal in the pulmonary area. Murmurs of this kind are frequently heard in early infancy and may radiate softly to the axillae, when they may be labelled as innocent with a high degree of confidence, and are less common later in childhood. In older children, distinction from an atrial septal defect or mild pulmonary stenosis can be difficult, and may warrant further investigation.

*Carotid bruit*

This medium-frequency, rough ejection systolic murmur heard over the carotid artery (right or left or bilateral) at the root of the neck is very common in children, being usually softer or inaudible below the clavicle.

*Venous hum*

A high-pitched, blowing, rather variable, continuous murmur, heard over the sternoclavicular junctions or over the neck and changing with the position of the head, is frequently heard in children. This murmur almost always disappears completely when the patient lies flat and may be eliminated by gentle compression of the neck veins.

It should be appreciated that innocent murmurs may be heard in around 50% of normal school-aged children and adolescents. In early infancy, the frequency of soft murmurs is probably around 80%. Because of the very high frequency of soft heart murmurs, it is essential that all doctors involved in caring for infants and children become familiar with the common innocent murmurs; they should be able to recognize them with confidence and be able to exclude organic heart disease (Fig. 15.1.5). Where doubt exists, patients should be referred for formal cardiological assessment.

### Cyanosis

The distinction between peripheral and central cyanosis is important. Central cyanosis is generalized. Examination of the tongue and mucous membranes will usually exclude central cyanosis. Where doubt exists about the presence of cyanosis the use of pulse oximetry is helpful.

## Manifestations of heart failure

Cardiac failure in infancy tends to be dominated by pulmonary congestion, which leads to dyspnoea/tachypnoea.

Dyspnoea contributes to feeding difficulties, reduced intake and increased metabolic rate. These may combine to cause failure to thrive. Chronic dyspnoea may lead to the appearance of Harrison's sulci, which are deformations of the rib cage at the site of the diaphragmatic attachments. Crepitations at the lung bases are more often a manifestation of superimposed infection rather than heart failure in infants.

Systemic venous congestion is manifest by liver enlargement and/or oedema. Liver enlargement results in a firm liver with its edge palpable below the costal margin. In infants, oedema is often diffuse and difficult to detect. It is often best seen around the face and eyes (periorbital oedema). Raised jugular venous pressure cannot be assessed easily in infancy.

Other evidence of cardiac failure may include persistent tachycardia, a chronic dry cough and profuse sweating, especially of the forehead and scalp.

## Investigations

### Chest X-ray

The chest X-ray provides information about heart size, shape and lung vascularity. The heart is enlarged when, on a posteroanterior chest film, the cardiothoracic ratio exceeds 0.5 in an adult or 0.55 in a child. In infancy, the cardiothoracic ratio may be as large as 0.6 (Fig. 15.1.6). If vascular shadows in the hilum are increased, this implies high pulmonary flow (pulmonary plethora; Fig. 15.1.6) or pulmonary venous congestion. Diminished vascular marking, with abnormally dark lung fields (pulmonary oligaemia), is associated with the decreased pulmonary flow occurring in some forms of cyanotic heart disease (e.g. tetralogy of Fallot). Individual cardiac chamber size is often difficult to assess on plain chest X-rays, although variations in cardiac contour may provide useful clues.

### Electrocardiography

The ECG can provide information about heart rate and rhythm, and about atrial or ventricular hypertrophy or hypoplasia.

In the newborn infant, right ventricular forces tend to dominate, whereas by the end of the first year of life left ventricular forces predominate. This evolution reflects changes in ventricular wall thickness, and evaluation of ventricular hypertrophy needs to take into account the normal values for children of each age group. Additionally, normal values for heart rate, PR interval, QRS duration, QT interval and T-wave axis vary at different ages.

### Echocardiography

This is the main modality for cardiac imaging and assessment of cardiac physiology in children. Current echocardiographic systems allow the sectional anatomy of the heart, as it beats in 'real time', to be displayed. This is referred to as two-dimensional echocardiography (Fig. 15.1.7).

Doppler echocardiography allows quantification of the direction and velocity of blood flow at individual sites. Colour Doppler imaging gives semiquantitative information about flow volume, direction and velocity. Pulse-wave and continuous Doppler techniques may be utilized to measure the speed of blood flow with more accuracy. This can provide useful quantitative information about the presence and severity of valvar stenoses, regurgitation and septal defects. Use of the Bernoulli principle allows the assessment of relative pressure differences within the heart and blood vessels. Newer systems also allow the same Doppler technique to be applied to the myocardium to assess heart function.

### Cardiac catheterization

Cardiac catheterization allows measurement of intracardiac pressures and shunts. It also allows for angiographic demonstration of abnormal anatomy.

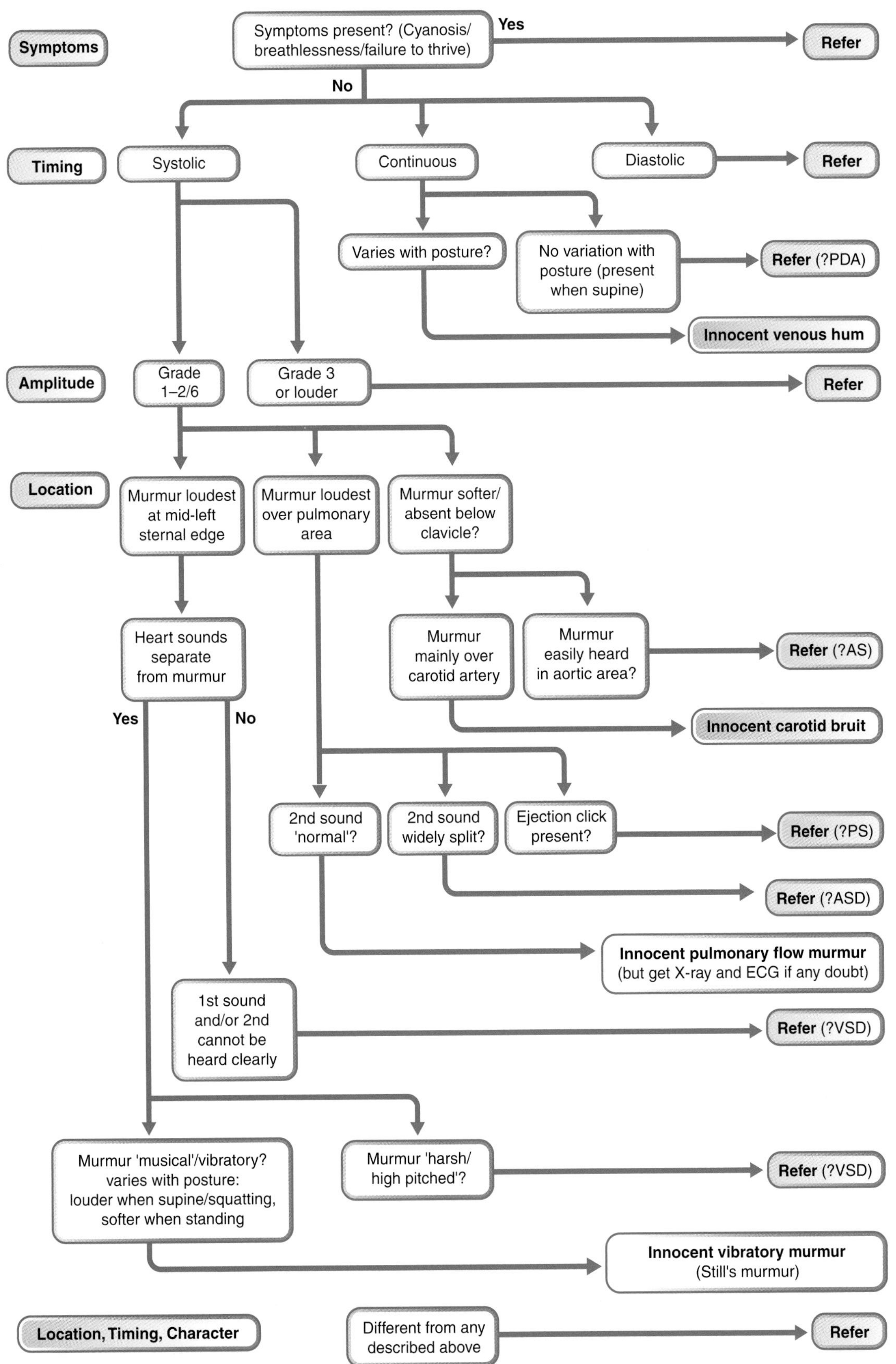


Fig. 15.1.5 An approach to the child with a murmur. AS, aortic stenosis; ASD, atrial septal defect; ECG, electrocardiography; PDA, patent ductus arteriosus; PS, pulmonary stenosis; VSD, ventricular septal defect.

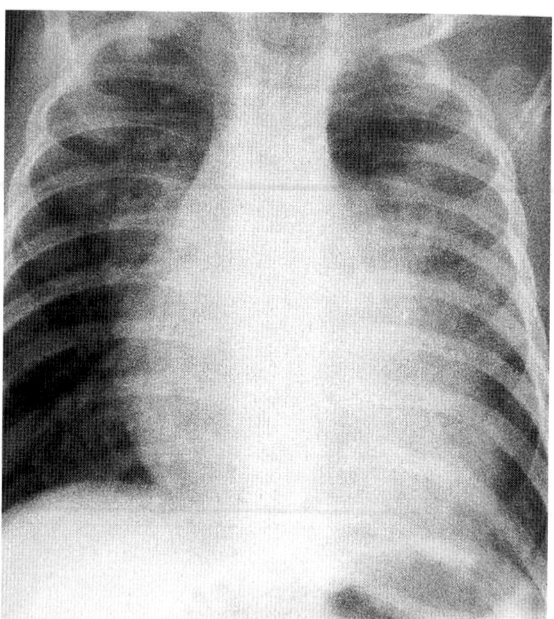

Fig. 15.1.6 Chest X-ray showing cardiomegaly and pulmonary plethora in a child with a large ventricular septal defect (see Chapter 15.2).

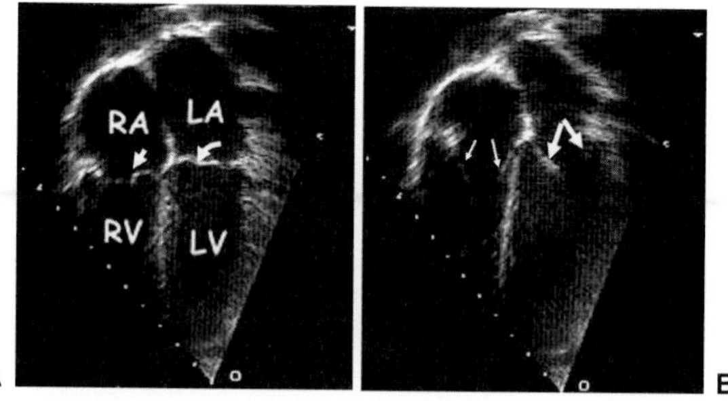


Fig. 15.1.7 Echocardiogram: 'four chambers view'. (**A**) Four chambers with the mitral valve (curved arrow) and tricuspid valve (straight arrow) closed during ventricular systole. (**B**) Same anatomy during diastole with the mitral (large arrows) and tricuspid (small arrows) valves open. The atrial and ventricular septa can be seen separating the left heart chambers (LA and LV) from the right-sided chambers (RA and RV).

As much of this can be obtained using echocardiography, the requirement for catheterization has diminished substantially. The number of diagnostic procedures performed has fallen further with the advent of the additional non-invasive imaging modalities of computed tomography (CT) and magnetic resonance imaging (MRI). In the vast majority of cases, a diagnosis can be made and treatment instituted on the basis of non-invasive investigations without cardiac catheterization. However, catheterization may be necessary for planning surgical treatment, especially in more complicated heart defects.

The number of catheters performed for therapeutic purposes, however, has increased as new devices have been developed. These procedures include balloon dilatation of valves (valvuloplasty) for pulmonary or aortic valve stenosis, or placement of an occlusion 'device' to close a persistent ductus arteriosus, atrial septal defect or VSD. Stenotic vessels can also be balloon-dilated (angioplasty) or may require to be helped open with stents. More recently, transcatheter techniques have evolved to implant pulmonary and aortic valves in suitable patients.

## Treatment

### Cardiac failure

The development of heart failure in a newborn should be regarded as an emergency requiring urgent hospitalization, usually at a major cardiac centre. The transportation of such patients can present a major challenge and may be best achieved by arranging for the patient to be accompanied by well trained medical and/or nursing personnel with appropriate resuscitation equipment.

#### ABC

The basics of resuscitation should be followed (see Chapter 5.2).

#### Respiratory support

In the presence of severe cardiac and/or respiratory failure, positive pressure ventilation may be helpful in allowing stabilization of the child's condition.

#### Circulatory support

Intravenous inotropic support may be required but should be started in consultation with experienced medical staff.

#### Correction of acidosis

Where respiratory or metabolic acidosis are present, these should be corrected by ventilatory support and/or circulatory support.

#### Prostaglandin

In infants developing symptoms in the newborn period, due to congenital heart disease, a 'ductus-dependent congenital defect' is often responsible. Infants with such defects (e.g. left heart obstruction, obstructed pulmonary blood flow) may benefit from infusion of prostaglandin $E_1$ to reopen/maintain patency of the ductus. Care should be used when starting prostaglandin because it has the side-effect of causing hypotension due to vasodilatation and can also induce apnoea.

### Diuretics

Frusemide is usually the diuretic of choice. This may be given parenterally initially. A potassium-sparing diuretic (e.g. spironolactone) is typically used in combination in order to prevent significant hypokalaemia.

### Angiotensin converting enzyme inhibitors

Inhibition of the angiotensin converting enzyme (ACE) results in a reduction in systemic vascular resistance and the amount of work that the heart has to perform with each contraction. These effects may be useful in the management of large left-to-right shunts (e.g. VSD) or in patients with heart failure due to reduced ventricular function (e.g. dilated cardiomyopathy).

### Oxygen

Oxygen should be administered if significant hypoxia is detectable, although in the presence of significant cyanotic congenital heart disease the administration of oxygen will seldom produce much improvement in oxygenation. Furthermore, even moderate central cyanosis when due to cyanotic heart disease is often well tolerated in the neonatal period.

### Feeding

Gavage feeding via nasogastric tube may be helpful if the infant is too breathless to feed adequately. Introduction of high-calorie/more concentrated feeds may be helpful. Infants with heart failure tend to tolerate small, frequent feeds better than larger feeds. In the presence of more severe congestive failure, feed volume should be reduced to 120 mL per kg per 24 h (or less) to avoid fluid overload.

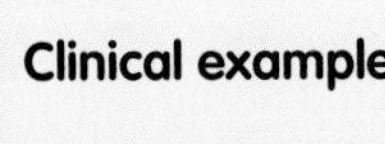

**Clinical example**

Stacey, aged 6 years, presented with fever, cough and breathing difficulty. She had been known to have a heart murmur since infancy, which was labelled as being 'innocent' by her paediatrician. Examination showed her to be febrile with a temperature of 39.6 °C, a red throat and crepitations over the lungs, with widespread rhonchi. A grade 2/6 murmur was audible at the upper sternal edge that extended from systole into early diastole. Her chest X-ray showed a normal cardiac contour with patchy opacity in the right lower zone. The ECG was normal. An echocardiogram showed a small patent ductus arteriosus (PDA) with no chamber enlargement.

Stacey had pneumonia following a viral respiratory infection. Her murmur was 'continuous', although audible only during systole and early diastole. It could easily be mistaken for a purely systolic murmur unless careful attention was paid to assessing the timing. For this reason (being judged to be a soft systolic murmur) it had been incorrectly labelled as innocent. The persistent ductus was an incidental finding and the normal heart size on X-ray, normal ECG and absence of chamber enlargement demonstrated by the echocardiogram all indicated that the shunt was small and hence not likely to be contributing to her current symptoms. Her pneumonia was treated with appropriate antibiotics and the PDA was reassessed and treated (probably with a catheter procedure to implant a coil or occlusion device) after she had recovered from her current illness.

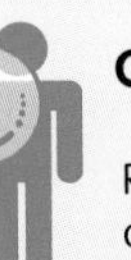

**Clinical example**

Ryan was a 2-month-old infant with recent onset of episodic cyanosis when distressed. He had been noted to have a heart murmur a few days ago but had been feeding well and gaining weight normally. His mother thought that his colour was normal most of the time, but when he cried his lips and fingers became purple. His chest X-ray was normal but the electrocardiogram indicated right ventricular hypertrophy. Pulse oximetry showed a saturation of 92% while he was asleep, but when upset the saturation was 65%.

This baby was likely to have a cyanotic heart defect, as evidenced by his low saturations on pulse oximetry – both at rest and more so when crying. Minor desaturation (with saturations above 85%) may be difficult to detect clinically and Ryan might appear to be pink when he was comfortable. However, when distressed, his oxygen demands would increase and he would become more obviously hypoxic, with reduced saturations and clinically apparent cyanosis. An echocardiogram was organized to establish the nature of his heart defect – the commonest problem to present like this being Fallot's tetralogy (see Chapter 15.2).

### Surgery

In many cases, surgical treatment offers the best means of alleviating the problem that has produced heart failure, and medical treatment should be pursued only in an effort to achieve stabilization of the infant's condition and allow a diagnosis to be reached so that planning of surgical management may proceed.

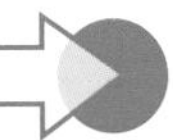

**Practical points**

- In developed countries, most heart disease in childhood is congenital, but various acquired disorders are important.
- Clinical assessment, including auscultation, remains vital and should not be omitted – even though investigations such as echocardiography may be necessary.
- Cardiac catheterization is seldom required to establish the diagnosis but is frequently used for therapeutic (interventional) procedures.
- Many serious heart defects, which lead to symptoms in the early days/weeks of life, are 'ductus dependent'. Use of prostaglandin $E_1$ infusion to reopen the ductus may be life-saving.

# 15.2 Heart disease

Michael Cheung

Congenital malformations affecting the heart and/or great vessels occur in a little under 1% of newborn infants. Eight defects are relatively frequent and together make up approximately 80% of all congenital heart disease (Table 15.2.1). The remaining 20% of defects comprise a large number of abnormalities, some being quite rare and/or complex malformations.

## Presenting features

The major presenting features are:

- presence of an abnormal murmur
- development of symptoms or signs of congestive heart failure
- central cyanosis
- any combination of the above.

## Acyanotic defects

These comprise approximately 75% of all congenital heart defects and can be subdivided into: (1) those that are associated with an isolated left-to-right shunt, and (2) obstructive heart defects.

Common defects with a left-to-right shunt are:

- ventricular septal defect (VSD)
- patent ductus arteriosus (PDA)
- atrial septal defect (ASD)
- atrioventricular septal defect (AVSD).

### Ventricular septal defect

These comprise around 30% of all cardiac defects. They vary from tiny defects, of pinhole size, to huge defects. Small defects are more common than large ones and are usually asymptomatic. Defects are frequently situated in the region of the membranous septum (perimembranous defects), but VSDs involving the muscular septum are also common (Fig. 15.2.1). Very tiny muscular defects may be demonstrated by echocardiography in infants with no clinical signs to suggest a septal defect.

#### Presentation and clinical findings

With a small VSD, there is usually a loud, harsh, high-pitched systolic murmur audible at the left sternal border, frequently associated with a thrill. The heart sounds otherwise may be normal and there are often no other abnormal findings. The murmur is usually 'pansystolic' in timing, indicating flow across the defect throughout systole. Alternatively there may be a short early systolic murmur, which is often well localized at the mid left sternal border and reflects a small muscular defect that becomes smaller during ventricular contraction.

With a larger VSD, left heart dilatation occurs, signs of cardiac failure may be present and the physical signs are different. These may include a parasternal heave, a displaced apex, and the systolic murmur may be softer and less harsh. Large shunts are associated with an apical diastolic murmur, owing to increased flow through the mitral valve. Infants with a large VSD have difficulty feeding due to tachypnoea and fail to thrive, owing to a combination of poor intake and increased metabolic demands. Tachypnoea, increased work of breathing and hepatomegaly are frequent clinical findings.

#### Investigation

With small defects, the chest X-ray and electrocardiogram (ECG) are frequently normal. With larger defects, the chest X-ray shows cardiomegaly and increased pulmonary plethora (see Fig. 15.1.6). The ECG often shows biventricular hypertrophy. The site and size of the defect can be documented well with echocardiography. Cardiac catheters to document degree of shunting are rarely done but may be performed to measure pulmonary vascular resistance and response to pulmonary vasodilators in patients thought to have pulmonary hypertension secondary to a left-to-right shunt.

#### Management

The natural history of a VSD varies. Small defects frequently undergo spontaneous closure, which may occur in 50% or more. Some moderate defects may also diminish in size and the shunt becomes minor.

**Table 15.2.1 Relative frequency of common congenital heart defects**

| Defect | Approximate frequency (%) |
|---|---|
| Ventricular septal defect (VSD) | 30 |
| Persistent arterial duct (ductus arteriosus; PDA) | 12 |
| Atrial septal defect (ASD) | 8 |
| Pulmonary stenosis | 8 |
| Aortic stenosis | 5 |
| Coarctation of the aorta | 5 |
| Tetralogy of Fallot | 5 |
| Transposition of the great arteries | 5 |

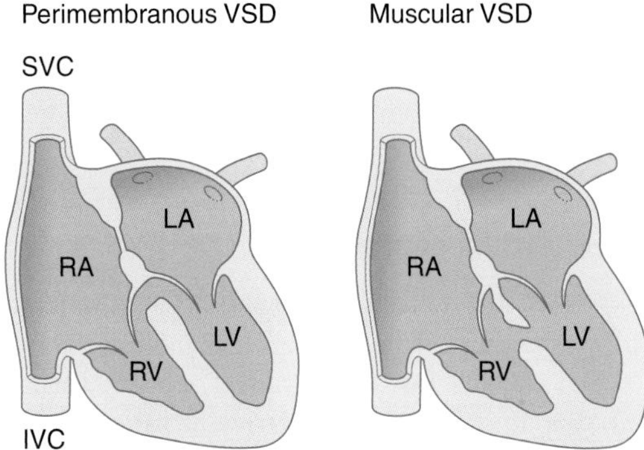


Fig. 15.2.1 Sites of ventricular septal defect (VSD). In the left panel, the defect is close to the membranous part of the ventricular septum (perimembranous VSD). In the right panel, the defect is in the muscular septum. IVC, inferior vena cava; LA, left atrium; LV, left ventricle; RA, right atrium; RV, right ventricle; SVC, superior vena cava.

Important complications include progressive aortic regurgitation, when the adjacent leaflet of the aortic valve is sucked (prolapses) into the defect, due to the Venturi effect of high-velocity left-to-right flow across the VSD. Aortic valve prolapse due to this mechanism does not occur with defects that are far away from the aortic valve. In some cases of VSD, infundibular pulmonary stenosis or right ventricular cavity muscle bundles may develop. Small isolated defects are generally left alone if the investigation shows no significant haemodynamic disturbance and the patient remains symptom-free.

Large VSDs are associated with a variable degree of increased pulmonary pressure. The natural fall in pulmonary artery pressure from birth means that large defects may not cause symptoms or significant signs in the first few days of life. As pulmonary vascular resistance naturally declines in the first few months of life there will be an increasing volume of pulmonary blood flow. Children with isolated large VSDs who are asymptomatic aged more than a few months of age are concerning, because this indicates that the natural fall in pulmonary vascular resistance has not occurred.

### Indications for closure of VSD

- Heart failure/failure to thrive unresponsive to medical therapy
- Pulmonary hypertension, which is still responsive with medical therapy
- Aortic valve prolapse
- Infective endocarditis.

VSDs may be closed by open heart surgery or by transcatheter techniques if suitable for the latter. Perimembranous VSDs are currently closed mainly by open heart surgery due to concerns regarding heart block following transcatheter closure.

## Patent ductus arteriosus

Failure of the ductus arteriosus (which connects the pulmonary artery to the descending aorta) to close in the newborn period may be due to severe prematurity or to a congenital abnormality. The duct typically closes in the first few days of life. The clinical findings depend on the size of the duct and the amount of blood flow across the vessel. Patients with a small PDA are usually asymptomatic, with the only abnormality being a continuous murmur audible at the upper left sternal border or left infraclavicular area.

Such murmurs may be present throughout the cardiac cycle ('machinery murmur'), but may disappear during diastole and be mistaken for a systolic murmur, especially if the duct is large and there is associated pulmonary hypertension.

With a large duct, the large left-to-right shunt causes left heart dilatation. Symptoms such as failure to thrive, dyspnoea and recurrent chest infections are similar to those of a large VSD. Bounding pulses may be palpable. The apex may be displaced and forceful, and an apical mid-diastolic murmur may be heard; as with a VSD, this is due to increased flow through the mitral valve.

The presence of cardiomegaly and pulmonary plethora on the chest X-ray indicates a large shunt, and left ventricular hypertrophy may be seen on the ECG. The diagnosis can be confirmed by echocardiography.

In symptomatic premature infants, medical treatment with indomethacin or other non-steroidal anti-inflammatory drugs, which inhibit prostaglandin synthesis, may be effective in promoting ductal constriction. Unfortunately, drug treatment is typically not effective in mature infants and in such patients intervention to close the ductus is indicated. This should be carried out at an early stage in symptomatic patients (including premature infants if indomethacin is ineffective) but may be delayed in asymptomatic patients. With small PDAs, intervention is indicated to eliminate the risk of infective endocarditis, rather than to treat cardiac failure or pulmonary hypertension. The risk of endocarditis occurring, however, is very small. The preferred method of duct occlusion is by a transcatheter approach. The type of device used depends on the size and shape of the PDA. Large ducts, especially those in small infants, may, however, require surgical ligation, typically from a left lateral thoractomy.

## Atrial septal defect

Defects of the atrial septum are usually in the central part of the septum and are termed 'secundum' ASD (Fig. 15.2.2). Unlike small VSDs and PDAs (which tend to be associated with loud murmurs), small ASDs may go completely undetected because the volume of blood flow across the defect is small and also the pressure gradient across the defect, and hence the velocity of blood flow, are both low. With larger defects, a significant shunt is present, and this is rarely associated with pulmonary hypertension. Even large ASDs seldom cause symptoms in early childhood. If patients with large defects reach adult life without surgery, they may develop atrial arrhythmias in middle adult life and often have reduced exercise capacity, even if arrhythmias are not a problem. Isolated ASDs hardly ever lead to Eisenmenger syndrome.

The characteristic findings in children with an ASD are related to the increased blood flow through the right side of the heart and right heart enlargement. A parasternal heave related to a dilated right ventricle

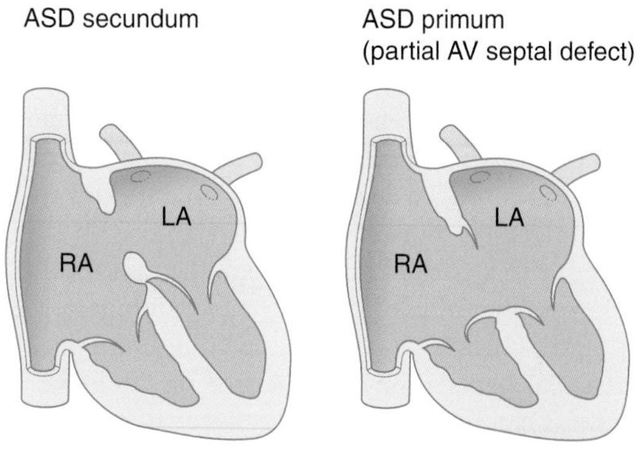

Fig. 15.2.2 Common types of atrial septal defect (ASD). Secundum defects are in the fossa ovale (mid-atrial septum). Primum defects are low in the atrial septum and abut on the atrioventricular (AV) valves, which are abnormal and often incompetent. LA, left atrium; RA, right atrium.

may be palpable. An ejection systolic murmur, due to increased pulmonary blood flow, is present in the pulmonary area but not usually louder than grade 2/6 and not harsh in character. A soft mid-diastolic murmur may be heard at the lower sternal border, secondary to increased flow across the tricuspid valve. The aortic and pulmonary components of the second heart sound are fixed and widely split (i.e. loss of the normal variation in separation during inspiration and expiration; see Fig. 15.1.2).

The chest X-ray characteristically shows cardiomegaly with pulmonary plethora. The ECG often shows features of partial right bundle branch block. The diagnosis may be confirmed by echocardiography.

Closure of the defect is recommended in patients where there is evidence of a significant shunt as indicated by right heart enlargement. In many cases a transcatheter procedure can be performed with placement of an 'occluder' device. This is a non-surgical option for patients with central defects of small to moderate size with good margins that are able to support the device without interfering with surrounding structures such as the mitral valve, right-sided pulmonary veins or the vena cavae. Surgical repair either by direct suture or patch closure may be required for defects that are unsuitable for a transcatheter approach.

## Atrioventricular septal defect

This category of defect accounts for approximately 3% of all congenital cardiac defects and includes a group of septal defects low in the atrial septum (primum ASD) that abut on the atrioventricular valves and may involve the upper part of the ventricular septum.

When the ventricular septum is intact (partial AVSD or primum ASD), only an atrial communication is present. In addition to the septal defect, the atrioventricular junction and valves are abnormal in all forms of AVSD. The left-sided atrioventricular valve in this condition typically has three leaflets rather than the usual two-leaflet mitral valve. This is sometimes described incorrectly as a cleft in the mitral valve and is associated with varying degrees of regurgitation. Children with a primum ASD or partial AVSD behave physiologically and symptomatically like those with an ASD. Those with significant regurgitation of the left-sided atrioventricular valve, however, develop symptoms much earlier in infancy and early childhood.

When a significant VSD coexists (complete AVSD; Fig. 15.2.3), the presentation resembles that of a VSD with difficulty feeding and failure to thrive. This defect is commonly associated with Down syndrome.

The chest X-ray usually shows quite marked cardiomegaly and pulmonary plethora, especially in the complete form of the defect. The ECG characteristically shows left-axis deviation accompanied by partial right

ASD primum
(partial AV septal defect)

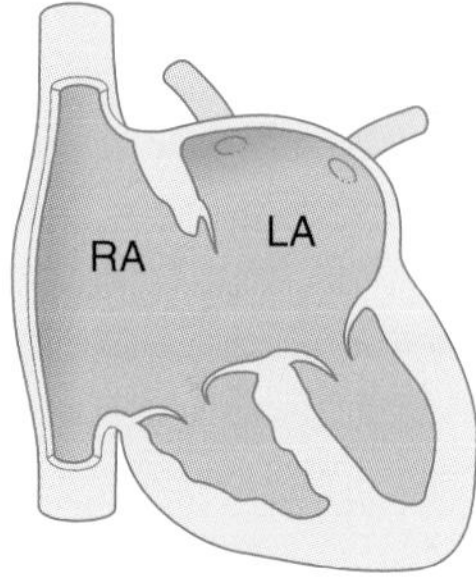


AV canal
(complete AV septal defect)

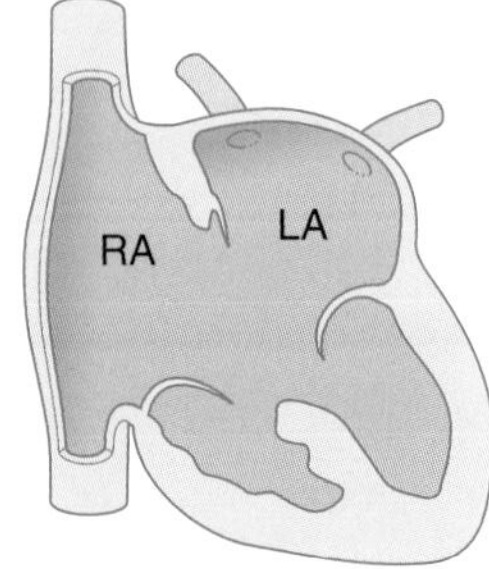


Fig. 15.2.3 Atrioventricular (AV) septal defect. The complete form is associated with a common AV valve and the septal defect allows communication between all four cardiac chambers. ASD, atrial septal defect.

bundle branch block. The presence of left-axis deviation distinguishes 'primum' ASDs from 'secundum' defects. Echocardiography confirms the diagnosis and will differentiate partial from complete atrioventricular defects.

Surgical repair is almost always required. When pulmonary hypertension is present, this is generally recommended in the early months of life (3–4 months) in order to obviate the risk of pulmonary vascular disease, particularly in children with Down syndrome. In patients with an isolated primum ASD, when pulmonary hypertension is absent, surgery may be delayed until the age of 2–4 years. Operation involves placement of a patch to close the ASD and repair of the left atrioventricular valve. Although there is an association with both types of AVSD, left ventricular outflow tract obstruction is more likely to occur with partial than complete AVSDs.

## Obstructive heart defects

The following defects have no shunt when they occur in isolation, and are obstructive lesions:

- pulmonary stenosis
- aortic stenosis
- coarctation of the aorta.

### Pulmonary stenosis

Pulmonary stenosis usually occurs at valve level and is the commonest of the pure obstructive malformations. The pulmonary valve often has thickened leaflets and partially fused commissures. In some cases the valve may be bicuspid. Other sites of pulmonary stenosis, occurring as isolated abnormalities, are less frequent. These include muscular subpulmonary obstruction involving the right ventricular outflow tract (infundibular stenosis) and supravalvular or branch pulmonary stenosis.

Most patients are asymptomatic in infancy and childhood because very severe ('critical') obstruction is uncommon and even moderate obstruction is generally well tolerated. An ejection systolic murmur is heard at the left upper sternal edge and radiates through to the back. An early ejection sound (ejection click) is usually audible at the left sternal border (Fig. 15.2.4) with valvar stenosis.

The size of the heart is usually normal on chest X-ray, but the main pulmonary artery is often prominent due to post-stenotic dilatation. The ECG is normal with mild obstruction but shows right ventricular hypertrophy in more severe cases.

Mild pulmonary stenosis is generally a benign condition and is often non-progressive. More severe pulmonary stenosis leads eventually to effort intolerance and cardiac failure. 'Critical' (very severe) pulmonary stenosis may present in early infancy with cyanosis due to right-to-left shunting through the foramen ovale or an associated ASD.

The diagnosis may be confirmed by echocardiography. Treatment involves a catheter technique known as balloon valvuloplasty. This involves manipulating a catheter-mounted balloon to lie across the pulmonary valve, typically using the femoral vein for access, and then inflating the balloon to open the valve more fully. This procedure is simple and effective in most cases, requires only a very short hospital stay and saves the patient an open heart operation. If this is not

Mild pulmonary stenosis

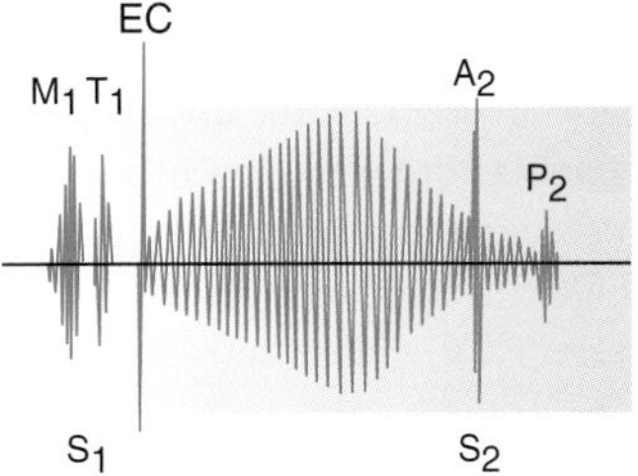


Mild aortic stenosis

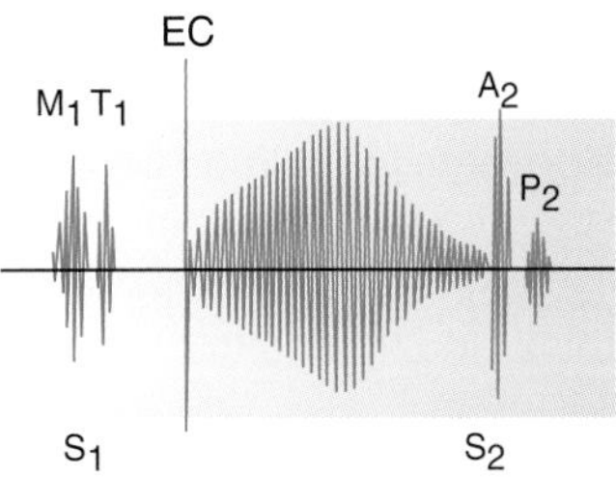


Fig. 15.2.4 Auscultatory findings in pulmonary and aortic stenosis. The ejection click (EC) is earlier in pulmonary stenosis and the second sound is widely split. In aortic stenosis the click is best heard at the apex.

effective, as is often the case when the valve leaflets are very thickened or the valve annulus is small, surgical valvotomy may need to be performed. Balloon valvuloplasty is not used for subpulmonary obstruction and is rarely effective in supravalve stenosis.

## Aortic stenosis

Valve stenosis with thickened, often bicuspid, leaflets and fused commissures is the most common form of aortic stenosis. Subaortic stenosis due to either a fibrous stricture or muscular obstruction in the left ventricular outflow tract, or supra-aortic stenosis (i.e. above the aortic valve) are less common causes of left heart obstruction.

Except in very severe cases, affected children are symptom-free in infancy and early childhood, and present with the chance finding of an ejection systolic murmur over the precordium and in the aortic area. Characteristically, with valvar stenosis the murmur is best heard to the right of the sternum and radiates to the carotids. A thrill is commonly present over the carotids and may also be felt in the aortic area. An ejection click is usually heard with valvar stenosis (see Fig. 15.2.4) and is often most easily audible at the apex or lower left sternal border. In more severe cases a forceful apical impulse due to left ventricular hypertrophy may be apparent. In subaortic stenosis the murmur is best heard at the left sternal edge and a click is not heard. Conversely, the murmur of supravalvar stenosis is often best heard over the carotid artery.

The natural history of aortic stenosis is generally one of gradual progression. With more severe obstruction, symptoms include dizziness and syncope on exertion, chest pain, effort intolerance and sudden death. In a small minority of cases, with 'critical' stenosis, severe congestive heart failure may appear in early infancy.

In mild and even moderate aortic stenosis, the chest X-ray and ECG may show little abnormality. In more severe cases the ECG shows left ventricular hypertrophy. Echocardiography allows assessment of the site and severity of the obstruction.

Treatment should be recommended if severe stenosis is present, even in the absence of symptoms. In cases of moderate stenosis the presence of symptoms as described above or ECG changes on exercise are an indication for treatment. Balloon aortic valvuloplasty is an alternative to surgery, but is more likely to induce aortic regurgitation. Surgical repair involves aortic valvotomy using cardiopulmonary bypass.

## Coarctation of the aorta

In this condition a stricture is present in the distal part of the aortic arch with the maximal site of obstruction usually close to the aortic end of the ductus arteriosus (Fig. 15.2.5). Coarctation of the aorta is often associated with other cardiac defects, including aortic stenosis, ventricular septal defect and mitral valve abnormalities. A bicuspid aortic valve is present in 40% of cases even in the absence of other malformations.

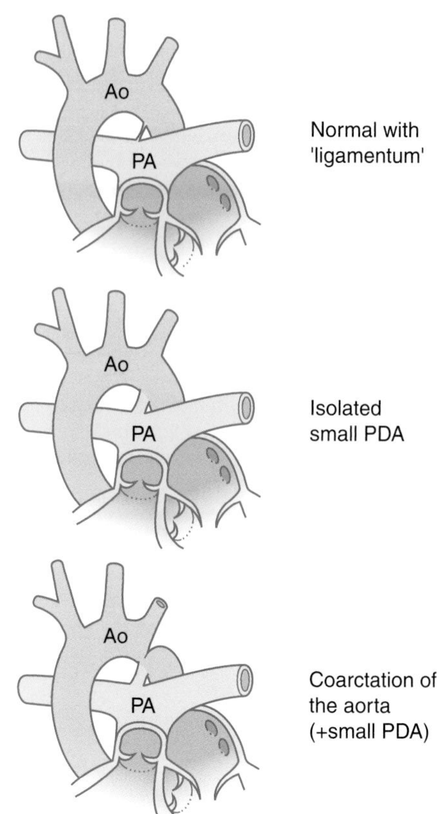


**Fig. 15.2.5** Aorta (Ao) and pulmonary artery (PA) showing persistent ductus and site of coarctation (often associated with patent ductus arteriosus, PDA).

Coarctation usually leads to the development of severe cardiac failure in the newborn period, with oliguria and acidosis, often in the first 2 weeks of life when the ductus closes. In around 30% of cases, presentation may be delayed until late in childhood or even adolescence or adult life. These older patients may present with asymptomatic hypertension, poor exercise capacity or lower limb claudication.

The characteristic physical findings are of diminished or absent femoral pulses. Simultaneous palpation of the right brachial pulse and a femoral pulse shows quite obvious delay in the pulses in older children and adults, but this is difficult to detect in young children. Upper limb hypertension may be present and there may be a significant difference in upper and lower limb blood pressure. Continuous murmurs may be audible over the back due to the development of collateral vessels.

The chest X-ray and ECG findings vary according to the age of presentation. In symptomatic infants cardiomegaly and pulmonary congestion are usually seen on the chest X-ray, and the ECG shows right ventricular hypertrophy. In older children the X-ray may show an abnormal appearance of the aortic knuckle and rib notching due to the presence of enlarged intercostal arteries, which act as collateral vessels to bypass the obstructed segment of aorta. This is seldom seen before the age of 8 years. The ECG may show left ventricular hypertrophy.

In infancy the onset of congestive heart failure occurs after closure of the ductus arteriosus. In the presence of ductal patency, the lower body is supplied by deoxygenated blood due to right-to-left flow through the duct from the pulmonary artery and into the descending aorta. Reopening the duct by the intravenous infusion of prostaglandin $E_1$ may be helpful in resuscitation. Basic principles of resuscitation should be followed in addition to this therapy. Surgery to relieve the obstruction is indicated when the neonate is in the best possible condition.

In other patients intervention may be deferred until later in childhood. In selected cases, with a localized coarctation shelf, balloon angioplasty (or placement of a stent) may be employed as an alternative to surgical repair. Patients who have required surgical relief of coarctation (especially those operated on in early infancy) and those who have had balloon angioplasty as a primary procedure may develop restenosis at the coarctation site. These areas of recurrent stenosis may be amenable to further balloon angioplasty or stent implantation.

Patients with coarctation who undergo repair in later childhood and as adults (i.e. those who escape detection during childhood) are at increased high risk of persisting systemic hypertension, left ventricular failure, aortic dissection and cerebrovascular accidents. Children successfully repaired in early childhood are less prone to these complications in later life.

### Hypoplastic left heart syndrome

A small subgroup of infants with both severe aortic stenosis and coarctation may present with associated hypoplasia of the left ventricle. In some cases the aortic valve and/or mitral valve are atretic (Fig. 15.2.6).

Presentation is similar to that for other forms of severe left heart obstruction, and these infants present with severe cardiac failure or shock in the first few days of life. All peripheral pulses are diminished or absent and manifestations of cardiac failure are severe.

The condition is invariably fatal without surgery. Medical treatment, including infusion of prostaglandin and other measures, may lead to improvement. Palliative surgery (the initial Norwood procedure and subsequent Fontan circulation) is possible and can produce long-term survival. Heart transplantation for this condition, in the newborn period, is offered to some families in North America.

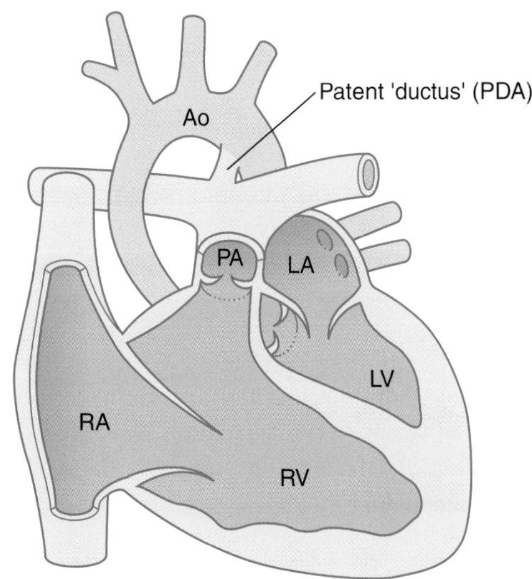


Fig. 15.2.6 Hypoplastic left heart syndrome showing hypoplasia of left ventricle, mitral valve, aortic valve and ascending aorta. The ductus provides the only effective route through which the systemic circulation can be maintained from the right ventricle with right-to-left shunting across the duct. Ao, aorta; LA, left atrium; LV, left ventricle; PA, pulmonary artery; PDA, patent ductus arteriosus; RA, right atrium; RV, right ventricle.

## Cyanotic defects

The presence of cyanosis in a child with congenital heart disease indicates that deoxygenated blood from the systemic venous circulation is being directed back into the systemic arterial circulation without going through the lungs (i.e. right-to-left shunt). Cyanotic defects account for approximately 25% of all congenital heart malformations. Such defects are almost always associated with the presence of a septal defect, coupled with additional abnormalities such that right-to-left shunting within the heart occurs.

Three major subgroups exist. In the first group (exemplified by tetralogy of Fallot) pulmonary blood flow is reduced as a result of a combination of obstruction to the right ventricular outflow tract and a septal defect below the obstruction through which blood may flow from the right ventricle to left. In tetralogy of Fallot the shunt is almost completely right to left, whereas in some other defects associated with low pulmonary flow the physiology is more complex, with right-to-left shunting at one level and left-to-right shunting at another (e.g. tricuspid atresia or pulmonary atresia).

In the second group of cyanotic defects bidirectional shunting is associated with very large communications between the left and right sides of the heart with free mixing of blood (e.g. 'single ventricle') and truncus arteriosus. In such defects pulmonary blood flow is usually high and pulmonary hypertension is a feature. Cyanosis is generally mild and may pass unnoticed.

A third group of cyanotic defects, best exemplified by transposition of the great arteries, may be considered as a 'plumbing problem'. In transposition, the aorta and pulmonary artery are connected to the wrong side of the heart and as a result systemic venous blood is directed straight through into the systemic circulation again (see below).

## Tetralogy of Fallot

Of the four components that comprise Fallot's tetralogy (VSD, pulmonary stenosis, right ventricular hypertrophy, overriding aorta), the important ones are pulmonary stenosis and the VSD (Fig. 15.2.7). The presence of severe pulmonary stenosis, which is typically infundibular muscular obstruction coupled frequently with valvar hypoplasia and commissural fusion, leads to right-to-left shunting into the aorta. The degree of outflow tract obstruction determines the degree of right-to-left shunt and, hence, the amount of pulmonary blood flow and the degree of cyanosis. Tetralogy may be associated with microdeletion of the long arm of chromosome 22.

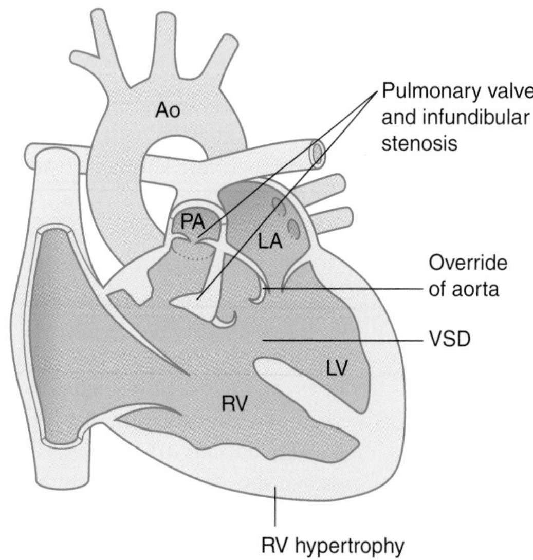


Fig. 15.2.7 Fallot's tetralogy, showing infundibular and valvar pulmonary stenosis and hypoplasia of the branch pulmonary arteries, all of which are frequent. Ao, aorta; LA, left atrium; LV, left ventricle; PA, pulmonary artery; RV, right ventricle; VSD, ventricular septal defect.

### Clinical features

Cyanosis is not usually obvious in the newborn period but appears later in infancy in most affected children. Oxygen saturations (with pulse oximetry) may be normal or mildly depressed in the early weeks of life. A harsh ejection systolic murmur is audible at the left sternal edge and/or in the pulmonary area (infundibular stenosis) and radiates through to the back. The second heart sound is often quite loud but may be single because the pulmonary closure sound is quieter (Fig. 15.2.8).

Cyanosis appears gradually during the first 6–12 months of life or rarely later, and is characteristically more obvious on crying or exertion. The development of intermittent episodes of severe cyanosis ('hypoxic spells'), which may appear spontaneously but are quite commonly precipitated by stress or exercise, is concerning. Such spells are characterized by marked pallor or cyanosis with some infants going floppy or losing consciousness. Hypoxic spells are associated with increased right-to-left shunting and a sharp reduction in pulmonary flow. In the past these have been attributed to infundibular 'spasm', but the physiology is more complex and spasm may not in fact occur. Initial treatment of spells, which are potentially dangerous, involves soothing and pacifying the distressed infant. In severe cases intramuscular morphine may be helpful. Older children often adopt a squatting posture at intervals or during these episodes. This manoeuvre increases systemic vascular resistance, reducing right-to-left shunting and leading to a transient rise in pulmonary blood flow with improved oxygenation. Placing an infant into the knee–chest position will achieve the same effect. Oxygen, intravenous fluid, correction of acidosis, beta-blockade and mechanical ventilation may be required in severe spells.

### Course and prognosis

Cyanosis generally progresses gradually, with diminishing exercise tolerance, finger clubbing and in severe cases growth retardation. Following surgery, children

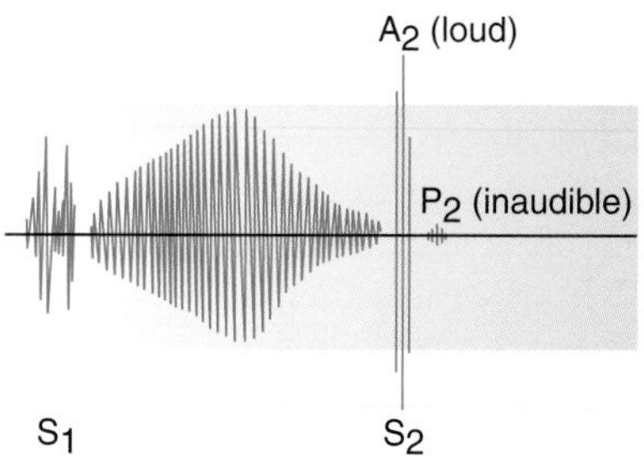


Fig. 15.2.8 Auscultatory signs in Fallot's tetralogy. The systolic murmur is 'ejection', owing to the pulmonary stenosis. The aortic closure sound is accentuated and pulmonary closure is so soft as to be inaudible. The second sound appears to be 'single'.

typically show catch-up growth. Development of cardiac failure is unusual but the severe cyanosis leads to compensatory polycythaemia, and cerebral thromboembolic complications (e.g. stroke) may occur. Infective endocarditis and cerebral abscess also are important complications.

### Investigations

The chest X-ray shows the heart size to be normal with an uptilted apex and concave pulmonary segment associated with reduced lung vascularity (oligaemia). In severe cases the cardiac contour may resemble the shape of a wooden clog – *coeur en sabot* – often referred to as 'boot-shaped'. The ECG usually shows right ventricular hypertrophy. Echocardiography is diagnostic. Cardiac catheterization is rarely performed but may be indicated if coronary anatomy is unclear on ultrasound imaging.

### Differential diagnosis

In infancy, before the onset of cyanosis, the murmur is often mistaken for that of a small VSD. Other cyanotic defects, such as tricuspid atresia, may be differentiated by ancillary investigations, such as ECG and echocardiography.

### Treatment

Total correction involving repair of the VSD and relief of the infundibular and pulmonary valve stenosis can be carried out even in early infancy if the anatomy is suitable. In those children who have small branch pulmonary arteries, it may be useful to delay repair by carrying out a palliative systemic–pulmonary artery shunt operation first to increase pulmonary blood flow. Most surgeons use a prosthetic tube graft to create an anastomosis between a subclavian artery and the ipsilateral pulmonary artery (modified Blalock–Taussig shunt).

Infants who are having significant hypoxic spells can be treated medically in the short term with beta-adrenergic blocking drugs, for example propranolol, to prevent spells while the child is awaiting surgery.

### Follow-up

The long-term problems following repair of tetralogy of Fallot are related to chronic pulmonary regurgitation, recurrence of right ventricular outflow tract obstruction, and the development of arrhythmias. Most patients with repaired tetralogy will require further procedures to replace the pulmonary valve. The approach to this depends on the age and size of the patient and the morphology of the outflow tract. The majority of patients currently undergo further open heart surgery to replace the valve. Selected patients may be suitable for transcatheter pulmonary valve replacement.

## Transposition of the great arteries

In this condition the aorta and pulmonary arteries arise from the incorrect ventricles (Fig. 15.2.9). There are therefore two parallel circulations with: (1) systemic venous blood flowing through the right side of the heart back into the aorta, and (2) pulmonary venous blood through the left side of the heart back into the pulmonary circulation. Survival is dependent on mixing of blood between these two parallel circuits via the foramen ovale, ductus arteriosus or a septal defect. Affected infants generally survive for several days or even weeks because of shunting through the foramen ovale and/or ductus arteriosus, but few live longer than a month without help, unless they have a coexisting septal defect, such as a VSD. Chromosomal defects are rarely present in patients with transposition of the great arteries.

### Clinical features

Cyanosis is present from the early hours of life and usually progresses gradually over the next few days. Metabolic acidosis may develop, because of tissue hypoxia, if the situation persists untreated. Apart from cyanosis the infant may appear completely normal. Palpation reveals a forceful right ventricular impulse at the left sternal edge, but on auscultation there is frequently no murmur audible.

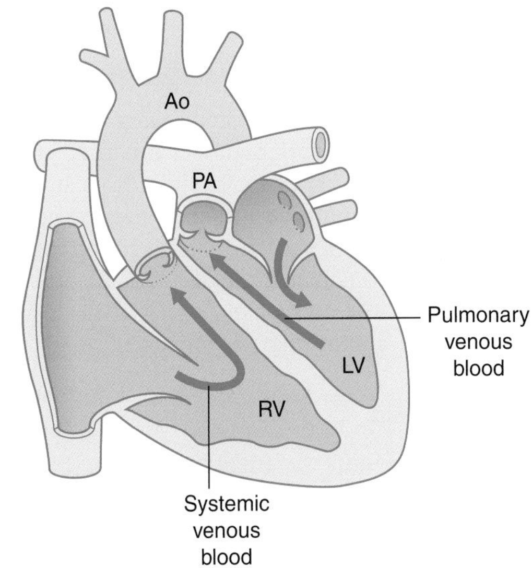


Fig. 15.2.9 Transposition of the great arteries. Systemic venous blood is ejected from the right ventricle (RV) to the aorta (Ao), while pulmonary venous blood passes from the left ventricle (LV) to the pulmonary artery (PA).

### Investigations

The chest X-ray shows a normal-sized or mildly enlarged heart with a contour that sometimes resembles 'an egg on its side'. Pulmonary vascular markings are usually increased. The ECG shows normal ventricular complexes, but may manifest T-wave abnormalities. The diagnosis may be established rapidly by echocardiography.

### Treatment

*Balloon atrial septostomy*
Cardiac catheterization may be required as an emergency procedure to improve systemic arterial oxygen saturation. Venous access is typically through the umbilical vein or femoral vein. An inflatable balloon-tipped catheter is passed into the left atrium via the foramen ovale under ultrasound guidance. The balloon is then inflated and forcefully withdrawn into the right atrium, in order to tear the atrial septum and create an ASD. This results in an increase in highly saturated pulmonary venous blood flowing into the right atrium and then into the systemic circulation.

*Surgery*
After successful balloon septostomy most infants will manage comfortably for many days or weeks. Surgical correction involves transecting the great arteries above the level of the sinuses and re-anastomosing them to the appropriate ventricle. It is also necessary to transfer the coronary arteries across from the aortic root (initially above the right ventricle) to the new aortic origin from the left ventricle. The arterial switch procedure is preferably performed in the first few weeks of life. After this time, the normal decline in pulmonary vascular resistance leads to atrophy of the left ventricle such that it becomes less accustomed to working at higher workload, which is problematic when restored to the systemic circulation postoperatively. If the operation is delayed and there is concern regarding the ability of the left ventricle to support the systemic circulation then strategies such as preparatory banding of the pulmonary artery or postoperative mechanical support may be employed.

## Tricuspid atresia

In this malformation the tricuspid valve is blocked completely and there is no communication between the right atrium and ventricle. Systemic venous blood passes via the foramen ovale or an ASD into the left side of the heart, and at ventricular or arterial level a left-to-right shunt exists (via a VSD or PDA). This allows blood to perfuse the pulmonary circulation, usually in reduced amounts.

### Clinical features

Cyanosis develops early. A systolic murmur is audible along the left sternal border.

### Diagnosis

The diagnosis may be suspected on the characteristic ECG pattern of left axis deviation, right atrial hypertrophy, left ventricular hypertrophy and right ventricular hypoplasia. Echocardiography confirms the diagnosis.

### Treatment

A palliative arterial shunt may be needed in infancy (see above under Tetralogy of Fallot). Later in childhood, cardiac surgery is usually feasible and involves the creation of a bidirectional cavopulmonary connection (bidirectional Glenn) by anastomosing the superior vena cava to the right pulmonary artery. Subsequently the inferior vena cava is also connected to the pulmonary arteries, to allow the majority of systemic venous blood to pass directly into the pulmonary circulation (Fontan operation). The Fontan procedure is used in several forms of congenital heart disease where there is either only one functional ventricle (e.g. hypoplastic left heart syndrome or pulmonary atresia with intact ventricular septum) or the cardiac anatomy is too complex to allow biventricular repair.

## Pulmonary atresia

In this condition the origin of the pulmonary artery from the right ventricle is completely obstructed or absent. Blood in the right side of the heart passes via an ASD, foramen ovale or VSD into the left ventricle and aorta. Pulmonary blood flow depends on collateral flow from the aorta via a PDA or other collateral channels.

### Clinical features

Cyanosis develops early and many infants have an easily audible continuous murmur due to the associated PDA or other collaterals feeding the pulmonary circulation from the aorta.

### Diagnosis

The diagnosis is usually confirmed by echocardiography, although it may be suspected strongly on clinical grounds coupled with ECG and X-ray findings. Other forms of cardiac imaging may be needed to clarify the pulmonary blood flow especially if multiple aortopulmonary collaterals (MAPCAs) are detected on echocardiography.

### Treatment

Initial medical therapy may involve prostaglandin infusion to maintain patency of the ductus. Early surgical treatment usually involves a systemic-to-pulmonary shunt procedure. At a later stage, which depends on the associated defects, surgical correction may be performed by opening up a way through from the right ventricle into the pulmonary arteries, often by insertion of a valved conduit and closure of the VSD.

## Truncus arteriosus

This defect is associated with the presence of a single artery, which branches shortly after arising from the heart to give rise to the pulmonary artery and aorta. The truncal valve usually sits astride a large VSD and receives blood from both right and left ventricles.

### Clinical features

Cyanosis is usually mild or absent and congestive heart failure often appears in the newborn period. Most infants will have a systolic murmur and in some cases a diastolic murmur may be heard that is due to regurgitation of the abnormal truncal valve.

### Diagnosis

The diagnosis can be made by echocardiography. Chest X-ray and ECG findings are usually non-specific.

### Treatment

The only effective treatment is surgical correction, which needs to be carried out in early infancy. The pulmonary artery is separated from the truncus and, after closure of the VSD leaving the aorta arising from the left ventricle, a valved conduit is placed to connect the right ventricle to the pulmonary arteries.

**Clinical example**

Aaron was 6 months old and had gained weight poorly since birth. Birth weight was 2.8 kg and his present weight was 4.1 kg. Several doctors had examined him but had failed to find a cause for his poor weight gain.

Examination showed a thin infant who was tachypnoeic with a respiratory rate of 60 per minute. All pulses were easily palpable and of large volume (bounding). The cardiac impulse was forceful, with the apex displaced towards the anterior axillary line. Auscultation revealed a grade 2/6 ejection systolic murmur of non-specific character audible over the precordium and in the pulmonary area. A soft diastolic murmur was also heard at the apex.

A chest X-ray showed a large heart and plethoric lungs. An ECG showed left ventricular hypertrophy.

The fact that the murmur had not been heard before suggested that it might have been soft or dismissed as being innocent. The signs suggested a significant ventricular septal defect or patent ductus arteriosus with pulmonary hypertension. It was not possible to make a definite diagnosis without echocardiography, which needed to be organized as soon as possible. The X-ray and ECG abnormalities indicated a major haemodynamic disturbance and the defect was likely to be large. Aaron's failure to thrive was likely to be the consequence of the cardiac abnormality.

The diagnosis, confirmed by echocardiography, was a large patent ductus arteriosus. The absence of a continuous murmur was due to the presence of severe pulmonary hypertension.

# Acquired heart disease in children

There are several forms of acquired heart disease in children.

## Kawasaki disease

This condition is described elsewhere (see Chapter 13.3.). It may lead to the development of coronary artery aneurysms, with risk of myocardial ischaemia or infarction.

## Myocarditis

This condition follows a viral infection, and the pathogenesis is immunologically mediated. A wide variety of common viruses have been implicated in this disease. The auscultatory signs are non-specific, with soft heart sounds, a gallop rhythm but no murmur in most cases. Congestive heart failure may develop rapidly or insidiously, and the condition is accompanied by ECG, X-ray and echocardiographic evidence of myocardial damage, ventricular dilatation and depressed myocardial function. In the past, the condition was frequently fatal, although some patients recovered. The use of immunoglobulin or immunosuppressive drug therapy (e.g. steroids, azathioprine, ciclosporin) may be of help, although the mainstay of therapy is supportive treatment.

## Cardiomyopathy

This term encompasses a group of conditions with heart muscle disease and myocardial dysfunction, often associated with progressive effort intolerance, arrhythmias and/or heart failure. The condition may result from an earlier episode of myocarditis, but in most cases the aetiology is unknown and no specific treatment is available. Some forms of cardiomyopathy may be inherited. In those patients where the condition progresses to end-stage heart failure, cardiac transplantation offers the only prospect of survival currently.

## Rheumatic heart disease

Rheumatic heart disease is now very uncommon in the developed world. The condition follows acute rheumatic fever, although a clear history of rheumatic fever may be absent in some cases. The host's abnormal immune response to certain streptococcal antigens results in an autoimmune disorder affecting the heart, synovial membranes and other tissues.

The main cardiac sequelae of rheumatic fever are the development of damage to heart valves, resulting in the development of mitral stenosis and/or incompetence and aortic stenosis/incompetence. Other valves are occasionally affected. In the acute phase, inflammation of the heart muscle (myocarditis) and pericardium (pericarditis) can also occur. Myocarditis may cause reduced ventricular function and also arrhythmias, typically causing heart block.

### Clinical manifestations

Rheumatic fever follows a streptococcal infection, usually tonsillitis.

Major criteria for diagnosis include:

- migratory polyarthritis affecting mainly large joints
- evidence of carditis with tachycardia, cardiac enlargement, the development of new murmurs and, in severe cases, cardiac failure
- choreiform limb movements – Sydenham chorea
- a transient demarcated skin rash on the trunk – erythema marginatum
- the development of nodules over bony prominences.

Minor criteria are:

- fever
- arthralgia
- previous history of rheumatic fever
- raised erythrocyte sedimentation rate (ESR) or C-reactive protein level
- prolonged PR interval on ECG.

All patients with suspected rheumatic fever should have throat cultures and be tested for evidence of streptococcal antibodies (antistreptolysin O (ASO) titre, anti-DNAase titre).

### Diagnosis

The diagnosis cannot usually be regarded as established unless evidence of a recent streptococcal infection is demonstrable (i.e. a positive throat culture or positive antibody titres). If such evidence is found, however, the presence of two minor criteria and one major criterion as listed above, or the presence of two or more major criteria, may be regarded as indicative of the presence of rheumatic fever.

### Treatment

Treatment involves bed rest and administration of aspirin in full anti-inflammatory doses. Steroids may also be administered in the presence of more severe carditis and will usually reduce the duration of the acute episode, although they probably do not affect the development of chronic valve disease. Supportive treatment for heart failure and rhythm disturbance may also be needed.

## Infective endocarditis

Turbulent blood flow predisposes the adherence of bacteria and establishment of infection. In addition to the generalized effects of infection, collections of infection have the potential to damage local structures, and vegetations may also embolize. The development of a transient bacteraemia is usually the precursor of such infection, although the source of the bacteraemia is often not clear.

Systemic symptoms include fever, rigors, anorexia and weight loss, which can typically occur over several weeks. Physical signs may include evidence of anaemia, sometimes with petechial haemorrhages, splinter haemorrhages in the nail beds, splenomegaly and finger clubbing. In many cases the manifestations are relatively subtle and a high index of suspicion is required if the diagnosis is to be reached. Any child with known structural heart disease, whether operated on or not, is at risk (though very unlikely with a PDA or a secundum ASD that has been closed surgically or with a device more than 6 months previously). Should such a patient become chronically unwell or have prolonged unexplained fever, infective endocarditis should be considered. Investigations should include a full blood count and ESR, multiple blood cultures and careful echocardiography. In the majority of children transthoracic echocardiography is sufficient to exclude or establish a diagnosis, which is in contrast to adult recommendations. Transoesophageal echocardiography may be necessary in some children where assessment is suboptimal on transthoracic imaging.

Occasionally, infective endocarditis may develop in a patient with no previously known cardiac defect. The responsible organism is most commonly *Streptococcus viridans* or *Staphylococcus* (both *aureus* and *albus*). Other organisms include enterococci, *Escherichia coli* and fungi, especially *Candida albicans*.

Treatment involves intravenous antibiotic therapy initially, usually for a total duration of antibiotic therapy of 6 weeks. Drug choice is guided by identification of the organism and sensitivity of the organism to antibiotics. Surgical removal of vegetations may be necessary if response to therapy is poor, significant damage to valve function occurs, or systemic complications occur.

Prophylaxis against endocarditis should be advised in all patients who are considered to be at risk, and should be administered on occasions when a bacteraemia is likely to result from surgical or dental procedures. Such procedures include dental extractions and other dental procedures involving significant gingival trauma, other oropharyngeal instrumentation and surgery on the bowel and genitourinary tract. Effective cover can usually be achieved with amoxicillin (in combination with an aminoglycoside to cover procedures on the genitourinary or gastrointestinal tract). A single dose of antibiotic, administered an hour prior to the procedure (oral dose) or at induction of anaesthesia (intravenous dose), is usually adequate.

## Cardiac arrhythmias

Phasic variation in heart rate (*sinus arrhythmia*) is normal in children. It is related mainly to respiration, although not exclusively.

### Supraventricular tachycardia

This condition is characterized by the sudden onset of very rapid tachycardia, usually with a rate of 200–300 beats per minute. Affected infants may become pale and appear mildly distressed with tachypnoea and poor feeding. Heart failure may develop and the appearance of supraventricular tachycardia in an infant requires urgent treatment. Older children are often aware of their rapid heart rate and observers may notice rapid pulsations in the neck.

The ECG between episodes will show evidence of pre-excitation in Wolff–Parkinson–White syndrome. In other forms of supraventricular tachycardia, the resting ECG may be normal. The ECG during the episodes will usually show a tachycardia with a narrow QRS complex. It is particularly useful for a 12-lead ECG to be recorded during attempts to terminate the tachycardia.

The acute episode may sometimes be terminated by vagal manoeuvres, such as the application of ice packs to the face or the Valsalva manoeuvre. Intravenous adenosine will usually terminate the episode, or alternatively a DC cardioversion may be needed if the patient is haemodynamically compromised.

Some patients have recurring and troublesome attacks over many years. If the episodes are infrequent, brief or can be easily terminated by Valsalva manoeuvres, some families may opt for conservative management. For the longer, frequent and haemodynamically significant episodes of tachycardia, chronic antiarrhythmic drug treatment or invasive transcatheter electrophysiological treatment may be needed.

### Ventricular tachyarrhythmias

Sustained ventricular tachyarrhythmias are uncommon during childhood; however, the presence of ventricular premature beats may be detected as irregularities in the pulse on routine examination or on a chance ECG. The presence of such premature beats in an otherwise normal child with no other evidence of structural defects or heart muscle disease may be benign, and even when premature beats occur frequently they very rarely lead to any symptoms or require treatment. It is important, however, to exclude family history of arrhythmia or cardiomyopathy. In older children, the suppression of ventricular ectopy on exercise stress testing is a reassuring sign.

### Long QT syndrome

There are families or individual children who have prolonged repolarization with increase in the corrected QT interval on the ECG. These patients are at risk of ventricular tachyarrhythmias (ventricular tachycardia or ventricular fibrillation), typically in association with sudden surges in adrenergic drive (e.g. exercise, morning alarm clock). Any patient developing dizziness or syncope on exertion should, therefore, be assessed with a view to excluding this condition, which often is familial and may lead to sudden death.

Treatment may involve antiarrhythmic medication and implantation of an automatic defibrillator.

### Heart block

Congenital complete heart block is an uncommon problem in the newborn period. It may be detected on antenatal assessment with fetal bradycardia. As ECG is difficult to perform, echocardiography can be used to distinguish complete heart block from sinus bradycardia. Among affected infants, 50% have no structural cardiac abnormality but a range of congenital anomalies may be associated with heart block. Those with otherwise normal hearts may have developed heart block due to the presence of maternal autoimmune antibodies causing damage to the conduction system, for example in association with maternal systemic lupus erythematosus or Sjögren syndrome. Some fetuses may develop hydrops and its associated complications *in utero*.

The heart rate is usually in the range of 40–70 beats per minute and the response of the newborn to bradycardia is variable. Children with symptomatic bradycardia may require administration of a positive chronotropic agent (e.g. isoprenaline) or positive inotropes whilst waiting for implantation of a temporary or permanent pacemaker.

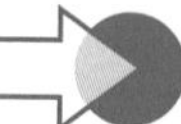

**Practical points**

- Ventricular septal defect (VSD) is the commonest congenital heart defect.
- Minor heart defects (small VSD/patent ductus arteriosus (PDA); mild pulmonary or aortic stenosis) may be well tolerated with no symptoms.
- Necessity for treatment depends on careful assessment of the severity of disturbance to cardiac function and risk of complications (including endocarditis). Some defects (e.g. small VSD; mild pulmonary stenosis) pose little threat and do not need intervention.
- Treatment for congenital heart defects was, in the past, usually surgical. In the current era, many of the simpler heart defects can be managed with catheter interventions – but choice of surgery versus catheter procedures still requires careful assessment of the risks and benefits of the different options.

PART 16

# HAEMATOLOGICAL DISORDERS AND MALIGNANCIES

# 16.1 Anaemia

Paul Monagle

## Definition

Anaemia is a common medical condition throughout all ages of childhood. However, the common causes vary with age. Anaemia refers to a reduction in haemoglobin (and hence red cell mass) below that which is considered normal for the patient in question. Normative haemoglobin data differs with age and, in teenage years, sex. Clinicians need to ensure that, when considering a diagnosis of anaemia, correct age-specific and, where applicable, sex-specific reference ranges are used. These reference ranges may vary according to the laboratory analyser in use. Thus each laboratory should report their own specific age-related reference ranges. An example of the age-related variation is shown by the reference ranges in Table 16.1.1. The majority of reference ranges in clinical use reflect 95% confidence intervals, so that 2.5% of individuals who are in fact 'normal' would be expected to consistently have haemoglobin levels just below the lower limit of the reported reference range.

## Physiology

The prime function of haemoglobin is tissue oxygen delivery. Hence anaemia threatens this critical bodily function. Acutely, severe anaemia can lead to hypoxic tissue injury, and chronic anaemia can lead to growth failure and organ dysfunction as a result of chronic hypoxia or failure of compensatory mechanisms. The physiology of tissue oxygen delivery is critical to understand, as it enables the clinician to understand the concepts of relative anaemia and to determine appropriate treatment of the anaemic patient.

$$\begin{aligned}&\text{Tissue oxygen delivery (mL/min)}\\&= \text{cardiac output}\,(\text{L/min}) \times \text{haemoglobin (g/L)}\\&\times \text{haemoglobin saturation (\%)} \times 1.34\,(\text{mL/g})\end{aligned}$$

where 1.34 is a constant and represents the amount of oxygen carried by 1g normal haemoglobin.

The key issues in this basic physiological equation are that:

- the parameters are multiplied, such that small decreases in cardiac output *and* haemoglobin *and* haemoglobin saturation lead to an overall large decrease in tissue oxygen delivery. Thus patients with cardiac disease may tolerate less reduction in haemoglobin before developing tissue hypoxia, and hence often have considerable urgency in treating their anaemia. No single haemoglobin (Hb) level can be used as an indication for transfusion therapy as these other factors need to be considered.
- in the presence of anaemia, cardiac output must be increased to maintain tissue oxygen delivery (Hb saturation cannot be increased above 100%). Failure of this compensatory mechanism or limitation of cardiac output by another disease will result in tissue hypoxia. Cardiac output is determined by cardiac stroke volume and heart rate. Therefore, heart rate is an important measure of the stress the anaemia is placing on the patient's cardiac reserve. All anaemic patients should have their vital signs, especially heart rate and respiratory rate, assessed as part of their initial medical evaluation, and these parameters should be used to monitor progress and response to therapy.
- Hb saturation is normally close to 100% in children without cyanotic congenital heart disease or significant lung pathology. Thus, in otherwise well children with severe anaemia, or children in whom the Hb saturation is measured as 99–100%, inspired oxygen therapy makes little if any contribution to improving tissue oxygenation. Recovery of red cell mass (and hence Hb) is the most effective therapy.
- in children with cyanotic congenital heart disease or pulmonary pathology, the natural compensation for reduced Hb saturation is to increase Hb concentration. Hence, if a child with cyanotic congential heart disease who usually has a relatively increased Hb was to develop a 'relative anaemia', they might develop symptoms of anaemia at Hb levels that would be considered normal in most children. Treatment of 'relative anaemia', if required, is based on the same principles as treatment of 'true anaemia'.

## Clinical presentations

Children with anaemia most often present with pallor (reflecting the reduced Hb) or signs of reduced exercise tolerance (reflecting inability to increase tissue oxygen delivery to meet the demands of exercise). Reduced exercise tolerance manifests differently according to age.

In infants, poor feeding is often described. In older children, shortness of breath on exertion or generalized lethargy are more common. Alternatively, incidental finding of anaemia when full blood examination has been performed for another indication is also very common.

Once the presence of anaemia has been confirmed, thorough history-taking and examination of the patient is required. Patient age and the duration of symptoms is important as a first step in determining the likely aetiology of the anaemia.

In addition, during the history and examination, other key considerations are:

- Is there evidence of cardiac decompensation or other adverse events as a result of the anaemia? This clearly makes appropriate therapy a matter of urgency.
- Are there clues to the aetiology of the anaemia?
- Is there evidence of multilineage cytopenias (neutropenia and thrombocytopenia)?
- Is there evidence of an associated, perhaps causative, disease?

Information that assists in answering these questions is shown in Table 16.1.2.

**Table 16.1.1 Normal haemoglobin values for age**

| Age | Haemoglobin (g/L) |
|---|---|
| Birth | 135–200 |
| 1 month | 100–180 |
| 2 months | 90–140 |
| 6 months | 95–135 |
| 1 year | 105–135 |
| 2–6 years | 110–145 |
| 6–12 years | 115–155 |
| >12 years (female) | 120–160 |
| >12 years (male) | 130–180 |

**Table 16.1.2 Relevant information required on history and examination for patients with anaemia**

| Critical question | Information obtained on history and examination |
|---|---|
| Cardiac decompensation | Exercise tolerance<br>Heart rate and respiratory rate<br>Signs of congestive heart failure<br>Altered conscious state, irritability, restlessness |
| Aetiology | Duration of symptoms (bone marrow failure and haematinic deficiency usually have a longer duration of symptoms)<br>Family history (hereditary spherocytosis, G6PD deficiency, haemoglobinopathies and others are inherited causes of anaemia. Maternal history (e.g. veganism may be associated with $B_{12}$ deficiency in infants)<br>Birth and neonatal history (blood loss at birth, birth asphyxia and maternal blood group compatibility are all important in assessing neonatal anaemia. Jaundice at birth may give a clue to an episodic haemolytic disorder in older children)<br>Presence or absence of jaundice (haemolysis)<br>Drug exposure: as a cause of haemolysis, or bone marrow suppression<br>Blood loss: trauma, recent surgery, iatrogenic in neonates, epistaxis, menstrual loss<br>Dietary history: iron deficiency can be predicted in infants less than 12 months of age fed cow's milk, or in toddlers who have failed to transfer to solid foods adequately |
| Multilineage cytopenias | Bruising or bleeding, especially petechiae (thrombocytopenia)<br>Infection, mouth ulceration (neutropenia) |
| Associated disease | Gastrointestinal symptoms (e.g. coeliac disease, inflammatory bowel disease)<br>Joint or bone pain (e.g. leukaemia, sickle cell disease, arthritis)<br>Renal disease<br>Malignancy<br>Infection: as a primary cause (e.g. malaria), a precipitant of acute deterioration in a more chronic anaemia, or a trigger to acute haemolysis<br>Neurological disorders, developmental delay/regression, failure to thrive may reflect functional $B_{12}$ deficiency in infants. Pica may be associated with iron deficiency<br>Eating disorders in older children<br>Bleeding disorders |

## Initial investigations

Progressive selective investigation, guided by the history, the clinical findings and the result of the blood count, is recommended. The first investigation will be a blood count, which automatically includes red cell indices (full blood examination (FBE) or complete blood count (CBC)), reticulocyte count and examination of the blood film. These initial investigations will usually allow classification of the anaemia. The presence or absence of polychromasia on the blood film, and the reticulocyte count, enable the anaemia to be classified as regenerative or aregenerative. This is a most important initial decision to be made. The red cell indices, in particular the mean corpuscular volume (MCV), and the blood film, enable the anaemia to be classified by red cell size into microcytic, normocytic and macrocytic. Finally, the blood film enables any specific red cell morphology to be determined, and confirms the platelet and leukocyte parameters. At this stage, a probable aetiology is likely and thus the direction of further investigations can be determined.

In the interpretation of these initial tests, there are a number of important considerations. First, sample integrity is vital, and preanalytical variables such as a clotted or inadequately mixed specimen can cause significant erroneous results. If the results do not match the clinical findings, repeat testing should always be considered. Second, MCV also varies with age. MCV is highest in the neonate (98–118 fL), falls to its lowest value between 6 and 24 months of age (79–86 fL, then increases progressively throughout childhood (75–92 fL). A low MCV indicates microcytosis and a high MCV indicates macrocytosis. Reticulocyte counts may be expressed as a percentage of the total red cell count (3–7% in the neonate, thereafter 0–1%), or more usually as an absolute count (normally 20–100 $\times 10^9$/L). If expressed as a percentage, the reticulocyte count can be misleading, so an absolute count is preferable. An increased reticulocyte count indicates active regeneration of red cells, seen after blood loss, haemolysis or in response to correct haematinic therapy. Blood loss and previous haematinic therapy can usually be excluded on history, so that an increased reticulocyte count is often suggestive of haemolysis. A low reticulocyte response in the presence of anaemia indicates a lack of marrow response, because of a deficiency of the necessary iron or vitamins or inappropriate therapy for the anaemia, or inability to respond, such as marrow aplasia or infiltration.

### Examination of the blood film

This is as important as the evaluation of the red cell indices, leukocyte count and platelets. The presence of abnormal red cell size, shape, inclusions, Hb content, and evidence of regeneration will usually suggest the cause of the anaemia and direct the next stage of investigation. The presence of abnormal leukocytes or abnormal platelet numbers may suggest a specific diagnosis such as leukaemia. Examples of a normal blood film and blood films in some conditions associated with anaemia are shown in Figure 16.1.1. Further investigations are suggested by the algorithms in Figures 16.1.2 and 16.1.3.

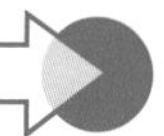

**Practical points**

**Determining the urgency of investigation of anaemia**

- Mild anaemia (Hb > 8 g/L) may still require urgent investigation and management, depending on the cause. Hence, until the cause of anaemia has been determined in a broad sense, discharge from emergency department/hospital should not be considered.
- Acute regenerative anaemia (blood loss or haemolysis) has the capacity rapidly to develop severe anaemia. Blood loss is usually obvious, so haemolysis must be excluded or the rate of haemolysis (multiple Hb levels over a number of hours) understood before a patient can safely leave hospital. Thus, a FBE, reticulocyte count, blood film examination and serum bilirubin are almost always indicated in initial investigations.
- Megaloblastic anaemia in infancy, irrespective of the level of anaemia, requires urgent investigation because of the potential for rapid neurological deterioration. Hence the MCV is a crucial piece of information in the initial FBE, as is the blood film examination. A history of failure to thrive and neurological impairment in infancy should lead to consideration of megaloblastosis, as anaemia is often not the presenting symptom. A FBE with careful consideration of the red cell parameters is always warranted in this circumstance.
- Anaemia as part of a multilineage failure may have a degree of urgency because of the potential for febrile neutropenia or thrombocytopenic haemorrhage.

## Specific disease entities

### Disorders of stem cell proliferation

#### Pluripotential stem cell failure (aplastic anaemia)

Normal marrow function is dependent on stem cell renewal and maturation of all cell lines. Failure of stem cell proliferation and differentiation results in aplastic anaemia. Both genetically determined and acquired forms occur (Table 16.1.3).

*Fanconi anaemia*

Fanconi anaemia, the commonest of the genetic forms of aplastic anaemia, is recessively inherited and is characterized by a variable phenotype, progressive marrow failure and an increased risk of malignancy.

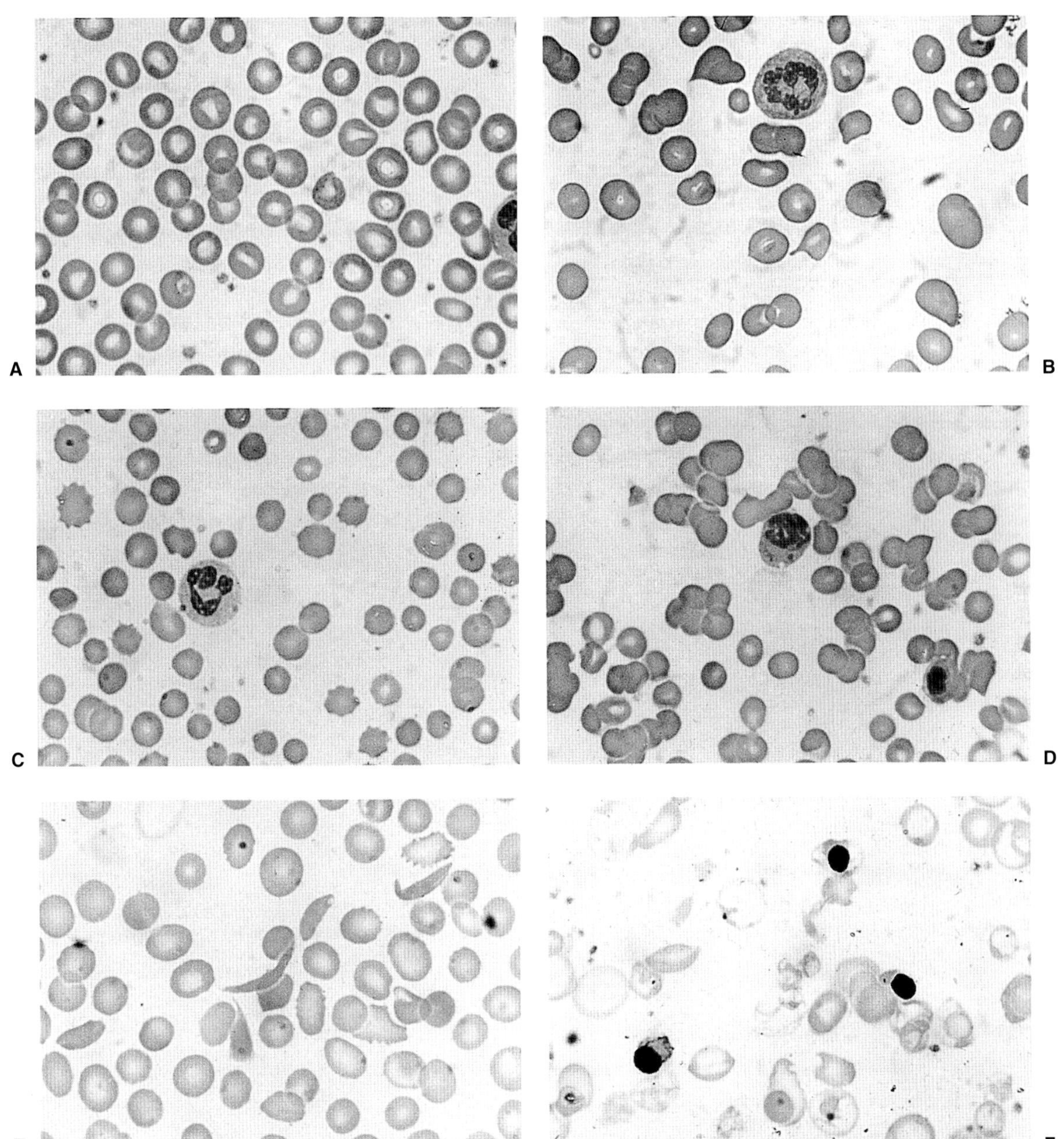


Fig. 16.1.1 Blood films. (**A**) Normal. (**B**) Macrocytosis – note hypersegmented polymorph. (**C**) Spherocytes in hereditary spherocytosis. (**D**) Autoimmune haemolytic anaemia showing red cell agglutination. (**E**) Sickle cell disease. (**F**) Thalassaemia major showing hypochromic microcytes and macrocytes, with nucleated red cells.

There appear to be multiple gene defects in this condition, which explains the diversity of clinical manifestations.

Approximately 75% of children have congenital abnormalities, with a wide range of defects. The commonest are café-au-lait spots, short stature, microcephaly and skeletal anomalies, with thumb and radial hypoplasia or aplasia being most characteristic. Renal anomalies, stenosis of auditory canals, micro-ophthalmia, hypogenitalism and a variety of anomalies of the gastrointestinal tract may also occur. The child shown in Figure 16.1.4 has many features of this disorder.

The diagnosis may be suspected at birth if there are congenital abnormalities. Haematological abnormalities are rare at birth. Pancytopenia develops gradually, usually by the age of 10 years. Onset is earlier in boys than

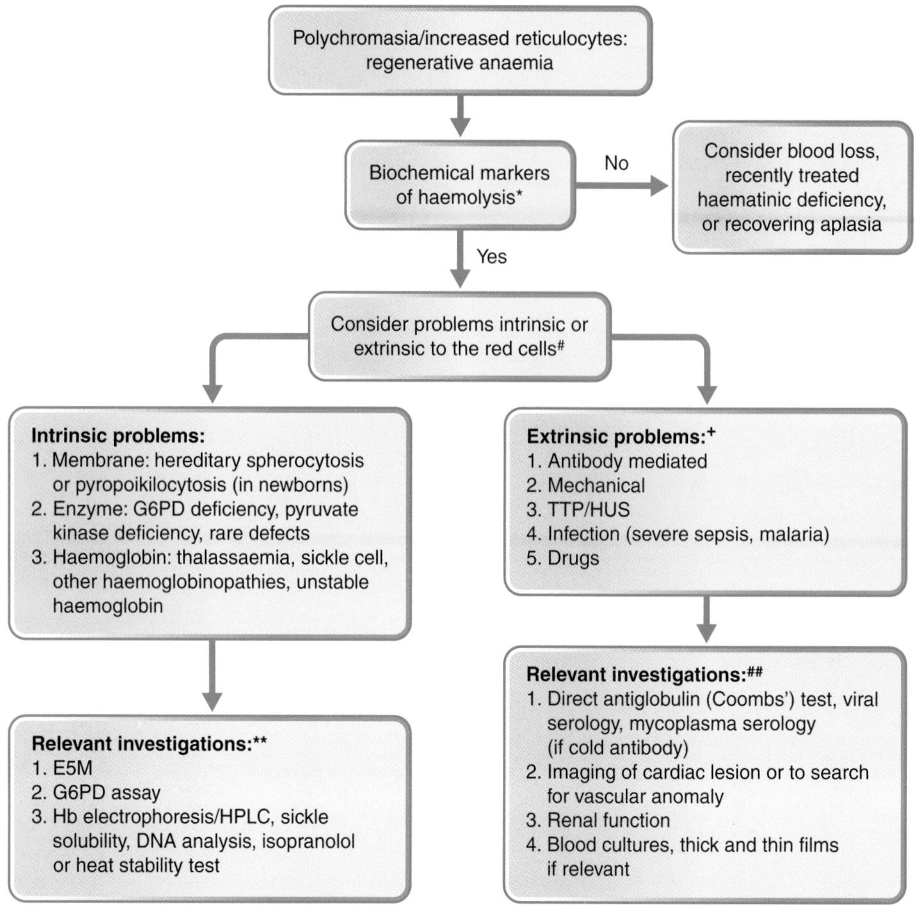

Polychromasia/increased reticulocytes: regenerative anaemia
Biochemical markers of haemolysis*
No
Consider blood loss, recently treated haematinic deficiency, or recovering aplasia
Yes
Consider problems intrinsic or extrinsic to the red cells#
Intrinsic problems:
1. Membrane: hereditary spherocytosis or pyropoikilocytosis (in newborns)
2. Enzyme: G6PD deficiency, pyruvate kinase deficiency, rare defects
3. Haemoglobin: thalassaemia, sickle cell, other haemoglobinopathies, unstable haemoglobin
Extrinsic problems:+
1. Antibody mediated
2. Mechanical
3. TTP/HUS
4. Infection (severe sepsis, malaria)
5. Drugs
Relevant investigations:**
1. E5M
2. G6PD assay
3. Hb electrophoresis/HPLC, sickle solubility, DNA analysis, isopranolol or heat stability test
Relevant investigations:##
1. Direct antiglobulin (Coombs') test, viral serology, mycoplasma serology (if cold antibody)
2. Imaging of cardiac lesion or to search for vascular anomaly
3. Renal function
4. Blood cultures, thick and thin films if relevant


Reasonable first line investigation screen in haemolytic patients includes FBE, reticulocyte count, serum bilirubin, E5M, G6PD assay, Hb HPLC, DAT, renal function, and in neonates urine and blood culture.

BEWARE: Severe intravascular haemolysis (G6PD, some antibodies, microangiopathic (TTP/HUS, mechanical, sepsis)) may release free Hb which falsely elevates the measured haemoglobin. Always check that the red cell count is proportional to the measured Hb. Methaemoglobinaemia in severe G6PD haemolysis may increase tissue hypoxia for any given measured haemoglobin. All acute haemolytic anaemias have the potential for life-threatening haemolysis to develop within hours and as such should be treated with extreme caution. In general, admission to hospital, close monitoring of vital signs and FBE until the tempo of the haemolysis is established is recommended. Folate deficiency in haemolysis may reduce the ability of the bone marrow to respond and worsen the anaemia as well as causing diagnostic confusion.

* Biochemical markers of haemolysis: in most cases the presence of an elevated unconjugated serum bilirubin is sufficient. Haptoglobins and LDH are frequently non contributory in small children.

# Blood film may be diagnostic. E.g. G6PD-blister and bite cells, spherocytosis (in neonates reflects either HS, ABO incompatability or severe sepsis), sickle cells.

** E5M requires less than 0.5 mL and is offered by many laboratories. G6PD assay may be elevated in the presence of a reticulocytosis so borderline results should be repeated after the acute event and at least 3 months post transfusion if the clinical and blood film findings are suggestive. Most laboratories perform HPLC to detect abnormal haemoglobins and use electrophoresis to identify abnormal bands. DNA testing should not be ordered acutely, but as a confirmatory test electively. HPLC and sickle solubility are most useful initial tests.

+ Antibody mediated haemolysis may be warm (usually IgG, spherocytes on film) or cold (usually IgM, +/– complement fixation, agglutination on film). Haemolysis due to mechanical, TTP/HUS or severe sepsis (DIC) are usually characteristically microangiopathic in blood film morphology.

## The Direct Antiglobulin (Coombs') Test (DAT) is crucial to perform in all haemolysing children as IgG mediated haemolysis can be life threatening, and so the diagnosis should not be missed.

Fig. 16.1.2 Further investigation and initial management of regenerative anaemia. DAT, direct antiglobulin test; DIC, disseminated intravascular coagulopathy; E5M, eosin-5-maleimide; FBE, full blood examination; G6PD, glucose-6-phosphate dehydrogenase; Hb, haemoglobin; HPLC, high-performance liquid chromatography; HUS, haemolytic–uraemic syndrome; Ig, immunoglobulin; TTP, thrombotic thrombocytopenic purpura.

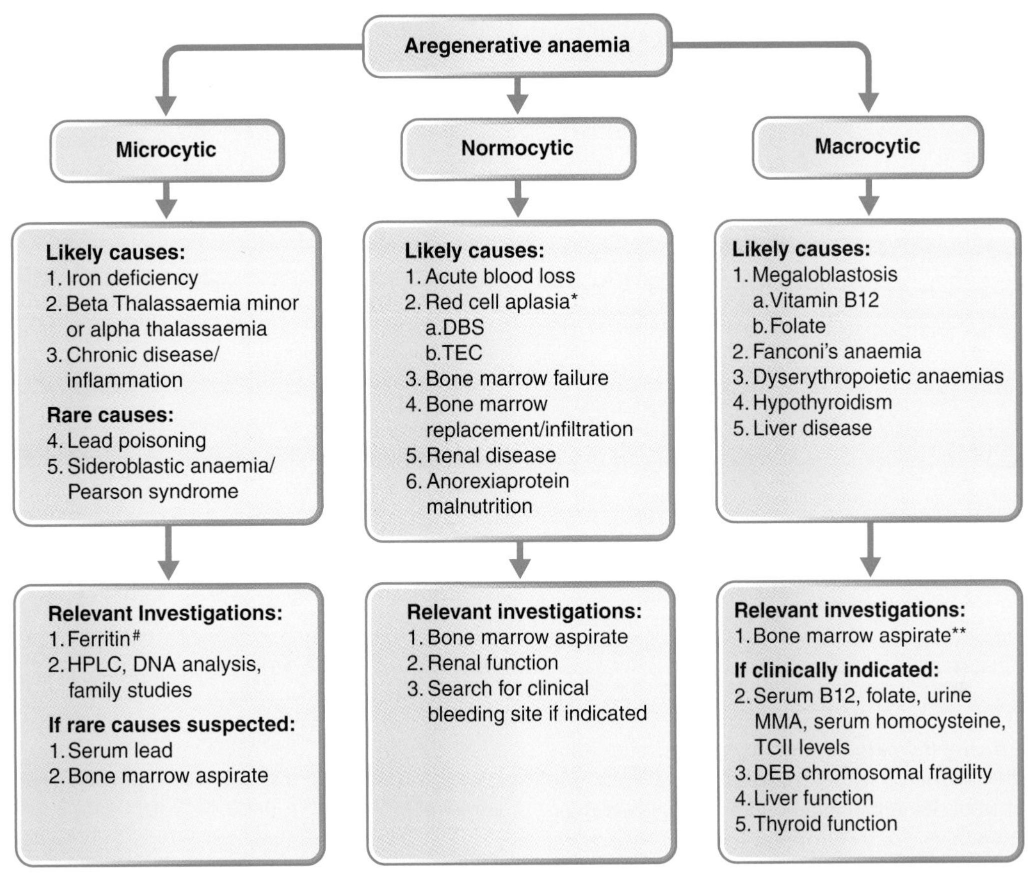

Aregenerative anaemia
Microcytic
Normocytic
Macrocytic
Likely causes:
1. Iron deficiency
2. Beta Thalassaemia minor or alpha thalassaemia
3. Chronic disease/ inflammation
Rare causes:
4. Lead poisoning
5. Sideroblastic anaemia/ Pearson syndrome
Likely causes:
1. Acute blood loss
2. Red cell aplasia*
a. DBS
b. TEC
3. Bone marrow failure
4. Bone marrow replacement/infiltration
5. Renal disease
6. Anorexiaprotein malnutrition
Likely causes:
1. Megaloblastosis
a. Vitamin B12
b. Folate
2. Fanconi's anaemia
3. Dyserythropoietic anaemias
4. Hypothyroidism
5. Liver disease
Relevant Investigations:
1. Ferritin#
2. HPLC, DNA analysis, family studies
If rare causes suspected:
1. Serum lead
2. Bone marrow aspirate
Relevant investigations:
1. Bone marrow aspirate
2. Renal function
3. Search for clinical bleeding site if indicated
Relevant investigations:
1. Bone marrow aspirate**
If clinically indicated:
2. Serum B12, folate, urine MMA, serum homocysteine, TCII levels
3. DEB chromosomal fragility
4. Liver function
5. Thyroid function


BEWARE: Megaloblastic anaemia in infancy (<2 years) is often accompanied by severe failure to thrive and neurodevelopmental regression. Often these patients deteriorate very rapidly once they have finally reached medical attention, and investigation is a matter of urgency so that replacement therapy can be commenced ASAP and long term neurological sequelae minimized. The bone marrow aspirate confirms megaloblastic tissue quickly, such that treatment can be commenced pending further investigations of the child and if a breastfed infant, investigation of the mother for Vitamin B12 or folate deficiency.

*Red cell aplasia may be isolated or part of a broader marrow dysfunction. The differential between transient erythroblastopenia of childhood (TEC) and Diamond-Blackfan Syndrome (DBS) is often difficult, even with thorough investigations.

# Investigation of iron deficiency in children needs to be appropriate. In children with a classic history of cow's milk intake before 12 months, or inadequate transition to solids, no investigations may be required after the blood film diagnosis, and treatment should be commenced. In otherwise normal children, ferritin is the most useful investigation and other iron studies are rarely contributory. Ferritin is an acute phase protein, so testing may need to be delayed if an acute febrile illness is coexistent. Full iron studies may be of value in children with complex medical problems.

** In the absence of clear renal, liver or thyroid disease, bone marrow aspirate is indicated for most significant normocytic or macrocytic anaemias. Bone marrow aspirates must always be examined in conjunction with the peripheral blood smear, and ancillary investigations. Hence consultation with a haematologist early in the investigation of such patients is often worthwhile. With the exception of megaloblastic anaemia, where bone marrow examination is often an emergency procedure to allow commencement of replacement therapy immediately, BMA can often be performed electively, and should never delay transfusion of a borderline or decompensating patient. In cases of suspected aplasia, bone marrow trephine may assist in assessing marrow cellularity.

Fig. 16.1.3 Further investigation of aregenerative anaemia. DBS, Diamond–Blackfan syndrome; DEB, diepoxybutane; HPLC, high-performance liquid chromatography; MMA, methylmalonic acid; TCII, transcobalamin II; TEC, transient erythroblastopenia of childhood.

girls. Macrocytosis is followed by thrombocytopenia, neutropenia, then anaemia. Bone marrow aspirate and trephine show hypoplasia or aplasia.

In contrast, infants with the thrombocytopenia–absent radius (TAR) syndrome are severely thrombocytopenic at birth and have radial anomalies without thumb abnormalities.

The diagnosis of Fanconi anaemia is established by special chromosome studies of lymphocytes. Chromosomes from patients with Fanconi anaemia

**Table 16.1.3 Causes of anaemia due to defective stem cell proliferation**

| Pathological process | Aetiology | Disease entity | Usual age of presentation |
|---|---|---|---|
| Pluripotential stem cell failure | Congenital | Fanconi anaemia | Variable, majority < 10 years |
| | Acquired<br>Drugs<br>Infection<br>Idiopathic | Aplastic anaemia | Any age |
| Erythroid stem cell failure | Congenital | Blackfan–Diamond syndrome | Neonate to 1 year |
| | Acquired<br>Idiopathic | Transient erythroblastopenia of childhood | <5 years |
| | Erythropoietin deficiency | Chronic renal failure<br>Hypothyroidism | |
| | Unknown | Chronic infection<br>Chronic inflammatory disease | |
| Bone marrow replacement | Malignant transformation of progenitors | Leukaemia | Infant–adult |
| | Marrow infiltration | Disseminated malignancy | |
| | Abnormal accumulation of metabolic substrates | Lipid 'storage' disease | |

show markedly increased spontaneous and alkylating agent (cells incubated with mitomycin C or diepoxybutane) induced chromosomal breaks, gaps, rearrangements, exchanges and endoreduplication. Antenatal diagnosis is possible.

Androgen therapy may produce long remissions of the anaemia but has little effect on thrombocytopenia and neutropenia. Its use is associated with masculinization and is therefore undesirable in young children, particularly girls. Granulocyte–macrophage colony-stimulating factor has been used with some success. Bone marrow transplantation offers the only possibility of cure of the aplasia. Supportive care with transfusions and antibiotics is required for patients without a marrow donor, but death from infection, bleeding or the development of leukaemia usually occurs within a decade of diagnosis.

**Clinical example**

John, aged 5 years, presented with pallor and bruising of several months duration. He had a past history of tracheo-oesophageal fistula and had always been small, with his height and weight on the third centile for age. His teacher had expressed concern about his hearing. On examination he was pale and had multiple bruises and several café-au-lait spots. He had a convergent squint and his external auditory canals were narrow. There was no hepatosplenomegaly or lymphadenopathy. A blood test showed a macrocytic anaemia with a Hb level of 80 g/L and a white cell count of $1.4 \times 10^9$/L with neutrophils $0.7 \times 10^9$/L. The platelet count was $25 \times 10^9$/L. A bone marrow aspirate showed hypocellular fragments, and trephine biopsy confirmed marrow aplasia. Cytogenetic studies on peripheral blood lymphocytes confirmed that John had Fanconi anaemia by showing an increased rate of spontaneous and mitomycin C-induced chromosome breaks. His sister was found to be HLA-identical with normal cytogenetic studies, and plans were made for elective bone marrow transplantation within the next few months.

*Acquired aplastic anaemia*

A number of agents may cause marrow failure, either in a dose-dependent fashion (irradiation and cytotoxic drugs) or in an idiosyncratic fashion. Some viral infections are associated with marrow suppression. No cause is identified in about 50% of children with marrow failure. Fanconi anaemia must be excluded by cytogenetic studies, as not all affected individuals have congenital abnormalities.

Common causes are:

- drugs: chloramphenicol, anticonvulsants, non-steroidal anti-inflammatory agents and cytotoxic drugs
- chemicals: benzene, organic solvents, insecticides
- viral hepatitis: usually non-A, non-B, non-C hepatitis, less commonly Epstein–Barr virus, cytomegalovirus, parvovirus or human immunodeficiency virus (HIV)
- preleukaemic: acute lymphoblastic leukaemia occasionally has a transient period of aplasia before the onset of the disease
- paroxysmal nocturnal haemoglobinuria.

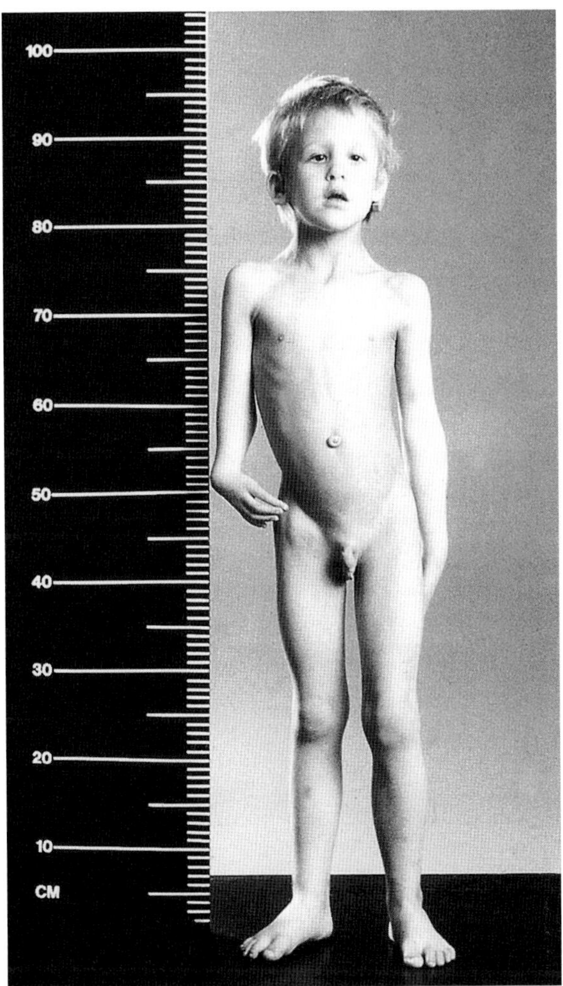


Fig. 16.1.4 Child with Fanconi anaemia. Note short stature, absent right radius and thumb, micro-ophthalmia and the presence of a hearing aid.

Presentation is with the gradual onset of pallor, lethargy and bruising. There may be a history of recent infection. Physical examination reveals little other than pallor, bruising, petechiae and oral mucosal bleeding. Importantly there is no enlargement of liver, spleen or lymph nodes, but there may be fever and focal infection associated with the neutropenia.

The blood shows a pancytopenia with a normocytic anaemia without regeneration. Bone marrow aspirate and trephine biopsies reveal absent or decreased haemopoiesis.

Initial management depends on the severity and clinical manifestations of the aplasia. Potentially causative agents must be removed. Infections are treated vigorously. Supportive red cell and platelet transfusions are given as required. The general principles of transfusion therapy in aplastic anaemia are to avoid HLA sensitization by using leukocyte-depleted cellular products, and to minimize alloimmunization by minimizing donor exposure through the appropriate selection of blood products. Early referral to a tertiary centre is vital. Although a small number of children will recover within a few weeks, bone marrow transplantation from an HLA-compatible sibling is generally regarded as the treatment of choice for severe aplastic anaemia, particularly in those aged under 5 years. Only 30% of children will have a matched sibling donor. For the remainder, antithymocyte globulin, together with granulocyte colony-stimulating factor and cyclosporine, produces improvement or complete recovery in about two-thirds of children. Onset of response may not occur for 2–3 months after initiation of therapy, and supportive care during this time is vital. For those failing to respond, unrelated donor transplantation is an option and a donor search should be initiated early.

*Red cell aplasia (erythroid stem cell failure)*

Isolated aplasia of red cells results in a normocytic normochromic anaemia without reticulocytosis. The platelets and white blood cells are normal. Congenital and acquired forms occur.

*Congenital red cell aplasia (Diamond–Blackfan syndrome).* This disorder is almost certainly heterogeneous, with sporadic, dominant and recessive forms occurring. Faulty ribosome biogenesis, resulting in pro-apoptotic erythropoiesis leading to erythroid failure, is hypothesized to be the underlying defect.

Normocytic anaemia may be present at birth and usually is evident by 2–3 months of age. However, diagnosis beyond 1 year of age is reported. Early treatment with steroids results in a reticulocytosis and an increase in Hb levels in about two-thirds of patients. In steroid responders, long-term low-dose steroids are recommended before total weaning is attempted. Some steroid-responsive patients are successfully weaned off steroids, but many remain steroid-dependent. Those failing to respond to steroids or requiring large doses will need regular blood transfusion and chelation therapy. Bone marrow transplantation has corrected the condition in steroid-resistant patients.

*Acquired red cell aplasia.* Pure red cell aplasia (PRCA) is primarily a disease of adults but cases have been documented in teenagers. A large number of disorders, including thymoma, malignancy, autoimmune disease, viral infection and drug administration, have been implicated. Therapy is directed primarily toward the cause but may include immunosuppression, plasmaphaeresis, thymectomy and splenectomy.

*Transient erythroblastopenia of childhood (TEC).* This self-limiting aregenerative anaemia occurs typically in children between 1 and 3 years of age. The aetiology remains unclear but antibodies directed against early red cell precursors have been documented in some children. Parvovirus B19 has not been isolated consistently.

The typical presentation is with pallor of gradual onset in an otherwise well child. The only abnormal clinical finding is pallor. The anaemia may be marked, without evidence of regeneration. A bone marrow aspirate will generally show absent or diminished erythropoiesis, but if spontaneous recovery is already occurring at the time of presentation there may be many early erythroid progenitors present.

As the onset of the anaemia is gradual, most children will have compensated well and tolerate quite marked degrees of anaemia. If, however, there is no evidence of recovery occurring by the time the Hb level falls to below 50 g/L, transfusion is likely to be required. Folic acid supplements should be given during the recovery phase. Spontaneous recovery usually occurs within 1–2 months and it is unusual for more than one transfusion to be required. Steroids have no role in the management of this disorder.

In some cases the distinction between Diamond–Blackfan syndrome (DBS) and TEC is extremely difficult. Neither the clinical scenario nor the bone marrow findings are absolutely diagnostic. In such cases, transfusion therapy without steroids may be useful initially to enable the patient every opportunity to recover. If steroids are introduced early, on the presumption of DBS, and recovery occurs, one is reluctant to cease steroid therapy quickly for fear of relapse, and a spontaneously recovering TEC could potentially receive unnecessary steroids for a prolonged period.

*Transient erythroid aplasia in chronic haemolytic anaemias.* An aplastic crisis may occur in patients with one of the chronic haemolytic anaemias, such as sickle cell disease, hereditary spherocytosis and autoimmune haemolytic anaemia. Infection with human parvovirus B19 has been documented as the usual cause. Folic acid deficiency may be a further precipitating factor.

Because of the shortened red cell survival, there is a precipitous fall in Hb concentration when erythroid proliferation ceases. Pallor and lethargy develop relatively quickly. The absence of jaundice, lack of increase in the degree of splenomegaly and absence of a reticulocyte response enables an aplastic crisis to be distinguished from increased haemolysis. Blood transfusion is likely to be required. Spontaneous recovery usually begins within 10–14 days.

### Marrow replacement

Infiltration with neoplasia, particularly leukaemia, is the commonest cause of marrow failure in childhood. Several other childhood malignancies (neuroblastoma, non-Hodgkin lymphoma, Ewing sarcoma and rhabdomyosarcoma) metastasize to the bone marrow. Progressive pancytopenia with a normocytic anaemia and an associated shift to the left in the erythroid and myeloid series develops. Nucleated red cells and immature granulocytes (left shift) may be seen in the peripheral blood (leukoerythroblastic blood picture). Replacement of marrow with storage cells (e.g. Gaucher disease), fibrous tissue (myelofibrosis) or bone (osteopetrosis) will have a similar result. Careful examination of the blood film looking for leukaemic blasts, and a bone marrow examination that will identify abnormal cells, are required in any child with pancytopenia.

## Dyserythropoietic/ineffective erythropoiesis

### Congenital dyserythropoietic anaemias

This group of rare hereditary disorders of erythropoiesis is characterized by ineffective erythropoiesis resulting in shortened red cell survival with associated jaundice, a variable degree of anaemia, with normocytic to macrocytic red cell morphology, and anisopoikilocytosis and fragmentation in some types (Table 16.1.4). Bone marrow findings are characterized by erythroid hyperplasia, multinuclearity and internuclear bridging. The aetiology is unknown. Some patients in whom haemolysis is severe require regular transfusions.

### Megaloblastic anaemia

Megaloblastic anaemias in childhood are rare but prompt diagnosis of the cause, especially in infants, is important to prevent potentially irreversible neurological damage, which may result from deficiencies of vitamin $B_{12}$ or its transport protein transcobalamin II.

*Vitamin $B_{12}$ deficiency*

Because the daily requirement for vitamin $B_{12}$ is low and body stores are generally high, dietary deficiency of vitamin $B_{12}$ is rare, occurring only after prolonged inadequate intake, as may occur in vegans. Breastfed infants of vitamin $B_{12}$-deficient mothers are at risk and may present with anaemia in the first year of life. The commonest causes of maternal deficiency are undiagnosed pernicious anaemia and veganism. In infants with megaloblastosis it is important to determine whether maternal deficiency, transcobalamin II deficiency or a cobalamin pathway defect is the cause. Maternal deficiency requires short-term parenteral therapy of the infant; however, transcobalamin II deficiency requires long-term high-dose parenteral $B_{12}$ injections. The majority of older children with vitamin $B_{12}$ deficiency have a malabsorptive problem, either specific to vitamin $B_{12}$, as in pernicious anaemia, or secondary to inflammation or loss of the ileum, the portion of the small bowel in which vitamin $B_{12}$ absorption occurs.

Vitamin $B_{12}$ deficiency results in an anaemia with oval macrocytosis, hypersegmentation of neutrophils

**Table 16.1.4 Anaemias that are due to ineffective erythropoiesis and dyserythropoiesis**

| Pathological process | Aetiology | Disease entity | Usual age of presentation |
|---|---|---|---|
| Impaired DNA synthesis (megaloblastosis) | Unknown | Congenital dyserythropoietic anaemia | Infancy to adulthood |
| | Vitamin $B_{12}$ deficiency | | |
| | Congenital | Transcobalamin II deficiency | Neonate to 12 months |
| | | Cobalamin pathway defect | Neonate to 12 months |
| | | Congenital pernicious anaemia | <3 years |
| | Acquired | Maternal $B_{12}$ deficiency | 3–12 months |
| | | Juvenile pernicious anaemia | <10 years |
| | | Ileal resection | Any age |
| | | Regional ileitis | Any age |
| | | Blind loop syndrome | Any age |
| | Folate deficiency | | |
| | Congenital | Rare metabolic abnormalities | Infancy |
| | Acquired | Dietary deficiency | Any age |
| | | Malabsorption (coeliac disease) | >6 months |
| | | Increased utilization (haemolysis) | Any age |
| Defective haem synthesis (microcytosis) | Iron deficiency | Dietary deficiency | Infancy, adolescence |
| | | Malabsorption | Any age |
| | | Blood loss | |
| | | Occult | |
| | | Overt | |
| Reduced/absent globin-chain synthesis | Gene deletion/ mutation | β-thalassaemia major | 6 months to 5 years |
| | | HbH disease (α-thalassaemia) | Any age |
| | | Thalassaemia traits | >6 months |
| Abnormal globin-chain production | Gene mutation/amino acid substitution | Haemoglobinopathies | Any age |
| | | Sickle cell disease | 1–4 years |

and thrombocytopenia. Bone marrow examination shows erythroid hyperplasia with megaloblastosis characterized by abnormally large erythroid and myeloid progenitors, in which nuclear maturation is delayed compared with cytoplasmic maturation. Intramedullary destruction of erythroid precursors leads to a mild unconjugated hyperbilirubinaemia. Raised serum homocysteine and urinary methyl malonic acid are useful to confirm the presence of intracellular vitamin $B_{12}$ deficiency.

Therapy depends on the cause of the vitamin $B_{12}$ deficiency. Dietary deficiency is treated by an initial dose of parenteral vitamin $B_{12}$, followed by dietary correction. Abnormalities of absorption, whether due to pernicious anaemia, ileal malabsorption or resection, require long-term intramuscular injection of the vitamin (hydroxycobalamin) at 1–3-month intervals according to the severity of the malabsorption.

*Folate deficiency*

Daily folate requirements are low, but body stores are small. Folate is heat-labile and, although ubiquitous in food, is often destroyed by cooking.

Extra folate is required at times of rapid growth, during pregnancy and in patients with haemolytic anaemia. Deficiency is most likely to occur under these circumstances. Dietary deficiency most commonly occurs in infants fed exclusively on goat's milk, which is deficient in the vitamin. Malabsorption occurs in generalized malabsorptive syndromes such as coeliac disease and Crohn's disease.

Some anticonvulsant drugs (e.g. phenytoin) may interfere with folate absorption, and megaloblastic changes are common among patients taking these drugs.

Inherited disorders of folate metabolism are rare and may present diagnostic difficulty.

Folate deficiency presents with a macrocytic anaemia without neurological abnormality. Oral administration of folic acid is effective in reversing deficiencies. Doses required are small, as 0.1 mg daily produces an optimal haematological response. In patients with increased requirements or malabsorption, higher doses of 0.5–5 mg daily are given. It is essential to exclude coexistent vitamin $B_{12}$ deficiency before treatment as the haematological picture may improve initially with folate therapy, but progression of the neurological effects of vitamin $B_{12}$ deficiency will still occur.

## Defective haem synthesis

### Iron deficiency

Iron deficiency is the commonest cause of anaemia in childhood, being particularly common in the first 2 years of life when iron requirements are increased because of rapid growth and dietary intake is often inadequate. Early adolescence is another risk period for development of iron deficiency because of rapid growth.

Low-birth-weight infants and infants having exchange transfusions or frequent blood sampling have low total body iron stores and are at high risk of early development of iron deficiency anaemia, as iron stores and dietary intake are inadequate to keep up with rapid postnatal growth. Breast milk and cow's milk have a similar iron content but iron bioavailability from breast milk is approximately 50%, compared with 10% from cow's milk. Breastfed term babies therefore are rarely iron-deficient in the first 6 months of life, but iron concentrations in breast milk decline postnatally and the iron content of breast milk is insufficient to meet the needs of the infant over the age of 6 months.

Oral iron supplementation (2 mg/kg daily) is given to low-birth-weight infants, generally from approximately 3 months of age. Iron-containing foods should be introduced by 6 months of age to all term babies. Most infant formulae are iron-fortified. Infants weaned early on to cow's milk (before 12 months of age), particularly those in whom milk continues to be the major component of the diet without the appropriate introduction of mixed solid feeding, are the group presenting most commonly with gross iron deficiency. In some, iron deficiency is exacerbated by the development of cow's milk protein enteropathy, leading to peripheral oedema secondary to hypoalbuminaemia in addition to anaemia.

Older children with diets poor in iron-containing foods (red meat, white meats, legumes, green vegetables, egg yolk) are also at risk. Blood loss must always be considered in an iron-deficient child or adolescent without an appropriate dietary history. Menorrhagia is an important cause of iron deficiency in adolescent girls. Occult blood loss is usually gastrointestinal in origin, from such diverse causes as cow's milk enteropathy, polyps, haemangiomas, Meckel's diverticulum and hereditary telangiectasia, but repeated epistaxes and chronic blood loss from the renal tract must be excluded.

Iron malabsorption is uncommon and is usually associated with malabsorption syndromes such as coeliac disease or chronic inflammatory bowel disease.

Iron deficiency initially leads to depletion of marrow iron stores without any haematological abnormality. When iron stores are exhausted, serum iron concentration and transferrin binding falls and there is reduced intracellular iron availability for haem synthesis, with a consequent reduction in Hb production, leading to microcytosis and the development of anaemia.

Symptoms of early iron deficiency with no or minimal anaemia may include poor attention span and irritability. As anaemia develops, cognitive deficits may increase and lethargy and pallor become apparent. Some chronically iron-deficient children exhibit pica (the ingestion of non-food items such as dirt and clay, and chewing of ice).

Examination reveals pallor, most easily detected in the palmar creases and conjunctivae. Signs of cardiac decompensation will occasionally be present if the anaemia is severe. Mild splenomegaly is found occasionally but is more common in thalassaemia minor, from which iron deficiency must be distinguished.

Therapy of iron deficiency involves correction of the underlying cause and replenishment of iron stores. Improvement in the dietary intake of iron-containing foods is the most important strategy in the majority of iron-deficient children. Reduction in the total milk content of the diet may be necessary to allow the child to develop an appropriate appetite. If a source of blood loss is identified, appropriate therapy is undertaken and iron supplements are given until the deficiency is corrected.

Therapeutic iron is optimally given orally in two to three divided doses daily in a dose of 6 mg per kg per day of elemental iron. Absorption is enhanced when iron is taken with vitamin C and between meals, but the side-effects of abdominal discomfort are reduced when iron is taken with food. Ferrous sulphate is cheaper and better absorbed than ferrous gluconate, although the gluconate is better tolerated. A reticulocyte response to iron should be seen within 7–10 days, but iron therapy should continue for 3 months to replenish iron stores. The stools are grey–black in individuals on iron.

**Clinical example**

Tan, a 15-month-old boy, had been breastfed for 10 months and then was given cow's milk. He had occasional solid foods only, and rarely had any foods with a significant iron content. He had become irritable, seemed to be low in energy and slept more than his parents thought was usual. When he was seen by his doctor because of an upper respiratory tract infection, he was noted to have pale conjunctivae and pale palmar creases.

Tan's Hb level was 51 g/L, his MCV was 51 fL, and his mean corpuscular haemoglobin concentration (MCHC) was 15 pg. The total WBC was normal and his platelet count was $432 \times 10^9$/L. The blood film showed microcytic and hypochromic red cells; there was no reticulocytosis and no basophilic stippling. The serum ferritin concentration was 4 μg/L (normal range 16–300).

Tan's anaemia had all the features of an iron-deficiency anaemia due to a deficient iron intake in his diet. A dietitian assisted in instructing his mother in ways to improve his diet by including foods such as red and white meats, green vegetables, legumes and egg yolks. Tan was given ferrous gluconate mixture at a dose of 6 mg/kg of expected weight per day, to be taken as two doses daily. His parents were asked to give this with orange juice to improve absorption. They were warned that the mixture could make Tan's stools a grey–black colour, but that this was not of concern. They were asked to brush his teeth after each dose to prevent any minor staining. They were warned of the toxic effects of iron if taken in overdose accidentally by an inquisitive toddler; the mixture was provided in limited amounts only in a bottle with a safety top, and they were asked to keep it in a secure place, preferably a locked cupboard.

The iron mixture was continued for 3 months. Tan's reticulocyte count rose in a few days, and his Hb level began to rise in 10 days. By 6 weeks of therapy, the Hb concentration was normal; the iron mixture was continued for another 6 weeks to ensure that his iron stores were replenished.

It is rarely necessary to use the parenteral route for iron administration but, in occasional children with poor absorption or poor compliance, intravenous infusions of iron may be required.

## Haemoglobinopathies

Haemoglobin is a compound protein made up of two pairs of globin chains with a haem molecule inserted into each. One of these globin chains is designated as the alpha (α) chain, the other variably being termed beta (β), delta (δ), epsilon (ε), gamma (γ) and zeta (ζ). ζ and ε chains are expressed only in early embryonic life, with ζ-chain production switching to α-chain production, and γ-chain production replacing ε-chain synthesis in the early weeks of gestation. In the perinatal period there is a further switch from γ- to β-chain production. The predominant fetal haemoglobin is HbF ($\alpha_2\gamma_2$). In children beyond 6 months of age and adults, the major haemoglobins are HbA ($\alpha_2\beta_2$) and HbA2 ($\alpha_2\delta_2$). A number of abnormalities of globin chain production or point mutations within globin genes may result in significant disease.

### Thalassaemias

These are genetic disorders characterized by reduced or absent production of one or more of the globin chains of haemoglobin.

The thalassaemias are found commonly in people originating from the Mediterranean region, the Middle East, the Indian subcontinent, south Asia and Africa. The inheritance is in a Mendelian recessive manner.

#### *β-Thalassaemia*

β-Thalassaemia occurs as a result of point mutations or deletions within one or both of the two β-globin genes, resulting in reduced or absent production of β-globin chains. The heterozygous state is termed thalassaemia minor and the homozygous state thalassaemia major.

*β-Thalassaemia minor.* Affected individuals are usually asymptomatic, with mild anaemia detected either during investigation of another illness or as a result of family screening. Mild pallor and splenomegaly may be noted, but the examination is often unremarkable. There is a mild microcytic hypochromic anaemia with occasional target cells. The differential diagnosis is iron deficiency, although both may coexist. The $HbA_2$ level is raised. If present, iron deficiency may mask the thalassaemia minor, preventing diagnosis until the iron deficiency is corrected.

*β-Thalassaemia major (Cooley anaemia).* This is caused by the inheritance of two abnormal β genes. At birth, the haemoglobin is normal but, as the γ–β switch occurs, there are no ($\beta^0$) or insufficient ($\beta^+$) β chains to balance α chains. Excess α chains precipitate, causing shortened red cell survival with destruction within the bone marrow (ineffective erythropoiesis) and spleen. HbA production is inadequate to compensate for the gradual fall in HbF as γ-chain production switches to inadequate β-chain production.

Children with thalassaemia major usually present between 3 months and 1 year of life with pallor and hepatosplenomegaly. There may be mild jaundice. Occasionally presentation is delayed to 4–5 years, with these children having increased skin pigmentation, frontal bossing and malar prominence due to chronic marrow expansion. The Hb level may be very low, with blood examination revealing hypochromia, red cell stippling, microcytosis, macrocytes, target cells and nucleated red cells (see Fig. 16.1.1F). An increased HbF level (usually 50–100%) confirms the diagnosis. Globin chain synthesis studies can differentiate between $\beta^+$ and $\beta^0$ thalassaemia.

Without treatment, the severe chronic anaemia leads to growth retardation, poor musculoskeletal development and increased iron absorption, resulting in skin pigmentation. Extramedullary haemopoiesis in liver and spleen together with hypersplenism result in organ enlargement and abdominal distension. Marrow expansion produces the characteristic facial appearance with frontal bossing, maxillary hypertrophy with exposure of the upper teeth, prominence of the malar eminences and a flattened nasal bridge. Skull X-rays show expansion of the diploic space, and the subperiosteal bone has a typical 'hair on end' appearance. There is cortical thinning of long bones, and fractures may occur. Death usually occurs within 10 years from cardiac failure, cardiac arrhythmias or infection.

Current treatment is with regular transfusion at 3–4-weekly intervals, aiming to suppress endogenous haemopoiesis (preventing marrow expansion) and to keep the Hb level above 100 g/L. Regular transfusion results in iron loading, and chelation therapy must accompany transfusion support to prevent the toxic effects of iron on the myocardium, liver, pancreas and gonads (cardiac arrhythmias, cardiac failure, diabetes mellitus, hepatic fibrosis, infertility). The recent availability of effective oral iron chelation therapy has dramatically improved the quality of life for these patients. Many centres now transfuse by erythrocytaphaeresis to reduce iron loading. All patients receive folic acid supplements and hepatitis B vaccination, and are encouraged to participate in all normal activities. Splenectomy, preceded by appropriate vaccinations, is occasionally required.

Bone marrow transplantation from matched siblings is producing high cure rates provided it is carried out before hepatic dysfunction develops, but long-term results are still to be evaluated.

With improvements in therapy, some patients are now surviving into the fifth decade. A proportion of adults have preservation of gonadal function and have had children.

*Haemoglobin E/β-thalassaemia.* Haemoglobin E ($\beta^{26Glu-Ly}$) occurs extensively throughout South-East Asia. Neither the heterozygous nor the homozygous state produces clinical abnormalities. The doubly heterozygous state of HbE with β-thalassaemia results in a clinical condition similar to thalassaemia major. Diagnosis is confirmed by blood examination and Hb electrophoresis. Clinical presentation and management are similar to that of a moderately severe β-thalassaemia.

*α-Thalassaemia*

There are four α-globin genes, and α-thalassaemia results from the loss of one or more of these. The loss of one gene produces neither haematological nor clinical abnormality (silent carrier). Loss of two genes results in hypochromia and microcytosis, but no anaemia, and is known as α-thalassaemia trait. α-Thalassaemia occurs with a very high incidence in Asian populations and is assuming increasing importance in our community.

*Haemoglobin H disease.* The loss of three α genes results in the formation of excess β chains, which form an unstable tetramer ($\beta_4$), accounting for 30–40% of the total haemoglobin. The clinical picture is similar to that of β-thalassaemia intermedia, with pallor, jaundice and moderate hepatosplenomegaly. There is a moderate anaemia (Hb level 80–100 g/L) and persistent reticulocytosis. The anaemia is aggravated by infections, pregnancy and oxidant drugs (e.g. phenacetin or primaquine), which should be avoided. No specific treatment is necessary other than folic acid supplements.

*Haemoglobin Barts (hydrops fetalis syndrome).* All four α genes are deleted and no α chains are produced. The haemoglobins present are HbBarts ($\gamma_4$) 70%, HbH ($\beta_4$) 0–20% and HbPortland ($\zeta_2\gamma_2$). Severe fetal anaemia develops, resulting in cardiac failure, hepatosplenomegaly and generalized oedema. The infants are generally stillborn or die shortly after birth. *In utero* transfusions may result in a liveborn infant, and exchange transfusion followed by ongoing transfusion support has led to the survival of a few patients. Bone marrow transplantation should cure these patients.

*Sickle cell disease*

Haemoglobin S (HbS) results from a single amino acid substitution in the β-globin chain ($\beta^{6Glu-Val}$). Under hypoxic conditions, deoxyhaemoglobin S polymerizes into fibre bundles, which distort the cell into a sickle shape. Sickling may be reversible on reoxygenation or may become irreversible. The sickle cell gene occurs in people from Africa, the Middle East and the Mediterranean region, as well as in the African American population.

The heterozygous carrier (*sickle trait*) is asymptomatic, with normal Hb and red cell morphology. Haemoglobin electrophoresis reveals a HbA of approximately 60% and a HbS level of 30–40%.

In the homozygous state (*sickle cell anaemia*) there is a normochromic normocytic haemolytic anaemia with target cells, sickle cells, nucleated red cells, fragments and spherocytes (see Fig. 16.1.1E). The diagnosis is confirmed by finding a raised HbS level (60–90%) on electrophoresis with approximately 2% $HbA_2$, the remainder being HbF. The higher the level of HbF the less severe the symptoms of the disease.

The doubly heterozygous *sickle trait–β-thalassaemia* is expressed with clinical features very similar to those of homozygous sickle cell disease. In contrast to sickle cell anaemia, the red cells are microcytic and hypochromic, and target cells are present. Sickling can be demonstrated and both HbS and $HbA_2$ levels are raised. Examination of the parents' blood confirms sickle cell trait in one and thalassaemia minor in the other. The management of this condition is similar to that for sickle cell anaemia.

The clinical course of the patient with sickle cell disease, or doubly heterozygous sickle/thalassaemia, is characterized by 'crises' as a result of sickling of red cells that obstruct the lumen of capillaries and small venules, causing infarction of surrounding tissues. Haemolytic 'crises' may also occur during infective illness.

Presentation is usually between the ages of 6 months and 4 years with pallor, jaundice, abdominal or limb pain and/or swelling of the hands and feet. Haemolytic crises are characterized by increased pallor and jaundice, infarctive 'crises' with acute pain, generally of limbs or back, and aplastic crises with an aregenerative anaemia. Splenic sequestration crises occur in young children predominantly under the age of 5 years. In this potentially life-threatening complication, red cells are trapped in splenic sinusoids, resulting in hypovolaemia, a rapid increase in splenic size and profound anaemia. Stroke is also common before 5 years of age. Patients with sickle cell disease have an increased risk of infection, particularly pneumococcal infection. Functional asplenia secondary to repeated splenic infarction occurs in most patients.

The emphasis in management is on avoidance of environmental factors known to precipitate a crisis. The following protective measures are recommended:

- good nutrition with regular folic acid supplements
- penicillin prophylaxis from infancy, with prompt treatment of infections
- appropriate immunization schedule
- maintenance of adequate hydration, particularly during hot weather
- prevention of vascular stasis. This may occur with tight clothing, the use of tourniquets applied during an operative procedure, and exposure to cold.

Vaso-occlusive crises require prompt control of pain, the maintenance of hydration and treatment of underlying infection. Severe crises (pulmonary syndrome or cerebral infarction) require blood transfusion to reduce the HbS concentration. Occasionally exchange transfusion may be required.

Patients with splenic sequestration require prompt restoration of intravascular volume and correction of acidosis.

Patients with frequent crises may be managed with hydroxycarbamide (hydroxyurea), which increases the proportion of HbF and reduces the number of sickle crises. Hydroxycarbamide is not usually commenced until at least 3 years of age, but usually 5 years. In more severe cases, regular blood transfusions to suppress endogenous HbS production are required. These patients also require iron chelation. Successful bone marrow transplantation has been reported.

### Genetic counselling

Current DNA techniques allow prenatal diagnosis of the thalassaemias and sickle cell disease. With increased community awareness and education, many couples who carry either a thalassaemia or sickle trait are now seeking antenatal counselling and prenatal diagnosis. This will have significant effects on the incidence of newly diagnosed homozygotes in the future.

## Anaemia due to increased red cell destruction (haemolysis)

Anaemia secondary to haemolysis (Table 16.1.5) occurs when bone marrow replacement does not keep pace with the rate of destruction.

**Table 16.1.5 Anaemias due to increased red cell destruction**

| Pathological process | Aetiology | Disease entity | Usual age of presentation |
|---|---|---|---|
| Oxidative cell damage | Enzyme defects of the glycolytic pathway | G6PD deficiency<br>Pyruvate kinase deficiency | Neonate to 10 years<br>Neonate to adult |
| Membrane abnormality (decreased red cell deformability) | Congenital – splenic destruction | Hereditary spherocytosis<br>Hereditary pyropoikilocytosis | Neonate to adult<br>Neonate |
| Antibody-mediated membrane damage | Fetomaternal Rh and ABO incompatibility<br>Autoantibodies ± complement reacting with red cell membrane<br>Infection<br>Drugs<br>Autoimmune disease | Haemolytic disease of newborn<br>Autoimmune haemolytic anaemia | *In utero* to 24 hours<br>Any age |
| Toxic membrane damage | Infection<br>Heavy metals | *Clostridium perfringens*<br>Wilson disease | Any age<br>Late childhood to adult |
| Mechanical membrane damage | Membrane damage | Disseminated intravascular coagulopathy<br>Haemolytic–uraemic syndrome<br>Cardiac prosthesis | Any age<br>Childhood |

G6PD, glucose-6-phosphate dehydrogenase.

Haemolysis may be intravascular or may occur by phagocytosis within the spleen or liver. Intravascular haemolysis occurs in some autoimmune haemolytic anaemias, acute haemolysis in glucose-6-phosphate dehydrogenase (G6PD) deficiency, and acute transfusion reactions. Free haemoglobin is released and combines with haptoglobin. The complex is cleared by the reticuloendothelial system of the liver and spleen. If the free plasma haemoglobin concentration exceeds the haptoglobin binding capacity, haemoglobinuria occurs. The colour of the urine may vary from pink through brown to almost black, depending on the amount of free haemoglobin excreted.

If haemolysis occurs predominantly in the reticuloendothelial system (autoimmune haemolytic anaemia, membrane abnormalities), there is little free haemoglobin in plasma. Haemoglobin is converted to bilirubin within phagocytes, transported to the liver bound to albumin, then conjugated and excreted into the bile. Jaundice is variable, depending on the rate of haemolysis and hepatic conjugation. To compensate for the reduced red cell survival, the bone marrow increases its output of red cells, releasing immature reticulocytes and, in acute severe haemolysis, nucleated red cells into the peripheral blood.

### Intracellular enzyme defects

Mature red cells lack a nucleus and intracellular organelles necessary for synthesis of proteins and generation of adenosine triphosphate (ATP) via oxidative pathways. Energy production for maintenance of the integrity of the red cell is via one of the two glycolytic metabolic pathways within it. About 95% of glucose metabolism is via the anaerobic Embden–Myerhof pathway and 5% through the hexose monophosphate shunt (pentose phosphate pathway). Enzyme defects in either pathway result in oxidative damage and haemolysis. Deficiencies or abnormalities of G6PD, the first enzyme in the hexose monophosphate shunt, are extremely common worldwide. All the documented enzyme deficiencies of the Embden–Myerhof pathway resulting in haemolytic anaemias are rare. Examples are pyruvate kinase deficiency and glucose phosphate isomerase deficiency.

#### *G6PD deficiency*

This X-linked enzyme deficiency is the commonest inherited disorder of the red cell. It is expressed fully in hemizygous males and in homozygous females. Heterozygous females show a variable level of enzyme activity due to variation in X-chromosome inactivation. There are more than 200 variant enzymes and the clinical expression of the disorder is variable, with four major clinical syndromes. Neonatal jaundice is common in the Chinese and Mediterranean variants; favism (acute haemolysis after ingestion of broad beans or inhalation of pollen) is a feature of the Mediterranean variant, whereas oxidative-stress-induced haemolysis (drugs, infection), although common to all variants, is the predominant feature in affected individuals of African descent. Individuals of northern European descent have chronic moderate haemolysis, whereas other variants experience haemolysis only with appropriate stress. Patients typically present severely anaemic with dark urine, having been well until 1–2 days prior to presentation. The precipitating factor is usually identifiable on history. Because of the rapidity of the fall in haemoglobin, there often is profound lethargy and restlessness at presentation.

Examination of the blood film shows polychromasia and anisocytosis, and typically 'blister' cells. The diagnosis is established by enzyme assay in mature red cells. Enzyme levels are higher in reticulocytes in some variants and a normal enzyme level at the time of an acute haemolytic episode does not exclude the diagnosis. Management is to avoid precipitating factors. Patients having acute crises may require blood transfusion, although a brisk reticulocyte response may result in rapid spontaneous recovery.

**Clinical example**

Thomas was an 8-year-old boy from Hong Kong. He presented with the onset of pallor over 24 hours and was passing very dark urine. He had recently been treated for tonsillitis. He had no past history of serious illness. On examination, apart from marked pallor, splenomegaly was present. His urine contained haemoglobin. Blood tests revealed a haemoglobin concentration of 40 g/L with a raised reticulocyte response. Blister cells were evident on the blood film. The G6PD assay was borderline normal and assays on the parents showed that Thomas's mother was heterozygous for G6PD deficiency. One month after this episode, Thomas was shown to have a severe deficiency of G6PD activity. The earlier borderline result was caused by the presence of many young red cells with high G6PD activity.

### Intrinsic membrane defects

Abnormalities of the red cell membrane result in alterations of cell shape, usually due to changes in transmembrane electrolyte flux. Changes in cell shape cause decreased deformability, splenic trapping and destruction within the spleen, resulting in chronic haemolytic anaemia. The commonest membrane abnormality is hereditary spherocytosis, most commonly a dominantly inherited condition.

### Hereditary spherocytosis

There is a marked variability in the severity of haemolysis in this condition. Neonatal jaundice is common. Some children present with anaemia in infancy, whereas others remain asymptomatic until a haemolytic or aplastic crisis occurs in association with a viral infection. Hypersplenism or gallstones may result in the presentation of a previously asymptomatic patient with well-compensated haemolysis. A positive family history is often obtained. Examination reveals pallor, often mild jaundice and a variable degree of splenomegaly. The diagnosis is suggested by the presence of spherocytes in the peripheral blood (see Fig. 16.1.1C). The best test currently to confirm the diagnosis is the E5M test. In this test, the dye eosin-5-maleimide reacts covalently with Lys-430 on the extracellular loop of band 3 protein. Reduced E5M staining is seen in patients with hereditary spherocytosis, congenital dyserythropoietic anaemia type II and South-East Asian ovalocytosis and cryohydrocytosis.

Folic acid supplements should be given. Blood transfusion may be required for anaemia resulting from inadequately compensated haemolysis and for aplastic crises, during which the haemoglobin level may fall precipitously. Aplastic crises usually are associated with parvovirus B19 infection. Haemolysis is abolished by splenectomy. Overwhelming postsplenectomy infection may occur, particularly in children less than 5 years of age. Pneumococcal, meningococcal and *Haemophilus influenzae* b immunizations should be given before splenectomy, and penicillin prophylaxis should be continued indefinitely after splenectomy.

Decisions about splenectomy should be based on the following:

- degree of haemolysis and anaemia
- age
- size of spleen
- presence of gallstones.

**Clinical example**

Angela was 9 years of age. In the neonatal period she required exchange transfusion for severe jaundice. She had always been pale and had a small appetite. With upper respiratory tract infections, her pallor increased and jaundice had appeared. At 2 years of age hereditary spherocytosis was diagnosed and folic acid supplements were commenced. Angela's father also had this condition. She presented with abdominal pain, pallor, icterus and splenomegaly of 6 cm. Ultrasound examination confirmed the presence of gallstones. Following pneumococcal and *Haemophilus influenzae* b vaccination, splenectomy and cholecystectomy with removal of gallstones was undertaken. Prophylactic penicillin was commenced after the surgery and would continue indefinitely.

#### Extrinsic membrane damage

Acquired membrane damage leading to haemolysis can result from antibody–antigen reactions, mechanical insults (e.g. intravascular prosthetic patches), burns, toxins (e.g. copper) and infective agents (e.g. *Clostridium perfringens*).

### Antibody-mediated haemolysis

The binding of immunoglobulin or complement, or a combination of the two, to the red cell membrane may result in premature cell destruction or immune haemolysis. The antibody involved may be immunoglobulin (Ig) G (warm antibody) or IgM (cold antibody). Immune haemolytic anaemias may be classified as follows.

*Isoimmune haemolysis in the newborn*

- Rhesus incompatibility (mother Rh negative, baby Rh positive)
- ABO incompatibility (mother group O, baby group A or B).

*Autoimmune haemolysis in children*

- *Idiopathic.* In many instances of IgG warm-antibody-mediated haemolysis, no definite aetiological agent is identified.
- *Postinfectious.* Many common infectious diseases, such as measles (IgG), infectious mononucleosis (IgM) and mycoplasmal infection (IgM) may be associated with acute haemolysis.
- *Drug related.* This is very uncommon in children. Some drugs (e.g. α-methyldopa) stimulate the production of antibodies that are directed against red cell antigens but not against the drug. A second mechanism involves a drug, such as penicillin, binding to the red cell membrane, with antibody to the drug being formed and attaching to the drug. The antibody-coated red cells then undergo destruction in the spleen. The third mechanism of drug-related haemolysis involves the deposition of antibody–antigen complexes on the red cell surface with activation of complement and brisk intravascular haemolysis.
- *Associated with connective tissue disease or malignancy.* This is rare in childhood but may be associated with systemic lupus erythematosus in adolescence.

Presentation of a child with immune-mediated haemolysis is usually acute with rapid onset of pallor, severe anaemia and dark urine. Jaundice may be present. Life-threatening anaemia may develop rapidly, with vasoconstriction, cardiac failure and hypoxia. Modest splenomegaly is often present.

The peripheral blood shows a predominantly normocytic anaemia with spherocytes (IgG), or rouleaux formation/red cell agglutination (IgM) (see Fig. 16.1.1D). As a compensating reticulocytosis develops, polychromasia and macrocytosis are seen. A positive direct antiglobulin test (DAT) confirms the diagnosis. The specificity of the positive DAT classifies the type of antibody involved. The commonest are warm IgG antibodies, but cold IgM antibodies are found in association with mycoplasmal infection and infectious mononucleosis.

Urgent blood transfusion may be required. In some cases the presence of strong autoantibody in recipient plasma makes the provision of compatible blood and the exclusion of underlying alloantibodies difficult. Transfused cells may be haemolysed rapidly and careful observation is required. Repeated transfusions may be necessary. Adequate hydration must be maintained to avoid renal tubular damage from haemoglobinuria. Where a warm antibody is identified, steroid therapy is instituted and maintained until the Hb concentration stabilizes, then tapered gradually. Haemolysis is usually self-limiting over the course of days to weeks. Occasional patients may have severe ongoing haemolysis, or frequent relapses. Plasma exchange, exchange transfusion or high-dose immunoglobulin may be useful but, if these measures fail, splenectomy may be life-saving.

### Blood loss

Blood loss, if acute, results in vasoconstriction, then tachycardia and finally hypotension. The haemoglobin, if measured very early in the course of a bleeding episode, will be normal or only slightly reduced. When there has been time for haemodilution to occur, the haemoglobin level falls. A compensatory reticulocytosis occurs after approximately 48 hours. Chronic blood loss results in iron-deficiency anaemia.

## Blood transfusion therapy

The majority of children with anaemia do not require transfusion therapy. The critical questions that must be addressed in deciding whether to transfuse are:

- Has the patient evidence of cardiovascular decompensation?
- Is the anaemia likely to be progressive and at what rate?
- What is the likely timing of spontaneous recovery?
- Are there alternative therapies that are likely to succeed?

Major acute blood loss due to trauma, acute haemolytic anaemias and chemotherapy-induced anaemia are the most likely causes of acute anaemia to require transfusion. The exact transfusion trigger will be a function of the physiological considerations discussed previously in this chapter. Major haemoglobinopathy and bone marrow failure syndromes may require chronic transfusion programmes. Nutritional anaemia rarely requires transfusion therapy in the absence of cardiovascular instability.

There are specific indications for exchange transfusion in neonates and, for example, older children with sickle cell disease.

### Risks of blood transfusion therapy

Parents worry about viral infections from blood transfusion, although this remains an extremely low risk. If the clinician has used the principles above to determine the need for transfusion, then the risks of not transfusing usually far outweigh the risks of transfusion. In terms of viral safety, Australia has one of the safest blood supplies in the world. Factors contributing to this are that every blood donor is a volunteer (unpaid) and must meet strict selection criteria, including answering a comprehensive questionnaire about their health and lifestyle, and undergoing a personal interview by trained staff at which they sign a declaration. Every blood donation is screened for syphilis, hepatitis B and C, HIV and human T-cell leukaemia/lymphoma virus (HTLV). Two types of test for hepatitis C and HIV are now performed – antibody testing and nucleic acid testing (detects viral materials directly and therefore infection at an earlier stage). Only blood that is negative for all these tests is released for use.

#### Current risks of transfusion transmitted infection

Australian Red Cross Blood Service (ARCBS) uses sophisticated mathematical models to calculate the current infection risks for blood transfusions in Australia, as shown in Table 16.1.6. These risks are very small compared to the risks of everyday living. The chance of being killed in a road accident in Australia is about 1 in 10 000.

#### Non-viral risks associated with blood and blood products

ABO incompatibility remains one of the most common fatal complications of blood transfusion and most cases are due to avoidable errors (most commonly

| **Table 16.1.6 Risks based on Australian Red Cross Blood Service (ARCBS) data, 1 July 2000 to 30 June 2003** | |
|---|---|
| Infection | Residual risk with tested blood per unit transfused |
| HIV | 1 in 7 299 000 |
| Hepatitis C | 1 in 3 636 000 |
| Hepatitis B | 1 in 1 339 000 |
| HTLV | Considerably less than 1 in 1 000 000 |
| Syphilis | Considerably less than 1 in 1 000 000 |
| Variant CJD | Unknown: possible and cannot be excluded |

CJD, Creutzfeldt–Jakob disease; HIV, human immunodeficiency virus; HTLV, human T-cell leukaemia/lymphoma virus.

associated with patient/sample identification). Table 16.1.7 gives estimates of risk based on reports from a number of countries, which are subject to the problem of underestimation due to lack of reporting and recognition of transfusion reactions (hence the broad ranges). The transfusion of autologous blood is not without risk and the same indications apply as for the use of homologous blood.

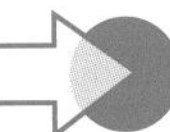

## Practical points

**Deciding if a patient needs a red cell transfusion**

- The actual haemoglobin level, although important, does not alone determine the need for a transfusion.
- Consider the cause and time course of the anaemia. Haematinic deficiencies rarely need transfusion. Acute blood loss (especially if ongoing) and acute haemolysis frequently need transfusion.
- Coexistent disease is important in determining the likely ability of the patient to cope with a degree of anaemia. Cardiac and lung function, as well as haemoglobin level, are important determinants of oxygen delivery. The ability to maintain oxygen delivery is the key question when considering most acute red cell transfusion questions.
- Reduced oxygen saturation measured by pulse oximetry may reflect lung disease, cyanotic heart disease or abnormal Hb with reduced oxygen affinity (e.g. methaemoglobin), and may reduce the transfusion threshold. In the absence of adequate cardiac output or Hb, normal pulse oximetry does not equate to adequate tissue oxygen delivery.
- Clinical signs of cardiac stress (increased heart rate) or hypoxia (restlessness, altered conscious state/behaviour) are critical indicators of the need for urgent transfusion. In children, hypotension is a late sign in acute blood loss. These factors should be monitored closely in anaemic patients. In a child with cardiovascular decompensation from anaemia, do not delay urgent transfusion therapy in favour of thorough investigation. A live child who remains a diagnostic dilemma is better than a dead child in whom you know the diagnosis.

**Table 16.1.7 Non-viral serious risks of blood transfusion (per unit transfused unless specified)**

| | Morbidity | Mortality |
|---|---|---|
| Bacterial sepsis | | |
| Red cells | 1 in 40 000–500 000 | 1 in 4 000 000–8 000 000 |
| Platelets | 1 in 10 000–100 000 | 1 in 50 000–500 000 |
| Haemolytic reactions | | |
| Acute | 1 in 12 000–38 000 | 1 in 600 000–1 500 000 |
| Delayed | 1 in 1000–12 000 | 1 in 2 500 000 |
| Anaphylaxis – IgA deficiency | 1 in 20 000–50 000 | |
| Fluid overload/cardiac failure | 1 in 100–700 per patient | |
| TRALI* | 1 in 5000–100 000 | 1 in 5 million |
| TA-GVHD† | Rare | 90% cases fatal |

*Transfusion-related acute lung injury (TRALI) is characterized by acute respiratory distress (within hours of transfusion) with non-cardiogenic pulmonary oedema. Full recovery in 48 hours is usual if the patient is well resuscitated/supported. TRALI is likely to be significantly under-reported.

†Transfusion-associated graft versus host disease (TA-GVHD) is due to viable engraftment of T lymphocytes and usually affects severely immunocompromised patients or recipients who share an HLA haplotype with a specific donor. Gamma-irradiation of blood products for specific at-risk groups of patients (refer to hospital guidelines) prevents this rare but usually fatal event.

# 16.2 Abnormal bleeding and clotting

Ben Saxon, Chris Barnes

Bleeding disorders range from those that are severe and potentially life-threatening through to mild disorders that may be difficult to distinguish from normal.

Abnormal bleeding is the result of a disorder of one of the following:
- the platelets
- the coagulation mechanism
- the blood vessel or its supporting tissue.

## Clinical approach to diagnosis

As a general rule, history-taking, physical examination and a small number of relatively simple laboratory tests will find most causes of abnormal bleeding. The history, with particular reference to the past and family history, will usually provide the most valuable information.

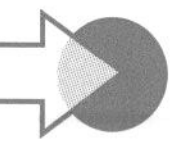

**Practical points**

**Bleeding disorder assessment**
- History to determine normal from abnormal is the most valuable tool.
- Simple coagulation tests such as platelet count, activated partial thromboplastin time (aPTT), prothrombin time (PT/ international normalized ratio (INR)) and fibrinogen will confirm the majority of diagnoses.
- Mucosal bleeding needs assessment for von Willebrand disorder.
- Assessment of other family members is often required.

### History

#### What is abnormal?

The main question to answer in the history is whether the bleeding symptoms are within or outside normal limits. Isolated bruises over the shins are common, whereas spontaneous petechiae are abnormal. Finger-induced epistaxis is common and not indicative of a bleeding disorder; however, recurrent nose bleeds lasting for more than 10 minutes or leading to anaemia are often related to a bleeding disorder. Table 16.2.1 gives some clinical guidance.

#### When did the bleeding start?

*Prenatal and neonatal*
- Congenital infection may result in a bleeding disorder.
- Mucosal bleeding occurs with haemorrhagic disease of the newborn.
- Umbilical stump bleeding is associated with factor XIII deficiency and dysfibrinogenaemias.
- Intracranial haemorrhage may occur with factor deficiencies and with neonatal alloimmune thrombocytopenia.
- Prolonged bleeding following circumcision is suggestive of haemophilia and may be the presenting feature of haemorrhagic disease of the newborn.

*Early childhood*
- Bleeding often implies a congenital defect.
- Bruising, muscle and joint bleeding is strongly suggestive of haemophilia.
- Petechiae and mucosal bleeding suggests a platelet problem or von Willebrand disorder.

*Sudden onset*
- Usually indicates an acute problem such as immune thrombocytopenic purpura.
- Non-accidental injury may have a haemorrhagic presentation with inadequate explanations for each specific bruise, which may have an unusual distribution (see Chapter 3.9). Skeletal trauma and other stigmata of non-accidental injury may be present.

#### Where is the bleeding?

Specific bleeding sites have characteristic associations:
- *Joint bleeding*: haemophilia A and B
- *Nasal mucosa*: local irritation; von Willebrand disorder and platelet dysfunction
- *Gums, periosteum, skin*: scurvy
- *Gastrointestinal*: haemorrhagic disease of the newborn in babies; liver disease in older children
- *Retro-orbital*: haematological malignancy or disseminated solid tumour.

**Table 16.2.1 What symptoms and signs may be related to a bleeding disorder?**

| Site | Within normal limits | May be abnormal and due to a number of causes | Often due to a bleeding disorder |
|---|---|---|---|
| Nose | Finger-induced | Unilateral | Recurrent, requiring medical intervention or causing anaemia |
| Oral | Blood on brush | Gum ooze < 30 min | Gum ooze > 30 min |
| Gut | Rectal fissure, blood in nappy | Haematemesis, melaena | |
| Menstrual loss | 4–7 days | 'Same as Mum' | Loss leading to anaemia or transfusion |
| Skin | Shins do not count | Bony prominences | Spontaneous bruising over soft areas, laceration bleeding > 30 min |
| Joints and muscles | | Trauma induced | Spontaneous |
| Intracranial | | Neonatal, trauma-induced | Spontaneous |

### What is the context of bleeding?

*Family history*
Haemophilia A and B are X-linked; most von Willebrand disorder subtypes and haemorrhagic hereditary telangiectasia are recessive and several platelet function disorders are dominantly inherited. Clinical penetrance in haemophilia carriers and von Willebrand disorder may be variable. It is important to review whether the family has a history of bleeding complicating surgical challenges and it may be helpful to explore any history of menorrhagia in family members.

*Other aspects of history*
Easy bruising, bruising at abnormal sites, prolonged bleeding following trivial trauma or bleeding following surgery and dental extractions are all indications for investigation. Bleeding may also occur in the presence of disorders such as systemic lupus erythematosus, liver disease, extrahepatic portal hypertension, gross splenomegaly, giant haemangiomas, reticuloendothelial malignancies and leukaemia.

*Drug ingestion*
Drugs may produce abnormal bleeding through:

- *depression of clotting factors*: anticoagulants, liver toxins
- *bone marrow depression*: chloramphenicol, cytotoxic agents, radiation
- *antigen–antibody reactions with platelet membranes*: quinine group of drugs
- *direct inhibition of enzymes in platelets*: aspirin effects on platelet cyclo-oxygenase.

## Physical examination

The following should be noted on physical examination.

### The type of skin bleeding

Petechiae alone strongly suggest a platelet or vessel problem, whereas ecchymoses alone suggest a factor deficiency. Combined petechiae and ecchymoses suggest a severe disorder, often of platelet origin.

### The site of the bleeding

Confirmation of history, defining the number of all different bleeding sites, and assessment of severity of bleed and functional implications are all important aspects for both diagnosis and management.

### Splenomegaly

Hypersplenism occurs when a large spleen removes platelets from the circulation, leading to bleeding. The problem is the underlying cause of the splenomegaly. Hepatomegaly, splenomegaly, lymphadenopathy and/or anaemia, in association with bleeding, strongly suggest leukaemia.

### Miscellaneous

Bleeding in association with eczema is a feature of Wiskott–Aldrich syndrome; telangiectasia and mucosal bleeding are typical of hereditary haemorrhagic telangiectasia. Hyperelastic skin, hyperextensible joints and bruising are associated with Ehlers–Danlos syndrome.

### Investigation of bleeding in childhood

The tests in Table 16.2.2 are the most important.

#### Other tests

Measurement of von Willebrand factor level (antigen), activity (ristocetin co-factor and/or collagen binding assay) and factor VIII level are required to diagnose von Willebrand disorder. The bleeding time has lost favour because of its scarring potential but is characteristically prolonged in thrombocytopenia (normal 2–7 min), von Willebrand disorder and platelet function disorders, and is normal in other coagulation disorders.

## Bleeding due to platelet disorders

Bleeding disorders resulting from platelet abnormalities are usually due to thrombocytopenia but may be due to qualitative platelet defects. The various types of inherited and acquired thrombocytopenia are listed in Table 16.2.3.

### Immune thrombocytopenic purpura

Immune thrombocytopenic purpura is the most common acquired bleeding disorder in children. It may be acute or chronic (defined as lasting longer than 12 months), episodic or continuous. Common to all clinical variations is the marked reduction in platelet life span due to immune-mediated splenic sequestration.

Features of typical acute immune thrombocytopenic purpura:

- 80–90% of paediatric immune thrombocytopenic purpura cases
- preceding viral illness is common
- peak age 2–5 years
- abrupt onset of bleeding
- mucosal and skin bleeding
- petechiae common
- otherwise normal examination – no lymphadenopathy or hepatosplenomegaly
- platelet count usually < $20 \times 10^9$/L
- normal red cell and white cell parameters.

There is no need for other investigations if these 'typical' features are present.

**Table 16.2.2 Interpretation of initial blood tests in children with abnormal bleeding**

| Test | Result | More common causes | Less common causes |
|---|---|---|---|
| Blood count | Isolated thrombocytopenia | ITP<br>NAIT | Congenital anomaly<br>Early SAA |
| | Pancytopenia | Leukaemia<br>SAA | Myelodysplasia<br>Osteopetrosis |
| | High white cell count and thrombocytopenia | Leukaemia<br>Infections | Myeloproliferative disorders |
| Blood film | Thrombocytopenia and red cell fragmentation | Microangiopathic anaemia (e.g. HUS, DIC) | |
| | Small platelets | | Wiscott–Aldrich syndrome |
| | Giant platelets | | Bernard–Soulier syndrome |
| Prothrombin time (PT/INR) | Isolated prolongation | Vitamin K deficiency<br>Warfarin therapy | Congenital factor VII deficiency |
| | Prolonged PT and aPTT | DIC<br>Septicaemia<br>Liver disease | Factor X, factor V, prothrombin or fibrinogen deficiency |
| aPTT | Isolated prolongation | Unfractionated heparin therapy<br>Haemophilia A or B<br>'Lupus anticoagulant' | Factor XI deficiency<br>Contact system* deficiency |
| Fibrinogen | Low | DIC | Congenital fibrinogen disorders |
| All tests | Normal | Non-accidental injury<br>Henoch–Schönlein purpura | |

*Contact system refers to factor XII, prekallikrein and high-molecular-weight kininogen.
aPTT, activated partial thromboplastin time; DIC, disseminated intravascular coagulation; HUS, haemolytic–uraemic syndrome; INR, international normalized ratio; ITP, immune thrombocytopenic purpura; NAIT, neonatal alloimmune thrombocytopenia; PT, prothrombin time; SAA, severe aplastic anaemia.

| Table 16.2.3 Inherited and acquired thrombocytopenias | | |
|---|---|---|
| | Disorder | Key Information |
| **Acquired** | | |
| Neonatal | Immune thrombocytopenia | Neonatal alloimmune or maternal autoimmune |
| | Intrauterine infection | TORCH |
| | Pre-eclampsia | |
| | Birth asphyxia | |
| | Giant haemangioma | 'Kasabach–Merritt syndrome' features platelet consumption |
| Any age | Immune thrombocytopenia (ITP) | The most common acquired thrombocytopenia |
| **Inherited** | | |
| With platelet dysfunction | Examples include Bernard–Soulier syndrome and Wiskott–Aldrich syndrome | Rare |
| Without platelet dysfunction | Examples include Fanconi anaemia and Alport syndrome | Rare |
| | Mediterranean macrothrombocytopenia | Large platelets, autosomal dominant |

TORCH, toxoplasmosis, other (e.g. HIV and parvovirus B19), rubella, cytomegalovirus, herpes simplex.

Differential diagnosis is predominantly that of evolving aplastic anaemia.

*Chronic immune thrombocytopenic purpura* occurs in 10–20% of cases and often has an insidious onset in children aged over 7 years; it affects girls more commonly than boys. *Recurrent immune thrombocytopenic purpura* is rare and is characterized by thrombocytopenia at more than 3-month intervals.

Treatment approaches to *immune thrombocytopenic purpura* are shown in Table 16.2.4.

## Bleeding due to qualitative platelet defects

The child with a functional platelet defect will have a normal platelet count but abnormal platelet function test results. These tests analyse aggregation of platelets in response to several stimuli. The more common disorders in this group are the 'aspirin-like' syndrome and platelet storage pool disorders. The most severe disorder is Glanzmann disease. Before undertaking platelet function studies, it must be ensured that there has been no ingestion of aspirin for at least 7 days.

### Clinical example

Chloe presented at the age of 4 years, 2 weeks after a viral upper respiratory infection, with a 3-day history of a petechial rash on her face and gum bleeding with toothbrushing. Examination revealed several fresh skin bruises along with the petechiae. There was no hepatosplenomegaly and the only palpable lymph nodes were slightly tender tonsillar nodes, 2 cm in diameter. The only abnormality on full blood examination was a platelet count of $9 \times 10^9$/L. Chloe was treated with prednisolone 4 mg/kg daily in three divided doses for 4 days as an outpatient, with alternate daily platelet counts. On the second day of treatment her platelet count was $65 \times 10^9$/L and the count became normal within 5 days. She had no further episodes of thrombocytopenia.

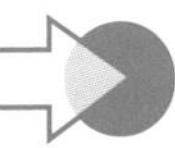

### Practical points

**Acute bleeding history**

- Splenomegaly, lymphadenopathy or hepatomegaly indicate a systemic illness (e.g. Epstein–Barr virus infection, leukaemia).
- Always examine the fundi for bleeding changes.
- Careful review of the blood film is important to exclude other causes of thrombocytopenia.
- Anaemia and reticulocyte response aid determination of severity and duration of bleeding.
- Assess for the presence of 'wet' purpura (mucosal bleeding) as some authorities claim that this may be associated with an increased likelihood of intracranial bleeding.

## Bleeding due to coagulation disorders

The coagulation system, as monitored by the available investigations, is shown in Figure 16.2.1. Initiation of coagulation and the production of a fibrin clot is shown in Figure 16.2.2.

**Table 16.2.4 Treatment options for acute immune thrombocytopenic purpura with either bleeding problems or if the platelet count is less than $10 \times 10^9$/L**

| Treatment option | Advantages | Disadvantages | Time course to resolution |
|---|---|---|---|
| **First-line therapies** | | | |
| Conservative | No drug side-effects | Longest time to platelet count $> 20 \times 10^9$/L<br>$< 1\%$ risk of ICH while awaiting platelet recovery | 75% remission in 4–6 weeks<br>15% take 4–6 months |
| Corticosteroids (standard dose*) | No blood product exposure | Steroid side-effects‡ common | 1 week |
| Corticosteroids (high dose†) | No blood product exposure<br>Rapid rise in platelets | Steroid side-effects‡ less common | Platelets $> 20 \times 10^9$/L: 2 days<br>Platelets $> 50 \times 10^9$/L: 3–4 days |
| Intravenous gammaglobulin (IVIG)§ | Rapid rise in platelets | Pooled blood product with at least two viral inactivation steps | Platelets $> 20 \times 10^9$/L: 1–2 days<br>Platelets $> 50 \times 10^9$/L: 3 days |
| **Second-line therapies** | | | |
| Anti-Rh(D) antibody | | Only useful in Rhesus-positive children<br>Similar efficacy to IVIG and steroids | |
| Splenectomy | Most useful in children > 5 years old with chronic ITP | Immunizations for meningococcus, *Haemophilus influenzae* and pneumococcus are mandatory<br>Lifelong antibiotic prophylaxis | Rapid in the majority |
| **Evolving therapies** | | | |
| Thrombopoietins | Patients with refractory chronic ITP may respond | Few short-term and long-term clinical data in paediatrics | Variable |
| Rituximab | Patients with refractory chronic ITP may respond | Profound B-cell immune suppression | Variable |

*Standard dose: prednisolone 2 mg/kg body weight daily for 21 days.
†High dose: prednisolone 4 mg/kg body weight daily for 4 days.
‡Steroid side-effects include gastric irritation, transient diabetes and other metabolic derangements, immune suppression, cushingoid body fat distribution, growth delay, osteopenia and rarely avascular necrosis of the femoral head.
§IVIG 0.8 g/kg body weight, repeat within 1–7 days if platelet count remains $< 10 \times 10^9$/L or any platelet count with problematic bleeding. Lower doses may be equally effective. IVIG side-effects include flu-like symptoms and rarely transient aseptic meningitis. Blood products may theoretically transmit viral and prion particles.
ICH, intracranial haemorrhage; ITP, immune thrombocytopenic purpura.

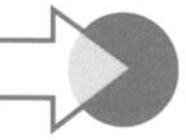

## Practical points

**Understanding coagulation**

- The aPTT and PT/INR are screening tests that represent how various 'factors' interact in the test tube; they are useful tests to determine which factor may be low.
- *In vivo* coagulation does not occur as a 'cascade', rather a series of positive feedback reactions starting with tissue factor and factor VII and culminating in a thrombin burst.
- Clotting occurs at the site of injury by thrombin cleaving fibrinogen to fibrin.
- Thrombin inhibits coagulation by binding with thrombomodulin on normal blood vessels.

## Clinical example

Albert was born at term, received intramuscular vitamin K, and developed a large bruise in his thigh. No circumcision was performed. He always seemed to have fingerprint bruises under his arms from being picked up. When he began sitting unaided he developed buttock bruising, and when he began walking he presented to the accident and emergency department with a swollen, hot right ankle. The joint had virtually no movement and ultrasonography confirmed a fluid-filled joint. The history was highly suggestive of haemophilia. The INR was normal, the aPTT was 90 seconds and the factor VIII level was less than 1%. Haemophilia A was diagnosed and prophylaxis with 25 U/kg recombinant factor VIII three times per week was commenced.

At the age of 4 years Albert fell from a chair on to his occiput after missing a dose of prophylaxis. Within 2 hours he had a falling level of consciousness and respiratory depression. Computed tomography diagnosed a subdural haematoma. Treatment with high-dose factor VIII and neurosurgical intervention led to an uneventful recovery.

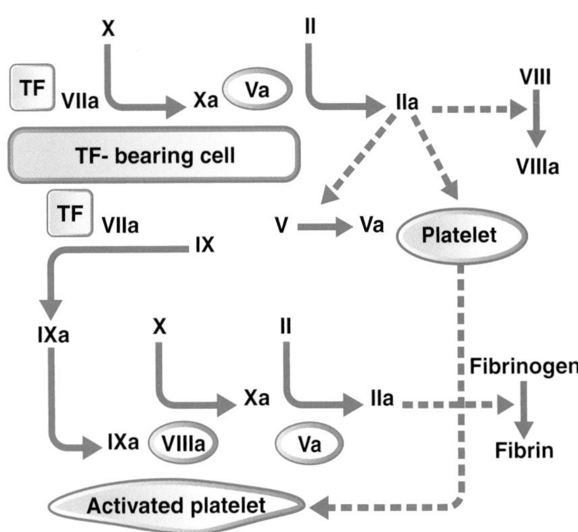


Fig. 16.2.2 Initiation of coagulation and the production of a fibrin clot. TF, tissue factor.

## Haemophilia

### Prevalence

- Haemophilia A (factor VIII deficiency): 5–10 males per 100 000 population
- Haemophilia B (Christmas disease, factor IX deficiency): 0.5–1 per 100 000
- Factor XI deficiency (haemophilia C): rare
- Other factor deficiencies: exceedingly rare.

### Genetics

Haemophilia A and B are both X-linked. Up to one-third of all new cases of haemophilia are due to new mutations. Female carriers sometimes have low levels of factor VIII or IX and may have a bleeding disorder.

### Severity

Severity is defined by plasma factor level and correlates with clinical severity:

- *severe*: < 2%, frequent spontaneous deep tissue bleeding
- *moderate*: 2–5%, infrequent spontaneous bleeding
- *mild*: 6–30%, bleeding with trauma and surgery, not spontaneously.

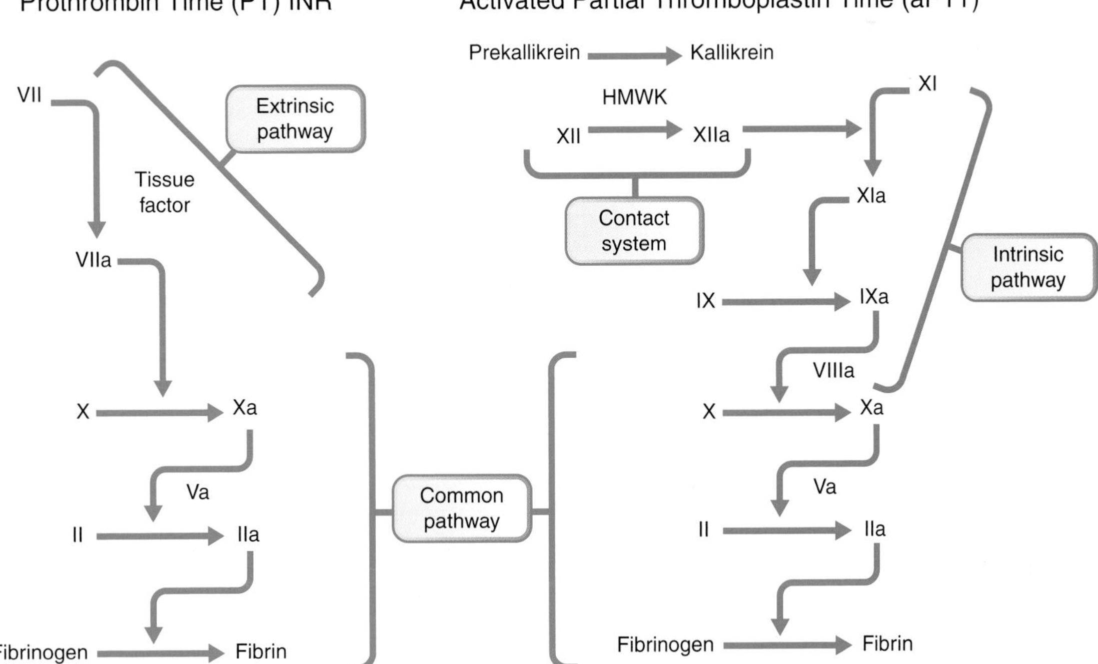


Fig. 16.2.1 The coagulation system as measured by initial blood tests: prothrombin time (PT) and activated partial thromboplastin time (aPTT). HMWK, high-molecular-weight kininogen; 'a' indicates activated factor. This figure does not represent *in vivo* coagulation, rather the coagulation factors (in test tubes) that influence the PT and aPTT. INR, international normalized ratio, is a function of the PT.

## Clinical manifestations

*Neonatal*

A positive family history or known carrier status allows for definitive diagnosis in the newborn period. Cord blood genetics are most reliable. Some laboratories perform factor VIII or factor IX assays on cord blood, but technical difficulties may arise and results should be interpreted with caution. There is prolonged bleeding following circumcision. Intracranial haemorrhage is suspicious of a bleeding disorder in the term neonate.

*Early childhood*

Skin and soft tissue bleeds are common in the first year and beyond. Haemarthroses usually only occur once the child is walking. The ankles are common bleeding sites in young children; elbow and knee bleeding (Fig. 16.2.3) occur more commonly in older children.

*Specific bleeds*

Bleeding into the forearm may occlude the neurovascular bundle and cause a Volkmann ischaemic contracture. Bleeding into the posterior pharyngeal wall may interfere with respiration and cause dysphagia. Iliopsoas bleeding may be complicated by femoral nerve compression. Intracranial vascular accident is the cause of death in 7% of patients with haemophilia. Haematuria is common in adolescents and is seldom serious.

*Chronic illness*

There is synovial hypertrophy and arthritis. Psychosocial problems arise as a result of chronic illness, lifestyle restrictions and the need for injections. HIV/AIDS occurred in more than 50% of patients receiving blood products in the years 1980–1985. Hepatitis C infection is also common prior to viral identification, screening and viral inactivation of plasma products. Variant Creutzfeldt–Jakob disease (vCJD) is a prion disease. It has been shown to be transmissible in blood products and is not removed by current viral inactivation processes. Fortunately there have been no cases of vCJD described in patients with haemophilia.

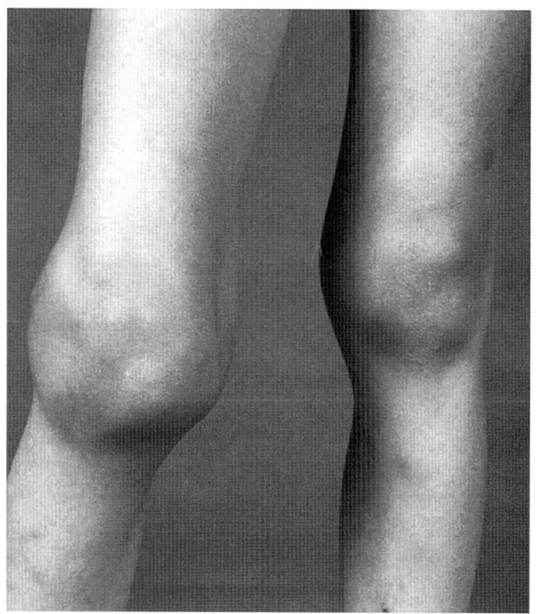

Fig. 16.2.3 Haemarthrosis of the right knee in a boy with haemophilia.

## Complications

Inhibitors are anti-factor VIII or anti-factor IX antibodies, which prevent regular doses of factor concentrate from working. Central lines may be required to ensure venous access in young children. These may be complicated by infection or large vein thrombosis.

## Management

*Correct or prevent the bleeding tendency*

- Mild and moderate haemophilia A often responds to desmopressin acetate infusions to increase plasma factor VIII levels.
- One unit of factor VIII per kilogram body weight given intravenously increases the factor VIII level by approximately 2%.
- Life-threatening bleeds require plasma factor levels greater than 80%.
- Most other bleeds require plasma factor levels of 30–60%.
- Prophylactic infusions of 25–40 U/kg three times a week 'convert' severe disease into moderate disease, thereby decreasing the risk of spontaneous bleeding.

*Choice of product*

- Most developed countries, including Australia, now offer recombinant product to all patients with haemophilia.
- Plasma-derived factor products are still available. These are screened for HIV and hepatitis B and C, and then undergo two viral inactivation steps in the processing.

*Orthopaedic*

- Rest, immobilization, ice, compression and elevation (RICE) are usually sufficient to control pain.
- Splinting followed by physiotherapy and exercises when pain has settled preserves function.

*Haemophilia centres*

- Provide a focus of education and training for patient and family.
- Multidisciplinary group with expertise in haemophilia management.

*Inhibitors*
- Inhibitors are found in up to 30% of patients.
- At least half of these are low-titre inhibitors, which can be treated by high-dose factor VIII.
- High-titre inhibitors require 'immune tolerance' therapy for eradication of inhibitor, and infusions of the factor VIII and IX bypass agent, recombinant factor VIIa, to treat bleeds.

**Clinical example**

Vanessa was a 13-year-old girl with menorrhagia since menarche. She had always had 'easy bruising' and required a transfusion after tonsillectomy due to excessive bleeding. She often bled from her gums after brushing her teeth. Her older sister and her mother both had heavy periods but neither had had severe postsurgical bleeding. Platelet count, INR and aPTT were all normal. Von Willebrand antigen was 30%, activity (ristocetin co-factor) 25% and factor VIII 35%. Vanessa was diagnosed with mild von Willebrand disorder.

### Von Willebrand disorder

This disorder has the following features:
- Quantitative (types 1 and 3) or qualitative (type 2) defect in von Willebrand factor (vWF), a molecule that assists platelet adhesion to the subendothelium
- Common: 125 per million population
- Type 1 is inherited as autosomal dominant with variable penetrance, is mild and is the most common
- Types 2 and 3 are rare
- Mucosal bleeding, excessive bruising and postoperative or post-traumatic bleeding
- Prolonged bleeding time but normal INR and aPTT, unless severe disease is present
- Abnormal vWF antigen and activity (ristocetin co-factor)
- Treatment for type 1 vWF is desmopressin (DDAVP), which releases stored vWF/factor VIII
- DDAVP may be repeated once stores have reaccumulated, usually after 12–24 hours
- Plasma-derived factor VIII products often contain vWF and may be used in those unresponsive to DDAVP
- Cryoprecipitate should be avoided due to lack of virus inactivation.

### Haemorrhagic disease of the newborn

Haemorrhagic disease of the newborn fortunately is now rare, since the introduction of routine vitamin K administration for all babies at the time of delivery. Features of haemorrhagic disease of the newborn:
- Coagulation factors requiring vitamin K for post-transcriptional modification:
  - factor II (prothrombin)
  - factor VII
  - factor IX
  - factor X
  - protein C and S

  These fall in neonates as a result of nutritional deficiency.
- Bleeding is usually from the gastrointestinal tract or following circumcision
- Occurs early, often on day 2–3
- Prophylactic vitamin K eliminates this disease
- Vitamin K 1 mg, given by the intramuscular route, stops bleeding rapidly.

## Disorders of bleeding due to vascular defects

The commonest vascular defects seen in childhood are:
- anaphylactoid purpura
- infective states
- nutritional deficiency.

### Anaphylactoid purpura (Henoch–Schönlein purpura)

The aetiology of this relatively common disorder is still not clear. It is readily recognized by the characteristic distribution of the rash over the buttocks, legs and backs of the elbows (Fig. 16.2.4). Frequently, it is accompanied by abdominal pain, melaena, joint

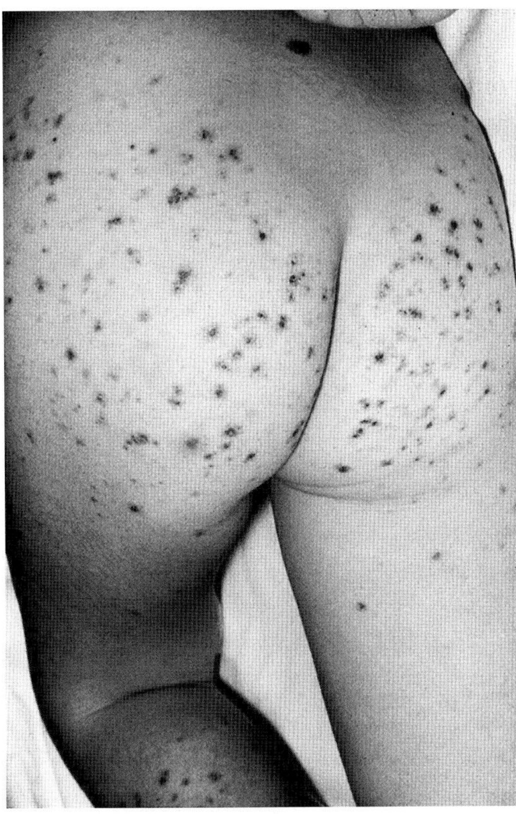

Fig. 16.2.4 Anaphylactoid purpura. The rash is typically distributed over the buttocks and backs of the legs.

swellings and occasionally glomerulonephritis. In anaphylactoid purpura, investigations for assessment of coagulation are normal. Thus, diagnosis must be made on the clinical picture alone.

The outlook for patients with anaphylactic purpura is excellent, except for an occasional child who develops a progressive renal lesion (see Chapter 18.1). It is important to document the child's blood pressure at presentation. There is a reasonable amount of scientific evidence to suggest that the use of corticosteroids may prevent long-term renal impairment but also reduce the duration of the acute symptoms of abdominal and joint pain.

### Infective states

The purpura associated with such disorders as meningococcaemia and dengue haemorrhagic fever result in activation of the coagulation mechanism producing disseminated intravascular coagulation. Management involves that of the infection and of the associated vascular collapse.

### Nutritional deficiency

Scurvy is uncommon and occurs in the artificially fed infant with inadequate vitamin C supplementation. The child is often pale, with skin bruises, is immobile in the frog position because of painful subperiosteal haemorrhages, and has gingival bleeding.

### Purpura fulminans (e.g. post-varicella infection)

This is a life-threatening and rare form of non-thrombocytopenic purpura that may follow such infections as scarlet fever, varicella, measles and some other viral infections. Typically there are rapidly spreading skin haemorrhages involving the buttocks and lower extremities. Congenital deficiencies of either protein C or protein S are the cause of neonatal purpura fulminans.

### Miscellaneous

Bleeding from vascular wall defects is a feature of a group of rare disorders. These include hereditary haemorrhagic telangiectasia, polyarteritis nodosa, other vasculitides and uraemia. Anoxia, and thus damage to the capillary wall, may cause purpura in the asphyxiated newborn. The bleeding that accompanies Cushing syndrome, Ehlers–Danlos syndrome and cutis laxa is the result of defects in vascular supporting tissue.

## Clotting due to coagulation disorders

### Physiology of anticoagulation

The formation of a fibrin clot is tightly regulated in its local environment by anticoagulants. Local thrombin binds thrombomodulin located on normal endothelium which activates protein C. Activated protein C (APC) with the co-factor, protein S, inhibits factors Va and VIIIa by cleaving the molecules. A mutation of factor V at one cleavage point prevents the APC inhibitory effect and is termed APC resistance. The mutation is called factor V Leiden. The other key coagulation inhibitor is antithrombin, a direct inhibitor of thrombin and also of factors Xa, IXa, XIa and XIIa. Heparins potentiate the effect of antithrombin greatly. The largest risk factor for paediatric thrombosis is not a protein deficiency but the presence of a central venous catheter.

Table 16.2.5 lists the causes and features of thrombosis in childhood.

**Table 16.2.5 Major causes of thrombosis in childhood**

| Cause | Clinical features | Diagnostic tests | Treatment |
|---|---|---|---|
| Venous access device | Blocked access/emboli, limb swelling | Echocardiography and contrast radiography | Heparin. Removal of device |
| Phospholipid antibodies | Superficial/deep vein thrombosis | Prolonged INR/aPTT, not corrected by normal plasma | Often no therapy; may require corticosteroids or heparin |
| Protein C and S homozygous | Purpura fulminans | Very low protein C or S | Protein C replacement + heparin |
| Protein C and S heterozygous | Superficial/deep vein thrombosis; rare cerebral, mesenteric and renal vein thrombosis | Low protein C or S | Heparin followed by long-term warfarin |

**Table 16.2.5 Major causes of thrombosis in childhood—cont'd**

| Cause | Clinical features | Diagnostic tests | Treatment |
|---|---|---|---|
| Factor V mutation (Arg506 to Gln), 'Factor V Leiden' | Early-onset vascular disease in family | Activated protein C resistance test | Heparin and long-term warfarin |
| Antithrombin deficiency | Venous thrombosis in adolescence | Decreased level of antithrombin | Antithrombin replacement, heparin and warfarin |
| Dysfibrinogenaemia | Rare thrombosis in childhood | Prolonged thrombin time and snake venom times | Replacement therapy |
| Homocysteinaemia | Arterial and venous thrombosis | Biochemical tests | Diet and short-term anticoagulants |

aPTT, activated partial thromboplastin time; INR, international normalized ratio.

# 16.3 Cancers

Antoinette Anazodo, Tracey O'Brien

Over the past 30 years we have seen dramatic improvements in the treatment and survival of childhood cancer. Survival rates have climbed from below 30% to more than 80%. This improvement is largely due to the use of clinical cancer trials conducted through collaborative national and international childhood cancer study groups and underpins the need for a continued cohesive approach to the treatment of rare diseases. Despite these remarkable improvements, 20–25% of children diagnosed with cancer are not cured with current therapies and many cured patients will be left with long-term complications of therapy. This clearly dictates the need for ongoing research to improve survival outcomes.

## Incidence and distribution of childhood cancers

Approximately 1 in 600 children will be diagnosed with cancer before the age of 15 years, and the incidence has slowly increased since the 1970s. The distribution of cancer types in children aged 0–14 years is shown in Table 16.3.1. The incidence varies by sex and ethnic origin, and the types of tumour also vary by age.

Acute leukaemia – acute lymphoblastic (ALL) or acute myeloblastic leukaemia (AML) – accounts for just over one-third of all childhood cancers. Primary brain or central nervous system (CNS) tumours account for another third and are the most common solid cancer tumours. Lymphomas (non-Hodgkin lymphoma and Hodgkin disease) make up 10% of all childhood malignancies. The most common abdominal tumours are neuroblastoma and Wilms' tumours, accounting for 6–8% of childhood cancers respectively. Bone tumours (e.g. Ewing sarcoma and osteosarcoma) and soft tissue sarcomas (e.g. rhabdomyosarcoma) account for a small proportion of childhood cancers. In adolescent patients, melanoma, bone sarcomas, thyroid cancers and germ cell tumours are more common.

## Aetiology of childhood cancer

When confronted with a diagnosis of childhood cancer, parents often ask: 'Why did this happen to my child?' or 'Did this happen because of something I have done or passed on to my child?' With the exception of several known predisposing genetic syndromes (Table 16.3.2), the proportion of paediatric cancers that have a clearly hereditary component is very small. Similarly, despite extensive epidemiological studies, few environmental agents have been linked consistently with childhood malignancy.

It is hypothesized that cancer initiation results from a series of genetic mutations resulting in the inability of a cell to respond normally to intracellular and/or extracellular signals that control cell proliferation, differentiation or death (apoptosis). Examples include mutations involving tumour suppressor genes (e.g. *RB1*, *p53* or *WT1*) or activation of cellular proto-oncogenes (e.g. *myc* or *abl*). The number of required genetic alterations may differ depending on the type of malignancy from as few as one to a complex cascade arising directly or indirectly from inherited gene mutations, environmental, chemical or radiation-induced DNA damage or random errors in DNA synthesis.

## Approach to management of a patient with suspected malignancy

Treatment types and duration vary for individual children and adolescents depending on the age at diagnosis, type of cancer, stage and specific biological differences of the tumour. Prompt referral to a paediatric oncology centre for diagnostic work-up and management is critical for all children and adolescents with a suspected malignancy. A centralized multidisciplinary team approach, utilizing skills of specialist medical, nursing and allied health practitioners is the 'gold standard' in delivery of excellence in care to children with cancer. A number of steps are involved before a child can start treatment:

- *Diagnosis* will be made by a combination of diagnostic tests, radiological imaging and biopsies that varies dependent on the cancer type. Examples of these will be shown later as we discuss specific tumour groups.
- *Staging investigations* are then needed to document whether the cancer has spread. These tests give important information about survival and allow clinicians to decide on the most suitable clinical trial.

| Table 16.3.1 Frequency of malignancy in childhood | |
|---|---|
| Malignant disease | Frequency (%) |
| Leukaemia | 35 |
| Primary central nervous system tumours | 20 |
| Lymphoma: non-Hodgkin and Hodgkin | 10 |
| Wilms' tumour | 6–8 |
| Neuroblastoma | 6–8 |
| Rhabdomyosarcoma, soft tissue sarcoma | 5 |
| Sarcoma of bone: Ewing and osteosarcoma | 4 |
| Histiocytosis | 5 |
| Teratoma | 2 |
| Retinoblastoma | 1 |
| Hepatic | 1 |
| Other | 5 |

| Table 16.3.2 Inherited/genetic syndromes associated with increased risk of childhood malignancy | |
|---|---|
| Cancer | Associated syndrome |
| Leukaemia | Trisomy 21, Bloom syndrome, Fanconi anaemia, ataxia telangiectasia, neurofibromatosis, Kostmann syndrome, Klinefelter syndrome, Li–Fraumeni syndrome, Diamond–Blackfan anaemia, Noonan syndrome |
| Central nervous system tumours | Neurofibromatosis, tuberous sclerosis, Li–Fraumeni syndrome, von Hippel–Lindau syndrome |
| Lymphoma | Immunodeficiency disorders |
| Wilms' tumour | Denys–Drash syndrome, Beckwith–Weidermann syndrome, WAGR syndrome |
| Rhabdomyosarcoma | Li–Fraumeni syndrome |
| WAGR, Wilms' tumour, aniridia, genitourinary anomalies and mental retardation. | |

- *Toxicity assessment* such as echocardiography, glomerular filtration rate and audiology are regularly carried out to ensure that treatment does not affect normal structures such as the heart, kidneys and hearing.
- *Treatment* usually involves combinations of four common treatment options, although scientists are researching new novel treatments that may improve survival:
  - Chemotherapy with drugs that kill rapidly dividing cancer cells. Unfortunately, these drugs cause side-effects by affecting normal cells such as bone marrow or hair follicles. Depending on the chemotherapy agent, the drug may be given intravenously, orally, intramuscularly or intrathecally (into the cerebrospinal fluid, CSF).
  - Surgery – some tumours can be removed by a surgical procedure at diagnosis; others are removed after chemotherapy to make the tumour smaller or easier to remove.
  - Radiotherapy is the medical use of ionizing radiation as a cancer treatment or part of treatment to control cancer cells. Some tumours are very radiosensitive (e.g. lymphomas), whereas others, such as osteosarcomas, are not radiosensitive.
  - Bone marrow transplant treats diseased bone marrow by ablating the marrow with a combination of chemotherapy and/or radiotherapy, coupled by replacement with a stem cell infusion (of bone marrow, peripheral stem cells or cord blood).

## Acute leukaemia

Leukaemia is the abnormal proliferation of lymphoblasts (ALL) or myeloblasts (AML) in the bone marrow. ALL accounts for 80% of all childhood leukaemia, with AML accounting for the majority of the remainder. In ALL, presentation peaks at age 2–5 years, whereas there is no peak in AML. Chronic leukaemia, including chronic myeloid leukaemia (CML) and juvenile myelomonocytic leukaemia (JMML), is rare, accounting for fewer than 5% of cases.

The cause of leukaemia is unknown, but the theory is that a abnormal stem cell develops capable of indefinite renewal. These cells occupy the marrow space, leading to reduced numbers of normal haematopoietic cells, resulting ultimately in pancytopenia. Secondary involvement of the reticuloendothelial system (leading to lymphadenopathy and hepatosplenomegaly), bone, joints and, rarely, CNS, testes and skin can occur.

A two-step pathogenesis for ALL (Greaves' hypothesis) has been suggested, with the initial event, occurring during fetal life, driving clonal expansion and a second trigger occurring during childhood, possibly resulting from viral stimuli of cellular proliferation. This theory stems from evidence that a significant proportion of children presenting with ALL have molecular evidence of leukaemic clones identified retrospectively at birth on newborn screening cards.

Leukaemia can be further classified into distinct categories:

- precursor B-cell ALL (early pre-B, pre-B, transitional pre-B): 80–85%
- mature B-cell ALL: 2–3%
- T-cell ALL: 10–15%.

Classification is on the basis of:

- Morphological characteristics – appearance of the blood film, bone marrow aspirate and bone marrow trephine under the microscope
- Cytogenetics – the study of tumour chromosomal material using techniques such as florescence *in situ* hybridization (FISH) and comparative genomic hybridization (CGH)
- Immunophenotyping – a technique used to identify surface markers and antigens on leukaemia and lymphoma cells to aid diagnosis and classification.

## Acute lymphoblastic leukaemia

### Presentation

The clinical presentation of ALL can be quite variable, but most children will present with a 3–4-week prodrome that may include pallor, increased bruising or bleeding, lethargy, anorexia, recurrent infection or fevers, anorexia, bone pain or reluctance to walk.

Common physical examination findings include pallor (80%), petechiae (50%), lymphadenopathy (35%), hepatomegaly or splenomegaly (50–60%). Rarely, skin infiltration (chloroma) and testicular infiltration (usually presenting as a painless swelling) are seen.

T-cell leukaemia, more common in older boys, presents with a mediastinal mass in 50% of cases. This can result in life-threatening airway compromise and obstruction of the superior vena cava. Some 30% of patients with T-cell ALL present with a leukocyte count greater than $100\times10^9$/L, and there is a higher incidence of CNS disease.

### Investigations

The peripheral blood film can be normal but will usually demonstrate the presence of leukaemic blasts with or without anaemia and thrombocytopenia. The white blood cell count (WCC) is frequently raised at diagnosis (leukocytosis), with a presenting WCC below $10\times10^9$/L in 25%, 10–$50\times10^9$/L in 50% and above $50\times10^9$/L in 25% of patients. A bone marrow aspirate and biopsy (trephine) are the ‘gold standard’ diagnostic tests and will show replacement of normal haematopoiesis by leukaemic cells (Fig. 16.3.1).

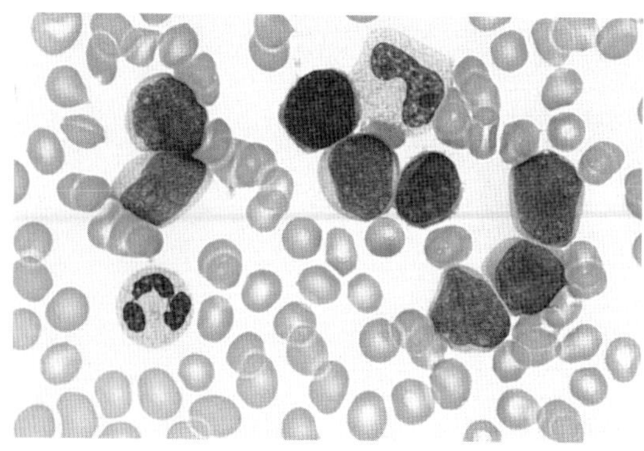

Fig. 16.3.1 Bone marrow aspirate in acute lymphoblastic leukaemia.

A lumbar puncture is also done during the staging work-up; approximately 5–10% of patients show leukaemic spread to the CSF.

### Classification and prognostic factors

Specific chromosomal translocations can also be identified, for example t(8;14) in B-cell ALL and the unfavourable t(9;22) or the *BCR-abl* gene (Philadelphia chromosome) identified in CML and 5% of paediatric patients with ALL.

Table 16.3.3 shows prognostic risk factors for ALL. Clinical features such as age and WCC at diagnosis are becoming less significant as protocols stratify treatment based on the response to treatment; for example, reduction of initial blast count following steroid therapy is an important prognostic factor, as is detection of minimal residual disease (MRD) by molecular methods after chemotherapy.

### Treatment

Current combination chemotherapy protocols for ALL result in cure of 80% of patients. Much of the required therapy can be given on an outpatient basis. Treatment consists of phases of therapy including induction, consolidation, CNS-directed therapy, re-induction, and continuation or maintenance therapy.

By the end of the first month of therapy (induction) with 3–4-drug combination chemotherapy (vincristine, asparaginase, prednisone, daunorubicin), remission will be achieved in more than 95% of patients. Further combination therapy is required to prevent relapse. The optimal total duration of therapy varies in clinical trials between 2 and 3 years.

CNS-targeted therapy using high-dose intravenous and intrathecal methotrexate has allowed cranial irradiation to be avoided except in patients with overt CNS disease or high-risk disease requiring a bone marrow transplant. This has reduced, but not eliminated, potential long-term cognitive, endocrine and growth complications.

**Table 16.3.3 Risk group classification for acute lymphoblastic leukaemia**

| Risk group | Clinical features | Molecular/genetic features |
|---|---|---|
| Low risk | Age 2–10 years, WCC < 50 × $10^9$/L<br>Not T-cell phenotype<br>No central nervous system or testicular disease<br>Rapid response to induction therapy | DNA index > 1.16<br>Absence of:<br>*t*(9;22) *BCR–abl*<br>*t*(4;11) *MLL/AF*$_4$<br>*t*(1;19)<br>*MLL* rearrangement<br>*t*(12;21) *TEL/AML1* |
| High risk and very high risk | Induction failure<br>Age < 12 months<br>Poor prednisone response<br>High MRD levels | *t*(9;22), *t*(4;11)<br>*MLL* rearrangements |

MRD, minimal residual disease; WCC, white blood cell count.

### Clinical example

Sally was a 3-year-old girl who presented with a 2–3-week history of intermittent fever, lethargy and poor appetite. Reluctance to walk and increased bruising were also noted for 1–2 days prior to presentation. Examination confirmed a pale child with truncal petechiae, limb bruising, cervical lymphadenopathy, splenomegaly and hepatomegaly. What was the differential diagnosis?

The presence of fever suggested infection, pallor suggested anaemia, and petechiae and bruising suggested thrombocytopenia. A blood count would confirm this. Lymphadenopathy and hepatosplenomegaly were consistent with infection (e.g. infectious mononucleosis, cytomegalovirus) or leukaemic infiltration. Reluctance to walk, fever and mild anaemia may be consistent with a primary joint problem such as juvenile rheumatoid arthritis or osteomyelitis. A blood count and film were warranted and a bone marrow aspirate was needed to confirm the diagnosis of acute leukaemia. Other paediatric malignancies that may present with bone marrow involvement should be considered, including lymphoma, neuroblastoma, rhabdomyosarcoma and Ewing sarcoma.

## Acute myeloid leukaemia

AML is a cancer of the myeloid white blood cells, which are produced in the bone marrow. AML accounts for 20% of acute leukaemia.

### Differential diagnosis

Like ALL, the differential diagnosis can include infection, juvenile rheumatoid arthritis, idiopathic thrombocytic purpura, aplastic anaemia and osteomyelitis.

### Presentation

Presenting symptoms and signs are similar to those of ALL, and can include pallor, bleeding, fever, anorexia, malaise and bone pain. Certain subtypes of AML have more distinctive presenting clinical features. Acute promyelocytic leukaemia (APML) can present with serious haemorrhage or disseminated intravascular coagulation (DIC), whereas acute monoblastic or myelomonoblastic leukaemia may present with skin infiltration (chloroma) or gum hypertrophy. CNS leukaemia is diagnosed in 5–15% of patients.

### Classification and prognostic factors

As well as bone marrow aspirate and trephines, it is important to exclude testicular disease in boys and CNS disease, as these are both sanctuary sites of disease.

In AML, characteristic morphological features include the presence of Auer rods as well as positive staining for myeloperoxidase and monocyte-associated esterases (Fig. 16.3.2). Classification into one of

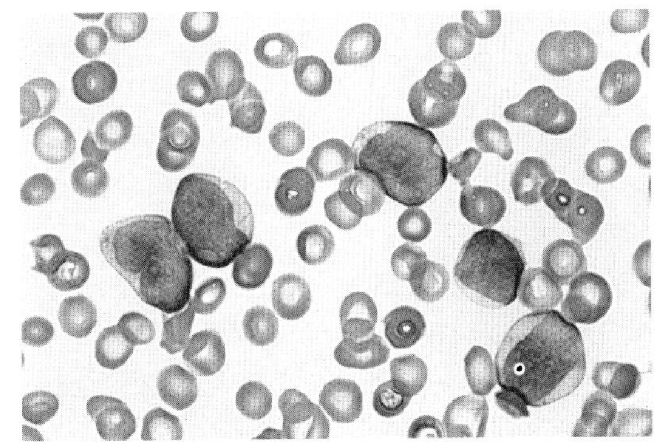

Fig. 16.3.2 Bone marrow aspirate in acute myeloid leukaemia, showing the presence of Auer rods.

eight morphological subclasses using the French–American–British (FAB) system is possible.

In addition to morphology and immunophenotype, genetic features of leukaemic cells can provide diagnostic and prognostic information. In AML, characteristic translocations are seen within FAB morphological subgroups; for example, M3 or APML is identified by the translocation t(15;17), and t(8;21) is a favourable cytogenetic abnormality seen in FAB M1 and M2.

### Treatment

In contrast to ALL, therapy for AML is of shorter duration but more intensive, often requiring frequent hospital admissions with aggressive supportive care, including blood products and antimicrobials during lengthy periods of marrow suppression.

Overall, the outlook for patients with AML is less optimistic, with survival rates reported of 50–75%.

> **Clinical example**
>
> Monica is an 8-year-old girl who presented with a 1-week history of lethargy, poor appetite, recurrent epistaxis and gum bleeding when brushing her teeth. Examination revealed anaemia, gum hypertrophy, bruising on the lower limbs and trunk, hepatosplenomegaly and inguinal lymphadenopathy.
>
> A full blood count confirmed anaemia and thrombocytopenia with a haemoglobin level of 8.2 g/L and platelets $12 \times 10^9$/L, and a white cell count of $1.6 \times 10^9$/L with circulating blast cells. Her coagulation profile was prolonged, consistent with mild disseminated intravascular coagulation.
>
> Bone marrow aspirate confirmed the diagnosis of acute promyelocytic leukaemia (Fig. 16.3.3), and this was confirmed by immunophenotyping and cytogenetics (Fig. 16.3.4). Lumbar puncture was performed to exclude CNS spread.

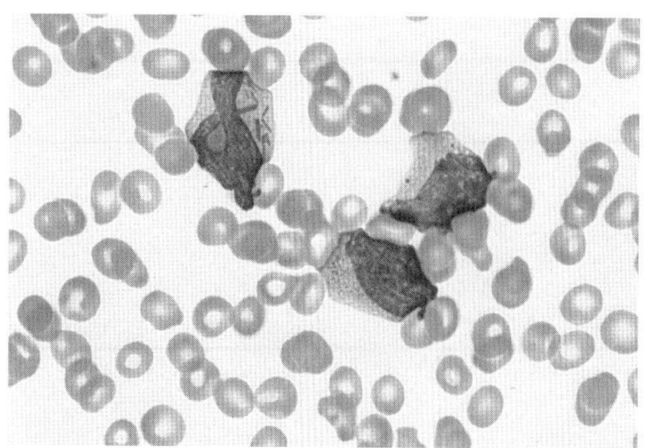

Fig. 16.3.3 Bone marrow aspirate in acute promyelocytic leukaemia.

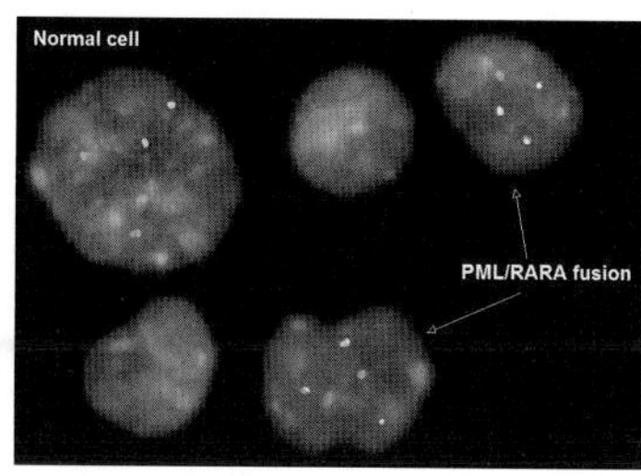


Fig. 16.3.4 Dual-colour fluorescence *in situ* hybridization with probes *PML* (15q22) and *RARA* (17q12), demonstrating the presence of a *PML–RARA* fusion resulting from the 15:17 translocation arrows in acute promyelocytic leukaemia.

APML is a subtype of AML which is caused by an accumulation of immature granulocytes called promyelocytes. This is due to the formation of a translocation t(15;17) fusion gene, which causes an arrest in the maturation of myeloid cells at the promyelocyte stage. Patients often present with a coagulopathy, which requires urgent careful management. In addition to standard AML therapy, these patients also need treatment with ATRA, which allows the maturation of promyelocytes.

### Haematopoietic stem cell transplant

For most patients with high-risk, relapsed or refractory leukaemia, haematopoietic stem cell transplantation is the treatment of choice. Stem cells can be sourced from the bone marrow, from peripheral blood or from the umbilical cord of a newborn infant. Siblings have a 25% chance of being an identical match. Patients lacking a sibling donor are reliant on volunteer bone marrow and cord blood donors sourced through international donor registries. Umbilical cord blood transplants are used with increased frequency because of the advantages of speed of availability and greater likelihood of matching.

## Brain and central nervous system tumours

Brain tumours or tumours of the CNS are the most common primary solid cancer, representing approximately 20% of all childhood malignancies. Brain tumours as a group are heterogeneous with regard to clinical presentation, location, histological type and natural history.

95% of CNS tumours occur within the brain, often in specific sites for different age groups. Posterior fossa tumours are more common in childhood, except during the first year of life, and in adolescence, when supratentorial sites predominate. Box 16.3.1 shows

**Box 16.3.1 Classification of central nervous system tumours**

1. Supratentorial
   a. Hemisphere: astrocytoma; glioblastoma; primitive neuroectodermal tumour
   b. Midline: craniopharyngioma; optic nerve glioma; pineal
2. Infratentorial
   a. Cerebellar and fourth ventricle: astrocytoma; medulloblastoma; ependymoma
   b. Brainstem: brainstem glioma
3. Spinal cord
   Astrocytoma; ependymoma

a working classification of CNS tumours. The most common histological subtypes are:

- astrocytomas (50%)
- primitive neuroectodermal tumours (21%)
- gliomas (15–20%)
- ependymomas (9%).

## Presentation

Early symptoms and signs of CNS tumours may be few and difficult to elicit (Box 16.3.2). Evidence of raised intracranial pressure is the most common presentation because posterior fossa and deep midline tumours usually obstruct CSF pathways.

**Box 16.3.2 Signs and symptoms of brain and central nervous system tumours**

**Raised intracranial pressure**
- Headache, often on waking
- Vomiting
- Papilloedema
- Tense fontanelle and increased head circumference in infants indicating hydrocephalus
- Drowsiness, bradycardia and hypertension (late signs)

**Posterior fossa signs**
- Truncal ataxia due to central cerebellar tumours
- Coordination difficulties and tremor due to lateral lesions
- Cranial nerve palsies, suggesting a brainstem lesion
- Defective upward gaze with tumours of the pineal region
- Deep midline tumours around the third ventricle
- Impaired visual acuity and visual field defects due to craniopharyngioma or optic nerve glioma
- Diabetes insipidus and growth failure
- Severe wasting and anorexia due to the diencephalic syndrome of a hypothalamic tumour

**Seizures**
- Uncommon as sole presenting symptom
- Consider tumour with focal seizures or progressively more difficult to control seizures

## Treatment

Treatment of brain tumours depends on the tumour type and location, and can include surgery, chemotherapy and radiation therapy. A number of factors affect outcome and survival, including age, tumour location and operability, histological subtype and presence or absence of metastatic dissemination.

Survival has improved considerably over time for some types of tumour, notably medulloblastoma. For other tumour subtypes, however, such as brainstem gliomas, outcome remains poor. Additionally, increasing attention is being paid to the longer-term toxicity of treatment. This is particularly true of radiation therapy, which, where possible, is spared in younger children because of the potential impact on cognition and growth.

**Clinical example**

Ben is an 18-month-old boy who developed a squint of his right eye, and his mother noted that his right eye had begun to bulge. In retrospect, he was also falling more frequently and bumping into things. He had a number of café-au-lait spots on his trunk and abdomen, but no subcutaneous nodules. He had proptosis and his right optic disc was pale.

An ophthalmology review showed he had no vision in his right eye and reduced vision in his left eye. Magnetic resonance imaging of his brain and orbit (Fig. 16.3.5) confirmed the presence of a bilateral optic tumour but no signs of raised intracranial pressure. Chromosomal analysis and family tree confirmed that Ben had neurofibromatosis type 1 (NF1), which is associated with optic gliomas.

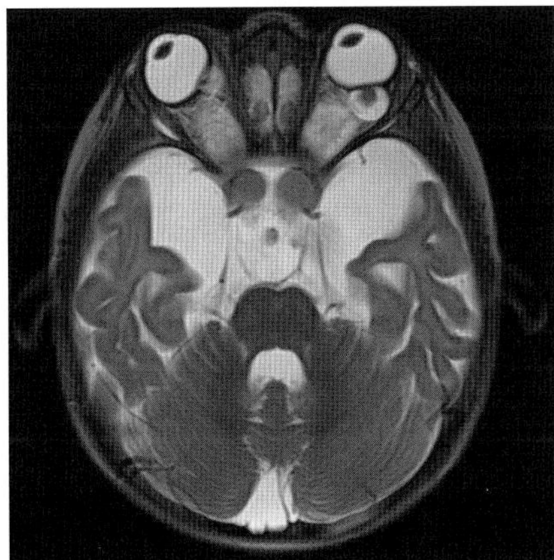

Fig. 16.3.5 Brain magnetic resonance image confirming the presence of a bilateral optic tumour with no evidence of raised intracranial pressure.

Neurofibromatosis type 1 (NF1) is an autosomal dominant disorder associated with benign and malignant tumours. The severity in individuals shows variable expression. There are two types; type 1 is associated with tumours of the optic nerve known as optic gliomas, neurofibromas, freckling of the groin and axilla, café-au-lait spots, skeletal abnormalities and Lisch nodules in the iris.

Optic gliomas are the most common tumours of the optic nerve. Biopsy is not required if radiology shows a classical appearance. Treatment with surgery and chemotherapy is highly variable. Optic gliomas are usually low-grade and slow-growing in children, and affected patients with NF1 have a more favourable prognosis.

## Lymphoma

Lymphoma is a tumour of the lymph tissues (lymph nodes, lymph vessels, spleen, bone marrow, thymus and tonsils), which are part of the immune system. The lymphatic system runs throughout the body, which means you can get a lymphoma almost anywhere in the body.

Lymphomas account for approximately 10% of childhood cancers and are the third most common form of malignancy in childhood. There are two basic types: non-Hodgkin lymphoma (NHL) and Hodgkin disease. Both are more common in boys than in girls. Although lymphadenopathy attributable to an infectious aetiology is common in childhood, any child with persistent adenopathy (>2–3 weeks) should be considered for a biopsy. The site of adenopathy (e.g. supraclavicular) or character (firm, large >2 cm) may indicate the need for earlier biopsy.

### Non-Hodgkin lymphoma

Childhood NHL has quite different features from its adult counterpart. Childhood NHL is more often disseminated, diffuse, not nodular, high-grade, immature T- or B-cell lineage with frequent spread to extranodal sites, marrow and CNS. In contrast, adult NHL is usually a low-grade malignancy with predominantly nodal involvement.

#### Presentation

NHL usually presents acutely or subacutely with very short symptom intervals. Nodal disease may be present, but is rare. Systemic symptoms such as fever, weight loss, and night sweats referred to as B symptoms are not as common as in Hodgkin disease. Specific symptoms depend on the site of involvement.

A mediastinal primary of T-cell immunophenotype accounts for 25% of NHL and often presents with acute superior vena caval and/or airway obstruction (a medical emergency) producing stridor and cough, usually with an associated pleural effusion and characteristically occurring in pre-teen or early teenage males.

Abdominal lymphoma accounts for 35–40% of NHL, is of B-cell immunophenotype, and characteristically presents either as a local tumour causing intussusception or as massive, diffuse abdominal disease, often with ascites. An acute abdomen is not infrequently misdiagnosed as appendicitis.

#### Investigations

Diagnosis and staging involves ultrasonography of palpable lymph nodes and computed tomography (CT) of the chest, abdomen and pelvis. Positron emission tomography (PET) has been useful in diagnosis and reassessment, but is not currently used in risk stratification in NHL.

Discussion about the appropriate biopsy site between oncologist and surgeons and interventional radiologist is important to minimize risk. Lymph node biopsy or resection, bone marrow aspirates and trephine samples are analysed for morphology, immunophenotyping and cytogenetics. CSF examination is also required.

When more than 25% of bone marrow is involved, disease is classified as T- or B-cell ALL. NHL in childhood can be classified as:

- lymphoblastic NHL – diffuse, poorly differentiated, primarily T-cell lineage
- small non-cleaved (undifferentiated) Burkitt or non-Burkitt subtypes, primarily of B-cell origin. A t(8;14) translocation is characteristic of Burkitt lymphoma
- large cell lymphoma – can be cleaved or non-cleaved and of B- or T-cell origin.

#### Treatment

Multiagent chemotherapy is the treatment of choice, although surgical resection may be part of the treatment. The intensity and duration depends upon the histological type and stage. Stages I and II have a more than 90% cure rate, and stages III and IV a 70–80% cure rate.

**Clinical example**

Luke is a 12-year-old boy who presented with acute cough, wheeze and sudden onset of faint stridor. Examination revealed supraclavicular adenopathy, a mass palpable in the suprasternal notch, decreased air entry and dullness to percussion note at the right base. Luke's face was suffused with venous distension.

Symptoms and signs suggested superior vena caval syndrome with airway obstruction. This constituted an oncological emergency. Chest X-ray confirmed a large mediastinal mass and a right pleural effusion. Urgent diagnosis and commencement of therapy (steroids) was required to prevent complete airway obstruction. Thoracocentesis and cytological analysis confirmed a diagnosis of T-cell lymphoblastic lymphoma. Precautionary admission to the intensive care unit was recommended. Full staging work-up required chest/abdomen/pelvis CT, nuclear medicine PET, bone marrow biopsies and lumbar puncture. Although uncommon, the diagnosis of an obstructive mediastinal mass should be entertained in children or adolescents with onset of wheezing, particularly when there is no prior history of asthma.

## Hodgkin disease

Hodgkin disease is commonly seen in adolescent and young adult patients, more commonly in boys than girls, and is rare before age 5 years. Epstein–Barr virus (EBV) can be identified in some Hodgkin cells, but the significance is not clear. There are five types of Hodgkin disease: classical Hodgkin disease is either mixed cellularity, nodular sclerosis, lymphocyte-depleted or lymphocyte-rich on histology, whereas nodular lymphocyte predominant is a separate entity.

### Presentation

A painless, progressive swelling of lymph nodes (above the diaphragm in two-thirds of patients) is the most common clinical presentation. Dissemination to spleen, liver, lungs, bones and bone marrow can occur. Patients with mediastinal disease may present with shortness of breath, cough, orthopnoea or chest pain. Constitutional symptoms (B symptoms) occur in one-third of patients. Adolescent or young adult patients who drink alcohol may complain of pain at the sites of nodal disease (10%).

### Diagnosis

The diagnosis and staging investigation are the same as for suspected NHL. PET has been useful in diagnosis and reassessment, and in reducing late effects by enabling risk stratification; patients with a good response to treatment continue on chemotherapy but no longer require radiotherapy.

### Treatment

Multiagent chemotherapy and radiotherapy clinical trials have achieved excellent cure rates, with survival greater than 90%. The emphasis has now turned to reducing late effects, preserving fertility, reducing rates of secondary cancers (associated with the use of radiation and etoposide) and reducing long-term organ morbidity (e.g. lung toxicity from bleomycin, cardiomyopathy from anthracyclines) without compromising cure rates.

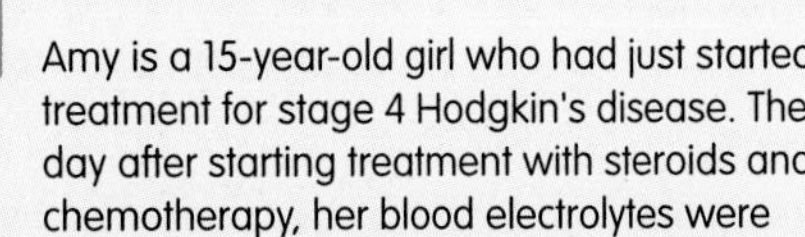

**Clinical example**

Amy is a 15-year-old girl who had just started treatment for stage 4 Hodgkin's disease. The day after starting treatment with steroids and chemotherapy, her blood electrolytes were markedly deranged, with increased potassium, urate and phosphate, low calcium and poor urine output. Her blood pressure was in the normal range, but was higher than her pre-treatment blood pressure.

Amy's fluid input was increased, she was started on rasburicase (recombinant urate oxidase) and her electrocardiogram (ECG) was monitored continuously for arrhythmias. Blood electrolytes and venous gases were measured frequently to ensure Amy did not develop renal failure.

Tumour lysis syndrome is the rapid development of metabolic abnormalities, from the release of intracellular contents into the bloodstream due to cell death, which can result in renal failure. Tumour lysis syndrome can result in significant renal impairment and life threatening electrolyte disturbances (hyperkalaemia, hyperphosphatemia and hypocalcaemia). This can happen spontaneously or at the start of treatment, and is commonest with leukaemias and lymphomas, although it can occur with large solid tumours.

Recognition of patients at risk and prevention by assessment of electrolytes, fluid balance, weight and blood pressure is important in the first 3–5 days after the start of treatment. Vigorous hydration with intravenous fluid, forced diuresis and allopurinol are standard. Dialysis is occasionally required. Allopurinol is a xanthine oxidase inhibitor that is given to reduce the conversion of nucleic acid by-products to uric acid and therefore prevent urate nephropathy. In patients with a high WCC or very bulky disease or renal impairment, recombinant urate oxidase converts poorly soluble uric acid to soluble allantoin, lowering plasma uric acid levels.

## Neuroblastoma

Neuroblastoma accounts for about 8–10% of childhood cancers. It is the most common extracranial solid tumour in childhood. Most cases occur in children under the age of 5 years, with a median age at presentation of 23 months. Neuroblastomas originate from primordial neural crest cells that normally give rise to adrenal medulla and sympathetic ganglia; they can develop at any site of the sympathetic nervous system. Some 70% arise in the abdomen, either in the adrenal gland or in retroperitoneal sympathetic ganglia, and 30% arise in cervical thoracic or pelvic ganglia.

### Presentation

The clinical manifestations of neuroblastoma vary depending on the primary site of disease, metastatic burden and metabolically active by-products. Variations in the location, degree of differentiation, clinical and biological behaviour of these tumours are diverse. Spontaneous regression and differentiation into benign neoplasms is seen at one end of the spectrum and highly aggressive tumours resistant to intensive chemotherapy at the other. Metastatic neuroblastoma in children older than 18 months has a poor prognosis. Unfortunately, more than 75% of patients present with metastatic disease at the time of diagnosis.

Common presentations include:

- Non-specific symptoms, such as pallor, irritability, bone pain and gait changes
- Abdominal disease – abdominal mass or abdominal pain
- Cervical or thoracic disease – cervical mass, cough, dyspnoea, dysphagia, Horner syndrome
- Paraspinal disease – presents with back pain, tenderness, limp, bladder and sphincter dysfunction
- Skin disease – subcutaneous nodules
- Paraneoplastic syndromes:
  - opsomyoclonus–myoclonus
  - excessive catecholamine secretion, causing sweating, flushing, pallor, headaches, palpitations and hypertension
  - vasoactive peptide secretion, causing intractable diarrhoea resulting in failure to thrive and hypokalaemia
- Common sites for metastatic disease are bone, lymph nodes and bone marrow.

### Investigations

- Haematological – full blood count (FBC) and coagulation
- Biochemistry – urea, electrolytes and creatinine (UEC), comprehensive metabolic panel (CMP), liver function tests (LFTs)
- Tumour markers – raised lactate dehydrogenase (LDH), ferritin, non-specific enolase (NSE)
- Urine catecholamines positive in 90% of patients
- Biopsy is required for histological diagnosis and biological samples that are required to stratify patients to risk groups.
- Staging investigations include CT/magnetic resonance imaging (MRI) of the primary tumour, bilateral bone marrow aspirate and trephine (core) biopsies, bone scan and meta-iodobenzylguanidine (MIBG) scan. MIBG is a radiolabelled compound taken up by cells of the sympathetic nervous system that demonstrates catecholamine synthesis. Approximately 90–95% of neuroblastomas show uptake of MIBG.

### Stage 4S disease

Stage 4S disease is seen in infants less than 18 months who have a localized tumour with metastatic disease to skin, liver or bone marrow, but not bone cortex disease. These infants generally have excellent survival, with tumours spontaneously regressing without the need for treatment.

### Prognostic factors

- Biochemical – NSE $<100$ ng/mL, normal ferritin, high vanillylmandelic acid/homovanillic acid (VMA/HVA) ratio and low LDH are good prognostic factors.
- Biological – The N-*myc* oncogene is present in increased numbers of copies in about 30% of neuroblastomas and correlates with poor survival. 17q gain and loss of heterozygosity are also poor prognostic factors, whereas hyperdiploidy is a good prognostic factor.

### Treatment

Low risk:

- usually surgery is enough
- usually infants
- >95% cure rate.

Intermediate risk:

- 90% cure rate
- treated with surgery and low-dose chemotherapy.

High risk:

- metastatic, N-*myc* amplified
- need surgery, intensive chemotherapy, transplant, radiation, maintenance therapy.

Novel cytotoxic agents, targeted radionucleotide therapy and immune-mediated therapy are all currently being investigated in clinical trials.

## Wilms' tumour (nephroblastoma)

Wilms' tumours account for 6% of childhood malignancies and are the fifth most common childhood malignancy. They represent the vast majority of primary renal cancers in childhood. Over 90% of children diagnosed with Wilms' tumour are under 5 years of age. Thanks to collaborative multicentre clinical trials, the overall survival of these patients exceeds 90%.

### Presentation

Children usually present with a painless abdominal swelling or an asymptomatic abdominal mass picked up by one of their parents. Occasionally the tumour may bleed or rupture, causing pain in 20% of patients. Malaise, gross or microscopic haematuria, fever, anorexia or hypertension occur in approximately 25% of patients. Some 8–10% of patients with Wilms' tumour have an acquired von Willebrand factor abnormality with prolonged coagulation studies at diagnosis.

Most Wilms' tumours are not associated with a genetic syndrome, but it is very important to take a three-generation family tree history and examine the child for genital abnormalities (hypospadias, crytorchidism), hemihypertrophy (asymmetry of the left and right side of the body) and aniridia (iris hypoplasia). Some examples of predisposing syndromes associated with Wilms' tumours include Beckwith–Wiedemann syndrome, Denys–Drash syndrome, congenital aniridia, hemihypertrophy and trisomy 18. These children are screened every 6 months by abdominal ultrasonography.

### Investigations

The common sites of blood-borne metastases are liver and lung. Extension to regional lymph nodes, hepatic adhesion, and tumour invasion of the renal vein and inferior vena cava, which can extend up to the right atrium, occur rarely.

Baseline investigations usually include a FBC, renal and liver function, coagulation screen and urinalysis. If tumour extension or involvement of the inferior vena cava is suspected, contrast-enhanced CT of chest, abdomen and pelvis is carried out for staging.

Biological studies on the tumour have identified heterozyygosity at 16q or 1p as an adverse prognostic factor increasing the chance of relapse and death.

### Treatment

Surgery can be performed at diagnosis or after response to some initial chemotherapy. The frequency and intensity of chemotherapy following surgery then depends on stage and histological subtype (favourable versus unfavourable or anaplastic). Radiotherapy is used in patients with stage III and IV disease. Cure rates exceed 90% for stage I–III and 85–90% for stage IV disease.

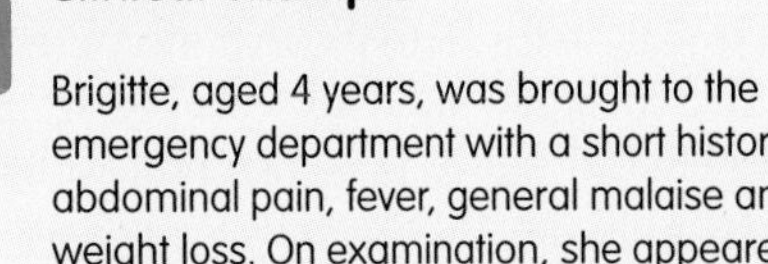

**Clinical example**

Brigitte, aged 4 years, was brought to the emergency department with a short history of abdominal pain, fever, general malaise and weight loss. On examination, she appeared to be an irritable child with tachycardia and mild hypertension. She had a distended abdomen with a large, poorly defined, palpable, hard mass in the periumbilical area. A plain X-ray showed calcification within the mass. A large primary adrenal mass was confirmed on CT. Open biopsy confirmed neuroblastoma, and the remaining staging examination (bone marrow biopsy, nuclear medicine bone scan and MIBG scan) demonstrated metastatic disease to the bone marrow and bone cortex of three vertebrae consistent with stage 4 disease. Tumour biology from lymph node biopsy and bone marrow aspirate confirmed the presence of increased copies of the N-*myc* oncogene, a bad prognostic indicator. Differential diagnosis of an abdominal mass in childhood includes neuroblastoma, Wilms' tumour, lymphoma, rhabdomyosarcoma and germ cell tumours.

## Sarcomas

Sarcomas are tumours arising from connective tissue. These cells originate from bone, cartilage and fat tissues, and are given a number of different names depending on the type of tissue from which they arise.

**Bone cancers (osteosarcoma and Ewing sarcoma)**

Primary bone tumours in childhood occur less frequently than bony metastases to the skeleton. Bone tumours are the sixth most common tumour type in childhood, but the third most frequent tumour type in adolescents and young adults. Osteosarcoma (OS) is more common than Ewing sarcoma.

### Osteosarcoma

Osteosarcomas are commonly located at the metaphyseal region of the distal femur, proximal tibia and proximal humerus, although they can be found in the pelvis, skull and jaw. They are more common in adolescents and young adults, with a peak in the second decade of life, but they also affect younger children. There is a slightly higher incidence in males and in patients of African descent.

The aetiology of osteosarcoma is not clear, but there is a known association with exposure to ionizing radiation, bone dysplasias such as Paget disease, and syndromes such as retinoblastoma, Rothumund–Thomson syndrome and Li–Fraumeni syndrome. Mutations in recessive oncogenes (the retinoblastoma susceptibility locus and *p53)* have been postulated to play a role in the tumorigenesis in osteosarcoma.

*Presentation*
Common presentation includes joint swelling, bone pain especially with activity that becomes constant, pain worse at night, and not relieved by painkillers (non mechanical pain). It is common to have associated history of trauma. Systemic symptoms and pathological fractures are rare.

The sentence should be unfortunately these patients can present with long symptom intervals. This may be because the failure to report symptoms, clinicians do not think about malignancies in this age group or they have a confounding history of trauma or musculoskeletal problems.

*Investigations*
Common sites of blood-borne metastases are lung and, less commonly, bones. Diagnostic workup should include a plain X-ray and MRI or CT of the primary lesions. Lung CT and bone scan are needed to identify potential disease spread, followed by a surgical biopsy for a definitive histological diagnosis. PET is still being evaluated in diagnosis and staging.

*Treatment*
Treatment consists of chemotherapy followed by surgical resection of tumour and then further chemotherapy. Most patients can have limb salvage surgery (surgery to spare the limb) rather than amputation surgery. Osteosarcomas are rarely sensitive to radiotherapy.

Cure rates for patients with non-metastatic disease at diagnosis are over 70%. The histological response of tumour following chemotherapy is a predictor of outcome; patients with a good response (defined as >90% necrosis) have a long-term survival rate greater than 80%, compared with poor or standard responders, whose survival rate is 40–60%. The survival of patients with metastatic disease at diagnosis remains poor (<50%). The addition of the immune-enhancing drug muramyl tripeptide (MEPACT) has increased survival from 70% to 78% in localized disease. Clinical trials are looking at the addition of immune enhancing drugs such a muramyl tripeptide (MEPACT) and Interferon.

### Ewing sarcoma

This is the second most common bone cancer, accounting for 10–15% of primary malignant bone tumours. In contrast to OS, the peak incidence of Ewing sarcoma tumours occurs between 15 and 19 years of age after which rates show a decline, but they are also seen in younger children and young adults. Ewing sarcoma is more common in males than in females and, unlike OS, it is very uncommon in patients of African descent.

Most of these tumours originate in the bone, although they can occasionally arise in soft tissue (extraosseous Ewing). These tumours usually appear in the middle of the bone (diaphysis), and the primary site of disease is either in the extremities (53%) or in the axial skeleton (47%).

*Presentation*
Like osteosarcoma, these patients usually present with a long history of pain (96%) and a palpable mass (61%). About 15% of patients have a pathological fracture at time of diagnosis. Approximately 25% of patients have evidence of metastatic disease at diagnosis. Common sites of spread are lung, bone and bone marrow (not seen in osteosarcoma).

*Investigations*
Diagnostic tests include plain X-ray of the lesion in two planes. The typical X-ray appearance of Ewing sarcoma shows a poorly defined, destructive or 'moth-eaten' pattern, often accompanied by a multilaminated 'onion skin' periosteal reaction with elevation (Codman's triangle).

MRI of the lesion is the 'gold standard' for local staging, but CT of the primary lesion may also be required, particularly to demonstrate cortical fractures. A bone scan, bilateral bone marrow aspirates and biopsies, and CT of the chest are performed at diagnosis to define the metastatic spread of disease.

A tumour biopsy is required in all patients to confirm the histological diagnosis. Molecular testing will identify a translocation involving t(11;22) or *EWS* (Ewing sarcoma gene) in more than 90% of Ewing tumours.

*Treatment*
Treatment consists of a combination of multiagent chemotherapy, surgery and radiotherapy. The majority of patients are able to have limb salvage surgery (surgery to spare the limb). Recent research has shown that intensifying chemotherapy by compressing chemotherapy cycles (from 28 to 21 days) with granulocyte colony-stimulating factor (G-CSF) support increases survival.

Several prognostic factors have been identified, including tumour site, tumour size, histological grade, response to therapy, and the presence or absence of overt metastatic disease at diagnosis. Currently, 60–70% of patients with localized disease will be cured. The survival rate for patients with metastatic disease remains less than 50%, underpinning the need for ongoing investigation into novel agents.

## Rhabdomyosarcoma and soft tissue sarcoma

Soft tissue sarcomas make up 5% of paediatric cancer; about 50% of these are rhabdomyosarcomas. Rhabdomyosarcomas occur in early childhood with a median age at diagnosis of 5 years, although a small number are seen in adolescent and young adult patients, who tend to present with more metastatic tumours.

There is a recognized association between rhabdomyosarcoma and familial syndromes, including neurofibromatosis and Li–Fraumeni syndrome. Li–Fraumeni syndrome includes clusters of soft tissue sarcomas, adrenocortical carcinoma and early-onset breast cancer, and results from germline mutations in the *p53* tumour suppressor gene. Rhabdomyosarcomas are included in the small, round, blue cell tumours of childhood and are thought to arise from mesenchymal cells committed to muscle differentiation. There are two major histological subtypes of rhabdomyosarcoma: embryonal (80%) and the more aggressive alveolar (20%).

*Presentation*

Differences in presentation are seen depending on the clinical site. The common clinical sites and presentation include:

- orbit, head and neck including parameningeal (40%) – proptosis, loss of or change in vision, rhinorrhoea and nasal obstruction
- extremities (20%) – painless mass, regional or distant lymphadenopathy
- genitourinary (20–25%) – bladder or bowel dysfunction, paratesticular mass or mass arising from cervix or vagina, change in menstruation pattern or menorrhagia
- trunk (10–15%).

*Investigations*

Approximately half of all patients will have irresectable tumours at diagnosis. Less than 25% of patients will have metastatic disease at diagnosis involving lung, bone marrow, bone or lymph nodes, but this increases in adolescent patients. MRI of primary tumour is the investigation of choice for children with rhabdomyosarcomas. Technetium-99m bone scan, CT of the lung and bone marrow biopsy are required to assess for metastatic disease.

*Treatment*

Therapy for rhabdomyosarcomas depends on the location and stage of disease, and is often multimodal, involving surgery, adjuvant chemotherapy and radiotherapy. Prognostic variables include metastatic disease at diagnosis, site of disease, surgical resectability, histological subtype and age. Early-stage disease is curable in more than 85% of patients. Patients with more aggressive disease have a poorer prognosis, ranging from 30% to 50% depending on risk factors.

**Clinical example**

Peter, aged 13 years, had a 4-month history of pain around the knee. In the last 2 weeks this had become severe and he was able to walk only short distances. Peter recalled a minor injury playing sport at the onset of his symptoms 4 months ago. Examination demonstrated swelling on the medial aspect of the proximal tibia with a diffuse, firm, non-tender mass present. The most likely diagnosis was a bone or soft tissue sarcoma. Plain X-ray of the tibia confirmed a soft tissue mass and destructive bony lesion with a 'sunburst' appearance, reflecting periosteal elevation in the metaphyseal region. CT and MRI were used to delineate anatomy, followed by biopsy, which confirmed osteosarcoma. A history of trivial injury is often associated with bone tumours, but there is scant evidence to suggest a causal relationship; more probably the injury serves as a trigger to seek medical attention.

## Rare tumours

A detailed review of all childhood malignancy is beyond the scope of this chapter. The reader is referred to more extensive paediatric oncology material for a review on retinoblastoma, hepatoblastoma, germ cell tumours, histiocytic disorders, nasopharyngeal carcinomas and other malignant diseases occurring in childhood.

## Late effects of cancer therapy

Survival for most childhood malignancies has improved, so that, in 2011, 1 in every 250 adults was a survivor of childhood or adolescent cancer. In additional to improving survival, clinical trials are now focusing on ways in which the potential late effects of cancer treatments can be reduced. The late effects of cancer treatment can affect every organ, and unfortunately 50% of survivors have at least one long-term problem following treatment. Systematic surveillance and management of late effects of therapy is now the focus of many childhood cancer units and cooperative study groups. Examples of potential late effects are:

- Psychosocial – effect of treatment on education and employment attainment, entry into certain jobs, relationships with peers, and health insurance
- Neurocognitive effects – secondary to surgery, chemotherapy or radiotherapy
- Endocrine effects – poor growth, pituitary dysfunction due to surgery, chemotherapy or radiotherapy, infertility, obesity
- Cardiac – cardiomyopathy secondary to anthracycline chemotherapy or heart damage due to radiotherapy
- Respiratory – pulmonary fibrosis secondary to chemotherapy (e.g. busulphan or bleomycin) or radiotherapy
- Effects on eyes, hearing or teeth – cataracts, keratoconjunctivitis, decreased tear production, failure of primary or secondary teeth to develop, discoloration or increased dental caries, hearing loss due to chemotherapy
- Second malignancy – due to chemotherapy, radiotherapy or an increased genetic susceptibility.

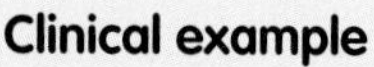

### Clinical example

Emily is a 12-year-old girl who was treated at age 13 months for stage 4 neuroblastoma with chemotherapy, surgery and total body irradiation. Eleven years after treatment she is a survivor of childhood malignancy but has a number of complications of treatment that require regular follow-up. Emily has short stature due to radiotherapy and chronic illness, and started growth hormone 1 year ago, which has increased her growth velocity. She has high-frequency hearing loss requiring bilateral hearing aids, and poor renal function secondary to cisplatin chemotherapy. She has bilateral cataracts and problems with her teeth due to radiotherapy. She enjoys school and will be starting in high school next term, but has delayed numeracy and literacy skills requiring extra educational support. The continual medical needs require a coordinated multidisciplinary team and have long-term financial and psychosocial effects on Emily and her family.

## Palliative care

Cancer is the most common cause of non-accidental death in childhood. Approximately 20–25% of children diagnosed with a malignancy die from their disease. Optimal palliation requires open and ongoing communication between all members of the health-care team, the child and family. Management of symptoms, including pain, dyspnoea, nausea/vomiting and bowel abnormalities, is important, as is optimization of psychological, social and spiritual needs. Open discussion regarding the desired place of death (e.g. home, hospital or hospice) should take place in advance. A child's understanding of death will vary depending on age and the individual, but many studies suggest that children as young as 6 years have an understanding of death and should be given the opportunity to talk openly about their illness. Following the death of a child, one of the essential roles of the treating team is to provide bereavement support for parents and siblings.

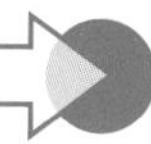

### Practical points

**Childhood cancer**

- Childhood cancer is rare, with excellent survival rates for most cancer types.
- A multidisciplinary team approach delivers best therapy to children with cancer.
- Acute leukaemia and brain tumours account for a significant proportion of all childhood cancers.
- Treatment depends on cancer type and stage and can include surgery, radiation, chemotherapy and immunotherapies.
- The long-term consequences of therapy must be considered, including the impact on growth, fertility, learning and development, as well as late organ toxicity and second cancers.

PART 17

# SEIZURE DISORDERS AND DISORDERS OF THE NERVOUS SYSTEM

# 17.1 Seizures and epilepsies

Jeremy Freeman, Simon Harvey

Few events are more alarming to parents than their child having a first febrile convulsion or epileptic seizure. Seizures occur in up to 5% of children, but fortunately most are single episodes of a non-serious nature. This chapter is concerned with the diagnosis of seizures and related disorders, less so with the treatment of epilepsy and co-morbid conditions.

## Terminology and classification

An epileptic seizure is a transient occurrence of signs and/or symptoms due to abnormal excessive or synchronous neuronal activity in the brain. Epilepsy is characterized by an enduring predisposition of the brain to generate epileptic seizures and by the neurobiological, cognitive, psychological and social consequences of this condition. For practical purposes, this definition has generally excluded individuals with single seizures, neonatal seizures, febrile seizures and seizures considered provoked by acute neurological insults or systemic illness. Children with conditions that do not meet the criteria for diagnosis of epilepsy make up the vast majority of those presenting with seizures.

The International League Against Epilepsy recognizes two major categories of epileptic seizures, based on clinical and electroencephalographic (EEG) features: focal seizures and generalized seizures. Focal seizures originate within neural networks involving one hemisphere of the brain and are more or less localized at onset, whereas generalized seizures start in and rapidly involve networks in both cerebral hemispheres. Several, pathophysiologically distinct generalized seizure types are recognized by their different clinical and EEG patterns, the most common being tonic–clonic, absence and myoclonic seizures. Focal seizures have common pathophysiological features and are not further classified, but can be distinguished by the region of brain involved and the resultant clinical manifestations; the terms 'simple' and 'complex partial' are no longer applied to focal seizures according to degrees of impaired consciousness, although this is still an important clinical distinction. Epileptic spasms are not definitively focal or generalized in nature, hence are given a separate category in the current seizure classification (Box 17.1.1).



The conditions that predispose to epileptic seizures (*the epilepsies*), are best characterized, when possible, by the cause of the particular condition and by the epileptic syndrome. An epileptic syndrome is an electroclinically distinctive condition identifiable on the basis of a typical age of onset, specific EEG findings, seizure types, and often other features that, when taken together, permit a specific diagnosis. The syndrome diagnosis often has implications for treatment, management and prognosis. One practical way of organizing the list of recognized syndromes is by age of onset (Box 17.1.2). Some of the recognized syndromes are known to be due to single-gene mutations, primarily of genes coding for neuronal ion channels. Some epilepsies are due to cerebral or cortical malformation, and others are associated with rare metabolic disorders. Some are due to prenatally or postnatally acquired brain injuries. Unfortunately, the causes of the most common syndromes remain unknown, although a polygenetic basis is most likely.

Prospective studies of new-onset epileptic seizures in childhood reveal that approximately 50% of patients with a first seizure have a recurrence. Epilepsy, with recurrent unprovoked seizures, has an incidence of about 60–80 in 100 000 and a prevalence of about 5 in 1000 in childhood, the incidence and prevalence being highest in infancy. Studies of new-onset epilepsy in childhood indicate a greater proportion with focal seizures than generalized and undetermined seizures. Prospective studies of treated and untreated new-onset epilepsy reveal that about 80% of children go into remission, some with subsequent seizure relapses, and about 20% of children have treatment-resistant epilepsy.

## Common epilepsies of infancy, childhood and adolescence

### Febrile seizures

Fever and seizures may occur together with infections of the central nervous system (CNS) and with febrile illnesses in children with epilepsy. However, fever and seizures most often coexist as a manifestation of the syndrome of *febrile seizures,* a condition in which some infants and young children have a presumed genetic predisposition to seize in the presence of fever. Although not included within the classical definition of epilepsy, the syndrome of febrile seizures shares features in common with certain epilepsies, including an age-limited

**Box 17.1.1 Classification of epileptic seizure type, based on clinical and EEG features**

**Generalized**
- Tonic–clonic
- Absence
- Myoclonic
- Clonic
- Tonic
- Atonic

**Focal**

**Uncertain**
- Epileptic spasms

**Box 17.1.2 Epileptic syndromes by age of onset***

**Neonatal period and infancy**
- Early myoclonic encephalopathy
- Early infantile epileptic encephalopathy with suppression burst (Ohtahara syndrome)
- Epilepsy of infancy with migrating focal seizures
- Benign familial neonatal and infantile epilepsy
- Generalized epilepsy with febrile seizures plus (GEFS+)
- Infantile epileptic encephalopathy with epileptic spasms (West syndrome)
- Benign myoclonic epilepsy of infancy
- Severe myoclonic epilepsy of infancy (Dravet syndrome)

**Childhood**
- Childhood absence epilepsy
- Benign childhood epilepsy with centrotemporal spikes (rolandic epilepsy)
- Early-onset benign occipital epilepsy (Panayiotopoulos syndrome)
- Late-onset benign occipital epilepsy (Gastaut type)
- Epilepsy with myoclonic–atonic seizures (Doose syndrome)
- Epilepsy with myoclonic absences
- Childhood epileptic encephalopathy with tonic seizures (Lennox–Gastaut syndrome)
- Autosomal-dominant nocturnal frontal lobe epilepsy
- Epileptic encephalopathy with continuous spike-and-wave during sleep
- Landau–Kleffner syndrome

**Adolescence**
- Juvenile absence epilepsy
- Juvenile myoclonic epilepsy
- Epilepsy with generalized tonic–clonic seizures alone
- Progressive myoclonus epilepsies

**Less specific age relationship**
- Epilepsies with focal seizures due to structural brain abnormalities (e.g. temporal lobe and frontal lobe epilepsy)
- Reflex epilepsies (e.g. photosensitive epilepsy)

*This table excludes consideration of common conditions presenting with seizures in childhood, but not fulfilling criteria for epilepsy. These include: benign neonatal seizures, febrile seizures, single seizures and acute symptomatic (provoked) seizures.

predisposition to seizures and a family history of seizures in more than 30% of children. Some families are described in which the same neuronal ion channel gene mutation is found in individuals with epilepsy and those with febrile seizures alone. Febrile seizures are not just a non-specific seizure susceptibility in infants.

Simple febrile seizures are defined as brief, generalized tonic and/or clonic seizures in which there is neither clinical nor laboratory evidence of CNS infection, the temperature is 38 °C or higher, and the child has no history of previous afebrile seizures, neurological deficits or developmental delay to suggest an underlying neurological problem. Most febrile seizures are associated with upper respiratory or urinary tract infections or viral exanthemas and occur once at the beginning of the illness. Complex febrile seizures are those that are prolonged, focal or multiple.

Febrile seizures occur in approximately 3% of the population, commencing between the ages of 5 months and 5 years, with most manifesting in the first 2 years of life. In approximately one-third of children febrile seizures are recurrent, the risk increasing to 50% if onset is in infancy or there is a family history of febrile seizures. Only 3% of children with febrile seizures develop epilepsy. The risk is increased when there is abnormal development or neurological impairment, when there is a family history of epilepsy or if the febrile seizures are complex. When epilepsy follows febrile seizures it is invariably a later manifestation of the same underlying seizure predisposition. Very rarely, later epileptic seizures may be the result of brain injury from prolonged and focal febrile seizures (febrile status epilepticus). Febrile seizures are not associated with increased mortality or later intellectual impairment.

## Treatment

The cause of the febrile illness is investigated and treated on its own merits. There is no role for EEG or brain imaging in febrile seizures. There is debate about the role of antipyretics and gentle cooling. Seizures have usually ceased before medical help is obtained; however, if a febrile seizure continues after 3–5 minutes, it should be terminated urgently, usually with buccal, intramuscular or intravenous midazolam. Meningitis or encephalitis should be strongly considered if the child has a history of vomiting, is younger than 6 months, has repeated seizures following presentation, has been treated with antibiotics, has not recovered promptly from the seizure or seems more ill than would be expected following a simple febrile seizure.

Antiepileptic medication does not diminish the likelihood of later epilepsy and is rarely prescribed for the syndrome of febrile seizures. Parents and carers need explanation and reassurance about the benign nature of the condition, the likelihood of further febrile seizures, and the management of subsequent febrile illnesses and seizures. Children with a history of prolonged febrile seizures may be prescribed emergency buccal midazolam.

## West syndrome

West syndrome, also known as *infantile spasms*, is the most common and important to recognize severe epileptic syndrome in infancy. The principal seizure type is epileptic spasms, which are essentially brief tonic seizures that typically occur in series over a minute or more, usually many times a day. Onset of spasms is usually between 3 and 8 months of age, and males are affected more often than females. Flexor or salaam spasms are the most common and consist of sudden drawing up of the legs, hunching forward of the neck and shoulders, and flinging out of the arms; opisthotonic or extensor spasms are less common. The EEG usually shows a diffusely disorganized pattern with high-voltage, multifocal epileptic activity, called hypsarrhythmia (Fig. 17.1.1). Development may be delayed prior to the onset of spasms, or there may be loss of visual attention and arrest or regression of development at seizure onset. The developmental regression that occurs in West syndrome is attributable to the epileptic disorder and the condition is therefore considered to be an *epileptic encephalopathy*. Differential diagnosis includes a variety of normal or benign infant behaviours, such as sleep jerks, colic, shuddering attacks, benign myoclonus of infancy and gastro-oesophageal reflux, as well as other less sinister myoclonic epilepsies of infancy.

West syndrome is an age-dependent manifestation of a severe disturbance in the immature CNS. An underlying cause is identified in about 80% of infants, including prenatal, perinatal or postnatal brain injury (stroke or infection), focal or diffuse brain malformations, tuberous sclerosis and metabolic conditions. In these cases, the outcome for seizures and development is usually poor. In children where no cause is identified, outcome is more variable; if there is a prior history of developmental delay and spasms are not quickly controlled with treatment, outcome is again poor. Overall, 70–80% of children with West syndrome develop some degree of intellectual disability and 30–50% develop intractable seizures. In many children with chronic epilepsy following West syndrome, the electroclinical picture evolves to that of the *Lennox–Gastaut syndrome* with refractory tonic and other seizures, generalized slow spike–wave and paroxysmal fast activity on EEG, and severe intellectual disability. The neurological sequelae of West syndrome are the result of both the underlying cause and the deleterious effects of the epileptic encephalopathy on the developing brain.

### Treatment

West syndrome needs urgent diagnosis, investigation and treatment. Treatable metabolic conditions need exclusion, and pyridoxine-dependent seizures should be considered in children with prior epileptic seizures. Corticosteroid therapy (oral prednisolone or intramuscular adrenocorticotrophic hormone, ACTH) is more efficacious than vigabatrin and other antiepileptic drugs for achieving rapid cessation of spasms. For children with no identified predisposing condition, corticosteroid therapy also leads to better developmental outcome. Vigabatrin is a second-line agent, except in children with tuberous sclerosis where it is often used first. Other antiepileptic medications are of lower efficacy or unproven

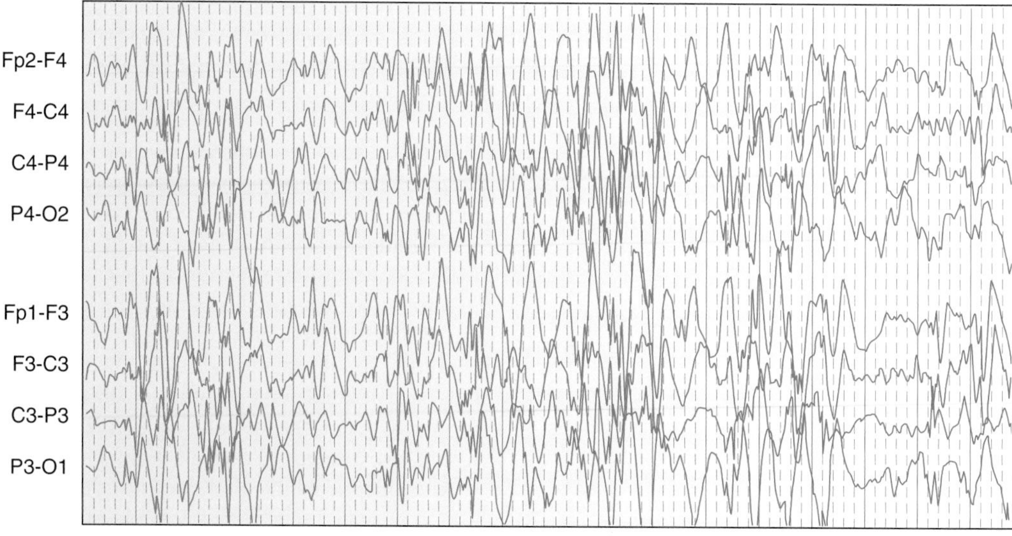


Fig. 17.1.1 The EEG pattern of hypsarrhythmia, showing diffuse, continuous, high-amplitude, irregular sharp waves, spikes, and slow waves on a disorganized background, typical of that seen in West syndrome.

benefit. In infants with unilateral strokes or malformations and drug-resistant seizures, epilepsy surgery may be considered. The aims of all treatments are to stop seizures, suppress the epileptic EEG disturbances and maximize neurological development.

### Clinical example

Baby Jonathan presented at the age of 5 months with episodes of stiffening and drawing up of his legs, thought to be colic. The attacks lasted only seconds but occurred in clusters up to 10 times each day, often after waking. During the attacks, his eyes rolled up, he appeared unaware and he would cry briefly. Jonathan's parents were also concerned that he seemed irritable, was not fixing on their faces and was no longer smiling. The pregnancy, birth and early developmental milestones had been unremarkable.

On examination, Jonathan made little eye contact and had poor head control. A cluster of typical symmetrical epileptic spasms occurred during the assessment. An EEG that day showed a modified hypsarrhythmic pattern, confirming West syndrome, and high-dose oral prednisolone was started promptly. MRI examination, metabolic testing and molecular karyotype were normal. Spasms ceased after the third day of prednisolone and there was improvement in visual attention in the following week. EEG after 2 weeks of treatment showed a marked reduction in epileptic activity with normal background activity. Prednisolone was tapered over the next 3 weeks and there was no recurrence of seizures after 1 month. Close observation for recurrent seizures, monitoring of developmental progression and repeat EEG were planned. The prognosis given to his parents was hopeful but not overly optimistic concerning developmental outcome.

## Absence epilepsy

Absence seizures are manifest by sudden cessation of activity with staring, usually lasting only 5–15 seconds. Blinking, upward deviation of the eyes, slight mouthing movements and some fidgeting hand movements (automatisms) may occur. The child is unresponsive, does not fall, is rarely incontinent and returns promptly to normal activity at the offset of the absence, with no memory of the seizure. The EEG shows generalized spike–wave activity during the seizure (Fig. 17.1.2). Usually, many attacks occur in a day. Absence seizures can generally be precipitated in the clinic room and during EEG recordings with hyperventilation. Differential diagnosis of absence seizures includes day-dreaming and focal seizures of temporal lobe origin.

Epilepsies with absence seizures usually present after 4 years of age and in otherwise normal children. There are two main syndromes described. In *childhood absence epilepsy* (formerly 'petit mal' epilepsy), absences begin before 10 years of age, tonic–clonic seizures are rare, the EEG shows runs of regular 3-Hz spike–wave activity, and prognosis for seizure remission is good. In *juvenile absence epilepsy,* onset of absences is later, sometimes in the teen years, the EEG may show faster and more irregular spike–wave activity, there may be associated tonic–clonic seizures, and prognosis for seizure remission is poorer.

### Treatment

EEG is needed to confirm absence seizures and characterize the epileptic syndrome; brain imaging is unnecessary. Sodium valproate, ethosuximide and lamotrigine are the medications used commonly to treat absence seizures. Treatment is usually for 2 years in typical

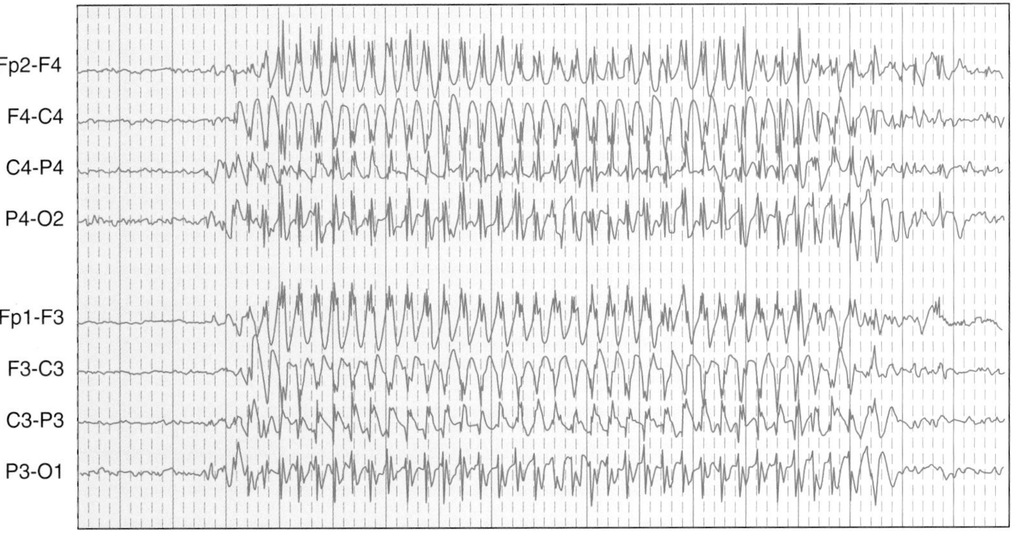


Fig. 17.1.2 The EEG of childhood absence epilepsy during an absence seizure, showing a paroxysm of generalized 3-Hz spike–wave activity.

childhood absence epilepsy, with an expectation of seizure remission, and through puberty into the teen years in juvenile absence epilepsy. Rare refractory cases may respond to treatment with a ketogenic diet.

**Clinical example**

Nadine, a 6-year-old girl, was noted by her parents to frequently 'blank out' while sitting at the dinner table and, most recently, to stop walking and talking while shopping with her mother. These episodes were occurring several times a day and seemed to last only a few seconds. Her schoolteacher had not noticed any problems. Hyperventilation in the clinic room provoked a typical episode lasting 12 seconds, during which Nadine was seen to stop hyperventilating, be unresponsive, fidget with her shirt and have slight bobbing of her eyes. Childhood absence epilepsy was confirmed with an EEG, which showed 3-Hz generalized spike–wave activity during spontaneous and hyperventilation-induced absence seizures. Sodium valproate was introduced slowly over 3 weeks, with no absences noted after the second week of treatment and none precipitated with hyperventilation when reviewed. Slight irritability and moodiness were reported by Nadine's parents as potential side-effects of treatment.

## Benign focal epilepsies of childhood

The benign focal epilepsies of childhood are some of the most common epileptic syndromes in children. They occur in otherwise normal preschool and primary school-aged children, and typically manifest with infrequent, sleep-related focal seizures and prominent focal epileptiform patterns on EEG. The two most common varieties are *benign rolandic epilepsy (benign childhood epilepsy with centrotemporal spikes)*, in which the seizure and EEG focus is low in the central sulcus (rolandic) region on one or both sides, and *benign occipital epilepsy,* in which the seizure and EEG focus is in the occipital lobe on one or both sides. The cause of the benign focal epilepsies is unknown; they are not due to underlying structural brain lesions, and current evidence of a genetic association is lacking. An age-limited, maturational disturbance in these brain regions is postulated. The EEG abnormalities of the benign focal epilepsies can be found in children with no history of seizures, sometimes leading to diagnostic errors.

In *benign rolandic epilepsy,* seizure onset is usually between 5 and 10 years of age and there is a male predominance. Focal seizures feature tingling or twitching of the mouth and preserved consciousness, often with associated drooling, choking noises and inability to speak. Seizures may progress to jerking of one side of the body, with or without impairment of consciousness. Some children have convulsions in which the focal onset is not recalled or witnessed. Attacks typically occur from sleep. EEG recordings that include sleep reveal frequent focal epileptiform activity over the centrotemporal regions on one or both sides (Fig. 17.1.3).

In *benign occipital epilepsy*, the presentation is usually before 6 years of age and there is a female predominance. The focal seizures are characteristically from sleep, beginning with staring, vomiting, head rotation, eye deviation, and may lead to hemiclonic or bilateral jerking. Again, the focal onset may be unwitnessed. Seizures can sometimes be prolonged and raise concern about encephalitis. Daytime attacks may occur with episodic visual distortions or hallucinations and migraine-like headaches. EEG recordings that include sleep reveal focal epileptiform activity over the occipital regions. In typical cases of benign focal epilepsy, brain imaging is unnecessary.

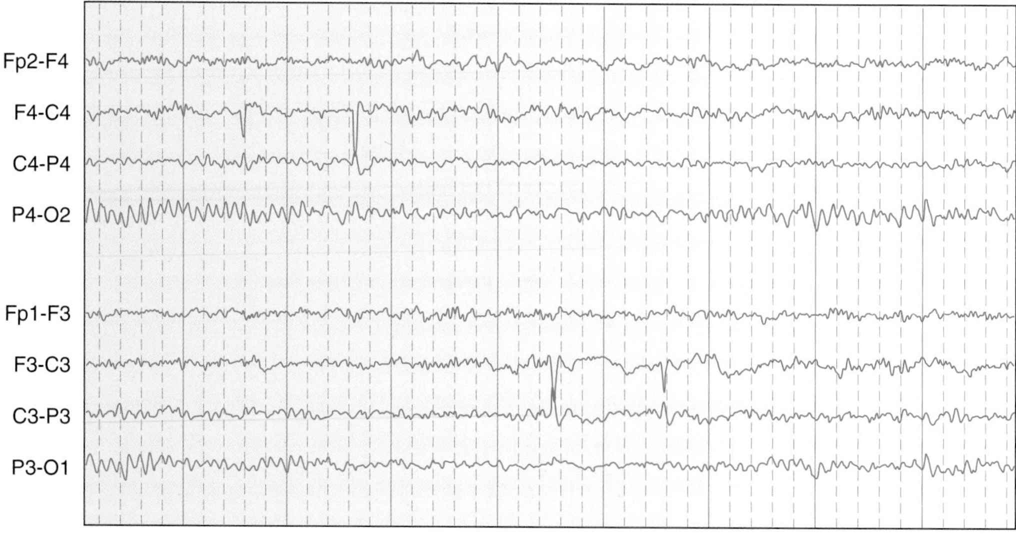


Fig. 17.1.3 The EEG of benign childhood epilepsy with centrotemporal spikes (rolandic epilepsy) showing independent bilateral focal epileptiform activity in the central regions.

### Treatment

Seizures tend to be infrequent in the benign focal epilepsies and many children have only one or two seizures in total. Because of this, and the tendency for nocturnal occurrence, treatment with antiepileptic medications is not always necessary. If warranted, treatment with sodium valproate or carbamazepine for 1–2 years is usually adequate. Prognosis is excellent, with absence of cognitive and behavioural problems, and remission of seizures by the teenage years – hence the term 'benign'. In rare instances, these epilepsies may manifest in an atypical way with more problematic seizures, continuous bilateral EEG disturbances, and deleterious effects on language and motor development; this tends to occur in children with pre-existing neurological problems.

**Clinical example**

Michael, a developmentally normal 8-year-old boy, presented to the emergency department of a regional hospital after being found seizing in his motel bed at 5 a.m. while holidaying with his family. The seizure was brief, had bilateral tonic–clonic movements, was associated with prominent gurgling noises, and was followed by a 10–15-minute period during which his speech was slurred and his face drooped on one side. The parents recalled hearing similar noises from Michael's bedroom once or twice previously and occasionally finding his pillow wet with saliva in the morning. Michael described waking from his sleep in this seizure, having a fuzzy feeling in his mouth and being unable to call out to his parents, who were sleeping in the same room.

An EEG arranged subsequently showed very frequent left central–temporal epileptiform discharges that became almost continuous in sleep. A diagnosis of benign rolandic epilepsy was made. Following much parental counselling and reassurance about the benign nature of this type of epilepsy, it was decided to not perform magnetic resonance imaging (MRI) and to defer treatment with antiepileptic medication. General safety and lifestyle advice was given about seizures, although it was appreciated that seizure occurrence in the day was unlikely.

## Epilepsies with generalized tonic–clonic seizures

Generalized tonic–clonic seizures begin with loss of consciousness, stiffening (tonic), temporary cessation of breathing and falling if standing, then gradually progress to a phase with generalized, rhythmic jerking (clonic), which is initially rapid but gradually slows. Generalized tonic–clonic seizures invariably cease spontaneously, usually within a few minutes, and are followed by a postictal period with depressed consciousness and headache, during which the person usually sleeps. There are no warning symptoms (auras), no significant focal features to the seizure, and no memory of the actual seizure. Generalized tonic–clonic seizures often occur during febrile illnesses in young children and either during sleep or following periods of sleep deprivation or stress in older children and adolescents.

The epilepsies with generalized tonic–clonic seizures are a heterogeneous group of disorders that typically begin in childhood or adolescence and sometimes feature additional absence and myoclonic seizures. Although the majority of the epilepsies with generalized tonic–clonic seizures are of unknown cause, genetic factors are strongly implicated and some examples of single-gene defects are known. In general, there is no structural brain or metabolic abnormality, usually normal intellect and often a family history of seizures. Sometimes there is a history of prior febrile seizures or absence seizures; in these cases, the later occurrence of tonic–clonic seizures represents an age-dependent expression of the same genetically determined seizure tendency. The routine EEG shows generalized spike–wave and polyspike–wave discharges. *Juvenile myoclonic epilepsy* typically begins in teenage years with generalized tonic–clonic seizures, early morning myoclonic jerks, and sometimes brief or subtle absence seizures. *Photosensitive epilepsy* is another syndrome with generalized tonic–clonic seizures, where the seizures and EEG abnormalities are almost exclusively related to flashing light stimulation.

The differential diagnosis of generalized tonic–clonic seizures includes: focal seizures that spread to become bilateral and convulsive; syncope, which typically involves clonic movements; and psychogenic seizures. A preceding aura, focal or asymmetrical features to the seizure, transient postictal unilateral weakness (Todd's paresis), focal neurological deficits on examination, or a history of a prior cerebral trauma or infection should suggest a focal basis for an apparently generalized tonic–clonic seizure. Seizures of brief duration with rapid recovery and seizures occurring in typical vasovagal settings (see below) should suggest syncope rather than epilepsy. Psychogenic seizures are highly variable in their manifestations and can occur in patients with epilepsy, making their diagnosis sometimes difficult; signs that suggest psychogenic seizures include eye closure during the event, resistance to passive eye-opening, and intermittent or waxing and waning motor activity.

### Treatment

Sodium valproate is the drug of choice for generalized tonic–clonic seizures, especially when there is generalized spike–wave on EEG or a history to suggest absence or myoclonic seizures. Carbamazepine is sometimes used for generalized tonic–clonic seizures, but there is a risk of exacerbating absence and myoclonic seizures in predisposed patients. Several other antiepileptic medications are also effective (Table 17.1.1).

**Table 17.1.1 Antiepileptic medications most effective in different seizure types**

| Seizure type | Antiepileptic medication |
|---|---|
| Focal | Carbamazepine, oxcarbazepine, levetiracetam, lamotrigine, sodium valproate, topiramate, gabapentin, pregabalin, lacosamide, zonisamide, benzodiazepines, phenytoin, phenobarbital |
| Generalized tonic–clonic | Sodium valproate, lamotrigine, topiramate, levetiracetam, carbamazepine, phenytoin, oxcarbazepine, benzodiazepines, phenobarbital |
| Absence | Sodium valproate, ethosuximide, lamotrigine |
| Myoclonic, atonic, tonic | Sodium valproate, lamotrigine, benzodiazepines, topiramate, levetiracetam |
| Epileptic spasms | Prednisolone/ACTH, vigabatrin |

Seizure control is usually possible with medication and lifestyle adjustments (e.g. avoiding sleep deprivation). Many children with tonic–clonic seizures alone outgrow their need for medication, but adolescents with juvenile myoclonic epilepsy usually require treatment into adult life.

**Clinical example**

Stephanie, a 13-year-old girl with a history of a single febrile seizure in infancy, presented to a regional hospital emergency department after having a generalized tonic–clonic seizure at school camp. The seizure occurred in the shower at 7 a.m., the morning after girls in Stephanie's cabin had stayed awake until 4 a.m. Stephanie was heard to fall in the shower and was found by a friend convulsing on the shower floor. She sustained a forehead bruise and hot water scalding on her back. There was no history of staring episodes or isolated jerking of the limbs. Stephanie recalled that on one occasion she had had to walk away from a computer game that her brother was playing because she felt sick and her head started jerking. There was no family history of epilepsy.

Subsequent EEG recording showed frequent bursts of generalized fast spike–wave activity at rest and during photic stimulation. A diagnosis of epilepsy with generalized tonic–clonic seizures and associated photosensitivity was made. Long discussions were held with Stephanie and her parents over the initial and subsequent consultations, highlighting safety and lifestyle factors. Sodium valproate was commenced after discussion of the high likelihood of further seizures. The potential for weight gain and mild hair loss as side-effects of treatment was also discussed, these concerning Stephanie more than the risk of further seizures. The family was given a guarded prognosis for seizure remission in the later teen years and regular review was arranged.

## Epilepsies with focal seizures due to structural brain abnormalities

Focal seizures can arise in any part of the brain and the manifestations of the seizure depend on the location and extent or spread of the seizure. An *aura* is the phase of a focal seizure without loss of consciousness that manifests as a feeling or experience rather than as a movement or behaviour. Epilepsies with focal seizures can be described in terms of the location of the seizure onset and the underlying pathology. Seizures begin at any age but onset in late childhood and adolescence is common, even when due to congenital malformations. In infants and young children, lesions may be multilobar or hemispheric. Where no lesion is identified on MRI there may be clinical, EEG or functional imaging features that suggest an occult lesion.

Seizures in *temporal lobe epilepsy* (TLE) characteristically manifest by motionless staring, fearful or bewildered facial expression, unresponsiveness, hand and mouth movements that resemble voluntary actions (*automatisms*), and postictal amnesia and confusion. In some patients there may be head-turning or stiffening or jerking of the limbs on one side during the seizure. Autonomic disturbances, such as facial flushing or pallor, salivation and sometimes vomiting, may occur; apnoea may be the predominant manifestation in infancy. An aura is often present but may not be described at the time or recalled in a young or developmentally delayed child; fear, unusual smells or tastes, abdominal discomfort and dizzy or dreamy states are the usual descriptions. Seizures may spread to become bilaterally convulsive. Seizures in TLE last longer than absence seizures, generally 30–60 seconds, and are followed by postictal confusion and sleepiness. They are usually infrequent and commonly occur in clusters over several days, alternating with seizure-free periods.

Seizures in *frontal lobe epilepsy* (FLE) often occur from sleep, are brief in duration, and typically manifest with prominent motor features such as unilateral or bilateral stiffening or jerking, asymmetrical tonic posturing with head deviation to one side, loud vocalization, and hyperkinetic automatisms such as tapping, cycling and running. Seizures may occur on a multiple nightly basis. Consciousness may be preserved even when there are bilateral motor features, or be lost when the seizure discharge spreads bilaterally.

The EEG in epilepsies with focal seizures may be normal, show non-specific abnormalities, or show localized epileptic patterns over the affected brain region. Video-EEG monitoring with recording of seizures is sometimes necessary to confirm the diagnosis and localize the seizures. The differential diagnosis of TLE, with episodes of staring and confused behaviour, includes day-dreaming, absence seizures, behavioural outbursts, migraine and psychogenic seizures. The differential diagnosis of FLE, with nocturnal convulsive or thrashing seizures, includes parasomnias and epilepsy with generalized tonic–clonic seizures. Benign focal epilepsies can usually be distinguished from TLE and FLE by their characteristic clinical and EEG features. If typical features of benign focal epilepsy are not present, the diagnosis cannot be made confidently, and brain imaging with MRI is needed to search for an underlying lesion.

### Treatment

Carbamazepine is the drug of first choice for epilepsies with focal seizures, including TLE and FLE. Seizures may be resistant to treatment and over time the patient may be tried on other medications (see Table 17.1.1). Cognitive, physical and behavioural problems may be present in some children and are usually manifestations of the underlying cerebral disturbance or lesion. These co-morbid problems may require specific assessment and intervention in their own right. Spontaneous seizure remission occurs in some patients, mainly when a lesion is not identified on MRI. In children with uncontrolled seizures that impact significantly on the life of the child and family, or are exerting detrimental effects on neurological development, epilepsy surgery should be considered.

**Clinical example**

Steven, a 9-year-old boy with a history of learning problems, was referred for management of refractory seizures. Seizures began at age 5 years, occurred in clusters each week, and were characterized by a scared feeling in the abdomen followed by cessation of activity, loss of responsiveness, stiffening of the right hand and rocking movements. Twice during illnesses, seizures became bilaterally convulsive. None of the three antiepileptic medications used over the years had controlled Steven's seizures.

MRI showed a lesion of benign appearance in the uncus of the left temporal lobe, thought to be a developmental tumour. Video-EEG recording of seizures showed electrical onset in the left temporal lobe region. Cognitive testing showed normal intellect but decreased verbal abilities. Left temporal lesionectomy was performed and the histopathology revealed a ganglioglioma. After a year free of seizures, Steven was gradually weaned off his medication. Learning and behavioural difficulties persisted but were better managed with understanding of their cause, abolition of seizures, and institution of specific behavioural and educational strategies.

## Non-epileptic episodic disorders

Not all episodes of neurological dysfunction in infancy and childhood are epileptic. Sleep disorders, movement disorders, circulatory disturbances, migraine and some normal behaviour may mimic epileptic seizures (Box 17.1.3). Disorders frequently misdiagnosed as seizures are breath-holding attacks in infancy and syncope in older children and adolescents, because of their paroxysmal nature with loss of consciousness and associated convulsive movements. In such attacks, the neurological manifestations are secondary to transient cerebral ischaemia and not to any intrinsic cerebral dysfunction.

### Breath-holding attacks

Attacks usually start in the first or second year of life and are reported in up to 4% of children. Crucial to the diagnosis is recognition that attacks are precipitated by either physical trauma, such as a knock or a fall, or emotional trauma such as fright,

**Box 17.1.3 Differential diagnosis of epileptic seizures**

- Normal behaviours (e.g. sleep jerks, day-dreaming, masturbation)
- Parasomnias (e.g. night terrors, sleepwalking)
- Breath-holding spells
- Syncope (e.g. vasovagal, cardiac arrhythmia/outflow obstruction)
- Migraine and migraine variants (e.g. benign paroxysmal vertigo/torticollis)
- Movement disorders (e.g. tics, tremor, clonus, shuddering attacks)
- Non-neurological (e.g. gastro-oesophageal reflux, hypoglycaemia)
- Psychiatric (e.g. rage attacks, psychogenic seizures)

anger or frustration, but precipitants are not always severe or noticed. Attacks usually commence with crying, but this may be brief or absent. Apnoea and bradycardia then occur, either suddenly or gradually, with cyanosis or pallor following. The attack may terminate without loss of consciousness or progress, with the child becoming unconscious, limp, and sometimes briefly stiffening or jerking in response to the cerebral ischaemia. Recovery is usually rapid, although some children are drowsy and lethargic after an attack with convulsive features. Attacks usually cease by the third or fourth year of life.

The pathophysiology of breath-holding attacks is not well understood, but affected children probably have an age-related dysfunction in cardiorespiratory reflexes. Iron-deficiency anaemia is an exacerbating factor in some children with frequent attacks or prominent convulsive features. Breath-holding attacks are not a cause of death, epilepsy, intellectual disability or cerebral damage and families should be reassured about their benign nature. EEG is unnecessary, but ECG may be considered if there are atypical features.

### Syncope

Syncope, or fainting, is common in childhood. As in adults, it is the result of decreased cardiac output and cerebral perfusion leading to loss of consciousness and falling. Brief tonic stiffening, clonic jerking or incontinence often accompanies the loss of consciousness and may lead to misdiagnosis as an epileptic seizure. Recovery is usually prompt following syncope. Light-headedness, dizziness, visual loss, and auditory or sensory changes may be recalled prior to loss of consciousness; these are manifestations of focal cortical ischaemia. Sweating and tachycardia during recovery are common, as a result of reflex sympathetic drive. However, a more important clue to the diagnosis than the recalled or observed clinical features is the situation in which the episode occurred. Syncope should be suspected as the basis of loss of consciousness or convulsing when attacks occur contemporaneously with vomiting illnesses, prolonged standing (e.g. classroom, church), hair-brushing, injury, venepuncture or other medical procedures, and witnessing medical or veterinary procedures. Syncope without a precipitant, or syncope during exercise or while in water, should prompt concern about a primary cardiac cause, such as prolonged QT syndrome or left ventricular outflow obstruction. No investigations, other than perhaps an ECG, are needed in syncope, and most patients and families need only explanation and reassurance. Recognition of precipitating situations and presyncopal symptoms is helpful in taking evasive action.

## Assessment of children with seizures

Three important and successive steps in the assessment of a child with suspected seizures are to:

- distinguish epileptic seizures from non-epileptic attacks
- determine the type(s) of seizure the child is having, most importantly whether they are generalized or focal, and determine whether unrecognized minor seizures are occurring
- determine the type of epilepsy and underlying aetiology in the child having recurrent seizures.

The diagnosis of epileptic seizures is made on clinical grounds with investigations used to confirm the diagnosis, help characterize the seizure disorder and determine the underlying cause. Detailed history from the patient and observers, sometimes combined with home video-recordings of attacks, are the basis of making a correct diagnosis. Children with epilepsy should be examined for dysmorphic features, neurocutaneous stigmata, focal neurological deficits, signs of raised intracranial pressure and markers of systemic disease.

Metabolic disturbance, especially hypoglycaemia and hypocalcaemia, should be considered in infants with seizures and children with no identifiable cause for their epilepsy. Pyridoxine dependency, although very rare, should be considered in refractory infant-onset epilepsy.

EEG is invaluable in the characterization of seizures and epilepsies, and should generally be requested in all children with definite afebrile seizures. EEG is of no value in the investigation of febrile seizures. In epilepsy, the EEG helps to distinguish focal from generalized seizures and aids diagnosis of specific epileptic syndromes, especially the epilepsies with generalized seizures and benign focal epilepsies of childhood. In this way, the EEG may assist in making the correct choice of antiepileptic medication and determining the need for brain imaging. It is important to note that the interictal EEG is normal in many patients with epilepsy, particularly those with focal epilepsies due to known or suspected structural brain abnormalities. Conversely, epileptiform abnormalities, particularly centrotemporal spikes and brief generalized spike–wave bursts in drowsiness, are seen in up to 5% of normal children without seizures, and more frequently in children with underlying neurological and developmental problems. EEG should therefore *never* be used to 'rule out' epilepsy in a child with undiagnosed attacks. In children with undiagnosed recurrent attacks, or children with epileptic seizures of uncertain type, video-EEG monitoring may be needed.

Brain imaging is indicated when one suspects an underlying cerebral abnormality. MRI should be requested in children with focal seizures or significant focal EEG abnormalities, except when they are characteristic of a benign focal (rolandic or occipital) epilepsy. MRI should also be performed in children with focal or generalized seizures who have significant developmental delay, abnormal neurological findings on examination, a history of a prior neurological insult, or poorly controlled seizures. Brain imaging is unnecessary in typical cases of benign focal epilepsy, epilepsies with absence seizures and epilepsies with generalized tonic–clonic seizures in otherwise normal children. Computed tomography (CT) is indicated only in children suspected of conditions that may require immediate intensive care or neurosurgical intervention, such as stroke, traumatic brain injury or raised intracranial pressure. To limit unnecessary irradiation, CT should *never* be requested in an otherwise well child.

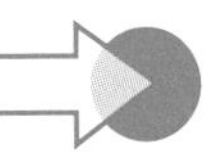

**Practical points**

**Diagnosis**

- A detailed description of the attacks and the situations in which they occurred, sometimes supplemented with a home video-recording, are the keys to correct diagnosis of epileptic seizures and non-epileptic events.
- The differential diagnosis of episodic staring includes day-dreaming or inattention, absence seizures, and focal seizures with impaired consciousness.
- The differential diagnosis of collapse and convulsing includes syncope, generalized tonic–clonic seizures, focal seizures and psychogenic attacks.
- EEG is helpful in characterizing seizures and epilepsies but should not be done to clarify the nature of undiagnosed events. Further history, home video-recording or video-EEG monitoring may be needed for undiagnosed episodic phenomena.
- Benign focal epilepsies and epilepsies with absences or generalized tonic–clonic seizures usually have characteristic epileptic patterns on routine EEG; if these are not present, consideration of non-epileptic episodes or epilepsy with focal seizures due to structural brain abnormality is required.
- MRI is performed when the seizures, EEG, history or examination suggest an underlying cerebral abnormality or cannot exclude one. MRI is not performed in benign focal epilepsies and in epilepsies with absences or generalized tonic–clonic seizures.
- Learning and behavioural problems in a child with epilepsy are often the result of the underlying neurological problem rather than being secondary to seizures or medications.

## General principles of treatment of seizures in children

Explanation and reassurance, provision of information about the child's specific seizure disorder, first-aid advice about how to manage future seizures, discussion of potential seizure precipitants, consideration of lifestyle modification, and safety advice regarding bathing, swimming, heights and driving are all important aspects of seizure management. The decision to treat a child with antiepileptic medication, and the choice and duration of treatment, depend on the type of epilepsy and several patient and family factors. Antiepileptic medications reduce the likelihood of seizures but do not alter the course of epilepsy; that is, seizures do not remit any sooner on treatment. The appropriate antiepileptic drug is usually indicated by the predominant seizure type (see Box 17.1.1).

Seizures can usually be controlled with one medication at an optimal dose. Children vary greatly in their dosage requirements and tolerance of antiepileptic drugs; patient age and associated disabilities are the main determinants. Except in status epilepticus and other situations with frequent or severe seizures, antiepileptic medications are usually started singly and in low dosage, then increased gradually to a dose where seizure control is obtained or side-effects appear. The duration of therapy depends on the type of epilepsy and its natural history, the degree of seizure control and the patient's lifestyle. Several years of freedom from seizures are desirable before antiepileptic drugs are ceased, and this is best done slowly over a period of months. Antiepileptic drug interactions are common, both pharmacokinetic and pharmacodynamic, some being advantageous (e.g. sodium valproate and lamotrigine) and others leading to side-effects (e.g. barbiturates and benzodiazepines).

Almost all antiepileptic drugs produce side-effects such as drowsiness and unsteadiness if given in excess. These effects are common when medications are commenced and the dose is increased but they often wear off after the maintenance dose is reached. Some antiepileptic medications have side-effects of an idiosyncratic type, such as rash or behaviour disturbance (Table 17.1.2).

Use of serum levels for monitoring some antiepileptic medications is particularly useful if seizure control is inadequate, side-effects attributable to toxicity are suspected or compliance is uncertain. Blood level monitoring is of particular value in young infants, in children with intellectual disability and in patients with impaired consciousness (i.e. patients who are not able to describe side-effects). Barbiturate and phenytoin levels correlate well with both seizure control and

**Table 17.1.2 Side-effects of antiepileptic medications**

| Medication | Side-effects |
|---|---|
| **Toxicity** | |
| Able to be produced by most antiepileptic medications, especially in combination | Drowsiness, ataxia, tremor, nystagmus, dysarthria, confusion, nausea, vomiting, sleepiness or insomnia, mood disturbance |
| **Idiosyncratic** | |
| Carbamazepine | Rash, leukopenia, hyponatraemia, irritability, weight gain |
| Clonazepam | Behaviour disturbance, increased bronchial and salivary secretions |
| Lamotrigine | Rash, severe hypersensitivity syndrome |
| Levetiracetam | Behaviour disturbance |
| Oxcarbazepine | Rash, hyponatraemia |
| Phenytoin | Rash, serum-sickness-type illness, extravasation injury |
| Phenobarbital | Rash, behaviour disturbance |
| Sodium valproate | Weight gain, alopecia, pancreatitis, behaviour disturbance, fulminant hepatitis (rare) |
| Topiramate | Kidney stones, weight loss, speech disturbance, oligohydrosis/hyperthermia |
| Vigabatrin | Peripheral vision impairment, behaviour disturbance, weight gain |
| Pregabalin | Weight gain, constipation, ankle oedema |
| Zonisamide | Rash, oligohydrosis/hyperthermia |

side-effects, less so for carbamazepine. However, there is little role for blood level monitoring with the other antiepileptic medications, including sodium valproate and the benzodiazepines.

In addition to regular prescription of antiepileptic medication to prevent seizures, some parents and carers are instructed in the use of rectal diazepam or buccally administered midazolam to treat prolonged or recurring seizures, in children with a tendency to prolonged or clustering seizures.

For children with uncontrolled epilepsy, in whom seizures continue despite correct diagnosis and correct prescription of antiepileptic medications, specialized treatments such as epilepsy surgery, a ketogenic diet and vagus nerve stimulation may be considered. Surgical treatment is reserved for children with well characterized and drug-resistant focal epilepsy in whom seizures are impacting greatly on quality of life or development. Surgery is most effective when the seizure focus is discrete, away from critical functional cortex and associated with a lesion on MRI. Epilepsy surgery is carried out only after detailed evaluation in a centre with special experience in paediatric epileptology. A ketogenic diet, with high fat and low carbohydrate and protein intake, is sometimes effective in refractory epilepsy, especially in younger children, and in epilepsies with absence and myoclonic seizures. Vagus nerve stimulation, a form of chronic brain stimulation for the treatment of refractory epilepsy, is being utilized increasingly in children with uncontrolled seizures where drugs and surgery are ineffective.

When treating epilepsy it is necessary to consider the whole child and family in their environment, and not only the seizures. Problems pertaining to education and vocation, problems related to adjustment to the diagnosis, and associated psychological and behavioural problems may be more difficult to manage than the seizures. Disentangling the effects of seizures, medications, underlying lesions and conditions, pre-existing states, family dynamics and psychosocial factors can often be difficult, and requires specialist involvement. It is beyond the scope of this chapter to cover these important areas.

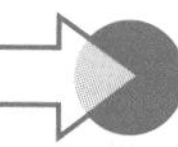

## Practical points

**Treatment**

- Explanation, reassurance, lifestyle modification and first-aid advice are important aspects of epilepsy management.
- For febrile seizures, reinforce that febrile seizure recurrence is common, epilepsy development is uncommon and neurodevelopmental sequelae are rare.
- In a child with epilepsy, the decision to treat, the choice of medication and the duration of therapy are determined by the type of seizure and epilepsy.
- As a general rule in antiepileptic drug therapy, 'start low and go slow' and withdraw medications slowly.
- Antiepileptic drug level monitoring is important with phenobarbital and phenytoin, often helpful with carbamazepine, but of limited value with sodium valproate and other drugs.
- If seizures continue despite treatment with antiepileptic medication, consider whether the diagnosis of epilepsy and the seizure/syndrome type are correct, whether the choice of medication is appropriate, and whether medication is being given and taken in appropriate doses.

# 17.2 Cerebral palsy and neurodegenerative disorders

Dinah Reddihough, Kevin Collins

## Cerebral palsy

> Cerebral palsy (CP) describes a group of permanent disorders of the development of movement and posture, causing activity limitation, that are attributed to non-progressive disturbances that occurred in the developing fetal or infant brain. The motor disorders of cerebral palsy are often accompanied by disturbances of sensation, perception, cognition, communication, and behaviour, by epilepsy, and by secondary musculoskeletal problems.
>
> (Rosenbaum P et al 2007 Dev Med Child Neurol Suppl 109:8–14)

The term is generally applied to children with permanent motor impairment due to non-progressive brain disorders occurring before the age of 5 years. There are many different causes, a wide range of manifestations of the motor disorder, and various associated problems.

Cerebral palsy is not a single disorder, but a group of disorders with diverse implications for children and their families. For some young people with mild cerebral palsy, the only motor deficit may be a minimal hemiplegia, causing clumsiness with certain movements. In other children with severe cerebral palsy, the motor deficit may be spastic quadriplegia with little or no independent movement. Because each child with cerebral palsy is different, individual assessment and treatment are essential.

### Prevalence

*Cerebral palsy is the most common physical disability in childhood.* The prevalence of cerebral palsy is between 2.0 and 2.5 per 1000 live births and has remained fairly stable since 1970 (Fig. 17.2.1).

### Aetiology

The cause of cerebral palsy is unknown in many children. Known risk factors include low birth weight, prematurity and multiple pregnancy. In a significant proportion of children who have cerebral palsy, there appears to have been no single event but rather a sequence of events or 'causal pathways' that have culminated in the motor damage.

#### Historical aspects

There has been a fundamental change in our understanding of aetiological factors during the past 20 years. Before this, most cases of cerebral palsy were thought to be caused by lack of oxygen during labour or at birth, and it was expected that improvement in obstetrics and neonatal care would lower cerebral palsy rates. However, despite an increased use of interventions such as caesarean section and electronic fetal monitoring, cerebral palsy rates have remained constant.

Current research suggests that about 8–10% of cases are associated with perinatal asphyxia, a condition in which there have been perinatal events likely to reduce oxygen supply, evidenced by significant acidosis, and failure of function in at least two organs (usually the brain and kidney). Perinatal asphyxia may not necessarily be the primary cause of the cerebral palsy and is generally not preventable. Because it is often impossible to ascribe clinical signs and symptoms to an event during birth, the term 'birth asphyxia' should be avoided.

#### Current knowledge about aetiology

When does the brain insult occur?

- Prenatal events are responsible for approximately 75% of all cases of cerebral palsy.
- Perinatal events contribute 10–15%.
- Postneonatal causes (occurring after 28 days of life) account for about 10% of all cases.

A prenatal cause is assumed in the absence of clear evidence for a perinatal or postnatal cause.

#### What are the prenatal causes?

*Malformations.* Disturbances of brain development, usually between 12 and 20 weeks' gestation, resulting in a variety of abnormalities. They may be identified

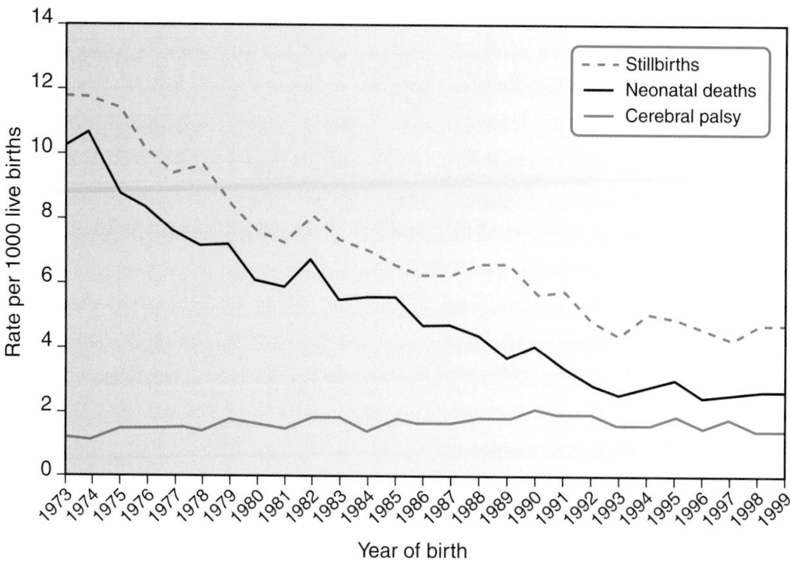


Fig. 17.2.1 Cerebral palsy, stillbirth and neonatal death rates per 1000 births in Victoria using published and unpublished data from the Victorian Cerebral Palsy Register and the Victorian Perinatal Data Collection Unit. (Source: Reid S, Lanigan A, Reddihough DS 2005 Report of the Victorian Cerebral Palsy Register.)

by brain imaging, magnetic resonance imaging (MRI) being the preferred investigation. Some malformations have a genetic basis.

*Vascular.* Vascular events such as middle cerebral artery occlusion (Fig. 17.2.2).

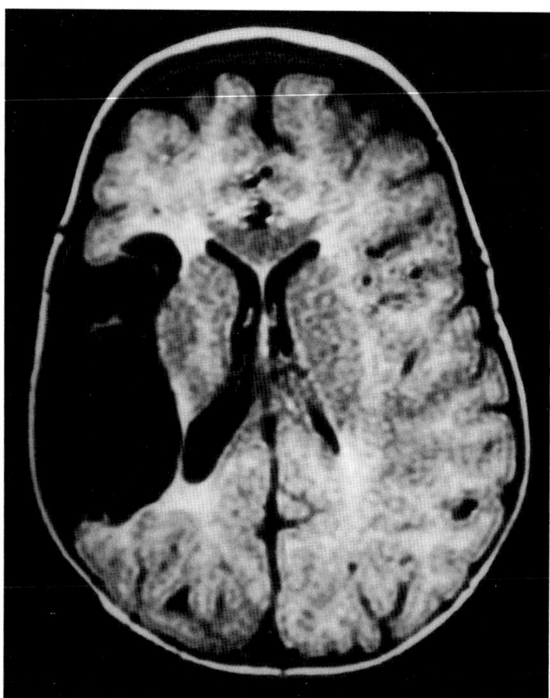

Fig. 17.2.2 Magnetic resonance image of the brain of a 2-year-old boy with left spastic hemiparesis, showing loss of brain tissue in right temporal and frontal lobes, consistent with an old (prenatal) right middle cerebral artery territory infarct.

*Infective.* Maternal infections during the first and second trimesters of pregnancy, including the TORCH group of organisms (*t*oxoplasmosis, *r*ubella, *c*ytomegalovirus and *h*erpes simplex virus). There is also evidence that maternal infections in the perinatal period may form part of the causal pathway to cerebral palsy.

*Genetic.* Uncommon genetic syndromes.

*Metabolic.* Iodine deficiency in early pregnancy, an important cause in many parts of the world.

*Toxic.* Lead, methylmercury ingestion and other toxins are rare associations.

## What are the perinatal causes?

*Problems during labour and delivery.* Obstetric emergencies such as obstructed labour, antepartum haemorrhage or cord prolapse compromising the fetus.

*Neonatal problems.* Conditions such as severe hypoglycaemia or untreated jaundice may be involved.

## Why are premature and low-birth-weight infants at risk of cerebral palsy?

Premature and low-birth-weight children have a higher risk of cerebral palsy. For those born at less than 33 weeks' gestation, the risk is up to 30 times higher than for those born at term. Some premature infants develop brain damage from complications of their immaturity, such as intraventricular haemorrhage, whereas others are damaged earlier in pregnancy. Intrauterine growth retardation is associated with cerebral palsy in both term and pre-term infants.

Periventricular white matter injury and the more localized pattern of periventricular leukomalacia is a common radiological finding in premature children with cerebral palsy. It is caused by an ischaemic process, usually occurring between 28 and 34 weeks' gestation, in the watershed zone that exists in the periventricular white matter of the immature brain. Periventricular white matter injury is also found in infants born at term, suggesting that the insult occurred early in the third trimester even though the pregnancy progressed to term.

### Why is multiple pregnancy a risk factor?

Multiple pregnancy is associated with pre-term delivery, poor intrauterine growth, birth defects and intrapartum complications and with an increased risk of both mortality and cerebral palsy. Intrauterine death of a co-twin is associated with a substantially increased rate of cerebral palsy.

### What are the postneonatal causes of cerebral palsy?

- Infections, for example, meningitis, encephalitis and septicaemia.
- Injuries may be accidental (such as motor vehicle accidents and near drowning episodes), or non-accidental. Improved road safety and mandatory fencing around home swimming pools are important preventative measures.
- Apparent life-threatening events and cerebrovascular accidents.
- Meningitis, septicaemia and infections such as malaria are important causes of cerebral palsy in developing countries.

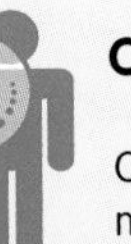

**Clinical example**

Caitlin is aged 2 years and 6 months. Her mother went into labour at 33 weeks' gestation after an uneventful pregnancy. The delivery was rapid. Apgar scores were 6 at 1 minute and 8 at 5 minutes. Her parents remember some panic in the labour ward and felt that more could have been done to slow the labour. Caitlin developed hyaline membrane disease and mild jaundice. In the early neonatal period she had difficulty sucking, which was attributed to her prematurity. She was slow in her motor development and did not sit until the age of 15 months. A diagnosis of cerebral palsy was made at that time.

When Caitlin was 2 years old, her parents requested an opinion as to whether subsequent children were likely to have cerebral palsy, believing that her prematurity and problems at birth were responsible for her condition. MRI of the brain demonstrated a brain malformation with bilateral clefts in the cerebral cortex, dating the problems to early pregnancy rather than the perinatal period.

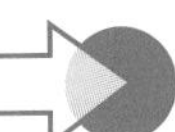

**Practical points**

- Cerebral palsy is a diverse disorder with multiple risk factors and aetiologies.
- When determining aetiology, distinguish risk factors from causes.
- Most cases of cerebral palsy relate to events long before birth.
- Perinatal asphyxia is responsible for only a small proportion of cases (approximately 8–10%).
- It is important to establish the cause of cerebral palsy if at all possible. It is helpful for families and essential for genetic counselling.
- Magnetic resonance imaging (MRI) should be undertaken if the cause is not apparent.

## Classification

Cerebral palsy is classified by motor type, topographical distribution and the severity of the motor disorder.

### Type of motor disorder

Cerebral palsy is a disorder of movement (difficulties with voluntary movement and/or abnormal movements), posture and muscle tone. Children with cerebral palsy have various types of movement disorder.

*Spastic cerebral palsy (70%).* This is the most common type. Spasticity involves increased muscle tone with characteristic clasp-knife quality. Children with spasticity often have underlying weakness. In spastic cerebral palsy, there is damage to the motor cortex or corticospinal tracts, in contrast to dyskinetic and ataxic cerebral palsy, which are associated with abnormalities of the basal ganglia and cerebellum, respectively.

*Dyskinetic cerebral palsy (10–15%).* This refers to a group of cerebral palsies with involuntary movements and is characterized by abnormalities of tone involving the whole body. Several terms are used within this group:

- *Dystonia* is the term used for sustained muscle contractions that frequently cause twisting or repetitive movements, or abnormal postures.
- *Athetosis* refers to slow writhing movements involving the distal parts of the limbs.
- *Chorea* is the term for rapid jerky involuntary movements.

*Ataxic cerebral palsy (less than 5%).* Children have a fine tremor, more noticeable when movements are initiated, and often have poor balance and hypotonia. Ataxia is associated with other neurological conditions that must be excluded before this diagnosis is made.

Some children have more than one type of motor disorder.

### Topographical distribution

The terms diplegia, hemiplegia and quadriplegia generally apply to children with spastic cerebral palsy as the extrapyramidal types (dyskinesia and ataxia) usually involve four limbs:

- The term *diplegia* is used where the predominant problem is in the lower limbs but signs are usually also present in the upper limb. Most of these children have normal intelligence. Spastic diplegia is the pattern most commonly seen in premature infants who have the radiological finding of periventricular white matter injury.
- Children with *spastic hemiplegia* usually have normal intelligence, frequently have epilepsy (50–70%) and visual deficits (homonymous hemianopsia), and may have sensory impairments in the upper limb.
- Children with *spastic quadriplegia* often have intellectual disability, epilepsy and visual impairment. Poor trunk control and oromotor difficulties may also be present.

### Severity of the motor disorder

The Gross Motor Function Classification System (GMFCS) provides information about the severity of the movement problems based on children's motor abilities and their need for walking frames, wheelchairs and other mobility devices. There are five levels: children in levels I and II walk independently; children in level III need walking frames or elbow crutches; and children in levels IV and V use wheelchairs. This classification system does not consider cognitive and other deficits.

Growth Motor Development Curves for each of the GMFCS levels are available and provide some guidance regarding prognosis for motor development.

The Manual Abilities Classification System (MACS) describes how children with cerebral palsy use their hands to handle objects in daily activities. It also has five levels, from level I, where children handle objects easily and successfully, to level V, where children are unable to handle objects and have severely limited ability to perform even simple actions.

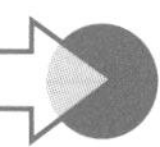

**Practical points**

- Cerebral palsy can be classified according to motor type, distribution and severity.
- GMFCS provides information about severity of gross motor function; MACS provides information about how children use their hands.
- Classifying motor severity using the GMFCS provides information about motor prognosis.
- Co-morbidities such as epilepsy are more common in certain types of cerebral palsy.

## Presentation

The diagnosis of cerebral palsy is not always easy, particularly in children born prematurely. Signs evolve during the first year of life. For example, spasticity is not usually present in the early weeks of life and involuntary movements are generally not seen in the first year of life. Conversely, abnormal neurological signs may disappear. Cerebral palsy may present as follows:

- Follow-up of 'at risk' infants, such as those born prematurely or those with a history of neonatal encephalopathy.
- Delayed motor milestones, particularly delay in learning to sit, stand and walk.
- Development of asymmetrical movement patterns, for example a strong hand preference in the early months of life.
- Abnormalities of muscle tone, particularly spasticity or hypotonia. Hypotonia in isolation may be an early sign of global developmental delay rather than cerebral palsy.
- Management problems, for example severe feeding difficulties or behavioural abnormalities such as unexplained irritability. These problems should be investigated carefully as many other conditions present with these symptoms.

## Examination and investigation

- Look for abnormalities in muscle tone, posture and deep tendon reflexes, along with persistence of primitive reflexes.
- Exclude other conditions that may present with motor delay including neuromuscular, neurodegenerative and metabolic disorders.
- Undertake an MRI brain scan where the cause or causes are uncertain or unknown.

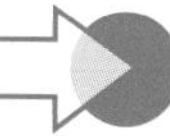

**Practical points**

- Observation of the child often provides more information than 'hands on' examination. It will provide information about the presence or absence of age-appropriate motor skills and their quality.

## Associated disabilities

The following associated disabilities may be present.

- Visual problems including strabismus, refractive errors, visual field defects and cortical visual impairment in about 40% of children with cerebral palsy.
- Hearing deficits in 3–10% of children with cerebral palsy. High-frequency hearing loss may be found in children with congenital rubella or other congenital infections.

- Communication disorders including receptive and expressive language delays and articulation problems.
- Epilepsy in up to 50% of children with cerebral palsy, most commonly in those with spastic hemiplegia and quadriplegia.
- Cognitive impairments – intellectual disabilities, learning problems and perceptual deficits are common. There is a wide range of intellectual ability and some children with severe physical disabilities may have normal intelligence.

*Some children with cerebral palsy have only a motor disorder.*

## Management

A team approach is essential, involving a range of health professionals and teachers, with input from the family of paramount importance. Caring for a child with cerebral palsy involves:

- management of the associated disabilities, health problems, and the consequences of the motor disorder
- developmental assessment and referral to appropriate services for the child and family.

### Management of the associated disabilities, health problems and consequences of the motor disorder

*Associated disabilities*

- All children require a *hearing* and *visual* assessment.
- Assessment and advice about *epilepsy* and prescription of antiepileptic medication when appropriate.
- Children benefit from a formal *cognitive* assessment and may need help with their educational programme. Assessment of cognitive abilities can be difficult when children have severe physical disabilities.

*Health problems*

- *Growth* should be monitored and dietary advice provided to ensure adequate nutrient and calorie intake. Failure to thrive and undernutrition frequently occur due to eating difficulties resulting from oromotor dysfunction. Nasogastric or gastrostomy feeds should be considered if there is difficulty in achieving satisfactory weight gains, or if the length of time taken to feed the child is excessive. Conversely, *obesity* may interfere with progress in motor skills and increase difficulties for caregivers as the child gets older.
- *Gastro-oesophageal reflux* occurs commonly in cerebral palsy. It can result in oesophagitis or gastritis, causing pain and poor appetite, and, if severe, aspiration can result.
- *Constipation* is common and results from immobility, low-fibre diet and poor fluid intake. Dietary and laxative advice is important.
- *Chronic lung disease* develops in some children with severe cerebral palsy due to aspiration from oromotor dysfunction or severe gastro-oesophageal reflux. Coughing or choking during mealtimes, or wheeze during or after meals, may signal the possibility of aspiration, but it may also occur without clinical symptoms or signs. There is no 'gold standard' test for aspiration, but barium videofluoroscopy may be helpful. Alternative feeding regimens, such as the use of a gastrostomy, should be considered if aspiration is present.
- *Hydrocephalus* requiring ventriculoperitoneal shunts is present in many children, particularly those born prematurely.
- *Dental problems* – children should have regular dental surveillance.
- *Osteopenia* causing pathological fractures may occur in children with severe cerebral palsy.
- *Emotional problems* may be responsible for suboptimal performance, with either academic or self-care tasks.

*Consequences of the motor disorder*

- *Drooling* (dribbling or poor saliva control). Speech pathologists can assist with behavioural approaches and methods to improve oromotor control. Medication (anticholinergics) and surgery are helpful for some children.
- *Incontinence*. Children may be late in achieving bowel and bladder control due to cognitive deficits or lack of opportunity to access toileting facilities because of physical disability and/or inability to communicate. Sometimes children have detrusor overactivity causing urgency, frequency and incontinence. If continence cannot be achieved, provide advice about incontinence aids.
- *Undescended testes* require the same treatment as in other boys with this problem (usually scrotal orchidopexy). The testes may be in the normal position at birth but ascend with time (secondary to chronic spasm of cremaster muscle).
- *Orthopaedic problems.* Children may develop contractures that require orthopaedic intervention. Surgery is undertaken mainly on the lower limb, but is occasionally helpful in the upper limb. Physiotherapists are essential in the postoperative rehabilitation phase.
  - *The hip.* Non-walkers and those partially ambulant (GMFCS levels III–V) are at risk of hip subluxation and dislocation. Early detection is vital and hip X-rays should be performed at regular intervals according to hip surveillance guidelines. If there is evidence of subluxation or

dislocation, children should be referred for an orthopaedic opinion. Dislocation causes pain and difficulty with perineal hygiene. Ambulant children rarely develop hip problems.
  - *The knee.* Flexion contractures at the knee may require hamstring surgery.
  - *The ankle.* Equinus deformity at the ankle is the commonest orthopaedic problem in children with cerebral palsy. Toe-walking is treated conservatively in young children, with orthoses, inhibitory casts and botulinum toxin A therapy. Older children benefit from surgery for a definitive correction of the deformity.
  - *Multilevel surgery.* Sometimes children require surgery at several different levels (for example, hip, knee and ankle). This involves a single hospitalization and is called 'single-event multilevel surgery'. It is of most benefit to children who walk independently or with the assistance of crutches. The usual age is between 8 and 12 years. An accurate assessment of the walking problems is undertaken in a gait laboratory. The aims of surgery are to correct deformities and to improve both the appearance and the efficiency of walking. A carefully planned intensive rehabilitation physiotherapy programme lasting for up to 1 year is required to maximize the benefits.
  - *The upper limb.* Procedures can be offered following careful assessment.
  - *Scoliosis.* Correction is sometimes necessary.
- *Spasticity* management is aimed at improving function, comfort and care and requires a team approach. Options include:
  - *Oral medications*, for example diazepam, dantrolene sodium and baclofen. These medications are not always effective or may cause unwanted effects.
  - *Inhibitory casts* aim to increase joint range. The main application is below-knee casts for equinus, but occasionally casts are used in the upper limb.
  - *Botulinum toxin A* is injected into muscles and reduces localized spasticity.
  - *Intrathecal baclofen* is administered by a pump implanted under the skin. This treatment is suitable for a small number of children with severe generalized spasticity and/or dystonia, and may enhance quality of life.
  - *Selective dorsal rhizotomy* is a neurosurgical procedure whereby specific posterior spinal roots are sectioned to reduce spasticity. It has been used mostly in young children aged between 3 and 7 years with spastic diplegia. An intensive rehabilitation period is required.

**Clinical example**

Tom was born at 26 weeks' gestation. He had many neonatal problems, including a severe (grade IV) intraventricular haemorrhage. The parents were informed that some degree of cerebral palsy was likely. At 4 months of corrected age, his mother noted that his right hand was fisted. The diagnosis of cerebral palsy was confirmed and a physiotherapy programme was commenced.

When Tom began to walk independently at 24 months of corrected age, his gait was noted to be asymmetrical with a tendency to walk on his toes on the right side. This problem was more apparent by 30 months and Tom fell more than would be expected for his age. He was fitted with an ankle–foot orthosis (AFO) and his walking pattern was much improved. After a further 10 months the problem had recurred. This time Tom appeared not only to walk in equinus, but he also was flexed at the knee. Hamstrings as well as calf muscles were tight. Botulinum toxin A injections were given to both muscle groups, with an excellent result. A new AFO was made as Tom had grown considerably over this time. When Tom was 5 years old, he required further botulinum toxin A injections. At 7 years of age, surgery was undertaken by the same orthopaedic surgeon who had been monitoring him since the age of 24 months. Now Tom is 10 years old and no treatment is currently planned, although the family has been advised that further surgery may be required following his adolescent growth spurt.

### Developmental assessment and referral to appropriate services for the child and family

*The role of the team.* Careful multidisciplinary assessment is essential to enable children to achieve their optimal physical potential and independence:
- Physiotherapists give practical advice to parents on positioning, handling and play, to minimize the effects of abnormal muscle tone and encourage the development of movement skills. They also give advice regarding the use of orthoses, special seating, wheelchairs and other mobility aids.
- Occupational therapists help parents to develop their child's upper limb and self-care skills, and also recommend suitable toys, equipment and home adaptations.
- Speech pathologists assist in the development of communication skills, including advising about augmentative communication systems for children with limited verbal skills. They provide guidance about feeding difficulties and saliva control problems.
- Orthotists, medical social workers, psychologists, special education teachers and nurses are helpful.

*Therapy approaches.* Therapy to address movement problems and to optimize children's progress in all areas of development is incorporated into early childhood intervention and school programmes. The two most commonly used approaches by therapists in Australia are:

1. *Neurodevelopmental therapy* (NDT or 'Bobath' therapy). This is a therapeutic approach to the assessment and management of movement problems with the goal of maximizing the child's functional ability. Family members receive education in NDT principles so that they can implement the programme at home, preschool and school.
2. *Programmes based on the principles of Conductive Education.* Conductive Education is a Hungarian system for educating children and adults with movement disorders. It provides an integrated group programme whereby children and parents learn to develop daily living, physical, social, cognitive and communication skills.

*Assistive technology.* Appropriate equipment tailored for the individual child can enhance communication, mobility, learning and socialization. Examples include powered wheelchairs, electronic communication devices, and computers for educational and recreational purposes.

*Trends in service provision.* Services are best provided within local communities. Therapists and special education teachers work with children at home and later in childcare centres, kindergartens and schools. Most children attend mainstream preschools and schools, but others benefit from attendance at centre-based early childhood intervention programmes and special schools. Parents should be made aware of all available options.

*Alternative therapies.* There are many non-mainstream (or 'alternative') treatments available. Sometimes great claims, usually not justified, are made for alternative approaches. Families can be reassured that any new treatment that is of value will be assessed and incorporated into mainstream practice. There is no evidence to suggest that alternative methods are superior to conventional treatments, and some may do harm. It is important to be aware of alternative approaches and to be prepared critically to examine their claims.

*Working with families.* Care of the child with cerebral palsy involves developing a trusting and cooperative relationship with the parents. The child is part of a family, and concerns in parents or siblings must be addressed. As with all children, a supportive home environment builds self-esteem and confidence. Parents may need practical support, such as provision of respite care, and may be helped by meeting other families in similar circumstances, or by attending parent support groups. Provision of information about financial allowances is an important aspect of care.

### Life expectancy

Children with mild and moderate cerebral palsy have a normal lifespan. Those with severe motor impairment, particularly those who are wheelchair-dependent and require tube-feeding, have a reduced life expectancy. Chronic lung disease is the most common cause of morbidity and mortality in this group.

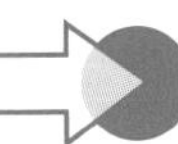

**Practical points**

- In the child with cerebral palsy, the associated disorders and health problems may require more attention than the motor disorder itself.
- A family-centred multidisciplinary approach provides optimal management of the child with cerebral palsy.

## Neurodegenerative disorders

This section addresses the problem of the child who presents because of concern about regression in development that has been normal previously, or with apparent worsening of a pre-existing neurological disorder or developmental delay. In infants and young children, concern may arise because of loss of gross and fine motor, personal social and language skills, as introduced in Chapter 2.2. Declining school performance may lead to referral of the older child.

An approach to this problem will be outlined, with examples of the many disorders that may present in this way. Some of these disorders are mentioned in Chapter 10.5. Broader management issues are covered in Chapter 3.8.

The diagnostic process is presented here as a series of questions.

### Is there evidence of regression or lack of progress in any area of development?

This is sought in a sequential history of progress in each area of development, supplemented by questions such as: 'How is your child's speech now, compared with this time last year? Is there any area where your child has gone backwards or shown no progress at all?'

An ongoing loss of former skills, as shown in the latter part of curve C in Figure 17.2.3, clearly raises concern about a progressive disorder, but this may be less certain during the earlier 'plateau' phase before actual regression appears. This is to be distinguished from the pattern of abnormally slow but consistent progress shown in curve A. This pattern is often found in children with an intellectual disability or cerebral palsy

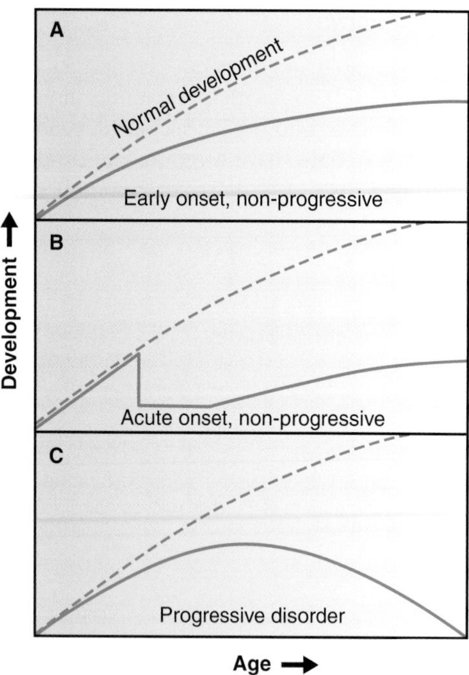


Fig. 17.2.3 Curves demonstrating the course of development over time in a child with static (**A** and **B**) and progressive neurological disease (**C**) compared with expected normal development. The actual age scale will vary, and a different curve may apply to each aspect of development in each child or disease process.

(due to a static brain disorder), who may fall behind other children in abilities, while continuing to acquire new skills, but at a slower pace.

A variation on this pattern, demonstrated in curve B, occurs in the child whose initially normal progress is interrupted by an acute injury or illness (for example, meningitis or encephalitis) causing brain damage with later slow development.

### Could the apparently progressive symptoms be due to a static disorder complicated by other factors?

Such factors may be amenable to treatment, and include the following:

- frequent seizures, especially subtle myoclonic and atonic episodes, which may severely impair alertness and coordination
- drug toxicity, particularly from antiepileptic drugs
- psychological or emotional factors, including depression, withdrawal and psychosis
- joint deformities due to soft tissue contractures in spastic cerebral palsy, leading to worsening of postural stability and gait.

Finally, the natural history of some conditions should be considered, including the evolution of spastic and dyskinetic cerebral palsy, and the tendency for some children with autism to show arrest or regression in social and language skills during the second year of life.

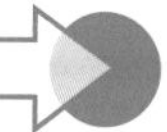

**Practical point**

- When evaluating a child whose development is delayed in any area, it is important to enquire specifically about regression or loss of skills, as parents do not always volunteer such information.

### If this is a progressive disorder, what is its distribution in terms of brain anatomy?

Important anatomical patterns to consider are as follows.

#### One lesion

Progressive hemiparesis, perhaps associated with focal seizures, suggests a cerebral hemisphere tumour, whereas spinal cord tumours may produce progressive weakness and spasticity affecting the lower limbs, either alone or with variable upper limb involvement, thus imitating diplegic cerebral palsy. This clinical pattern, sometimes with associated ataxia, is also seen in slowly progressive hydrocephalus, even in the absence of a cerebral neoplasm. The triad of cranial nerve palsies, corticospinal tract signs and ataxia suggests a brainstem glioma. Most other childhood tumours of the nervous system raise clear concern because of symptoms of raised intracranial pressure, but the insidious visual loss associated with optic nerve glioma and craniopharyngioma often is not recognized as a progressive problem until late in its course.

#### One functional system or group of systems

The prototype of 'system degenerations' is Friedreich ataxia. In this disorder, abnormalities of spinocerebellar, corticospinal and sensory tracts arise in the second decade of life. In other cerebellar ataxia syndromes there is involvement not only of neural pathways but also of other body organs, as with ataxia telangiectasia, in which chromosomal breaks, immunological defects and skin lesions occur. A system disorder involving basal ganglia or extrapyramidal motor function may be inferred from the signs of dystonia, rigidity and choreoathetosis. An important example in this category is Wilson disease, which is treatable by removal of copper from the body.

Peripheral neuromuscular diseases, which also may be regarded as system disorders, are discussed separately in Chapter 17.3.

### A multifocal process, with several discrete lesions in the brain

This is exemplified by recurrent cerebral infarctions associated with cyanotic congenital heart disease. In the absence of cardiac disease, repeated cerebral vascular occlusions are suggestive of moya-moya disease, a well-recognized but poorly understood syndrome. Angiography shows progressive occlusion of the major cerebral arteries, with a network of fine collateral vessels in the basal ganglia.

Among a group of disorders, known collectively as mitochondrial encephalomyelopathies, one form (MELAS) may present with repeated stroke-like episodes and multifocal brain lesions, associated with abnormal mitochondria in muscle, increased lactate levels in blood and cerebrospinal fluid, and deletions of the nuclear or mitochondrial DNA controlling mitochondrial enzyme activity.

Homocystinuria, an inborn error of amino acid metabolism, may present with recurrent cerebral venous or arterial thromboses. Although multiple sclerosis is a major cause of multifocal lesions in young adults, it seldom begins in childhood.

### A diffuse degenerative disorder of the nervous system

Diseases causing widespread loss of neurological function are generally separated into those that begin by affecting predominantly cortical grey matter, or nerve cell bodies, and those in which white matter, or nerve sheath myelin, is primarily involved. Although this distinction is of clinical value, many disorders are not easily classified in this way.

*Diffuse disorders of grey matter.* These tend to cause seizures (often myoclonic) and early loss of intellectual function, with progressive impairment of language, comprehension and memory. In addition, involvement of nerve cells in the retina leads to a variable pattern of visual loss. This clinical syndrome is seen in several of the lipid storage disorders, of which Tay–Sachs disease is the best known. Subacute sclerosing panencephalitis is an infrequent complication of measles, and evolves as a sequence of behavioural change, intellectual decline, myoclonic jerks and later rigidity.

*Diffuse disorders of white matter.* By involving corticospinal tracts, these tend to present with early motor impairment and spasticity, and may masquerade initially as cerebral palsy. Impaired vision, when present, reflects optic pathway disease. Peripheral nerve myelin also may be involved, with clinical effects, as in Krabbe disease and metachromatic leukodystrophy, both of which are lipid storage disorders.

The above three questions can generally be answered after a careful clinical history and examination, but the remaining steps in diagnosis require knowledge of a growing number of recognized but rare diseases. In practice, this will involve specialist consultation.

### Which disorders are known to occur in children of this age, and to produce the other clinical features present in this child?

Individual neurodegenerative diseases tend to have a characteristic age of onset. It is useful to consider broad age ranges (early infancy, late infancy and later childhood) in narrowing the diagnostic field. Next, by matching possible diagnoses against associated clinical findings, such as enlargement of liver and spleen, ocular abnormalities or unusual facial features, the physician may further refine the search and select the most relevant diagnostic tests.

**Clinical example**

Vincent, aged 6 years, was referred to a paediatric neurologist because the teachers at his special school were concerned about his deterioration over several months, with loss of speech and comprehension of language, impaired coordination and increasingly hyperactive, aggressive behaviour. He had been diagnosed as having developmental delay at age 3 years because of limited speech and overactive behaviour. On examination, in addition to the developmental and behavioural findings, he had slightly coarse facial features with thickened eyebrows, an enlarged liver and a mild thoracic kyphosis. These features raised the clinical suspicion that he had *Sanfilippo disease*, one of a group of disorders in which a deficiency of lysosomal enzymes leads to an accumulation of mucopolysaccharides in the tissues and excretion in the urine. The diagnosis was confirmed on specific blood and urine tests. Much professional support was needed by Vincent's parents, confronted with the prospect of their son's progressive dementia and immobility as well as the autosomal recessive inheritance of his condition.

A diagnosis is often reached merely by answering these questions. If not, it is useful next to turn from clinical features to pathophysiology.

### Are any other, less evident, diagnoses suggested by a systematic review of known mechanisms of disease?

The previous selective clinical correlations can be investigated further by considering in turn the major categories of:

- disease process, including metabolic errors, neurocutaneous disorders, slow virus infections and chronic intoxications

- biochemical substrates, such as lipids, vitamins and minerals
- cellular organelles, including lysosomes, peroxisomes and mitochondria, with their respective disorders.

This search may yield a further short list of possible diagnoses, known to the clinician but not considered, usually because of limited experience with them.

### Are there any treatable disorders among the diagnoses being considered in this child?

This important question may alter the priority of investigation, as a potentially treatable disorder, however unlikely, must be rigorously excluded at an early stage. The major groups to recognize are the following:

- Neoplasms and other space-occupying lesions involving the brain, and especially the spinal cord or optic nerves, where they are often not suspected until late, after irreversible damage.
- Subacute and chronic infections of the nervous system, such as tuberculous or cryptococcal meningitis and HIV infection.
- Intoxications: lead poisoning, glue sniffing, prescribed medications and, occasionally, chronic drug administration by a disturbed parent.
- Inborn errors of metabolism. The use of a modified diet in phenylketonuria is well known, but may also be of value in other rare disorders. Removal of toxic agents, for example copper in Wilson disease, may be possible. In seizures due to pyridoxine dependency and in other vitamin-dependency syndromes, large doses of vitamins may effectively compensate for the metabolic defect.
- Deficiency states, especially of vitamins required for normal growth and function of the nervous system or the musculoskeletal system, including vitamin $B_{12}$ and vitamin D.

Effective treatment is not yet available for most degenerative neurological disorders of childhood, but accurate diagnosis remains the basis for genetic counselling, and for offering a realistic prognosis. A specific diagnosis or 'answer' is of great value to parents in coping with the distress of having a child with a disability.

# Neuromuscular disorders 17.3

Monique Ryan, Andrew Kornberg

Neuromuscular disorders of childhood have become a focus of increasing attention in recent years. Although many of these conditions are difficult to diagnose without sophisticated investigations, and they are generally incurable, this group of disorders cannot be ignored because of the significant morbidity and mortality associated with them, their genetic implications and the arrival of potential therapies. Early diagnosis is important in the rational management of these disorders as it allows provision of accurate prognostic and genetic information. Accurate diagnosis in this wide array of disorders is dependent on a careful clinical assessment followed by confirmatory and appropriate investigations. Recent advances have unravelled the molecular biology of many neuromuscular conditions, but the clinical assessment of patients remains the cornerstone of diagnosis and management.

The management of neuromuscular disorders requires recognition, diagnosis, therapy and counselling.

## Recognition that a child's presenting symptoms or signs may be due to peripheral neuromuscular disease

> Please listen to the patient; he's trying to tell you what disease he has.
>
> (Michael H. Brooke 1977 *A Clinician's View of Neuromuscular Disease*. Williams and Wilkins: Baltimore)

Although the hallmark of neuromuscular disorders is weakness, parents do not come into the consulting room saying, 'I'm worried because my child is weak'. The physician needs to recognize that the presenting symptoms or signs relate to the neuromuscular system before the diagnostic process begins. Failure of this recognition results in diagnostic delay. Although this failure may not affect the ultimate prognosis, it adds considerably to patient and parental frustration. A tragedy occurs when opportunities for prevention are missed and a second affected child is born to the immediate or extended family.

Common presenting complaints of neuromuscular disorders include:

- difficulty walking and running
- poor at sports
- clumsy or poorly coordinated
- not able to keep up with peers
- frequent falls
- tires easily.

Another trap in the recognition of neuromuscular disease in childhood is that classical neurological signs, readily demonstrated at the end of a disease process in adult patients, are often absent in children at the beginning of the disease process. For example, adults with Charcot–Marie–Tooth disease very often have pes cavus, distal muscle wasting and generalized areflexia. In children, Charcot–Marie–Tooth disease presents with an abnormal walk or run, clumsiness and frequent falls. Foot deformity is a presenting symptom in a minority. In addition, although areflexia is the rule in adult patients, about 10% of children with Charcot–Marie–Tooth disease have normal reflexes at presentation. Not understanding the age-dependent symptoms and signs of neuromuscular disorders will lead to failure to recognize them in childhood.

Other modes of presentation include a family history of neuromuscular disease; weakness, hypotonia, respiratory or feeding difficulty in the neonatal period; delayed motor milestones; abnormal gait (particularly toe-walking); and orthopaedic abnormalities such as foot deformity or scoliosis. Some patients present with non-neuromuscular problems, such as intellectual disability or delayed language development, for example in Duchenne muscular dystrophy.

## Diagnosis of neuromuscular disease based on anatomical, electrophysiological, biochemical, histopathological or DNA identification

After recognizing that the symptoms are due to neuromuscular disease, the differential diagnosis is based on a logical anatomical approach. Although this may appear overly simplistic, as some disorders may affect more than one anatomical area or be multisystemic, this approach will provide a broad differential diagnosis that leads on to definitive diagnosis.

The anatomical localization is based on the clinical findings listed in Table 17.3.1 and includes disorders affecting the:

- anterior horn cell
- anterior and posterior nerve roots
- peripheral nerve (motor, sensory, autonomic)
- neuromuscular junction
- muscle.

**Table 17.3.1 Clinical clues helpful in establishing the site of the lesion in neuromuscular disease**

| Clinical feature | Anterior horn cell | Peripheral nerve | Neuromuscular junction | Muscle |
|---|---|---|---|---|
| Weakness | Proximal | Distal | Cranial/proximal | Proximal |
| Hypotonia | ++ | + | +/– | ++ |
| Hyporeflexia | +/– | Early | +/– | Late |
| Fasciculations | +++ | + | – | – |
| Sensory abnormalities | – | +/– | – | – |
| Myotonia | – | – | – | +/– |
| Autonomic dysfunction | – | +/– | – | – |
| Muscle enlargement | – | – | – | +/– |

The use of a timeframe of symptoms, such as acute, subacute or chronic, will also provide an important frame for the differential diagnosis.

The definitive diagnosis rests on a combination of:

- clinical history and examination
- family history
- serum muscle enzymes, particularly creatine kinase (CK)
- electrophysiology (e.g. nerve conduction studies, electromyography, repetitive nerve stimulation)
- histology of muscle and/or nerve
- metabolic studies (e.g. muscle glycogen, carnitine assay, mitochondrial studies)
- DNA studies.

## Anterior horn cell disorders

### Acute

#### Poliomyelitis

This disorder is rare in developed countries, but should still be considered where there is acute onset of weakness of a single limb, or with patchy asymmetrical distribution, particularly if this is associated with fever, vomiting, neck or back stiffness, and muscle pain or spasms. Sensory abnormalities are absent.

### Chronic

In childhood the chronic disorders characterized pathologically by degeneration of anterior horn cells and associated clinically with progressive muscle weakness are called the spinal muscular atrophies (SMAs). The important SMA syndromes and their classification are listed in Table 17.3.2.

#### Spinal muscular atrophy type I (Werdnig–Hoffmann disease)

This autosomal recessive disorder occurs in approximately 1 in 6000 live births, making it the most common fatal autosomal recessive disorder of early childhood. The earliest symptom may be decreased fetal movements in late pregnancy. Presentation is invariably before 6 months of age and is either at birth with hypotonia, weakness, joint deformity and respiratory difficulty, or more commonly later with marked hypotonia and limb weakness, poor feeding, poor cough and cry. The onset is sometimes relatively rapid and when first seen the child is usually severely weak (Fig. 17.3.1). Weakness, although generalized, is maximal proximally in the shoulder and hip girdle muscles. Intercostal muscle weakness leads to chest deformity, a poor cough and a weak cry. The respiratory

**Table 17.3.2 Clinical classification of childhood-onset proximal spinal muscle atrophy**

| Designation | Symptom onset (months) | Course | Age at death (years) |
|---|---|---|---|
| I (severe) | 0–6 | Never sits without support | < 2 |
| II (intermediate) | < 18 | Never stands without aid | > 2 |
| III (mild) | > 18 | Stands alone | Adult |

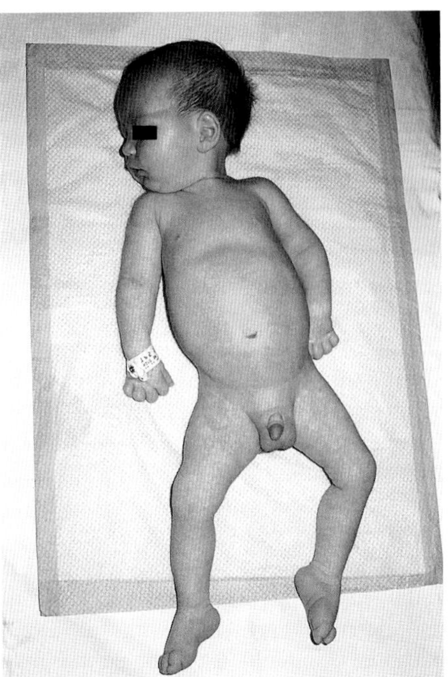

Fig. 17.3.1 Child with spinal muscular atrophy type 1, showing profound hypotonia and weakness.

pattern becomes diaphragmatic. Deep tendon reflexes are absent. Fasciculations of the tongue are an important clinical clue, but this can be a difficult sign to be certain about and one can only be confident if the baby is relaxed and there are no 'voluntary' movements of the tongue. Facial weakness in SMA is very mild and the extraocular movements remain full, giving the baby an alert appearance. Death, usually from pneumonia and respiratory failure, occurs by 18 months of age in 95% of patients, with those with onset in the first 2 months of life having the shortest survival.

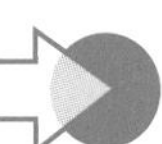

**Practical points**

- Tongue fasciculations can be seen with certainty only when the tongue has no voluntary movement, i.e. is at rest in the floor of the mouth and the child is not crying or actively moving the tongue.
- The presence of deep tendon reflexes makes it extremely unlikely that the child has type 1 SMA and an alternative diagnosis should be considered.

SMA is caused by homozygous deletions of the *SMN1* gene, causing loss of SMN protein production in motor neurons of the anterior horn of the spinal cord. Prenatal diagnosis and carrier testing of relatives are available.

Various therapeutic strategies are being trialled. Most are designed to upregulate SMN protein expression via a variety of mechanisms.

### Spinal muscular atrophy type 2

The genetic abnormality in SMA types 2 and 3 is allelic to that of SMA type 1, but these are milder forms of the disease. The clinical onset of SMA type 2 is almost invariably before 3 years of age, with hypotonia, weakness and delayed motor milestones. The clinical picture is one of severe generalized weakness and wasting, with proximal predominance. Deep tendon reflexes are decreased or absent and often there are fasciculations of the tongue. The facial muscles may be mildly weak but eye movements remain normal and the patient is usually normal intellectually. Many patients have a fine, rapid tremor of the hands. Children with SMA type 2 never walk unsupported. Survival varies from 18 months through to adult life. Major management problems include the prevention of orthopaedic deformity, especially scoliosis, and the management of the respiratory complications of muscle weakness. Prompt treatment of chest infections prolongs survival, and many children and adults with SMA type 2 benefit from nocturnal non-invasive ventilatory support. Patients with a later onset and a moderately benign clinical course are classified as SMA type 3 (Kugelberg–Welander syndrome). Most have onset in the first two decades, with only a few in the third decade, and survival is usually for many decades. Persons with SMA type 3 are able to walk at some point, and many remain ambulant into adulthood.

## Peripheral nerve disorders

A number of peripheral neuropathies with various time courses (acute, subacute or chronic) occur in childhood. They may be inherited or acquired; they may involve motor, sensory or autonomic fibres, or commonly a mixture of all three. Pathologically, they may be associated with combinations of demyelination and axonal degeneration. Some central nervous system degenerative disorders, such as Krabbe disease and metachromatic leukodystrophy, also affect the peripheral nerves. The most common nerve disorders of childhood are Guillain–Barré syndrome (GBS) and Charcot–Marie–Tooth disease (CMT). Chronic inflammatory demyelinating polyneuropathy (CIDP), while uncommon, is important because it is responsive to immunotherapies.

### Acute neuropathies

#### Guillain–Barré syndrome

GBS is the most common acute neuropathy in clinical practice and can occur at any age, although it is rare in infancy. An infection, commonly of the upper respiratory tract or gastrointestinal tract

(*Campylobacter jejuni*), precedes the neurological syndrome in at least 50% of cases. Typical GBS is a monophasic illness with symmetrical, ascending weakness involving proximal and distal muscles. Paraesthesia and muscle pain may be presenting complaints but sensory impairment is usually minimal. Severe back pain and stiffness may occur, especially in young children. The deep tendon reflexes are lost early in the course of the illness. Cranial nerve involvement, particularly of the facial nerve, is relatively common. Autonomic involvement can cause wide fluctuations of the blood pressure as well as cardiac arrhythmias and bladder dysfunction. Respiratory failure occurs in about 30% of patients. GBS typically progresses over less than 4 weeks, with most patients reaching their maximal deficit within 2 weeks of onset. Artificial ventilation is occasionally required. Recovery continues over weeks to months, with most children returning to normal function. Some more severely affected children have residual weakness, most commonly of ankle dorsiflexion. Fatigue is common during the recovery period.

Diagnosis is based on the clinical features, with increased cerebrospinal fluid (CSF) protein with only a few, if any, cells in the CSF. Spinal magnetic resonance imaging (MRI) and/or nerve conduction studies are useful in difficult diagnostic situations. All children with suspected GBS should be admitted to hospital for monitoring of their respiratory status, blood pressure and cardiac rhythm. Management of GBS requires special expertise in medical and nursing care, and affected children should be referred to centres used to dealing with this condition. Supportive therapy is very important. Intravenous gammaglobulin or plasmapheresis, if used early, may hasten recovery, but is not always required for milder cases.

### Chronic neuropathies

#### Chronic inflammatory demyelinating peripheral neuropathy (CIDP)

This rare but treatable autoimmune neuropathy presents subacutely or as a chronic neuropathy. The course can be monophasic but is more commonly relapsing/remitting. Acute presentations can occur and may cause confusion with GBS. Symptoms and signs of weakness, often most prominent proximally, bring the child to medical attention. The diagnosis is confirmed by nerve conduction studies, increased CSF protein and, if there is diagnostic doubt, pathological abnormalities on nerve biopsy. CIDP is treated with intravenous immunoglobulin, corticosteroids and other immunosuppressive agents.

#### Charcot–Marie–Tooth disease (hereditary motor and sensory neuropathy)

CMT is the most common form of genetic neuropathy, affecting about 1 in 3000 people. The numerous forms of CMT are classified on the basis of their clinical presentation, neurophysiological findings and genetic cause. Autosomal dominant, X-linked and recessive forms of CMT are recognized. Approximately 60% of affected persons have onset of symptoms in the first decade of life.

Pes cavus, loss of foot dorsiflexion and eversion, hyporeflexia and sensory loss are typical findings in childhood CMT. However, relatively asymptomatic children may present because of a family history, whereas others present with gait disturbance, particularly toe-walking, frequent falling or poor coordination. Weakness and wasting in the legs may progress slowly, and distal weakness in the arms is sometimes seen. Enlarged peripheral nerves can occasionally be palpated. Parents of children with suspected CMT should also be examined as they may have mild clinical changes suggestive of the diagnosis.

The diagnosis can be confirmed by nerve conduction studies, although DNA studies (targeted, or a chromosomal microarray) are generally the usual first step in diagnosis. In CMT1A, the most common form of CMT, DNA studies show a duplicated region on chromosome 17p involving the *PMP22* gene.

There is as yet no cure for CMT, but physiotherapy, occupational therapy, orthotics and orthopaedic surgery are often helpful in minimizing weakness and functional problems.

**Clinical example**

Claudine, a 5-year-old girl, was seen by her paediatrician because of frequent falls and an unusual gait. He found areflexia and bilateral foot drop without proximal weakness. There was an extensive family history (with an autosomal dominant inheritance pattern) of a chronic neuropathy, presumed to be a form of CMT, although Claudine's mother was asymptomatic.

Examination of Claudine's mother revealed minor sensory loss in the feet and hyporeflexia. Both mother and child underwent chromosomal microarrays (molecular karyotypes), which showed a duplication at 17p11 including the *PMP22* gene, confirming the diagnosis of CMT1A.

Children with neuromuscular disease often do not have all the clinical features seen in adults, and sometimes it is the family history that gives the vital clue. The severity of CMT varies considerably and some adults are asymptomatic and undiagnosed. Careful clinical examination of a parent and further diagnostic studies sometimes unmask the apparent missing link. The absence of foot deformity or sensory disturbance in a child does not exclude CMT.

## Neuromuscular junction disorders

### Acute

#### Infant botulism

Infant botulism results from production of *Clostridium botulinum* toxin in the gastrointestinal tract. It differs from botulism associated with food poisoning, in which there is ingestion of preformed toxin from contaminated food. In infant botulism, botulinum spores are ingested. The disease usually occurs in infants under 9 months of age because of immaturity of the immune system within the infant gut.

Constipation for days or weeks typically precedes the onset of floppiness, weakness and ptosis, which develop over hours or 1–2 days at most. Feeding and swallowing difficulty, a poor cough, weak cry, hyporeflexia and respiratory insufficiency are typical. Extraocular movements may be impaired and dilated; sluggishly reacting pupils are often seen and can be helpful diagnostically. Deterioration may be rapid, with many patients requiring artificial ventilation for up to 2 months while the neuromuscular junctions regrow.

Diagnosis is clinical, supported by isolation of the organism and its toxin from faeces. Treatment is supportive. Botulinum antitoxin has been used but has not been shown to be helpful. Human intravenous botulism immune globulin (BabyBIG) may have a place in therapy if the child is treated early. The prognosis is excellent, with full recovery unless complications from cerebral hypoxia intervene. Prompt recognition and transfer to a facility capable of long-term ventilatory support is essential.

### Chronic

#### Autoimmune myasthenia gravis

Myasthenia gravis is an autoimmune disorder caused by antibodies directed against post-synaptic acetylcholine receptors of the neuromuscular junction. Onset occurs at any time from the second year of life. Symptoms develop quickly in most patients, and there can be rapid progression to respiratory failure if myasthenia gravis remains untreated. Symptoms and signs are similar to those in adults. Ptosis, ophthalmoplegia, diplopia, difficulty chewing and swallowing, and slurred speech with or without predominantly proximal limb muscle weakness of recent onset should raise the suspicion of myasthenia gravis. Fatigability, the hallmark of myasthenia, is usually prominent, but this is not invariable. In some children muscle weakness may be confined to the extraocular muscles. Suspicion of myasthenia gravis should trigger an urgent diagnostic assessment.

Diagnosis is based on clinical observation of fatigability, often best seen in the upper eyelid, response to intravenous or intramuscular anticholinesterase agents such as edrophonium or neostigmine, repetitive nerve stimulation testing and assay of acetylcholine receptor antibodies. Symptomatic relief may be obtained by oral administration of an anticholinesterase, commonly pyridostigmine. Corticosteroids, thymectomy, intravenous immunoglobulin and plasmaphaeresis have a role in selected circumstances. Although myasthenia gravis is a serious long-term and potentially fatal disorder, the disease remits in some children.

#### Transient neonatal myasthenia gravis

Transient neonatal myasthenia gravis occurs in about 10% of offspring of mothers with myasthenia gravis. It is due to placental transfer of anti-acetylcholine receptor antibodies from a myasthenic mother to her fetus during pregnancy. Affected children present in the first few days of life with feeding difficulties, respiratory difficulty, weakness or hypotonia. Myasthenic symptoms in the mother may be minimal. Appropriate supportive measures and anticholinesterase medication are used until the syndrome resolves over the ensuing weeks.

#### Congenital myasthenic syndromes

Congenital myasthenic syndromes are genetic disorders of the neuromuscular junction. They are not autoimmune disorders. Detailed electrophysiological and morphological testing, available in only a few laboratories, is usually required to diagnose and characterize these disorders definitively. Hypotonia, limb weakness, facial weakness, ptosis, ophthalmoplegia and apnoeic episodes, particularly with infections, may be seen, but the emphasis varies with the particular syndrome. Some show improvement with time despite life-threatening episodic apnoea in infancy, whereas others cause persisting weakness and ophthalmoplegia. Some affected children respond to anti-anticholinesterase preparations, and others respond to fluoxetine, ephedrine or 3,4-diaminopyridine. As these are not autoimmune disorders, the immunomodulatory therapies normally used in myasthenia gravis are not indicated for children with congenital myasthenic syndromes.

# Muscle disorders

## Acute myopathies

Acute muscle disorders are uncommon in childhood. Probably the most common is benign acute myositis, a disorder of mid-childhood, typically affecting boys. Symptoms include calf pain and difficulty walking after a viral illness. Affected children often toe-walk or adopt a wide-based, stiff-legged gait. Muscle tenderness is generally isolated to the gastrocnemius–soleus muscles. Creatine kinase levels are raised but no other significant biochemical changes are seen, and most children recover completely within 1 week.

Rhabdomyolysis with myoglobinuria appears occasionally after an upper respiratory tract infection or after exercise, and is probably related to an underlying metabolic disorder of muscle. Rhabdomyolysis can also follow snake bite or be triggered by medications. The dominantly inherited, sometimes fatal, syndrome of malignant hyperthermia during anaesthesia also causes muscle necrosis and myoglobinuria. This disorder is associated with central core disease (see below) and a number of other inherited myopathies.

## Chronic myopathies

### Congenital myopathies

The congenital myopathies are a group of inherited disorders that are clinically non-specific but that have distinctive findings on morphological analysis of the muscle biopsy. Common congenital myopathies include central core disease (Fig. 17.3.2) and nemaline myopathy.

These myopathies, usually inherited, are characterized by onset of weakness and hypotonia at or shortly after birth, or occasionally later in childhood or adulthood. Weakness may be mild or severe and is usually only slowly progressive. Pathologically there are structural changes in the contractile apparatus within muscle fibres caused by changes in muscle-specific genes. The identification of these disorders allows important genetic and prognostic information to be given to the family, and enables appropriate monitoring for disease-specific complications such as cardiac involvement, scoliosis, hip dysplasia and development of contractures.

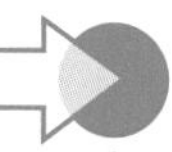

**Practical points**

- In a family exhibiting autosomal dominant inheritance of a muscle disorder consistent with a congenital myopathy, central core disease should be considered a possibility and precautions taken against malignant hyperthermia if an anaesthetic is given (e.g. for muscle biopsy).

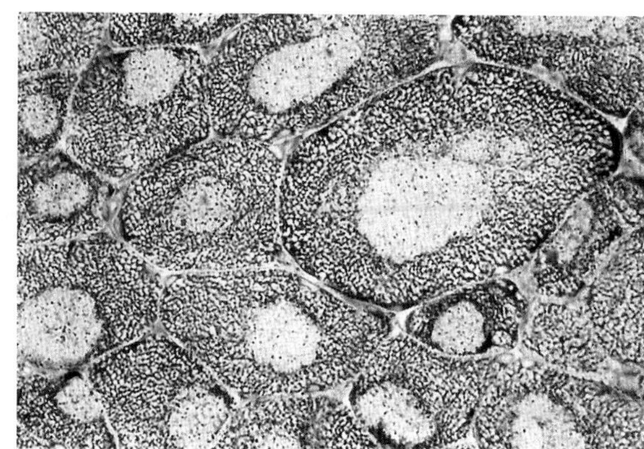

Fig. 17.3.2 Muscle biopsy in central core disease.

### Muscular dystrophies

The muscular dystrophies are a group of inherited disorders of muscle characterized by weakness presenting from birth to late adulthood, with the common feature being the pathological appearance of dystrophic muscle (Fig. 17.3.3). These disorders primarily affect skeletal muscle but other tissues may be involved; for example, congenital muscular dystrophies may be associated with developmental abnormalities in the brain.

The various forms of muscular dystrophy share a common pathogenesis of muscle plasma membrane instability secondary to the lack, or abnormality, of proteins and glycoproteins linking the subsarcolemmal cytoskeleton to the extracellular matrix (Fig. 17.3.4). Absence or dysfunction of these structural proteins makes the muscle fibre more prone to damage. Muscle fibre death is followed by fibre regeneration with gradual accumulation of connective tissue and fat, resulting in the eventual development of muscle weakness.

Many of the muscular dystrophies share common clinical features, although their severity varies. The age of onset, pattern of weakness, family history and relatively specific findings on examination are important in diagnosing specific forms of muscular dystrophy.

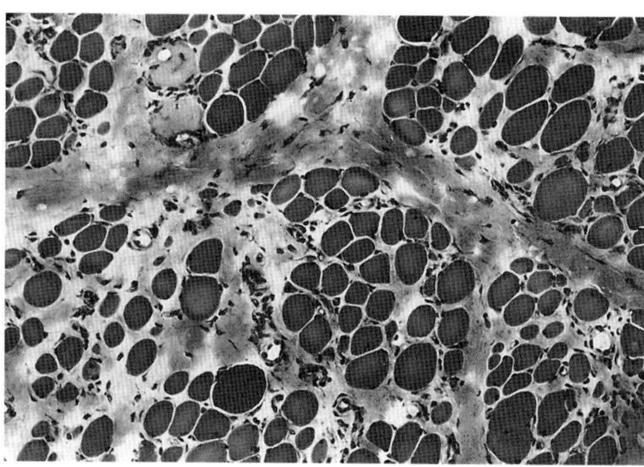

Fig. 17.3.3 Dystrophic muscle biopsy.

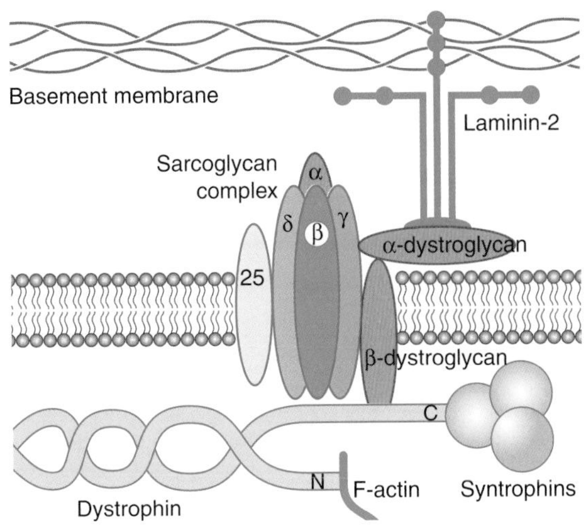


**Fig. 17.3.4** Subsarcolemmal cytoskeleton.

Some of the muscular dystrophies are named because of their pattern of weakness, but these labels will probably change with the identification of specific protein defects.

The clinical features of the more common muscular dystrophies are described below.

*Duchenne muscular dystrophy*

Duchenne muscular dystrophy (DMD) is the most common muscular dystrophy, occurring in 1 in 3500 boys. It is an X-linked disorder and occurs nearly exclusively in males. It is a disease of devastating proportions because it is progressive, it has significant genetic implications, there are no curative treatments available and it has serious medical complications, causing death from respiratory or cardiac failure in or after the second decade of life.

DMD is caused by a mutation on chromosome Xp21, causing loss of dystrophin, a muscle protein important for stabilizing the contractile apparatus within muscle fibres. Two-thirds of patients have a family history of muscular dystrophy or are isolated cases with an unsuspecting female carrier mother. In one-third of cases boys are affected as a result of a spontaneous mutation.

Development in the first year of life is usually normal. The first symptoms are usually recognized from 18 months to 4 years of age, with delayed walking being the most common presenting complaint. Approximately 50% of children with DMD walk later than 18 months of age. Abnormal walking or running, toe-walking, difficulty in climbing, difficulty in getting up from the floor or chair, and frequent falls are other prominent early features. Although many are intellectually normal, a significant proportion of boys with DMD have developmental problems other than motor delay, such as static intellectual impairment or delayed language development. The mean IQ of boys with DMD is approximately 85.

Proximal muscle weakness accounts for the motor difficulties. This can be demonstrated on formal muscle strength testing or by functional tests looking at ability to arise from the floor, climb stairs and run. On arising from the floor, boys with DMD usually use a Gowers' manoeuvre (Fig. 17.3.5). A Gowers' sign is not specific for DMD and is seen in other disorders with proximal muscle weakness. Enlargement (pseudohypertrophy) and firmness of the calf, quadriceps and triceps muscles is also common in DMD (Fig. 17.3.6).

There is some variability in the course, but the following generalizations apply to most children with DMD. Between the ages of 4 and 6 years there is an apparent improvement in mobility, with children acquiring new motor skills. This is because normal muscle development (and regeneration) outstrips the degenerative process. After this period of improvement a decline in function occurs, with increasing proximal limb weakness. The trunk muscles are also weakened. This leads to a waddling gait, increasing lumbar lordosis and increasing equinovarus foot deformities. Independent mobility is lost, usually between 8 and 13 years of age, with the child becoming wheelchair-bound, after which scoliosis generally develops. During the second decade of life there is a gradual decline in pulmonary function, related to scoliosis and progressive muscle weakness. Death is usually due to respiratory complications, although cardiac failure secondary to cardiomyopathy can occur. Cardiac arrhythmias may be a terminal event.

The diagnosis of DMD should be based on the family history (if any), clinical features, serum CK, DNA testing and muscle biopsy. Pathological confirmation of the diagnosis is essential except where the diagnosis has been confirmed in another family member or by a genetic testing, which shows a deletion in more than 70% of cases. Less common mutations, such as nonsense mutations or duplications, may be seen only on advanced forms of genetic testing. Measurement of the CK level is a reliable screening test and is invariably grossly increased in a child with DMD, even from the neonatal period. Conversely, a normal CK test result after the neonatal period excludes the later development of DMD.

Effective genetic counselling can be offered only if the first case in the family is diagnosed before other affected males are born. The early diagnosis of DMD can be facilitated by using the following criteria for ordering serum CK estimations in males:

- known or suspected family history of muscular dystrophy
- male not walking before 18 months of age without obvious cause
- unexplained gait disturbance (particularly toe-walking)
- unexplained mental retardation
- unexplained language delay.

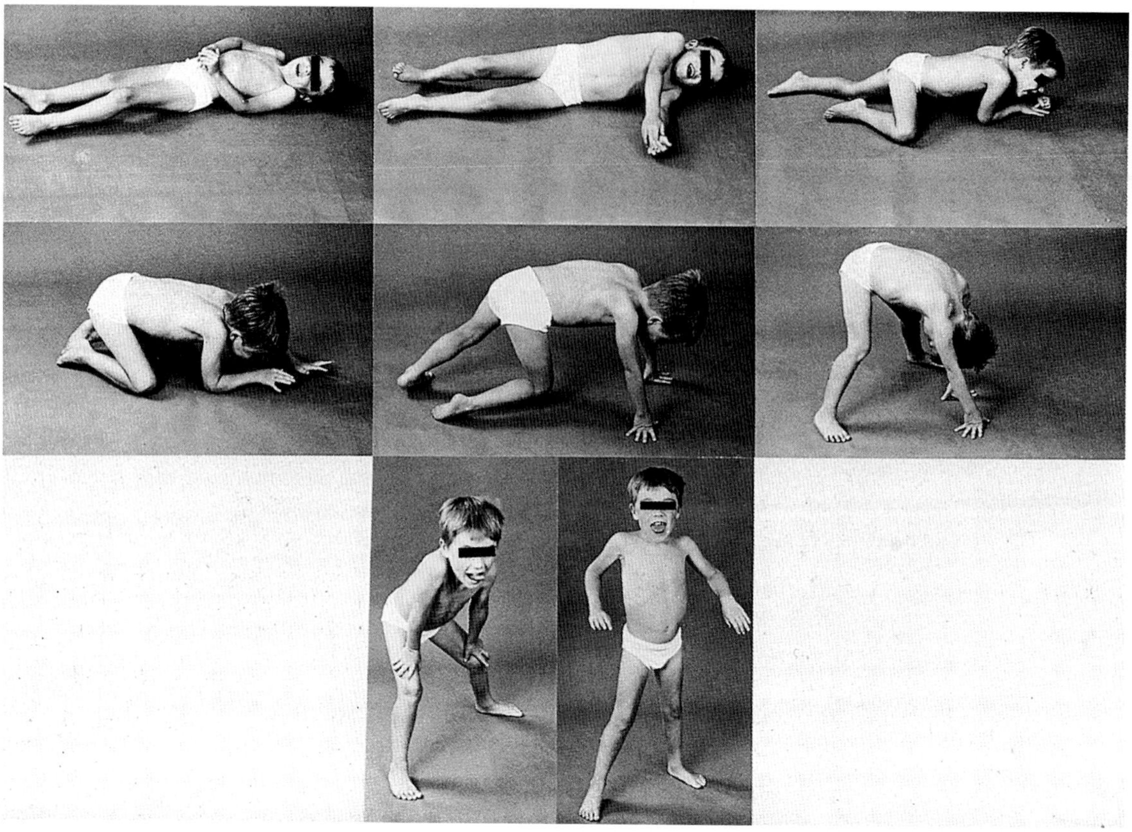

Fig. 17.3.5 Gowers' sign in a patient with Duchenne muscular dystrophy, illustrating the sequence of manoeuvres required to rise from the supine position. (Reproduced with permission from Williams 1982.)

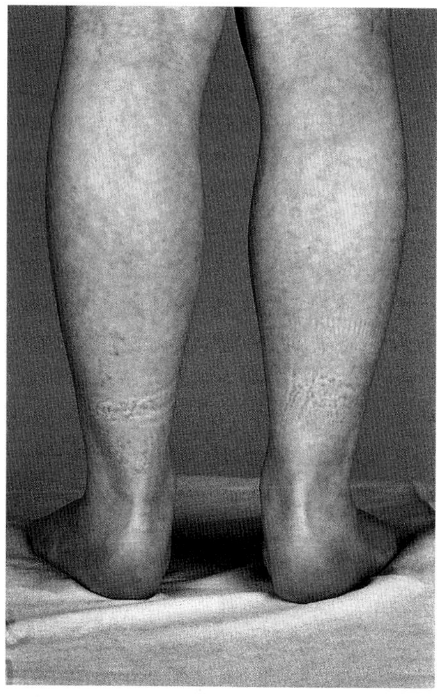

Fig. 17.3.6 Pseudohypertrophy of muscles.

Detection and counselling of female carriers is a most important aspect of family management. The male offspring of a known carrier have a 50% risk of having DMD, and 50% of female offspring will be carriers. Females may still be carriers even though there is no other family history. Only 60% of known carriers have a raised CK level and hence a normal level does not exclude the carrier state. Antenatal diagnosis by deletion testing or linkage analysis is available.

Currently there is no cure for DMD. Management involves a very positive approach to meeting the emotional, social and educational needs of the affected boy and his family, together with judicious use of physiotherapy, occupational therapy, orthotic devices, and surgery for scoliosis and joint contractures. Corticosteroid therapy improves muscle strength in this condition, prolonging independent ambulation and helping preserve respiratory and cardiac muscle function. Daily oral steroid therapy is generally initiated at age 4–6 years, or when boys show evidence of decreasing muscle strength and increasing fatigability and falls. Early treatment with angiotensin-converting enzyme (ACE) inhibitors prevents and slows development of cardiomyopathy in DMD. Adolescents and young adults with DMD often benefit from treatment with non-invasive ventilatory support for nocturnal hypoventilation caused by respiratory muscle weakness. These treatments, and improved physiotherapy, occupational therapy and orthopaedic management, have had a significant impact on life expectancy in DMD, which is now into the third or fourth decade of life for boys diagnosed in the last decade.

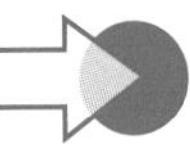

**Practical point**

- The most common reason for the late diagnosis of Duchenne muscular dystrophy is not thinking of the diagnosis in a young male with delayed motor, mental or language development.

*Becker muscular dystrophy*

Becker muscular dystrophy is allelic to DMD but much less common. It is less severe than DMD and has a variable age of presentation.

*Facioscapulohumeral syndrome*

Facioscapulohumeral (FSH) muscular dystrophy is a relatively common autosomal dominant myopathy that predominantly affects the shoulder girdle, in particular the periscapular, humeral and facial muscles. It is a relatively mild disorder with very slow progression. Onset is most commonly in adolescence or early adult life, although FSH occasionally presents in early childhood.

Facial muscle weakness is generally one of the first symptoms. Patients have difficulty closing the eyes, blowing out the cheeks, whistling or sucking through a straw. Shoulder girdle weakness usually begins at the same time as the facial weakness and can be quite asymmetrical. Symptoms include difficulty lifting the arms above the head. There is obvious winging of the scapulae in adult patients, but this may not be obvious in children. On abduction of the shoulders, the scapulae move upwards and give the shoulders a characteristic appearance. Foot drop is not uncommon. The infantile form of FSH dystrophy is associated with more severe weakness.

The locus for autosomal dominant FSH has been mapped to the distal arm of chromosome 4.

Treatment is symptomatic. Sensorineural hearing loss and Coats' disease, a proliferative retinopathy, are associated with early-onset FSH dystrophy. Aggressive treatment of these associated disorders is important.

## Myotonic disorders

Myotonia is the common feature of this clinically heterogeneous group of myopathies. Myotonia is the inability of muscles to relax after voluntary contraction or stimulation. Myotonia can be detected during attempted relaxation of a voluntary contraction, such as after shaking hands or eyelid closure, by percussion of a muscle or by electromyography. Older children may describe myotonia as stiffness or cramping.

Many of these disorders are due to defects of muscle ion channels. In some instances different mutations within the one gene can cause myotonia and/or periodic paralysis.

### Myotonia congenita (Thomsen disease)

There are autosomal dominant and autosomal recessive forms of this disorder. Onset is in infancy or early childhood with symptoms due to myotonia, such as stiffness, difficulty initiating rapid movements and sometimes feeding difficulties. Muscle hypertrophy is common. The myotonia decreases with continued activity and may be aggravated by cold. Symptoms improvement occurs with increasing age. Symptomatic treatment of myotonia with quinine or mexiletine is sometimes required.

### Myotonic dystrophy (Steinert disease)

Myotonic dystrophy is an autosomal dominant disorder, but the affected parent may be relatively asymptomatic and may not be diagnosed prior to the birth of their more significantly affected children. The disease is due to an excessive number of repeats of the CTG sequence on chromosome 19. The spectrum of clinical severity in myotonic dystrophy is extremely broad. This is a severe multisystemic disease that is diagnosed on genetic testing. Antenatal diagnosis is available and cascade testing of other family members is often required when an affected infant is born to a family.

*Juvenile type*

The clinical features are similar to those seen in adults, with ptosis, facial and distal muscle weakness and wasting, and myotonia. Cataracts, frontal alopecia, testicular atrophy, cardiac arrhythmias and cardiomyopathy may occur in adult life.

*Congenital type*

Congenital myotonic dystrophy is invariably inherited from the mother, and is more severe than in the mother because of expansion of the CTG repeat sequence during meiosis. Congenital myotonic dystrophy presents at birth with hypotonia, marked weakness, arthrogryposis, feeding and respiratory difficulties. Intellectual disability is virtually invariable if the child survives the neonatal period. Affected children have persisting weakness and are at risk of ongoing respiratory insufficiency, endocrine problems and cardiac involvement in later life. Myotonia is not present at birth in this disorder, but can generally be elicited by late childhood.

**Clinical example**

Mrs McGill, aged 25 years, had myotonic dystrophy, as did her father, sister and brother. She had a son and twin daughters who were normal at birth and who remained asymptomatic. Her next child, Tessa, was 4 weeks premature and at birth was very hypotonic, had respiratory difficulty and required gavage feeding. There was marked bilateral facial weakness, talipes equinovarus and mild flexion deformity at the knees. The respiratory and feeding difficulties gradually resolved, but the facial muscle weakness remained and Tessa later showed delay in motor and language milestones. There was no clinical myotonia when she was seen at 3 years of age.

Tessa had typical features of the congenital form of myotonic dystrophy, which typically occurs when it is the mother who is the affected parent. Some babies are stillborn, whereas others do not survive the neonatal period. Tessa was affected only moderately and will survive into adult life, but will almost certainly require special schooling. The dominant inheritance is clear from the family history. Mrs McGill and her husband wanted to know whether the other children might develop the disease. Although they were asymptomatic at the time, there was still a chance that they had inherited the abnormal gene. DNA testing for the triplet expansion on chromosome 19 could be used to allow antenatal diagnosis.

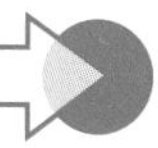

**Practical point**

- Facial diplegia with respiratory difficulty or pharyngeal incoordination in a neonate should raise the suspicion of congenital myotonic dystrophy.

### Inflammatory myopathy

Dermatomyositis, the only common chronic inflammatory myopathy of childhood, presents with proximal weakness that is often very insidious in onset, a pinkish (heliotrope) facial rash, irritability and exercise intolerance. Diagnosis is often delayed. The serum CK level is moderately increased. Muscle ultrasonography or MRI can be useful, but a muscle biopsy is generally required for diagnosis. Long-term immunosuppressive therapy is often required. Complications of childhood dermatomyositis (which unlike its adult counterpart is not associated with malignancy) include gastrointestinal involvement, calcinosis and joint contractures.

### Metabolic myopathies

A large number of individually uncommon metabolic disorders may produce episodic, acute or chronic muscle weakness, hypotonia, stiffness or cramping, exercise intolerance or myoglobinuria. Symptoms are sometimes accentuated or precipitated by exercise, rest after exercise, fasting or excessive carbohydrate intake.

The underlying metabolic defects are usually of glycogen metabolism (e.g. Pompe disease), lipid metabolism (e.g. carnitine deficiency, carnitine palmitoyltransferase deficiency), potassium metabolism (e.g. the periodic paralyses associated with hyper-, hypo- or normo-kalaemia) or mitochondrial function (e.g. myopathies due to abnormalities of respiratory chain enzymes).

Knowledge of the underlying metabolic causes of many of these disorders is increasing and the hope is that, once the underlying pathophysiological processes have been elucidated, more specific and effective therapies will become available.

## The 'floppy' infant syndrome

Hypotonia, or floppiness, is a common observation in infancy and has many different causes. Muscle tone is assessed by observation of posture, and assessment of the resistance of joints to passive movements and of range of movement. Normal muscle tone depends not only on the peripheral neuromuscular system but also on spinal cord and higher centres. Neonatal hypotonia is more often due to disorders of the central nervous system than to peripheral neuromuscular disorders.

When an infant or young child is found to be significantly hypotonic, an important question is whether the hypotonia is 'central' or 'peripheral' in origin. Hypotonia of neuromuscular origin usually is associated with significant weakness (e.g. Werdnig–Hoffmann disease), with decreased or absent reflexes, whereas central hypotonia is usually not associated with significant weakness (e.g. Down syndrome or Prader–Willi syndrome). In practice, the differentiation in early childhood can sometimes be quite difficult. Apart from the absence of significant weakness, clues to a central cause of hypotonia may be:

- a history of adverse perinatal events
- abnormal behaviour in the neonatal period
- delayed mental development
- seizures
- abnormality of head size or shape
- the presence of normal or brisk deep tendon reflexes.

Hypotonia of peripheral neuromuscular origin is usually, but not invariably, accompanied by hyporeflexia in an alert baby with normal mental development.

## Acknowledgements

We would like to thank Dr Lloyd K. Shield, who has been our mentor and the person who kindled our interest in neuromuscular disorders.

# Neural tube defects, large heads and hydrocephalus

17.4

Peter Flett, Ray Russo

## Neural tube defects

The neural tube is the embryological structure from which the brain and spinal cord develop. The term neural tube defect (NTD) refers to a group of malformations involving the brain and/or spinal cord in association with varying degrees of absence or malformation of the overlying tissues: meninges, bone, muscle and skin. *Anencephaly* occurs when the neural tube fails to close at the head, and the brain and skull bones do not develop normally. *Myelomeningocele* (*myelo* meaning 'cord'; *meninges,* coverings of the spinal cord; *cele,* 'sac') involves all the tissue layers including the skin and bone, and is an outpouching of the spinal cord through the posterior bony vertebral column that has failed to form. *Meningocele* is an outpouching of the meninges or coverings of the spinal cord only, and not the cord itself. The term *spina bifida* refers to the normal bony projection over the spine being divided or 'bifid'. *Spina bifida occulta* is the failure of the formation of the posterior elements of the vertebrae but without any outpouching of the meninges or spinal cord. It occurs in 5–10% of the population and is most often asymptomatic. X-rays of the spine documenting the incomplete vertebral arch confirm the diagnosis. Accompanying associated features may include dermal hyperpigmentation, a fatty swelling, a tuft of hair or a dermal sinus on the back. *Spina bifida cystica* refers to myelomeningocele and meningocele. Myelomeningocele is the more serious and commoner type of spina bifida cystica. *Spinal dysraphism,* which includes spina bifida occulta, meningocele and myelomeningocele, is part of the family of NTDs that encompasses abnormalities of the cranium and its contents (anencephaly, encephalocele and cranial meningocele) as well as abnormalities of the spine.

### Incidence

The incidence has varied in different countries, the highest rates being recorded in the past in Northern Ireland, the west of Scotland and south Wales. In South Australia, the total incidence of NTDs during 1966–1991 was 2.01 per 1000 births and the incidence of myelomeningocele was 0.97 per 1000 births, with no upward or downward trend. Despite the total incidence remaining stable, prenatal diagnosis and termination of pregnancy resulted in an 84% fall in the birth prevalence of all NTDs during the years studied. Screening by serum α-fetoprotein (AFP) measurements or mid-trimester ultrasonography, or both, detected more than four-fifths of cases in 1986–1991 in South Australia.

Recurrence risks in families such as close relatives have been documented extensively. Recurrence risk statistics suggest a polygenic or environmental aetiology. The risk of recurrence following the birth of the first child with a NTD is approximately 4–8%, or 1 in 25. A woman is at equal risk of either spina bifida or anencephaly in future pregnancies, regardless of whichever of these NTDs occurred in the previous pregnancy. The risk increases to at least 10% after the birth of two affected children.

NTDs are found commonly in spontaneous first-trimester miscarriages. They are also more common in females than in males, in lower socioeconomic groups, different ethnic groups, and in women taking certain anticonvulsant drugs.

### Embryology and pathogenesis

The human neural tube closes just before the 30th day following fertilization and thus any influence affecting the closure of the neural tube must be present before this early stage of pregnancy. The typical motor, sensory and sphincter dysfunctions of spina bifida and myelodysplasia are the most evident clinical manifestations but represent only one aspect of this complex teratological anomaly. There is a high incidence of gross and microscopic brainstem, cerebellar and cerebral malformation. The aetiology of NTDs is still debated. Polygenic inheritance and environmental and teratogenic factors have been implicated. It has been demonstrated unequivocally that vitamin supplementation with folic acid reduces the incidence of recurrence in high-risk populations. Dietary factors may therefore play a major part in low-risk populations. Many other potential aetiological causes have been examined also during the last 20 years.

## Antenatal diagnosis, antenatal counselling and fetal surgery

The presence of abnormally high levels of AFP in the amniotic fluid has a high correlation with myelomeningocele. AFP is a component of fetal cerebrospinal fluid (CSF) and it probably leaks into the amniotic fluid from the open NTD. Closed lesions often do not cause increased AFP levels. The false-positive rate for the determination of myelomeningocele is less than 0.5% and the false-negative rate is 2%. AFP is synthesized by the yolk sac, hepatic cells and gastrointestinal tract of the fetus and is normally excreted in the amniotic fluid in fetal urine. The detection rate for open NTDs using maternal serum screening is approximately 80%, with a low false-positive rate. Ultrasonography can detect or confirm the extent of the NTD.

Offering counselling for the family with an antenatal diagnosis of a NTD is important, especially as the family will probably consider their options about whether to continue with the pregnancy or elect for termination. Great care should be taken about the information conveyed. Preferably, it should be given by a specialist experienced in caring for children with a NTD, in an appropriate environment and with time available to answer the family's questions about all the facets of raising a child with this diagnosis. The antenatal scan can offer some guidance, but it must be remembered that ultrasound scan findings cannot predict all aspects of functioning (physical and cognitive) accurately. In addition, families can be offered further counselling through community-based organizations (e.g. the Spina Bifida and Hydrocephalus Association). All families should be made aware of preventative measures (periconceptional folate) and offered genetic counselling if they wish to have other children in the future.

Fetal surgery (for closure of the myelomeningocele lesion) at 20–30 weeks' gestation, after which the fetus is returned to the uterus, has been developed with the hope of preventing significant complications in the affected child. Early studies have demonstrated good cosmetic closure of the lesion but the complication rate (primarily due to the fetus being delivered prematurely) was found to be high. The primary outcome is a significant reduction of the development of hydrocephalus in the treatment group.

## Clinical features

NTDs may be classified as in Box 17.4.1.

**Box 17.4.1 Classification of neural tube defects**

**Anencephaly**
- At birth, presents as an opened, malformed skull and brain
- Most babies are stillborn
- No effective treatment is possible
- Death usually occurs within hours or days

**Cranium bifidum**

*Cranial meningocele*
- The underlying brain is normal
- A meningeal sac protrudes through a skull defect

*Encephalocele*
- A midline sac protrudes that may contain brain
- Hydrocephalus is common

**Spina bifida occulta (Fig.17.4.1)**
- One or more vertebral arches are incomplete posteriorly but the overlying skin is intact
- Diagnosed incidentally, for example as the result of X-ray of the spine
- Spinal cord usually normal; however, abnormalities of the spinal cord can occur
- Ectodermal abnormalities may be associated with pigmented naevus, angioma, hirsute patch, dimple or dermal sinus on overlying skin
- The ectodermal component may communicate with the dura; may pose some risk of intraspinal infection (if associated with a dural sinus)
- The fatty swelling may be a lipomeningocele

**Spina bifida cystica**
- *Meningocele* (Fig. 17.4.2), where the spinal cord is not involved:
- Herniation consists of meningeal cyst filled with cerebrospinal fluid, in absence of other malformations, neurological signs are normal
- Not associated with hydrocephalus
- Constitute less than 10% of all cases of spina bifida cystica
- *Myelomeningocele* (Figs 17.4.3 & 17.4.4), in which vertebral column skin, meninges and spinal cord are involved:
- Almost always obvious at birth
- May occur anywhere along the length of the spinal column, with lumbar and lumbosacral regions being the most frequent anatomical levels
- Abnormal spinal cord tissue and nerve roots may be readily apparent macroscopically
- There may be spinal abnormalities such as kyphosis at the site of the lesion
- Functional deficits almost always include:
  - Arnold–Chiari type 2 malformation and hydrocephalus
  - paraplegia, with motor and sensory impairment; intellectual impairment and neuropathic sphincter disturbance (bowel and bladder)

**Sacral agenesis**
- Genetic disorder, marked by total absence of coccyx and lower two or three sacral vertebrae
- Functional deficits include flaccid neurogenic bladder, motor and, to lesser extent, sensory deficits of lower extremities

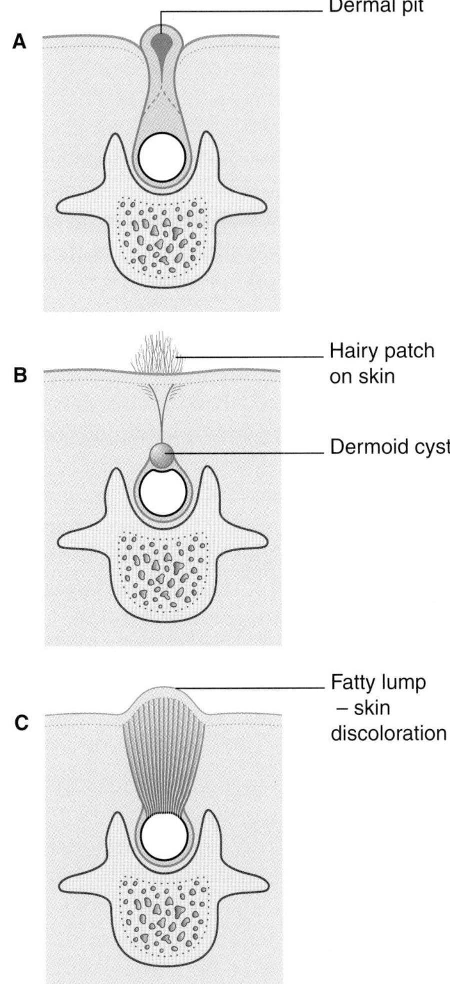


**Fig. 17.4.1** Schematic representation of spina bifida occulta. (**A**) Dermal sinus. (**B**) Intraspinal cyst pressing on the cord. (**C**) Lipomatous mass infiltrating the cord elements.

## Management of myelomeningocele

A team approach that includes the parents is essential for the proper management of myelomeningocele. An important factor, which compounds the disability, is that the defect is apparent at birth. Information given to the parents and the manner in which it is conveyed will influence their reaction at this most vulnerable time and will affect the future of the child and the family. Medical specialists in this team include the neurosurgeon, orthopaedic surgeon and urologist. The medical team leader is most appropriately a paediatrician or paediatric rehabilitation specialist with special skills in the field of child development and rehabilitation. The medical team leader will coordinate care but, importantly, will also manage and advise on the multiple problems experienced by the children and their families. These include disability issues, school integration, interventions to improve functional outcome, and various activities to support the parents and child through the many problems, both physical and psychological, that invariably arise. The physiotherapist, occupational therapist, speech pathologist, dietitian, orthotist, psychologist and medical social worker, together with trained hospital and community-based nursing staff and teachers, are important members of this team. The team has three major goals:

- to promote good health in the short and long term
- to promote maximum function in the child so that, as nearly as possible, normal developmental sequences and timing can be followed to enable maximal independence for the child and family
- to support good family functioning to assist the child to reach their maximum potential within the family and community.

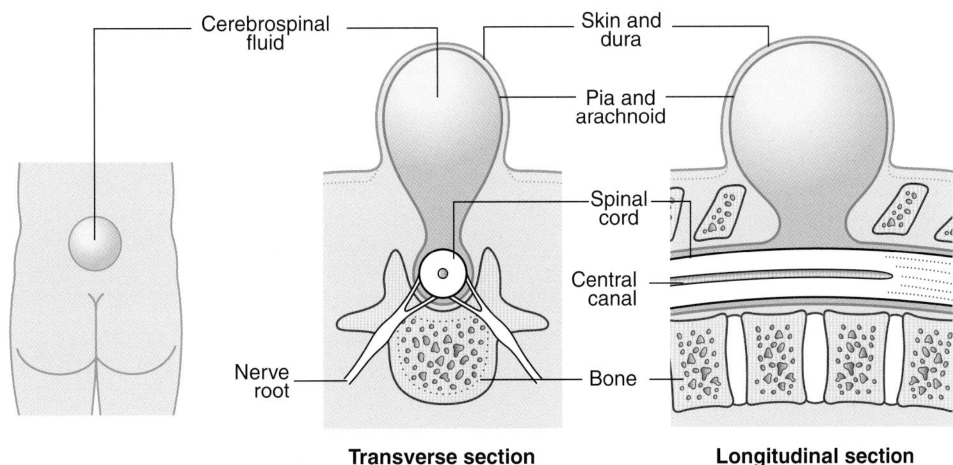


**Fig. 17.4.2** Meningocele: diagrammatic representation.

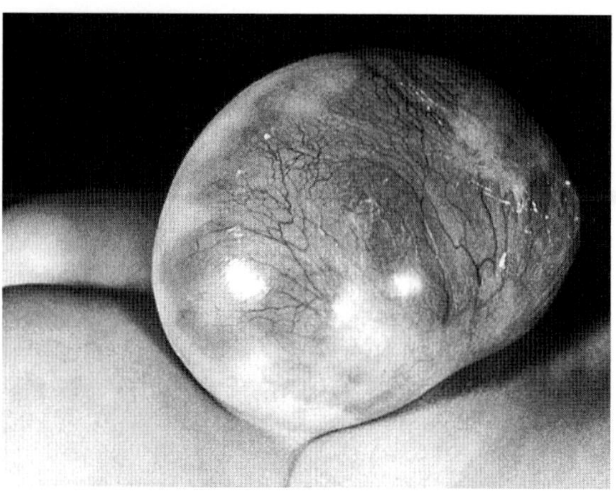

Fig. 17.4.3 A lumbosacral myelomeningocele.

### Specific problems in the management of the newborn with spina bifida

It is possible to predict with considerable accuracy the potential for future impairment in a number of areas. These include ambulation and subsequent mobility, probable bowel and bladder function, and hydrocephalus, with its probable sequelae. It is much more difficult to predict the effects that these impairments will have on the lifestyle of the individual and family. Also, it is possible to recognize early those lesions that are inoperable because of massive bony deformity and extensive skin loss, which would prevent closure of the defect. The specific problems are as follows:

1. Children with high lesions (thoracic and thoracolumbar), significant hydrocephalus at birth, major kyphosis or other significant problems (either congenital or acquired) have a significantly increased mortality rate in early life and substantial morbidity if they survive. In these circumstances, in discussion with the family, supportive care only may be recommended. If the infant survives the perinatal period, elective surgical care may be indicated. In the absence of such adverse factors, in discussion with the family, early surgical repair/removal of the lesion usually is recommended.
2. Careful serial evaluation of head circumference and ventricular size by ultrasonography or computed tomography (CT) will indicate whether hydrocephalus is developing. Once it is established that progressive hydrocephalus is present, a shunt procedure is recommended.
3. Baseline orthopaedic, urological and neurosurgical assessments provide the basis for ongoing discussions with the family and management of the condition. Occasionally, active urological intervention is required for urinary retention.
4. It is critical to begin to establish an empathetic, therapeutic relationship with the parents in the newborn period that forms the foundation for ongoing support throughout childhood.

### Ongoing management

#### Management of physical disability and mobility

Physiotherapists play an essential role in reducing deformities and encouraging mobility. Foot deformities are common at birth as a result of unopposed muscular activity *in utero*. Splinting and passive stretching are the mainstays of treatment in early life. Persistent foot deformities may require corrective orthopaedic surgery. Surgery also may be needed for dislocated hips, particularly if the child is likely to walk. At times, three-dimensional gait analysis (3DGA) is beneficial for surgical decision-making and can assist in planning for this intervention.

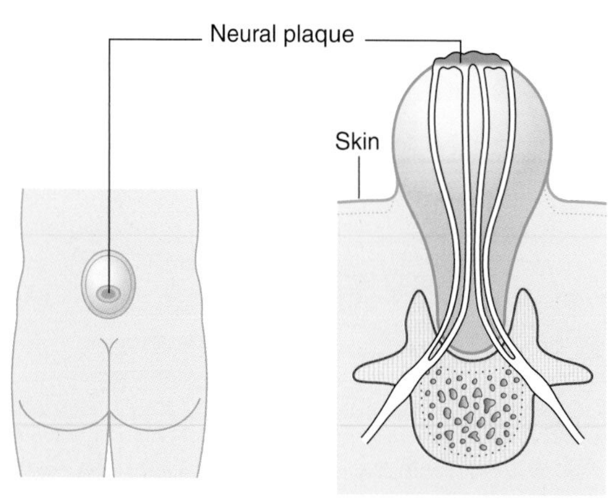


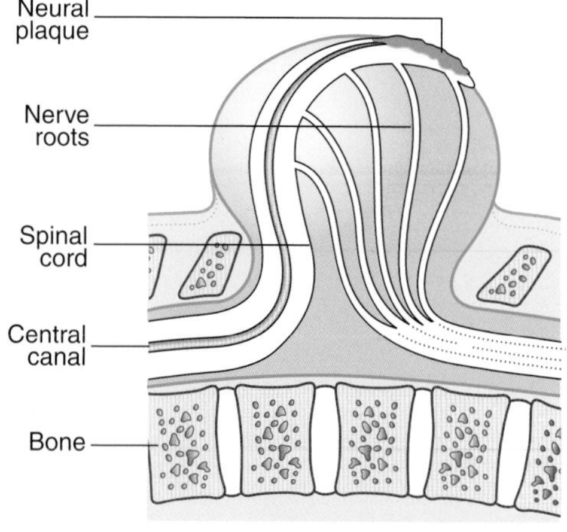


Fig. 17.4.4 Myelomeningocele: diagrammatic representation.

The outlook for walking depends on the level of the spinal cord lesion, intelligence and motivation. Most children with a lesion at L4 or lower will walk, with or without splints and crutches. Children with higher lesions may walk with orthotics in early childhood, but most will choose wheelchair mobility by mid to late childhood.

### Spinal deformities

A significant proportion of children will develop scoliosis and many of these will require spinal instrumentation. Spinal jackets are not well tolerated and have a very limited role in the management of paralytic scoliosis.

### Neuropathic fracture

Fractures of the lower limbs, due to osteopenia, are common in children with myelomeningocele. Fractures may occur with minimal trauma. Encouraging children to walk, or stand in a standing frame on a regular basis may improve the mineralization of long bones and lessen the likelihood of further fractures. However, nutrition, calcium and vitamin D from sunlight may also be important factors in management.

### Sensory deficit and skin care

Pressure ulcers or burns in anaesthetic areas are common. Parents are encouraged to check anaesthetic areas daily for the presence of pressure sores. Early recognition and treatment is essential to prevent long periods of morbidity and hospitalization.

### Neuropathic bladder

Almost all children with myelomeningocele have a neuropathic bladder. Failure to empty the bladder may lead to recurrent urinary tract infections, vesicoureteric reflux, renal calculi and hydronephrosis. Hypertension and renal failure may be seen in a small number of cases. Management of the neuropathic bladder is by clean intermittent catheterization performed four or five times daily by the parents, and later by the child. This is usually commenced at around 3–4 years of age, or earlier if repeated urinary infections occur. Prophylactic antibiotics may be required for recurrent urinary infections. Bladder augmentation and/or artificial sphincter operations may be indicated if the clinical situation dictates. The use of anticholinergic medications and of oxybutynin to increase bladder capacity may be tried. Regular assessment of renal function is essential throughout the person's life.

### Neuropathic bowel

Most children have limited or absent rectal sensation, and have little or no bowel control. Constipation with megacolon, faecal impaction and overflow incontinence is the major risk in spina bifida. Faecal softeners may be needed in infancy. Some children can attain continence simply by regular toileting, whereas others may need high-fibre diets, faecal softeners, suppositories or microenemas. Aperients are avoided whenever possible. Refractory cases may require regular bowel washouts. Another technique that may increase independence is the anterograde colonic enema (ACE). This surgical procedure creates a stoma on the anterior abdominal wall through which a catheter can be passed to allow for easier access for the provision of an enema. The advantage is that the enema is completed independent of others and can assist greatly in the management of refractory neuropathic bowel.

### Sexual function

Many people with spina bifida achieve satisfactory sexual relationships. In females, pregnancy has been achieved in many individuals and is generally a positive experience. Predictably, there are a number of potential difficulties with pregnancy and confinement. Urinary tract infections, worsening pressure sores, worsening mobility and spinal problems are particularly common. In males, the situation is more complex. Difficulties range from impotence to retrograde ejaculation and infertility. Sexual counselling is important in adolescence.

### Tethered spinal cord

Following repair of a myelomeningocele, the lower end of the spinal cord may become tethered to the site of repair. As the child grows, this may cause progressive neurological deterioration in motor or sensory function, or in bladder control. Regular monitoring of the neurological state is essential particularly during the rapidly growing phase. MRI is performed to demonstrate the tethering process. If the neurological deterioration is significant, or the child experiences significant pain, consideration should be given to neurosurgical release of the tethered cord.

### Arnold–Chiari malformation

This has been described (Fig. 17.4.5). It is present in a significant number of children with myelomeningocele and is elegantly demonstrated by MRI. Symptoms are variable: they may be quite minor (e.g. strabismus or mild difficulties with chewing and swallowing) or they may be severe, with laryngeal stridor and apnoeic

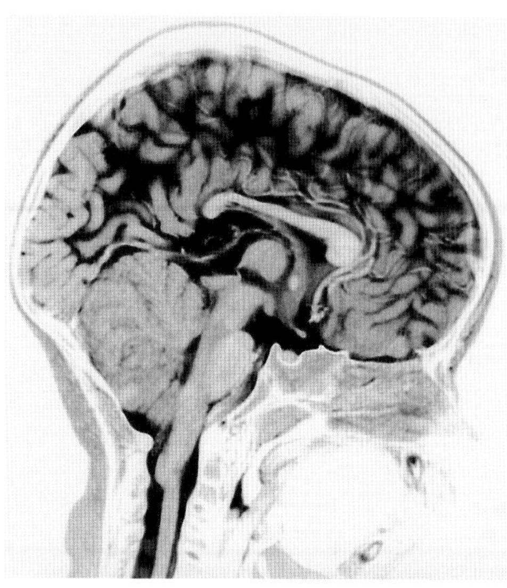

Fig. 17.4.5 Magnetic resonance image of a child with a spina bifida showing the Arnold–Chiari malformation. Note the herniation of the cerebellum into the upper cervical canal.

spells. Life-threatening episodes may necessitate neurosurgical intervention to decompress the posterior fossa. Related feeding difficulties can often be managed by full evaluation of feeding and swallowing function, adjustment of the diet (e.g. giving foods of a pureed consistency) and, at times to prevent life-threatening aspiration events, discontinuing oral feeding and using alternative means of feeding (e.g. gastrostomy).

### Education

Children with myelomeningocele often have intellectual disability and/or specific learning problems, requiring assistance at school. This is often evaluated by a clinical psychologist to determine the child's strengths and weaknesses to assist the school in maximizing the learning progress of the child. Overall intelligence is generally in the low average range, with a wide range of abilities. Verbal IQ is usually considerably higher than performance IQ, and many children have apparently very good expressive language but with a paucity of meaning and content of speech (often referred to as 'cocktail party syndrome'). Difficulties with mathematical concepts are very common, as are problems with abstract reasoning. Many children have a poor attention span and distractibility, but also poor memory. Problems with fine motor control and visual perceptual difficulties are frequently present. Most children with spina bifida attend normal schools, with varying levels of assistance for physical and cognitive/learning difficulties from support teachers. Schools may require modification to provide access and suitable toilet arrangements.



### Social and emotional adjustment and transition to adulthood

A child with a chronic disability places severe strains on the emotional and financial resources of a family. Members of the team must be alert to signs of distress and be ready to provide the necessary support. During the teenage years, the usual problems of adolescence are superimposed on the difficulties associated with the disability, and these young people need sensitive counselling. For the families, parent groups provide valuable practical and emotional support.

### Adults with spina bifida

There are now increasing numbers of young adults with spina bifida. A coordinated approach to management is still desirable but more difficult to attain, because of the wish of the young people to be independent and to break away from what they perceive as overprotection by the medical fraternity. Ongoing health-care issues in adult life include urological, gastroenterological, musculoskeletal, sexual health, skin, neurological, cognitive impairment, other chronic health issues, and also vision and hearing. There is recent evidence to support continuing high mortality throughout adult life in persons with open spina bifida, and many deaths are unexpected.

## Prevention of neural tube defects

NTDs (spina bifida, anencephaly and encephalocele) result from defective closure of the neural tube in early pregnancy. The human neural tube closes just before the 30th day post-fertilization and thus any influence affecting the closure of the neural tube must be present before this early stage of pregnancy. Primary prevention of this group of conditions may now be feasible. Research has suggested a relationship between maternal diet and the birth of an affected infant. Medical evidence has confirmed that folic acid (a water-soluble vitamin found in many fruits, leafy green vegetables, wholegrain breads, cereals and legumes) may prevent the majority of NTDs.

A randomized controlled clinical trial carried out by the UK Medical Research Council demonstrated a 72% reduction in risk of recurrence by periconceptional (i.e. at least 1 month before and for 3 months after conception) folic acid supplementation of 4 mg daily. Other epidemiological research, including work done in Australia, suggests that primary occurrences of NTD births may also be prevented by folic acid, either as a supplement or in the diet, and this has been confirmed in a randomized controlled trial from Hungary, which found that a daily multivitamin supplement containing 0.8 mg folic acid was effective in reducing the occurrence of NTDs in first births.

The National Health and Medical Research Council of Australia has recommended the following:

- *All women planning a pregnancy or likely to become pregnant* should be offered advice about folate and encouraged to increase their dietary intake of folate-rich foods, particularly in the month before and in the first 3 months of pregnancy.

In addition:

- *Low-risk women* (no family history of NTDs, not on anticonvulsants) should be offered periconceptional folic acid supplementation (0.5 mg daily). Generally, periconceptional supplementation with other vitamins is not necessary. When supplements are used, the potential risks of vitamin overdose should be considered. In particular, large therapeutic doses of vitamin A may predispose to birth defects.
- *Women with a close family history of NTDs* (e.g. they or their partner has spina bifida, they have already had an affected child, they have a sibling or other close relative with a NTD) should:
  - be referred for genetic counselling
  - be advised to take periconceptional folic acid supplementation 5 mg daily (the 4-mg formulation is not available in Australia)
  - continue to be offered prenatal diagnosis with AFP estimation and tertiary-level ultrasonography, by an operator experienced in anatomical scans, at 16–18 weeks' gestation. Although the risk of recurrence is reduced significantly if folic acid supplementation is used appropriately, there is a residual risk of about 1% in women taking supplements who have previously had an affected infant.
- *Women on anticonvulsant drugs* should take folic acid supplementation only under the supervision of and with close monitoring by their physician.
- Because of the increased risk of NTDs in the offspring of women taking some anticonvulsants (notably sodium valproate), these women also should be counselled and offered prenatal diagnosis.

### Fortification of staple foods with folic acid/folate

Fortification of bread-making flour with folic acid was introduced in Australia in September 2009. Mandatory addition of folic acid to flour in the USA and Canada has been in place now for more than 10 years. After mandatory wheat flour fortifications in the USA, there was a 30% reduction in NTDs. Folic acid fortification of flour is inexpensive.

### Education, research and monitoring

- There should be educational programmes, for health professionals and the public, on how to achieve adequate folate intake with diet and supplementation to prevent NTDs.
- There should be continued research into the mechanisms of action of folic acid and the minimum dose of folic acid required for prevention.
- Close monitoring of both the prevalence of NTDs (including terminations of pregnancy) and the increase in folate intake should be undertaken to evaluate the effectiveness of any health promotion campaigns.
- Further research should be monitored, and these recommendations reviewed in the light of any developments.

In Australia, health promotion campaigns have been undertaken to inform health professionals and women about folate and the prevention of NTDs. For example, folic acid (folate) in fruit and vegetables is easily destroyed by cooking and prolonged storage. It is wise to eat fruit and vegetables that are fresh, and either raw or lightly cooked. For good health and enough folate per day, one would need to aim for at least two servings of fruit, five servings of vegetables, and seven servings of bread and cereals every day. The safety of increased folate ingestion before and during early pregnancy appears to be confirmed. Furthermore, an intake of folate from fortified food is unlikely to be high enough to constitute a hazard for those people in the community with unknown and untreated vitamin $B_{12}$ deficiency, which can worsen their symptoms if folate is given to these individuals without also giving vitamin $B_{12}$.

## Large heads (macrocephaly)

Macrocephaly can be defined as head circumference more than two standard deviations above the mean on growth charts.

The more common causes include:

- normal variant (often familial)
- an oversized, overweight brain (as in megalencephaly)
- hydrocephalus (progressive or 'arrested')
- a tiny cerebrum (as with large chronic subdural effusions or hygromas in infancy)
- no cerebrum (as in hydranencephaly).

Normal variants tend to be diagnosed by exclusion, based upon careful history (including family history), measurement of head circumferences including those of the parents and siblings, and of neuroradiological investigations.

Head enlargement in megalencephaly can be a late manifestation of many cerebral degenerative disorders such as lysosomal storage diseases or leukodystrophies. Megalencephaly also occurs in a wide variety of other clinical disorders and syndromes, such as neurocutaneous syndromes and cerebral gigantism (Sotos syndrome). It can be unilateral (hemimegalencephaly) or bilateral, and may also be familial and associated with a wide spectrum of developmental symptoms and signs including normal development.

Hydranencephaly is a condition of uncertain aetiology. The cerebral cortex is represented by a thin membrane composed of glial cells, with islands of cerebral cortex sometimes scattered in this tissue. The third ventricle, basal ganglia, brainstem and cerebellum are present but may reveal morphological abnormalities. The head size is usually normal at birth but increases rapidly within a few weeks of life. Neurological function may initially be normal, shortly after gross neurological abnormality is evident (rigid muscle tone, tremors, and persistent and exaggerated primitive reflexes). Optic atrophy is common and the head transilluminates readily. The child sleeps excessively, is irritable, feeds poorly and has unstable thermoregulation. Electroencephalography reveals a flat tracing or few low voltages over islands of cerebral cortex.

## Hydrocephalus

Hydrocephalus (Greek: *hydro* meaning 'water', and *cephale,* 'head') refers to a group of conditions characterized by:

- an increase in CSF volume
- ventricular dilatation
- increased intraventricular pressure.

Hydrocephalus occurs when there is an imbalance between the formation and absorption of CSF. Impaired absorption is almost always due to some degree of obstruction along the CSF pathways. If the passage of CSF is obstructed within the ventricular system, the resultant hydrocephalus is labelled *non-communicating,* whereas if obstruction exists in the surface pathways, the hydrocephalus is described as being *communicating.* The rate of this volume change varies from patient to patient and depends in large part on the degree of obstruction. The lesions that commonly produce hydrocephalus are listed in Box 17.4.2.

In supratentorial lesions, CSF obstruction is a late event, so that neurological or endocrinological abnormalities often precede symptoms of raised

**Box 17.4.2 Lesions producing hydrocephalus**

**Non-communicating**

*Aqueduct stenosis or atresia*

- Commonest site of intraventricular obstruction in infants with congenital hydrocephalus
- May occur as an isolated anomaly or be associated with myelomeningocele and the Arnold–Chiari malformation
- Histologically, subependymal gliosis around the aqueduct is demonstrable
- May be slowly progressive in some, not being clinically apparent for several years before obstructive symptoms appear
- Sporadic
- Familial
  - Inherited as a sex-linked trait; features include a short flexed thumb, mental retardation and other cerebral abnormalities

*Obstruction at the fourth ventricle*

- Dandy–Walker syndrome
  - Cystic dilatation of the fourth ventricle, with cerebellar hypoplasia; other structural brain anomalies may also occur
  - Associated with atresia of the exit foramina of the fourth ventricle
  - Hydrocephalus may be present at birth or may develop subsequently
  - Diagnosis is suggested in typical cases by the shape of the skull and the presence of cerebellar signs
- Arachnoiditis

*Obstruction due to intracranial mass lesions*

- Should always be considered in any child where head enlargement develops in late infancy or childhood
- Neoplasm, cysts
  - Childhood tumours usually arise in the posterior cranial fossa and include medulloblastoma, astrocytoma and ependymoma
  - Intracranial pressure develops early, because of their close proximity to the fourth ventricle
  - Ataxia, incoordination, nystagmus and papilloedema are suggestive of the diagnosis
  - Differential diagnosis includes craniopharyngioma, gliomas, pinealomas and arachnoid cysts
- Haematoma
- Galenic vein aneurysm

**Communicating**

*Arnold–Chiari malformation*

With myelomeningocele (type 2) (see Fig. 17.4.3)

Without myelomeningocele (type 1)

- Consists of:
  - downward displacement and elongation of the hind brain
  - herniation of the medulla, cerebellar vermis and inferior part of the fourth ventricle into the upper cervical canal
- CSF flow is impaired, usually within the subarachnoid space
- Hydrocephalus usually develops in early infancy
- Frequently associated with cranium bifidum, myelomeningocele and hydromyelia

*Encephalocele*

Meningeal adhesions

- Postinflammatory
- Posthaemorrhagic
- May be secondary to neonatal meningitis (post inflammatory adhesions), or intraventricular or subarachnoid haemorrhage
- Hydrocephalus is common, and is usually communicating (but may be non-communicating)
- Neurological deficit, developmental delay and seizures are usually the result of the infective process, but the hydrocephalus, if not relieved, will aggravate the brain injury

*Choroid plexus papilloma*

- A rare cause of hydrocephalus
- Hydrocephalus is produced by excessive fluid secreted by the tumour, sometimes with obstruction to CSF flow
- Recurrent haemorrhage from the tumour may play a role
- Total excision of the tumour usually leads to a resolution of the hydrocephalic process

intracranial pressure. Less commonly, cerebral tuberculoma, torular meningitis or an aneurysm of the vein of Galen may simulate intracranial neoplasms. The latter should be suspected if, in addition to hydrocephalus, a loud intracranial bruit, high output failure and vascular naevi are also present in the patient.

**Clinical example**

Ivan, a 5-year-old boy, presented with a 2-month history of early morning headache and vomiting. This was associated with a decline in his school performance and he was noted to be increasingly unsteady on his feet. The significant findings on examination included a wide-based, unsteady gait, horizontal nystagmus and severe bilateral papilloedema. Computed tomography (CT) revealed the presence of a large mass in the cerebellar vermis, which was distorting the fourth ventricle.

Ivan underwent a craniotomy and the tumour arising in the cerebellar vermis was excised. Following the operation the symptoms of raised intracranial pressure subsided and serial CT scans showed a resolution of the dilated lateral and third ventricles.

With this patient, excision of the obstructing mass was an effective form of treatment for a significant degree of non-communicating hydrocephalus. The presenting symptoms were in part due to raised intracranial pressure and in part due to interference with cerebellar function.

## Approach to clinical diagnosis

The clinical appraisal of the hydrocephalic child involves:

- establishment of the diagnosis and aetiology
- neurological and developmental examination
- a search for other associated malformations.

It is essential to determine the age and rapidity of onset of hydrocephalus and its rate of progression. In most clinical situations, in infants with hydrocephalus, the child presents with a large head, which may already be apparent at birth or at a few months of age. Despite the obviously large head, many babies thrive and may develop normally, apart from poor head control. Other infants with hydrocephalus, however, feed poorly, are irritable, vomit excessively and fail to gain weight. In infants with congenital hydrocephalus, the birth weight, nature of delivery and neonatal course should be noted. In addition, enquiry as to whether there has been a similar illness in an older sibling or possible intrauterine infection is relevant.

Hydrocephalus that develops in an older and previously normal child suggests the possibility of a posterior fossa neoplasm. Because ventricular dilatation is generally subacute in children with cerebellar tumours, symptoms of raised intracranial pressure are often associated with changes in behaviour, a clumsy gait, abnormal articulation, tremors and incoordination. If an increase in ventricular pressure occurs abruptly, attacks of nausea, vomiting, head retraction and extensor spasms are prominent. In very ill children, symptoms of a primary illness, such as cranial infection and haemorrhage, may obscure symptoms of intracranial hypertension. It is important in all cases to ascertain any neurological symptoms, determine the time of onset of head enlargement and assess the developmental progress of the child.

An acute increase in intracranial pressure should prompt consideration of the possibility of drug intoxication (tetracycline, vitamin A, nalidixic acid), lead encephalopathy, subdural haematoma and Reye syndrome.

In children with myelomeningocele and shunted hydrocephalus, raised intracranial pressure is usually secondary to a blocked shunt. Children may present with features typical of a blocked shunt (irritability, headache, somnolence, vomiting, loss of consciousness), but may also present with atypical features such as seizures or unusual behaviours. Diagnosis requires exclusion of other underlying causes, and a high index of suspicion prompting the clinician to question shunt dysfunction.

**Clinical example**

William was an 11-year-old boy with spina bifida and shunted hydrocephalus. During the course of the clinical consultation as part of long-term follow-up of his condition, he complained that he had been experiencing some facial pain on the right side of his face for the past 3 days. He had a decreased appetite and his mother noted that he had been confused about his daily routine, which surprised her.

On examination, William had a flaccid lower limb paralysis and was wheelchair-mobile. He had mild hyperreflexia in his upper limbs and nystagmus of gaze, both longstanding problems associated with his condition. His shunt appeared to empty, but was slow to refill. His fundi did not show evidence of papilloedema. There was no history of recent trauma or infection to explain his facial pain, and it was decided that he should have a CT scan to exclude hydrocephalus as a cause. This revealed enlarged ventricles and William was taken to theatre that day by the neurosurgical team to revise his shunt.

In this situation, the classical signs of raised intracranial pressure were not present and the diagnosis of shunt dysfunction required a high index of suspicion. This boy might well have progressed to developing further signs later, but by then the risk of an adverse outcome would probably have increased.

## Physical examination

Classically, in the infant, hydrocephalus is recognized by a progressive increase in occipitofrontal head circumference out of proportion to other bodily dimensions. A single head circumference measurement that greatly exceeds the 97th percentile strongly suggests the existence of hydrocephalus. Where head enlargement is equivocal, and neurological abnormality is absent, serial head measurements will often indicate the need for further diagnostic studies. It must be emphasized that, once enlargement of the skull is clinically obvious, the ventricles are already grossly dilated and the cerebral cortex is thinned.

Clinical signs that frequently precede obvious enlargement of the head include:

- a large and bulging fontanelle
- thinning of the bones of the calvarium
- widening of the coronal, sagittal and lambdoidal sutures.

With advancing hydrocephalus:

- the scalp thins and becomes shiny and pale
- there is upward retraction of the eyelids
- the eyes are fixed in a downward gaze (the 'setting sun' sign)
- hair appears sparse
- superficial scalp veins become distended
- the brow overhangs the small, triangular face.

Despite the enormous head size, papilloedema is uncommon in congenital hydrocephalus. The shape of the skull should be noted. A large protruding occiput is typical of a Dandy–Walker cyst, whereas an asymmetrical head may be due to unilateral obstruction at the foramen of Monro. In addition, auscultation for cranial bruit should be performed over the eyeballs and over the calvarium.

Many mildly affected hydrocephalic children have remarkably normal development and minimal neurological deficit. Gross abnormalities in a child with mild hydrocephalus are usually related to the underlying disorder that caused the hydrocephalus. However, prolonged stretching and compression of neural structures will lead ultimately to profound neurological injury. Where the increase in intracranial pressure is rapid and there has been no compensatory increase in head size, the highly irritable child frequently gives a short, high-pitched 'cerebral cry'. During these screaming episodes, decerebrate posturing may be evident. In the older child with 'arrested' hydrocephalus, it is important to evaluate the mental and psychological status. These children are frequently talkative, jovial and euphoric ('cocktail party syndrome'), but their capacity for concentration, language comprehension and abstract thinking is often lacking. Manifestations of longstanding hydrocephalus include a variety of endocrinological and metabolic disorders such as precocious puberty, diabetes insipidus and abnormal thermoregulation. NTDs, skeletal defects and cutaneous naevi are known to coexist with obstructive hydrocephalus.

## Investigations

The child's assessment, based on the history and examination, will often enable a diagnosis of hydrocephalus to be made with some degree of certainty. However, in all cases, investigations are required to confirm the diagnosis, determine the extent of the disorder and, if possible, define the aetiology. Investigations are also of assistance in deciding the need or otherwise for active treatment and also as a means of assessing the success or otherwise of treatment.

The widespread use of ultrasonography (Fig. 17.4.6) has in recent times greatly facilitated the assessment of infants with suspected hydrocephalus. Real-time ultrasound imaging through the open fontanelle provides a clear demonstration of the ventricles and may define other structural anomalies well. This non-invasive risk-free investigation can be undertaken with little or no sedation and can be repeated as often as required. When the fontanelle closes, satisfactory imaging can no longer be obtained. Ultrasound examination during pregnancy can indicate whether the fetus has hydrocephalus.

In the older child, and occasionally in infants where more detail is required, computed tomography (CT) (Fig. 17.4.7) is typically the initial investigation. This

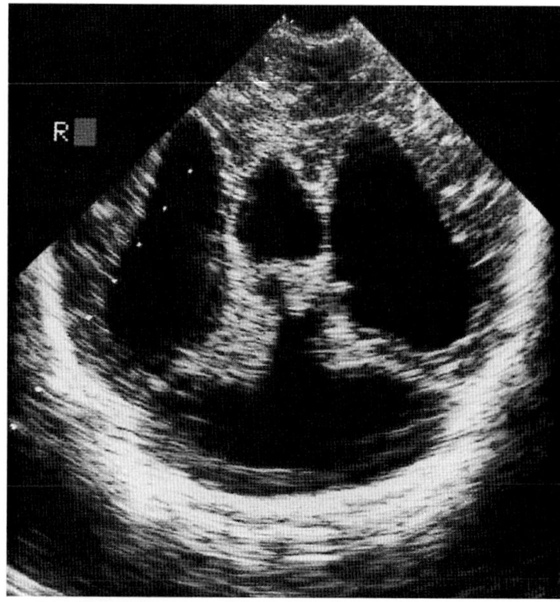


Fig. 17.4.6 Frontal view of a real-time ultrasound study showing markedly dilated lateral ventricles on either side of a large posterior fossa cyst in a patient with Dandy–Walker malformation.

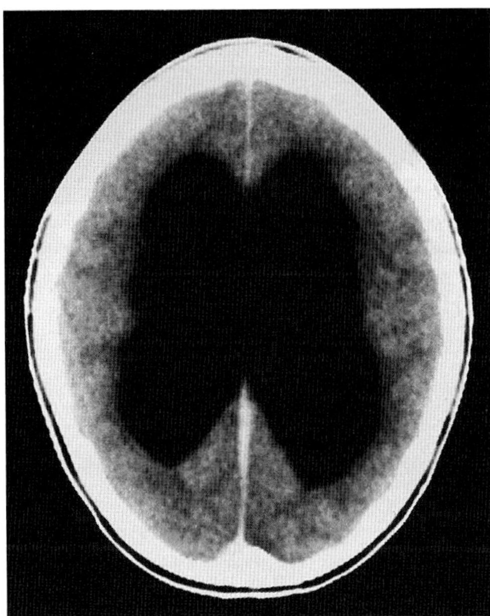

Fig. 17.4.7 Computed tomogram demonstrating gross ventricular dilatation in hydrocephalus.

technique provides excellent detail of the intracranial anatomy, and the images may be enhanced by the injection of contrast material. Many children can have CT without sedation, whereas others require sedation or occasionally a general anaesthetic. The radiation involved in a single scan is of an acceptable degree.

Magnetic resonance imaging (MRI) (see Fig. 17.4.5) is rarely undertaken as a primary investigation but may be of value in defining the cause of the condition. Small tumours in the region of the aqueduct causing obstruction to CSF flow may not be visualized by CT but are clearly defined on MRI.

## Treatment

The indications for treatment are based on a clear understanding of the natural history of the disorder. Three patterns may be described:

- the process continues, followed by neurological deterioration
- the process progresses to a point, and then stabilizes ('compensated hydrocephalus')
- the process is temporary.

In the majority of patients, the ventricles will continue to enlarge and the overlying brain will become stretched, compressed and thinned. If the process starts in infancy before the skull bones have developed significant attachment to each other, massive head enlargement will result, and under these circumstances significant brain injury will result. This type of progression will be detected by the presence and persistence of signs of raised pressure, an excessive rate of head growth and, less commonly, by the finding of neurological abnormality and developmental delay. Serial imaging will confirm progression of ventricular dilatation. In this group treatment is essential if brain injury is to be avoided or minimized.

In a lesser number of patients limited enlargement of the ventricles will occur and then cease. The term 'arrested hydrocephalus' has been applied to this group. The ventricles remain somewhat larger than normal but there are no clear signs of raised intracranial pressure and brain function appears normal. The head may be large but the rate of growth will either be normal or only slightly excessive, and serial images will show no significant alteration in ventricle size. With this pattern, decisions regarding treatment are less well defined. If the degree of dilatation is mild to moderate there is no good evidence that treatment will influence the outcome favourably. Under these circumstances, frequent assessment is required to ensure that stability is maintained.

With the widespread use of head imaging techniques, it has become apparent that hydrocephalus may be a temporary state in certain circumstances. Posthaemorrhagic hydrocephalus in the low-birth-weight infant is often of this type, as is the disorder complicating certain forms of meningitis. In these patients it appears likely that the CSF pathways have regained their patency. These patients are usually defined by repeating imaging. Such studies would show reduction in size of ventricles to normal and this satisfactory state would be associated with the disappearance of all physical signs of progressive hydrocephalus. Obviously, no long-term treatment is required in this group but intermittent removal of CSF by either a lumbar puncture or a ventricular puncture may help to resolve the process and prevent any excess ventricular dilatation during the period before effective CSF flow is established via normal pathways. On occasions, a reservoir may be inserted into a lateral ventricle to facilitate such intermittent removal. In addition, drugs that reduce CSF production, such as acetazolamide and isosorbide, have been used with the same intent.

### *Operative treatment*

The definitive treatment of hydrocephalus is a surgical procedure. The usual method of treatment is by a shunt that diverts the CSF to some other site in the body. In some cases of non-communicating hydrocephalus, ventriculostomy may successfully re-establish normal CSF pathways.

*Ventriculoperitoneal shunt.* This is the operation performed most frequently in paediatric patients with hydrocephalus. A Silastic catheter is placed in a lateral ventricle through a burr-hole and the other end of the tube is passed subcutaneously to the abdomen and then placed in the peritoneal cavity. A valve is interposed and an adequate length of tube is placed in the peritoneal cavity to allow for growth. The peritoneum absorbs CSF effectively.

*Ventriculoatrial shunt.* In this procedure the lower end of the shunt is passed via a neck vein to the right atrium. The catheter is designed so that CSF can pass from the catheter tip but blood cannot flow back into the lumen. The turbulent blood flow in the atrium prevents thrombus formation around the catheter. This operation is not undertaken often in childhood as maintenance may involve the lengthening of the atrial catheter on several occasions.

*Complications of ventricular shunts*

The operation is generally well tolerated with infrequent early difficulties. Common complications include meningitis, ventriculitis and shunt obstruction.

The most common presentation of a child with a blocked shunt is that of a vague illness. Irritability and vomiting are frequent and headache may be present. The symptoms are very similar to those of many childhood illnesses, and difficulties are often experienced in trying to decide whether the symptoms are a consequence of shunt malfunction or an unrelated illness. Definite signs of raised intracranial pressure, if present, are of great assistance but are often not ascertained readily. Palpation of the shunt mechanism may also frequently be inconclusive. Thus, when assessing a child with potential shunt dysfunction, a neurosurgeon should always be consulted.

The treatment of shunt obstruction is usually a simple procedure and involves the replacement of the defective component. However, a small number of patients suffer from repeated episodes of obstruction, and management can be difficult and may involve many variations of shunt equipment and surgical technique.

**Clinical example**

Sara, a 6-year-old child with a past history of having had a ventriculoperitoneal shunt inserted in infancy for congenital hydrocephalus, presented at the outpatient clinic for review having missed a previous planned attendance. Her mother stated that Sara was generally well but was concerned by her visual function. Sara insisted on sitting immediately adjacent to the television set and had been moved to the front of her class to enable her to see the blackboard.

When examined, Sara appeared to be generally well, but head measurement indicated an excessive rate of growth. Her visual acuity was markedly diminished in each eye and funduscopy revealed severe secondary optic atrophy. On palpation the shunt tubing was disconnected and an immediate CT scan showed very large ventricles. The shunt was revised immediately, but unfortunately there was no improvement in Sara's poor vision.

The shunt had obviously been malfunctioning for a prolonged period of time and had resulted in chronic raised intracranial pressure. Sara had not complained of any symptoms but the presence of intracranial pressure produced marked optic atrophy over this interval of time. If Sara had attended for the planned reviews, the abnormality might well have been recognized and corrected before visual deterioration resulted.

# 17.5 Headaches

Ian Wilkinson, Gopinath Musuwadi Subramanian

Headache occurs in most children at some time. In a number of these, frequent headaches are a disabling problem. In one study in primary schools in Australia, 23% of parents believed that their children suffered from 'frequent headaches'. A population study of 4–18-year-olds in the USA, published in 2009, found that 17% had suffered from frequent or severe headaches in the previous 12 months.

Many processes result in headache. These will be considered in two major classes: 'cranial' headaches, where the cause of pain is a process directly involving the brain and associated structures, including meninges, cerebral blood vessels and scalp; and 'extracranial' headaches, where the primary cause is remote from the brain.

The mechanisms of headache are multiple, but it should be recognized that the brain itself is insensitive to pain. Some neurosurgical operations for intractable epilepsy are actually performed on the brain with the patient awake.

This chapter deals particularly with recurrent or chronic headaches and not with those that accompany acute events such as trauma, intracranial bleeds or infections of the nervous system.

## Cranial causes

Migraine and stress or tension types are the most common of chronic or recurrent headaches with origins in and around the brain. The migraine subset is numerically the biggest in Australian children. Stress and tension components often interact with a predisposition to migraine. Pure stress and tension headaches are less common than in adults. Often headaches in children that are classified as 'stress' or 'tension' start out as migraine headaches but, as a consequence of recurrent pain, disability and fear of the next headache, develop strong features suggesting that stress or tension is the primary cause. Of the different headache types in children, migraine, because of its great prevalence and associated morbidity, will receive most attention in this discussion.

### Migraine

#### Epidemiological features

Migraine is:

- the commonest cause of recurrent headaches
- showing increasing prevalence. In a 1974 Finnish study using rigid criteria, 1.9% of 7-year-old children suffered from migraine headaches. In 1992 the study was repeated with the same criteria and the prevalence had increased to 5.7%.
- more common with increasing age of the child
- more common in males before puberty but in females after puberty
- a leading cause of referrals to paediatricians and child neurologists.

#### Clinical manifestations

Childhood migraines result from the same biological process as those in adults but clinical manifestations may be quite different. Some of these differences relate to the difficulty a child has in describing or explaining the features; for example, young children may not be able to describe throbbing, or lateralization, or sensory associations. Nevertheless, there are some features, such as dizziness and vomiting, that are clearly more common in children.

'Classical' migraine (which is a relatively uncommon type of migraine even in adults) includes aura, or transitory neurological dysfunction, especially of the visual system, and may involve sophisticated hallucinations such as fortification spectra, which often precede the onset of headache and then disappear as the headache commences. This classical sequence may occur in older children and adolescents but often instead there is a description of sensory hallucination that occurs with, or during, the headache. This may be a visual disturbance described in unsophisticated terms, such as 'flashing lights', 'seeing things double' or 'blurry, like looking through a curtain', or something more complex and bizarre-sounding, and often very frightening. Such hallucinations include the appearance that objects are too big or too small, or that things moving in the environment appear to be going too fast or too slow, or that body images are distorted. It is suggested that Lewis Carroll drew on personal migraine experiences in writing *Alice in Wonderland* when describing Alice's distorted body perception after she ate the magic substance.

Such hallucinations can involve the auditory process, for example things sounding too loud or someone speaking too fast. At times, the aura for a child defies description but may involve a sense of unreality or depersonalization.

What can make the migraine process more difficult to unravel in a child is the not uncommon situation where the actual sensory hallucination is not accompanied (during that event) by a headache. This is referred to as migraine dissociée, and there may be more alarm and distress for a child or parent than when there is an accompanying headache.

Other variations from adult migraine involve the location of the pain. Whereas in adult migraine attacks the pain can often be lateralized (a true 'hemicrania' – one origin of the word migraine), this is frequently not the case in young children, who will simply point to their forehead (without lateralization) as being the location. As the child grows older a description of pain that is unilateral and sometimes located in one or other temple becomes more common. The pain is more often in the frontal half of the head, and pain that is located only posteriorly raises the possibility of more sinister causes of headache.

A description of the quality of the pain in migraine in children is often difficult for them. The pain tends to be more of an aching type 'like a tummy ache' rather than sharp 'like a needle'. A combination of the two may be described. Further, in adults with pure migraine attacks it is frequent for the pain to be described as throbbing, implying involvement of vascular structures. Children with migraine may well experience throbbing pain but may not be able to describe it as such, although, as the child becomes older, he or she may describe it as 'beating like a drum' or 'like a hammer'.

Although many adults do not acknowledge headaches as being migraine unless they are severe and resulting in cessation of usual activities, in children there can be a great range in the severity of migraine events, from the situation where the child is able to continue in school or at play, to the level where all activity must cease and the child retreats to bed in misery.

Adults with migraine attacks may not change greatly in external appearance, but children are often extremely pale.

Nausea and vomiting may occur in association with adult migraine and not uncommonly continue throughout and exacerbate the headache, resulting in treatment with an antiemetic. During the attack, abdominal pain, nausea and vomiting are extremely common in children, but the sequence may be that a single vomit, often followed by a sleep, terminates the attack.

Formulating rigid diagnostic criteria for childhood migraine has proven very controversial and strict requirements for certain features to be present in combination before a diagnosis can be made may be counterproductive in clinical practice. In practice, children with headaches with some of the previously mentioned features, occurring intermittently and with symptom-free periods, who are normal to neurological examination, may be considered to suffer from migraine.

The single feature that has caused most disagreement between those studying children with headaches and those studying adults is a requirement for the headache to be of a certain duration. A diagnosis of migraine had originally required, by International Headache Society criteria, a duration of at least 4 hours. Eventually it was conceded that childhood migraine attacks may last as little as 1 hour.

Classical teaching about headaches due to tumours and other situations of raised intracranial pressure has been that they are present upon awakening, or actively cause the patient to waken. Although in reality this is not always the case, a contrast remains with childhood migraine, where the onset is more commonly later in the day, perhaps approaching midday or during the afternoon or evening.

Childhood migraine is a very cyclical condition. Patients may have a bout of recurrent headaches that lasts for weeks or months, followed by a period of remission that may last for a year or more, to be followed by another bout. Hot weather may be a factor in relapses.

## Types of migraine

In the International Classification of Headache Disorders (ICHD, second edition, 2004) there are six categories and 17 subcategories of migraine. Precise classification is necessary in migraine research but is not always so important in clinical diagnosis and management, and there is often overlap between different types in children. To categorize according to the presence or absence of 'aura' in children can be very difficult. The 'aura', in children who can describe it, may often occur during the headache and not precede it, and frequently involves some sense of disequilibrium, perhaps true vertigo. Visual auras are often basic, such as blurring or double vision, and unsophisticated.

There are some conditions that are considered to be part of the migraine phenomenon, although appearing to have little relationship with adult migraine types:

- Unexplained attacks of vomiting, without associated headache, may also be precursors of migraine. These attacks can be very puzzling diagnostically and often very debilitating, possibly recurring after a predictable interval and sometimes requiring intravenous fluids and hospitalization. With the passage of time, headaches may become more of a feature of these attacks, which are labelled 'cyclical vomiting'.

- Recurring episodes of unexplained abdominal pain defying diagnosis despite multiple investigations can also be very debilitating. There may be a family history of migraine and as time goes by the child's pain, known as 'abdominal migraine' may become associated with and eventually replaced by migraine headaches.
- In early childhood, usually before the age of 5 years, patients may experience recurrent episodes of sudden onset of true vertigo. These are extremely distressing and cause the child to seek a cuddle, or lie on the ground to relieve the feeling of spinning. These events last a few minutes, sometimes hours, and may be associated with pallor, nausea and vomiting, and possibly nystagmus. In some studies up to 80% of these children, who are described as having 'benign paroxysmal vertigo', subsequently develop migraine headaches.

The most recent ICHD (2004) now includes a section entitled 'Childhood periodic syndromes that are common precursors of migraine', incorporating (1) cyclical vomiting, (2) abdominal migraine and (3) benign paroxysmal vertigo.

In infancy, 'paroxysmal torticollis', where the head becomes tilted strongly to one or either side for periods of hours or days, may be a precursor of migraine, although simultaneous headache may not be apparent. A similar process involving the trunk has been described. These infants have been demonstrated to be at greater risk of later developing migraine headaches.

*Hemiplegic migraine* may present with unilateral weakness, and possibly unilateral sensory disturbance, and this often precedes the actual headache.

Expressive or receptive language difficulties also may be a presenting feature of some attacks, with the headache not occurring till an hour or so later.

In *acute confusional migraine* the patient is quite disoriented and distressed, with short-term memory loss. This condition raises concerns about more sinister neurological processes, or drug intoxication, often leading to invasive investigations. Again, the headache may not become apparent until later in the event.

**Clinical example**

Jarrod, aged 13 years, was sitting in class when he developed tingling in his right arm. He tried to put his arm up to tell the teacher but it was too weak. When he tried to call his teacher, he could not find the words to say. He became very distressed and confused. An ambulance took him to hospital where he was found to have a right hemiparesis. He had developed a headache on the left side and underwent computed tomography of his head, and lumbar puncture. Both were normal. The weakness, numbness and confusion resolved over the 3 hours from onset, but the headache lasted for 6 hours. It was discovered that his father had suffered similar attacks of hemiparesis and headache when he was a teenager. This is an example of familial hemiplegic migraine.

## Aetiology

The causative mechanisms for migraine are very complex and much researched, and it is beyond the scope of this textbook to go into great detail.

At a chemical level, both noradrenergic and serotonergic transmitter pathways are implicated, and this has relevance to drug therapy.

Certainly genetics plays a major role and as many as 90% of children with migraine will have parents or siblings with the same condition.

Many different mechanisms of inheritance have been postulated. In recent years there has been clear evidence that *familial hemiplegic migraine* is associated with mutations on three different chromosome sites (chromosomes 19, 1 and 2), although they all present with similar clinical features. The sites on chromosomes 19 and 2 disrupt calcium and sodium channel function respectively.

In 1944 Leao described 'spreading depression of activity in cerebral cortex'. The slow spread of this electrical change across the visual cortex was synchronous with the spread of the visual aura accompanying the migraine attack. It was thought that this spreading depression was produced by ischaemic changes resulting from vasoconstriction, and that the subsequent vasodilatation of innervated blood vessels produced the pain response.

This vascular theory of migraine held sway for 50 years, but in the last decade a new theory has arisen, which proposes that the cortical depression results from an abnormal excessive depolarization of neurons, which spreads across the cortex producing neurological dysfunction. This has been well demonstrated during the march of depolarization across the motor cortex that accompanies the spreading weakness of hemiplegic migraine, but can also occur in sensory and cerebellar cortex.

This *neurogenic theory* postulates that the depolarization producing the motor or sensory dysfunction sends afferent (or inward) messages into brainstem centres that interact, reach a critical threshold, and then send efferent (or outward) messages via the trigeminovascular system to blood vessels in pain-sensitive structures, which undergo dilatation as well as sterile inflammatory change, resulting in headache.

Given that some children are at risk genetically of developing migraine, it is clear that there may be provoking factors for individual attacks. These include head injuries, not necessarily severe ones. The head injury may be the commencing point for recurrent bouts of migraine headache, and this may have legal ramifications. Other provoking factors are:

- intercurrent systemic infections, particularly with fever
- strenuous physical exercise
- hot weather
- dehydration

- worry and stress, either domestic, social or educational in origin. While these factors remain, they may greatly complicate treatment. The distinction from 'stress' or 'tension' headaches without an underlying migraine basis may be very difficult
- foodstuffs. This is a very controversial area, with evidence for and against. Citrus fruit, cheese, chocolate and processed meat have been implicated
- food additives, such as monosodium glutamate, sodium nitrite, benzoic acid, tartrazine.

### Treatment

Treatment can be divided into the following tiers:
- avoidance of triggers
- non-specific analgesia for attacks
- specific anti-migraine medication for attacks
- prophylactic medication
- non-medication treatments.

Avoiding specific triggers in childhood migraine can be difficult. In many, they do not exist. In Australia, hot weather and exercise are common precipitants that are part of a normal childhood lifestyle. Ensuring adequate hydration in the above situations may be helpful.

The role of restrictive diets is controversial. If it is evident that certain foodstuffs or drinks regularly provoke attacks then they should be avoided. Placing children on very limited diets is not only unpleasant and difficult to enforce, but may even have nutritional consequences.

The use of non-specific analgesics in attacks is the simplest means of treatment. The most commonly used is paracetamol, best given in an initial dose of 20 mg/kg. Unfortunately, children may not seek medication, or as a result of being at school may not be able to access medication, until the attack is advanced. The paracetamol may not be effective at this time, or may be vomited. There may be a role for rectal paracetamol in this latter situation.

A recent study has indicated that ibuprofen in a dose of 10 mg/kg may be more effective than paracetamol. Other non-steroidal anti-inflammatory drugs (NSAIDs) may be helpful.

In recent years aspirin has been avoided in childhood because of concerns about its relationship with Reye syndrome, a rare but severe acute encephalopathy with potentially fatal outcome. Nevertheless, aspirin in doses of 15 mg/kg may be employed in older children with recurrent headaches.

The use of codeine and powerful narcotics in childhood headache is not usually necessary and is potentially hazardous, although restricted infrequent use of combinations of paracetamol and codeine in older children may be necessary and effective.

Ergotamine has long been a useful antimigraine drug in adults, particularly at the beginning of the attack. Although some studies have shown efficacy of oral dihydroergotamine in children, ergotamines have had limited use because children often delay seeking treatment and also because they may produce side-effects such as vomiting and abdominal discomfort.

Triptans are serotonin agonists with multiple methods of action against migraine attacks, and may be useful in children and adolescents. Sumatriptan has been the most employed in this age group, and the nasal spray, either 10 or 20 mg has been shown to be effective in patients aged 12–17 years. It should be administered as early as possible in the course of the attack.

Sumatriptan and other triptans have little proof of efficacy when given orally or subcutaneously to children and adolescents.

Antiemetics such as promethazine, prochlorperazine and metoclopramide may be useful in situations where the migraine attack is associated with pernicious vomiting, but this is unusual in children, and often a vomit followed by a sleep brings about the end of the particular attack. Antiemetics may produce significant drowsiness, and metoclopramide in particular may be associated with acute dystonic reactions.

Prophylactic treatment to prevent migraine attacks may be indicated when there is significant suffering and disruption of the patient's lifestyle. It is difficult to define what frequency of attacks should dictate a decision to implement prophylaxis; opinions vary between two and four events per month. The decision process should combine the frequency of the attacks with the negative impact on the young person's lifestyle. Many commonly used medications may have significant side-effects.

One of the problems in managing migraines in this age group is the difficulty in obtaining proof that individual medications are effective. Controlled trials are complicated by the cyclical nature of migraine in the young, with bad bouts being followed shortly afterwards by periods of temporary or permanent remission, and by the very high placebo response rates.

A 2008 revision of a Cochrane database study again concluded a lack of evidence for the benefit of prophylaxis in childhood migraine. The only proven treatments were for propranolol (in a study, subsequently contradicted) and flunarizine in repeated studies. Unfortunately flunarizine is not readily available in Australia, although it is used widely in Europe.

Nevertheless, the following medications are commonly used in clinical practice:
- Cyproheptadine, an antihistamine with serotonin-blocking and calcium channel-blocking properties. Side-effects include drowsiness (which may be minimized with a single night-time dose regimen) and increased appetite. Effective doses range from 0.1–0.3 mg per kg per day, given either once or twice daily.

- Propranolol, a β-adrenergic blocking drug, also blocks release of serotonin from platelets. It is contraindicated in asthma. Doses range from 0.5 to 2.0 mg per kg per day in two or three equal doses. The value of propranolol and similar drugs has been proven in adults, but trials in children have produced conflicting results.
- Pizotifen, with antiserotonin and antihistamine properties, has side-effects of increased appetite, weight gain and drowsiness. The last may be avoided by a single night-time dose. Doses are limited by the single-size pill format (0.5 mg) but range from one to three at night.
- Clonidine, a vasoactive drug, has been trialled in a range of conditions in children but lacks good evidence for use in migraine and has significant potential side-effects.
- Amitriptyline, originally marketed as an antidepressant, has been used for migraine prophylaxis in children. It may be particularly useful where there are stress and depressive features, but care must be taken to avoid provoking cardiac arrhythmias.

In recent years there has been increasing evidence that drugs introduced as anticonvulsants may have a role in psychiatric treatment, and also in prevention of migraine headaches. Sodium valproate has been shown to be effective in some studies but may be associated with unacceptable weight gain. Topiramate is approved in Australia for migraine prophylaxis but can affect alertness and cognition, and may be associated with weight loss.

Many of the preventative medications, early and recent, have channel-blocking effects and this may explain their benefit, as increasingly there is evidence for channelopathies as underlying the pathogenesis of migraine.

Because of the high remission rates in children, prophylactic medications should not be used continuously for more than 6 months without attempting to wean patients from them.

Non-medication treatments may at times be successful, but again there is a paucity of controlled trials in children. Biofeedback and relaxation techniques have been used, particularly in Europe and North America. Acupuncture has proved to be successful in adults but is a potentially painful procedure. Homeopathic formulations are enjoying increased popularity in many conditions but lack evidence in childhood migraine. Chiropractic treatments are controversial, lack controlled trials and may be dangerous in young children.

Although discussion in this section has focused on migraine, the non-specific medications and treatments cited may be useful in all headache types.

### Prognosis

Childhood migraine is often cyclical, with bad bouts followed by prolonged remissions, sometimes followed by relapses in later childhood or adult life. Various studies have indicated an overall 30–40% 10-year remission rate. It is not uncommon when taking a family history to find that parents, when pressed, remember having childhood migraines long since in remission. Similarly, in apparent adult-onset migraine, a long forgotten history of severe childhood headaches may eventually be recalled. Other children, like adults, will have a history of infrequent migraines throughout their developing years.

**Clinical example**

Jason, aged 8 years, presented in March with headaches that had occurred about twice a week for the previous 3 months, although he had had some after playing soccer the previous winter. The headaches commenced after lunch at school, were frontal and throbbing, and Jason looked very pale. Paracetamol sometimes helped him but often he would vomit, go to sleep, and then awake without headache and eat his evening meal. His mother had a history of migraine. Neurological examination in Jason was normal. After daily treatment with cyproheptadine for 2 weeks, Jason's headaches ceased. The history is consistent with childhood migraine.

## Tension-type headache

In adults, tension-type headache (TTH) represents the most common type of primary headache. This is not true in children, where TTH affects 15–20% of adolescents and an even smaller proportion of younger children. The term TTH replaces the previous terms 'muscle contraction headache' and 'tension headache', etc. The International Headache Society classification describes the typical features of TTH as non-throbbing but as an oppressing or tightening pain that is usually bilateral and is present anywhere in the cranium or suboccipital regions. The headache is usually of mild to moderate intensity and lasts for 30 minutes to several days. The absence of vomiting and nausea, and the absence of photophobia and phonophobia, are distinguishing features from migraine. On a pain scale, TTH is placed on the lower end of continuum whereas migraine with aura is placed on the severe end.

A TTH may occur periodically (episodic), or fewer than 15 days a month, the most common being once or twice a month, to be distinguished from a headache that occurs daily or for more than 15 days a month, also known as chronic TTH. The latter is described under the chronic headaches.

There is no single cause for TTH. As the name suggests, the most common cause for such a phenomenon is stress, and this is present usually in the environment of the child which includes the school, family, friends, peers, etc. A small proportion is passed on as an inherited trait that runs in families.

The rule of targeted history-taking and focused examination is very important to exclude organic causes as clinical features of a TTH can be non-specific. A quick run through into the psychosocial environment and the daily functioning of a child is useful as this will provide the most common triggering for such headaches.

The treatment of TTH is usually a combination of non-drug and drug strategies. Among the non-drug strategies the initial focus should be on lifestyle changes (sleep, dietary changes), physiotherapy, stress management and relaxation techniques, and, most importantly, counselling. The drug strategies for TTH are no different to those for symptomatic treatment of headache, and are usually successful with over-the-counter pain medications.

The overall prognosis for TTH is better than that for migraine headaches, with at least one-third becoming completely symptom-free on longer follow-up studies, and the majority much improved.

## Chronic daily headache

Patients with daily, or near-daily, recurring headaches form a very challenging subgroup among children and adolescents presenting with headache. A proportion of these would have been labelled as having 'stress and tension headaches' before the current classification became accepted. There has always been a need for precise categorization of chronic headaches.

Chronic daily headache (CDH) is formally defined as occurring when headaches are present for more than 3 months, during which the patient has more than 15 headaches per month that last for more than 4 hours per day.

According to the ICHD (2004), the chronic forms of primary headache are subgrouped into four types based on the existing and past clinical features.:

1. Transformed/chronic migraine
2. Chronic tension-type headache
3. New-onset daily persistent headache
4. Hemicrania continua.

The most common is transformed or chronic migraine. This group of children or adolescents has a history of infrequent migraine headache in the past and may not even have a label until the new daily pattern occurs. The severe and daily occurrence of headache may obscure the diagnosis, but the past history and migraine features suggest the diagnosis. The second group is of patients with an occasional TTH who transform to a daily headache pattern without any history of migraine headache features in the past. The third group is of those with new daily persistent headaches. As the name suggests, there is no history of remembered headache in the past, and over a few days these children present with unrelenting headache. There are studies highlighting that specific trigger factors are remembered as the initiating factor to the headache. The last category, hemicrania continuum with autonomic features accompanying the unilateral headache, is the least common form.

To qualify for a label of CDH, the subject over a period of time presents with a baseline headache with fluctuating severe headache, which is never accompanied by symptoms related to increased intracranial pressure; clinical examination is normal; imaging is negative; overall secondary or organic pathology should be ruled out, so the diagnosis is arrived at by exclusion.

Various theories exist regarding pathogenesis of CDH, but none offers a complete explanation. Nevertheless, the scenarios listed are common. The aetiology in selective cases may be amply clear in that the symptom of headache may be used in a conscious and malingering fashion to avoid a specific situation, or in a manner as seeking desperately for help. A more common situation is where the child has suffered headaches infrequently in the past but extraneous factors bring a crescendo effect, resulting in a chronic headache. Further along is a situation where the child or adolescent is a part of a high-functioning family unit. The subject balances a delicate and demanding combination of school, additional tutoring, sport and performing arts, etc. really well until a major event such as a protracted viral infection or a surgical illness or a minor head injury occurs. Very commonly, the child experiences headache among other symptoms during the acute phase. A slow convalescence leads to a protracted or a delayed catch-up of premorbid functioning. Failure to catch up or fear of permanently losing the skills achieved earlier may lead to recurrence of headache and other generalized fatigue symptoms following the acute illness. This scenario fits new-onset chronic headache. In others, a psychiatric disposition or related diagnosis increases the risk of suffering anxiety, stress or somatic complaints leading to chronic headache. On the same note, family dynamics, past or present, and lifestyle issues including sleep and diet have been implicated. In some cases, there are no antecedents and headache presentation may be frustratingly difficult for the clinician attempting to come to grips with the nature of these headaches. Although subgroups are useful to classify, a mixed bag of two different headaches is not uncommon and may coexist.

Evaluation includes thorough history-taking to include antecedent events, evolution of symptoms and the impact of illness on the child at home in the family, and at school. Headache is rarely the only symptom in CDH. The clinician should ask for other symptoms including dizziness, abdominal pain, fatigue, syncope, concentration and attention issues, personality and mood changes, and sleep hygiene. School grades, school absences and peer interaction should be documented. Medication use and overuse should be assessed. Headache diaries help maintain and document events, triggers and treatment response. Family history should focus on parent relationships, interactions and separation, etc. Often, there is nothing abnormal to note on clinical examination. A wide list of differentials ranges from common to rare diagnoses, but detailed history-taking and normal clinical examination eliminates several of them. Most often, a key feature to note during consultation is the scenario of encountering a child or adolescent who appears completely indifferent to his or her presenting symptoms, ranging through to an individual manifesting intense anxiety. At times, parental anxiety dominates the consultation. Investigations have often already been performed and results are available, the patient having been tested for infection, nutritional markers and immunological problems, etc.

Children with CDH complain of two types of headache. One is a continuous baseline headache that waxes and wanes and is present 24/7. The other is a severe intermittent headache occurring with a period of exacerbation lasting for hours to days on top of the baseline headache.

Investigations for chronic headache are almost always negative. More often than not, brain imaging is performed on the grounds of excluding a host of rare conditions, from malignant tumours to brain infection. Radiological investigations rarely contribute to a positive diagnosis, but a normal result may be the only way to alleviate anxiety. In the situation of a conversion reaction, it may reinforce to the patient that there really may be an organic problem. A counter effect may result and this needs to be thought through and discussed with the family, in order to avoid unnecessary screening tests.

A lumbar puncture may also be required if the history and clinical features suggest a longstanding headache and the investigation of headache has given normal imaging results. The presence of high cerebrospinal fluid (CSF) opening pressure can be diagnostic of idiopathic intracranial hypertension, which may be disguised.

Treatment is often difficult. It should be emphasized to the family that any medication intervention, current or future, may not yield dramatic relief but that the goal in such a situation is to reduce the frequency of the severe headaches and make the baseline headache less intense. Acute headache management should go along with daily preventive medication management if an underlying migraine basis is identified. Pain management of other chronic headache on similar lines is often practised, with little evidence. In the latter situation, treatment should also be tailored to treat co-morbidity – as a priority, rather than placing emphasis just on headache treatment. Where the headache appears secondary to, or aggravated by, a psychiatric disorder, consultation with a child psychiatrist is strongly advised.

Acute pain management for intense CDH is often less effective in the longer period. Most patients will have tried various forms and combinations of over-the-counter analgesics. A significant proportion in the long term does not report benefit, which leaves two categories of medication users. One group avoids using any form of pain medication because of lack of therapeutic effect. The other group is at risk of overuse following an attempt to control pain, resulting in escalation of doses and medication frequency. This group is also at risk of rebound headache when medications are discontinued. In a rare situation, emergency or acute-care presentation may require a cocktail of management – opioids, antiemetics and sedatives. At times, selective agents such as ketorolac, dihydroergotamine or triptans may be useful.

Prophylactic medications should be given consideration in patients where chronic headache symptoms impair social/school functioning or personal well-being, and in those patients at risk of medication overuse.

Evidence-based medicine on current medications of chronic daily headache is limited by the impressive response rate from placebo arm of trials. This leaves clinicians to consider the better known and used choices. The key to successful treatment should focus on considering a medication option as one of the treatment arms and not as a cornerstone of management. A slow titration to an effective dose may be time-consuming and the therapeutic effect may take weeks to manifest.

The authors' line of practice is to use cyproheptadine, pizotifen, amitriptyline and propranolol as options. The choice is based on considering co-morbidities (weight gain is an undesirable effect with the first three agents mentioned above), and the suitability or unsuitability of the side-effect profile (avoid the last agent in children with asthma) from medication. Once an effective dose has been achieved, maintenance treatment can be tailored to the next 3–6 months, with an attempt to wean subsequently.

Several non-pharmacological therapies may have a role. These include: muscle relaxation, stress avoidance, biofeedback, hypnosis and acupuncture. These therapies are resource-intensive and are non-conventional management options. These are most often self-referred and belief-centred.

**Clinical example**

Chloe is an 8-year-old girl presenting with recurring headaches. For the last year she has been complaining of a headache several times a week. Her headaches occur mostly on school days but have not been severe enough to cause her to miss school. She rarely mentions having a headache during weekends or vacations. She has never had a headache that awakened her from sleep. When asked, she does not recall where her head usually hurts.

There is no history of nausea, vomiting, visual or auditory symptoms. The patient's general health has been good. There is no family history of headache. Her parents mention that she is average at schoolwork, required speech therapy at school entry, and has trouble learning mathematics and English. She enjoys outdoor activities with her siblings.

Chloe's neurological examination reveals no focal deficits. She is well spoken and appeared to interact well during the consultation. A school counsellor has assessed her and identified that Chloe has difficulty interpreting complex sentences, solving simple word problems, and subtracting two-digit numbers.

The history is consistent with chronic daily headache.

### Headaches due to raised intracranial pressure

The possibility of childhood headaches being caused by raised intracranial pressure, especially due to tumours, is often a cause for great concern in the treating physician as well as the child and family. In reality, only a very small number of childhood headaches are due to raised pressure. Even when there is increased pressure, the ability of the child's skull to expand may mitigate some of the effects.

Although headaches due to raised intracranial pressure have classically been described as worse in the morning upon awakening, or causing the patient to awaken, and associated with vomiting, this is not always the case.

Raised intracranial pressure can be a result of abnormal fluid collections, solid masses or vascular malformations.

Fluid can collect abnormally either within ventricles, within the substance of the brain or over the surfaces:

- Build-up of fluid within the ventricles is referred to as hydrocephalus (see Chapter 17.4). This often presents in infancy, and the ability of the skull to expand, coupled with the inability of the child to report the pain, may be the reason that headache is not always a presenting feature. In older children, the onset of hydrocephalus is often associated with a mass lesion obstructing the intracerebral CSF pathways, and this may result in major headaches.
- Intracranial abscesses are uncommon in children in Western society. Children with cystic fibrosis or cyanotic heart disease are at increased risk. Abscesses can develop by spread from infections of the paranasal sinuses. Headaches resulting from abscesses are often associated with systemic manifestations such as fever, and tend to build up in severity over days or weeks.
- Arachnoid cysts occur in a number of different locations, often adjacent to the surface of the brain. They result from fluid collecting within a split arachnoid membrane and usually are asymptomatic, but can produce headaches.
- Fluid, including blood, can collect in the subdural or extradural spaces, often as a result of trauma. Accompanying headaches are often crescendo in frequency and severity, and may be associated with focal signs.
- Headaches due to tumours are most often due to mass effect, or obstruction of CSF pathways, and are less likely to be due to direct local involvement of pain-sensitive structures. Intracranial tumours in children are usually primary and are most frequently found in the posterior fossa, where they readily obstruct fluid pathways. It is not uncommon that there is a substantial delay in detection of the tumour in such headaches.
- Aneurysms are uncommon in children, but arteriovenous malformations or cavernous angiomas are found in this age group. These may produce headache owing to their size, or obstruction of fluid pathways.

The signs associated with raised pressure often involve the eyes.

Papilloedema may take days to develop, even in the presence of grossly increased pressure. Abnormalities of ocular movements, particularly failure of abduction with resultant paralytic convergent strabismus, or failure of upward gaze, can occur. Sluggish pupillary light reflexes may be found. Deep tendon reflexes are often brisk. There may be neck stiffness. Bradycardia and systemic hypertension are later effects.

Treatment of such headaches usually involves surgical approaches, either directly to the mass or to drain fluid from the ventricles or brain surface via a shunt. Oedema surrounding a mass may be treated with corticosteroids or osmotic diuretics, but these are temporary measures only.

### Idiopathic intracranial hypertension (previously known as benign intracranial hypertension)

This condition, sometimes also referred to as 'pseudotumour cerebri' because the clinical features can mimic a tumour, occurs in children and adults. It results from a build-up in intracranial pressure, without a space-occupying lesion, probably due to an imbalance between production and reabsorption of CSF. It is potentially serious as it can eventually result in visual loss. There is often an association with adolescent females, who may be overweight but otherwise apparently healthy. This may have a hormonal basis.

Specific causes of intracranial hypertension in individual cases include:

- recurrent middle ear infections, sometimes associated with mastoiditis, where the draining cerebral venous sinuses near the ear become obstructed
- head trauma
- oral contraceptives
- the use or withdrawal of corticosteroids
- excessive amounts of vitamin A
- tetracyclines
- growth hormone treatment.

In some cases a specific cause is not found and the old entity of 'benign intracranial hypertension' should probably be divided into idiopathic and symptomatic categories.

The clinical features include:

- headache, which tends to be daily, often worse in the morning but not necessarily severe
- abnormalities of the eyes, most commonly papilloedema (which may be asymptomatic), possibly lateral rectus palsies due to pressure on the abducens nerves, and enlarged blind spot
- nausea and vomiting
- raised pressure at lumbar puncture, to values of 20–40 cm$H_2O$ or more
- normal CSF laboratory findings.

In the presence of papilloedema or other eye signs it is prudent to perform a structural study, preferably magnetic resonance imaging (MRI), before performing the lumbar puncture. Magnetic resonance venography (MRV) may be helpful in demonstrating obstructed venous sinuses.

Cerebral images are usually otherwise quite normal, without a space-occupying lesion or dilatation of the ventricles. Even in the presence of a normal scan result, it is reasonable to examine the CSF for malignant cells, as in rare cases undifferentiated tumours can present with raised intracranial pressure in the presence of apparently normal scan findings.

Treatment is varied but includes:

- repeated lumbar punctures to remove fluid; this is quite traumatic and not always effective. Occasionally a single puncture may bring resolution
- acetazolamide, which potentially reduces production of CSF by interfering with the carbonic anhydrase enzymes, or more powerful diuretics, such as furosemide, if acetazolamide fails
- steroids
- shunting procedures to remove fluid from the cranial cavity. These should be reserved for drug-resistant cases
- decompression procedures on the optic nerves
- anticoagulation if there are thrombosed draining venous sinuses.

Patients must be seen by an ophthalmologist, to monitor visual function, as prolonged papilloedema can lead to optic nerve damage.

The prognosis for idiopathic intracranial hypertension is generally good. The process, particularly where no underlying cause is demonstrated, often remits spontaneously.

**Clinical example**

Lisa, 14 years old, developed daily headaches. These were often present by the time she had breakfast, and were distressing, but she could get to school most days. The pain continued throughout the day and was all over her head. She had noticed some visual difficulty. The problem started after she was placed on an oral contraceptive for dysmenorrhoea.

On examination, Lisa was obese. There was papilloedema but no other neurological abnormality. Her blood pressure was normal. Cranial tomography was normal and a lumbar puncture resulted in the fluid pressure rising out of the top of the tube. The fluid was normal in the laboratory.

Lisa responded to cessation of the contraceptive and treatment with 250 mg acetazolamide each morning.

The history is consistent with idiopathic intracranial hypertension.

### Seizure-related headaches

In adults, severe headaches are common following a major seizure. In young children, postictal headaches tend to be less debilitating. Children may describe a headache during an actual epileptic event, while conscious. This can be associated with focal discharges, possibly from the temporal lobe, and may be only a brief event, not always associated with other clinical features. Electrical discharges in the occipital region may give visual hallucinations, vomiting and headaches not always associated with motor convulsions. This condition may be familial and often difficult to diagnose.

## Extracranial causes

Headache is a frequent associate of systemic illness, without there being a primary pathological process in the nervous system:

- The most frequent association is with systemic febrile illnesses not directly involving the nervous system.
- Connective tissue disease, especially 'mixed connective tissue disease', may lead to vascular-type headaches.

- Systemic hypertension is much less common in children, and hypertensive encephalopathy is not seen frequently. Nevertheless, in persistent severe hypertension in children a major encephalopathy may develop, with headache, seizures and altered consciousness. Acute glomerulonephritis may present in this way.
- Metabolic pathway disturbances such as urea cycle defects can produce headaches, especially during biochemical decompensation.
- Hypoglycaemia is a potent trigger for migraine but can also result in non-specific headaches and may be a result of poor diabetic control.
- Hunger without demonstrable hypoglycaemia sometimes provokes headaches.
- Although controversial, allergic disorders can be associated with migraines and other headaches.
- Obstructive sleep apnoea and other sleep disorders not uncommonly produce a clinical picture of daytime headaches and somnolence.

In these situations treatment of the underlying cause is preferable to symptomatic relief.

## Overrated causes of childhood headaches

Children with recurrent headaches are frequently initially referred to optometrists or ophthalmologists. The basis for these headaches is often migraine.

Glaucoma (rarely seen in children) and iritis may produce aching in and around the orbit. Convergence insufficiency and other ocular muscle imbalances are common findings in children. Headaches may be attributed to these problems but the evidence is not convincing.

Minor refractive errors detected on examination, but with doubtful clinical relevance, may be blamed incorrectly as a cause of childhood headache. Spectacles or ocular movement exercises may result in apparent temporary relief of the headaches, but not infrequently they return.

### Clinical example

Reuben is 9 years old. He had recurring, but not daily, frontal headaches. His mother took him to an optometrist near their home who found he had mild hypermetropia and dispensed spectacles. The headaches settled for a few months then recurred. An ophthalmologist thought that the refractive error was minor and could find no other abnormality.

Reuben's father revealed a history of similar headaches until he went to high school. Reuben started cyproheptadine at night. The headaches resolved after a month and had not recurred after 8 months of treatment. The story was consistent with migraine.

Acute sinusitis is a potential cause of headache in children, often associated with other features such as fever, purulent nasal or postnasal discharge, local tenderness and puffiness around the eyes. The pain can be widespread in the skull, and the location can be confusing. This is a potentially dangerous condition, occasionally leading to intracranial abscesses.

More frequently seen is the situation where recurrent frontal migraine headaches are attributed to chronic sinusitis and referral for a plain radiographic series is the first investigation. These are frequently negative. With the increasing availability of computed tomography (CT) and MRI performed for other reasons, it is not uncommon that asymptomatic fluid collections are detected in paranasal sinuses, usually with no clinical consequences.

The frontal and other sinuses are not formed in early childhood and may not be capable of harbouring infections until the end of the first decade.

## Headaches found in adults that are unusual in children

- Giant cell or temporal arteritis is a potentially serious cause of headaches in the elderly and can lead to visual impairment or cerebrovascular accidents if not treated. Fortunately, it is not a condition of childhood.
- Acute angle-closure glaucoma is another cause of pain in the ocular region. It is uncommon for this to occur in isolation in childhood.
- Cluster headaches are a condition of adult life and can result in some of the most severe headaches known. They can be very resistant to treatment, but are not usually seen in children.
- Headaches due to arthritic changes in the neck, often chronic disabling headaches, generally relate to long-standing degenerative processes and are not common in children.

## Investigations

Childhood headaches are frequently over-investigated. In general, blood investigations have little yield. Plain radiography of the skull may demonstrate signs of chronically raised pressure, or sinusitis, but is of little use in most situations.

CT can demonstrate hydrocephalus, other fluid collections and tumours, although it is not ideal for visualization of the middle or posterior fossae, and is associated with significant radiation exposure and risk of subsequent malignancy. MRI is more likely to detect tumours and masses, particularly in the middle and posterior fossae. Magnetic resonance arteriography (MRA) or venography (MRV) is quite sensitive for detecting vascular abnormalities and is relatively non-invasive. Lumbar puncture is the diagnostic test for idiopathic intracranial hypertension.

Electroencephalography (EEG) is sometimes useful in situations where headaches coexist with clinical seizures, or in the situation described above where there is an association with significant visual aura and vomiting, but is otherwise not often useful.

Specialist consultation is frequently more rewarding and less expensive then laboratory investigation.

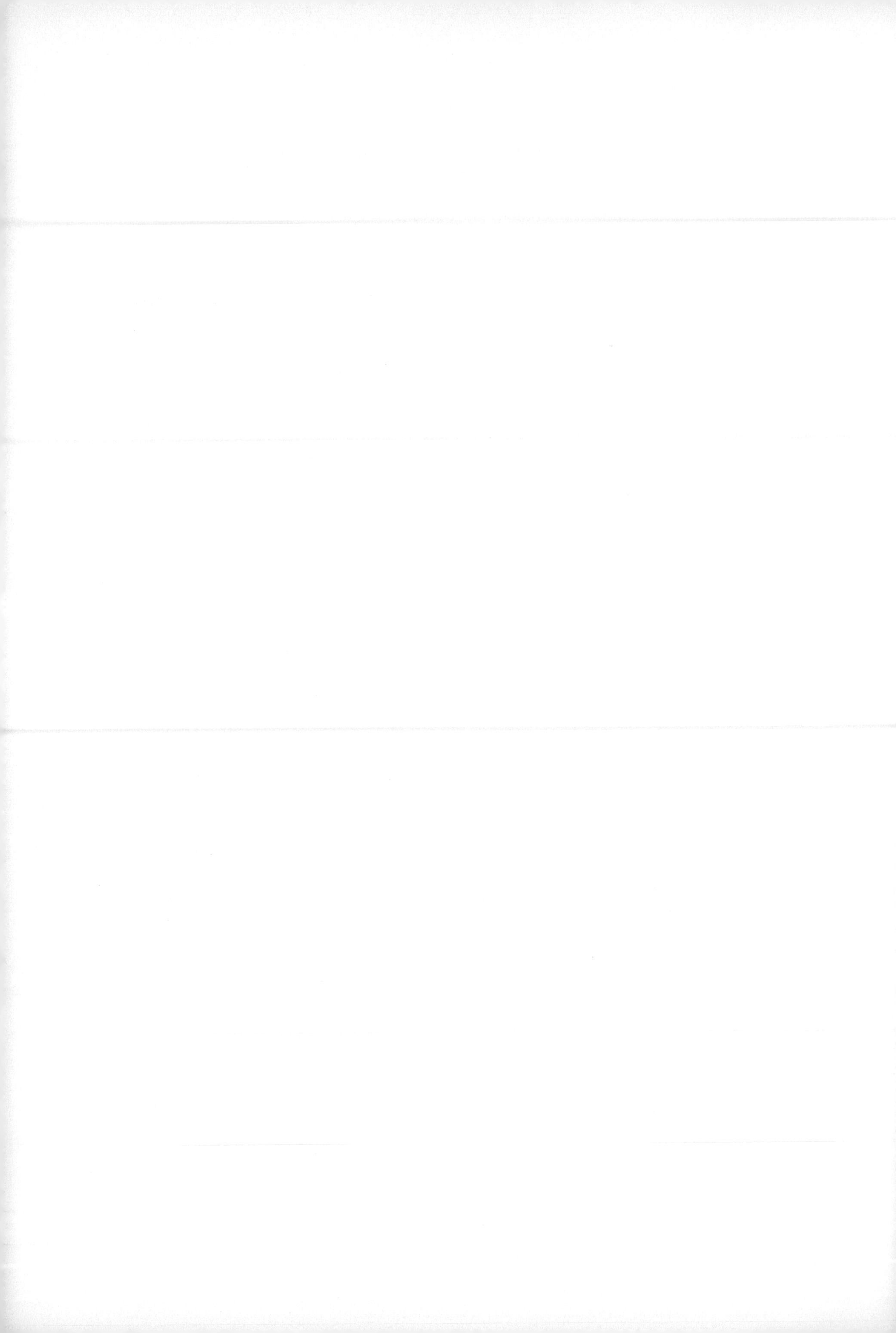

# PART 18

# URINARY TRACT DISORDERS AND HYPERTENSION

# 18.1 Urinary tract infections and malformations

Colin Jones, Joshua Kausman

## Urinary tract infections

Urinary tract infection (UTI) is the second most common bacterial infection affecting children. UTI can cause septicaemia or chronic ill-health with failure to thrive, and is often an indication of an underlying urinary tract malformation.

### Epidemiology

Epidemiological studies have shown that 2% of boys and 8% of girls have had a UTI by the age of 7 years; 75% of UTIs occur under the age of 1 year in males and 50% under the age of 1 year in females. The prevalence of UTI in febrile infants under the age of 3 months presenting to emergency departments is 20–30%, and boys outnumber girls. After the age of 3 months, the prevalence of UTI in febrile children falls to around 8% in female and 2% in male children. The incidence of UTI in uncircumcised boys is 4–10 times that in circumcised boys in the first 3 months of life. Common clinical patterns of UTI are described in Table 18.1.1.

### Diagnosis

The frequency of symptoms of UTI in a recent series of 304 children less than 5 years of age presenting to a Sydney hospital emergency department is listed in Table 18.1.2. The presentation varies with age because of the developmental status of the child. Although a wide range of symptoms can occur, an infant will probably have an acute illness with fever and vomiting or a chronic illness with failure to thrive, reflecting the systemic response to infection at this age. The preschool child, who has usually achieved continence, will often show wetting or frequency, complain of generalized abdominal pain and sometimes indicate dysuria. The teenage girl will usually present with symptoms of cystitis (fever, frequency, dysuria, strangury and accurately localized pain) or pyelonephritis (fever, often with rigor, and loin pain and tenderness). At any age, symptoms of fever, vomiting and systemic unwellness occur with pyelonephritis.

#### Urinalysis and microscopy

Microscopy for bacteria with Gram stain has the highest accuracy for rapid detection of UTI (sensitivity 91%, specificity 96%) but requires laboratory facilities. The finding of a positive urinary dipstick test for leukocyte esterase is sensitive for urinary infection (approximately 80% of urine infections detected) and urinary nitrite testing is specific (97% of positive tests indicate infection). Taking the prevalence rates for urine infection at different ages (see Epidemiology) into account, positive tests for both nitrites and leukocyte esterase in a child under 3 months of age predicts a 90% chance of a urine infection. Negative rapid test results are found in 10% of infants with infection. This is not good enough to use negative tests to exclude urinary infection for clinical purposes, because the diagnosis would be missed in a significant number of ill infants. In a child aged 3 years or more or in a circumcised male, the prevalence of urine infection is much lower and the finding of negative tests (leukocyte esterase and nitrites) is reassuring as there is then only a 1% chance of urine infection. Thus, negative test results are quite useful in this older age group in excluding urinary infection and at least justifying withholding antibiotic treatment until the results of urine culture are available.

Microscopy will usually reveal leukocytes and non-glomerular red cells (red cells that appear normally haemoglobinized and of uniform size and shape under phase-contrast microscopy) in freshly examined urine. The presence or absence of bacteria on microscopy can be unreliable: the presence of bacteria on microscopy of a fresh, well collected specimen (e.g. by suprapubic aspiration of urine) can be sensitive and specific for UTI, particularly if the white cell count is high (more than 10 white cells/μl). The finding of epithelial squamous cells indicates a poorly collected sample, and the absence of leukocyturia in a sample with mixed growth or low colony count on culture may indicate a contaminated sample.

Urinary nitrite tests are frequently used to monitor the urine of children prone to recurrent UTI (e.g. continent children with vesicoureteric reflux). Nitrite testing of early morning urine on a weekly basis has been reported to detect UTI in asymptomatic children, enabling treatment to be initiated earlier than would otherwise occur.

**Table 18.1.1 Common clinical patterns of urinary tract infection**

| | Infant | Toddler and young child | Adolescent |
|---|---|---|---|
| Presentation | Males more common than for females, especially under 3 months<br>High fever<br>Systemically unwell<br>Commonly recurs | Common for females, uncommon for males<br>Mild fever, wetting, dysuria and smelly urine<br>Frequent recurrences | Common for females, rare for males<br>Pyelonephritis or cystitis |
| Precipitating factors | *Males*: High-grade VUR (often associated with significant congenital renal malformation), physiological phimosis<br>*Females*: Low-grade VUR, usually associated with no or minor renal malformation<br>*Both*: Immature voiding pattern with high voiding pressure and detrusor hyperactivity | Low-grade VUR – ?associated with development of acquired renal injury<br>Dysfunctional elimination symptoms<br>Detrusor dyssynergia<br>Infrequent voiding<br>Constipation<br>Vulvovaginitis | Often history of VUR<br>Sexual activity<br>Vulvovaginitis |
| Prevention of recurrence | Prophylactic antibiotic | Treatment of precipitating factors identified | Counselling<br>Adjustment of sexual habit (void post-intercourse, antibiotic at time of sexual activity) |

VUR, vesicoureteric reflux.

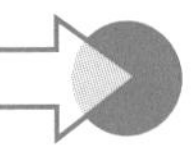

**Practical points**

**Dipstick testing**

- Positive leukocyte esterase is a reasonably sensitive test but is not at all specific for urinary tract infection (UTI).
- Positive nitrites are less sensitive but quite specific for UTI.
- Negative testing for leukocyte esterase and nitrites does not exclude UTI, especially in babies. Some 10% of babies with UTI will have negative dipstick testing.
- Always send urine for culture if UTI is suspected.
- Negative dipstick testing may reasonably be used in making the decision to withhold antibiotics from children over 3 years of age while awaiting urine culture results.

### Urine culture

Urine culture is the 'gold standard' for diagnosis, but management decisions often have to be made before the results are available.

The five common forms of urine collection are compared in Table 18.1.3.

*Microbiology*

*Escherichia coli* accounts for 80–90% of pathogens isolated. *Proteus* species are the cause of infection in 30% of boys over 1 year of age. Coagulase-negative *Staphylococcus* species are common in teenagers and *Klebsiella* is frequent in the neonatal period. *Pseudomonas* species are frequently isolated in children with more complicated anatomical malformations and in those who have had surgical procedures, especially where foreign materials (e.g. urinary stents) have been left *in situ*. Enterococci cause around 5% of UTIs and are the most common organism found that is resistant to gentamicin. Approximately 5% of children have two organisms isolated. Viral causes of infection have been thought to be rare in children who were not immunosuppressed, but recent urinary polymerase chain reaction (PCR) testing for adenovirus has shown a number of children with classical symptoms and often macroscopic haematuria have this cause.

## Initial treatment

Once the urine culture has been obtained, a decision on acute treatment must be made. Intravenous therapy is required if: the child is systemically unwell (dehydrated, signs of septic shock such as hypotension, tachycardia and decreased conscious state); vomiting and unable to retain oral medications; and in infants under the age of 6 months generally, because oral absorption is unreliable. In the child in whom an infection is likely on the basis of urinalysis and presentation, and the child is reasonably well (generally older and not vomiting), oral antibiotics may be commenced, with review once the culture is through in 24–48 hours. In the child in whom urinary infection is a possibility and the child is not unwell, culture results should be awaited before starting treatment.

**Table 18.1.2 Frequency of symptoms in children under 5 years with symptomatic urinary tract infections**

| Symptom | % |
|---|---|
| History of fever | 79.6 |
| Axillary temperature >37.5 °C | 59.5 |
| Irritability | 52.3 |
| Anorexia | 48.7 |
| Malaise/lethargy | 44.4 |
| Vomiting | 41.8 |
| Diarrhoea | 20.7 |
| Dysuria | 14.8 |
| Offensive urine | 13.2 |
| Abdominal pain | 13.2 |
| Family member with past history of UTI* | 11.2 |
| Previous unexplained febrile episodes | 10.5 |
| Frequency | 9.5 |
| Urinary incontinence† | 6.6 |
| Macroscopic haematuria | 6.6 |
| Febrile convulsion | 4.6 |

*First-degree relative.
†Defined as a noticeable increase in the frequency of daytime wetting.
UTI, urinary tract infection.
Source: Craig JC, Irwig LM, Knight JF et al 1998 J Paediatr Child Health 34:154–159.

The intravenous antibiotics and oral antibiotics used acutely are listed in Table 18.1.4. Intravenous antibiotics are usually ceased within 2–3 days once culture results have been obtained and the child has improved clinically. Acute treatment is completed with oral antibiotics, usually of 5 days' duration.

## Prophylactic antibiotics

After acute treatment the child may be placed on prophylactic antibiotics given once each night. The antibiotics usually used for prophylaxis are listed in Table 18.1.4. These antibiotics are excreted in the urine, achieve high urinary concentrations and are well tolerated over long periods of time without inducing excessive microbiological changes in the gut (leading to the emergence of resistant organisms or candidiasis). They are usually given until the results of imaging tests are available. Long-term antibiotic prophylaxis to reduce the risk of further UTI is an area of medical controversy: systematic review of higher quality studies has shown that about 16 children need to be treated with prophylactic antibiotics to prevent one UTI.

## Investigations

The investigation necessary after a first UTI is an area of medical controversy. After several decades where the trend was to perform several detailed investigations, many centres are now more conservative and reserve more invasive investigations, and those involving irradiation, for special situations.

Investigations are aimed at excluding obstructive urinary tract lesions and determining whether there are significant underlying urinary tract malformations. Nearly all centres perform renal ultrasonography. This enables the presence, site, size and shape of the kidneys to be determined. In the age group under 5 years, only 15% of abnormalities found on dimercaptosuccinic acid (DMSA) scan ('scars/dysplasia') will be seen on ultrasound examination. The ureters are not visualized unless enlarged. The finding of hydronephrosis or hydroureter leads to further nuclear medical imaging (discussed below) to diagnose obstructive lesions of the urinary tract. An idea of bladder function can be determined by measuring the post-void residual volume (normally less than 20 mL in children under 7 years).

Radiological examination of the urethra and bladder by means of micturating cystourethrography (MCU) is performed in some centres as a routine on infants (less than 1 year of age) and selectively at older ages where visualization of the bladder surface and urethra is required. This investigation is performed less frequently than in the past because the demonstration of vesicoureteric reflux (VUR; see below) does not alter management at many centres. The patient and parental acceptability of the test is poor and against the ethos of 'pain- and anxiety-free' paediatric procedures. The authors generally have MCU performed under general anaesthesia in children older than 6 months.

Nuclear medicine investigations with technetium-99m-labelled radioisotopes are useful for a number of purposes. These investigations carry radiation toxicity of less than one-tenth of a routine chest X-ray.

The diethylenetriamine penta-acetic acid (DTPA) radionuclide is injected intravenously, is filtered by the glomerulus and then is neither secreted nor absorbed by the tubule of the kidney. Like creatinine or insulin, it can be used to obtain an accurate measure of the glomerular filtration rate.

**Table 18.1.3 Comparison of methods of urine collection**

| Urine collection method | Advantages | Disadvantages | Recommended use |
|---|---|---|---|
| Paediatric bag | Widespread use in primary care paediatrics<br>Considered convenient<br>Avoids invasive procedure | Contamination with skin flora common so that only results of $<10^8$ cfu/L (excluding infection) are useful | Collection of urine from infant or toddler at low risk for UTI (not febrile and no known urological abnormality) for urinalysis: if positive for leukocytes or nitrites, another urine collection method should be used for culture<br>Should not be used where immediate antibiotic treatment is required |
| Clean catch | Non-invasive<br>Good correlation with SPA/MSU/CSU results | Perceived to be difficult to collect (majority can be collected within 1 h) | Method of choice in infants and toddlers<br>$>10^8$ cfu/L indicates infection, although presence of squamous epithelia and lack of pyuria indicates contamination |
| Midstream urine collection (MSU) | Non-invasive<br>Widespread patient acceptance | Poor technique (failure to withdraw foreskin or wash labia) results in contamination<br>Difficult with phimosis or for obese females | Method of choice in toilet-trained child<br>$>10^8$ cfu/L indicates infection, although presence of squamous epithelia and lack of pyuria indicates contamination |
| Catheter sample (CSU) | Usually results in collection of sample of urine; reasonable for diagnosis especially if first drops of urine discarded | Invasive – poor acceptance by parents and can establish fear in child of future clinic visits<br>Difficult with phimosis | Second choice to SPA in infants and toddlers with high risk of UTI (febrile and proven urological abnormalities) where treatment is required before culture available<br>$>10^3$ cfu/L may indicate infection, although presence of squamous epithelia and lack of pyuria indicates contamination |
| Suprapubic aspirate of urine (SPA) | 'Gold standard' as avoids contamination<br>Less invasive than CSU collection | 'Dry tap' relatively common (ultrasound confirmation of full bladder can minimize this) | Method of choice in infants and toddlers at high risk of UTI<br>Useful in obese females with recurrent contaminated MSUs<br>Any growth significant |

cfu, colony-forming unit on bacterial culture; UTI, urinary tract infection.

**Table 18.1.4 Antibiotic treatment of urinary tract infection**

| Antibiotic | Dose | Organisms sensitive* (%) |
|---|---|---|
| **Acute** | | |
| *Intravenous* | | |
| (sick, <6 months old, pyelonephritis) | | |
| 1. Benzyl penicillin | 50 mg/kg (max. dose 2 g) 6 hourly | Covers *Enterococcus* |
| and | | |
| 2. Gentamicin | 7.5 mg/kg daily for age <10 years, 6 mg/kg daily for age >10 years (max. dose 360 mg)<br>Monitoring: trough level <1 mg/L taken on 3rd day and serum creatinine 3rd day | ≥95 |
| *Oral* | | |
| Trimethoprim | 4 mg/kg (max. dose 150 mg) 12 hourly | ≥85 |
| or | | |
| Co-trimoxazole | (40 mg/200 mg per 5 mL)<br>0.5 mL/kg (max. dose 20 mL) 12 hourly | ≥85 |
| or | | |
| Cefalexin | 15 mg/kg (max. dose 500 mg) 8 hourly | 95 |
| or | | |
| Augmentin† | 10–25 mg/kg 8 hourly | 95 |
| **Prophylactic** | | |
| Co-trimoxazole | (40 mg/200 mg per 5 mL)<br>0.25 mL/kg nightly | ≥85 |
| Nitrofurantoin | 1–2 mg/kg nightly | ≥85 |
| Cefalexin‡ | 5 mg/kg nightly | ≥95 |

*Percentage of bacteria causing urinary tract infection diagnosed in the emergency department of major Australian hospitals that are sensitive to antibiotics.

†Amoxicillin alone only covers 60% of organisms encountered, so Augmentin is preferred.

‡The suspension forms of the cephalosporins and penicillins lose activity after a few weeks.

The mercapto-acetyl-triglycine (MAG3) scan has largely replaced the DTPA scan because, in addition to some glomerular filtration, the isotope is secreted mainly by the proximal tubular cells into the urine so that the signal to background ratio is higher than in the DTPA scan. This is particularly useful in children with renal impairment or infants in the first 3 months of life when the glomerular filtration rate is low. Both of these investigations are useful for diagnosing the presence of obstruction to urinary flow from the kidneys to the bladder, for determining the 'split' of kidney function (between the right and left kidneys), and for estimating overall renal function.

The DMSA radionuclide is filtered by the glomerulus and taken up by the proximal tubular cells. Scanning takes place when it has been taken up by these cells, which are in the renal cortex. Lack of uptake gives a defect on the scan and this can be due to either transient impairment of the tubular cell function (e.g. following acute inflammation with pyelonephritis for a period of up to 3–4 months) or absence of kidney tissue (renal 'scarring/dysplasia').

Delayed uptake of any of these three radionuclides may occur in conditions where perfusion to the kidney is abnormal (e.g. renal artery stenosis in a unilateral case or dehydration in a bilateral case).

The ongoing management depends on the results of investigations. A flow diagram of possibilities is shown in Figure 18.1.1.

## Urinary tract infection and normal renal ultrasound findings

If the child responds to antibiotics, there is no need to perform another urine culture at the end of treatment. In the case of an infant, some would continue prophylactic antibiotics for 6–12 months. In the case of an older child with recurrent infections and normal baseline investigations, ultrasonography would be repeated and an examination for precipitating factors (see Table 18.1.1) such as constipation or a functional voiding disorder (daytime wetting) would be undertaken. Sexual activity should be considered in teenagers.

UTI

Ultrasound

Dilation of urinary tract
Hydronephrosis
Hydroureter

Small kidney (s)
or
Renal Injury

Normal

MAG 3 scan

Assess renal function – blood pressure, protein excretion, estimate GFR

+/- MCU *

Obstruction

No obstruction

Long term medical/renal follow up

Urology referral for possible cystoscopy, retrograde pyelogram and corrective surgery

MCU
or
Repeat US *

Manage urinary infections
+/- prophylactic antibiotics
+/- treat precipitating causes

DMSA scan 1- 2 years after last UTI

Renal Injury

Normal

Follow up for hypertension

Discharge

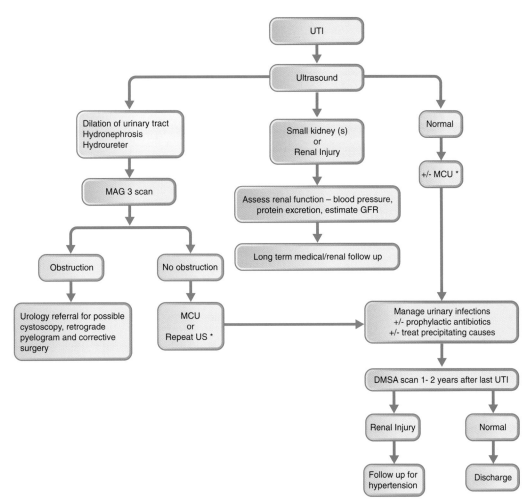

* Some centers will perform an MCU to diagnose vesicoureteric reflux but in other centers the test is not routinely performed. Until the last decade MCU was routine in children with UTI under the age of 1-2 years.

Bladder studies (urodynamic assessment of bladder volume and pressure, uroflow studies of micturition and post voiding residual volume) should be considered in all children with recurrent infection

Fig. 18.1.1 Flow diagram of ongoing management following a proven urinary tract infection (UTI). A normal ultrasound result does not exclude scarring. This age is chosen for convenience. Boys uncommonly have recurrent infections after 1 year; girls commonly have recurrent infection until about 3 years. Follow up includes a yearly blood pressure check. A normal dimercaptosuccinic acid (DMSA) scan result normalizes the risk of developing hypertension. MCU, micturating cystourethrography; MSU, midstream urine collection; US, ultrasonography; VUR, vesicoureteric reflux.

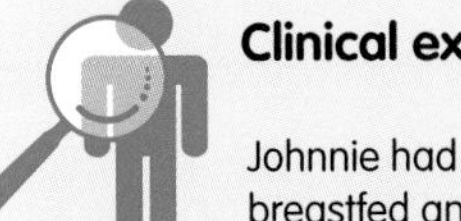

## Clinical example

Johnnie had a birth weight of 3.3 kg. He was breastfed and weighed 5.1kg at 2 months of age. For the next month he put on no weight and his mother noted that he was irritable, fed poorly and had the occasional vomit. The family doctor took a bag sample of urine and found more than $10^8$/L colony-forming units of an organism growing on culture the next day. The doctor arranged for a suprapubic aspirate of urine to be performed at the emergency department. This was done after a bladder scan showed a moderately full bladder. Johnnie was admitted to hospital and received treatment with gentamicin and penicillin given intravenously for 48 hours before an *E. coli* sensitive to co-trimoxazole was identified. He was discharged to complete 3 days of oral co-trimoxazole therapy and then to commence night-time co-trimoxazole prophylactic antibiotic treatment. MCU and renal ultrasonography were performed in the next few days.

The ultrasound scan showed bilateral hydronephrosis and hydroureter. MCU showed a mildly trabeculated bladder with bilateral vesicoureteric reflux; the urethra was abnormal in appearance with dilatation of the posterior urethra, suggesting a diagnosis of posterior urethral valves (Fig. 18.1.2). Prophylactic antibiotic treatment was continued and Johnnie was referred to both a paediatric urologist (for cystoscopy and evaluation of the urethra and bladder) and a nephrologist (for renal function assessment).

### Clinical example

Amy, a 14-year-old girl, presented to her local doctor on three occasions over 6 months with culture-proven UTIs. There was no family history of urinary infections, Amy had never had a UTI before, and there was no evidence of a wetting disorder. Further history revealed the onset of sexual activity at about the same time as the UTIs started.

Amy was counselled regarding contraception and sexually transmitted diseases, and she and her parents were offered counselling regarding her sexual activity. She was advised to have a 300-mL glass of water with a citravescent sachet immediately before or just after sexual intercourse. However, 1 month later Amy re-presented with another UTI. She was then advised to take nitrofurantoin (100-mg capsule) immediately after sexual intercourse. She was seen for review 3 and 6 months after this treatment, reported no further symptoms and remained compliant with the treatment. Because she was frequently changing sexual partners, Amy was advised to continue on the treatment.

### Asymptomatic infection

Up to 4% of adolescent girls have asymptomatic bacteriuria. A number of these children will have vesicoureteric reflux or reflux-associated nephropathy (see below). There is no evidence that treatment of asymptomatic bacteriuria is beneficial, and colonization frequently recurs after treatment, sometimes precipitating symptomatic infection caused by a more pathogenic organism.

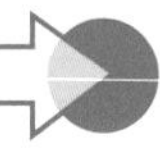

### Practical points

**Management of urinary tract infection in infancy**
- Suspect in a febrile infant with vomiting or failure to thrive
- Urine sample:
  - Acutely unwell: suprapubic aspiration (SPA), or catheter-specimen urine (CSU)
  - Not unwell: clean catch
- Unwell: commence treatment with intravenous gentamicin and intravenous penicillin initially, changing to oral antibiotic to finish course when improved
- Prophylactic antibiotic until renal ultrasound findings evaluated
- Long-term follow-up essential unless DMSA scan results normal

**Management of recurrent urinary tract infection in childhood**
- Characterize symptoms as pyelonephritis or cystitis
- Identify precipitating factors: wetting, vulvovaginitis, phimosis or balanitis, constipation
- Bladder abnormality
- Individualize therapy to minimize development of symptomatic urinary infection
- Longer-term follow-up essential unless DMSA result normal

## Abnormalities of the urinary tract

### Vesicoureteric reflux

This is a disorder in which urine passes in a retrograde direction from the bladder through the vesicoureteric junction into the ureter. It is a common disorder, affecting 40% of children under 1 year of age who are investigated for a first UTI. The diagnosis is made by MCU or by an indirect MCU done without urinary catheterization.

VUR is a familial trait affecting between 30% and 50% of first-degree relatives of index cases. This developmental abnormality is characterized by the distal end of the ureter running less obliquely through the wall of the bladder and having less muscle around it. In some cases, it is associated with renal malformation (variously referred to as renal scarring, dysplasia, reflux-associated nephropathy), excessive dilatation and tortuosity of the ureter, occurrence on the contralateral side, and abnormalities of bladder function including premature detrusor contractions (causing urgency symptoms and wetting) and poor bladder emptying. Higher grades of VUR are associated with higher recurrence rates of UTI.

The treatment of VUR has been controversial. Controlled trials (Box 18.1.1) have shown no advantage of either anti-reflux surgery or antibiotic prophylaxis in preventing urinary infections, hypertension, renal injury or renal failure. In fact, it is not clear whether these treatments are better than no treatment or episodic treatment of urinary infection alone. Much of the renal injury leading to renal failure in a small number of patients with VUR is congenital and the significance of acquired injury is debated. Thus, the aim of treatment of VUR is prevention of symptomatic UTI,

**Box 18.1.1 Management of vesicoureteric reflux (VUR): evidence and controversies**

Evidence-based analysis of surgical versus antibiotic treatment of VUR shows:
- No difference in overall rate of urinary tract infection (but reduced rate of pyelonephritis with surgery)
- No difference in occurrence of 'new scarring' or extension of 'old scarring'
- No difference in incidence of renal failure
- No difference in incidence of hypertension

Continuing controversies:
- Whether VUR surgery or antibiotics make any difference to development of acquired renal injury
- The frequency of acquired or congenital renal injury as a cause of reflux nephropathy
- The effectiveness of prophylactic antibiotic therapy
- The significance of smaller renal scars

not prevention of renal injury. Attention to reducing and treating precipitating factors for UTI, the use of antibiotic treatment in a prophylactic or episodic manner, and the selective use of anti-reflux surgery for patients with intractable symptoms form the basis of treatment.

VUR often resolves spontaneously (of a cohort of children with reflux, 20% will have resolution occurring spontaneously each 3-year period, with less severe degrees of reflux resolving earlier than more severe degrees). Resolution of reflux is often not associated with resolution of urinary infection, which can be expected to occur periodically throughout life in affected females, particularly with sexual activity and pregnancy.

## Reflux-associated nephropathy

Once thought to be due to the combination of VUR and infection, this abnormality of the kidney is most often congenital in origin. It is found in approximately 10% of children with VUR. The importance of this lesion lies in the possibility of development of hypertension, which is rare in early childhood but occurs in up to 15% of cases by the age of 20 years. Bilateral extensive reflux-associated nephropathy is a cause of renal failure occurring from mid childhood.

## Posterior urethral valves

This abnormality is also referred to as congenital obstructive posterior urethral membranes (COPUMs). It affects males and causes obstruction to urine flow at the level of the posterior urethra. The bladder is often thick-walled and trabeculated; there may be associated VUR with tortuous and dilated ureters draining grossly hydronephrotic kidneys. Antenatal ultrasonography demonstrating hydronephrosis and megacystis is a common presentation, as is urinary infection in early infancy, but some children present later with dribbling and wetting.

Diagnosis is made on the urethrogram phase of the MCU (see Fig. 18.1.2), and confirmation is obtained by cystoscopy. Treatment involves complex surgical procedures performed in the setting of a team approach to the patient, involving medical staff and continence physiotherapists. Preparation for end-stage renal failure treatment is often necessary.

## Bladder abnormalities

Bladder malfunction is strongly associated with UTIs and often overlooked in clinical management. Table 18.1.5 describes common bladder abnormalities and their management.

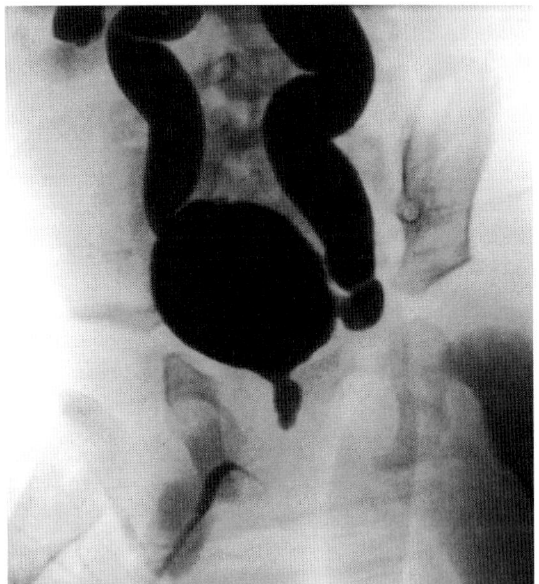


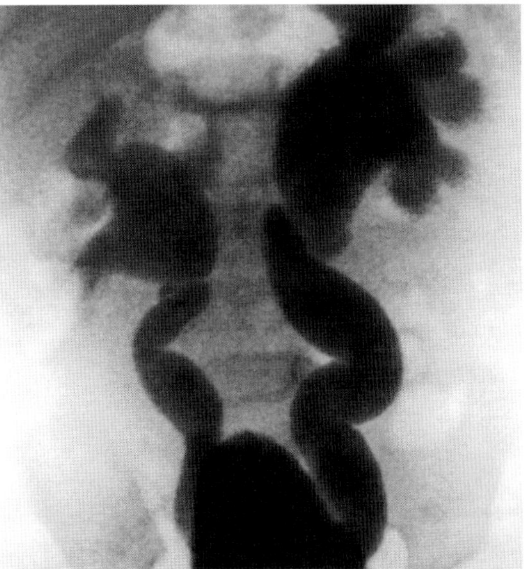


Fig. 18.1.2 **(A)** Micturating cystourethrogram (from the Clinical example) showing a dilated posterior urethra, mildly irregular appearance of the edge of the bladder ('trabeculation') and bilateral vesicoureteric reflux into dilated tortuous ureters. **(B)** Hydronephrosis with 'clubbing' of the calyces.

## Duplication

A kidney is said to be duplex if two separate collecting systems are identified. The ureters may join before entry into the bladder, or they may have separate openings into the bladder. The upper pole ureter enters the urinary tract more distal to the lower pole ureter and may enter the urethra, giving rise to incontinence, or may be obstructed at its lower end (ureterocele), in which case the upper pole of the kidney will be abnormal. The lower pole ureter often has vesicoureteric reflux.

**Table 18.1.5 Common bladder abnormalities**

| Bladder abnormality causes | Urodynamic assessment | Symptoms | Treatment |
|---|---|---|---|
| Small bladder<br>Primary<br>Posterior urethral valves<br>Bladder exstrophy<br>Neurogenic | Low volume<br>High pressure | Day and night wetting<br>UTI<br>Hydroureter | Frequent voiding<br>Bladder augmentation |
| Large bladder<br>Primary<br>Neurogenic<br>Vesicoureteric reflux | Large volume<br>Low pressure<br>High residual volume | Infrequent voiding<br>UTI<br>Wetting | Frequent voiding<br>Drainage by vesicostomy, CIC or catheterizable conduits |
| Detrusor dyssynergia syndrome<br>Primary<br>Vesicoureteric reflux | Premature detrusor contractions | Urge symptoms<br>Wetting<br>UTI | Anticholinergic drugs<br>Frequent voiding<br>Usually resolves |
| Neurogenic<br>Cord injury*<br>'Non-neurogenic'† | All of the above found | Wetting with 'overflow'<br>UTI<br>Obstructive nephropathy | Bladder drainage by vesicostomy, CIC or catheterizable conduit<br>Bladder augmentation |

*Cord injury may be clinically apparent (spina bifida) or determined by ultrasonography in a neonate when the cord can be imaged, or by MRI at later ages.

†Non-neurogenic neurogenic bladder is a term used for the clinical and investigational features of a neurogenic bladder in a child who does not have demonstrable spinal pathology.

CIC, clean intermittent catheterization; UTI, urinary tract infection.

### Other causes of urinary obstruction

#### Pelviureteric junction (PUJ) obstruction

This is now most commonly diagnosed following the evaluation of hydronephrosis detected on antenatal scanning of the fetus. At least 9 out of 10 such cases will resolve spontaneously over the first year of life. Periodic renal ultrasound observation, sometimes supplemented by diuretic renography using DPTA or MAG3 radioisotopes, is used to follow these infants. Pelviureteric junction obstruction may present in later childhood with renal colic and these patients usually require surgery.

*Vesicoureteric junction (VUJ) obstruction*

This often presents following investigation of UTI, with the ultrasonography showing a dilated ureter and MAG3 scan showing delayed passage of urine from the ureter to the bladder with a widened ureteric image. Treatment is stenting of the VUJ or reimplantation of the ureter.

*Renal calculi*

These may present following UTI, in which case the calculus is usually a triple phosphate (magnesium, calcium and ammonium) stone and the infecting organisms often urea-splitting (such as *Proteus mirabilis*), or renal colic. Other stones occasionally encountered are composed of cystine (autosomal recessive cystinuria), calcium oxalate and, uncommonly, uric acid.

*Antenatal renal abnormalities*

The advent of almost routine antenatal scanning at 18 weeks' gestation has led to the detection of approximately 1 in 200 infants having an increased renal pelvis diameter (>4 mm at 18 weeks). The postnatal diagnoses are shown in Table 18.1.6.

#### Management

Antenatal ultrasound imaging should be repeated in the third trimester of pregnancy. The presence of bilateral severe hydronephrosis with an enlarged bladder in the male infant suggests the diagnosis of posterior urethral valves. The presence of oligohydramnios suggests reduced urine output, and this is associated with the development of pulmonary hypoplasia and a higher risk of renal failure.

After birth, the infant should be placed on prophylactic trimethoprim until the diagnosis is determined. If

| Table 18.1.6 Antenatal renal abnormalities: postnatal diagnoses | |
|---|---|
| Diagnosis | % |
| Non-refluxing non-obstructive hydronephrosis | 55 |
| Vesicoureteric reflux | 15 |
| Pelviureteric junction obstruction | 5 |
| Multicystic kidney | 5 |
| Vesicoureteric junction abnormalities | 5 |
| Duplex | 5 |
| Agenesis | 5 |
| Posterior urethral valves | 2 |

the child is unwell or if significant severe abnormalities are suspected, imaging of the kidneys and urinary tract should be performed immediately. In contrast, if the baby is well and without severe urinary tract dilatation, postnatal ultrasound imaging is undertaken towards the end of the first week of life when the baby is well hydrated. Further investigations, usually looking for reflux or obstruction, are performed, depending upon the results of this ultrasound examination.

## Cystic renal disease

Common forms of cystic renal disease and the modes of presentation are listed in Table 18.1.7. Solitary cysts are uncommon in childhood and may be an indication of evolving polycystic kidney disease.

**Table 18.1.7 Forms and presentation of cystic renal disease**

| Cystic renal disease | Incidence | Genetics | Clinical features |
|---|---|---|---|
| Autosomal dominant polycystic kidney disease | 1–2 in 1000<br>M=F | Three gene defects cause it; 50% risk in subsequent children | Usually discovered because of family history<br>Uncommon cause of hypertension or loin/abdominal discomfort in childhood<br>Progresses to renal failure later in life |
| Autosomal recessive kidney disease | 1–2 in 10 000 births<br>M=F | One gene defect identified; 25% risk in subsequent pregnancies | Often present in infancy with enlarged hyperechogenic kidneys, oliguria, respiratory distress associated with pulmonary hypoplasia<br>Later may develop hypertension, renal impairment<br>Associated with hepatic fibrosis causing portal hypertension in mid-childhood |
| Cystic renal dysplasia | Common | Polygenic; low recurrence risk | Often asymptomatic<br>Associated with vesicoureteric reflux<br>May be bilateral |
| Multicystic dysplastic kidney | Relatively uncommon | Unknown; low recurrence risk | Enlarged, completely cystic non-functioning kidney without blood flow<br>Contralateral kidney usually normal but may be associated with vesicoureteric reflux or pelviureteric junction obstruction |

# 18.2 Glomerulonephritis, renal failure and hypertension

Steven McTaggart

## Haematuria

### Isolated microscopic haematuria

Asymptomatic isolated microscopic haematuria is common and can be detected on a single occasion in 0.5–2% of school-aged children. The majority of these children will not have significant kidney disease and, in the absence of symptoms or other abnormalities on urinalysis, further investigation is required only if haematuria is documented in at least three different specimens taken over a period of 2–3 weeks.

Persistent microscopic haematuria is usually benign, provided there is no infection or proteinuria, renal function is normal and no structural abnormality is present on ultrasonography. Possible diagnoses include idiopathic hypercalciuria, thin membrane disease or a mild proliferative glomerulonephritis such as immunoglobulin A (IgA) nephropathy (see below). A family history of microscopic haematuria is suggestive of thin basement membrane disease, which is often inherited in an autosomal dominant fashion.

### Glomerulonephritis

The clinical features of glomerulonephritis are:

- haematuria
- acute fluid overload – oedema, pulmonary oedema, congestive cardiac failure
- hypertension
- renal impairment – oliguria, raised plasma creatinine level.

Acute presentation with these clinical features is seen most commonly in post-streptococcal glomerulonephritis. Other forms of glomerulonephritis in childhood may have a less severe onset (Box 18.2.1). Most forms of glomerulonephritis result from an immunologically mediated injury involving either deposition of circulating immune complexes in the glomerulus or a specific antibody to the glomerular basement membrane.

#### Post-streptococcal glomerulonephritis

This disorder follows 7–14 days after group A β-haemolytic streptococcal throat infection and 3–6 weeks after streptococcal skin infection. It is hypothesized that streptococcal antigens deposit in glomeruli with activation of the complement system. The pathological appearance consists of proliferation of mesangial and endothelial cells with neutrophil infiltration (Fig. 18.2.1). Crescents may be present. Immunofluorescence shows IgG and C3, and electron-dense deposits (humps) are demonstrated by electron microscopy.

Clinically this disorder usually presents with macroscopic haematuria, acute fluid overload and hypertension in a school-aged child. Lassitude, fever and loin pain also may be present. Physical examination may reveal hypertension, papilloedema, facial and leg oedema. Serum urea, creatinine and potassium concentrations are often raised, and urinalysis shows red blood cell casts and dysmorphic red cells. Mild normocytic normochromic anaemia is common and is due to haemodilution from fluid overload. The anti-streptolysin O titre (ASOT) and anti-streptococcal DNase B are raised in 90% of cases. Activation of the classical complement pathway leads to low serum levels of C3, which generally returns to normal within 6–12 weeks.

The *major complications* of acute post-streptococcal glomerulonephritis are secondary to acute kidney injury resulting in salt and water retention. Fluid overload is responsible for hypertension and in severe cases can result in hypertensive encephalopathy or left ventricular failure. Fluid overload is best managed initially with furosemide 2–4 mg/kg daily, fluid restriction and a low-salt diet. More severe hypertension may be treated with oral nifedipine or prazosin. Bed rest is necessary only when the blood pressure is increased. A course of oral penicillin for 10 days eradicates any existing streptococcal infection, but does not alter the natural history of this condition.

The period of oliguria lasts for up to 10 days and dialysis is indicated in cases where the blood urea rises above 50–60 mmol/L, or when hyperkalaemia or pulmonary oedema is not controlled by diuretics and fluid restriction. The long-term prognosis is excellent, with only 1% developing chronic kidney disease. Microscopic haematuria may continue for up to 2 years, but proteinuria should clear within 6 months. Renal biopsy is not indicated unless there is uncertainty of diagnosis with the initial investigations or the period of oliguria lasts for longer than 3 weeks.

**Box 18.2.1 Causes of acute nephritis**

- Post-infectious glomerulonephritis
- Henoch–Schönlein purpura
- IgA nephropathy
- Lupus erythematosus
- Membranoproliferative glomerulonephritis
- Vasculitis

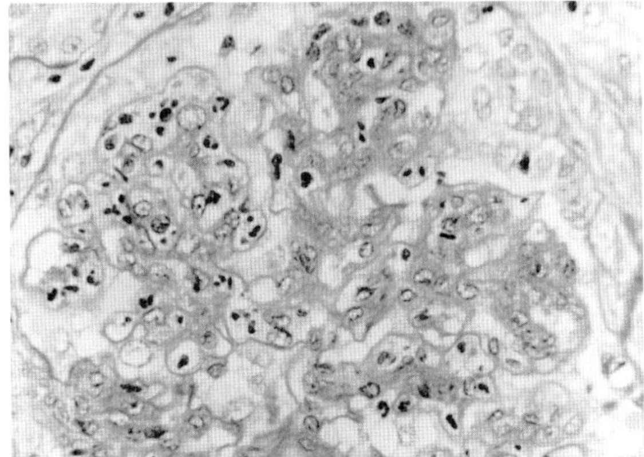

Fig. 18.2.1 Mesangial proliferation and neutrophil infiltration in post-streptococcal glomerulonephritis (periodic acid–Schiff stain, original magnification ×800).

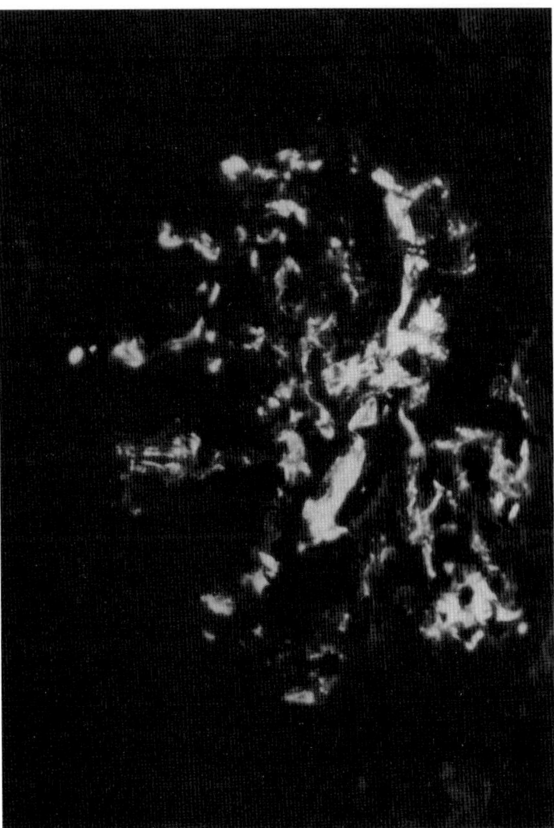

Fig. 18.2.2 Immunofluorescence shows mesangial IgA deposits (original magnification ×600).

Other infectious agents including viral and bacterial organisms rarely can produce an illness similar to post-streptococcal nephritis. These organisms include staphylococci and *Pneumococcus*, and Echo, Coxsackie and Epstein–Barr viruses.

## IgA nephropathy

This glomerulopathy is present in 50% of children who have recurrent episodes of macroscopic haematuria. The episodes of haematuria often occur simultaneously with intercurrent viral infections and may be associated with flank pain. Other presentations include abnormal urinalysis on medical examination and, rarely, an acute glomerulonephritis with renal failure. Renal biopsy shows a focal proliferative glomerulonephritis with IgA in the mesangium (Fig. 18.2.2). Although the prognosis for most children with IgA nephropathy is good, long-term studies show that about 10% progress to chronic renal failure by 15 years after onset of disease. Bad prognostic features include impaired renal function at presentation, heavy proteinuria and hypertension.

## Henoch–Schönlein purpura

This disease is a vasculitic illness involving predominantly small vessels in the skin, large joints and gastrointestinal tract (see Chapter 16.2). The illness is preceded by upper respiratory tract infection in 30–50% of patients. These children present with a petechial or purpuric rash that is localized over lower limbs and buttocks, abdominal pain and arthritis. A mild nephritis with microscopic haematuria and proteinuria is seen in 50–70% of cases. Rarely, blood pressure and serum creatinine levels are raised. Renal histology shows a proliferative glomerulonephritis with IgA in the mesangium. The prognosis is good, with less than 5% developing chronic kidney disease.

## Lupus erythematosus

Systemic lupus erythematosus (SLE) presents in childhood in 20% of cases and is more common in children from Asian countries. Facial rash, arthritis and fever are common presenting symptoms. Serum C3 complement is usually low and anti-nuclear antibodies can often be detected, especially to double-stranded DNA. Renal biopsy is indicated if haematuria and proteinuria are present. The type of glomerular disease in SLE can vary from a mild focal proliferative glomerulonephritis to a diffuse crescentic glomerulonephritis. The treatment is complex but generally involves various combinations of immunosuppressant medications such as prednisolone, azathioprine, cyclophosphamide or mycophenolate. The amount of immunosuppression is dependent on clinical severity of kidney disease and renal histology. This disorder is discussed further in Chapter 13.3.

### Alport syndrome

This is a familial disorder in production of type IV collagen and is inherited as an X-linked dominant (85% of cases), autosomal dominant or autosomal recessive condition. In males, this disorder presents in the first 10 years of life with microscopic or macroscopic haematuria and proteinuria, and is followed by onset of renal failure in the teenage years. High-tone nerve deafness and eye abnormalities are the other features of the syndrome.

## Proteinuria

### Isolated proteinuria

Transient proteinuria can be seen in many conditions including fever, exercise and seizures, and disappears when the condition resolves. Proteinuria that is detected in the standing position but not when recumbent is known as orthostatic or postural proteinuria; this occurs in 10% of children and is more common in adolescence. Testing with urinary dipsticks or urine protein : creatinine ratio shows negligible amounts of protein in first daytime void and increased protein excretion during the day. This phenomenon is benign but proteinuria in an overnight urine specimen will usually require biopsy to determine the cause.

### Nephrotic syndrome

Nephrotic syndrome is defined as:

- proteinuria (>40 mg per m² per h or protein/creatinine ratio >250 mg/mmol)
- hypoalbuminaemia (<25 mg/dL)
- oedema, and
- hyperlipidaemia.

The annual incidence in children is approximately 2–4 per 100 000. The major conditions associated with a primary nephrotic syndrome are listed in Box 18.2.2.

### Minimal change nephrotic syndrome

The majority of children present between the ages of 1 and 4 years with generalized oedema (Fig. 18.2.3). Renal biopsy is not initially indicated if clinical features suggest minimal change disease (Box 18.2.3).

Unless large pleural effusions, gross ascites or severe genital oedema are present, strict bed-rest is not necessary and the child should be allowed normal ward activity. A low-salt diet is encouraged. Fluid intake is generally not restricted because of the risk of hypovolaemia, but mild fluid restriction may be beneficial in some children with significant oedema. Prednisolone 2 mg/kg or 60 mg/m², daily, induces remission in 90% of cases. The prednisolone dose is then reduced over 6 months, with later doses being given on alternate days to reduce side-effects. If

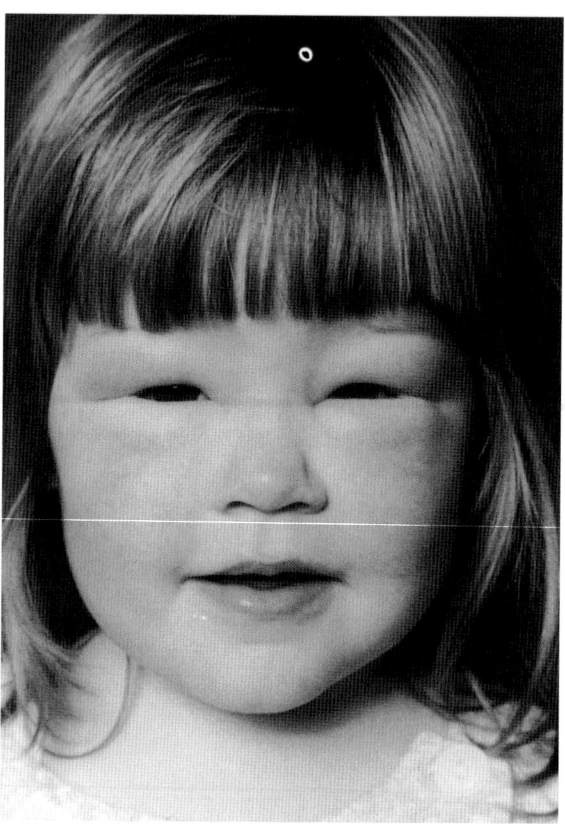

Fig. 18.2.3 Child with facial oedema due to the nephrotic syndrome.

**Box 18.2.2 Classification of primary nephrotic syndrome**

- Minimal change disease
- Focal segmental glomerulosclerosis
- Membranoproliferative glomerulonephritis
- Membranous glomerulopathy
- Congenital nephrotic syndrome

**Box 18.2.3 Clinical features of minimal change nephrotic syndrome**

- Age 1–10 years
- Blood pressure normal
- Renal function normal
- Microscopic haematuria 30%
- Complement levels normal

remission, as defined by complete loss of proteinuria, has not occurred by 4 weeks, the nephrotic syndrome is steroid-resistant and a renal biopsy is then indicated to exclude other pathology, particularly focal segmental glomerulosclerosis.

Approximately 70% of children have relapses, which are more likely to occur in association with viral upper respiratory tract infections. Frequent relapsers (four or more episodes per year) may be treated with regular prednisolone 5–15 mg, given on alternate days. Children with significant steroid side-effects require specialist assessment for consideration of alternative immunosuppressive regimens.

The *major complications* of the nephrotic syndrome are infections, hypovolaemia and thromboembolism. *Infections* such as peritonitis and septicaemia can be caused by both Gram-positive and Gram-negative organisms. The susceptibility to infections is related to loss of opsonins and immunoglobulins in the urine. If the patient develops a serious infection, the initial antibiotic treatment should cover both Gram-positive and Gram-negative organisms until cultures and sensitivity results are available. *Hypovolaemia* is due to loss of plasma water into the tissues with a consequent fall in the circulating blood volume. It occurs in 5% of cases and should be suspected if a child develops oliguria (<100 mL/day), poor peripheral perfusion, abdominal pain, tachycardia or postural hypotension. This complication is confirmed by a high haematocrit and a low urine sodium (<10 mmol/L). The preferred treatment is intravenous 20% albumin (1 g/kg over 3–6 h), which may need to be repeated, according to response. Intravenous furosemide (2 mg/kg) is given in the middle and at the end of the infusion to promote a diuresis.

*A hypercoagulable state* exists for a number of reasons. These include haemoconcentration and loss of antithrombin III in the urine. Renal vein thrombosis and pulmonary embolism are relatively rare occurrences that require prompt treatment with anticoagulants. The avoidance of bed-rest and the treatment of hypovolaemia may account for the decreasing incidence of these complications.

Approximately 90% of children with relapsing nephrotic syndrome cease relapsing by 16 years of age. Even those children who continue to relapse into adult life usually remain steroid-sensitive. It is very rare for a child with a steroid-sensitive minimal-change lesion nephrotic syndrome to progress to chronic kidney disease.

**Clinical example**

Sasha, a girl aged 5 years, presented with nephrotic syndrome at 2 years. At presentation serum albumin was less than 15 g/L, 24-hour urine protein 2.5 g/day and urine microscopy 30 red blood cells per mm$^3$. Blood pressure and complement were normal. Prednisolone 60 mg/m$^2$ per day induced remission in 10 days. In the next 2 years Sasha had six relapses with upper respiratory tract infections and was then managed with prophylactic prednisolone. In the last 6 months she had had two further relapses while still on maintenance prednisolone. She was now cushingoid and her height percentile had fallen from the 25th to below the 10th percentile. She commenced a 10-week course of cyclophosphamide (2.5 mg/kg daily).

Sasha had steroid-dependent nephrotic syndrome with significant steroid side-effects requiring a change in therapy.

## Focal segmental glomerulosclerosis

This glomerulopathy comprises 5–10% of children with nephrotic syndrome. The presentation is often similar to a minimal-change lesion but with steroid resistance. Renal biopsy (Fig. 18.2.4) shows segmental sclerosis or hyalinosis, whereas other glomeruli may be completely sclerosed. Immunofluorescence shows IgM and IgG in the affected segmental lesions. Mutations in podocin, a podocyte structural protein, are found in 10–30% of sporadic cases of steroid-resistant focal segmental glomerulosclerosis.

The majority of children with this lesion are resistant to immunosuppressive medications. Those children who remain nephrotic require treatment with diuretics (furosemide, spironolactone), mild fluid restriction and a low-salt diet. Approximately 60% progress to end-stage kidney disease over 10 years. This glomerulopathy has a 30% recurrence risk in a transplanted kidney, and in some cases plasmaphaeresis is beneficial.

## Congenital nephrotic syndrome

Congenital nephrotic syndrome (CNS) is defined as nephrotic syndrome occurring in the first 3 months of life. Nephrotic syndrome in this age group is often due to genetic causes, most commonly due to a mutation in the podocyte slit-diaphragm protein nephrin. This form

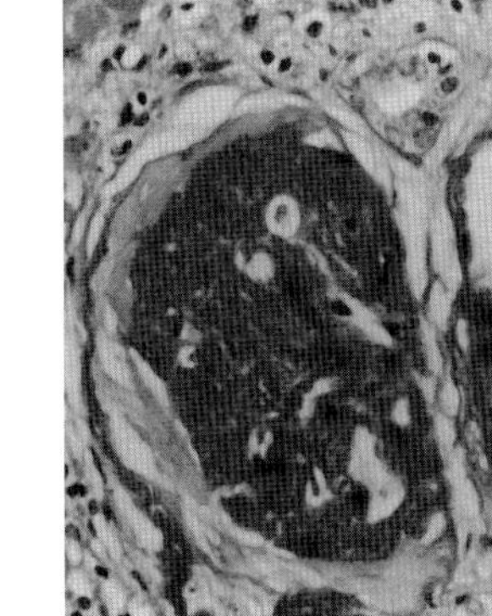

Fig. 18.2.4 Segmental and global sclerosis (periodic acid–Schiff stain, original magnification ×500).

of nephrotic syndrome is most common in Finland and is often referred to as congenital nephrotic syndrome of the Finnish type (CNF). Oedema is noted in the first weeks of life, with placentomegaly and prematurity being common precursors. There is no specific treatment and the natural history involves progression to end-stage kidney disease and transplantation. CNS with other histological patterns includes focal segmental glomerulosclerosis (often due to podocin mutations) and diffuse mesangial sclerosis, which may be part of a multisystem syndrome such as Denys–Drash syndrome. Nephrotic syndrome can also result from congenital infections such as syphilis and cytomegalovirus.

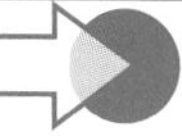

**Practical points**

**Glomerular disease**

- Microscopic haematuria without proteinuria is rarely associated with significant renal disease.
- Control of hypertension and fluid overload is the key to management of acute post-streptococcal glomerular nephritis.
- Non-postural proteinuria is an important diagnostic and prognostic finding and requires specialist assessment.
- Children with typical features of nephrotic syndrome that respond to prednisolone treatment do not require a renal biopsy.
- Children with frequently relapsing (2 relapses within 6 months of initial episode or ≥4 per year) or steroid-dependent (relapse on prednisolone) nephrotic syndrome require specialist referral.

## Acute kidney injury

The causes of acute kidney injury are listed in Table 18.2.1.

### Haemolytic–uraemic syndrome

Haemolytic–uraemic syndrome (HUS) is the most common cause of acute intrinsic kidney failure in childhood and is characterized by the triad of:

- microangiopathic haemolytic anaemia
- thrombocytopenia
- acute renal insufficiency.

It has been broadly classified into two groups: the typical or epidemic form, also known as diarrhoea-associated ($D^+$) HUS, and the atypical or sporadic form, diarrhoea-negative ($D^-$) HUS.

Diarrhoea-associated disease most commonly presents in children under the age of 3 years with bloody diarrhoea. Over the next few days, the child becomes pale, oliguric and unwell. Examination of the blood film shows fragmented red blood cells and thrombocytopenia. Urinalysis reveals haematuria and proteinuria. The serum creatinine level is usually raised and hypertension may be severe.

Pathogenesis is related to verocytotoxin production by *Escherichia coli*, usually serotype O157:H7, although other serotypes are also involved. The toxin crosses the damaged gut mucosa and adheres to endothelial cells in arterioles, with consequent swelling and widening of the subendothelial space with fibrin deposition. Management is supportive and dialysis is often necessary. Most children (90%) make a complete recovery. Bad prognostic signs are oliguria lasting for more than 2 weeks, cerebral involvement and age of onset over 5 years.

Non-diarrhoeal HUS ($D^-$) is associated with a variety of systemic disorders and may follow pneumococcal pneumonia. Recurrent HUS is often a recessively inherited disorder in regulation of the alternative pathway of complement activation.

## Chronic kidney disease

The incidence of chronic kidney disease in children is 2–4 per million total population per year. The commonest causes include:

- structural abnormalities of kidneys and renal tract (reflux nephropathy, obstructive uropathy)
- renal dysplasia/hypoplasia
- chronic glomerulonephritis.

The principles of management are as follows:

- Control of hypertension.

**Table 18.2.1 Causes of acute kidney injury**

| Pre-renal | Renal | Post-renal |
|---|---|---|
| Hypovolaemia<br>Gastroenteritis<br>Haemorrhage<br>Hypoalbuminaemia | Kidney disease<br>Glomerulonephritis<br>Haemolytic–uraemic syndrome<br>Interstitial nephritis | Posterior urethral valves<br>Neurogenic bladder<br>Ureterocele<br>Calculi |
| Peripheral vasodilatation<br>Sepsis | Myoglobinuria, haemoglobinuria<br>Nephrotoxic drugs | Tumours<br>Uric acid (tumour lysis syndrome) |
| Decreased cardiac output<br>Congestive cardiac failure | | |

- Adequate nutrition. Salt and fluid intake will vary with the type of renal disease but children with obstructive uropathy or renal dysplasia may require supplemental salt and water for adequate growth.
- Growth retardation may also be improved by growth hormone. Resistance to endogenous growth hormone is caused by low free insulin-like growth factor-1 levels.
- Prevention of renal osteodystrophy. Hyperphosphataemia should be treated vigorously with a low-phosphate diet and dietary phosphate binders in an attempt to prevent secondary hyperparathyroidism. Vitamin D supplementation with calcitriol (1,25-dihydroxycholecalciferol) is given in early renal failure to prevent rickets.
- Administration of alkali may be required to control acidosis (2–4 mmol/kg daily).
- Anaemia is corrected by erythropoietin. This is administered subcutaneously at intervals from weekly to monthly. Iron supplementation is necessary.

### Clinical example

Edward, aged 30 months, had chronic renal failure from birth from urethral valves and dysplastic kidneys. He had a poor appetite and required nasogastric feeding from 3 months. X-ray of the wrist at 18 months showed rickets requiring treatment with calcitriol. At 24 months he developed anaemia (haemoglobin 9.5 g/L) and commenced weekly subcutaneous darbepoietin-α. Edward had grown 2 cm in the last 12 months. Investigations showed a haemoglobin concentration of 11.3 g/L, serum sodium 136 mmol/L, potassium 4.5 mmol/L, urea 42 mmol/L, creatinine 650 μmol/L, calcium 2.4 mmol/L, phosphate 2.4 mmol/L, alkaline phosphatase 850 U/L. The parathyroid hormone level was increased.

Edward had now reached end-stage kidney disease and needed to commence peritoneal dialysis. Growth hormone was indicated for growth failure. He continued to take calcium carbonate at mealtimes in addition to calcitriol for renal osteodystrophy and erythropoietin for anaemia.

Dialysis and transplantation are now standard for young children with end-stage renal failure. Young children tolerate peritoneal dialysis better than haemodialysis, and the use of automated machines for overnight dialysis facilitates normal daytime activities and is preferred for school-aged children. Both deceased donor and living-related transplants are performed in children, with good results. Approximately 80% of children survive for at least 10–15 years after entering dialysis/transplant programmes.

## Hypertension

Hypertension is defined as average systolic and/or diastolic blood pressure that is equal to, or greater than the 95th percentile for sex, age and height on three or more occasions. Blood pressure of 120/80 mmHg or above in adolescents, or between the 90th and 95th percentile in children at any age, is labelled as prehypertension. When measuring blood pressure, the cuff bladder length should cover 80–100% of the circumference of the upper arm, as a smaller cuff may lead to a falsely high reading. In borderline hypertension, 24-hour ambulatory blood pressure recordings are useful to distinguish persistent blood pressure increase from 'white coat hypertension'. Normal blood pressure for children varies with sex, age and height, and raised levels on screening (Table 18.2.2) should be confirmed by reference to standard tables.

The major causes of hypertension are given in Box 18.2.4. Renal disease accounts for approximately 80% of cases prior to adolescence.

**Table 18.2.2 Screening values for hypertension in children: look up standard tables if…**

| Age (years) | Systolic BP (mmHg) | Diastolic BP (mmHg) |
|---|---|---|
| 3–5 | ≥100 | >60 |
| 6–8 | ≥105 | >70 |
| 9–11 | ≥110 | >75 |
| 12–14 | ≥115 | >75 |
| ≥15 | ≥120 | ≥80 |

Source: Mitchell CK, Theriot JA, Sayat JG et al 2011 J Paediatr Child Health 47:22–26.

**Box 18.2.4 Causes of hypertension – REDCAT**

**R** Renal parenchymal disease
- Acute glomerulonephritis
- Chronic glomerulonephritis
- Reflux nephropathy
- Obstructive uropathy
- Haemolytic–uraemic syndrome
- Polycystic kidneys

Renovascular (renal artery stenosis, renal vein thrombosis)

**E** Essential hypertension
**D** Drugs (corticosteroids, ciclosporin)
**C** Coarctation of aorta
**A** Adrenogenital syndrome, hyperaldosteronism
**T** Tumours (Wilms' tumour, phaeochromocytoma, neuroblastoma)

The investigation of hypertension should commence with a good history and examination. The history should specifically include enquiries about urinary tract infections, neonatal umbilical artery catheterization, medication use, and hypertension or early stroke in any relatives. Examination of hypertensive children focuses on identification of secondary causes and assessment of end-organ damage (Fig. 18.2.5). Initial investigations include serum biochemistry, urinalysis and renal ultrasonography.

Treatment of hypertension depends on the severity, presence of symptoms and underlying cause (Table 18.2.3). Children with a hypertensive emergency usually present with signs and symptoms involving the:

- nervous system – encephalopathy, facial palsy, retinopathy
- heart – left ventricular hypertrophy or congestive cardiac failure
- kidneys – raised serum creatinine level, proteinuria.

An acute hypertensive emergency requires immediate intervention with intravenous drugs (sodium nitroprusside, labetalol, hydralazine, diazoxide), which can produce a controlled reduction in blood pressure. The aim is to decrease blood pressure by 25% over the first 8 hours, with gradual normalization over the subsequent 24–48 hours. Severe hypertension without imminent serious clinical sequelae is managed as a hypertensive urgency, and blood pressure may be reduced gradually over 24–48 hours with oral drugs (e.g. nifedipine or minoxidil).

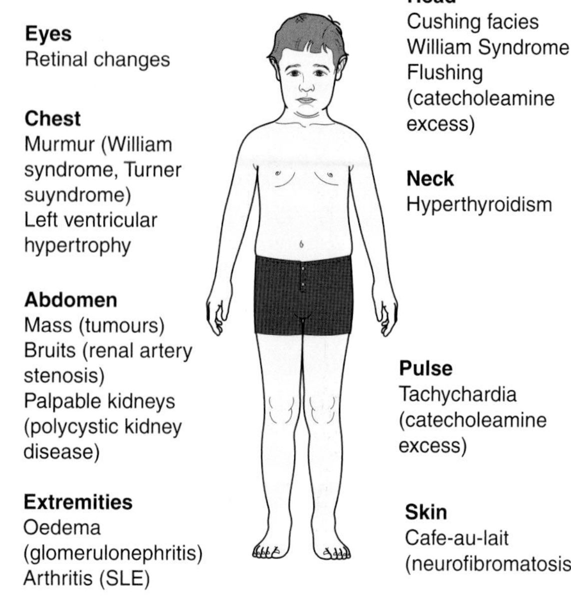


Fig. 18.2.5 Examination of the hypertensive child. SLE, systemic lupus erythematosus.

Medications used for treatment of chronic hypertension in children are similar to those used in adult patients. Angiotensin-converting enzyme (ACE) inhibitors are commonly used as initial therapy, except in patients with renal artery stenosis.

**Table 18.2.3 Management of hypertension**

| | Frequency of BP measurement | Therapeutic lifestyle changes | Pharmacological therapy |
|---|---|---|---|
| Prehypertension | Recheck in 6 months | Weight management counselling if overweight; introduce physical activity and diet management | None unless compelling indications such as chronic kidney disease, diabetes mellitus, evidence of end-organ damage |
| Stage 1 hypertension (between 95th and 99th percentile plus 5 mmHg) | Recheck in 1–2 weeks or sooner if patient is symptomatic; evaluate if persistently raised on 2 additional occasions | As above | Initiate therapy if symptomatic, presence of above indications, or persistent hypertension despite non-pharmacological measures |
| Stage 2 hypertension (>5 mmHg above 99th percentile) | Evaluate or refer for investigation within 1 week or immediately if patient is symptomatic | As above | Initiate therapy |

## Clinical example

Sally, aged 6 years, had a blood pressure recording of 140/100 mmHg at the time of tonsillectomy. Urine analysis, renal function and renal ultrasound findings were normal; echocardiography showed left ventricular hypertrophy; a mercapto-acetyl-triglycine (MAG3) scan showed that the left kidney contributed 44% and the right kidney 56% of total function; renal angiography showed a mid-aortic syndrome with bilateral renal artery stenosis from fibromuscular hyperplasia.

Sally's blood pressure was controlled with metoprolol 7.5 mg daily and amlodipine 5 mg daily. Left balloon angioplasty to 3–4 mm was performed, and Sally is awaiting a similar procedure on the right renal artery.

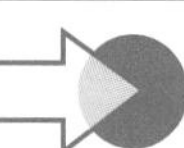

## Practical points

**Hypertension**

- Hypertension is defined as repeated systolic blood pressure and/or diastolic blood pressure measurements ≥95th percentile for sex, age and height. Some hypertensive children may have a normal blood pressure at presentation if they are in cardiac failure.
- 'White coat' hypertension is common in children and can be excluded by 24-hour ambulatory blood pressure monitoring.
- All hypertensive children should be evaluated for target organ damage and have investigations to identify secondary causes of hypertension.
- Intravenous treatment to achieve a slow, controlled reduction of blood pressure is indicated for hypertensive emergencies.
- The goal for antihypertensive treatment is reduction of blood pressure to ≤95th percentile.

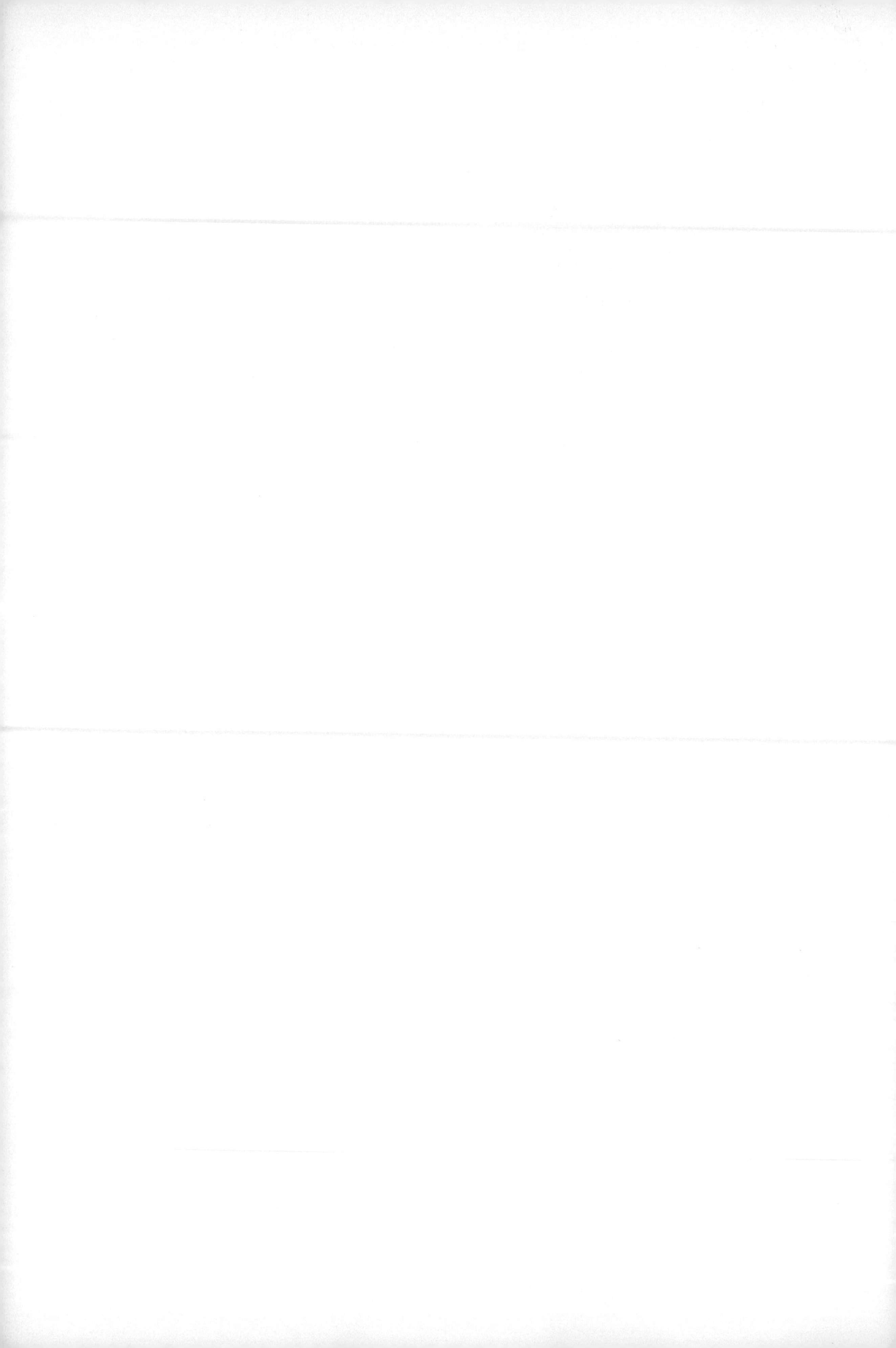

PART 19

# ENDOCRINE DISORDERS

# 19.1 Growth and variations of growth

Sarah McMahon

Growth is a multifactorial process influenced by genetic, nutritional, hormonal, psychosocial and other factors, including the general health of a child. As such, growth mirrors the psychosocial and physical wellbeing of a child and adolescent.

Physiological and pathological processes exert effects on growth and development at different stages of life. The three major determinants of growth are:

- genetic factors
- nutritional factors
- hormonal factors.

## Genetic factors

The genetic background of individuals is the major determinant of growth potential: tall parents generally have tall children, whereas short parents have short children. Although children's heights at maturity resemble those of their parents, little is known about the exact location of the individual height controlling genes, how many genes are involved or how they direct cellular growth. Major genetic disturbances such as chromosomal abnormalities are often reflected in poor growth patterns. For example, with loss of a sex chromosome in 45,XO Turner syndrome, as shown in Figure 19.1.1 (see also Chapter 10.3), adult stature is severely compromised. Other less severe chromosomal abnormalities also may result in abnormalities in stature.

Many inherited genetic conditions can also result in growth disturbance. The most striking of these are the skeletal dysplasias, which often follow an autosomal dominant mode of inheritance. The classical example of a skeletal dysplasia is achondroplasia, described in Chapter 10.3. Chromosomes may also influence tall stature, as seen in the case of an individual with an extra sex chromosome, for example Klinefelter syndrome XXY, which frequently leads to an adult height above that anticipated from the family pattern.

## Nutritional factors

Nutrition is the second most important factor determining normal growth in childhood and adolescence. Malnutrition is the world's primary cause of poor growth. In developed countries, both undernutrition and overnutrition may have long-lasting effects on growth patterns. Undernutrition, particularly intrauterine or at significant postnatal periods, may affect both the weight and height growth patterns and also the development of body organs. For example, children who are born small for gestational age and who experience significant catch-up growth in the first few months of life have been shown to have an increased risk of cardiovascular morbidity and mortality as well as type 2 diabetes later in life.

Many situations throughout childhood can cause poor nutrition and affect the growth of the child. Undernutrition due to poor quality and low quantity of food may lead to poor growth, particularly if prolonged. In addition, chronic disease may also lead to poor nutrition. Finally, emotional deprivation also has a profound influence on growth. On the other hand, overnutrition may lead to obesity with advanced linear growth and early pubertal maturation.

## Hormonal factors

Those of significance in growth are:

- growth hormone (GH)
- thyroid hormone
- testosterone and adrenal androgens
- oestrogens.

### Growth hormone–insulin-like growth factor I axis

The major hormonal influence involved in growth regulation at all ages is the growth hormone–insulin-like growth factor I axis (GH–IGF-I). GH is secreted by the anterior pituitary gland in a pulsatile pattern. Major peaks of secretion occur particularly at night. GH is bound to a specific growth hormone-binding protein and subsequently acts on a broad range of tissues via cell surface receptors, resulting in a range of metabolic and growth-related effects. Many of these effects are mediated via IGF-I, which is produced by the liver and many other tissues. The secreted IGF-I then acts either locally on adjacent tissues (paracrine action) or via endocrine mechanisms (i.e. via the circulation). IGF-I levels are age-dependent, being

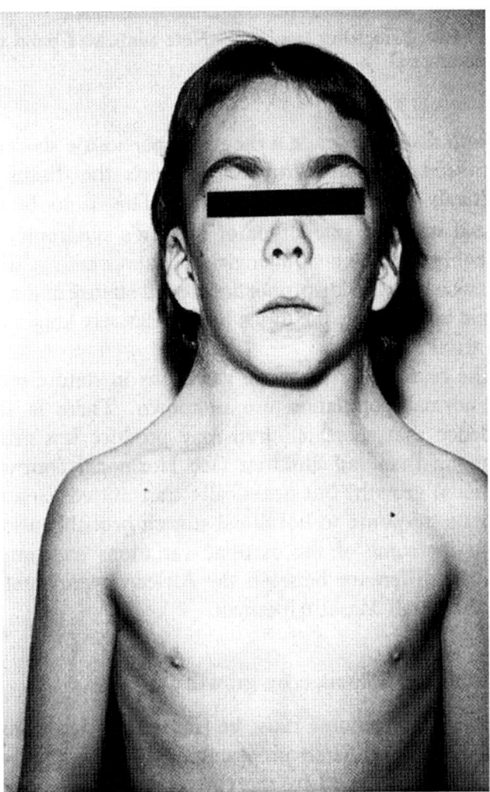

Fig. 19.1.1 Turner syndrome. Note webbing of the neck and widely spaced nipples.

low in the fetus, rising through infancy and childhood, peaking during puberty and then falling to adult levels. IGF-I is very sensitive to nutritional status and its measurement is of limited diagnostic value in the assessment of short stature. It circulates bound to one of its major binding proteins (IGFBPs).

### Thyroid hormone

Thyroxine is very important for postnatal growth. Children with untreated hypothyroidism may show both intellectual impairment and profound growth retardation, with delayed bony maturation (see Chapter 19.2).

### Testosterone and adrenal androgens

These hormones are anabolic and growth promoting. In males, testosterone and GH act synergistically to promote the adolescent growth spurt. Excess androgens in childhood may be produced as a consequence of adrenal enzyme disorders (congenital adrenal hyperplasia), precocious puberty and tumours, or may come from exogenous treatment. Some androgens are aromatized to oestrogens and will rapidly cause bone age advancement and may limit the potential for final height.

### Oestrogens

Oestrogens in small doses may synergize with GH to cause growth promotion. In higher doses, oestrogens will inhibit growth and promote early fusion of the bony epiphyses.

## Phases of growth

There are three main phases of growth: fetal growth, childhood growth and the pubertal growth spurt.

### Fetal growth

Fetal growth is the most rapid phase of growth. Initial embryonal/fetal growth is characterized by rapid differentiation of body organs, whereas late fetal growth involves continued rapid enlargement in tissues and organs, and growth in length. The most rapid linear growth velocity of all ages occurs in the weeks before birth. Factors controlling fetal growth include placental supply of nutrients and oxygen, and a range of local growth factors including insulin-like growth factors (IGFs). Pituitary GH probably plays a relatively small part in this phase of growth, whereas thyroxine is involved in brain and bone growth in the fetus. Pituitary gonadotrophins (luteinizing hormone (LH) and follicle-stimulating hormone (FSH)) regulate testicular testosterone synthesis in the male fetus, which is essential for normal growth of the male phallus. Thus a male infant with hypopituitarism may have a micropenis at birth.

### Childhood growth

During the first years of life, linear growth velocity is still very rapid (on average 8–12 cm/year) but plateaus through childhood to an average of approximately 5–6 cm/year. The growth velocity immediately before the pubertal growth spurt may be lower than this and represents a transient phase of poor growth. If the onset of the pubertal growth spurt is delayed, this phase of poor growth may be prolonged. During the childhood growth phase the limbs grow faster than the trunk, so the ratio of upper to lower body segments (divided at the pubic symphysis) diminishes from approximately 1.7 : 1 during infancy to 1 : 1 by age 10. It may fall to around 0.8 by mid-puberty. The arm span : height ratio increases during childhood and reaches 1 : 1 during puberty.

Factors controlling this phase of growth include genetic determinants, nutrition, absence of chronic disease and normal secretion of hormones, the most important of which are GH and thyroxine.

### Pubertal growth spurt

Puberty is associated with the onset of sex hormone production in boys and girls under the influence of pulsatile release of gonadotrophins (FSH/LH) from the pituitary gland. In girls, ovarian oestrogen secretion leads to the earliest pubertal sign of breast development at an average age of 10–11 years, followed by pubic and axillary hair growth in response to adrenal and ovarian androgens. The earliest sign of puberty in boys, at an average age of 11 years, is testicular enlargement (volume ≥4 mL measured with an orchidometer). Penile and scrotal growth follow, with development of pubic and axillary hair in response to testosterone synthesis. In boys testosterone also leads to muscle growth, whereas in girls oestrogens cause pelvic broadening and fat redistribution, leading to a female body shape. In both sexes, the onset of puberty is followed by a peak linear growth velocity, at an average age of 11.5 years in girls and 13.5 years in boys.

The hormonal changes of puberty include an increase in the amplitude of GH pulses, probably due to sex hormone effects. IGF-I levels rise during puberty in association with the high GH levels. Oestrogens have direct effects at the skeletal growth plate, ultimately leading to fusion of the bony epiphyses and cessation of growth at an average age of 15 years in girls and 17 years in boys. The pubertal growth spurt may be influenced by genetic factors and may also be affected adversely by poor nutrition or chronic disease, both of which can cause pubertal delay.

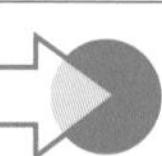

**Practical points**

**Puberty**

- The earliest sign of puberty in females is breast budding, at an average age of 10–11 years.
- The earliest sign of puberty in males is testicular enlargement, at an average age of 11 years.
- Pubic and axillary hair development usually follow the onset of breast development in girls and of testicular enlargement and genital development in boys.
- The pubertal growth spurt occurs at an average age of 11.5 years in females and 13.5 years in males.
- The growth spurt in puberty is the most rapid phase of postnatal growth.

## Assessment of growth

### Percentile charts

Any health professional who deals with children must have a working knowledge of normal variations in growth and development, and must be able to use a percentile chart. Childhood and pubertal growth patterns can be appreciated by examining growth charts, including linear height and weight charts (Fig. 19.1.2) as well as height velocity charts, indicating annual rate of growth (Fig. 19.1.3).

These charts demonstrate the range of normal growth, expressed either as percentiles or as standard deviations (SD) from the mean for age. The percentile curves are derived from the normal distribution (bell-shaped curve) of the data. The median is the 50th percentile and indicates that 50% of the measurements of a normal group of children are above and 50% are below that point. The 50th centile 'final' height value for males is 176 cm and for females is 163 cm. Children whose height or weight are 2 SD above or below the mean fall approximately between the 3rd and 97th percentiles (Fig. 19.1.2). There will be three normal children in every 100 who will be at or below the 3rd centile and three in every 100 who will be at or above the 97th centile.

Assessment of growth velocity (Fig. 19.1.3) is of far greater clinical significance than single measurements of height, and should be based on sequential measurements taken at 3-monthly intervals during a period of 6–12 months. When measured over this time period, a normal child will tend to follow the same height percentile (Fig. 19.1.2). A child with an organic or endocrine disease will tend to deviate from the percentile and may move across percentile lines. Thus serial measurement of children is the key to the assessment of their growth status.

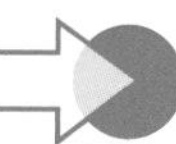

**Practical points**

**Growth**

- There is a wide variation of normal growth.
- Some 3% of normal children will be above the 97th percentile and 3% will be below the 3rd percentile.
- Assessment of growth velocity (growth over time) is of more value than a single growth measurement.
- The average growth rate during childhood is 5–6 cm/year.

### Bone age

Bone age is an index of physiological maturity, indicating the state of bony epiphyseal maturation. A bone age is obtained by performing an X-ray of the left wrist and hand, and is interpreted according to an atlas of age- and sex-specific standards. The bone age indicates the average age of children at a similar stage of bony maturation and is a guide to the remaining growth potential of the child. In normal children, the bone age will be within 1.5–2 years of the chronological age.

### Mid-parental height

The mid-parental height (MPH), also known as the target height, allows the height of any individual child to be considered in relation to the heights of

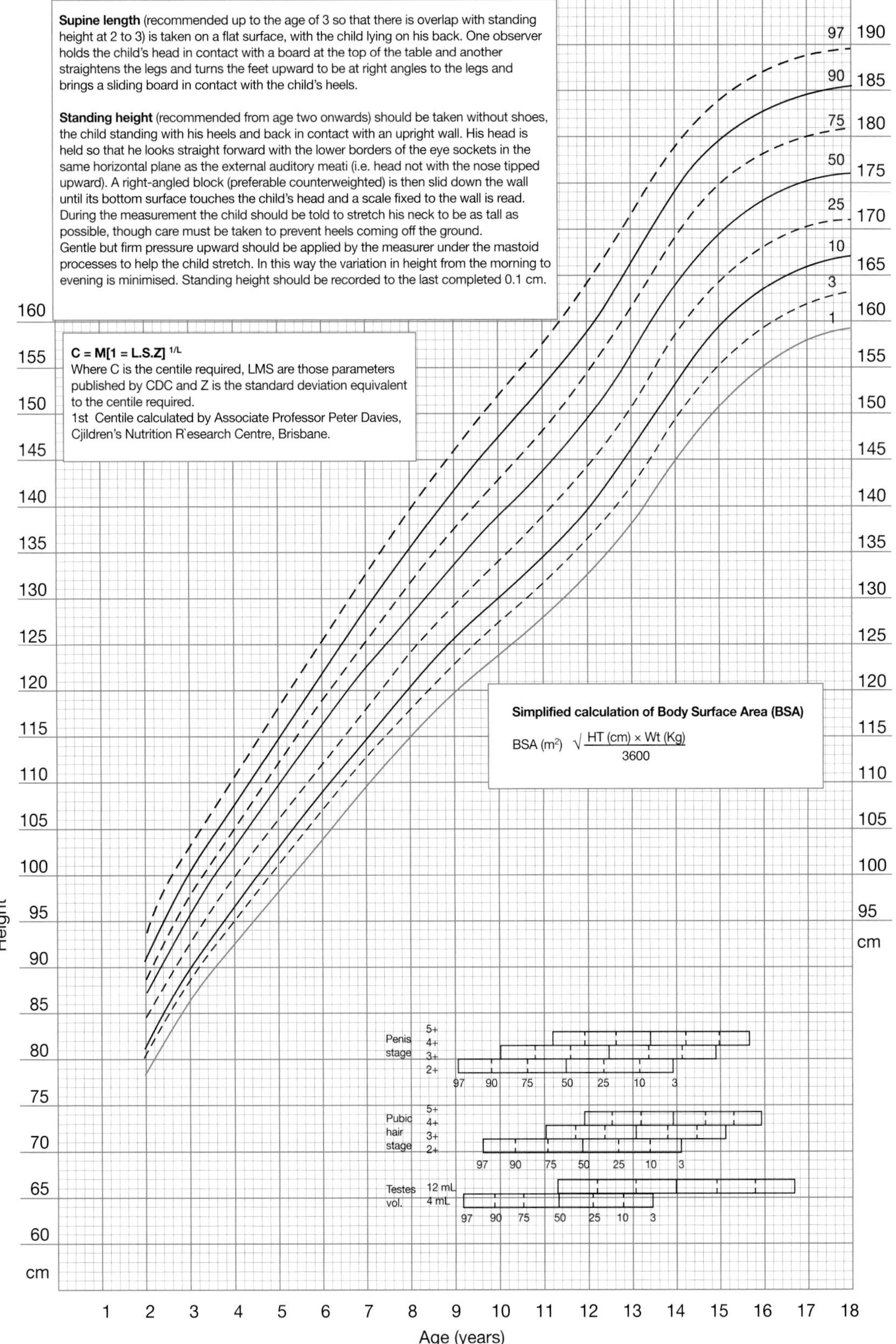


Fig. 19.1.2 Male height centile chart. A similar chart is available for females. CDC, Centers for Disease Control. (Reproduced with permission from Pfizer.)

**High velocity**

The standards are appropriate for velocity calculated over a whole year period, not less, since a smaller period requires wider limits (the 3rd and 97th centiles for a whole year being roughly appropriate for the 10th and 90th centiles over six months). The yearly velocity should be plotted at the mid=point of a year. The centiles given in black are appropriate to children of average maturational tempo, who have their peak velocity at the average age for this event. The blue line is the 50th centile line for the child who is two years early in maturity and age at peak height velocity, and the grey line refers to a child who is 50th centile in velocity but two years late. The arrows mark the 3rd and 97th centiles at peak velocity for early and late maturers.

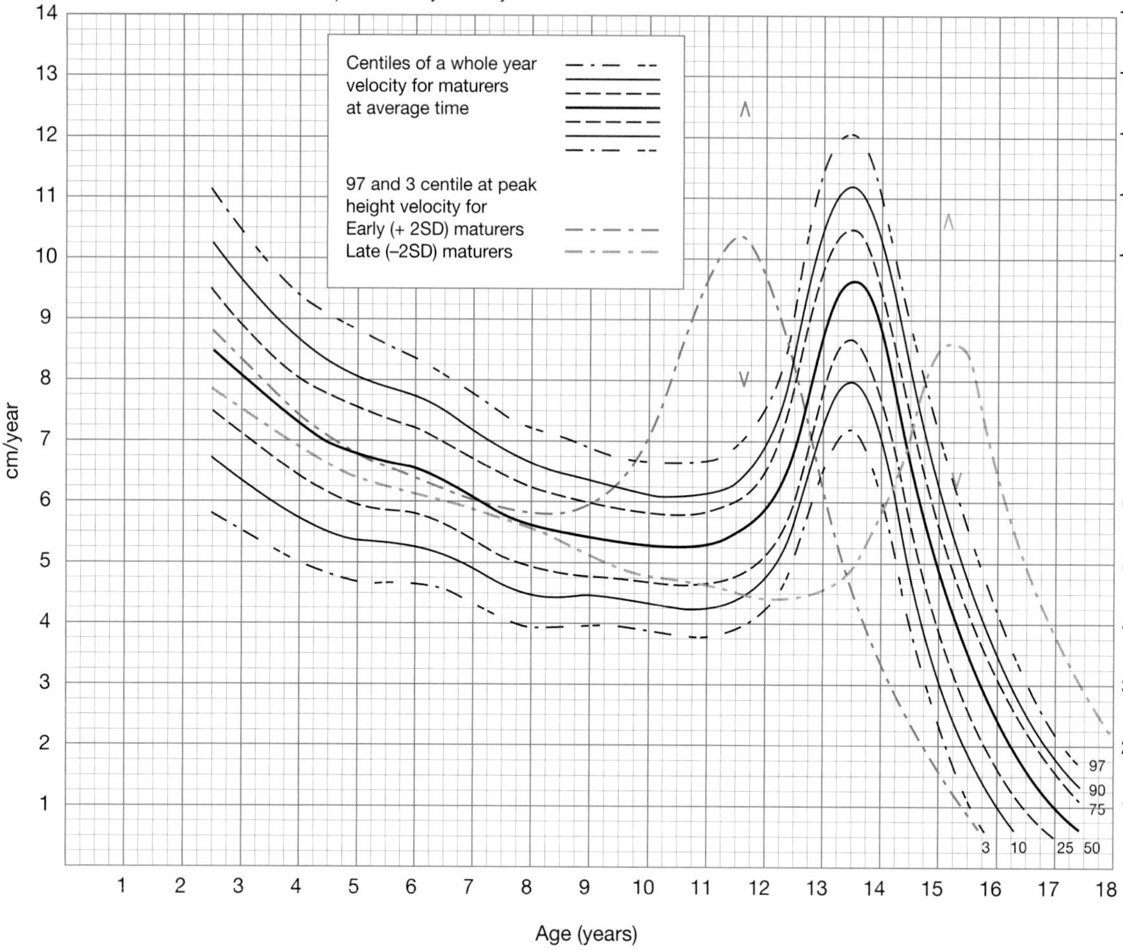

Fig. 19.1.3 Male height velocity chart. A similar chart is available for females. (Reproduced with permission from Pfizer.)

his/her biological parents. The mid-parental height (in centimetres) can be calculated using the following formulae:

$$\text{For boys: MPH} = (\text{father's height} + (\text{mother's height} + 13))/2, \pm 7.5\text{cm}$$

$$\text{For girls: MPH} = (\text{mother's height} + (\text{father's height} - 13))/2, \pm 6\text{cm}$$

## Short stature

The management of a child with short stature requires consideration of a number of issues. It is important to realize that the majority of short children will have no pathology but will either be following a familial pattern or have a variant of normal growth. The main causes of short stature in order of frequency of diagnosis are summarized in Box 19.1.1. As can be seen, endocrine causes of short stature are the least common.

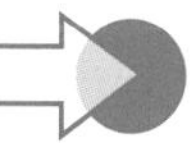

**Practical points**

**Short stature**

- The majority of short children are normal and healthy.
- The most common causes of short stature are familial short stature and constitutional delay of growth.
- Chronic disease is a major cause of short stature and is characterized by a decrease in both height and weight velocity.

**Box 19.1.1 Causes of short stature**

- Genetic/familial short stature
- Constitutional delay
- Small for gestational age
- Chronic illness – inflammation and malnutrition
- Skeletal dysplasia
- Chromosomal abnormality/syndrome
- Psychosocial
- Endocrine

## Variations from normal

### Familial (genetic) short stature

Important features of familial short stature are as follows:

- Height will track parallel to and below the 3rd centile.
- The growth rate (growth velocity) is usually normal.
- The adult height percentiles of both parents should be plotted on the child's growth chart to assess whether the child's height is appropriate for the heights of the parents.
- Pubertal development usually occurs at the appropriate time.
- Markers of physical maturation such as bone age tend to be consistent with chronological age.

### Constitutional delay in growth and puberty

Constitutional delay in growth and puberty is a very common variation of growth and leads to short stature during childhood with an adult height prognosis consistent with the mid-parental height expectation. Important features are:

- affects boys more commonly than girls, and boys are more likely to present to medical attention
- often there is a family history of a parent being short as a child, with delayed puberty and eventual catch-up with peers
- these children are the so-called 'slow growers and late bloomers'
- markers of physical maturation such as bone age are delayed
- the delay in puberty and associated delay in fusion of bony epiphyses means that both the pubertal growth spurt and the completion of growth will be delayed
- these children (most often boys) tend to grow into their late teenage years or early twenties.

## Pathological causes

### Small for gestational age

Babies may be born small for gestational age (SGA) as a result of a number of fetal, maternal and environmental factors (see Chapter 11.2). Some SGA children fail to demonstrate catch-up growth in the first 2 years of life and remain small.

### Chronic disease

Chronic disease is a major cause of growth failure:

- Usually the growth failure is associated with a similar fall off in weight velocity.
- An endocrine problem is unlikely to be the cause of poor growth if both the weight and height are affected.
- Nutritional insufficiency may contribute to the growth failure of chronic disease as a result of inadequate or inappropriate intake, poor absorption or impaired or excessive tissue utilization.

### Skeletal disorders

Skeletal disorders are usually familial, involving intrinsic cartilage or bone defects. Examples include achondroplasia, hypochondroplasia and the mucopolysaccharidoses. The major distinctive feature of these disorders is body segment disproportion, with increased upper to lower body segment ratios. The limbs are usually short, leading to a reduced arm span : height ratio. Weight gain is usually normal. These disorders in their mild form are relatively common and often overlooked. More information is given in Chapter 10.3.

### Iatrogenic

High-dose corticosteroid treatment may cause poor growth in children with conditions such as severe asthma, cystic fibrosis, arthritis, inflammatory bowel disease, nephrotic syndrome and malignancies such as leukaemia. Marked growth failure is associated with weight gain. Irradiation to the head and spine may result in hypothalamic–pituitary dysfunction and poor spinal growth. Poor growth of the trunk is characterized by an increased arm span : height ratio and a reduced upper to lower body segment ratio.

### Chromosomal abnormalities and syndromes

Turner syndrome and its variants are the most common chromosomal cause of short stature. This condition must be excluded in any girl with short stature, because the typical phenotypic features may not be seen, particularly in the mosaic forms of Turner syndrome. The most common associated abnormality is ovarian dysgenesis resulting in failed pubertal development in 95% of cases. Other commonly seen features include a webbed neck (see Fig. 19.1.1), small ears, increased carrying angle, bicuspid aortic valve, coarctation of the aorta, horseshoe kidney,

**Box 19.1.2 Features of Turner syndrome**

**General**
- Short stature
- Delayed puberty
- Primary amenorrhoea

**Lymphatic abnormalities**
- Neck webbing
- Low posterior hairline
- Lymphoedema
- Nail convexity/dysplasia

**Skeletal abnormalities**
- Micrognathia
- High arched palate
- Short 4th/5th metacarpals
- Increased carrying angle
- Madelung deformity
- Kyphoscoliosis
- Broad chest

**Metabolic**
- Autoimmune thyroid disease
- Impaired glucose tolerance/type 2 diabetes
- Abnormal liver function test results

**Miscellaneous**
- Recurrent middle ear infections
- Sensorineural hearing loss
- Bicuspid aortic valve
- Coarctation of the aorta
- Renal abnormalities (e.g. horseshoe kidney)
- Naevi

dysplastic nails and recurrent otitis media. All or none of these dysmorphic and clinical features may be present. The full range of features is summarized in Box 19.1.2.

Common dysmorphic syndromes presenting with short stature include Noonan syndrome and Russell–Silver syndrome.

### Psychosocial

Psychosocial causes of short stature cover the spectrum from severe deprivation to overt abuse, and may be associated with nutritional deficiencies. Fall-off in weight gain is usually as striking as failure of linear growth. Short stature due solely to psychosocial deprivation is uncommon.

**Clinical example**

Natalie's parents were concerned about her growth and saw a paediatrician when she was 4 years old. Her birth weight and length were around the 25th centile. At 2 years her length was on the 10th percentile, but then her growth had seemed to slow, particularly after the age of 3 years.

On assessment by the paediatrician at 4 years of age, her height was 6 cm below the 1st percentile. She had had a few middle ear infections in the last 2 years but had otherwise been well. Her early development was normal. Her cardiovascular examination was normal. She had widely spaced nipples but no other dysmorphic features. Initial investigations including full blood count, electrolytes and liver function tests, thyroid function tests and a coeliac screen were normal. Her bone age was the same as her chronological age. Her karyotype was consistent with Turner syndrome.

Natalie was referred to a paediatric endocrinologist who advised them that Natalie's growth could be improved with GH injections. It was very likely that she would eventually need hormonal induction of puberty and would have infertility owing to the gonadal dysgenesis associated with Turner syndrome. Natalie's parents were also informed that she would need ongoing care into adulthood to monitor for other health issues such as hypertension, hyperlipidaemia, type 2 diabetes, and aortic dilatation and dissection, all of which occur more commonly in women with Turner syndrome.

Natalie was referred to other specialists regarding other problems associated with Turner syndrome. Renal ultrasound imaging was normal and her heart was structurally normal. She continued to have middle ear infections and required insertion of grommets. She was commenced on GH injections 6 days per week and responded well. By the age of 7 years her height was on the 5th percentile.

### Endocrine

Endocrine causes of short stature are the least common pathological cause and include hypothyroidism, GH deficiency (possibly associated with other pituitary hormone deficiencies), Cushing syndrome (hypercortisolism) and adrenal insufficiency. These conditions are more likely to be associated with weight gain than a fall-off in weight centiles.

## Assessment

### Issues to determine

Assessment of short stature involves determination of the following issues:
- Is she or he short?
- Is she or he growing slowly (could this be pathological)?
- What is the underlying cause?

- What is the adult height prognosis?
- How is s/he coping with the short stature?
- Is any specific therapy warranted?
- Is any supportive therapy indicated?

The approach to the assessment of short stature should include history, examination, investigations if necessary, therapy and follow-up.

### History

When taking the history, the following should be sought:

- What is the height compared to peers?
- How long has the child been short?
- Who is concerned about the short stature and is there teasing at school?
- What is the school performance?
- What are the birth details and past medical history?
- Was there unexplained neonatal hypoglycaemia (suggesting pituitary hormone deficiency) or early illnesses?
- Determine milestone development, specific disease symptoms and nutritional status.
- Has puberty commenced?
- Are previous growth measurements available (child health record or measurements from local doctor or school)?
- What are the current heights and ages of pubertal onset of the parents and siblings?
- Is there a family history of specific diseases?

### Examination

On examination ensure/look for:

- accurate height (using a stadiometer) and weight, and body proportions (arm span, upper and lower segments)
- assessment of pubertal status – the characteristic pubertal changes in males and females are illustrated in Figures 19.1.4 and 19.1.5 (further issues regarding puberty are considered later in this section)
- general physical examination including evidence of chronic disease, nutritional state and dysmorphic features suggesting a syndrome
- any sign of goitre or clinical signs of hypothyroidism, including dry hair and skin, bradycardia and delayed reflexes
- evidence of 'midline brain development syndromes', which may result in hypopituitarism. This includes cleft palate, single central incisor and small male genitalia (associated with gonadotrophin deficiency *in utero*). The combination of neonatal hypoglycaemia and small genitalia suggests hypopituitarism
- visual fields and optic fundi to exclude the possibility of a pituitary lesion, in particular craniopharyngioma.

## Management

The single most important aspect of the assessment and management of short stature is to plot the current and previous heights and weights and parental heights

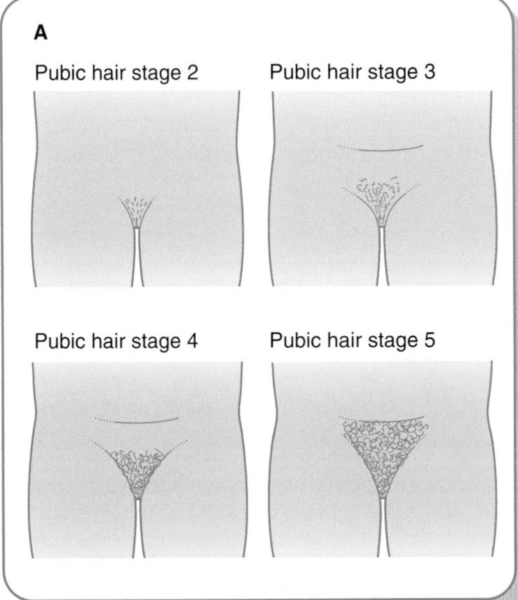


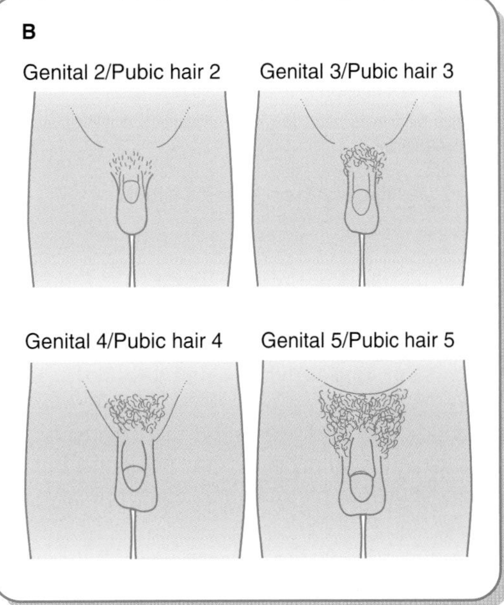


Fig. 19.1.4 (**A**) Pubertal pubic hair changes in the female. (**B**) Pubertal genital and pubic hair changes in the male.

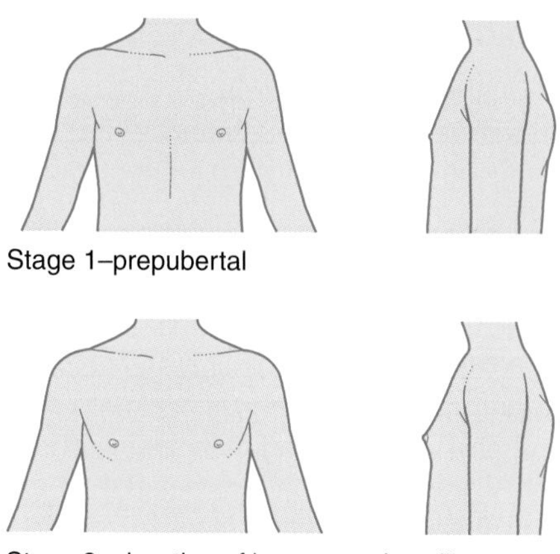

Stage 1–prepubertal

Stage 2–elevation of breasts and papilla

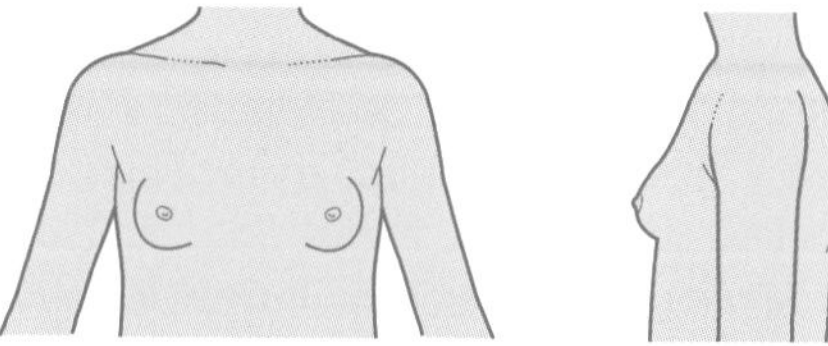

Stage 3–further enlargement and elevation of breast and areola but no separation of contour

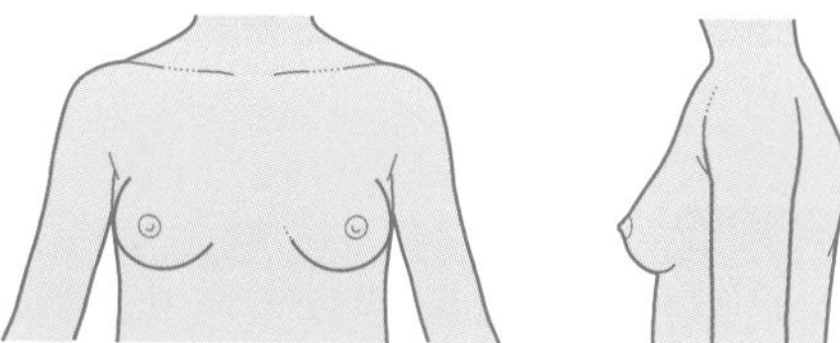

Stage 4–areola and papilla form a secondary mound above level of the breast

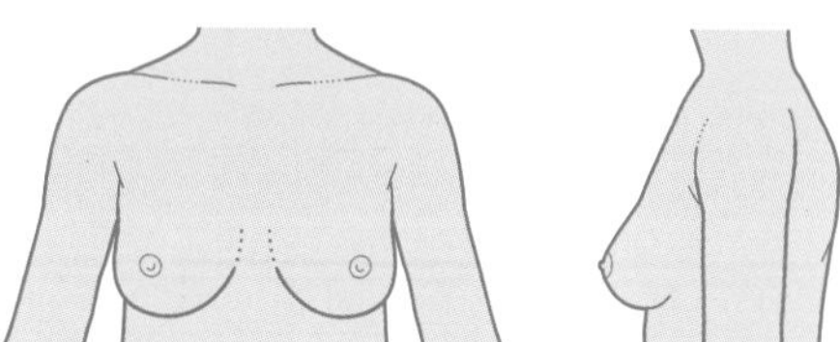

Stage 5–areola recedes to the general contour of the breast

**Fig. 19.1.5** Pubertal breast changes in the female.

on a percentile chart in order to answer the following questions:

- Is the child short and below the 3rd height centile? Is this appropriate for mid-parental height?
- Is the child growing slowly and is there evidence that the height is falling across the percentile lines? This can be further plotted on a height velocity chart (see Fig. 19.1.3).

A height velocity below the 25th centile for bone age is potentially abnormal in a short child. A reliable height velocity requires at least 6 months of growth data, and preferably 12 months with consistent measurements at 3–4-monthly intervals over that time. Examination of the growth data plus the points obtained in history and examination should allow distinction between a variation of normal and a pathological cause of short stature.

## Investigations

Investigations should be performed if there is any evidence of specific chronic disease, if there is a suggestion of chromosomal abnormality or if the growth velocity is subnormal. The following investigations may be performed:

- bone age X-ray
- full blood count
- urea, creatinine and electrolytes
- calcium and phosphate
- thyroid function tests
- C-reactive protein (CRP) and iron studies
- chromosomes (girls only)
- screening test for coeliac disease (total immunoglobulin (Ig) A and tissue transglutaminase antibodies)
- urinalysis ± microscopy and culture.

It is important to note that all girls with unexplained short stature should have a karyotype to exclude the possibility of Turner syndrome.

If puberty is markedly delayed it may be worthwhile measuring gonadotrophins (FSH/LH) and testosterone or oestradiol.

The listed investigations provide a screen for underlying chronic disease, infection or nutritional deficiency as well as hypothyroidism and Turner syndrome. Other investigations may be indicated by specific physical findings. In a child with unexplained combined weight and height fall-off, a malabsorptive disorder should be excluded and consideration should be given to measuring tissue transglutaminase antibodies as a possible indicator of the presence of coeliac disease. If these are raised, a small-bowel biopsy may be necessary (see Chapter 20.3).

### Clinical example

Ben was a 14-year-old boy whose mother complained that he did not seem to be growing at all. She said to her general practitioner that she had not needed to buy Ben any new clothes for the past 3 years. She remembered that her older son was always growing out of his clothes at this age. She was also concerned because Ben did not seem to have as much energy as other boys his age, and he ate much less than she would have expected at this age, based on her experience with her older son.

Further history revealed that Ben had always been a very healthy boy in the past, with no significant medical problems. He had become a fussy eater during the past couple of years. He said that many foods he had previously eaten now made him feel sick in the stomach and gave him stomach cramps. When asked if he had diarrhoea, Ben said 'no', but when asked how many times he went to the toilet he admitted that he needed to go at least six times a day, and that this pattern had developed only in the last year. Ben said he thought this was normal.

Physical examination confirmed that Ben's height and weight were almost the same as when he was 11 years old. Apart from being a little pale, there were no other abnormal physical findings on general examination. Ben was pre-pubertal.

Baseline investigations included a full blood count and CRP estimation. These showed that Ben had a low haemoglobin level and his CRP was 30 mg/L. All the other baseline tests including electrolytes, liver function tests, renal function, screening tests for coeliac disease and thyroid function tests were normal. Ben's bone age was significantly delayed. At 14 years of age his bone age was only that of 10 years.

The history of poor growth and the abdominal symptoms together with the low haemoglobin and raised CRP level suggested the possibility of a chronic gastrointestinal problem such as inflammatory bowel disease. Ben was referred to a paediatric gastroenterologist and had an endoscopy and colonoscopy, which demonstrated that he had Crohn's disease. After appropriate management his symptoms improved. He started to gain weight and over the next 12 months his growth also improved.

## Investigation for growth hormone deficiency

GH deficiency may be suggested by association with midline defects or by the presence of other pituitary hormone deficiencies, including secondary hypothyroidism or gonadotrophin deficiency. Biochemical GH deficiency is an indication for magnetic resonance imaging (MRI) of the central nervous system (CNS) and biochemical testing for other pituitary deficits. Specific underlying causes of GH deficiency include idiopathic (most common), pituitary or hypothalamic tumours or structural abnormalities, cranial irradiation and genetic GH deficiency (e.g. gene defects of pituitary transcription factors).

Specific tests to determine the presence of GH deficiency include:

- Physiological tests of GH sufficiency, such as:
  - measurement of IGF-I and IGFBP-3 levels. These tests are used for screening for GH deficiency prior to proceeding to more involved pharmacological tests. As yet the data are not sufficiently reliable to recommend that these tests be performed as a single diagnostic entity in a clinical setting. They may, however, be useful when considered in combination with other clinical information, results of MRI brain scans and GH tests
  - overnight sleep studies of GH secretion
  - exercise GH tests – performed in the fasting state on a bicycle ergometer with blood for GH levels taken before and 30 minutes after exercise. This is a screening test with 20% of normal children failing to reach cut-off levels
- Pharmacological tests of GH sufficiency, including:
  - glucagon stimulation test
  - arginine stimulation test
  - clonidine stimulation test.

Although no one test is superior to another, the glucagon stimulation test is at present the preferred pharmacological test of GH secretion. The glucagon stimulation test also provides information about the hypothalamic–pituitary–adrenal axis.

For the purposes of defining GH deficiency and assessing eligibility for human GH as a pharmaceutical benefit in Australia, biochemical GH deficiency is defined as failure to achieve a peak serum GH concentration of more than 10 mU/L in response to two stimulation tests, at least one of which is a pharmacological test, or in response to one test in the presence of other evidence suggestive of GH deficiency, such as structural CNS abnormalities or low plasma IGF-I and IGFBP-3 levels.

### Treatment

Short stature is considered by some children and their families to be a physical and psychosocial disability. The major growth-promoting agent used in the treatment of short stature is biosynthetic GH. This has been available commercially in Australia since 1985.

GH can be administered only by subcutaneous injections, usually given 6–7 days per week. Despite the availability of biosynthetic GH, the annual cost of GH therapy remains very high.

The Commonwealth Department of Health and Ageing has provided guidelines for the use of GH in Australia. Current indications include:

- short stature (less than 1st percentile) and slow growth (growth velocity below 25th percentile for bone age)
- biochemical GH deficiency associated with short stature and slow growth
- growth retardation secondary to an intracranial lesion or cranial irradiation
- Turner syndrome
- chronic renal insufficiency
- Prader–Willi syndrome.

### Psychological support and counselling

Psychological support and counselling are undoubtedly the most important part of the management of short stature and can be provided by either health professionals or lay support groups. Often, reassurance regarding the normality of the child and the reassurance of a reasonable height prognosis is all that is required.

## Tall stature

Tall stature is a relatively infrequent presenting problem compared with the number of children who present because of short stature. In general, very few tall children have an organic disease process as a basis for their condition. The most common reason for tall stature is genetic tall stature. Compared with 20 years ago, relatively few teenagers and their parents are concerned about tall stature, as it is now more socially acceptable for girls to be tall. As with short stature, there is no clear demarcation between normal and tall stature. A child whose height is above the 97th percentile for age should be considered tall.

### Causes

The following may be causes of tall stature:

- familial or normal variant
- precocious puberty
- syndromes – Marfan, Klinefelter, triple X, homocystinuria, Sotos
- endocrine causes: hyperthyroidism and pituitary gigantism.

#### Familial/normal variant tall stature

Most tall children are normal in all respects and their height is genetically determined. Some children with early but otherwise normal pubertal development will appear tall in relation to their peers and family during adolescence, but will have a predicted final height within the accepted normal range. These early developers have an advanced bone age and are at the opposite end of the spectrum to the short children with constitutional delay, who have delayed puberty but who will also reach a normal adult height consistent with their mid-parental height.

#### Precocious puberty

Precocious puberty is defined as pubertal development at less than 8 years of age in girls and less than 9 years in boys. Because of rapid acceleration of bone maturation and early epiphyseal fusion, many children with precocious puberty are excessively tall in early to mid childhood but finish up as relatively short adults. It is important to recognize precocious puberty, as treatment can be provided to switch off the premature activation of the hypothalamic–pituitary–gonadal axis. It is also important to ascertain whether the appearance of precocious puberty may be due to an aberrant source of androgen or oestrogen production, such as an adrenal or ovarian tumour.

#### Syndromes causing tall stature

Marfan syndrome may present with the classical picture of arachnodactyly, ligamentous laxity, chest deformity, cardiac abnormalities, high arched palate and subluxation of the lenses. Often, however, one sees tall, thin children with some marfanoid features but who are difficult to classify. Children with homocystinuria have a marfanoid phenotype but have intellectual impairment. Homocystinuria may be diagnosed by a study of urinary and serum amino acids. Tall girls with intellectual impairment should also be screened for the triple X syndrome, and tall boys with disorders of pubertal maturation, with small testes, gynaecomastia and sometimes behavioural disturbance, should have chromosomal analysis. They may have either XYY syndrome or Klinefelter syndrome (XXY).

#### Endocrine causes of tall stature

Hyperthyroidism is relatively uncommon in childhood and is an infrequent cause of tall stature. The clinical features of hyperthyroidism are discussed in Chapter 19.2. Pituitary gigantism is extremely rare but should be suspected if the history and examination suggest pituitary involvement in association with tall stature. Children with pituitary gigantism will have an abnormally rapid growth rate as well as tall stature, in contrast to genetically tall children who grow above but parallel to the 97th percentile but have a normal growth velocity.

### Approach to diagnosis and treatment

The approach to diagnosis in a tall child consists of a full history, including a history of family heights and pubertal maturation patterns. In addition, it is important to ascertain whether there are associated abnormalities or developmental delay that may suggest one of the chromosomal or syndromal disorders causing tall stature.

A full physical examination is essential, with emphasis on accurate height measurement, body shape, limb proportions and pubertal status. Neurological assessment should include fundoscopy, assessment of visual fields and intellectual function, and should determine any evidence of hyperthyroidism.

In most instances, a tall child will have a normal growth velocity with height tracking above but parallel to the 97th centile. An accurate height measurement and bone age assessment by an experienced radiologist or paediatric endocrinologist will enable an adult height prediction to be made.

In the past, sex steroids were used to reduce the final height in both males and females where the estimate of final height was thought to be excessive. High-dose oestrogen treatment was used in tall girls. However, recent studies have suggested an increased risk of psychological problems and impaired fertility in women treated with high-dose oestrogen for tall stature in adolescence. Currently this treatment is not advocated.

## Variations of pubertal development

### Early normal puberty

In many countries, including Australia, children appear to be starting puberty younger than previous generations. This is called the secular trend in growth and development. The earlier age of puberty is probably due to effects of improved nutrition and living circumstances, and absence of chronic disease. Many girls present just before 8 years of age with breast development. After assessment by a specialist, no specific treatment is usually required. Interestingly, although there has been a trend towards earlier onset of breast development, the average age of menarche (onset of periods) remains approximately 12.8 years for white girls.

**Table 19.1.1 Causes of delayed puberty**

| Cause | Clinical examples |
|---|---|
| **Associated with normal or low serum gonadotrophin levels** | |
| Constitutional delay | Usually familial: associated with a delayed bone age |
| Chronic illness | Cystic fibrosis, inflammatory bowel disease, juvenile idiopathic arthritis |
| Endocrine causes | Hypopituitarism (congenital and acquired), isolated gonadotrophin deficiency, Kallman syndrome, hypothyroidism, hyperprolactinaemia |
| Inadequate nutrition | Anorexia nervosa, excessive exercise |
| **Associated with raised serum gonadotrophin levels*** | |
| Gonadal dysgenesis | Turner syndrome, Klinefelter syndrome |
| Anorchia | |
| Gonadal damage | Vascular damage, irradiation, chemotherapy, mumps (boys), torsion, autoimmune disease, galactosaemia (girls) |

*This usually signifies primary gonadal dysfunction.

### Delayed puberty

Delayed puberty is very common and occurs in approximately 2% of the adolescent population. Delayed puberty is defined as the absence of pubertal changes over the age of 13 years for girls and over the age of 14 years for boys. In general, adolescents have a heightened awareness of body image and are often preoccupied with the normality or otherwise of their pubertal development. Boys in particular may suffer major psychological effects resulting from delayed puberty as they may experience bullying, may be left out of sporting teams and may be less generally able to compete with their peers due to poor muscular development. The most common causes of delayed puberty are familial or constitutional delay in puberty for which there is often a family history, particularly in the parents, uncles or aunts of a teenage boy. Puberty may also be delayed in the presence of any chronic illness of childhood or adolescence. The causes of delayed puberty are usually considered on the basis of the serum gonadotrophins (LH/FSH) and are outlined in Table 19.1.1.

#### Diagnosis and management

Assessment of delayed puberty requires a complete history, including a family history of pubertal maturation patterns. It is important to look carefully for the possibility of occult chronic disease, such as inflammatory bowel disease, which may become apparent initially as a delay in the onset of puberty. If the history is suggestive of familial or constitutional delayed puberty, and this is confirmed by physical examination, no further investigation may be necessary. If the diagnosis is not clear, the following investigations may need to be performed:

- full blood count
- urea/creatinine and electrolytes
- liver function tests
- CRP, iron studies
- screening test for coeliac disease (total IgA and tissue transglutaminase antibodies)
- thyroid function tests
- chromosomes
- bone age X-ray
- serum FSH and LH, testosterone or oestradiol
- serum prolactin.

#### Treatment

Indications for treatment of delayed puberty are primarily psychological. Induction of pubertal development in boys through the judicious use of intramuscular or oral testosterone preparations may be useful in alleviating the psychological stress caused by delayed puberty. Pubertal development at a normal time is also important for peak bone mass accumulation. Treatment of delayed puberty should be carried out only by paediatricians and endocrinologists experienced in this area, as excessive administration of sex steroids can adversely accelerate bony epiphyseal maturation and affect long-term height outcome.

### Psychological support and counselling

Psychological support and counselling are an extremely important part of the management of pubertal delay and in some instances may be all that is required while waiting for the onset of spontaneous pubertal development. It is very important to reassure the adolescent and their family that they are normal and that appropriate pubertal and sexual development will occur or can be relatively easily assisted with hormonal intervention. Such reassurance and support can profoundly improve an adolescent's self-esteem.

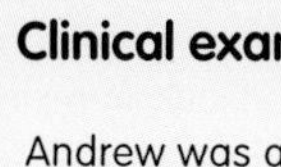

**Clinical example**

Andrew was a 15½-year-old boy. His father was concerned he was growing poorly and was underdeveloped for his age. Andrew's father had also been a late developer, and was bullied at school and left out of the rugby team because of his size. He reported that he was still growing when he left school and became an apprentice mechanic.

Further history revealed that Andrew was a healthy young man who had always grown along the 3 rd percentile, but from 14 years of age his height had fallen away from the 3 rd percentile line. He was a very keen sportsman and had always been a very fast runner but could no longer compete successfully with boys his age. Because of this he had recently taken up golf, which he and his father played together every Saturday. Andrew's physical examination confirmed that he was completely pre-pubertal, with an otherwise normal physical examination.

The most likely diagnosis was constitutional delay in puberty. Andrew was not distressed at all by his delayed puberty, and his father was reassured when the diagnosis was explained. During the next 3 years, Andrew's growth rate increased and he went through a delayed but otherwise normal puberty, eventually being the same height as his father.

## Precocious puberty

Precocious puberty is an uncommon problem and occurs much less frequently than delayed puberty. Precocious puberty is defined as pubertal development before age 8 years in girls and 9 years in boys. True or central precocious puberty is associated with raised gonadotrophin levels. True precocious puberty is much more common in girls than boys, and girls are less likely to have an identifiable underlying pathological cause than boys. Girls with this disorder will have accelerated growth and accelerated development of breasts and pubic hair. Boys with true precocious puberty have evidence of enlargement of both testes as well as accelerated linear and genital growth and pubic hair development. Various intracranial pathologies (including hypothalamic or pituitary tumours) can cause precocious puberty by triggering early activation of the hypothalamic–pituitary–gonadal axis.

Gonadotrophin-independent precocious puberty may be seen with congenital adrenal hyperplasia, adrenal, testicular or ovarian neoplasms, and tumours that secrete non-pituitary gonadotrophin such as human chorionic gonadotrophin (hCG). The McCune–Albright syndrome is also a cause of gonadotrophin-independent precocious puberty.

If precocious puberty is suspected, referral should be made to a paediatric endocrinologist, who will organize appropriate investigations. These may include measurement of serum FSH and LH, testosterone or oestradiol levels, dynamic tests of gonadotrophin secretion such as gonadotrophin-releasing hormone (GnRH) testing, bone age assessment, and MRI of the brain and pituitary gland. Treatment of precocious puberty should be managed by a paediatric endocrinologist experienced in this area. Treatment options include GnRH agonists, medroxyprogesterone acetate or anti-androgens. Consideration for treatment for precocious puberty will include factors such as the age of the child and the rate of progression of the pubertal development.

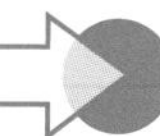

**Practical points**

**Delayed puberty**

- Delayed puberty is a common pubertal problem.
- Delayed puberty is defined as absence of pubertal development in girls older than 13 years and boys older than 14 years.
- Constitutional delay in puberty is the most common cause, particularly in boys, often with a positive family history.
- Chronic disease may cause delayed puberty.

## Conditions resembling precocious puberty

### Premature thelarche

Isolated breast development, either unilateral or bilateral, is relatively common in girls under 2 years of age but may occur at any time throughout childhood. By definition, premature thelarche has no other features of precocious puberty. All cases should be referred for assessment by a paediatrician or endocrinologist. In most cases, observation and follow-up is all that is required.

### Premature adrenarche

The appearance of isolated pubic hair development under the age of 8 years in a girl may occur as a variant of normal but may also be associated with an adrenal disorder such as a non-classical form of congenital adrenal hyperplasia. Careful assessment for any associated signs of virilization, such as clitoral enlargement, hirsutism or acne, should be performed. The appearance of pubic hair in a boy before the age of 9 years rarely occurs as a normal variant and should always be investigated. In all cases of premature pubic hair development, referral should be made to a paediatrician or paediatric endocrinologist so that appropriate investigation of adrenal androgens can be performed.

### Isolated premature menarche

Girls with this rare condition of unclear aetiology by definition have no other features of pubertal development. Most girls will have fewer than three episodes of bleeding and then puberty will eventually occur at a normal time. Before making the diagnosis of premature menarche, the specialist must eliminate all other causes of premature oestrogen secretion and/or any local causes of vaginal bleeding.

## Pubertal gynaecomastia

Gynaecomastia is very common in adolescent boys, occurring in 40–70% of 14-year-olds. In most instances the breast development is minor, transient and regresses. Rare causes of marked pubertal gynaecomastia include Klinefelter syndrome, adrenal and gonadal tumours, and drugs such as cimetidine, nifedipine, spironolactone and marijuana use. Hormonal therapy does not influence the natural history of pubertal gynaecomastia. If significant breast enlargement is causing psychosocial difficulties, it may be necessary to refer a teenage boy to a plastic surgeon for consideration for subareolar mastectomy.

## Asymmetrical breast development

Asymmetrical breast development can occur in both males and females. In males, it is clearly a variant of pubertal gynaecomastia. In females, asymmetry may be apparent at the beginning of breast budding or may evolve subsequently through breast development.

It is important to consider an underlying chest wall or pectoral muscle abnormality. In rare cases, an underlying vascular abnormality or lipoma may cause one breast to appear larger than the other. This can usually be readily determined by a physical examination and confirmed by ultrasonography.

In most cases, however, asymmetrical breast development is a physiological variant of puberty, and reassurance and monitoring are usually all that is required. For self-esteem and cosmetic reasons, advice should be given to teenage girls about temporary use of breast prostheses or padded bras to equalize the breast form. In most situations, the asymmetry resolves with full pubertal development. On rare occasions, however, referral to a reconstructive surgeon for breast reduction or augmentation may need to be considered.

# 19.2 Thyroid disorders

Fergus Cameron, Justin Brown

Normal thyroid function throughout infancy, childhood and adolescence is essential for a normal developmental and physiological outcome. Thyroid disease is one of the most common groups of endocrine disorders in childhood and adolescence, with approximately 1–2% of all children having a thyroid disorder at some time. Therefore, knowledge of thyroid disease and its management is fundamental to paediatric medicine.

## Thyroid physiology

The thyroid gland removes iodide from the bloodstream, combines it with tyrosine and releases iodinated tyrosine to the peripheral tissues. The thyroid gland is able to trap iodide and synthesize iodothyronine from 70 days' gestation. Release of thyroxine, however, does not occur until 18–20 weeks' gestation. Thyroid gland growth is regulated by thyroid-stimulating hormone (TSH) released from the anterior pituitary gland, which is in turn regulated by thyrotropin-regulating hormone (TRH) released from the hypothalamus. These regulating hormones are in turn controlled by negative feedback from tri-iodothyronine ($T_3$), the active metabolite of the major thyroid hormone thyroxine (or tetra-iodothyronine, $T_4$).

The thyroid gland is extremely effective at trapping serum iodide, with a concentration gradient from thyroid to serum of 30–40-fold. This gradient increases in times of iodide deficiency. Once trapped, iodide is oxidized to iodine and organification occurs. Organification is the iodination of thyroglobulin-bound tyrosyl residues to form mono-iodotyrosine (MIT) and di-iodotyrosine (DIT).

Organification and iodide oxidation (to iodine) are catalysed by thyroid peroxidase. Thyroid peroxidase couples the iodotyrosines to form iodothyronines within the thyroglobulin molecule, resulting in $T_4$ and $T_3$. In the absence of iodine deficiency, the $T_4$:$T_3$ synthesis ratio is 10–20:1. In adults, the release rate of $T_4$ to $T_3$ is 3:1. Once released, both hormones bind to thyroxine-binding globulin (TBG). Some 80% of circulating $T_3$ results from de-iodination of $T_4$ in peripheral tissues. Thyroid hormones bind to a nuclear receptor. $T_3$ binds to this receptor with 10 times the affinity of $T_4$. Once bound, thyroid hormones regulate gene transcription, increasing cytoplasmic proteins, which stimulate mitochondrial activity, thus increasing metabolic rate.

Disorders of thyroid function in childhood can be divided into the following categories:

- hypothyroidism
- hyperthyroidism
- thyroid masses.

## Hypothyroidism

### Congenital

Screening for congenital hypothyroidism has been performed in most developed countries for the past 15–20 years. In Australia, screening for congenital hypothyroidism, phenylketonuria and cystic fibrosis occurs on day 3–5 of life. Because of such screening the clinical picture of 'cretinism' (the later effects of congenital hypothyroidism, including severe intellectual disability) thankfully is now rarely seen.

#### Incidence

The incidence of congenital hypothyroidism is 1 in 3000–5000, with some geographical variation.

#### Aetiology and genetics

Some 75% of cases are due to dysgenesis (agenesis, ectopia), 10% to dyshormonogenesis, 5% to hypothalamic–pituitary deficiency (central hypothyroidism) and 10% to transient hypothyroidism (iodine exposure, maternal antithyroid antibodies, etc.). Although thyroid disease appears to be sporadic in the majority of children born with hypothyroidism, evidence for a genetic component is increasing. Hypothyroidism is familial in up to 2% of cases, and children with congenital hypothyroidism have a higher incidence of associated abnormalities (cardiac, renal, hip dysplasia) than the general population.

Studies in mouse models with congenital defects of thyroid development have provided the basis for molecular genetic studies in humans with congenital hypothyroidism. Mutations have been described in a number of genes, resulting in absent, misplaced, hypoplastic or unresponsive glands (Table 19.2.1). In some instances, a specific phenotype can be recognized, and prognosis is affected. For example, in individuals with the *NKX2.1* mutation, neurological outcome is poor despite early thyroxine treatment.

Hypothyroid patients with normally located and normally sized glands have defects in thyroid hormone biosynthesis. Recessive mutations in thyroglobulin, thyroid peroxidase, pendrin (causing Pendred syndrome – sensorineural deafness and hypothyroidism) and sodium/iodide symporter (*NIS*) genes have been described. Mutations in the TRH receptor gene, TSH β subunit and transcription factors regulating pituitary development have also been described in some individuals with central hypothyroidism.

### Clinical picture

Often the condition is subclinical and is detected on routine screening. Clinical features that should be looked for are jaundice, dry skin, a hoarse cry, puffy face, prominent tongue, listlessness, umbilical hernia, hypothermia, bradycardia and failure to thrive.

### Investigation results

An unconjugated hyperbilirubinaemia (due to glucuronyl transferase deficiency) is common. A raised level of TSH detected on testing of a heel-prick drop of blood collected on filter paper on day 3–5 of life is seen in primary hypothyroidism.

### Management

Confirmatory investigations are needed if the screening tests suggest an abnormality: repeat $T_4$ and TSH; thyroid scan (showing absent, lingual or increased uptake of radioisotope), X-ray distal femoral epiphysis (absence implying prolonged/prenatal hypothyroidism), and assessment and imaging of the pituitary gland if indicated. Treatment involves commencement of therapy (thyroxine replacement at 8–10 μg/kg daily). Thyroid imaging results for congenital hypothyroidism of varying causes are shown in Figure 19.2.1.

### Prognosis

Normal intellectual and physical development is likely if treatment is commenced promptly and monitored closely. Overtreatment may result in craniosynostosis.

## Acquired

Acquired hypothyroidism in the child or adolescent is relatively uncommon. In iodine-sufficient regions of the world the most common cause is autoimmune

**Table 19.2.1 Mutations in genes involved in thyroid development resulting in congenital hypothyroidism**

| Gene | Thyroid gland imaging | Clinical features | Genetics | Comments |
|---|---|---|---|---|
| *PAX-8* | Hypoplastic and cystic | Mild to moderate CH | Autosomal dominant | |
| *TTF-2* | Thyroid agenesis | Developmental delay, cleft palate, choanal atresia, spiky hair | Familial | Rare 'Bamforth syndrome' |
| *NKX2.1/TTF-1* | Normal, hypoplastic, agenesis | CH, lung disease, hypotonia, developmental delay and choreoathetosis | Sporadic; heterozygous loss-of-function mutations | Poor neurological outcome despite thyroid replacement |
| *TSH-R* | Normal to severely hypoplastic; normally located | Compensated hypothyroidism to severe CH | Recessive, inactivating mutations in compound heterozygotes | Heterozygous carriers may be relatively common; activating mutations cause congenital hyperthyroidism |

CH, congenital hypothyroidism; TSH-R, TSH receptor; TTF, thyroid transcription factor.

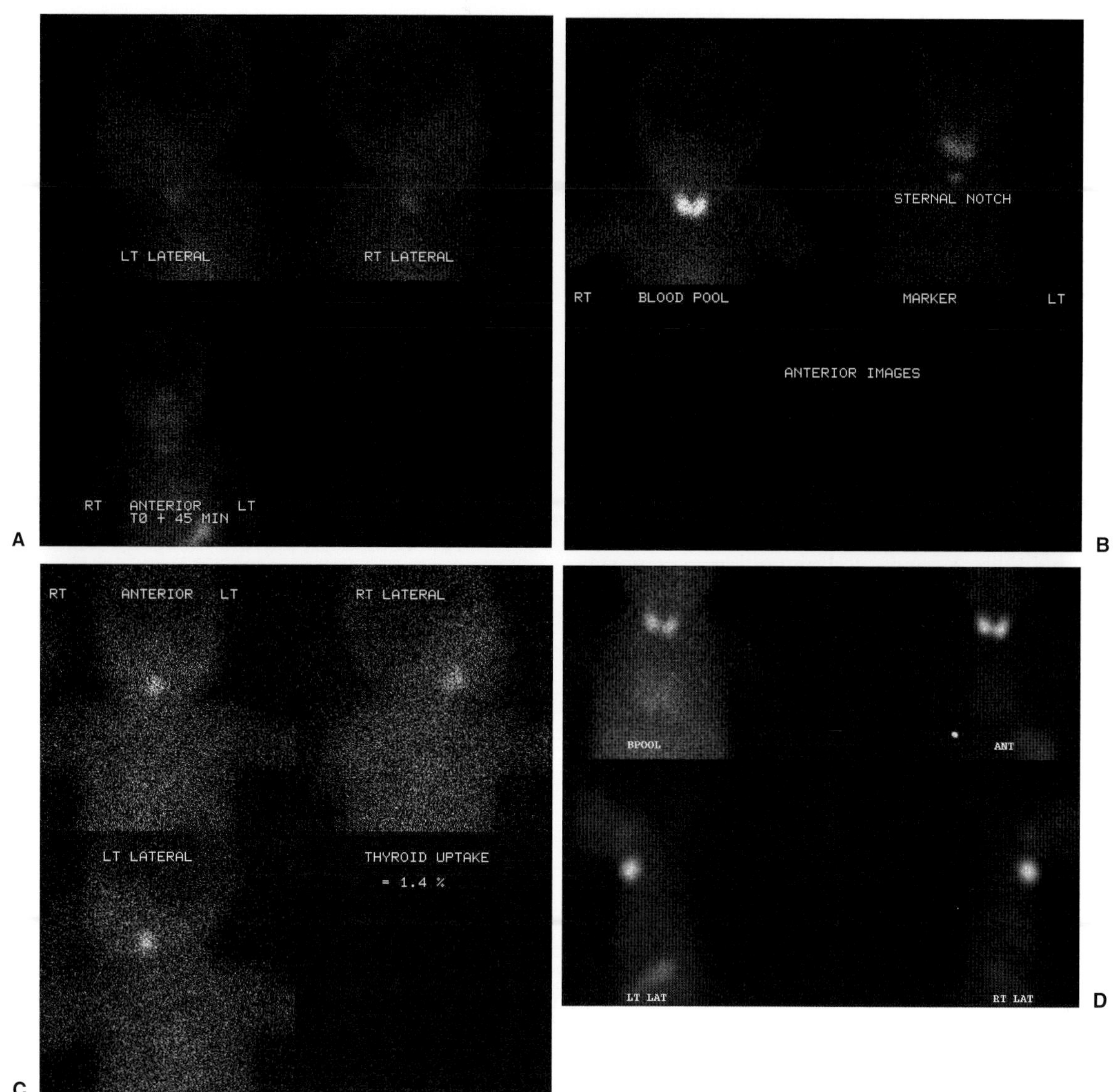


Fig. 19.2.1 Thyroid uptake scan appearances in congenital hypothyroidism. (**A**) Thyroid agenesis. No functioning thyroid tissue present in the neck or in the usual ectopic sites. (**B**) Dyshormonogenesis. The radioangiogram reveals relatively increased thyroid perfusion. The uptake of pertechnetate in 20 min is 14% (normal = 2–5%). The thyroid scan reveals a diffuse goitre normally located in the neck. (**C**) Lingual thyroid. There is no evidence of perfused thyroid tissue in the neck. The thyroid scan reveals a prominent midline lingual thyroid. The uptake of pertechnetate in 20 min is 1% (normal = 2–5%). (**D**) Normal thyroid. The radioangiogram of the head, neck and upper torso is unremarkable. The uptake of pertechnetate in 20 min is 5% (normal = 2–5%). The thyroid scan reveals a normally located bilobed gland.

thyroiditis. Accordingly, acquired hypothyroidism is seen twice as commonly in females as in males, usually manifesting in early puberty.

## Prevalence

Between the ages of 1 and 18 years, the prevalence is 1.2%. Acquired hypothyroidism is rare prior to 4 years of age.

## Aetiology

The causes in order of frequency are as follows: primary hypothyroidism – chronic lymphocytic, autoimmune (Hashimoto) thyroiditis, late-appearing congenital dyshormonogenesis, exogenous factors (e.g. high-dose iodine exposure (Wolff–Chaikoff effect), radiation) and severe iodine deficiency; and central hypothyroidism – congenital and acquired hypopituitarism.

### Clinical picture

The most common presentation is growth retardation and goitre. In addition, the triad of short stature, obesity and mental dullness indicates hypothyroidism until proven otherwise. Growth impairment usually affects mainly the limbs so that body proportions predominantly remain infantile. Other features include hypothermia, bradycardia, slow reflex relaxation, constipation, dry hair and skin, pallor, facial puffiness ('myxoedema') and dental delay. The onset is often insidious, with delays of up to 4–5 years being reported between the onset of growth retardation and the diagnosis of hypothyroidism. Although delayed puberty usually occurs, some cases of precocious puberty have been reported.

Autoimmune thyroiditis may be associated with other autoimmune diseases (autoimmune polyglandular syndromes) such as type 1 diabetes, autoimmune adrenalitis (Addison disease), vitiligo and pernicious anaemia. Occasionally, autoimmune hypothyroidism can be preceded by a period of transient hyperthyroidism.

### Investigation results

Goitre (detected either clinically or sonographically) is common in acquired hypothyroidism. Blood tests show a low circulating $T_4$ and (usually) a high circulating TSH level. Bone age is delayed and there may be positive thyroid autoantibodies (in autoimmune thyroiditis). There is patchy uptake of isotope on thyroid scan (in autoimmune thyroiditis). Hypothalamic or pituitary anomalies may be seen on computed tomography (CT) or magnetic resonance imaging (MRI) (in tertiary or secondary disease).

### Management

Replacement thyroxine (usually 50–100 µg/day in a single dose) is required. An appropriate individual dose is determined by measuring serum TSH at 6 or more weeks after commencing therapy.

### Prognosis

Severely hypothyroid children often show dramatic clinical changes with treatment. These include: weight loss, rapid growth, loss of primary teeth, some transient hair loss and increased energy/alertness. The long-term neurodevelopmental outcome is good, given that the rapid growth phase of the brain in the first 2 years of life has usually been protected. Despite short-term rapid catch-up growth, restoration of full growth potential often does not occur, because of rapid advancement of bone age in the first 18 months of treatment. Long-term treatment is usually required.

## Hyperthyroidism

### Congenital

This is always due to maternal thyrotoxicosis and is a rare clinical event. However, if unrecognized and untreated, neonatal hyperthyroidism may be fatal.

### Incidence

Maternal thyrotoxicosis is uncommon (1–2 cases per 1000 pregnancies). Neonatal disease occurs in 1 per 70 cases of pregnancies affected by thyrotoxicosis.

### Aetiology

Neonatal hyperthyroidism is the result of the transplacental passage of TSH receptor-stimulating antibodies from a mother with either active or inactive Graves disease. Measurement of maternal antibody status, rather than thyroxine levels, is predictive of the likelihood of neonatal hyperthyroidism.

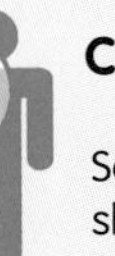

**Clinical example**

Sarah had been struggling at school ever since she started year 7. At the age of 13 years, her parents had become concerned that she was having difficulty settling into her new school as she was always complaining of feeling tired and having 'tummy pains'. Sarah's parents were at a loss to explain why she was behaving this way as she was a good student at primary school and had lots of friends. More recently Sarah's parents had noted that her weight had increased dramatically (they attributed this to her lack of activity, as she didn't seem to eat all that much), so much so that she now had a very 'fat' neck. She was also complaining of feeling cold all the time and was constantly wearing extra clothes even when the weather was warm. Her parents were concerned that she had a body image problem as a consequence of her recent weight gain. The school counsellor felt that Sarah might be depressed and her parents were most concerned.

On examination Sarah was moderately overweight with cool hands and she had a resting pulse rate of 50 bpm. She had dry hair and skin. She had a smooth, uniformly enlarged thyroid gland. Her reflexes showed a markedly delayed relaxation phase.

Investigations revealed that Sarah had a serum TSH level of 35 IU/mL (high) associated with a $T_4$ of 5 nmol/L (low). Her bone age was equivalent to that of 10 years and a plain X-ray of her abdomen showed faecal loading. Her antithyroid microsomal antibody titre was positive.

Sarah was commenced on 100 µg thyroxine per day. Within 2 weeks she was reporting much improved energy levels and affect. At 1-month review she had lost 5 kg in weight, her school performance had improved and her goitre was showing some signs of shrinkage.

### Clinical picture

Neonates may present with any of the following: irritability, poor weight gain, tachycardia, cardiac arrhythmias, flushing, hypertension, goitre, exomphalos, jaundice and hepatosplenomegaly. Although presentation soon after birth is more common, if the mother has been taking antithyroid drugs, presentation may be delayed until day 8–9 after birth, when the antithyroid medication has been eliminated from the neonate's circulation.

### Investigation results

High circulating $T_4$ or $T_3$ levels and low TSH levels are detected in the neonatal blood sample.

### Management

Immediately after diagnosis, sedation and treatment with either beta-blockade or digoxin may be required. Subsequent treatment with antithyroid medication (carbimazole, methimazole) is usually required. A therapeutic response should be seen within 24–36 hours after commencing treatment. Owing to concerns regarding hepatotoxicity, first-line treatment with propylthiouracil in childhood is no longer recommended.

### Prognosis

Mortality rates of up to 25% have been reported. The half-life of thyroid-stimulating antibodies in the fetal circulation is approximately 12 days; however, the clinical course may extend for a period of up to 12 weeks.

## Acquired

Hyperthyroidism in childhood and adolescence is less common than either euthyroid goitre or hypothyroidism. As with acquired hypothyroidism, it is most commonly due to autoimmune disease and is usually seen in young adolescent females.

### Incidence

Females are affected 6–8 times more commonly than males. Some ethnic groups (such as Asian females) have a greater reported incidence of autoimmune hyperthyroidism.

### Aetiology

Autoimmune hyperthyroidism (Graves disease) is the most common form of acquired hyperthyroidism in childhood and adolescence. Less frequent causes include the acute toxic phase of autoimmune hypothyroidism (Hashimoto disease; hashitoxicosis) and a toxic thyroid nodule (rare). There is often a family history of autoimmune thyroid disease (either Graves or Hashimoto disease). The primary defect is the presence of stimulating autoantibodies (thyroid receptor antibodies) that mimic the action of TSH. Overstimulation of the TSH receptor leads to thyroid growth and excess thyroxine production. There is often an associated ophthalmopathy due to the deposition of proteoglycans in the extraocular muscles and retro-orbital spaces.

### Clinical picture

The clinical features of hyperthyroidism result from sympathetic drive causing a hypermetabolic state. Many of the florid signs of thyrotoxicosis that are seen in adults are less pronounced in children. Symptoms include deteriorating school performance, weakness/fatigue, restlessness/sleeplessness, polyuria, hunger, heat intolerance, excessive sweating, anxiety and diarrhoea and weight loss. Clinical signs include: goitre or localized thyroid mass, tremor, tachycardia and brisk reflexes. Approximately 30% of children will have associated proptosis and other signs of thyroidal ophthalmopathy (lid lag, lid retraction and ophthalmoplegia).

### Investigation results

Suppressed serum TSH levels are seen and are associated with increased $T_4$ or $T_3$ levels. There will also be raised levels of thyroid autoantibodies (TSH receptor antibody-positive in Graves disease). The bone age is advanced and there is sonographic evidence of thyromegaly. Generalized and localized increased uptake of isotope is seen in Graves disease and toxic adenoma respectively.

### Management

In the setting of autoimmune hyperthyroidism there are three treatment options. The first of these, antithyroid medication, is the most commonly used. Carbimazole and methimazole have traditionally been used most commonly in Australia and Europe, whereas propylthiouracil has been more commonly used in North America. Propylthiouracil is no longer recommended as first-line treatment because of the risk of severe hepatotoxicity. Both types of medication block organification and are similarly efficacious, with comparable side-effect profiles. Beta-blockade (with propranolol) may also be used in the first 2–4 weeks of therapy to gain symptom control. This is contraindicated in children who suffer from asthma. Treatment with organification blocking drugs is continued for 2 years in the first instance. Other treatment options include thyroidectomy (subtotal or total) and radioactive iodine. In the setting of toxic adenoma, surgery is usually the preferred treatment option.

### Prognosis

After 2 years of medical therapy, approximately 20–50% of patients can be expected to enter spontaneous remission, with resolution of thyroid autoantibody status. Among those patients who do not remit spontaneously, long-term drug therapy is both safe and effective. In the advent of poor compliance with medical therapy, lack of control or increasing thyromegaly, a second treatment option – surgical subtotal or complete thyroidectomy – is considered. This results in 20% of patients becoming euthyroid, 50% of patients becoming hypothyroid and 30% of patients becoming thyrotoxic in the long term. Other paediatric and adult centres use a third treatment option, that of radioactive iodine. This treatment results in total thyroid ablation and requires subsequent lifelong thyroxine replacement therapy.

**Clinical example**

Tina, aged 15, had noticed increasing anxiety levels recently. She was quite bright academically and had set high standards for herself at school. Her parents were concerned that her anxiety was associated with some recent difficulties in concentrating during classes. Her teachers complained that she 'fidgeted' all the time and was quite restless. Despite a healthy appetite ('she eats more than anyone else in the family') Tina had been losing weight and had frequent loose bowel actions. Her mother also reported that, despite it being winter, Tina refused to wear appropriate cold weather clothing, preferring a T-shirt most of the time.

On examination, Tina appeared quite anxious and had very prominent eyes (proptosis). She had difficulty in sitting still on the examination couch and squirmed around quite a lot. Her resting pulse was 110 bpm and she had a fine tremor when her hands were held out. Her palms were very sweaty. She had a firm, smooth goitre with an audible bruit. Her reflexes were very brisk and she had difficulty standing from a squatting position.

A provisional diagnosis of Graves disease was made. This was confirmed by finding that Tina's serum TSH levels were unrecordably low in the face of a $T_4$ level of 52 nmol/L (high). Her anti-TSH receptor antibody titre was raised. Thyroid ultrasonography demonstrated a uniformly enlarged thyroid with no focal changes.

Tina was commenced initially on both carbimazole and propranolol. Her symptoms had largely abated within 3 weeks and her propranolol was ceased at this time. Ophthalmological review confirmed the presence of proptosis, with no other thyroidal eye signs being present. Over the following year Tina's goitre diminished in size; however, her proptosis remained unchanged. She was initially treated with carbimazole for 2 years. At this time she was still TSH receptor antibody-positive and it was decided to continue treatment for a further 2 years.

## Thyroid masses

### Goitre

The commonest cause of goitre on a worldwide basis remains iodine deficiency. In developed countries this had become rare until recent times, with the iodization of table salt and some infant milks. Recently, iodine deficiency has been reported again in Australian populations, presumably due to low-salt diets encouraged for cardiovascular health reasons.

#### Incidence

Goitres or diffuse enlargement of the thyroid gland occur in 4–5% of all children. They are more common in girls during puberty and are often not detected.

#### Aetiology

In Australia the main causes in order of frequency are: Hashimoto thyroiditis (majority are euthyroid), Graves disease, mild dyshormonogenesis, tumour (benign/malignant), acute/subacute thyroiditis and iodine deficiency. Foods that inhibit thyroxine synthesis and can lead to goitre (goitrogens) include cabbage, soybeans and cassava.

#### Clinical picture

Most often the goitre is asymptomatic and is frequently detected on routine examination undertaken for other reasons. Thyroid hypofunction or hyperfunction will present with the signs and symptoms described above. Occasionally, pressure symptoms related to the enlarged thyroid (dysphagia, stridor or neck discomfort) may be the presenting feature. Thyroidal tenderness is seen in acute/subacute thyroiditis. Regional lymphadenopathy associated with a goitre or thyroid nodule is suggestive of malignancy and is an ominous sign.

#### Investigation results

Sonography, serum thyroid function tests and serum thyroid antibody levels will distinguish most causes of goitre. Fasting urinary iodine levels will also help to define iodine status. Thyroid scanning will show increased uptake with mild dyshormonogenesis and patchy distribution in Hashimoto thyroiditis.

#### Management

Smoothly enlarged goitres with normal thyroid function can be managed simply by observation and iodine supplementation if required. Goitres with functional consequences will require either thyroxine supplementation or suppressive medication.

### Prognosis

This depends on the cause of the goitre. As most cases of asymptomatic goitre result in no disturbance of thyroid function, the prognosis is usually good.

## Thyroid nodules

Nodules within the thyroid gland are palpable, localized swellings. They may be single or multiple. The Chernobyl nuclear reactor disaster in 1986 led to a markedly increased incidence of benign and malignant thyroid nodules in children from the surrounding iodine-deficient areas.

### Incidence

Fewer than 2% of children have thyroid nodules. Of these, approximately 2% are malignant. If the nodule is single the risk of malignancy increases to 30–40%, higher than in adults.

### Aetiology

Benign nodules include cysts, cystic adenomas and variations of Hashimoto thyroiditis. Malignant nodules are carcinomas and occur in the following order: papillary/mixed, follicular, medullary and anaplastic. In one series of children with thyroid cancers reported in the 1950s, 80% had a history of having received head/neck radiotherapy. However, head/neck irradiation is now used less commonly and the aetiology of most thyroid cancers remains obscure. Radiation-exposed children need close follow-up, and regular ultrasound surveillance substantially increases the detection of thyroid malignancy. Medullary carcinomas may be sporadic, familial (autosomal dominant mode of inheritance) or part of a multiple endocrine neoplasia (MEN2) complex. Patients with MEN2 have been found to have mutations in the *RET* proto-oncogene.

### Clinical picture

The most common presentation is the lobular, irregular thyroid gland seen in Hashimoto thyroiditis. Nodules are usually asymptomatic and are often detected coincidentally upon routine examination. Rarely, nodules may be hyperfunctional ('toxic adenoma'). Medullary carcinomas may be associated with phaeochromocytoma (in later life) and parathyroid hyperplasia (MEN2A), or multiple mucosal neuromas, Marfan-like habitus and phaeochromocytoma (MEN2B). It is very rare for children with MEN2 to present with clinical disease. They are usually detected as part of a kindred subjected to genetic screening.

### Investigations

Nodules may be detected both sonographically and by thyroid scanning. The finding of multiple hot nodules associated with positive thyroid antibody titres and/or disturbed thyroid function is against a diagnosis of malignancy. Alternatively, a single cold nodule with or without serum calcitonin levels (associated with medullary carcinomas) is suggestive of malignancy. Fineneedle aspiration is not widely used in the diagnosis of thyroid nodules in children.

### Management

If there is any doubt as to the nature of any thyroid nodule it is appropriate to proceed to open biopsy. Solitary benign nodules are usually excised. Papillary thyroid cancers are treated with total thyroid excision, with subsequent radioactive iodine therapy if metastases are thought to be present. Medullary thyroid cancers are unresponsive to radioactive iodine and early total thyroidectomy remains the treatment of choice. In individuals with *RET* proto-oncogene mutations from families with a strong history of medullary carcinomas, prophylactic thyroidectomy is considered.

### Prognosis

Most thyroid nodules are benign and have an excellent prognosis. In the case of papillary carcinomas, serial thyroid scans for the first 3 years after surgery will detect any residual thyroid tissue or tumour recurrence. In patients suffering from medullary carcinomas, serial measures of serum calcitonin levels are the monitoring strategy of choice.

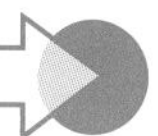

**Practical points**

- Normal thyroid function is essential for normal growth and development.
- Thyroid disorders are common and affect up to 2% of children and adolescents.
- Neonatal screening for congenital hypothyroidism allows early detection and treatment, resulting in normal development in the majority of affected infants.
- Symptoms of acquired hypothyroidism may be subtle in childhood and adolescence. Short stature may be the only presenting feature of hypothyroidism.
- Hyperthyroidism is much less common than hypothyroidism and non-specific associated symptoms may result in delay in diagnosis.
- Thyroid malignancy in isolated thyroid nodules is much more common in children than in adults.

## Summary

Disorders of the thyroid gland can have many manifestations: hypofunction, hyperfunction, pressure symptoms and incidental tumours. Given the importance of normal thyroid function for both neurological and physical development, and the potential for malignancy in thyroid nodules, a clinical awareness of potential thyroid problems in paediatrics is essential. Once detected, most thyroid problems can be successfully managed, with excellent clinical outcomes.

# 19.3 The child of uncertain sex

Jan Fairchild

Disorders of sexual development are congenital conditions in which the development of chromosomal, gonadal or phenotypic sex is atypical. This includes infants with a genital appearance that does not permit gender assignment:

- bilateral non-palpable testes
- perineal hypospadias with a bifid scrotum
- hypospadias and unilateral non-palpable gonad
- clitoromegaly
- posterior labial fusion
- a phenotypical female with a palpable gonad
- and those with discordant genitalia and sex chromosomes.

The birth of a child with a disorder of sexual development presents a psychosocial crisis for the family and may indicate an underlying medical condition such as congenital adrenal hyperplasia, which could be life-threatening if undiagnosed and untreated.

Disorders of sexual development (DSDs) are rare (1 in 4500), often complex, and always require urgent expert consultation. Optimal care requires an experienced multidisciplinary team.

## Normal sexual differentiation

An understanding of normal sexual differentiation is essential in the evaluation of the child with a disorder of sexual development. Normal sexual development in the embryo consists of three related sequential processes:

1. Establishment of chromosomal sex at fertilization, with XY as male and XX as female
2. Determination of gonadal sex, when the bipotential gonad develops into a testis or an ovary
3. Development of phenotypic sex, as a result of gonadal differentiation and gonadal hormone production.

### Internal genitalia

Up until about 7 weeks, male and female embryos develop in an identical fashion, with bipotential gonads and both wolffian and müllerian internal genital ducts present (Fig. 19.3.1).

In males, the presence of the sex-determining region on the Y chromosome (*SRY* gene) directs the bipotential gonad to become a testis. At least four other genes are also required for normal testicular development. By 7–8 weeks the testis has recognizable tubules and starts producing androgens, including testosterone from the Leydig cells and müllerian-inhibiting substance (MIS) from the Sertoli cells. Circulating hormone levels are low and masculinization of the internal genital ducts occurs by locally acting (exocrine) secretion of these hormones down the wolffian duct.

High levels of testosterone promote the ipsilateral development of the wolffian duct to become the epididymis, vas deferens and seminal vesicle. High levels of MIS lead to ipsilateral müllerian duct regression. This process occurs during a critical period between 8 and 12 weeks. The Leydig cells also produce a relaxin-like factor that, together with MIS and androgens, masculinizes the gubernaculum. The gubernaculum holds the testis near the inguinal ligament during early development and from 25 weeks it begins to elongate, steering the testis towards the scrotum.

**Clinical example**

A healthy, full-term infant was born with ambiguous genitalia. On examination there was an enlarged clitoris (2 cm in length), posterior fusion of the labia, with a single opening visible, and no gonads were palpable. The genitalia were noted to be hyperpigmented. There was no history of consanguinity but a previous male sibling had died at 2 weeks of age after a vomiting illness.

Initial investigations confirmed that the baby's chromosomes were 46,XX and pelvic ultrasonography showed the presence of a normal uterus and ovaries. The 17-hydroxyprogesterone level at 48 hours of age was markedly increased, confirming the diagnosis of congenital adrenal hyperplasia due to 21-hydroxylase deficiency. Treatment with hydrocortisone was commenced. Daily electrolytes were normal until the 6th day of life, when hyperkalaemia developed, confirming the salt-wasting form of the condition. Fludrocortisone therapy was then added. The child was referred to a paediatric surgeon for consideration of corrective genital surgery. She will require lifelong replacement therapy and monitoring.

The hyperpigmentation was due to the adrenocorticotrophic hormone (ACTH) excess and resolved with adequate replacement therapy. It was likely that the previous male sibling had also had the condition, as it is inherited as an autosomal recessive trait. The genitalia of affected males are usually normal at birth apart from some hyperpigmentation, and affected male infants typically present with a salt-wasting crisis in the first few weeks of life. It is often confused with pyloric stenosis, which also presents at this age with vomiting and dehydration.

In females, the absence of testosterone and MIS leads to wolffian duct regression and müllerian duct preservation. The müllerian ducts develop into the uterus, fallopian tubes and upper vagina.

## External genitalia

Up until about 8 weeks, the external genitalia of male and female embryos also have an identical appearance. Both sexes have a genital tubercle, two genital swellings and two genital folds (Fig. 19.3.2).

In males, between 8 and 12 weeks, androgen action on the external genitalia results in the development of normal male genitalia. Circulating levels of testosterone are insufficient for this action but testosterone is converted in the periphery to dihydrotestosterone (DHT) by the enzyme 5α-reductase. Dihydrotestosterone binds to the androgen receptors much more strongly than testosterone, thereby amplifying its effect. The genital tubercle develops into the glans penis, the genital swellings fuse

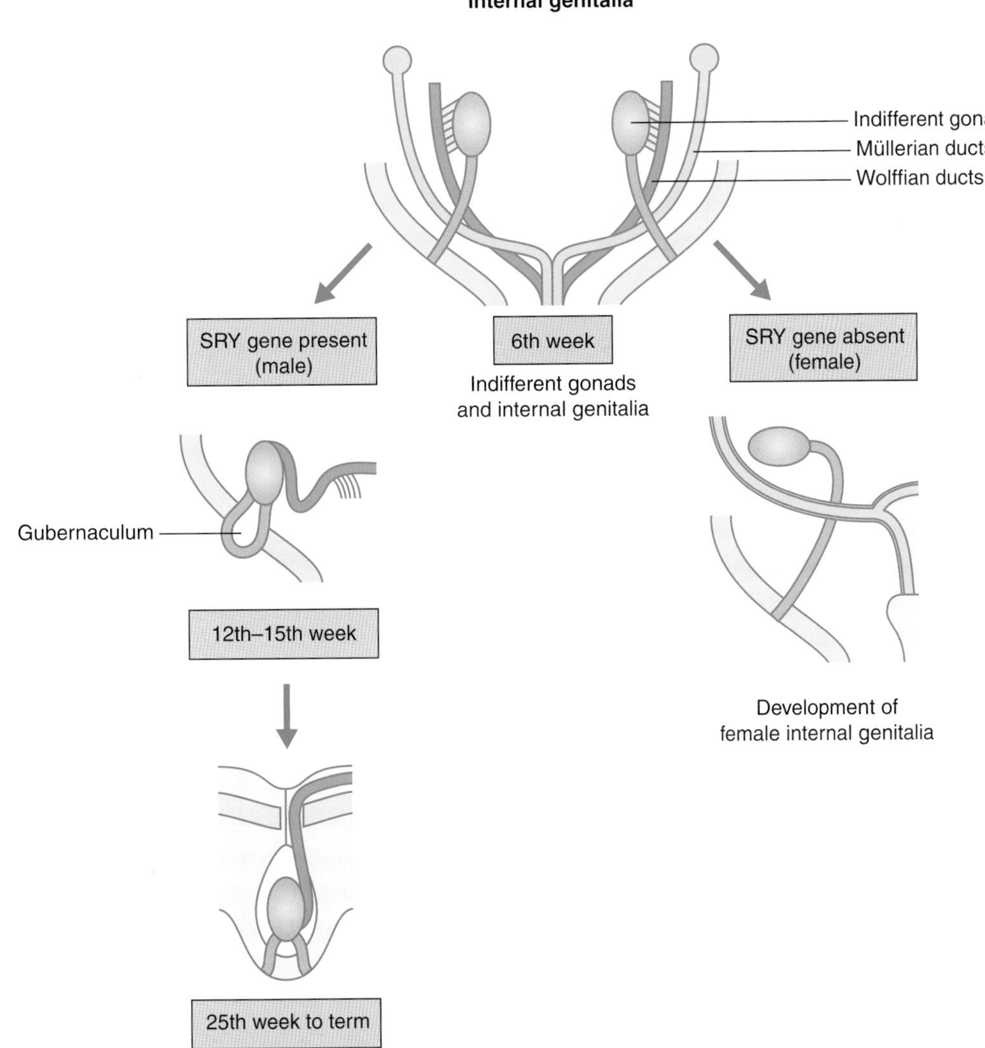


Fig. 19.3.1 Normal prenatal development: internal genitalia.

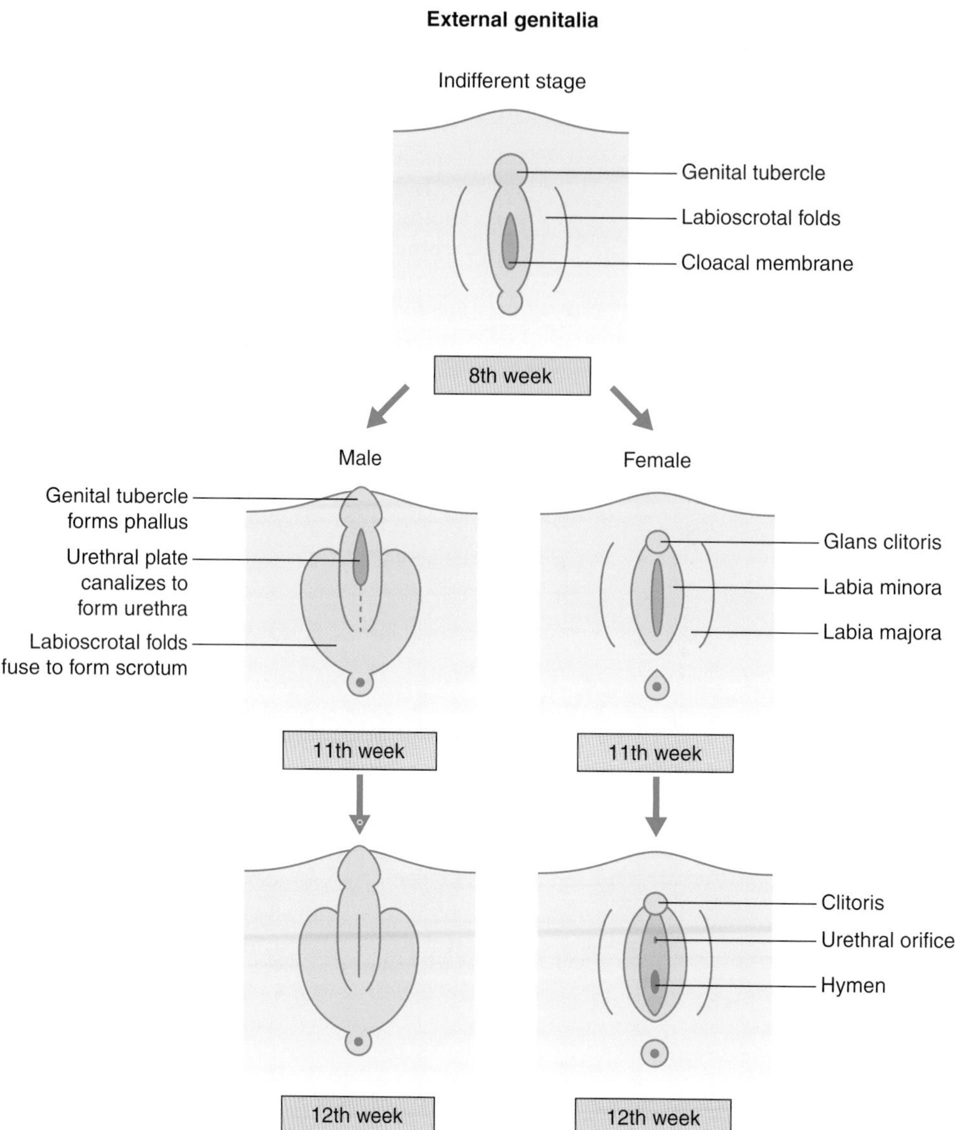


Fig. 19.3.2 Normal prenatal development: external genitalia.

to form the scrotum, and the genital folds elongate and fuse to become the shaft of the penis and the penile urethra. The prostate forms in the wall of the urogenital sinus. With the exception of the phallus, circulating androgens masculinize the external genitalia only during a critical period between 8 and 12 weeks.

In females, in the absence of androgen, the genital tubercle forms the glans clitoris and the short female urethra. The genital swellings remain unfused and become the labia majora. The genital folds become the labia minora and the vaginal plate, a thickening of the posterior wall of the urogenital sinus, canalizes to form the lower vagina.

## Evaluation of the child with a disorder of sexual development

The initial evaluation of the child with a disorder of sexual development should include a history, physical examination, urgent karyotype, ultrasound imaging of the internal anatomy, and assessment of adrenal and gonadal function.

### History

A careful history should include:

- prenatal exposure to androgens
- maternal virilization during pregnancy

- family history of females who are childless or have amenorrhoea (complete androgen insensitivity)
- family history of unexplained infant deaths (congenital adrenal hyperplasia)
- consanguinity.

### Physical examination

The physical examination should include:

- careful inspection of the external genitalia and palpation to determine the presence, location and symmetry of the gonads
  - if both gonads are palpable and symmetrical they are almost always testes
  - gonadal asymmetry implies one testis present, suggesting a mixed chromosomal pattern
  - if both gonads are impalpable, the gonadal and duct status is unknown.
- standardized measurement of the phallus
  - a normal term male infant has a stretched penile length of ≥2.5 cm
  - a normal term female infant has a clitoral length ≤9 mm
- general examination looking for:
  - dysmorphic features or non-genital abnormalities that may point to a specific disorder
  - hyperpigmentation and/or systemic illness which may suggest congenital adrenal hyperplasia.

**Clinical example**

A full-term infant with normal birth weight (3.1 kg) was noted to have a small penis (stretched penile length 1.5 cm, normal >2.5 cm) and undescended testes. Karyotype was 46,XY. The infant had had two episodes of hypoglycaemia treated with intravenous dextrose and on general examination was noted to have a small cleft in the palate. Hypoglycaemia is unusual in a full-term infant of normal birth weight, and in the presence of a midline defect raises the possibility of hypopituitarism. A diagnostic blood sample taken at the time of the hypoglycaemia revealed low levels of cortisol, growth hormone and free thyroxine, confirming the diagnosis. The baby was commenced on hydrocortisone and thyroxine with resolution of the hypoglycaemia. He was given a short course of testosterone at 6 months of age, which resulted in an increase in his penile length to 2.5 cm. Growth hormone therapy was commenced when his growth rate slowed at 12 months of age.

Micropenis and cryptorchidism can occur with either gonadotrophin deficiency or growth hormone deficiency and is a useful clinical sign of congenital hypopituitarism in male infants.

### Initial investigations

The initial investigations that should be undertaken are:

- urgent karyotype, including fluorescence *in situ* hybridization (FISH) with *SRY* probe – this permits classification of the infant into one of three diagnostic categories and determines further evaluation
- ultrasonography to determine the presence of gonads, uterus and vagina
- investigations to exclude congenital adrenal hyperplasia:
  - serum electrolytes and blood glucose series
  - serum 17-hydroxyprogesterone and other adrenal steroids.

### Further evaluation

This will be guided by the initial investigations and may include:

- evaluation of adrenal function with an ACTH stimulation test and assessment of urinary steroid profile
- evaluation of gonadal function with MIS, gonadotrophins, sex steroids and a human chorionic gonadotrophin (hCG) stimulation test to confirm a normal rise in gonadal hormones with stimulation, with the testosterone/DHT ratio reflecting 5α-reductase activity
- surgical procedures: genital skin biopsies for androgen receptor assay, panendoscopy and/or laparotomy to delineate internal genitalia ± gonadal biopsy.

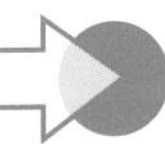

**Practical points**

**Initial evaluation of the child with a disorder of sexual development**

- History: androgen exposure, family history of DSD or infant deaths, consanguinity.
- Examination: determine the presence of palpable gonads, hyperpigmentation, systemic illness, non-genital abnormalities.
- Investigations: include an urgent karyotype, assessment of adrenal secretion, ultrasonography to assess internal anatomy.
- Assignment to one of the three diagnostic categories will determine further evaluation: virilized XX, undervirilized XY or mixed chromosome pattern.

## Diagnostic categories for disorders of sexual development

The results of the karyotype, in particular the sex chromosomes, will allow the infant to be classified into one of three diagnostic categories which will determine further evaluation:

- virilized XX
- undervirilized XY
- mixed chromosome pattern.

### Virilized XX

In the virilized XX child, the gonads are ovaries and the internal genitalia are female; therefore no gonads are palpable (Fig. 19.3.3). The external genitalia are virilized to a variable degree, from mild clitoromegaly to complete labial fusion with urethral tubularization to the tip of the enlarged phallus (Fig. 19.3.4). If the exposure occurred after 12 weeks there will be isolated clitoromegaly without labial fusion.

Causes of the virilized XX state may be:

- androgen excess from the fetal adrenals:
  - congenital adrenal hyperplasia (most common cause)
- androgen excess from the mother:
  - maternal ingestion of androgens
  - androgen-producing tumour
  - placental aromatase deficiency.

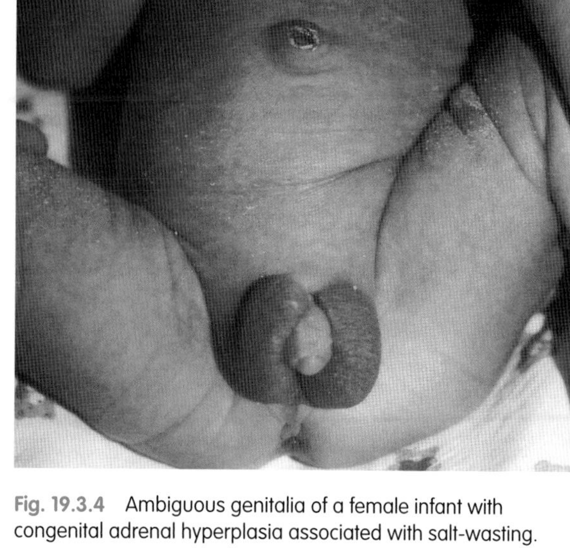

Fig. 19.3.4 Ambiguous genitalia of a female infant with congenital adrenal hyperplasia associated with salt-wasting.

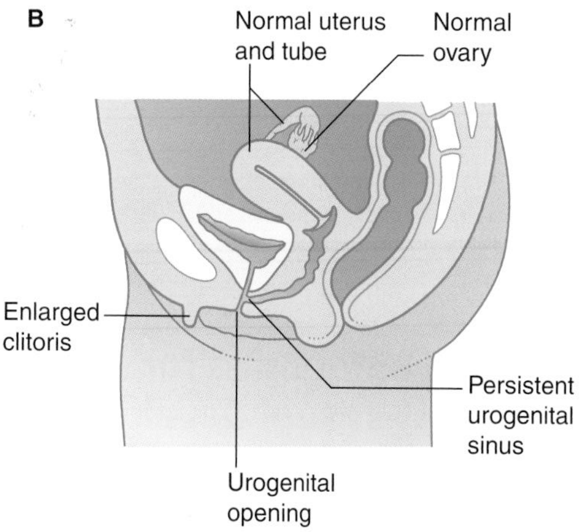


Fig. 19.3.3 Schematic illustration of normal and ambiguous female genitalia as in congenital adrenal hyperplasia. Note the urogenital sinus leading to a single opening and the enlarged clitoris induced by androgens. (Adapted from Moore and Persaud, 1993.)

### Undervirilized XY

The undervirilized XY child usually presents with a small phallus, posterior hypospadias, poorly developed, bifid scrotum and testicular maldescent.

The causes of the undervirilized XY state may be:

- inadequate androgen production:
  - hypoplastic testes (luteinizing hormone (LH) deficiency)
  - dysplastic testes
  - testosterone synthesis defects
  - inability to convert testosterone to DHT ($5\alpha$-reductase deficiency)
- impaired response to androgen:
  - androgen insensitivity syndrome.

#### Clinical example

A 16-year-old girl presented for investigation of primary amenorrhea. On examination she was found to be a tall girl for her family. She had breast development at stage 5 but sparse pubic hair (stage 2–3) and no axillary hair. She also had an inguinal mass, which was occasionally painful when knocked during sport. Investigations revealed a 46,XY karyotype, no uterus on pelvic ultrasonography and serum levels of testosterone characteristic of normal men.

A diagnosis of complete androgen insensitivity was made. Gonadectomy was performed as there is a high incidence of germ cell cancer and oestrogen replacement therapy was commenced. Psychological support was important in helping her come to terms with the diagnosis.

### Mixed chromosomal pattern

#### Ovotesticular disorder of sexual development

In ovotesticular DSD, both testicular and ovarian tissues coexist. The gonads are usually ovary and testis, or ovary and ovotestis. The chromosomes are usually 46,XX, although 46,XY mosaicism can occur. Asymmetry of the gonads, internal and external genitalia is the hallmark of this condition.

#### Mixed gonadal dysgenesis

In mixed gonadal dysgenesis there is also gonadal asymmetry with a testis on one side and a streak gonad on the other. The testis may be dysgenetic and the streak gonad usually contains ovarian stroma without oocytes. The chromosomes are commonly 45,XO/46,XY, and these infants may have the phenotypic features of Turner syndrome, but other mosaic patterns can occur. The risk of gonadoblastoma is high in dysgenetic testes and gonadectomy in the first decade of life is recommended.

### DSD with unambiguous genitalia

It is important to note that some patients with DSD have unambiguous genitalia. These patients have complete sex reversal with a phenotype the reverse of what would be expected from their genotype. Examples of this would be an XY child with complete gonadal dysgenesis or complete androgen insensitivity syndrome.

DSD may be missed if the diagnosis of hypospadias is made without due care. This diagnosis should never be made without full investigations, unless both testes are descended in a fused scrotum.

## Management

The birth of a child with a disorder of sexual development presents a unique set of challenging and often difficult management issues. A multidisciplinary team approach involving the paediatrician, paediatric endocrinologist, surgeon, geneticist, psychologist, social worker and adolescent gynaecologist is required for optimal management.

### Initial management

The initial management of the child with a disorder of sexual development requires attention to medical and psychosocial issues. Evaluation of the child must be carried out urgently, so that a decision about the sex of rearing can be made as quickly as possible and life-threatening medical conditions can be identified. Urgent expert consultation should always be sought.

The birth of a child with a disorder of sexual development is a psychosocial crisis for the family and must be handled sensitively. Every effort should be made to encourage the parents to bond with their baby. Gender assignment must be avoided before expert evaluation. The parents should be honestly informed that the sex their baby is meant to be is not yet known, but reassured that this will be determined as soon as possible. Instruct all staff to refer to the infant as 'your baby', not he, she or it. The parents will require guidance as to how to deal with family and friends, and the support of an experienced social worker or psychologist is invaluable. The parents should be advised not to name the baby or register the birth until sex assignment has been decided.

#### Congenital adrenal hyperplasia

The urgent medical issue is the exclusion of congenital adrenal hyperplasia and the attendant risk of adrenal crisis. Congenital adrenal hyperplasia is the most common cause of XX virilization and one of the causes of XY undervirilization. Serum electrolytes and blood glucose should be monitored closely and serum sent for urgent measurement of 17-hydroxyprogesterone and other adrenal steroids.

Congenital adrenal hyperplasia refers to a group of autosomal recessive disorders resulting from the deficiency of one of the five enzymes required for the synthesis of cortisol in the adrenal cortex. The most common enzyme deficiency is 21-hydroxylase deficiency, accounting for more than 90% of cases. The deficiency of cortisol results in ACTH-mediated adrenal hypertrophy and excessive production of cortisol precursors, which are diverted to the synthesis of androgens. Concomitant aldosterone deficiency leads to salt-wasting in 75% of cases.

Symptoms and signs of a salt-wasting adrenal crisis include vomiting, diarrhoea, hypovolaemia, hyponatraemia with hyperkalaemia, hypoglycaemia and cardiovascular collapse, and can occur within the first few days to weeks of life. If symptoms or signs of adrenal crisis are present, stress doses of hydrocortisone and intravenous fluid therapy with normal saline and 5% dextrose should be started immediately.

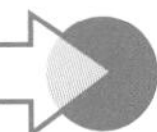

**Practical points**

**Management goals for the child with a disorder of sexual development**

- Gender assignment must be avoided before expert evaluation.
- An accurate and expeditious diagnosis is essential – and requires urgent expert consultation.
- Rational sex assignment is important.
- Therapy is directed towards achieving successful sex assignment.
- Psychological support for the family is required.
- Genetic counselling is an integral part of management.

### Gender issues

The issue of timing and approach to genital reconstruction is controversial and evolving. An evidence-based approach is hampered by the lack of long-term outcome studies involving large numbers of patients. Gender assignment and sex of rearing should be based on the most probable adult gender identity and potential for adult function. It involves consideration of the diagnosis, degree of virilization, capacity to respond to androgen, potential for adult sexual function and fertility as well as the parent's social and cultural background. There are no data demonstrating a link between early genital surgery and psychosexual orientation and, although early surgery may make life easier for the parents and the child, these irrevocable decisions may complicate the lives of adults. Decisions about sex of rearing and genital reconstruction should be made only by an informed family after careful evaluation and counselling by an experienced multidisciplinary team.

### Long-term management

Once gender has been assigned, every effort should be made to encourage the child's sex of rearing. Both the child and parents will benefit from long-term psychosocial support, and many individuals and their families derive benefit from support groups.

Specific management of the gonadal tissue in infants of uncertain sex may be required to reduce the risk of gonadal malignancy, torsion and infertility. Abdominal gonads bearing Y-chromosome material should be brought into the scrotum or removed surgically. The age of surgery will vary according to the underlying condition.

Sex steroid replacement should be provided consistent with the sex of rearing and age of the child to ensure adequate growth and pubertal development, and to prevent osteoporosis.

# Diabetes 19.4

Jennifer Couper, Timothy W. Jones

## Diabetes mellitus

Diabetes mellitus is caused by a deficiency in the secretion or action of insulin. It is one of the most common chronic diseases of childhood and adolescence, and causes considerable morbidity due to acute metabolic derangements and chronic, long-term microvascular and macrovascular complications. In childhood and adolescence the most common form of diabetes is type 1 diabetes (previously known as insulin-dependent diabetes). The incidence of type 1 diabetes has doubled over the last 20 years in Australia, now at 22 cases per 100 000 population. This trend is also seen in Europe and North America. The sex ratio is equal. Diabetes is uncommon in infancy. In parallel with the overweight and obesity epidemic, there has been increased recognition of type 2 diabetes in youth in Australia and New Zealand, especially in Aboriginal and Polynesian populations. Other less common forms of diabetes result from pancreatic disease (such as cystic fibrosis-related diabetes) and a rare group of specific genetic causes of deranged insulin secretion.

## Pathogenesis of type 1 diabetes

There are two major factors in the pathogenesis:

- genetic predisposition
- environmental triggers or protectors.

### Autoimmune destruction of beta cells

Type 1 diabetes is caused by autoimmune destruction of the beta cells (insulin-producing cells) of the islets of Langerhans. T-cell infiltration of the islets and circulating autoantibodies precede the development of diabetes by months to years. This preclinical phase, when blood glucose is normal and circulating antibodies to target antigens are present, provides clues for prevention or postponement of the onset of clinical diabetes. There is an increased frequency of certain HLA types (HLA DR3/DQ2 and DR4/DQ8) in type 1 diabetes.

Environmental factors that are potential candidates in the initiation or progression of autoimmunity include the heavier childhood population with associated insulin resistance, vitamin D insufficiency, and enteroviruses. Congenital rubella is a proven, very rare, environmental trigger.

## Metabolic effects of insulin

Insulin is the hormone of energy storage and anabolism. It allows glucose to enter cells and be stored as glycogen in the liver and muscle, and as triglyceride in fat. Insulin deficiency prevents glycogen and triglyceride storage and causes their breakdown, as well as that of protein. In addition, insulin deficiency promotes hepatic gluconeogenesis. The combined effect of glycogen breakdown, enhanced gluconeogenesis and failure of glucose entry into cells results in a rise in blood glucose levels. When the renal threshold is exceeded, glycosuria occurs. The osmotic effect of the glycosuria causes polyuria and eventually dehydration. Breakdown of triglyceride (lipolysis) releases free fatty acids into the circulation. In the liver these are converted to ketoacids (ketogenesis), with eventual development of ketoacidosis.

## Clinical presentation

When the autoimmune process has destroyed approximately 90% of the beta-cell mass, persistent hyperglycaemia causes the initial symptoms of polyuria, polydipsia, weight loss and fatigue. In routine practice, symptoms are usually present for 1–3 weeks before the diagnosis is made; however, a child with a suspected diagnosis of diabetes should be investigated immediately. A raised postprandial blood glucose to above 9 mmol/L may be detected months before symptoms develop and before the fasting blood glucose concentration rises.

As insulin deficiency progresses, diabetic ketoacidosis develops and, if not treated, results in death. Ketoacidosis initially causes vomiting and later, rapid, deep breathing (Kussmaul respiration). The hyperventilation is a compensatory mechanism to correct metabolic acidosis by removing carbon dioxide. Chemical breakdown of acetoacetic acid in the body yields acetone, which can be detected on the patient's

**Box 19.4.1 Type 1 diabetes: clinical features at presentation and useful investigations at diagnosis**

**Clinical presentation**
- Polyuria and polydipsia
- Enuresis and nocturia
- Weight loss and fatigue
- Thrush
- Vomiting (with increasing ketosis)
- Kussmaul breathing and coma (with increasing acidosis)

**Investigations**
- Urinalysis for glucose and ketones
- Random blood glucose (postprandial)
- Blood electrolytes and acid–base
- Blood or other cultures and blood count (if infection suspected)
- Islet antibodies (if type 2 diabetes suspected)

breath. Abdominal pain may mimic an acute surgical abdomen. Dehydration due to continuing urinary losses caused by the osmotic diuresis may progress to shock. The acidosis, dehydration and changes in plasma osmolality cause initial irritability, then confusion, drowsiness and eventually coma. A summary of the clinical features and useful investigations at the time of presentation of type 1 diabetes is presented in Box 19.4.1.

**Clinical example**

For 2 weeks, a mother noticed that her 4-year-old son, Harry, was irritable, thirsty and wetting the bed at night, having previously been dry. After being generally less well for 24 hours he became lethargic and began vomiting. On presentation at the emergency department, he was noted to be drowsy, dehydrated and had deep sighing respirations (Kussmaul breathing). The diagnosis of diabetic ketoacidosis was confirmed when he was found to have a blood glucose level of 22 mmol/L, blood ketones were 5.2 mmol/L, serum sodium 126 mmol/L, potassium 5.2 mmol/L, bicarbonate 10 mmol/L, pH 7.15 and the base deficit 26. He was treated with intravenous isotonic fluids, intravenous potassium and intravenous insulin.

Harry was discharged 4 days later, on two injections of insulin per day, a diabetes food plan and home blood glucose testing. During the hospital admission, his family received education from the diabetes educator and dietitian, and the education programme was continued on an outpatient basis. A community diabetes educator visited Harry's kindergarten to educate the staff about hypoglycaemia.

## Differential diagnoses

The diagnosis of type 1 diabetes in childhood is not usually difficult, provided the clinician is aware that this condition can occur even in the very young. The most common misdiagnoses are to mistake:

- polyuria for urinary frequency due to urinary tract infection
- the respiratory pattern of metabolic acidosis for a respiratory tract infection or asthma
- vomiting and abdominal pain for gastroenteritis or an acute abdomen.

Children with intercurrent infections, acute asthma or hypernatraemic dehydration may have transient hyperglycaemia and glycosuria that resolves with the intercurrent illness. Only very rarely do these children develop type 1 diabetes. Islet cell autoantibodies can be tested to determine whether the child is at risk of developing type 1 diabetes.

## Treatment of diabetic ketoacidosis

The aims of therapy are:

- emergency isotonic fluid replacement (10–20 mL per kg per h), if shock is present
- correction of dehydration slowly over 48 hours, using normal (isotonic or 0.9%) saline
- replacement of electrolyte losses and slow correction of acidosis: supplemental potassium of 40–60 mmol/L in intravenous fluids is required to maintain normal serum potassium levels after commencing insulin therapy
- correction of insulin deficiency with an infusion of soluble insulin.

Treatment should be undertaken in a centre equipped with paediatric intensive care facilities; the child may need to be transported there by an expert retrieval team. Frequent biochemical monitoring of the blood glucose, electrolytes and blood gases is required. The initial rate of insulin infusion is 0.1 unit per kg per h, and should be adjusted to produce a slow fall in the blood glucose level. Rapid reductions in the blood glucose or serum sodium concentration alter the plasma osmolality quickly and may increase the risks of the rare but life-threatening complication of cerebral oedema. Cerebral oedema is the commonest cause of death in children with diabetic ketoacidosis.

### Stabilization of newly diagnosed type 1 diabetes

When ketones clear, subcutaneous insulin is begun with regular food intake. Most children are stabilized on two to four daily injections of ultra-short- and intermediate- or long-acting insulins. Within days to weeks of the introduction of insulin, some recovery of the remaining viable beta cells may occur. During this period of partial remission (also known as the 'honeymoon' phase), insulin requirements fall. This phase may last for weeks or months but, as the underlying autoimmune destruction of beta cells is still in progress, insulin requirements eventually rise permanently. The process of islet destruction may continue for years, providing a potential window of opportunity to increase viable beta cells by immune modulation during the pre-clinical phase and the first years after diagnosis.

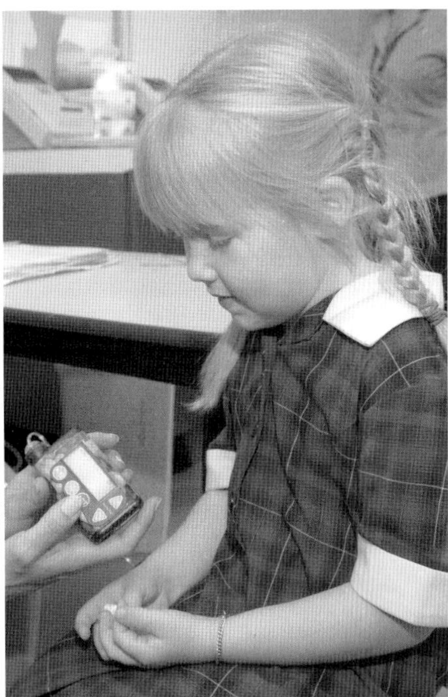

Fig. 19.4.1 Child with insulin pump.

## Management

### Aims of management

Type 1 diabetes is a permanent disorder. The long-term aims are for the child to achieve normal physical and psychological development, to lead a fulfilling life with as little restriction on lifestyle and occupation as possible, and to minimize the risk of long-term microvascular and macrovascular complications.

### Management principles

Because of the complexity of diabetes management, an interdisciplinary team is essential for adequate treatment of a child with diabetes. The team members should have expertise in both paediatric care and diabetes, and would normally include a paediatrician, diabetes nurse educator, dietitian, social worker and psychologist.

The adequacy of diabetes care to maintain good metabolic control during childhood is a crucial determinant of long-term outcomes. Good metabolic control is often difficult to achieve, especially in the age group under 5 years and in adolescents. The aim is to keep preprandial and postprandial blood glucose levels as close to normal as possible. Children are asked to measure their capillary blood glucose four or more times per day. The key influences on the blood glucose levels are:

- insulin
- diet
- exercise.

#### Insulin

Insulin therapy is individualized. Generally prepubertal children require around 0.8 units/kg body weight per day. Insulin is usually given as two to four subcutaneous injections daily or via a continuous subcutaneous insulin infusion (insulin pump) (Fig. 19.4.1). This requirement increases with more variability during puberty. Preschool children may be sensitive to short-acting insulin and, therefore, receive predominantly intermediate-acting insulin. Regimens using bolus doses of ultra-short-acting insulin analogue before meals and longer-acting insulin analogue before bed, or insulin pump regimens (basal insulin infusion subcutaneously and bolus doses of insulin with meals and snacks), are especially suitable for the adolescent needing more flexibility in the treatment schedule. These regimens and newer delivery systems improve metabolic control and reduce hypoglycaemia, provided compliance is excellent and there is accompanying blood glucose monitoring.

The dose of insulin is adjusted according to blood glucose measurements, anticipated carbohydrate intake, and exercise. Glycosylated haemoglobin (HbA1c) levels indicate the level of control during the preceding 6–8 weeks and provide the most meaningful guide when blood glucose levels are erratic. The target range for HbA1c is a value less than 7.5%, and has fallen considerably during the last 10 years. Target blood glucose levels are generally 4–8 mmol/L. Target HbA1c and blood glucose levels may need to be higher in preschool children or in children with a history of recurrent severe hypoglycaemia.

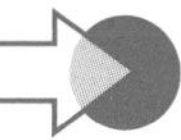

**Practical points**

**Poor metabolic control with high HbA1c**

- Is the prescribed insulin dose adequate?
- Is insulin omission a potential problem?
- Is food intake excessive or inappropriate?
- Consider education/dietary/psychological review.
- Consider an eating disorder, especially in girls.
- Consider increasing doses, changing insulin types and intensifying the insulin schedule if insulin omission is not a problem.

### Diet

Carbohydrate raises the blood glucose level, which must be balanced by the glucose-lowering effect of insulin and exercise. This balance is usually achieved by having the diet supply carbohydrate throughout the day in meals and snacks. However, toddlers usually have a grazing pattern of food intake and older adolescents may not need three snacks per day. Children and adolescents receiving insulin pump therapy have more flexibility with timing of meals and the amount of carbohydrate intake.

The usual diabetes diet is relatively high in complex carbohydrates, low in simple carbohydrates (sugar) and low in saturated fats. The glycaemic index is a classification of foods based on their postprandial blood glucose response and is a more predictable guide than merely measuring the carbohydrate content of foods. Individual and flexible food plans are essential to encourage adherence to the diet. It is also necessary to account for pre-existing family and cultural customs. Regular review by an experienced dietitian is necessary to cope with changing requirements as the child grows.

### Exercise

Exercise increases glucose uptake by the exercising muscles and lowers the blood glucose level. This effect is seen only if the diabetes is well controlled and serum levels of insulin are adequate (exercise undertaken during poor control and with low insulin levels may paradoxically raise blood glucose levels). To offset the hypoglycaemic effect of exercise, the child may need extra carbohydrate food or a small reduction in the preceding insulin dose. Regular exercise does not *per se* improve metabolic control, but may do so indirectly in some individuals by modifying appetite and by improving wellbeing and self-esteem.

## Outpatient management

For most children with diabetes, the initial hospitalization or day stay admission at diagnosis for stabilization and education is their only hospital admission. The early education programme can be provided by the diabetes educator and dietitian as an outpatient. Follow-up visits are usually every 3 months once the child is stabilized, to assess:

- general wellbeing
- history of hypoglycaemia
- home blood glucose monitoring
- insulin schedule
- food plan
- school progress
- height and weight
- injection sites
- size of the thyroid gland
- presence of skin infections
- signs of accompanying insulin resistance (increasing waist circumference, acanthosis nigricans).

The blood glucose profile is examined in the logbook kept by the patient, or downloaded from the patient's blood glucose monitor, and the adequacy of the dietary and insulin regimen is assessed. Continuous interstitial glucose monitoring (Fig. 19.4.2) may be useful for fine-tuning of the insulin schedule after a change to a new insulin schedule or insulin pump, or when there are concerns about undetectable nocturnal hypoglycaemia. The glycosylated haemoglobin (HbA1c) measures glycaemic control during the lifespan of the red cells (120 days). HbA1c can be measured in capillary blood within minutes in the outpatient clinic setting.

With the combined efforts of the family, the child and the diabetes management team, most children grow and develop normally, achieve their educational potential, and have a satisfying childhood and adolescence. However, fewer than 50% of children in Australia achieve target HbA1c levels below 7.5%.

### Co-morbidities

Several autoimmune disorders develop more frequently in type 1 diabetes. These are coeliac disease, autoimmune thyroid disease (which may result in hypothyroidism or hyperthyroidism) and rarely Addison's disease. Screening for these conditions is part of routine management.

### Long-term microvascular and macrovascular complications

Long-term vascular complications are:

- nephropathy
- retinopathy
- neuropathy
- cardiovascular disease
- peripheral vascular disease.

It is extremely rare for children and adolescents to show clinical signs of vascular complications, but subclinical signs may be detected from adolescence onwards. These form the basis of complication screening programmes and early intervention. It is recommended that from 5 years' duration of type 1 diabetes, the patient has an annual review including:

- measurement of resting blood pressure
- assessment of urinary albumin/creatinine ratio on an early morning sample
- fundoscopy on dilated pupils by an ophthalmologist, or retinal photography.

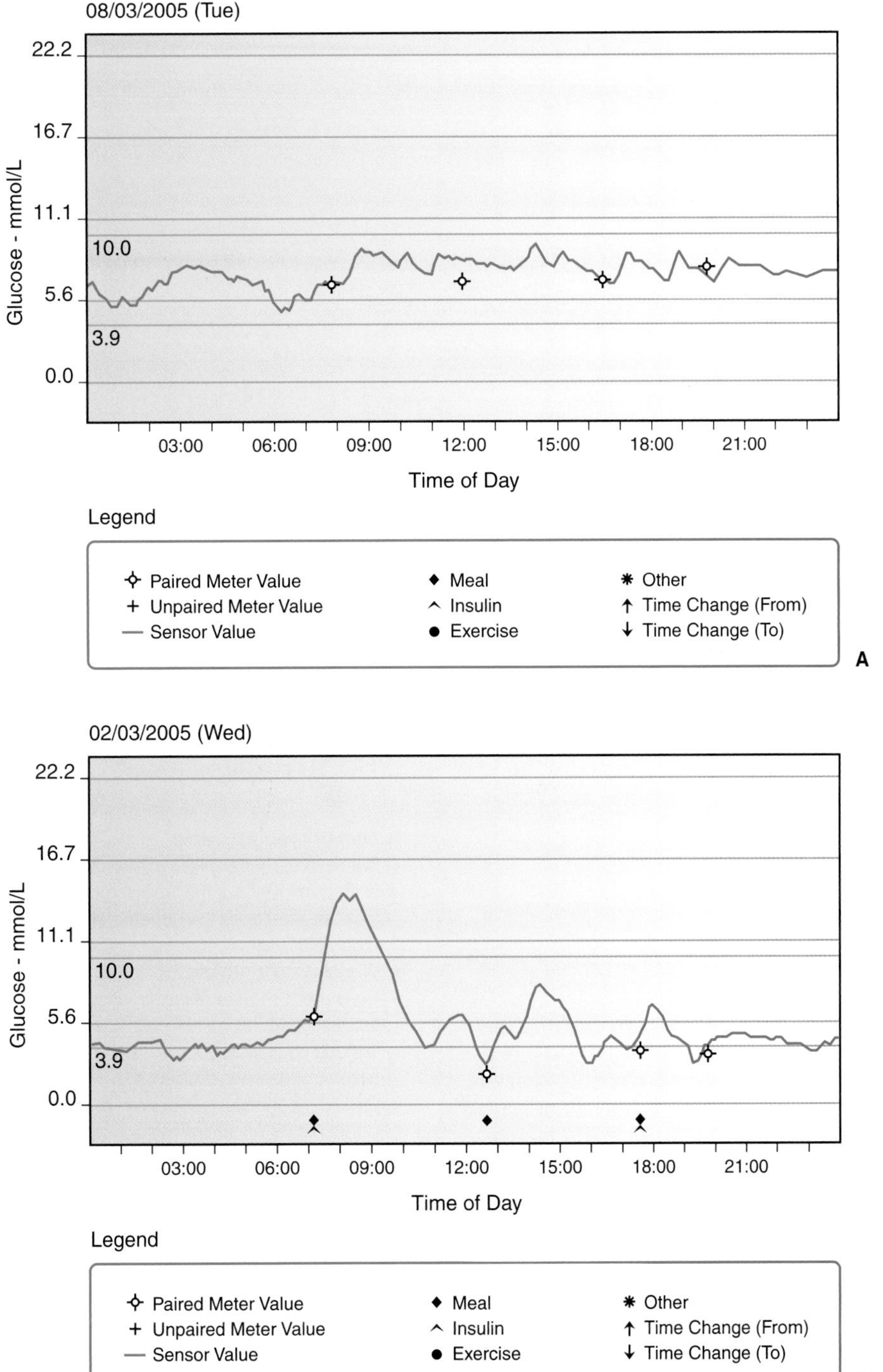


Fig. 19.4.2 Continuous interstitial glucose monitoring obtained from an indwelling subcutaneous sensor in three patients with type 1 diabetes. In (**A**), the pattern of results shows that the patient is in the remission phase. In (**B**), excellent control is seen, but the a.m. rise in glucose concentration requires an increase in a.m. ultra-short-acting insulin.

*Continued*

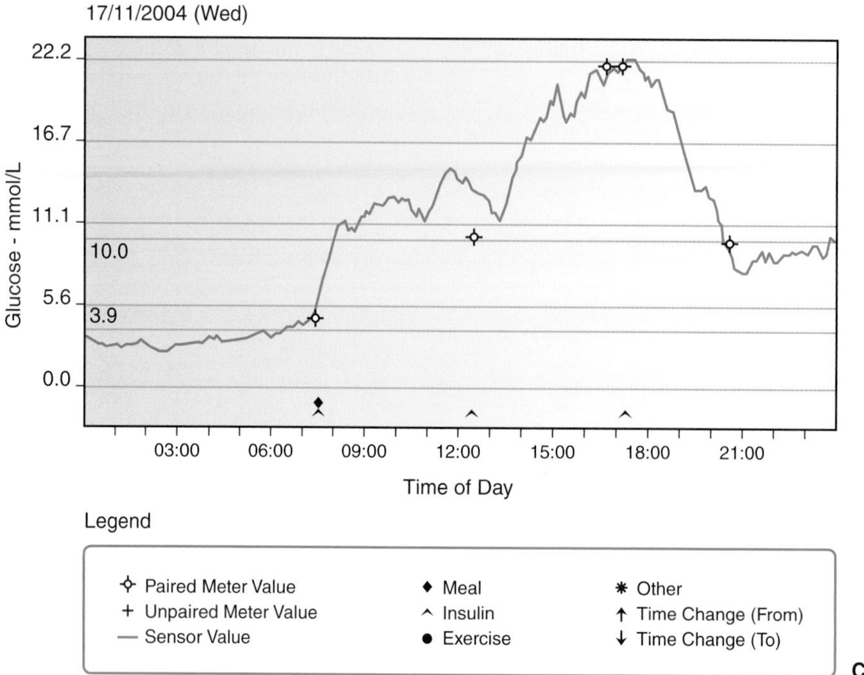


**Fig. 19.4.2, cont'd** In (**C**), the results show asymptomatic nocturnal hypoglycaemia and daytime hyperglycaemia. This requires adjustment of night-time long-acting insulin and daytime ultra-short-acting insulin.

Serum lipids can be measured every few years, particularly if there is a family history of a lipid disorder or of premature cardiovascular disease.

The major risk factors for the development of long-term vascular complications are:

- level of metabolic control
- duration of type 1 diabetes
- smoking
- hypertension
- dyslipidaemia
- family history.

It should be reinforced for the patient and their family that any improvement in their metabolic control, even if still not ideal, will reduce their risk of developing complications. There are current international guidelines to introduce angiotensin-converting enzyme (ACE) inhibitors for hypertension (above 95th centile for age and sex) and persistent microalbuminuria, and statin therapy for raised low-density lipoprotein (LDL) cholesterol.

## Special problems in management

### Hypoglycaemia

For parents, the occurrence of severe hypoglycaemia in their child (loss of consciousness or a convulsion) is one of the most distressing aspects of diabetes. No long-term harmful effects generally result from a severe hypoglycaemic episode. However, the risk remains, particularly if the adolescent uses other drugs such as alcohol, and hypoglycaemic unawareness may develop with recurrent episodes of severe hypoglycaemia.

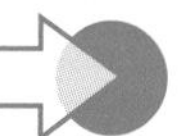

**Practical points**

**Recurrent hypoglycaemia**

- Is it severe, moderate or mild; is it daytime or nocturnal?
- Is there hypoglycaemic unawareness and at what blood glucose level does the patient detect symptoms of low blood glucose?
- What is the HbA1c level?
- Consider a change of insulin dose, insulin type or insulin timing schedule.
- Exclude coeliac disease, Addison's disease and autoimmune thyroid disease.
- Consider continuous interstitial glucose monitoring, particularly if nocturnal hypoglycaemia is suspected.
- Consider continuous subcutaneous insulin infusions (insulin pump therapy).

Hypoglycaemia may occur if the insulin dose is excessive, if insufficient food is eaten or if extra exercise is undertaken. Severe hypoglycaemia is most common during the night, when the glucose threshold for counter-regulatory hormone responses is lower. Minor hypoglycaemic episodes are relatively frequent and reflect the difficulties in achieving stable control with current insulin delivery to the systemic rather than enteroportal circulation. Insulin analogues (ultra-short-acting and basal) and insulin pump therapy have reduced the risk of hypoglycaemia. All patients with type 1 diabetes should carry some rapidly absorbable carbohydrate (e.g. glucose tablets or glucose-containing sweets) for immediate treatment of hypoglycaemic symptoms.

The clinical features of hypoglycaemia can be divided into:

- stimulation of the sympathetic nervous system – anxiety, palpitations, tachycardia, pallor, perspiration, headaches and abdominal pain
- effects on the central nervous system – lethargy, dizziness, ataxia, weakness, confusion, personality changes, visual disturbance, unconsciousness, localized and generalized convulsions.

These clinical features appear rapidly in a previously well child and there is no difficulty in differentiating hypoglycaemic coma from the coma of diabetic ketoacidosis.

The emergency treatment for the unconscious hypoglycaemic child is:

- lay them on their side and check the airway
- do not give oral fluids
- give intramuscular or subcutaneous glucagon (0.5 mg for children <5 years of age; 1 mg for older children and adults) or intravenous glucose (2.5 mL 20% dextrose per kilogram of body weight).

All families with a diabetic child should have glucagon at home and should be able to give it subcutaneously. The response to therapy is seen within minutes. For the less severely affected child, mild hypoglycaemia can be treated with oral glucose.

### Management of sick days

Children with well controlled diabetes are no more prone to infections than the non-diabetic child. However, the infection, especially if associated with fever, may cause a temporary insulin resistance and increased insulin requirements, or, in the case of enteric infections with vomiting/diarrhoea, reduced insulin requirements.

Advice to parents when child is sick at home:

- measure blood glucose levels frequently
- measure blood ketone levels regularly
- give frequent small doses (10–20% of daily requirements) of short-acting insulin every 3–4 hours if blood glucose and/or ketone levels are rising
- low doses of glucagon can help prevent hypoglycaemia in the child with vomiting
- regular phone contact with the diabetes doctor or educator.

### Growth and delayed puberty

Because insulin is the principal hormone of energy storage and anabolism, poor diabetic control can cause growth disturbances and pubertal delay. Hashimoto thyroiditis, coeliac disease or, less commonly, adrenal insufficiency can also cause pubertal and growth delay.

### Psychological stresses

The relevance of psychological wellbeing to good diabetes control is of such importance that the social worker and psychologist are integral members of the management team. Stress is common to all families with diabetes, and psychosocial support is essential. Patient and parent support groups and diabetes camps also nurture self-esteem and confidence. Family dysfunction, teenage rebellion and other emotional problems may cause a more profound instability, and psychological counselling may be required for the child and family. Clinicians must be alert to the higher incidence of mood disorders and eating disorders in adolescents with type 1 diabetes than in the normal adolescent population.

### Adherence

Excellent diabetes control in childhood and adolescence is difficult in the best of circumstances. It becomes impossible when the child or the family cannot adhere to diet, monitoring or injections of insulin. Problems in adherence are not unusual periodically and represent a natural rebellion against the never-ending discipline that characterizes diabetes management. The usual cause of recurrent diabetic ketoacidosis and chronic poor metabolic control in adolescence is insulin omission. Patience and counselling are necessary, especially in adolescence, when normal risk-taking behaviour and growing independence may not combine well with diabetes.

**Clinical example**

Michelle, a 14-year-old girl with a 5-year history of diabetes, had three episodes of diabetic ketoacidosis in 3 months. Her blood glucose logbook showed the values to be 4–10 mmol/L, although a glycosylated haemoglobin level (HbA1c) was 10.8% (normal range 4–6%). Her insulin dose was 0.9 units per kg per day and the recorded blood glucose levels appeared spurious.

Admission to hospital for stabilization confirmed increased blood glucose levels. Management required appropriate increases in insulin dose, education and counselling. The dietitian suspected that Michelle might also have had an eating disorder complicating her insulin omission, and psychological review was arranged.

Sometimes it is necessary for someone else (e.g. the parents or a community nurse) temporarily to take over responsibility for the insulin injections when there is a serious problem with insulin omission.

### Factors limiting management

Factors to consider when diabetes is proving difficult to manage are:

- difficulties in family functioning
- psychological stresses
- adherence problems
- eating disorders (particularly in adolescent girls)
- exaggerated fear of hypoglycaemia held by the family or patient.

## Future directions

Families frequently ask about research and management advances, and it is important that they have access to up-to-date information through regular seminars and reliable websites.

Oral and transdermal insulins are under investigation. Technical advances in interstitial glucose monitoring (continuous glucose monitoring systems) and insulin pump delivery are advancing the availability of a closed loop system that can monitor glucose levels and adjust insulin delivery.

Specific immunomodulation of the autoimmune process is being trialled in subjects with preclinical and newly diagnosed diabetes, in an attempt to prolong the life of beta cells.

Transplantation of isolated islets of Langerhans in adults using less beta-cell toxic immunosuppressive drugs has shown promise and is available for some adult patients with hypoglycaemic unawareness. Whole-pancreas transplants have been performed successfully in conjunction with renal transplantation. However, prevention of rejection of both types of transplant requires lifelong immunosuppression and the supply of human pancreas tissue is not plentiful. Stem cells and islet regeneration are other major research directions.

## Type 2 diabetes

The true incidence of type 2 diabetes in youth is not known, as patients are frequently asymptomatic. Characteristics of type 2 diabetes at diagnosis are shown in Box 19.4.2.

The distinction between type 1 and type 2 diabetes in childhood may be difficult to make on clinical grounds alone (for example, many children with type 1 diabetes are overweight and have a family history of type 2 diabetes), although children with type 2 diabetes often have acanthosis nigricans of the axilla and/or neck (Fig. 19.4.3A,B). Measurement of islet antibodies

**Box 19.4.2 Characteristics of type 2 diabetes at diagnosis**

- Obesity
- Acanthosis nigricans
- Family history of type 2 diabetes
- Absent or mild ketosis (although ketosis and ketoacidosis can occur)
- Absence of islet antibodies
- Raised C-peptide/insulin levels
- Microvascular complications, hypertension and lipid abnormalities may be present
- Hyperandrogenism may be present
- More common in Aboriginal and Polynesian populations

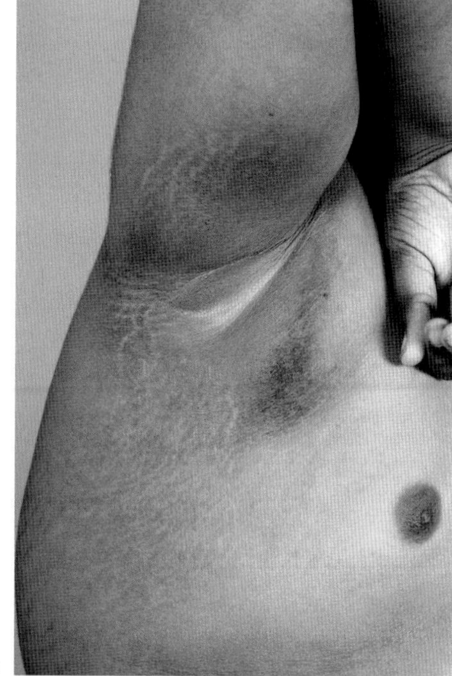

A

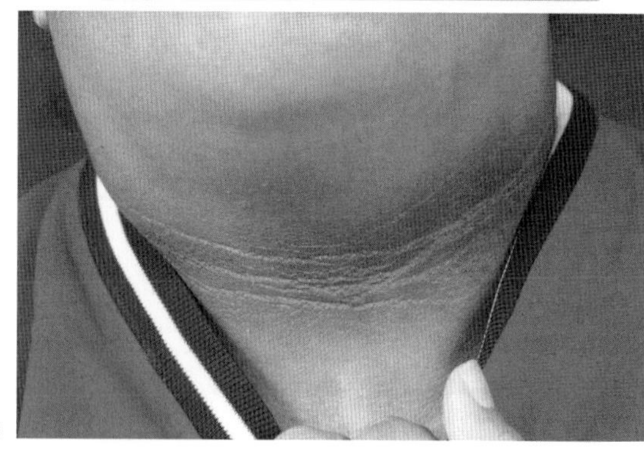

B

Fig. 19.4.3 Acanthosis nigricans of axilla (**A**) and neck (**B**).

to show their absence is usually necessary to confirm the diagnosis. The distinction is important, as patients with type 2 diabetes are treated with a weight-reducing diabetes diet and metformin as first-line measures. Insulin may still be required, especially during intercurrent acute infections when ketoacidosis can occur. Screening for microvascular and macrovascular complications should begin from the time of diagnosis in type 2 diabetes. Insulin resistance is always present and there may be other features of the metabolic syndrome such as dyslipidaemia, hypertension, non-alcoholic hepatosteatosis and hyperandrogenism in girls.

# 19.5 Bone mineral disorders

Colin Jones, Joshua Kausman

Hypocalcaemia, rickets and hypercalcaemia are the most common manifestations of disorders of calcium, phosphate and vitamin D metabolism. Disorders of magnesium metabolism are rare but share many features of calcium disorders.

## Calcium, magnesium and phosphorus (Table 19.5.1)

Calcium and phosphate form the major structural components of bone, in the form of hydroxyapatite. The majority of magnesium is also found in bones. A large proportion of each mineral in bone is freely exchangeable with the extracellular fluid (ECF). Calcium and phosphate ions, under normal circumstances, are present in supersaturated solution. A rise in phosphate will lead to the deposition of more calcium phosphate into bone as hydroxyapatite and cause hypocalcaemia. The distribution of calcium and phosphate between bone and the ECF is determined by hormonal regulation of the concentrations of these minerals. The most important hormones are 1,25-dihydroxyvitamin $D_3$ (activated vitamin D) and parathyroid hormone (PTH). The actions of these hormones are summarized in Figure 19.5.1.

The ionized ECF forms of calcium and magnesium are responsible for physiological effect. The ionized form of calcium should be measured to confirm that abnormalities in concentration are present, because the equilibrium between the ionized and protein-bound forms can change. For instance, an increase of 0.1 pH unit decreases the ionized calcium by 10%, and hypoalbuminaemia reduces total serum calcium but not the ionized calcium concentration, because 90% of bound calcium is bound to albumin.

### Clinical example

Kylie, a 6-year-old girl, has nephritis with a metabolic acidosis (pH 7.32, [HCO3⁻] = 15 mmol/L, $P\text{CO}_2$ 30 mmHg). She has an albumin of 20 g/L, serum total [$Ca^{2+}$] = 1.0 mmol/L and serum [phosphate] = 3.6 mmol/L. Is it safe to correct the acidosis with intravenous $NaHCO_3$? From Table 19.5.1, if the serum albumin was normal, 46% of the total serum $Ca^{2+}$ would be ionized. However, the serum albumin concentration is reduced by 50%, thus the amount of calcium bound to albumin will be reduced by 50% (the proportion of total calcium bound to albumin will be reduced to approximately 20%), leaving the ionized proportion of total serum calcium increased from the normal 46% to approximately 66% = 0.66 mmol/L. Increasing the pH to 7.4 could reduce the ionized portion and precipitate overt symptoms of hypocalcaemia. Thus, the calcium concentration should be corrected before giving $NaHCO_3$.

## Hypocalcaemia

In the neonatal period, hypocalcaemia is conventionally a total serum calcium concentration below 1.8 mmol/L (ionized calcium 1.0 mmol/L). Beyond this age, a total plasma calcium below 2.1 mmol/L (ionized calcium 1.2 mmol/L) constitutes hypocalcaemia. Clinical signs usually occur only with total serum calcium below 2 mmol/L (ionized calcium 0.75 mmol/L), although some patients can tolerate much lower levels and remain asymptomatic. The signs of hypocalcaemia are due to neuromuscular excitability. Jitteriness, apnoea, laryngeal spasm causing stridor and convulsions are frequent in infants. Tetany, carpopedal spasm and the Chovstek (facial twitch on percussion of the facial nerve near the temporomandibular joint) and Trousseau (tetany produced by inflating the sphygmomanometer with above systolic blood pressure for up to 2 min) signs are seen mainly in older children. Intracerebral calcification and cataracts are complications. The electrocardiogram (ECG) may show a prolonged QT interval.

Some causes of hypocalcaemia are listed in Box 19.5.1.

Early neonatal hypocalcaemia is common in premature infants and infants of diabetic mothers. In premature infants, it is possibly an exaggerated response to the normal interruption of the maternofetal calcium transfer; the serum calcium falls following delivery to a nadir, reached at a few days of age, and then increases to normal levels at 1–2 weeks of age. Signs are seen within hours of birth, become most severe about 48 hours after birth and then improve spontaneously. Hypocalcaemia can be

**Table 19.5.1 Distribution, serum concentrations, dietary requirements and sources of calcium, magnesium and phosphate**

| | Calcium | Magnesium | Phosphorus |
|---|---|---|---|
| **Body distribution (%)** | | | |
| Bone* | 99 | 60 | 80 |
| Intracellular | — | 40 | 20 |
| **Serum status (%)** | | | |
| Ionized† | 46 | 55 | 85 |
| Complexed | 14 | 25 | 5 |
| Protein bound | 40 | 20 | 10 |
| **Serum levels (mmol/L)** | | | |
| Cord blood‡ | 2.4 | 0.7 | 1.6 |
| Neonatal | 2.1–2.7 | 0.75–1.1 | 2.0–3.3 |
| Adult | 2.2–2.6 | 0.75–1.1 | 1.0–1.3§ |
| **Dietary intake, RDI (mg/day)** | | | |
| 0-6 months | 210 | 30 | 100 |
| 7–12 months | 270 | 75 | 275 |
| 1–3 years | 500 | 80 | 460 |
| 4–8 years | 700 | 130 | 500 |
| 9–18 years | 1300 | 240–410 | 1250 |
| **Milk content (mg/L)** | | | |
| Human | 300–500 | 40 | 100–300 |
| Cow | 1500 | 130 | 1000 |
| **Other food sources** | Tinned fish, dairy products | Green vegetables, seeds, nuts | Meats, dairy products |

RDI, recommended dietary intake.
* Ionic exchange occurs readily between extracellular fluid (ECF) and bone, enabling ECF concentrations to be kept fairly constant.
† The ionized form of phosphorus at pH 7.4 is $HPO_4^{2-}$ (70%) and $H_2PO_4^-$ (20%).
‡ Cord blood concentrations are higher than maternal blood concentrations, indicating that active transport mechanisms are involved in transplacental transfer. Parathyroid hormone-related peptide (PTHRP) is probably involved in these processes.
§ Levels of phosphate decline slowly during childhood and reach adult levels on completion of bone growth.

aggravated by early phosphate-rich formula feeding or hypoxic–ischaemic injury. Treatment of symptomatic infants involves intravenous (IV) calcium administration and commencement of diet, following the guidelines in Box 19.5.2.

Late neonatal hypocalcaemia usually presents as tetany after the first few days of life. The main cause is transient hypoparathyroidism, as demonstrated by high plasma phosphate and low serum PTH concentrations in the face of hypocalcaemia. A similar clinical picture is seen in infants of mothers with hyperparathyroidism and in infants with congenital heart disease. Treatment may involve calcium infusion, calcitriol, oral calcium supplementation and a low-phosphate formula. The infant can often be weaned from this treatment after a few weeks. Persistence of the hypocalcaemia beyond this time should prompt a search for other causes of hypoparathyroidism, such as DiGeorge syndrome (aplasia of the parathyroids, thymic aplasia with T-cell immunodeficiency and cardiovascular abnormalities), hypomagnesaemia or idiopathic congenital hypoparathyroidism. An abnormality of the calcium-sensing receptor on the parathyroid cells (an activating mutation decreasing PTH release) is also a cause. Treatment is based on the use of calcitriol, often in combination with phosphate restriction.

Late-onset hypoparathyroidism may occur with destructive injury of the parathyroids (copper deposition in Wilson disease, iron deposition in haemosiderosis, or autoimmune type I polyglandular syndrome). In this latter condition, children, usually girls, present with tetany or convulsions, and may have candidiasis and adrenal insufficiency or other autoimmune disorders such as alopecia, malabsorption, thyroiditis and diabetes. Pseudohypoparathyroidism is due to end-organ resistance to PTH, and blood levels of PTH are high. Mental deficiency and skeletal abnormalities (particularly a short fourth metacarpal) may be associated. Treatment is the same as for hypoparathyroidism.

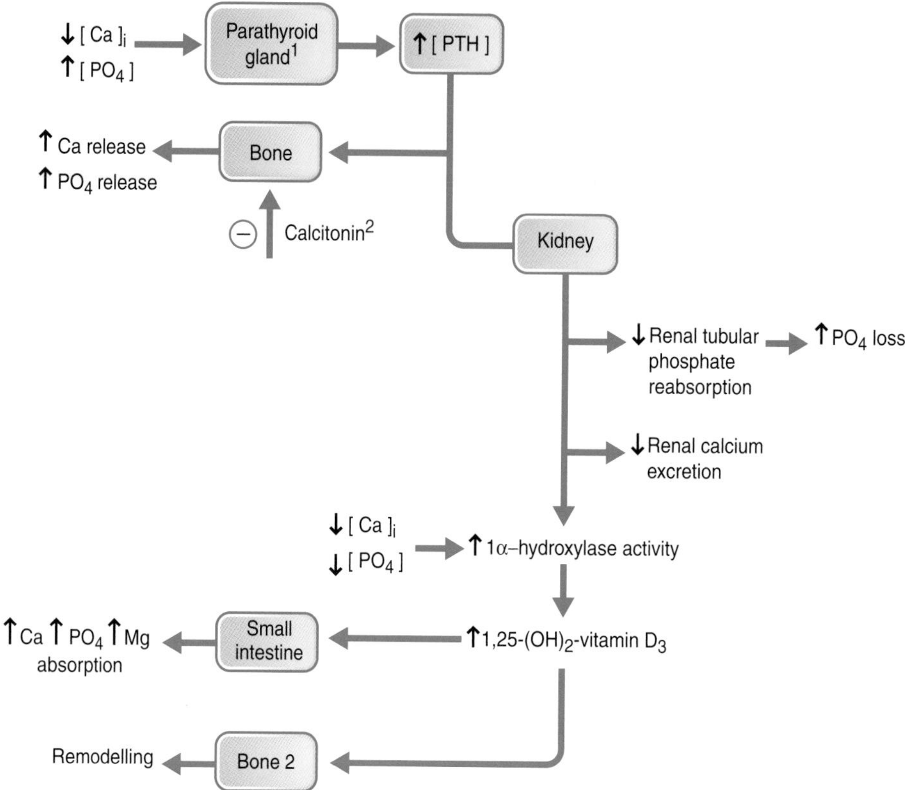
↓[Ca]i
↑[PO4]
Parathyroid gland1
↑[PTH]
↑Ca release
↑PO4 release
Bone
Calcitonin2
Kidney
↓Renal tubular phosphate reabsorption
↑PO4 loss
↓Renal calcium excretion
↓[Ca]i
↓[PO4]
↑1α–hydroxylase activity
↑Ca ↑PO4 ↑Mg absorption
Small intestine
↑1,25-(OH)2-vitamin D3
Remodelling
Bone 2
1. Calcium-sensitive receptors on the parathyroid cells lead to PTH production increasing with a rise and decreasing with a fall in ionized calcium concentrations.
2. Calcitonin is a hormone produced in the medullary (parafollicular) cells of the thyroid gland in response to an increase in calcium concentrations. It inhibits resorption of bone.

**Fig. 19.5.1** Hormonal control of calcium, magnesium and phosphate. PTH, parathyroid hormone.

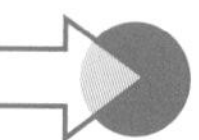

## Practical points

**Hypocalcaemia**

- Suspect symptomatic hypocalcaemia with tetany, unexplained stridor, irritability or convulsions.
- Confirm diagnosis with total and ionized calcium concentrations and draw blood for estimation of magnesium, phosphate and parathyroid hormone concentrations.
- Treat symptomatic hypocalcaemia with IV 10% calcium chloride 0.2 mL per kg per dose given slowly into a well-placed IV line, and monitor the ECG.

Hyperphosphataemia can cause hypocalcaemia acutely (as seen in tumour lysis syndrome, where cell death following the initiation of chemotherapy for bulky tumours results in the release of phosphate). Acute renal failure with retention of phosphate is associated with hypocalcaemia. The primary treatment in these conditions is to reduce serum phosphate concentrations through dietary restriction of phosphate, the use of phosphate binders (such as calcium carbonate) and dialysis. Rickets due to vitamin D deficiency or disorders of vitamin D metabolism can cause hypocalcaemia (see below).

## Clinical example

Kylie has induction treatment for T-cell lymphoma. She develops hypocalcaemia associated with a raised serum phosphate level in the days after this treatment. How should the hypocalcaemia be managed? The administration of intravenous calcium, combined with the elevated serum phosphate, would exceed the solubility product of calcium phosphate and lead to its metastatic deposition. The calcification would occur in blood vessels and soft tissues. Such an approach might, in fact, be necessary if Kylie had symptomatic hypocalcaemia (convulsions), but it would be preferable to lower the serum phosphate concentration first. This can be achieved by implementing a low-phosphate diet and administering oral phosphate binders (such as calcium carbonate) which bind the phosphate in the gut (calcium complexes phosphate and is not absorbed by the intestine). It would be uncommon to use dialysis or haemofiltration, but these treatments would also lower serum phosphate concentrations.

**Box 19.5.1 Causes of hypocalcaemia**

Neonatal
- Early neonatal – prematurity, IDM, IUGR, birth asphyxia
- Late neonatal – DiGeorge syndrome, phosphate load, low magnesium, IDM

Pseudohypocalcaemia
- Hypoalbuminaemia

Vitamin D deficiency
- Nutritional deficiency
- Disorders of vitamin D metabolism
  - 1α-hydroxylase deficiency
  - vitamin D-dependent rickets

Parathyroid hormone-associated
- Hypoparathyroidism
  - idiopathic
  - autoimmune polyglandular disease (with mucocutaneous candidiasis, or Addison disease)
  - calcium-sensing receptor activating mutations or antibodies
  - hypomagnesaemia
  - destructive lesions of the glands
  - hypoplasia
  - PTH receptor defect – pseudohypoparathyroidism
- Hyperphosphataemia
  - tumour lysis
  - renal failure

Pancreatitis

Medical treatment
- Large blood transfusion/exchange transfusion

IDM, infant of diabetic mother; IUGR, intrauterine growth retardation; PTH, parathyroid hormone.

**Box 19.5.2 Treatment of hypocalcaemia**

**Emergency**
- Patients with hypocalcaemia and symptoms should be treated with intravenous calcium*
- ECG monitor (bradycardia)
- IV calcium chloride 10% 0.2 mL per kg per dose (max 1 g) repeated 4–6-hourly or followed by infusion 1 mmol (=1.5 mL 10% $CaCl_2$) per kg per day
- Correct concurrent hypomagnesaemia (magnesium chloride 0.2 mmol/kg over 1 h)

**Maintenance**
- Treat underlying condition (see text)

*Note: Extravasation of IV calcium causes skin and subcutaneous tissue necrosis.

## Rickets

Rickets is impaired mineralization of osteoid tissue in the growing child. The mineralization defect affects the epiphyseal growth plates where cartilage cells proliferate and unmineralized osteoid tissue accumulates, resulting in widening metaphyses, weak bones and development of deformity, particularly in the weight-bearing bones. In established bones there is continued bone resorption but failure of mineralization results in soft, rarefied bones (this is osteomalacia, which is the same disease as rickets, in the adult).

Causes of rickets are deficiency of the effect of vitamin D and phosphate depletion. Figure 19.5.2 outlines the causes of vitamin D deficiency and abnormal metabolism of vitamin D in relation to the physiological production of the active product, 1,25-dihydroxyvitamin $D_3$.

The recommended dietary intake of vitamin D is 400 international units (IU) per day. With exposure to a small amount of afternoon sunlight, vitamin D supplementation is unnecessary. Breast milk contains 20–50 IU/L, yet rickets is uncommon in breastfed infants in the first year of life, provided the mother does not have osteomalacia. Most commercial milk formulas have 400 IU/L vitamin D.

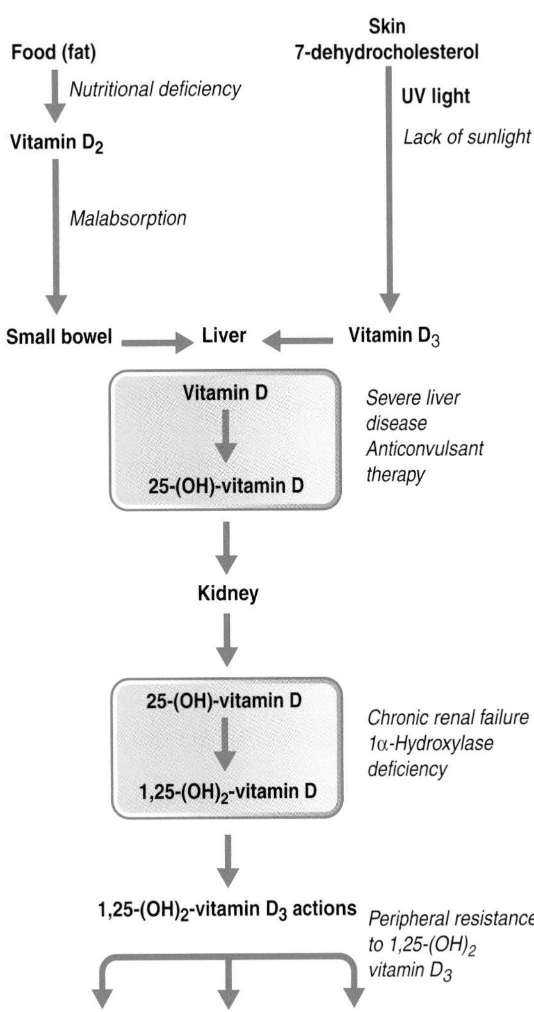


Fig. 19.5.2 Vitamin D metabolism and rickets.

In the past 30 years, the incidence of vitamin D deficiency has increased in Australia. This increase has been seen in the children of migrants from the Middle East, southern Europe and Asia, especially where the mother wears a hejab. Reduced sunlight and darkly pigmented skin combined with a range of social factors, including poor housing, lack of adequate infant welfare services for non-English-speaking migrants and unusual feeding patterns, have combined to make rickets more prevalent.

Malabsorption associated with gastrointestinal, hepatic or pancreatic disease can cause vitamin D deficiency. In approximately 50% of cases, hypocalcaemia is present at the time of diagnosis. Severe liver disease and prolonged use of anticonvulsant therapy with diphenylhydantoin or phenobarbital (through an increased hepatic turnover of vitamin D) can cause rickets.

1α-Hydroxylase deficiency (type I vitamin D-dependent rickets, characterized by normal or high 25-dihydroxyvitamin $D_3$ and low 1,25-dihydroxyvitamin $D_3$ levels) and peripheral resistance to 1,25-dihydroxyvitamin $D_3$ (type II vitamin D-dependent rickets, characterized by high concentrations of 1,25-dihydroxyvitamin $D_3$) present as severe hypocalcaemic vitamin D deficiency that fails to respond to treatment with vitamin D.

The clinical features of these forms of rickets are quite variable: young children may present with tetany and convulsions, older children incidentally when a chest X-ray is performed for an intercurrent chest infection. Early signs in nutritional rickets include weakness of the outer table of the skull (craniotabes), thickening of the costochondral junctions (the 'rachitic rosary'), and widening of the wrists and ankles. Later, asymmetry of the head with delayed closure of the anterior fontanelle, frontal and occipital bossing of the skull, development of a Harrison groove, scoliosis and lumbar lordosis, delayed dentition, and bowing and bending of the legs develop. Muscular weakness, ligament laxity and fractures are common.

The radiology of the ends of long bones is characteristic, showing widening of the space between metaphysis and epiphysis (Fig. 19.5.3). The metaphyseal ends of the long bones are widened, and appear cupped and frayed. The biochemical changes are a normal or low serum calcium, a low serum phosphate, a high serum alkaline phosphatase and a high PTH level.

Treatment of nutritional vitamin D deficiency is with oral vitamin D at a dose of 3000–5000 units per day for 6 weeks. In some cases treatment precipitates uptake of calcium into bones ('hungry bones') to such an extent that hypocalcaemia is accentuated and large doses of calcium supplement may be required to maintain normocalcaemia for the first week(s). In the longer term, adequate calcium intake (600–1500 mg/day) needs to be maintained, as does an adequate intake of vitamin D, 400 IU/day to age 4 years. In cases where poor compliance may be suspected, 'stoss therapy' using 50 000–150 000 IU vitamin D every 6 weeks may be used. Radiological improvement is usually apparent within 4 weeks. Some cases are refractory and require longer treatment periods. If there is no response, tests for 1α-hydroxylase deficiency, peripheral resistance to 1,25-dihydroxyvitamin $D_3$ or hypophosphataemic rickets should be undertaken.

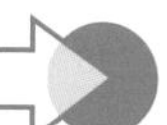

**Practical points**

**Rickets**

- Suspect with bowing of the long bones, exaggerated lumbar lordosis, splayed wrists and other rachitic changes in an irritable child.
- Examine for signs of hypocalcaemia and treat symptomatic hypocalcaemia.
- Suspect nutritional vitamin D deficiency in breastfed infants of mothers where covering clothing is worn at all times, children of dark skin colour, children with malabsorption or liver disease.
- Suspect another cause with failure to respond to vitamin D, low PTH concentrations and very low phosphate concentrations.

### Hypophosphataemic rickets

X-linked dominant hypophosphataemic (vitamin D resistant) rickets is caused by failure of phosphate resorption in the renal tubule and lack of an appropriate increase in 1α-hydroxylase activity (low phosphate concentrations normally increase the activity of this enzyme, which produces 1,25-dihydroxyvitamin $D_3$). In 50% of cases it is familial; the rest of the cases are due to new mutations. Clinically, the rickets affects the lower limbs predominantly, and investigations show the calcium and PTH concentrations are normal, whereas the phosphate concentration is quite low. Males are usually no more severely affected than females. Treatment consists of large amounts of dietary phosphate supplementation and large doses of calcitriol.

Chronic phosphate deficiency (e.g. renal Fanconi syndrome, dietary phosphate deficiency) from any cause will result in rickets.

## Renal osteodystrophy

This condition predictably occurs when the glomerular filtration rate in chronic renal failure decreases to less than 25% of normal. It occurs as a result of a combination of events, including an increase in plasma phosphate and decreased 1α-hydroxylation of 25-hydroxyvitamin $D_3$ in the kidney, leading to a fall in 1,25-dihydroxyvitamin $D_3$ production. This leads to hypocalcaemia and an increase in PTH concentration. The combination of

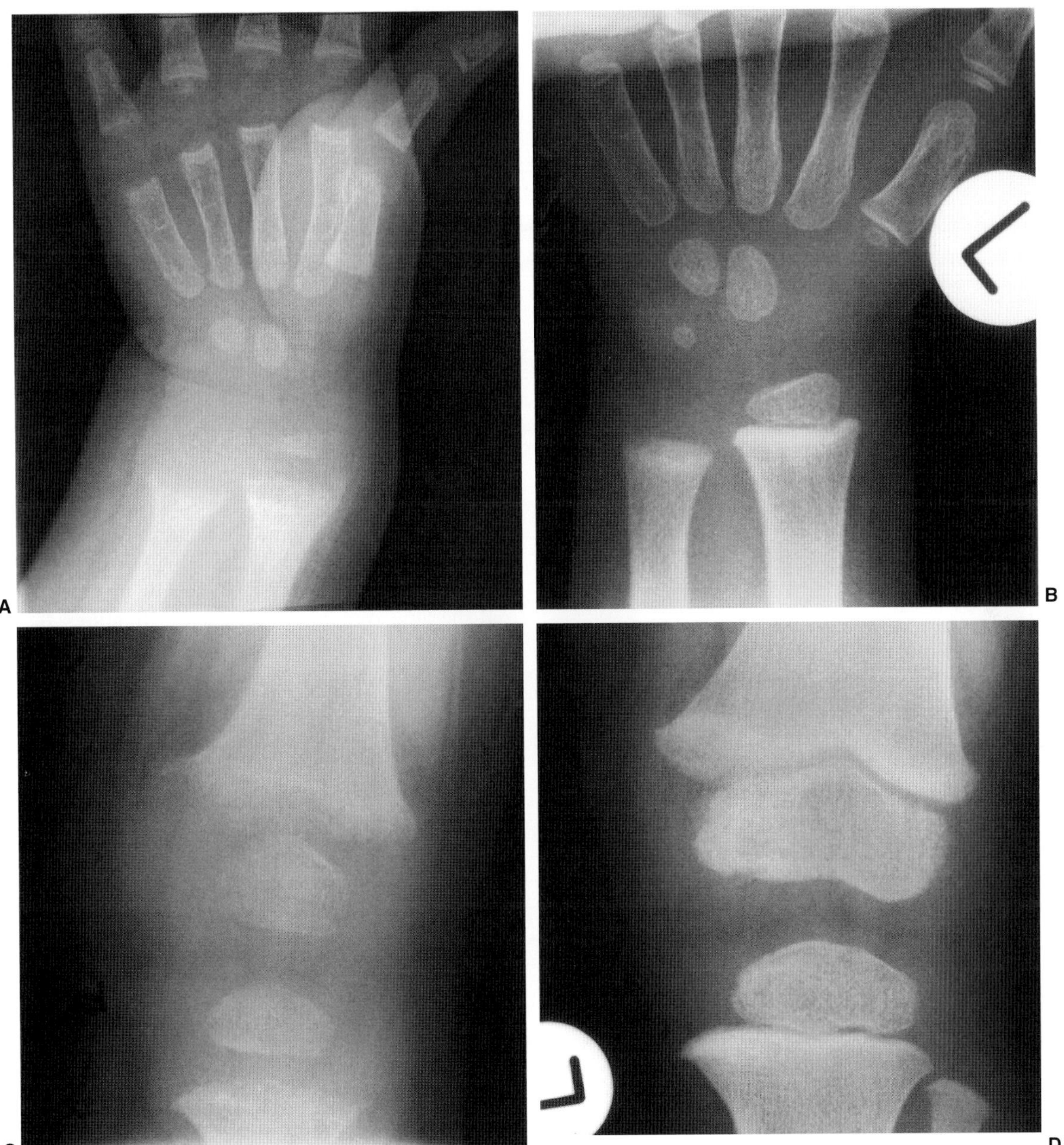


Fig. 19.5.3 X-rays of the wrist (**A**) and knee (**C**) of a child with nutritional rickets at 18 months of age when the diagnosis was made, and 8 months later (**B, D**) after treatment was finished.

rickets and secondary hyperparathyroidism can result in gross skeletal deformation. Treatment consists of a graded range of measures beginning with dietary phosphate restriction, use of phosphate binders (calcium carbonate) and addition of calcitriol.

## Hypercalcaemia

Hypercalcaemia is a total serum calcium above 2.7 mmol/L (ionized calcium > 1.3 mmol/L). Symptoms of hypercalcaemia include nausea and vomiting, polyuria and polydipsia, hypertension and failure to thrive. Ensuing hypercalciuria may cause nephrocalcinosis and urinary calculi. The ECG may show a shortened QT interval.

A list of causes of hypercalcaemia is given in Box 19.5.3. Most of these are rare. Primary hyperparathyroidism occurs with some frequency in the second decade of life and is due to hyperplasia or adenoma of the parathyroid glands. It may occur as part of the multiple endocrine neoplasia syndromes (type I hyperparathyroidism associated with prolactinoma or gastrinoma; type II with hyperfunction of the adrenal, parathyroid and medullary

**Box 19.5.3 Causes of hypercalcaemia**

Neonatal
- Hyperparathyroidism
- primary
- maternal hypoparathyroidism
- maternal pseudohypoparathyroidism
- Idiopathic infantile hypercalcaemia
- Williams syndrome
- Familial hypocalciuric hypercalcaemia
- Subcutaneous fat necrosis

Vitamin D excess
- Iatrogenic
- Ectopic production — sarcoidosis, tuberculosis, lymphoma

Parathyroid hormone excess
- Primary hyperparathyroidism
  - multiple endocrine neoplasia (MEN) syndromes
- Familial hypocalciuric hypercalcaemia
- Abnormalities related to PTH receptor or PTH-related peptide (PTHRP)

Other
- Bone disease, trauma and immobilization
- Thyrotoxicosis and hypothyroidism

cells of the thyroid). Investigations reveal high PTH concentrations, and X-ray appearances include subperiosteal resorption of bone (particularly the phalanges), 'salt and pepper' appearance of the cranium and cyst formation in long bones. Treatment of symptomatic disease usually involves subtotal parathyroidectomy.

Familial hypocalciuric hypercalcaemia is an autosomal dominant, usually asymptomatic, condition caused by an inactivating mutation of the parathyroid calcium-sensing receptor.

Idiopathic hypercalcaemia of infancy is a condition in which there is increased absorption of dietary calcium. The condition usually resolves by the end of the first year of life. Occasionally it is associated with cardiovascular abnormalities (supravalvular aortic stenosis) and dysmorphic facial 'elfin' features (Williams syndrome). The genetic defect for Williams syndrome involves the elastin gene, and cases may be diagnosed using fluorescence *in situ* hybridization (FISH) studies.

Treatment is directed at the cause of the hypercalcaemia. Severe symptoms may necessitate initiation of a diuresis using sodium chloride infusion, dietary phosphate supplements to bind calcium, glucocorticoids to reduce intestinal calcium absorption in vitamin D excess and bisphosphonates to prevent calcium release from bone. A low-calcium milk formula is used to treat idiopathic hypercalcaemia of infancy.

## Hypercalciuria

The normal upper limit of urinary calcium excretion is 0.15 mmol per kg per day or <0.7 mmol per mmol creatinine. Hypercalcaemia usually causes hypercalciuria

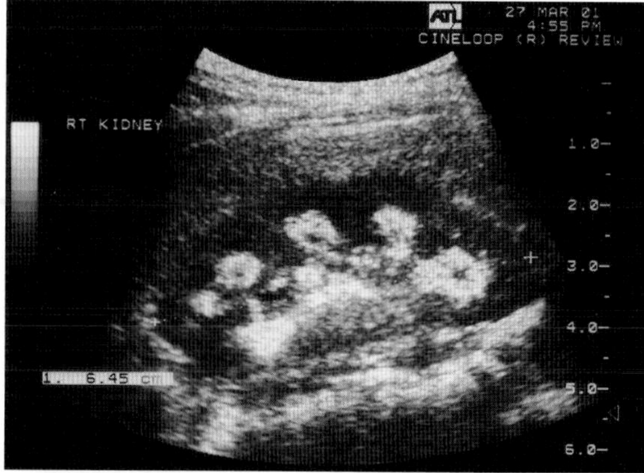


Fig. 19.5.4 Renal ultrasound image showing nephrocalcinosis of the medullary pyramids in a 4-year-old child with idiopathic nephrocalcinosis.

(see Box 19.5.3), with the notable exception of familial hypocalciuric hypercalcaemia. Normocalcaemic hypercalciuria is caused by furosemide or corticosteroid therapy, immobilization of limb fractures, distal renal tubular acidosis and some rare syndromes.

Idiopathic hypercalciuria is common and appears to be an autosomal dominant condition with incomplete penetrance. On a calcium-rich or calcium-sufficient diet there is intestinal hyperabsorption of calcium and the PTH and 1,25-dihydroxyvitamin D concentrations are normal. On a lower calcium diet, 'renal' loss of calcium occurs and higher levels of PTH and 1,25-dihydroxyvitamin D are found. Excessive bone resorption occurs in some patients and can cause osteoporosis. Thus, the therapeutic safety of a low calcium diet is limited because of the risks of development of osteoporosis. Hypercalciuria can cause nephrocalcinosis (Fig. 19.5.4) and urinary calculi. Where treatment is necessary, thiazide diuretics have proven useful.

## Osteoporosis

Osteoporosis is decreased mineral content of the skeleton. Measurement of bone mineral density has improved over the last decade with the use of dual-energy X-ray absorptiometry (DEXA). DEXA must be interpreted carefully, in consideration of the size of the bone where measurements are taken and the age of the patient, especially with regard to pubertal development of the child. Osteoporosis is apparent radiologically only when approximately half of the bone mineral content has been lost. Causes of osteoporosis are given in Box 19.5.4.

Idiopathic juvenile osteoporosis is a rare condition that occurs in mid-childhood with gross demineralization of the skeleton that can result in extensive fractures (particularly vertebral crush fractures). The disease remits spontaneously with the onset of puberty.

**Box 19.5.4 Causes of osteoporosis**

Calcium deficiency
- Nutritional
- Malabsorption

Malignancy
- Leukaemia

Glucocorticoid excess
- Iatrogenic
- Cushing disease

Homocystinuria
Osteogenesis imperfecta
Immobilization
Idiopathic juvenile osteoporosis

## Osteopetrosis

Osteopetrosis is a rare familial disorder of the skeleton in which there is a defect in bone and cartilage resorption, and hence of bone remodelling. This leads to a dense but brittle type of bone, which fractures easily. Infants usually present early in life with a severe leukoerythroblastic anaemia, symptoms of compression of cranial nerves (particularly optic atrophy leading to blindness) and marked hepatosplenomegaly. The bones show a characteristic dense and poorly modelled X-ray appearance.

## Magnesium disorders

Causes of hypomagnesaemia are given in Box 19.5.5. The symptoms of hypomagnesaemia resemble those of hypocalcaemia, with increased neuromuscular irritability. Severe hypomagnesaemia interferes with the release of PTH, and consequently hypomagnesaemia and hypocalcaemia often coexist.

Hypermagnesaemia occurs rarely in the absence of renal failure. The exception is the neonate born prematurely to a mother given magnesium sulphate for pre-eclampsia.

**Box 19.5.5 Causes of hypomagnesaemia and hypermagnesaemia**

**Hypomagnesaemia**
- Malabsorption, prolonged intravenous therapy
- Diuretic therapy
- Renal tubular acidosis
- Hereditary disorders of renal tubular resorption

**Hypermagnesaemia**
- Neonate of mother given magnesium sulphate for pre-eclampsia
- Medications containing magnesium given to patients with renal failure

PART 20

# GASTROINTESTINAL TRACT AND HEPATIC DISORDERS

# 20.1 Abdominal pain and vomiting

Spencer Beasley, Andrew Day

Acute abdominal pain and vomiting are common symptoms in children and a frequent reason for children to be taken to the doctor. Their causes are many and diverse; those that require surgery must be distinguished from those with a medical origin. Although there is considerable overlap of age in many disorders, other conditions occur only within a specific age range; for example, pyloric stenosis is not seen after the age of 3 months.

## Abdominal pain in the first 3 months of life

Abdominal pain without other symptoms is unusual in early infancy. Severe pain may be accompanied by other symptoms such as vomiting, abdominal distension or constipation. When pain is associated with other symptoms, it is more likely to have a surgical cause (e.g. malrotation with volvulus).

Infantile colic is a very common condition that usually commences in the first few weeks of life. The cause is poorly understood. The term 'colic' is sometimes used because of the common assumption that this pattern of behaviour is due to colicky abdominal pain but this explanation is controversial, and there are other more likely hypotheses including an irritable temperament (see Chapter 4.1). The term 'infant irritability' is now more commonly used.

The infant with irritability/colic:

- has attacks of screaming
- draws up the legs
- is unable to be comforted.

Significant vomiting is absent, bowel actions are passed normally and the infant is otherwise thriving. There are no specific abnormal findings on examination, or evidence of acute surgical problems such as a strangulated inguinal hernia. The symptoms usually disappear by the fourth month of age; until then, treatment is supportive.

In a vulnerable or unstable family situation, repeated irritability may place the infant at risk of abuse.

## Abdominal pain later in the first year

The main surgical cause of abdominal pain between 3 and 12 months of age is intussusception. Vomiting is a frequent accompanying feature, such that, when the colicky abdominal pain is not pronounced, intussusception must be distinguished from other causes of vomiting in this age group (see below).

### Intussusception

In intussusception, the distal ileum (the intussusceptum) telescopes into adjoining distal bowel (the intussuscipiens), resulting in intestinal obstruction. It can occur at any age but is most likely in the infant between 3 and 18 months who suddenly develops screaming attacks of pain with vomiting. During each episode of pain the infant becomes pale and may draw up the legs.

The spasms of pain tend to last for 2–3 minutes and occur at intervals of about 10–20 minutes, although after a while the pain becomes more persistent. Vomiting is an early symptom. The passage of a few loose stools early on represents evacuation of the bowel distal to the obstruction. The small volume and limited duration of loose stools in intussusception helps differentiate it from acute gastroenteritis. Congestion of the intussusceptum may lead to the passage of blood-stained or 'redcurrant jelly' stools. Many infants with intussusception present with little more than pallor, lethargy and vomiting, and may have little evidence of abdominal pain. Should these symptoms be ignored, the infant may progress to develop signs of septicaemia or shock.

The infant with intussusception looks pale, lethargic, anxious and unwell. A vague mass may be felt in the right or left upper quadrants of the abdomen but, once abdominal distension has developed, the mass becomes obscure and difficult to palpate (Fig. 20.1.1). The apex of the intussusceptum may be palpable on rectal examination in a few, and the examining glove may be blood-stained. A plain X-ray of the abdomen will often be normal but may show an unusual

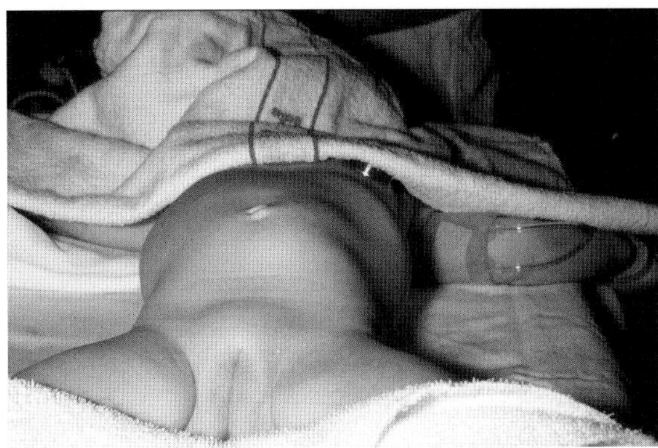

Fig. 20.1.1 Abdominal mass evident on left side of the abdomen in this toddler presenting with characteristic features of intussusception.

bowel gas distribution or features of bowel obstruction. Ultrasound examination may be helpful in making the diagnosis. Where intussusception is suspected clinically or confirmed on ultrasonography, a gas or barium enema must be performed (unless the child has peritonitis). The enema will demonstrate the position of the apex of the intussusception (Fig. 20.1.2).

### Treatment

Intussusception can be reduced non-operatively by gas enema or by hydrostatic reduction under ultrasonographic control: these techniques are successful in 80–90% of patients. If gas enema facilities are not available, a barium enema under continuous fluoroscopic control is a less effective but satisfactory alternative. Peritonitis and septicaemia, which suggest the presence of dead bowel, are the only contraindications to attempted enema reduction. A dehydrated child should have intravenous fluid resuscitation and be wrapped in warm blankets before commencing an enema reduction. The success of enema reduction is recognized when there is sudden or rapid flow of gas or barium into the ileum. If partial reduction is achieved, and the child remains in good clinical condition, a further enema should be attempted after several hours (so called 'delayed repeat enema'), and in about half of these patients it will be successful. Recurrence of intussusception occurs in about 9% of children after enema reduction, usually within days. Surgery is reserved for:

- those in whom enema reduction has failed
- those who have clinical evidence of necrotic bowel, such as peritonitis and septicaemia
- those in whom there is evidence of pathological lesions at the lead point.

### Differential diagnosis

Gastroenteritis is often confused with intussusception but becomes obvious on clinical grounds by the volume and persistence of the fluid stools. The plain radiological appearance of the abdomen may be similar in both conditions. Where doubt persists, ultrasonography or a gas or barium enema is indicated. Other causes of intestinal obstruction include volvulus secondary to malrotation, a band from a Meckel diverticulum, a duplication cyst or a strangulated inguinal hernia. Examination of the groin will detect the irreducible tender lump of a strangulated hernia.

## Acute abdominal pain in older children

Children often present with abdominal pain and in most no specific cause is found. Constipation and mesenteric adenitis are probably the most common non-surgical identifiable causes.

### Acute appendicitis

Appendicitis may occur at any age, although it is rare under 5 years of age. Early diagnosis is difficult in the young child (under 5 years) and in developmentally delayed children; many of these children have established peritonitis or an appendix abscess at presentation. Delays in the diagnosis of acute appendicitis in childhood is related in part to its variable symptomatology. For example, there may be relatively little abdominal pain, vomiting may be absent and diarrhoea may be a misleading feature.

Nevertheless, the most important and consistent feature is localized abdominal pain. The pain may be intermittent and colicky initially, or situated in the epigastrium or periumbilical region, but soon shifts to the right iliac fossa. Constant pain that is worse with movement is the result of peritoneal irritation ('peritonism'). Vomiting occurs in the majority of children, and some may pass a loose stool. The temperature is usually normal or slightly raised, but occasionally may be in excess of 38 °C.

Physical examination of the abdomen should be directed at showing that movement of adjacent peritoneal surfaces exacerbates the pain. The child's cooperation makes assessment easier, and repeated examination of the abdomen may be required to make the diagnosis. A child with appendicitis usually will exhibit tenderness and guarding localized to the right

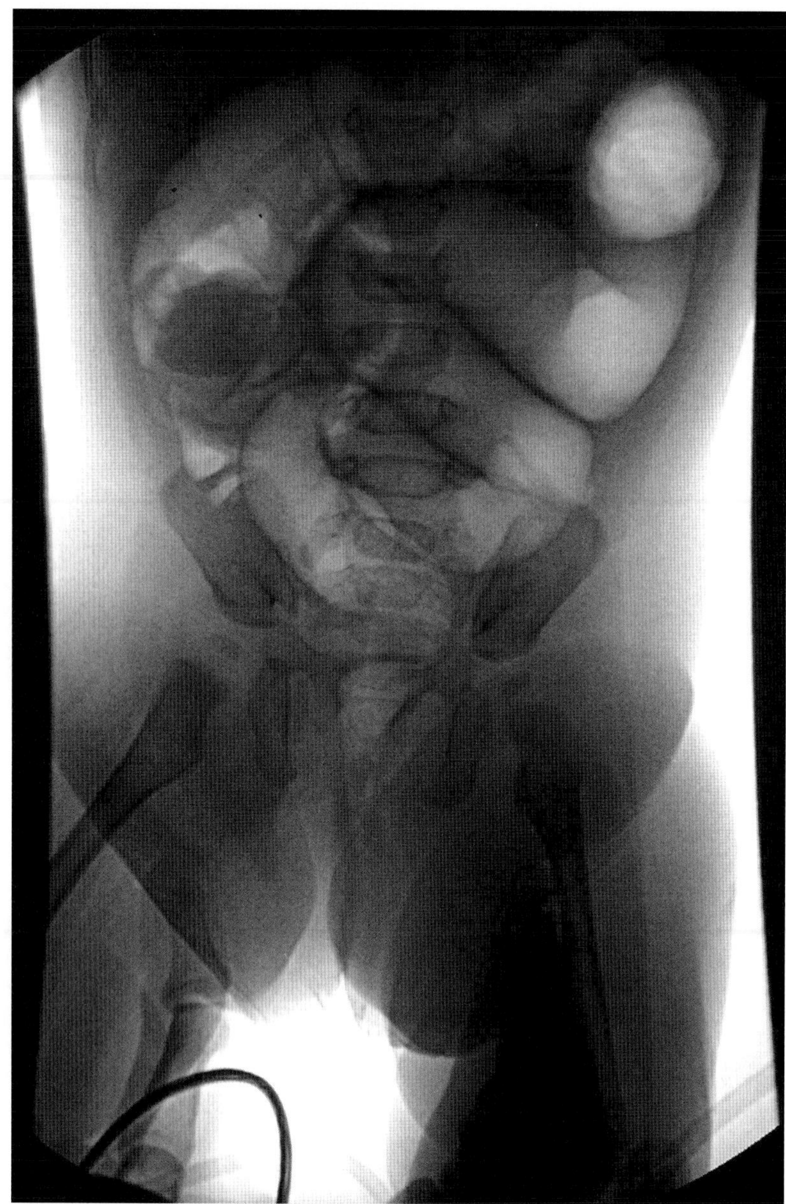

Fig. 20.1.2 Abdominal X-ray demonstrating air enema with apex of intussusception in the right lower quadrant.

iliac fossa. Gentle palpation and percussion tenderness, performed while observing the child's face, will provide the most reliable evidence of abdominal tenderness and involuntary guarding. Rebound tenderness is an unreliable sign in children, and attempts to elicit the sign may cause unnecessary pain and destroy the child's confidence in the doctor. Rectal examination is required rarely and is primarily indicated if a pelvic appendix or pelvic collection is suspected. It should not be performed when examination of the ventral abdominal wall has already enabled a confident diagnosis of acute appendicitis to be made. Bowel sounds may be normal or reduced and contribute little to the diagnosis.

Peritonitis should be suspected when the child is acutely ill with abdominal pain and fever and is reluctant to move. On examination, there will be generalized abdominal tenderness and guarding.

Laboratory studies are rarely helpful in making the diagnosis but the urine should be checked routinely. Ultrasonography has a role when the diagnosis is uncertain.

**Clinical example**

Mark, a 10-year-old boy, had 36 hours of constant lower abdominal pain, which steadily became more severe. He vomited once initially, and was 'off his food'. Movement made the pain worse. On examination, he was afebrile but appeared flushed. He was tender to gentle palpation in the right iliac fossa and had percussion tenderness in the same region. The urine contained a few white and red cells but no bacteria. No other investigation was performed. At laparoscopy an acutely inflamed appendix was removed.

## Differential diagnosis

Mesenteric adenitis is the most difficult disorder to distinguish from acute appendicitis. In general, localization of pain and tenderness is variable and less specific, and the temperature may be higher. Guarding is rarely present in mesenteric lymphadenitis.

Other conditions that may mimic acute appendicitis are relatively uncommon. Meckel diverticulitis has symptoms identical to those of appendicitis, such that differentiation is possible only at laparoscopy or laparotomy. Pain in the right iliac fossa may represent radiation from torsion of the right testis or a strangulated inguinal hernia, and highlights the importance of examination of the genitalia in all boys with lower abdominal symptoms (see Chapter 9.1). Acute abdominal pain may occur with renal colic, pyelonephritis and, at times, acute glomerulonephritis. Pain and tenderness is usually referred to the loin. Urine analysis and radiology will confirm the diagnosis. In Henoch–Schönlein purpura, the abdominal pain is often severe and colicky, and may be accompanied by vomiting. The characteristic skin lesions over the buttock and legs may be inconspicuous or absent when the child is first examined.

In the appropriate ethnic group, sickle cell anaemia is a prominent cause of acute abdominal pain and should be considered in a pale child with splenomegaly.

Children with cystic fibrosis frequently experience episodes of abdominal pain from faecal impaction (called 'meconium ileus equivalent'), a well-known manifestation of this disease. The symptoms resolve following a bowel washout.

It is unusual for constipation in an otherwise normal child to produce sufficient abdominal pain to suggest a surgical emergency. A plain X-ray of the abdomen will demonstrate the extent of faecal accumulation (Fig. 20.1.3). It should be remembered, however, that the diagnosis of constipation can almost exclusively be made on clinical grounds. Abdominal X-ray is not a standard tool in assessing for constipation and should be reserved solely for other indications or more complex cases.

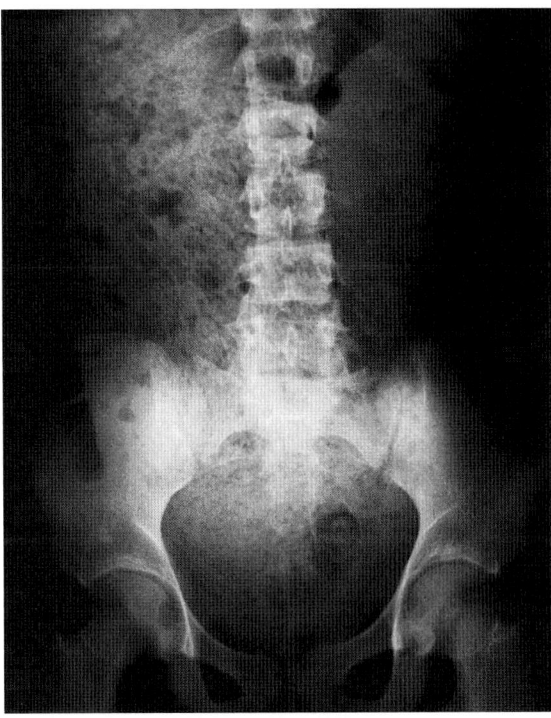

Fig. 20.1.3 Plain X-ray of the abdomen demonstrating gross faecal overload in a child with severe constipation causing abdominal pain. The child also had regular soiling.

Less common causes of abdominal pain include urinary tract infection, haemolytic–uraemic syndrome and diabetes. Ovarian torsion may present with pain and vomiting in girls. Acute hepatitis, cholecystitis and pancreatitis, although all rare in childhood, may also cause abdominal pain.

In pancreatitis, vomiting is prominent and epigastric tenderness with guarding may be marked. These children often look ill and obtunded. Pancreatitis is most commonly due to viral illnesses or may follow a blunt injury to the abdomen, (e.g. a handlebar injury), and several weeks later may produce a pancreatic pseudocyst. The diagnosis is suggested by increased levels of plasma or urinary amylase or plasma lipase, and is confirmed by ultrasonography initially, followed by magnetic resonance imaging (MRI) if indicated clinically. The management of acute pancreatitis involves correction of shock, intravenous fluid administration, bowel rest, nasogastric suction to keep the stomach empty, and analgesia.

Right lower-lobe pneumonia may masquerade as appendicitis. The child is usually febrile, with an increased respiratory rate, and has a cough. Signs of pneumonia may be difficult to elicit clinically, so that a chest X-ray will be required.

A general summary of disorders associated with abdominal pain is listed in Box 20.1.1.

**Box 20.1.1 Causes of abdominal pain in childhood**

**Common**
- Appendicitis
- Mesenteric adenitis
- Constipation
- Intussusception
- Urinary tract infection
- Torsion of the testis

**Uncommon**
- Volvulus secondary to malrotation
- Meckel diverticulitis
- Renal colic
- Pyelonephritis
- Acute glomerulonephritis
- Glandular fever
- Peptic ulceration
- Reflux oesophagitis
- Inflammatory bowel disease (e.g. Crohn's disease)
- Drug ingestion (e.g. salicylates, non-steroidal anti-inflammatory drugs, corticosteroids, some antibiotics, imipramine, phenytoin, iron)
- Abdominal migraine
- Lower-lobe pneumonia

**Rare**
- Sickle cell anaemia
- Henoch–Schönlein purpura
- Pancreatitis
- Cholecystitis
- Acute hepatitis
- Diabetes mellitus
- Haemolytic–uraemic syndrome
- Torsion of the ovary

### Peptic ulceration

The abdominal pain of peptic ulceration is epigastric and may be worse prior to meals. Nausea and vomiting may occur. Haematemesis and melaena suggest the diagnosis; alternatively it may be made following investigation of iron deficiency anaemia.

Acute gastritis and acute duodenitis produce abdominal pain with epigastric tenderness. A positive urea breath test is suggestive of *Helicobacter pylori* infection. Culture of biopsy specimens taken during endoscopic examination of the upper gastrointestinal tract will confirm *H. pylori* (see Chapter 20.4). Treatment with a combination of antibiotics (e.g. ampicillin and clarithromycin) and acid suppressors (e.g. omeprazole) is usually successful, but relapse may occur if the treatment course is incomplete.

### Gastro-oesophageal reflux disease and reflux oesophagitis

Physiological gastro-oesophageal reflux is very common in infancy and resolves with growth. This requires an expectant approach with reassurance and only rarely requires investigation or specific therapy. Gastro-oesophageal reflux disease (GORD), defined as reflux associated with symptoms or complications, can also begin in infancy. It may also resolve over time, but may persist into later childhood, with symptoms of belching, acid rise and intermittent vomiting. Substernal and epigastric pain ('heartburn') may suggest reflux oesophagitis. Oesophageal pH monitoring measures lower oesophageal pH over a period of 24 hours and can be used to quantify the reflux episodes and to establish the relationship of reflux to symptoms (see Chapter 20.4). Oesophagoscopy and biopsy may confirm oesophagitis and also exclude other causes (such as eosinophilic oesophagitis) of symptoms.

Initial management of GORD involves the administration of acid suppressors (e.g. $H_2$-receptor antagonists or proton pump inhibitors). However, when medical therapy is unsuccessful or when significant complications of GORD are present (e.g. episodes of reflux aspiration), surgical management of the GORD by laparoscopic fundoplication may be indicated.

## Recurrent abdominal pain in children

Recurrent bouts of abdominal pain is a fairly common paediatric presentation and one that may cause great anxiety to parents. The following clinical example is illustrative of this syndrome.

**Clinical example**

Thomas, aged 7 years, was brought in by his mother, who stated that for the last 4 months he had had severe bouts of abdominal pain. The attacks occurred at any time, but were more frequent at breakfast time. He was never awakened at night by them. Vomiting was not a feature, and his bowels had been regular. The pain usually was localized to the periumbilical region and usually lasted less than 1 hour. His parents felt that Thomas was pale and had a poor appetite. He was of normal height and weight. Physical examination was unremarkable. The urine was clear. Further questioning elicited the fact that the bouts of abdominal pain had occurred periodically since the age of 3 years.

Doctors will be impressed by the concern exhibited by parents of these children, who vividly describe the severe pain the child experiences; but there is a disparity between the parents' description and the physical findings on examination of the abdomen. Investigation almost invariably produces negative results. Enquiry into the personality of the child and into the home situation may reveal that the child is anxious or stressed, but often the pain occurs for no apparent reason. Sometimes the episodes of pain appear to be related to stress within the family, or occur on school days only.

A diagnosis of non-organic recurrent abdominal pain (RAP) can be made only after careful appraisal of the child in relation to the environment, and when the physical examination is normal. Most children need no investigations apart from urine culture. Further investigation is required if the abdominal pain is associated with abdominal tenderness or distension, symptoms that wake the child from sleep, bile-stained vomiting, persistent diarrhoea, fever, weight loss or urinary symptoms. Differentials to consider when such symptoms are present include inflammatory bowel disease, coeliac disease, malrotation with intermittent volvulus, and abdominal migraine. Appropriate investigations would depend on the pattern of symptoms, but may include full blood count, erythrocyte sedimentation ratio (ESR), C-reactive protein (CRP), liver chemistry and albumin, screening for coeliac disease, markers of malabsorption (such as iron, folate, and vitamins D and $B_{12}$), stool testing, and endoscopic studies of the upper and lower gastrointestinal tract. The urine should also be examined. If the vomitus is bile-stained, malrotation with volvulus should be excluded by an urgent barium meal.

The general status of the patient must be assessed. Retardation of height and growth may occur in chronic inflammatory bowel disease and malabsorption syndromes. Pallor may be associated with anaemia or conditions such as lead poisoning, sickle cell anaemia and other haemolytic diseases. Abdominal migraine may be seen in children with a family history of classical migraine; as time goes by the child's abdominal pain may become associated with and eventually be replaced by classical migraine headaches.

### Management of recurrent abdominal pain

Parents will find it helpful to realize that the problem has been taken seriously by the doctor, and the doctor must understand the parents' perception of the abdominal pain. With this knowledge and the negative physical findings, reassurance can be given more positively. Once parents are convinced that there is no significant organic basis to the RAP, they are usually much relieved. The child should be encouraged in all activities and self-esteem improved. Recurrent pain tends to disappear by the age of 12 years but in females may recur at the time of menarche. However, some children with recurrent pain in childhood present in adult life with symptoms of irritable bowel syndrome.

## Vomiting in the neonatal period

In the first 24 hours of life, neonates frequently vomit small amounts of mucus and blood swallowed during labour. If this vomiting does not clear spontaneously, gastric lavage with normal saline will usually relieve it. In the early weeks of life, many normal newborn babies regurgitate after feeds. Also known as 'spitting up' or 'possetting', this is a benign feature of physiological immaturity in the upper gut and resolves with time.

### Systemic infection

Vomiting is one of the many non-specific signs of infection in the neonate. Thus, unexplained vomiting should be an indication to culture the blood, urine and cerebrospinal fluid. Urine will usually be obtained by suprapubic aspiration in this age group.

### Bowel obstruction

In duodenal obstruction, vomiting appears early and is bile-stained because the site of the obstruction is almost always at the second part of the duodenum, just distal to the ampulla of Vater. In duodenal atresia, there may be other abnormalities such as Down syndrome and imperforate anus. The bile-stained vomiting commences from birth. The diagnosis is made on plain X-ray of the abdomen (see Chapter 11.5). Where there is bowel obstruction beyond the duodenum (e.g. small bowel atresia, Hirschsprung disease and meconium ileus), vomiting commences slightly later and is associated with increasing abdominal distension (see Chapter 11.5). A strangulated inguinal hernia may cause a bowel obstruction when a loop of ileum becomes trapped within the hernial sac at the external inguinal ring. The diagnosis becomes evident when a tender irreducible lump is observed in the groin (see Chapter 9.1).

### Malrotation with volvulus

Volvulus in a neonate or infant with malrotation causes a high bowel obstruction and produces bile-stained vomiting. The volvulus may cut off the blood supply to the midgut and lead to small bowel infarction, septicaemia and death if not identified and managed promptly. Any infant with bile-stained vomiting, otherwise unexplained, should be assumed to have malrotation with volvulus until proven otherwise. A barium meal will confirm the diagnosis. An urgent laparotomy is required to untwist the bowel (Fig. 20.1.4) and to perform a Ladd procedure to broaden the mesentery of the small bowel; this will prevent subsequent volvulus.

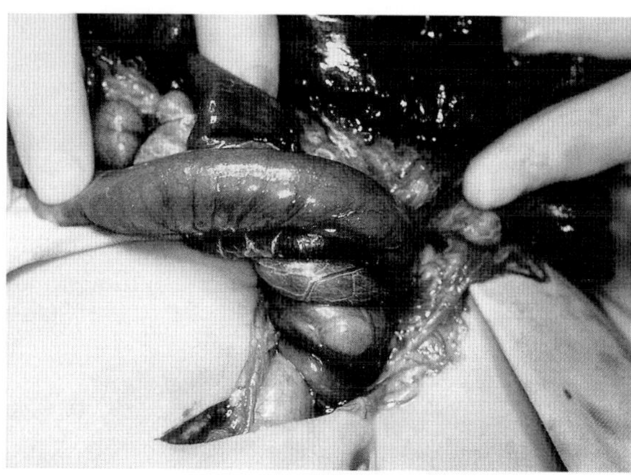

Fig. 20.1.4 Malrotation with volvulus. The small bowel is twisted upon its mesentery.

### Hypoglycaemia

Vomiting may be the only symptom of hypoglycaemia in the neonatal period. It is more common in 'small for dates' babies and in infants of diabetic mothers, but may be seen in any stressful situation in the neonatal period, including low birth weight, neonatal meningitis, septicaemia and severe Rhesus isoimmunization. Symptomatic hypoglycaemia does not usually occur with a blood glucose in excess of 2 mmol/L.

### Renal disease

In the neonatal period, urinary infection and renal insufficiency may present with vomiting and poor weight gain, reflecting an underlying urinary tract abnormality. Initial urological investigation will include urine culture, renal ultrasonography, micturating cystourethrography, and estimation of electrolytes, urea and creatinine. Renal tubular lesions occasionally present in the neonatal period with vomiting.

### Adrenal insufficiency

Congenital adrenal hyperplasia, in which there is deficiency of the enzyme 21-hydroxylase (see Chapter 19.3), presents with ambiguous genitalia in the female. If this is not recognized (as in the male), it may lead to unexplained vomiting, dehydration and collapse early in the second week of life. If the adrenal insufficiency is of the salt-losing type, the diagnosis is further suspected by finding low levels of sodium and increased levels of potassium in the serum, and is confirmed by appropriate hormonal studies.

### Inborn metabolic errors

Although individually rare, there are a number of inborn errors involving, separately, amino acid, carbohydrate and organic acid metabolism. Most are inherited recessively, and a number can now be treated. Frequently, the presentation is with unexplained vomiting, lethargy, collapse, seizures and coma (see Chapter 10.5).

## Vomiting in infancy

Vomiting is a common non-specific symptom in infancy, and disease of almost every system may present with vomiting.

### Infection

Vomiting is frequently associated with acute infections such as tonsillitis, otitis media, pneumonia, meningitis and urinary tract infection. Physical examination will exclude many of these but early signs may be minimal in meningitis and pneumonia, such that a lumbar puncture and chest X-ray will be required if these are suspected. In infants with urinary tract infection, dysuria, frequency of passing urine and loin pain cannot be relied upon for diagnosis, and the urine must always be examined (see Chapter 18).

### Lesions of the gastrointestinal tract

Conditions that produce vomiting in infancy are different from those seen in the neonatal period, except for duodenal obstruction from volvulus complicating malrotation, and GORD. Failure to recognize malrotation with volvulus may result in infarction of the entire midgut (see Chapter 11.5). Bowel trapped in a strangulated inguinal hernia in an infant will also produce vomiting. The diagnosis can be made easily if the inguinal orifices are examined (see Chapter 9.1).

### Gastro-oesophageal reflux disease

See Chapter 20.4.

### Pyloric stenosis

This is one of the most dramatic causes of vomiting in infancy. Typically, the onset is sudden, commencing between the second and sixth week of life. Males are affected five times more often than females and there is a definite familial incidence. Before the onset of vomiting, these infants feed well and are thriving. The vomiting is forceful and rapidly becomes projectile. The infant loses weight and becomes dehydrated. Despite vomiting, these infants remain hungry and are keen to feed even immediately after vomiting. The vomitus is not bile-stained but may contain altered blood. The diagnosis is made clinically by feeling the thickened pylorus ('pyloric tumour') in the midline in the epigastrium between the rectus abdominis muscles or in the angle between the right rectus and the liver edge. The pyloric tumour is palpable as a hard mobile mass about the size of a small pebble or olive. Peristaltic waves passing from the left costal margin to the right hypochondrium ('golfball waves') may be visible long after the last feed. Palpation of the tumour is sufficient to establish the diagnosis. Pyloric stenosis can also be shown on ultrasonography (which reveals a thickened pylorus) and barium meal (which shows delayed gastric emptying and a narrow pyloric canal). These infants develop a hypokalaemic, hypochloraemic metabolic alkalosis which, together with dehydration, must be corrected before surgery. Pyloromyotomy is curative (Fig. 20.1.5).

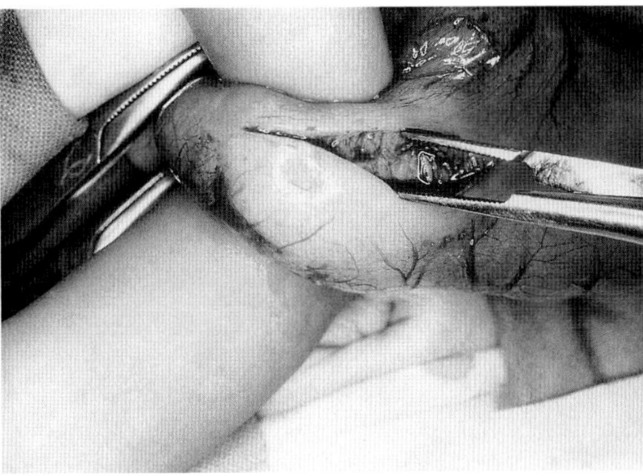

Fig. 20.1.5 Thickened pylorus in pyloric stenosis as seen during pyloromyotomy.

### Gastroenteritis

Vomiting in association with fluid stools is suggestive of gastroenteritis, particularly if the stools contain mucus or blood. However, these features may be seen in a variety of other medical and surgical disorders, which include intussusception and appendicitis. The diagnosis and management of gastroenteritis is discussed in Chapter 20.2.

### Malabsorption

In the majority of malabsorption syndromes vomiting is not a feature. Vomiting can be a presenting symptom in some children with coeliac disease (gluten enteropathy; see Chapter 20.3).

### Intussusception

Vomiting commences early in intussusception and is the most consistent symptom. The general features, diagnosis and treatment have been discussed above.

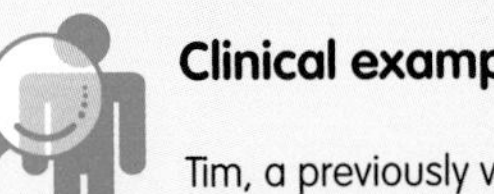

**Clinical example**

Tim, a previously well 22-month-old infant, suddenly became unwell with onset of vomiting and a temperature of 38.5 °C. Within 12 hours he started passing frequent, loose motions. Associated with this he appeared to have bouts of abdominal pain. On the second day the vomiting stopped but the diarrhoea persisted at a rate of more than eight stools per day. On presentation to the emergency department, Tim's weight was 13.6 kg, compared with 14.5 kg 3 weeks previously. He was clinically assessed to be 5–8% dehydrated and was treated with an oral rehydration solution via a nasogastric tube. A provisional diagnosis of acute gastroenteritis was made. His temperature gradually settled over 24 hours and oral feeds were introduced once rehydration was complete. His stools returned to their normal pattern after 5 days. Rapid stool testing for rotavirus antigen was positive.

### Strangulated inguinal hernia

Strangulation of an inguinal hernia is common in infants and young children. All irreducible inguinal hernias should be assumed to be strangulated. In practice, the vast majority of so-called irreducible hernias can be reduced manually by skilled hands (see Chapter 9.1).

## Vomiting in older children

Vomiting in older children is usually associated with infection, particularly viral or bacterial infection of the respiratory and gastrointestinal tracts. Nevertheless, there are some other less frequent, but important, causes of vomiting.

The possibility of an intracranial neoplasm should always be considered in a child with unexplained vomiting. There may be signs of increased intracranial pressure with midline cerebellar tumours, tumours involving the fourth ventricle, and tumours involving the pons or medulla. Initially, vomiting tends to occur in the morning before breakfast. There may be remissions for several days but the vomiting invariably returns.

### Migraine

In the older child, the association of severe paroxysmal frontal headache with pallor and vomiting is suggestive of migraine (see Chapter 17.5). A positive family history is common. In the younger child, attacks of pallor or vomiting may be the only symptom. The diagnosis of migraine is made on clinical history but, where it is difficult to exclude an intracranial space-occupying lesion clinically, cerebral computed tomography may be required.

### Acute appendicitis and peritonitis

In acute appendicitis in childhood, vomiting is a frequent early symptom but is usually preceded by pain. The general features of appendicitis have been described above. In the young child (under 5 years), vomiting with or without diarrhoea may be the only apparent symptom. Physical examination in this age group can be difficult and unreliable; the child will prefer to lie still, as movement worsens the pain. This pain and the fear of its exacerbation by palpation may make the child appear uncooperative. It is only by repeated examination of the abdomen and an ongoing high index of suspicion that the diagnosis will be made before widespread peritonitis has developed.

### Poisoning

Vomiting and respiratory and circulatory collapse in a previously well child should raise the possibility of poisoning (see Chapter 5.3). Non-accidental poisoning is becoming more frequent.

### Psychological causes of vomiting

Psychogenic vomiting may occur in any age group. It can be associated with attempts to force-feed a toddler or schoolchild, after punishment, and as an attempt to avoid situations perceived as threatening, such as going to preschool or school. Almost any stressful situation may precipitate vomiting in a tense or anxious child. The absence of abnormal physical signs will be a feature.

### Cyclical vomiting syndrome

Cyclical vomiting is a clinical syndrome of persistent periodic vomiting of childhood. The severity varies, but ketosis and metabolic acidosis may develop rapidly. The aetiology is unknown and attacks usually cease spontaneously. Children with cyclical vomiting are often tense and anxious, and may develop migraine or psychosomatic disease later in life. However, cyclic vomiting syndrome is a diagnosis of exclusion; it is essential to exclude other important causes of recurrent vomiting, such as intermittent volvulus from malrotation, neurological causes and metabolic disease.

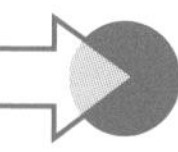

#### Practical points

- Intussusception, the primary surgical cause of abdominal pain between 3 and 12 months of age, usually presents with vomiting, abdominal pain, pallor and lethargy.
- Although appendicitis may occur at any age, it is rare in preschool children; in this age group its presentation may be atypical, making early diagnosis a challenge.
- Recurrent abdominal pain commonly occurs in children; it is often benign and self-resolving. Warning signs of a significant underlying organic cause include weight loss, night pain, pain worse with movement and bile-stained vomiting.
- Vomiting is a very non-specific symptom in infancy and early childhood, and may indicate infection.

# Infective diarrhoea and inflammatory bowel disease

## 20.2

Jeremy Rosenbaum, George Alex

The basic pathological mechanisms causing diarrhoea include osmotic, secretory and inflammatory processes (Table 20.2.1). Often more than one mechanism occurs simultaneously resulting in diarrhoea.

Diarrhoea is defined as a measured stool volume greater than 10 mL per kg per day. Both the consistency of the stool (loose or watery) and frequency (usually more than three stools in a 24-hour period) are important defining features of diarrhoea.

Acute diarrhoea usually lasts less than 10 days and can have a major impact on the individual's fluid and electrolyte status. The commonest cause of acute diarrhoea in children is an enteric infection (acute gastroenteritis). This can be driven by all three of the pathological mechanisms mentioned above.

Chronic diarrhoea is defined as symptoms being present for more than 2–3 weeks. This requires further investigation as several important causes such as inflammatory bowel disease need to be excluded to avoid possible systemic complications and negative effects on the nutritional state of the child. This can also have a significant effect on the nutritional state of a child (see Chapter 20.3).

## Acute gastroenteritis

### Viral gastroenteritis

Rotavirus infection (Fig. 20.2.1) is the most common cause of acute gastroenteritis in children worldwide, with a peak incidence between 6 and 24 months of age. It is also a major cause of mortality in developing countries and is responsible for the majority of cases where hospital admission is required. In Australia, before routine infant rotavirus immunization was introduced in 2007, approximately 10 000 children aged under 5 years were hospitalized each year due to rotavirus infection, 115 000 visited a general practitioner, 22 000 required an emergency department visit and, on average, one Australian child died each year from the complications of dehydration and shock. Since 2007, these numbers have fallen dramatically. Infants in developing countries are more susceptible to severe infection causing life-threatening diarrhoea because of pre-existing malnutrition and poor access to primary care. Similarly, Indigenous Australian children require hospitalisation due to rotavirus gastroenteritis about three to five times more commonly than non-Indigenous children.

The mucosal damage caused by rotavirus (Fig. 20.2.2) occurs primarily in the small intestine. It results in villus destruction and loss of digestive enzymes found on the tips of villi. This causes impaired digestion of carbohydrates, impaired intestinal absorption of fluid and electrolytes, and fluid loss from the intestine. The need for structural repair places considerable nutritional demands on malnourished children. Repeated asymptomatic reinfection helps maintain immunity.

The other major viral cause of hospital admissions is the enteric adeno family of viruses. Norovirus is also implicated in winter outbreaks of vomiting. Other less common viruses, such as calicivirus, astrovirus and other small viruses, have also been implicated in gastroenteritis requiring hospitalization. Cytomegalovirus (CMV) enteritis should be considered in immunocompromised patients.

### Bacterial and parasitic gastroenteritis

Bacteria cause fewer episodes of acute gastroenteritis in developed countries than viruses. The main causes of bacterial infection are *Campylobacter jejuni, Salmonella* spp., *Shigella* spp. and various types of *Escherichia coli*, each accounting for a small percentage. *Clostridium difficile*, known to cause pseudomembranous colitis following systemic antibiotic therapy, is usually hospital-acquired and becoming increasingly resistant to first line treatment options.

In developing countries, *E. coli* (enterotoxigenic, enteropathogenic and enteroinvasive), *Shigella* spp. and *Entamoeba histolytica* are especially important: *E. coli* because of the large number of episodes it causes, *Shigella* because it causes prolonged, debilitating illness and antibiotic-resistant strains are emerging, and *Entamoeba* because it causes severe life-threatening dysentery. These organisms are rarely acquired in industrialized countries.

**Table 20.2.1 Classification of diarrhoea**

| | Osmotic | Secretory | Inflammatory |
|---|---|---|---|
| Clinical features | Ceases when enteral feeding is ceased | Continues when enteral feeding is ceased | Presence of blood and mucus in the faeces |
| Stool volume | <200 mL/day | >200 mL/day | Variable, usually <200 mL/day |
| Faecal sodium | <60 mosmol/L | 90 mosmol/L | Variable |

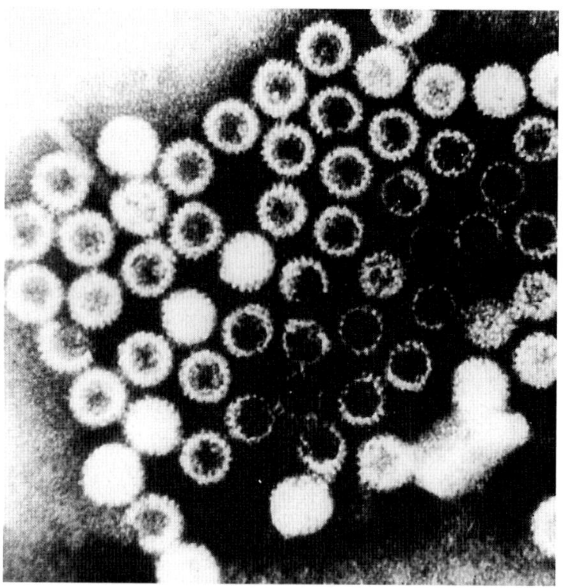

Fig. 20.2.1 The rotavirus (electron micrograph).

The parasite *Giardia lamblia* is a rare cause of acute dehydrating diarrhoea, but a common cause of persistent diarrhoea with flatulence and bloating. It is most common in toddlers and young children, and also in their parents and caregivers. It is also common in people who have travelled overseas especially to developing countries where drinking water supplies may be contaminated. Another parasite, *Cryptosporidium,* is another rare cause of acute diarrhoea in some infants admitted to hospital and should be considered in immunocompromised patients.

## Clinical features

Acute gastroenteritis is a relatively common cause of presentation to medical attention, but it should remain a diagnosis of exclusion, because several systemic disorders and surgical emergencies can present with diarrhoea and/or vomiting (Box 20.2.1) and should be considered in the differential diagnosis.

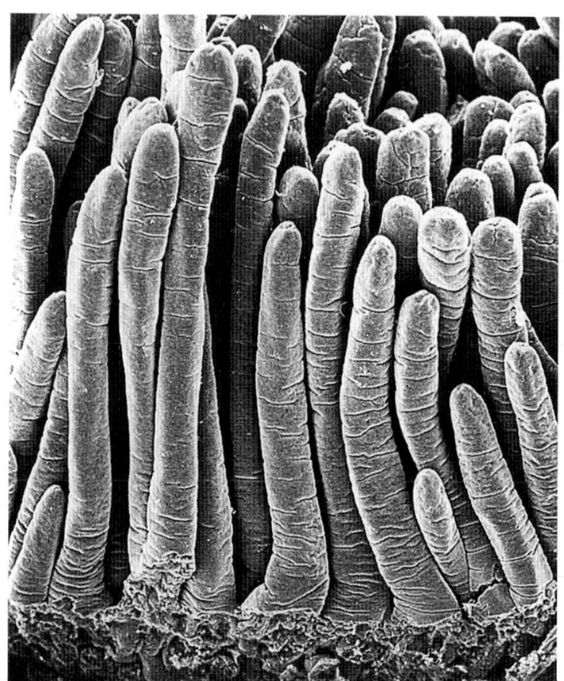

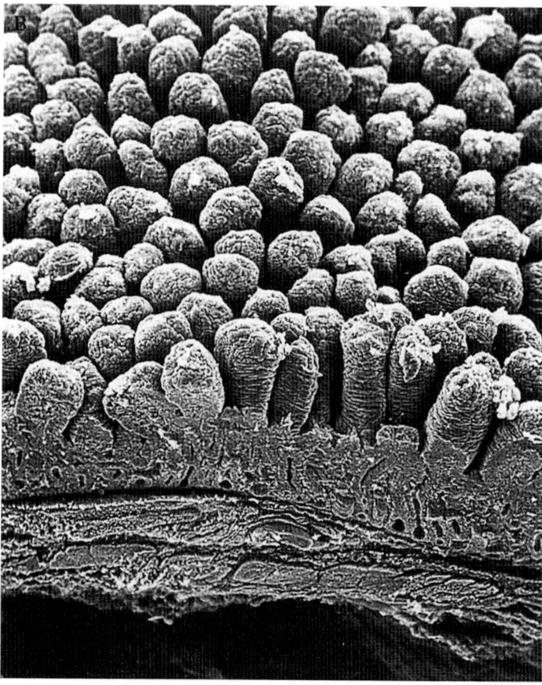

Fig. 20.2.2 Scanning electron microscope appearances of (**A**) normal and (**B**) rotavirus-infected calf jejunum. Villi are short, the epithelium is damaged, and crypts are deep. (Courtesy of DGA Hall, Institute for Animal Health, Compton, UK. With permission from Walker et al 1991.)

**Box 20.2.1 Differential diagnosis of acute diarrhoea and vomiting in infants and children**

**Enteric infection**
- Rotavirus
- Other viruses
- Bacterial
  - *Salmonella* spp.
  - *Shigella* spp.
  - *Escherichia coli*
  - *Campylobacter jejuni*
- Protozoa
  - *Cryptosporidium*
  - *Giardia lamblia*
  - *Entamoeba histolytica*
- Food poisoning
- Staphylococcal toxin

**Systemic infection**
- Urinary tract infection
- Pneumonia
- Septicaemia

**Surgical condition**
- Appendicitis
- Intussusception
- Partial bowel obstruction
- Hirschsprung disease

**Other**
- Diabetes mellitus
- Antibiotic diarrhoea
- Haemolytic–uraemic syndrome

Symptoms of acute gastroenteritis are watery diarrhoea (up to 10–20 stools daily) with or without vomiting and fever (to 39–40°C). Vomiting is often the predominant feature early in the illness, followed by diarrhoea. If both occur concurrently, there is an increased risk of dehydration. Maintaining hydration is easier after the cessation of vomiting. Blood, mucus and the passage of small frequent bowel actions accompanied by abdominal pain suggest a diagnosis of colitis due to bacterial gastroenteritis ('bacterial dysentery'), amoebic dysentery or, potentially, inflammatory bowel disease.

## Investigations

Stool samples should be sent for microscopy, bacterial culture and sensitivities (MC + S). Samples should also be sent for ova, cysts and parasites (OCP) and viral studies, which may include enzyme-linked immunosorbent assay (ELISA), polymerase chain reaction (PCR) and viral culture. Appropriate treatment should not be withheld pending results. Sending several stool samples from different bowel actions increases the positive yield of the test and is recommended.

## Management

Once the diagnosis of acute gastroenteritis is made on thorough clinical history and physical examination, the next step is to assess the degree of dehydration and institute an appropriate plan for rehydration. This should be combined with nutritional support that aids the patient during the recovery phase.

## Dehydration

The risk of dehydration is inversely related to age, with young infants being at greatest risk because they have a high surface area : body volume ratio, resulting in increased insensible fluid loss. They also tend to have more severe vomiting and diarrhoea than older children and adults.

Fluid loss is usually assessed on the basis of percentage body weight loss. Physical signs of dehydration are not usually apparent until 4% of body weight is lost.

The signs of dehydration traditionally described are outlined in Box 20.2.2. The three signs that discriminate best between dehydration and adequate hydration are deep breathing, decreased skin turgor and poor peripheral perfusion.

## Electrolyte loss

Dehydration is usually isotonic (water and electrolytes being lost in equal amounts). Hypertonic hypernatraemic dehydration (fluid loss > electrolyte loss) occurs in 5–10% of children with acute gastroenteritis, and hypotonic hyponatraemic dehydration (electrolyte loss > fluid loss) can occur if the colon (a major site of sodium resorption) is out of circuit (e.g. in short gut syndrome).

**Box 20.2.2 Assessment of dehydration**

**Mild (≤5% body weight loss)**
- Dry mucous membranes
- Decreased peripheral perfusion*
- Thirsty, alert, restless

**Moderate (6–9% body weight loss)**
- Exaggeration of the above
- Lethargic but irritable
- Rapid pulse, normal blood pressure
- Sunken eyes, sunken fontanelle
- Oliguria is usually obvious
- Pinched skin retracts slowly (1–2 s)*

**Severe (≥10% body weight loss)**
- General appearance:
  - Infants: drowsy, limp, cold sweaty, cyanotic limbs, comatose
  - Older children: apprehensive, cold, sweaty, cyanotic limbs
- Rapid feeble pulse, low blood pressure
- Sunken eyes and fontanelle
- Pinched skin retracts slowly (>2 s)*
- Deep acidotic breathing*

*These are the only signs proven to discriminate between hydration and dehydration.

If corrected too rapidly, hypernatraemic dehydration can cause convulsions due to rapid shifts of water into cells. Hyponatraemic dehydration can also cause significant neurological morbidity and mortality and, in contrast to the hypernatraemic state, requires vigorous replacement of sodium. Nasogastric rehydration has a much lower risk of these electrolyte complications than intravenous rehydration.

## Rehydration guidelines

See also Chapter 6.1.

### No dehydration

- Nutritional intake and fluids should not be modified and should be encouraged to keep up with ongoing losses, avoiding the need for rehydration via nasogastric or intravenous route.

### Mild to moderate dehydration

- Oral rehydration solution (ORS) is the cornerstone of successful rehydration and is recommended globally for the management of acute diarrhoea.
- The success of ORS is based on the principle that intestinal sodium transport is enhanced by glucose transport in the small intestine and that this sodium-coupled mechanism for glucose transport remains intact during acute gastroenteritis.
- To facilitate optimal absorption of sodium, glucose and water, the sodium and glucose must be in the range recommended (Table 20.2.2).
- Rehydration of deficit should take place over 4–6 hours and can be given orally or, if either vomiting or fluid refusal is a problem, by nasogastric tube. Ondansetron can be administered once in this setting but not in children <6 mo or <8 kg.
- If unable to maintain oral intake then maintenance fluids should be continued either by NGT or intravenous route with monitoring of potential ongoing losses during this time. (see Box 20.2.3).

**Box 20.2.3 An infant of 10 kg estimated at 8% dehydration has fluid requirements equal to**

Maintenance 100 × 10 kg = 1000 mL
Deficit 8% of 10 kg = 800 mL
Total = 1800 mL
Using oral rehydration the deficit can be replaced in 6 h rather than 24 h, so in the above example the infant would be offered fluid as follows:

**First 6 hours**
Deficit = 800 mL
Maintenance 6/24 of 1000 = 250 mL
Total = 1050 mL (175 mL/h)

**Next 18 hours**
Maintenance 18/24 of 1000 = 750 mL (45 mL/h)
Another simple method that gives about the right answer is to calculate the fluid deficit, double it, and give that volume over 6–12 h.

### Rapid nasogastric rehydration

- 25ml/kg/hr for 4 hours
- Suitable for the majority of patients with gastroenteritis and moderate dehydration

### Slower nasogastric rehydration

- Slower rehydration is preferred for the following patients:
- Infants < 6 months
- Co-morbidities present.
- Children with significant abdominal pain.
- Replacing deficit over first 6 hours and then daily maintenance over the next 18 hours.

### Severe dehydration (≥10%)

- If circulatory insufficiency is present, intravenous therapy is required. The usual requirement is to fill the vascular compartment quickly to restore circulation. This will require rapid rehydration, often using boluses of normal saline (10–20 mL/kg) by intravenous or intraosseous infusion.

**Table 20.2.2 Oral rehydration preparations available in Australia**

| | Na | K | Cl | Citrate | Glucose |
|---|---|---|---|---|---|
| World Health Organization | 90 | 20 | 80 | 10 | 90 |
| Hydralyte | 45 | 20 | 45 | 30 | 90 |
| Gastrolyte | 60 | 20 | 60 | 10 | 90 |
| Repalyte | 60 | 20 | 60 | 10 | 90 |

Concentration expressed as millimoles per litre (mmol/L).

**Box 20.2.4 A 10-kg child with 15% dehydration and shock**

Total fluid deficit = 15% of 10 kg = 1.5 L = 1500 mL
Assume a total of 40 mL/kg (400 mL) normal saline needed to restore circulation
Remaining deficit = 1500 − 400 = 1100 mL
Maintenance fluid requirement is 100 mL per kg per day = 10 × 100 = 1000 mL
Fluid in next 24 h = remaining deficit + maintenance = 1100 + 1000 = 2100 mL = 90 mL/h
Therefore, give 400 mL normal saline quickly, then 90 mL/h 5% dextrose in N/2 saline with KCl 40 mmol/L for the next 24 h.

- Once dehydration is corrected and normal organ perfusion is restored, ORS can be used in conjunction with intravenous fluids. The latter is rarely required for longer than 24 hours.
- In severe dehydration, replace deficit over first 6 hours and then daily maintenance over the next 18 hours with regular reviews of losses.
- Clinical observations must be highlighted; these allow the physician to reassess the patient's state of hydration and also help confirm the diagnosis of acute gastroenteritis.
- All patients with dehydration require regular checks on pulse, blood pressure, temperature and respiration. In addition, a strict fluid balance chart must be kept. The child should be weighed on admission and, in severe cases, after 6 and 24 hours, with an increase in weight being a reliable sign of rehydration. However, in some patients, weight may not fall even in the presence of severe dehydration, especially if the child has an ileus, so other signs of dehydration must also be sought (Box 20.2.4).

## Recommendations on nutritional management

In babies and young infants, breastfeeding should continue through rehydration and maintenance phases of treatment. Similarly, formula feeds should be restarted after rehydration. Use of special formulas or diluted formulas is unjustified unless problematic diarrhoea persists (see complications of acute gastroenteritis).

## Pharmacotherapy

- Infants and children with acute gastroenteritis should not be treated with antidiarrhoeal agents.
- Antibiotic treatment may be indicated in non-typhoid *Salmonella* gastroenteritis in infants (especially those aged <3 months) and children who are immunocompromised or who are systemically unwell. It may also be indicated in *C. jejuni* infection in compromised hosts and *Yersinia enterocolitica* in children with sickle cell disease.
- Pathogens for which antimicrobial therapy is indicated include *Shigella*, *Entamoeba histolytica* and *Giardia lamblia*.
- Certain types of probiotic may have a modest effect in acute infective gastroenteritis; however, their routine use is not recommended until further large-scale trials have been undertaken.
- The antiemetic ondansetron is being used increasingly to treat vomiting associated with gastroenteritis. It should be administered only once in this setting and does not change the natural history of the disease, but can improve tolerance of enteral rehydration. It is not recommended for children aged less than 6 months or weighing less than 8 kg.

## Prevention of acute gastroenteritis

A simple and effective method of prevention of this condition is via handwashing when in contact with an index case, as the faecal–oral route is the most common form of transmission.

Two live attenuated oral rotavirus vaccines, Rotarix® and RotaTeq®, have been used in Australia since 2007 to immunize all babies aged 2–6 months. Rotavirus vaccines are even more valuable in developing countries, where the burden of rotavirus disease is far higher.

Vaccines against typhoid and cholera infection are also available. Anti-*E. coli* colostrum tablets are also available to help prevent the most common type of traveller's diarrhoea, and *E. coli* vaccines are under development.

## Complications of acute gastroenteritis

### Sugar malabsorption

Sugar malabsorption is commonest in infants less than 6 months of age and presents with persistent diarrhoea after feeds are reintroduced. With exposure to carbohydrates, stools are often watery, frothy and tend to excoriate the buttocks.

If sugar intolerance is suspected, the napkin should be lined with thin plastic material, or a rectal examination should be performed and the fluid stool collected and tested for reducing substances. It is pointless to test solid stool material.

To test for lactose intolerance, mix 5 drops of liquid stool with 10 drops of water and add a Clinitest tablet. A positive test of more than 0.5% indicates lactose or glucose malabsorption, but not sucrose, which is not a reducing sugar.

Diarrhoea due to lactose malabsorption resolves rapidly on a lactose-free diet, which should be continued for approximately 4 weeks. A very small proportion of infants continue to have diarrhoea despite the exclusion of lactose and sucrose. Under these circumstances, a carbohydrate-free feed is given temporarily, with glucose and fructose (different transport mechanisms across the enterocyte) added to tolerance.

**Clinical example**

Tim, a previously well 22-month-old infant, suddenly became unwell with vomiting and fever (38.5°C). Within 12 hours he started passing frequent, loose motions. Associated with this he appeared to have bouts of abdominal pain. On the second day the vomiting stopped but the diarrhoea persisted at a rate of more than eight stools per day. On presentation to the emergency department, Tim's weight was 13.6 kg, compared with 14.5 kg 3 weeks earlier. He was clinically assessed to be 5–8% dehydrated and was treated with an oral rehydration solution via a nasogastric tube. A provisional diagnosis of acute gastroenteritis was made. His temperature gradually settled over 24 hours and oral feeds were introduced once rehydration was complete. His stools returned to their normal pattern after 5 days. Rapid stool testing for rotavirus antigen was positive.

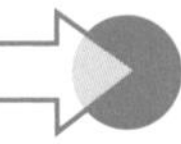

**Practical points**

**Acute gastroenteritis**

- Commonly caused by viruses and self-limiting.
- Assess dehydration carefully and correct appropriately, but reassess constantly.
- Not all children with diarrhoea and/or vomiting have gastroenteritis; be wary of other conditions that may mimic it.
- Proper hand-washing is the best measure to avoid transmission.
- Rotavirus vaccines are safe and effective.

## Inflammatory bowel disease

Chronic diarrhoea is defined as the presence of diarrhoea for more than 2–3 weeks. It can follow a bout of acute gastroenteritis, but usually begins insidiously. Many causes of chronic diarrhoea are associated with malabsorption of nutrients and are dealt with in detail in Chapter 20.3.

Inflammatory bowel disease (IBD) constitutes Crohn's disease and ulcerative colitis (UC). These conditions should be considered in the differential diagnosis of patients with chronic diarrhoea, particularly with blood and mucus, once infectious agents have been excluded. The incidence of inflammatory bowel disease has increased in recent years and Australia has among the highest rates reported in the world. Current opinion regarding aetiology favours the hypothesis that IBD results from a complex interaction between immunological, genetic and environmental factors. There is a positive family history of IBD in up to 20% of cases. The microbiota of the gut and its interaction with the host's immune system has been the focus of much attention recently with its importance becoming increasingly apparent.

Children may experience the same symptoms, clinical presentations, complications and response to treatment as adults with IBD, but often with more aggressive disease characteristics. This chapter will highlight some of the features of IBD that have particular importance to the paediatric patient.

### Crohn's disease

Crohn's disease is a lifelong condition that can present in several ways with variable involvement of any length of the gastrointestinal tract from mouth to anus. The disease causes transmural, granulomatous inflammation of affected areas, interspersed with normal areas. Numerous genes have been implicated in contributing to this complex disease including *NOD2* (also called *CARD15*), a gene that is involved in the regulation of intestinal epithelial cells, which are important in their role as mucosal barrier. Many other genes have been associated, but none in causation. Further advances in genetics will undoubtedly contribute to our understanding in the years to come.

The disease can be classified broadly into inflammatory, fistulizing or stricturing disease:

- Upper gastrointestinal Crohn's disease (oesophageal, gastric and small bowel) may present as nausea, vomiting, abdominal pain, diarrhoea and/or weight loss.
- Colonic involvement presents with passage of blood or mucus per rectum.
- Perianal involvement includes skin tags, fissures, fistulas and abscesses.
- Oropharyngeal involvement includes orofacial granulomatosis (lip and gum swelling) and recurrent mouth ulcers.
- Extraintestinal manifestations include growth retardation, anorexia, fatigue, delayed puberty, erythema nodosum, arthritis, clubbing, decreased bone mineral density, hepatitis and uveitis.

Crohn's disease can have an insidious onset with patients often having a prodrome of several months prior to the diagnosis being made. Patients may be referred by their local doctor for non-specific abdominal pain or other specialty units for consideration of Crohn's disease; for example, haematology for iron deficiency anaemia, endocrinology for growth retardation or pubertal delay, and rheumatology for arthritis.

### Ulcerative colitis

UC is characterized by continuous inflammation of the colon including the rectum. It involves only the lining of the intestine (unlike Crohn's disease which affects all layers of the intestinal wall). As the inflammation continues, the mucosa of the intestine begins to slough off, leaving pits (ulcerations). UC can present acutely or insidiously with a prodrome of several months. If there is a short history of colitic symptoms, it is essential to exclude infectious agents. Children with UC usually present with lower abdominal pain, urgency, tenesmus, diarrhoea and rectal bleeding. Additionally:

- systemic symptoms are less marked than in Crohn's disease
- the child can develop extra-intestinal manifestations of disease such as arthritis and sclerosing cholangitis
- pyoderma gangrenosum occurs more commonly in UC, but is still rare.

### Investigations

Several laboratory tests will support the diagnosis of IBD. These include anaemia, thrombocytosis, raised erythrocyte sedimentation rate (ESR), hypoalbuminaemia, and the presence of white and red blood cells on stool microscopy; however, endoscopy and biopsy are the 'gold standard'.

Antibody testing can help differentiate Crohn's disease from UC. Anti-*Saccharomyces cerevisiae* antibody (ASCA) positivity and anti-neutrophil cytoplasmic antibody (p-ANCA) negativity suggest Crohn's disease, and vice versa. However, these tests are not accurate enough to use for screening or diagnostic purposes.

Gastroscopy and colonoscopy (with ileoscopy) is essential, taking biopsies at all levels of the gut, whether or not there is macroscopic disease. Biopsies from a normal-appearing stomach or duodenum may contain granulomas, making the diagnosis of Crohn's disease more likely. Pathological findings above the ileum exclude the diagnosis of UC.

Magnetic resonance imaging (MRI) is a very useful way of visualizing the small bowel for evidence of disease and has less radiation exposure in comparison with the previously favoured barium follow-through. Occasionally, computed tomography (CT) is very useful in identifying abscesses and gut perforation. Ultrasound is safe and cheap and can provide helpful information about bowel wall thickness and abcess formation for example.

Wireless capsule endoscopy is a relatively new and evolving technology that is also inflammatory markers such as being used increasingly to image the small bowel mucosa, allowing more accurate mapping of disease distribution and activity.

Faecal markers of inflammation such as, faecal calprotectin, are a new way of measuring intestinal inflammation and are slowly becoming part of routine clinical practise. These tests may also have a future role in differentiating functional from inflammatory bowel conditions.

### Treatment

Treatment strategies for IBD often depend on the extent and severity of disease at the time of presentation. Medications are selected based on tolerance and side-effect profile. Adherence considerations are important, especially in adolescent patients, as perceived treatment failure can potentially lead to unnecessary treatment escalation.

#### Aminosalicylates

5-Aminosalicylates (5-ASAs) can be used both orally and topically (as enemas) to manage colonic disease in UC. They are often used in mild UC to achieve remission and as maintenance therapy.

#### Corticosteroids

- Used in the dose range of 1–2 mg/kg prednisolone for moderate to severe UC or Crohn's disease, usually for a 2–3-month period with a gradual dose reduction.
- Can adversely affect growth and have many unpleasant cosmetic and systemic side-effects.
- Associated with decreased bone mineral density and contribute to osteoporosis risk.
- Corticosteroids such as budesonide have fewer side-effects and are particularly useful for ileal and right-sided colonic disease, but are expensive, thus preventing their widespread use.
- Steroid enemas are helpful in the management of distal colonic and rectal inflammation.
- The minimum amount of steroids is used in order to avoid their numerous side effects and complications.

#### Exclusive enteral nutrition

- Utilizes polymeric and/or elemental feeds, which are equally effective but are generally not palatable and may require nasogastric infusion. All other oral intake is ceased during this treatment, which usually lasts 6–8 weeks.
- Provides a similar remission rate to corticosteroids in the treatment of childhood Crohn's disease (not UC) and improves growth and inflammatory markers.
- Exact mechanism of effect is unknown but generally thought to exert its beneficial effects by avoiding certain dietary antigens/substrates, alterations in gut flora, enterocyte nutrition and modulation of endogenous growth factors.
- Maintaining compliance with this treatment strategy is difficult, so discontinuation is a major cause of treatment failure.

### Immunomodulators

Thiopurine drugs such as azathioprine and 6-mercaptopurine/6MP are now a mainstay of treatment for IBD. They are effective for maintaining remission but not for inducing remission. They can be used in steroid-dependent children with either UC or Crohn's disease, but take 12–14 weeks to be clinically effective. They can cause nausea, pancreatitis and myelosuppression, and patients must be monitored. Methotrexate is also used as a maintenance agent; it can be administered orally and subcutaneously, which can be useful if compliance is a problem.

### Biologicals

The anti-tumour necrosis factor (TNF)-α class of drugs are very effective at inducing and maintaining remission in both adults and children. In the past, several issues limited use of these drugs in children, including cost, adverse effects such as severe allergic reactions, and concern over long-term safety. However, their use is becoming more frequent for several reasons, including more severe disease, failure of other medications and increasingly impressive safety data. These agents are traditionally administered intravenously at regular time intervals (8-weekly) although some newer agents have different dosing schedules and administration methods. Tolerance or resistance to anti-TNF-α treatment can develop in some patients, and the management of treatment failure in this population group is a challenge and the focus of much research.

### Other pharmacological treatments

- Antibiotics such as metronidazole and ciprofloxacin are useful in perianal and colonic Crohn's disease. Metronidazole has been shown to reduce recurrence rates at the anastomotic site following resection.
- Tacrolimus and cyclosporin, are sometimes used in the most severe disease or for rescue therapy in acute fulminant colitis.

*Immunosuppression*

Patients with IBD are often on one or more of these immunosuppressant medications. Therefore, they are at increased risk of infection and are vulnerable to opportunistic infections, such as CMV, tuberculosis or fungal infection. This must be considered during a febrile illness especially. These patients may also have reduced host response to immunizations whilst on these therapies.

## Surgery

Up to 80% of patients with long-term Crohn's disease will require surgery at some stage during their disease. This may be to treat a stricture, abscess or fistula. Unfortunately surgery will not prevent recurrence of the disease, so it is important to maintain a conservative approach to bowel resection. Nutritional deficiencies can result from resection of a significant length of small bowel, especially if the terminal ileum is involved. Appropriately timed surgery in children with Crohn's disease may accelerate growth and advance puberty, allowing a reduction in drug therapy.

In contrast to Crohn's disease, only a minority of patients with UC require surgery during the course of their lifetime. However, the impact of a colectomy and stoma can be significant, especially during childhood and adolescence when physical and psychological growth and development are taking place. There are several reasons to consider colectomy or subtotal colectomy in patients with UC, including fulminant colitis not responding to therapy, toxic megacolon, severe growth or pubertal failure, and/or disabling chronic symptoms. Total colectomy results in a permanent ileostomy but cures the individual of their disease and associated risks. Another option is a subtotal colectomy and ileal pouch–anal anastomosis (IPAA). This procedure is associated with pouchitis (50%), increased stool frequency and faecal incontinence in some cases.

## Cancer risk

There is an increased risk of cancer in IBD, which is greatest in children with UC, particularly those with pancolitis for more than 10 years. It is increased further in persons with coexisting sclerosing cholangitis.

Population-based studies demonstrate that the risk of colorectal cancer is 5.7 times that of the general population in both UC and Crohn's colitis, but patients with Crohn's disease that spares the colon do not have an increased risk.

Endoscopic screening is indicated after 8–10 years of disease. Unfortunately, as we are seeing younger patients in increasing numbers, cancer surveillance is becoming increasingly relevant to paediatric gastroenterologists.

To avoid colonic cancer, patients with longstanding extensive colitis face either prophylactic colectomy or regular surveillance colonoscopy. Neither option is perfect; a more reliable, cheaper process of screening would be ideal.

## Clinical example

Sarah presented at the age of 14 years with a 3-month history of recurrent abdominal pain and diarrhoea. Her stools were described as watery with variable amounts of blood and mucus. Clinical examination revealed mild pallor and, on abdominal examination, there was tenderness in both the left and right iliac fossa. Blood tests revealed a microcytic anaemia (haemoglobin 90 g/dL and mean corpuscular volume (MCV) 69 fL) and an ESR of 25 mm/h. Stool microscopy showed both red and white blood cells. Repeated stool cultures for viruses and bacteria, and testing for *Clostridium difficile* toxin, were negative. At colonoscopy, there was a pancolitis and a normal ileum. A provisional diagnosis of ulcerative colitis was made, subsequently supported by the histopathology. Sarah was treated initially with high-dose steroids and was later maintained on sulfasalazine, with good clinical response.

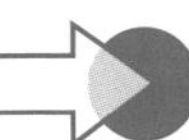

## Practical points

**Inflammatory bowel disease**

- Potentially a multisystem chronic relapsing disease.
- Assessment of the distribution of the disease may require multiple modalities (i.e. endoscopy and biopsy and imaging modalities).
- Treatment is individually tailored, based on the site and severity of disease.
- Be aware of long-term malignant risk, especially in ulcerative colitis, and also side-effects of various medications used.

# 20.3 Chronic diarrhoea and malabsorption

Shoma Dutt, Edward O'Loughlin

Malabsorption can be defined as the failure to absorb nutrients. A wide range of intestinal, pancreatic and hepatic disorders can be associated with malabsorption. To understand how one approaches the problem of malabsorption in the clinical setting, an understanding of the normal physiology of nutrient digestion and of salt, water and macronutrient and micronutrient absorption is essential. This information is available in general physiology texts.

## Diagnostic approach

A large number of children have loose stools without having underlying gastrointestinal disease. In young children this is called 'toddlers' diarrhoea'. A major clinical challenge is to differentiate well children with loose stools from children who have gastrointestinal disease. The diagnosis of the majority of children with malabsorption can be established with thorough clinical assessment, stool examination and simple ancillary tests.

### Clinical assessment

Initial assessment can reveal whether a child is ill. If so, immediate evaluation will be required. In the well child, a 'wait and see' approach may be more rewarding than immediate investigation.

Malabsorption does not present as malabsorption *per se*. Rather, individuals with malabsorption can present with a wide array of symptoms and physical signs (Table 20.3.1). Diarrhoea is the most common presentation and may be accompanied by loss of appetite, decreased physical activity, lethargy and growth failure. Children with coeliac disease may have decreased appetite, and are often cranky and irritable. In contrast, children with pancreatic insufficiency often develop a voracious appetite. In children with failure to thrive, a detailed dietary history is required. Occasionally, parents manipulate the child's diet in an attempt to control the diarrhoea, which can lead to significant dietary insufficiency with attendant weight loss. Assessment of the age of introduction of various foods into the diet may give insight to the underlying diagnosis. Onset of symptoms 3–6 months after the introduction of wheat products suggests the possibility of coeliac disease. Onset shortly after the introduction of cow's milk suggests cow's milk protein intolerance. History of overseas travel is important, as some unusual infections, such as amoebic dysentery, can cause chronic bloody diarrhoea.

The nature of the loose stool is important to ascertain, as it provides important clues to the pathophysiology and thus aetiology. Diarrhoea can be thought of in terms of fatty stools (steatorrhoea), watery diarrhoea (osmotic because of carbohydrate malabsorption or secretory disorders) and bloody diarrhoea. Box 20.3.1 provides a differential diagnosis of chronic diarrhoea and malabsorption categorized by the nature of the stool.

Assessment of general health is important, as many gastrointestinal disorders exhibit extraintestinal manifestations. Cystic fibrosis (see Chapter 14.6), Shwachman syndrome and immunodeficiency disorders (see Chapter 13.2) are associated with infections, particularly sinopulmonary infections. Delayed pubertal development can accompany many chronic disorders but is particularly prevalent in Crohn's disease (see Chapter 20.2).

Family history may be of note. Cystic fibrosis, primary disaccharidase deficiencies and abetalipoproteinaemia are recessively inherited. Coeliac disease and inflammatory bowel disease are more frequently observed in first-degree relatives.

Physical examination includes assessment of growth, nutritional status and pubertal development. Plotting percentile charts is mandatory. A child who is growing normally is unlikely to be suffering from serious gastrointestinal disease. Plotting longitudinal measurements, if available, is very important as it may give clues to the onset of disease and could indicate the diagnosis. Other physical signs of malabsorption and specific nutritional deficiencies include: loss of muscle bulk and subcutaneous fat; peripheral oedema (hypoproteinaemia); bruising (vitamin K deficiency); glossitis and angular stomatitis (iron deficiency); finger clubbing (cystic fibrosis, Crohn's disease, coeliac disease); skin rashes in coeliac disease (dermatitis herpetiformis) and inflammatory bowel disease (erythema nodosum, pyoderma gangrenosum); and specific skin disorders associated with zinc, vitamin A and essential fatty acid deficiencies (Fig. 20.3.1). Rickets is uncommon in our community, although biochemical vitamin D deficiency is quite common and is prevalent in patients with malabsorption, such as in cholestatic liver disease, and coeliac disease. It is important to examine carefully as there are many extraintestinal manifestations of gastrointestinal disease and malnutrition.

**Table 20.3.1 Some symptoms and signs of nutrient deficiencies**

| Nutrient | Symptom or sign of deficiency |
|---|---|
| Protein | Growth failure<br>Muscle wasting<br>Hypoproteinaemic oedema |
| Fat | Weight loss<br>Muscle wasting<br>Manifestation of deficiency of vitamins A, D, E, K |
| Carbohydrate | Weight loss |
| Salt/water | Electrolyte disturbances<br>Growth failure (chronic salt deficiency)<br>Dehydration (acute loss) |
| Vitamins | |
| A | Night blindness<br>Skin rash<br>Dry eyes (xerophthalmia) |
| D | Rickets<br>Hypocalcaemia |
| K | Bruising (coagulation defects) |
| E | Anaemia<br>Peripheral neuropathy |
| $B_{12}$ | Megaloblastic anaemia<br>Irritability<br>Hypotonia<br>Peripheral neuropathy |
| Folate | Megaloblastic anaemia<br>Irritability |
| Minerals | |
| Iron | Microcytic anaemia<br>Delayed development |
| Calcium | Rickets<br>Irritability<br>Seizures |
| Zinc | Diarrhoea<br>Skin rash (mouth, perineum, fingers and toes)<br>Poor growth |

**Box 20.3.1 Differential diagnosis of chronic diarrhoea and malabsorption categorized according to type of stool**

**STEATORRHOEA**

***Pancreatic insufficiency***
- Cystic fibrosis
- Shwachman syndrome
- Chronic pancreatitis
- Malnutrition (developing world)
- Isolated lipase deficiency

***Inadequate bile salt concentration***
- Biliary atresia
- Cholestatic syndromes
  - congenital
  - acquired
- End-stage liver disease
- Bacterial overgrowth syndrome
- Bile salt malabsorption (ileal resection)

***Inadequate absorptive surface***
- Coeliac disease
- Surgical resection (short gut syndrome)
- Milk protein intolerance
- Immunodeficiency

***Enterocyte defect***
- Abetalipoproteinaemia

***Defective lymphatic drainage***
- Intestinal lymphangiectasia
- Constrictive pericarditis

**WATERY DIARRHOEA**

***Osmotic***

*Disaccharidase deficiency*
- Lactase
- Sucrase–isomaltase

*glucose–galactose malabsorption*

*Excessive intake*
- Sorbitol
- Fructose

***Abnormal water and electrolyte transport***

*Congenital electrolyte transporter defects*
- Congenital chloride diarrhoea
- Congenital sodium diarrhoea

*infection*

*mucosal disease*
- Coeliac disease
- Milk protein intolerance
- Inflammatory conditions (inflammatory bowel disease)
- Immunodeficiency disorders
- Autoimmune enteropathy

*bile salt malabsorption*
- Congenital
- Ileal resection

*bacterial overgrowth syndromes*
- Gastrointestinal motility disorders
- Anatomical (blind loop)

## Stool examination

Stool examination is very simple and provides very important information. The presence of numerous white and red cells indicates colitis. This is usually due to bacterial or parasitic infection, to chronic inflammatory disorders of the large bowel, or to milk protein intolerance when identified in infants. Leukocytes are not increased in the stool of individuals with small bowel or pancreatic disease. Cysts of parasites such as *Giardia lamblia* indicate giardiasis.

Oil droplets seen on stool microscopy are always abnormal outside the newborn period and usually indicate fat maldigestion, as occurs with pancreatic insufficiency, for example in cystic fibrosis. Mucosal disease, such as coeliac disease, in general does not interfere

**Box 20.3.1 Differential diagnosis of chronic diarrhoea and malabsorption categorized according to type of stool—Cont'd**

**BLOODY DIARRHOEA**
***Infection***
- Bacterial
- Parasitic

**INFLAMMATORY BOWEL DISEASE**
- Crohn's disease
- Ulcerative colitis
- Milk protein intolerance

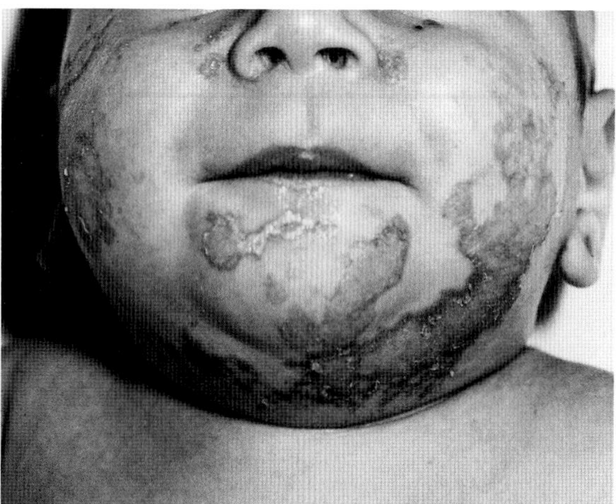

Fig. 20.3.1 Exfoliative rash of zinc deficiency.

with fat digestion because pancreatic function is usually normal. Mucosal disease interferes with the absorption of triglyceride products. These products are observed as fatty acid crystals on polarizing microscopy.

The presence of carbohydrate in the stool can be detected with Clinitest tablets. This is a commercially available bedside test in which the reaction between stool sugars such as lactose causes a colour change when added to the tablets. Greater than 500 mg/dL (0.5%) indicates carbohydrate malabsorption. Measurement of stool electrolytes and osmolality in the stool water is also a very useful test. When the sum of the stool electrolytes (i.e. sodium + potassium + chloride + bicarbonate) equals measured osmolality, a secretory diarrhoea is present. If the sum of the electrolytes is substantially less than the measured osmolality (> 100 mosmol/L), this indicates an osmotic diarrhoea.

## Malabsorption with chronic diarrhoea

Diarrhoea is the most common presentation of malabsorption. Diarrhoea can be defined as increased frequency, fluidity and volume of stool. The following discussion will provide a systematic approach to the child with malabsorption and diarrhoea based on the type of stool, i.e.:

- fatty
- watery or
- bloody.

Some illustrative cases will be provided and a summary of this approach can be seen in Figure 20.3.2.

### Fatty diarrhoea (steatorrhoea)

The differential diagnosis of fat malabsorption is quite wide ranging (see Box 20.3.1); however, if one understands the normal physiology of fat digestion and absorption, the differential diagnosis is much less daunting. Conditions that cause steatorrhoea can also be associated with protein maldigestion and/or malabsorption, although symptoms most commonly relate to the malabsorption of fat. The presence of fat in the stool is also more readily observed than protein.

**Clinical example**

Mary was 9 months old. She presented with poor weight gain, chronic diarrhoea and a history of recurrent respiratory illnesses, including one admission at age 3 months with 'bronchiolitis'. Loose stools were found each time her nappy was changed. On occasion her mother had noted oil drops in the stool. Despite the poor weight gain, Mary had an excellent appetite and was described as a voracious eater. She consumed a mixed diet, including infant formula, appropriate for age. Cereal was introduced at age 6 months. Mother also commented that she tasted salty when she kissed Mary.

On examination, Mary was found to be a thin wasted girl. Her height was on the 50th percentile and her weight was less than the 3rd percentile. She had mild finger clubbing, peripheral oedema, pallor of the tongue and palmar creases, but no signs of chronic liver disease. There was no abdominal distension of note, although she had a fine scaling rash over her trunk. Respiratory examination was normal. No other abnormal physical signs were present.

Results of investigations included haemoglobin 85 g/L (normal range 110–140) with a normocytic normochromic film, normal white cell count and differential; albumin 24 g/L (normal range 34–44) and normal liver function test results. Stool microscopy revealed copious fat droplets. Three-day faecal fat excretion estimation demonstrated an output of 35% of ingested fat (normal < 7% of intake).

Mary's diarrhoea was due to fat malabsorption, as evidenced by her mother's observation of fat droplets in the stool.

Mary's sweat test demonstrated a sweat chloride of 80 mmol/L (a result > 60 mmol/L is diagnostic of cystic fibrosis). Genetic testing indicated that she was homozygous ΔF508 (the commonest mutation), consistent with her relatively severe symptoms. Introduction of pancreatic exocrine replacement therapy, a high-fat diet and vitamin supplements alleviated her diarrhoea and eventually corrected Mary's failure to thrive, anaemia and skin rash.

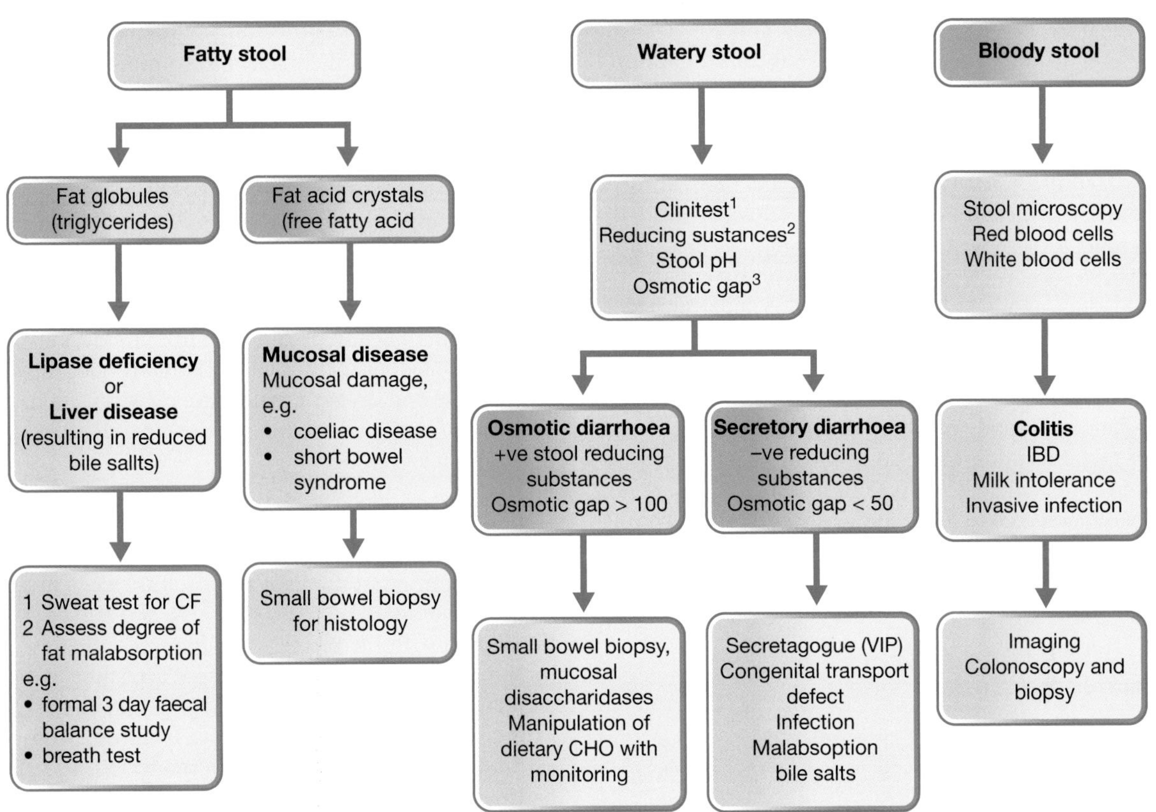


Fig. 20.3.2 Algorithm for investigation of patient with chronic diarrhoea. 1, Stool collection must be fresh as stool osmolality increases after excretion due to continued bacterial fermentation of faecal carbohydrates (breastfed infants can exhibit up to 0.5% reducing substances). 2, Sucrose is a non-reducing sugar, and not measurable as a reducing substance unless hydrolysed by boiling or acid. 3, Osmotic gap in stool fluid = Serum osmolality (280) – [2 × ([Na] + [K])]. CF, cystic fibrosis; CHO, carbohydrate; IBD, inflammatory bowel disease; VIP, vasoactive intestinal polypeptide.

## Fat and protein digestion and absorption

Ingested fat in the form of triglycerides, cholesterol and phospholipids is, to a large extent, digested in the lumen of the small intestine and absorbed in the jejunum. This requires bile salts, which form micelles and solubilize the fat; pancreatic enzymes, such as lipase and co-lipase, which digest the fat; and an intact intestinal mucosa, which is required for absorption of the products of digestion. Following digestion in the micelles, breakdown products diffuse across the enterocyte apical membrane and are reconstituted in the cell into chylomicrons. These are small packets of triglyceride, phospholipid and cholesterol that associate with carrier proteins, such as β-lipoprotein, essential for cellular trafficking of the chylomicrons. After the chylomicrons are reconstituted, they exit the mucosa into the lymphatic system and subsequently pass into the systemic circulation. Some small-chain triglycerides can bypass this system and enter the portal venous system directly.

Protein digestion begins in the stomach by the action of pepsin and acid. However, most protein hydrolysis occurs in the lumen of the jejunum by the action of pancreatic proteases. These are secreted as inactive precursors. Chymotrypsin is converted to trypsin by the action of the small intestinal enzyme enterokinase. Activated trypsin further activates chymotrypsin and other proteases, such as carboxypeptidase. The products of protein hydrolysis are amino acids and oligopeptides. The latter are further hydrolysed to mono-, di- and tri-peptides by brush border hydrolases and are absorbed by specific membrane transporters. Di- and tri-peptides undergo hydrolysis to amino acids in the cytoplasm of the enterocyte. Isolated protein maldigestion/malabsorption is extremely rare. It usually occurs in association with malabsorption of other macronutrients.

## Fat malabsorption

Diseases of the pancreas and the small intestine are the usual causes of steatorrhoea in children. Chronic liver disease may cause steatorrhoea but this is in the setting of severe and obvious liver disease (such as the patient who is cirrhotic and jaundiced) and is not usually a diagnostic problem.

Steatorrhoea causes bulky stools and can lead to other nutritional deficits. Fat is responsible for approximately 40% of caloric intake in the Western diet. Thus, fat malabsorption can lead to failure to thrive due to an energy-deficient diet. Some vitamins are fat-soluble and require normal fat digestion for their absorption. These include A, D, E and K. Thus patients with steatorrhoea may also develop signs of fat-soluble vitamin deficiency, as described above. Essential fatty acids such as arachidonic acid are also malabsorbed in patients with pancreatic malabsorption. A scaling skin rash is one physical manifestation of essential fatty acid deficiency.

Pancreatic and intestinal diseases associated with fat malabsorption can also result in protein and carbohydrate maldigestion/malabsorption. Thus it is not uncommon to find a mixed picture of malabsorption. Protein maldigestion/malabsorption results in hypoproteinaemia. The main physical manifestations are growth failure, peripheral oedema and ascites.

## Pancreatic disease

*Cystic fibrosis*

See also Chapter 14.6.

Cystic fibrosis:

- is the commonest cause of pancreatic malabsorption in the Caucasian population
- has an incidence in the population of approximately 1 per 2000
- is an inborn error in epithelial chloride secretion – cystic fibrosis transmembrane conductance regulator (CFTR).

Organs affected include:

- gastrointestinal tract and liver
- sinopulmonary tract
- pancreas
- exocrine portion of the sweat glands
- vas deferens
- sweat duct (CFTR absorbs rather than secretes chloride in this organ).

Because of the fluid and salt transport defects, patients with cystic fibrosis produce more viscous secretions in lung, gut, pancreas and vas deferens, leading to:

- chronic suppurative lung disease
- nasal polyps
- pancreatic insufficiency (approximately 85% of patients)
- intussusception
- meconium ileus and distal intestinal obstruction syndrome
- infertility
- raised sweat sodium and chloride, which can lead to heat prostration in warmer climates.

Chronic liver disease will develop in 10–15% of children with cystic fibrosis.



Malabsorption in cystic fibrosis frequently results in malnutrition and there may be symptoms and signs of specific nutrient deficits such as hypoalbuminaemic oedema, night blindness due to vitamin A deficiency, or skin rash due to essential fatty acid deficiency. Median life expectancy is 30 years, with death usually from respiratory failure or haemorrhage from portal hypertension and oesophageal varices.

Many mutations have been identified in the CFTR. Depending on what part of the channel is affected by the mutation, the phenotype can vary from mild to severe disease. Individuals with milder mutations have milder lung disease and do not usually have malabsorption, as pancreatic function is normal (pancreatic sufficient).

Newborn screening:

- can detect cystic fibrosis in the neonatal period
- involves measurement of immunoreactive trypsinogen and/or *CFTR* mutations
- is the commonest mode of presentation when it is performed.

In children with the severe phenotype who are missed by screening, or in countries where screening is not performed, presentation is usually in the first year with chronic diarrhoea and failure to thrive, with or without respiratory symptoms. In milder phenotypes, patients may not present until adult life with respiratory disease or infertility.

Diagnostic investigations for cystic fibrosis are:

- raised sweat sodium and chloride ('sweat test') – simplest and cheapest
- *CFTR* mutation analysis.

Treatment is usually undertaken in a tertiary referral multidisciplinary clinic and involves:

- physiotherapy, inhalation therapy and antibiotics for chest disease
- pancreatic enzyme supplements
- nutritional support and fat-soluble vitamin supplementation
- specific therapy may be required for the other intestinal/liver complications.

*Shwachman syndrome*

The features of Shwachman syndrome are:

- agenesis of the pancreatic acinus
- short stature
- dysplasia of the metaphysis of the long bones
- cyclical neutropenia.

There is no specific diagnostic test; treatment includes pancreatic enzyme replacement and treatment of infections.

*Chronic pancreatitis*

Causes of chronic pancreatitis include:

- protein energy malnutrition
- hereditary pancreatitis (*SPINK1*, *PRSS* and *CFTR* gene mutations)
- idiopathic fibrosing pancreatitis (rare).

## Small bowel disease

*Coeliac disease (gluten enteropathy)*

Coeliac disease is a disorder characterized by intestinal injury induced by the cereal protein gluten. Gluten is a glycoprotein found in wheat, barley and rye, and, to a lesser extent, oats. In susceptible individuals, the ingestion of gluten induces a cell-mediated injury of the intestinal mucosa resulting in severe villous atrophy, crypt hyperplasia and infiltration of the epithelium with lymphocytes (intraepithelial lymphocytes). In Western countries, the incidence of coeliac disease in the general population may be as high as 1 in 70, although not all affected individuals develop the classical manifestations of coeliac disease. At risk populations include individuals with type 1 diabetes mellitus, a positive family history of coeliac disease and other autoimmune disease (thyroiditis, hepatitis), and syndromes such as trisomy 21 and Turner syndrome. A changing pattern in the presentation of coeliac disease has been noted with the advent of accurate screening serological tests.

Modes of presentation include:

- 'Classical' coeliac disease (Fig. 20.3.3):
  - between 9 and 18 months of age
  - anorexia, weight loss, abdominal distension and wasting
  - chronic diarrhoea with or without iron deficiency anaemia, hypoproteinaemic oedema, fat-soluble vitamin deficiency (vitamins A, D, E, K)

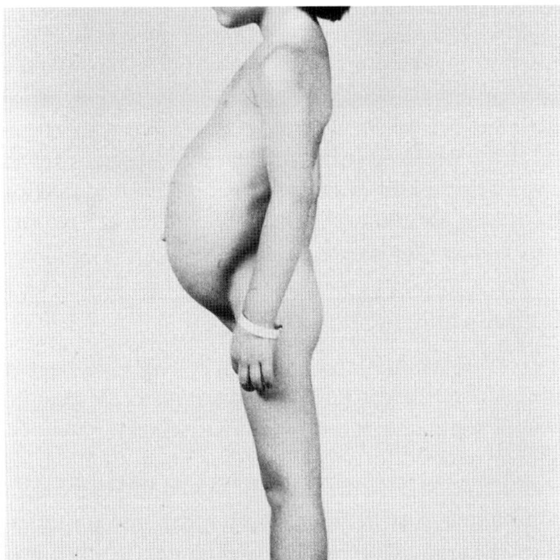

Fig. 20.3.3 Typical physical appearance of a young child with coeliac disease. Note the protuberant abdomen, buttock and shoulder girdle wasting and oedema of the lower limbs. (Courtesy of Professor K. Gaskin.)

- The older child with:
  - growth failure
  - chronic diarrhoea
  - iron deficiency
- Positive antibody screening (now the commonest form of assessment leading to diagnosis).

Examples of antibodies used to screen when there is suspicion of coeliac disease include:

- anti-gliadin
- anti-endomysial
- anti-tissue transglutaminase
- deamidated anti-gliadin antibodies.

Anti-endomysial and anti-tissue transglutaminase antibodies have a sensitivity and specificity greater than 95% in clinical trials but probably less in the clinical setting. These are mostly immunoglobulin (Ig) A-based tests and a false-negative result may occur with IgA deficiency (the deaminated anti-gliadin antibody is IgG based). However, it is important to note that these are screening tests only. There is a close association with human leukocyte antigen (HLA) DQ2 and DQ8 phenotypes. HLA DQ2 and DQ8 typing may be useful in assessing the risk of coeliac disease in close family members. These phenotypes are common in the general population and cannot be used to diagnose coeliac disease. However, their absence makes coeliac disease very unlikely.

The following are important points in the approach to the diagnosis of coeliac disease in childhood:

- Small bowel biopsy is mandatory for the diagnosis (Fig. 20.3.4).
- Small bowel biopsy should be performed while the patient is on an unrestricted diet.
- There is no place for an empirical trial of a gluten-free diet.
- Definitive diagnosis is important, as treatment is a lifelong gluten-free diet.

The patient should be monitored for a clinical response to treatment with a gluten-free diet, and antibody titres should be expected to fall with response.

*Enterocyte defect*

Abetalipoproteinaemia is a recessively inherited defect in chylomicron assembly. Patients develop steatorrhoea early in life with:

- fat-soluble vitamin deficiencies
- low serum cholesterol and triglyceride levels.

Small bowel biopsy reveals fat-laden enterocytes.

*Impaired lymphatic drainage*

Obstructed lymphatic drainage prevents chylomicrons from migrating from the gut to the systemic circulation. The main cause is intestinal lymphangiectasia. This can lead to:

- fat malabsorption
- low serum cholesterol and triglyceride levels
- hypoproteinaemia and lymphopenia (loss of lymph into gut lumen)
- abnormal mucosal biopsy.

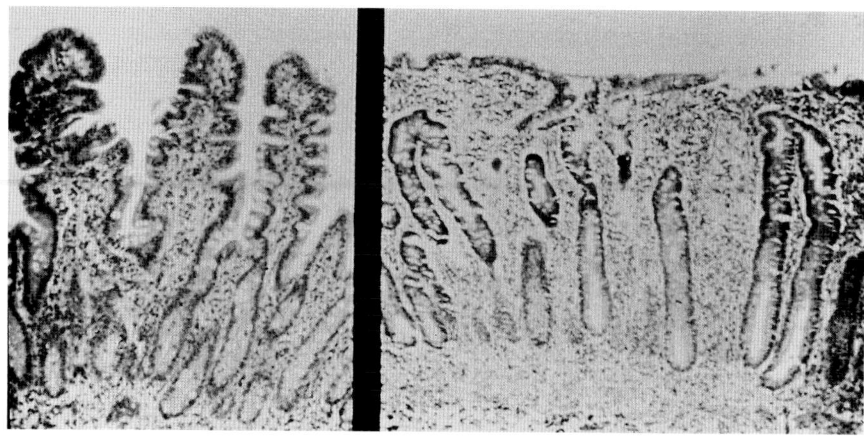

Fig. 20.3.4 Micrographs of normal intestine (left) demonstrating normal crypt villus structure, and coeliac disease (right) with marked crypt hyperplasia and villous atrophy.

*Other causes of reduced mucosal surface and reduced contact time*

Miscellaneous inflammatory and surgical conditions can lead to loss of absorptive surface or reduced contact between chyme and the mucosa. Such conditions include:

- milk protein intolerance (severe)
- infections such as rotavirus infection
- severe immunodeficiency disorders
- autoimmune enteropathy
- short gut syndrome (surgical removal)
- motility disorders causing very rapid intestinal transit.

**Clinical example**

George was 9 years old. He presented with a 6-month history of intermittent bloating, abdominal pain and diarrhoea up to 6–7 times per day. He had lost 1kg in weight in the past 2 months. He reported that dairy products such as milk and ice-cream made his symptoms worse. He had no past history of significant illness. George was the oldest son of Greek migrants. His mother reported that she could not drink milk, as it made her feel sick.

On examination, George was well looking. His weight was on the 50th percentile and his height on the 10th percentile. There was no abdominal distension, organomegaly, signs of chronic liver disease or evidence of nutritional deficiency such as anaemia or peripheral oedema. Examination of his anus did not reveal any evidence of perianal disease.

Investigations included a normal full blood count, differential white cell count and erythrocyte sedimentation rate (ESR). The C-reactive protein level was less than 1 g/L. Lactose breath hydrogen measurement following oral ingestion of 50 g lactose increased 100 parts per million above baseline levels within 60 minutes of ingestion of lactose (normal rise 20 parts per million), indicating lactose intolerance.

George was diagnosed as having lactose intolerance. His history suggested ontogenic lactase deficiency. This was confirmed by small bowel biopsy, which demonstrated normal morphology, and by disaccharidase measurement, which revealed very low lactase activity but normal sucrase and maltase activities. Treatment was a low-lactose diet.

## Watery diarrhoea

### Carbohydrate digestion and absorption

Dietary carbohydrates are primarily starch (polysaccharides, amylose and amylopectin), disaccharides (sucrose, in table sugar; lactose, in milk) and some monosaccharides such as fructose.

Starch polymers are large molecules composed of long chains of glucose. These chains are broken down by the action of salivary and pancreatic amylase, which release a disaccharide (amylose), trisaccharide (maltotriose) and a series of branched oligosaccharides (α-limit dextrins). These molecules are further digested by the brush border enzymes, sucrase–isomaltase and glucoamylase, to the monosaccharide glucose.

The disaccharides sucrose and lactose are metabolized by disaccharidases on the intestinal brush border. Sucrase breaks sucrose down to glucose and fructose, and lactase breaks down lactose into glucose and galactose. Glucose and galactose are absorbed by the enterocyte sodium–glucose co-transporter (SGLT), which absorbs the monosaccharides in an energy-dependent fashion. Fructose is absorbed by facilitated diffusion (non-energy-dependent) by glucose transporter type 5 (GLUT-5).

### Carbohydrate malabsorption

The presence of non-absorbed osmotically active nutrients in the gut lumen results in osmotic retardation of water absorption, leading to watery diarrhoea. This is referred to as osmotic diarrhoea. Osmotically active compounds are usually low-molecular-weight compounds such as monosaccharides and disaccharides. Osmotic diarrhoea is usually due to maldigestion and/or malabsorption of carbohydrates, but can be caused by the ingestion of laxatives such as sorbitol or magnesium chloride. Unabsorbed carbohydrate present in the lumen of the large bowel is fermented to short-chain fatty acids such as butyrate. This results in a highly acidic stool, which can cause perianal excoriation. The colon can absorb the anionic forms of these acids in exchange for bicarbonate, causing a mild hyperchloraemic acidosis.

While stating the obvious, it is important to appreciate that one cannot malabsorb a nutrient that has not been ingested. Thus, it is useful to obtain a dietary history in patients suspected of osmotic diarrhoea. One needs to ascertain the nature of the carbohydrates being ingested, and in some instances the age of introduction of the carbohydrate, which can then be compared with the age of onset of symptoms. For example, the onset of osmotic diarrhoea commensurate with the introduction of fruit into the diet suggests the diagnosis of congenital sucrase–isomaltase deficiency.

## Disaccharidase deficiencies and monosaccharide malabsorption

*Congenital*

*Ontogenic lactase deficiency:*

- occurs in most of the non-Caucasian population of the world
- is dominantly inherited
- is physiological (due to the disappearance of lactase)
- presents in late childhood.

Ingesting lactose causes diarrhoea, bloating, excessive flatus and weight loss. Treatment is a low-lactose diet.

*Congenital sucrase–isomaltase deficiency* is caused by inactivating mutations in the sucrase–isomaltase gene. These mutations:

- are recessively inherited
- lead to similar symptoms as for lactase deficiency with the ingestion of sucrose
- cause onset of symptoms at the time of weaning when fruit is introduced to the diet.

Treatment is a low-sucrose diet.

*Congenital monosaccharide malabsorption* refers to defective glucose/galactose malabsorption. Features are:

- mutations in *SGLT1*
- recessively inherited
- present in the neonatal period.

Treatment is substitution of fructose for glucose–galactose.

*Acquired*

Except for ontogenic lactase deficiency, acquired disorders are much more common than inherited deficiencies. Lactase is more susceptible to injury than sucrase.

Causes of disaccharidase deficiencies include:

- viral gastroenteritis
- coeliac disease
- chronic giardiasis
- milk protein enteropathy
- small bowel bacterial overgrowth syndrome
- immunodeficiency disorders
- autoimmune enteropathy.

Monosaccharide transporters are less susceptible to injury because, unlike disaccharidase enzymes, they are deeply embedded in the brush border membrane. However, severe enteropathies can occasionally result in monosaccharide malabsorption. Examples include:

- congenital villous atrophy (which presents in newborns)
- severe postinfectious enteritis
- milk protein intolerance
- autoimmune enteropathy.

Monosaccharide malabsorption is life-threatening and requires a level of care found only in tertiary paediatric centres. The treatment is to remove the offending carbohydrate from the diet and substitute an alternative. In acquired disorders, treatment may also be required for the primary mucosal disease.

## Disorders of fluid and electrolyte transport

In the normal child approximately 5 litres (depending on size!) of fluid and electrolytes enters the upper gastrointestinal tract per day. One litre is ingested and the remaining volume is from normal secretions into the lumen. The majority of this fluid is absorbed before reaching the colon. Stool weights range from 75 to 150 g per day, of which approximately 75% is water. Small increases in stool water, as little as 30–40 mL daily, are enough to produce diarrhoea.

Water is absorbed by osmosis through aquaporins and paracellular pathways in the mucosa. Electrolytes are absorbed by a variety of active transport or passive transport processes. Anions such as chloride and bicarbonate can be absorbed or actively secreted. This varies according to the region of small or large intestine. Regulation of gastrointestinal fluid and electrolyte transport is closely integrated by humoral and neural factors involved in fluid and electrolyte homeostasis. Abnormal fluid and electrolyte transport can be due to inherited defects in specific electrolyte transporters, but more commonly it is due to mucosal damage or inflammation.

*Congenital*

Congenital sodium diarrhoea and congenital chloride diarrhoea are rare inherited disorders of Na/H exchange and Cl/HCO exchange, respectively. They cause:

- diarrhoea *in utero*, which results in polyhydramnios
- profuse diarrhoea, obvious from birth
- systemic electrolyte disturbances.

*Acquired*

Isolated water and salt malabsorption is very rare in childhood in the developed world. However, defective salt and water transport can contribute to diarrhoea in:

- disorders that damage or inflame the mucosa of small or large intestine
- bile salt malabsorption (bile acids irritate the colonic mucosa and act as potent stimulants of secretion).

Excessive salt and water loss in the stool may lead to dehydration and electrolyte disturbances. Treatment may require salt and water replacement in addition to treatment of the underlying disease.

### Bloody diarrhoea (see also Chapter 20.2)

Chronic bloody diarrhoea is usually caused by inflammatory disorders of the colon such as:

- milk colitis in infants
- infections, such as with bacteria or parasites
- inflammatory bowel disease in older children. The two major forms are:
  - ulcerative colitis
  - Crohn's disease.

Blood is not always obvious in the stool. However, the presence of leukocytes on stool microscopy (Fig. 20.3.5) indicates the presence of colitis. Malabsorption of fluid and electrolytes by the inflamed colonic mucosa is a major factor contributing to diarrhoea. Malabsorption of nutrients is uncommon in milk colitis and inflammatory bowel disease. In contrast, excessive blood and protein loss from the inflamed intestinal mucosa can cause iron deficiency anaemia and hypoproteinaemic oedema. This is called protein-losing enteropathy, and can be assessed by measuring stool $\alpha_1$-antitrypsin levels.

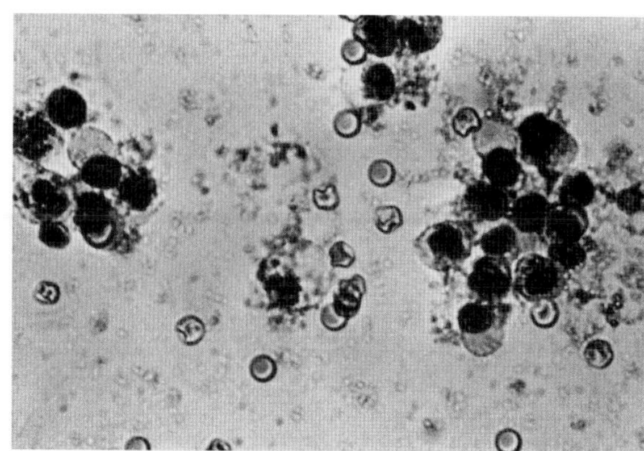

Fig. 20.3.5 Microscopic appearance of leukocytes in a stool smear. The large dark structures are polymorphonuclear leukocytes; the small round objects are red blood cells.

## Nutrient malabsorption with little or no diarrhoea

Children present with symptoms and signs of nutrient deficiency with little or no accompanying diarrhoea. This is often due to dietary insufficiency (e.g. inadequate iron intake), but can sometimes be due to malabsorption of the specific nutrient.

### Vitamin $B_{12}$

Vitamin $B_{12}$ is ingested in animal protein and is liberated by pepsin in the stomach. In the stomach, the free vitamin $B_{12}$ binds to a binding protein (R protein) that has greater affinity for the vitamin than intrinsic factor (carrier protein). Intrinsic factor is produced by epithelial cells in the gastric mucosa. The vitamin $B_{12}$–R protein complex moves to the duodenum where trypsin cleaves the complex, releasing free vitamin $B_{12}$, which then binds to intrinsic factor. The intrinsic factor–vitamin $B_{12}$ complex moves to the ileum where it is absorbed into the enterocytes by carrier-mediated transport. On entry into the enterocyte, vitamin $B_{12}$ is separated from intrinsic factor and subsequently exits the enterocyte into the circulation bound to transcobalamin, which carries the vitamin to sites distant from the intestine.

#### Clinical example

John was 9 months old. He presented with a 6-week history of poor weight gain, irritability and pallor. His mother was also concerned about his development. He was able to sit but could not pull himself to standing. His language had not progressed from babbling, which was in stark contrast to his older sibling, who had several single words at this age. John had a poor appetite but no diarrhoea. He was originally breastfed and his mother ingested a normal diet during pregnancy and lactation.

On examination, John was a pale irritable boy. He had moderate abdominal distension but no organomegaly. He could sit up unsupported but was mildly hypotonic and would not weight-bear. There were no focal neurological signs.

Investigation results included: haemoglobin 65 g/L (normal range 120–150) with a megaloblastic blood film, serum $B_{12}$ 50 pmol/L (normal range 120–600) and red blood cell folate 350 nmol/L (normal range 200–1000). A Schilling test revealed urinary excretion of ingested radioactive vitamin $B_{12}$ (after parenteral administration of a non-radioactive flushing dose of 1 mg vitamin $B_{12}$) of 1% (normal 8%), with no enhancement of urinary excretion with the addition of intrinsic factor.

John's Schilling test result suggested a defect in the ileal vitamin $B_{12}$ transporter, as the test was abnormal and did not recover with the addition of intrinsic factor. His age of presentation and lack of previous intestinal surgery suggest a congenital defect. His symptoms and megaloblastic anaemia corrected with administration of parenteral vitamin $B_{12}$.

Both congenital and acquired disorders can lead to vitamin $B_{12}$ malabsorption.

### Congenital disorders

Congenital defects in:
- ileal vitamin $B_{12}$ transporter
- intrinsic factor
- transcobalamin

can lead to vitamin $B_{12}$ malabsorption and deficiency. This usually presents in the second 6 months of life, after the vitamin $B_{12}$ accumulated during intrauterine life is exhausted.

Symptoms are due to megaloblastic anaemia and the central nervous system effects of deficiency. Babies born to vegan mothers (who ingest no animal product and thus can themselves be vitamin $B_{12}$-deficient) and weaned on to a vegan diet can present with a similar picture, although usually in the first 6 months, as they are deficient from birth. Dietary history is important to differentiate between dietary deficiency and malabsorption.

### Acquired disorders

Acquired disorders that lead to $B_{12}$ malabsorption are:
- surgical resection of the ileum
- atrophic gastritis
- gastric surgery
- autoimmune pernicious anaemia (blocking antibodies to intrinsic factor)
- pancreatic insufficiency (failure to hydrolyse vitamin $B_{12}$–R protein)
- small bowel bacterial overgrowth (competition for vitamin $B_{12}$ by bacteria).

## Iron

Iron absorption occurs in the duodenum and proximal jejunum. An apical enterocyte carrier called the divalent metal cation transporter mediates uptake into the enterocyte. Iron is exported to the circulation via a basolateral process that has not yet been fully defined. In non-breastfed children, only 5–10% of dietary iron is absorbed. The efficiency of iron absorption is greater in breastfed infants because the iron carrier transferrin is present in breast milk. Iron absorption is finely regulated at the level of the enterocyte so that absorption does not exceed requirements. Excessive iron accumulation can lead to multiple organ damage (haemochromatosis).

Iron deficiency is the commonest nutritional deficiency in humans and is usually due to:
- inadequate dietary intake
- excessive gastrointestinal blood loss (bleeding lesions or inflammation).

*Acquired disorders*

Iron deficiency anaemia can occasionally be the primary presenting feature of small intestinal disease such as:
- coeliac disease
- milk protein intolerance
- Crohn's disease.

## Miscellaneous nutrients

### Calcium

Calcium absorption occurs in the duodenum and proximal jejunum and is largely under the regulation of vitamin D:
- Hypocalcaemia can be associated with a wide variety of digestive disorders affecting intestinal calcium uptake or the biosynthesis and availability of vitamin D (see Chapter 19.5).
- It commonly presents with tetany of the fingers and occasionally seizures.

### Zinc

Zinc is absorbed by the small intestine. Zinc deficiency can be due to:
- low breast milk zinc levels in solely breastfed infants
- an inherited defect in zinc absorption (acrodermatitis enteropathica)
- conditions associated with steatorrhoea
- intestinal inflammatory disorders.

Zinc deficiency can cause diarrhoea but the most dramatic manifestation is an erythematous scaly rash on the fingertips and around the perineum and mouth (see Fig. 20.3.1).

### Magnesium

Magnesium is absorbed in the proximal small intestine. Magnesium malabsorption leading to deficiency can be:
- inherited (primary hypomagnesaemia)
- secondary to other conditions leading to malabsorption.

Hypomagnesaemia causes similar symptoms to calcium deficiency.

### Isolated protein malabsorption

Enterokinase deficiency:
- is a very rare disorder
- presents with diarrhoea, growth failure and severe hypoproteinaemia.

### Amino acids

Defective amino acid absorption due to mutations in amino acid transporters can occur in:
- Hartnup disease
- cystinuria
- lysinuric protein intolerance.

These defects are rare disorders affecting amino acid transport in gut and kidney, and in other organs in the last case. They do not involve gastrointestinal symptoms and there are no nutritional consequences because of compensatory absorptive mechanisms for peptide and amino acid absorption.

## Summary of the diagnostic approach to suspected malabsorption

Initial clinical assessment and stool examination will suggest the diagnosis in most children. Stool microscopy and measurement of stool-reducing substances can be performed in the clinician's office and are readily available 'bedside' tests. If the diagnosis is not immediately obvious, the clinician will be in a position to investigate a limited differential list with simple and well-directed diagnostic tests.

In patients with steatorrhoea, the following will be useful but are not necessarily indicated for every patient:

- full blood count and differential white cell count
- serum triglycerides/cholesterol
- sweat test
- small bowel biopsy
- X-ray of long bones.

In patients with carbohydrate maldigestion/malabsorption, the following might be indicated:

- breath hydrogen testing – challenge with the carbohydrate of interest (e.g. lactose)
- small bowel biopsy/mucosal disaccharidase activities
- occasionally with monosaccharide malabsorption inpatient dietary manipulation with close observation of stool output.

In patients with bloody diarrhoea (if stool culture is negative for pathogens) consider:

- gastroscopy and colonoscopy
- biopsy of small bowel and colon
- sometimes radiology looking for inflammatory bowel disease in jejunum/ileum.

Sometimes highly specialized investigations are required to establish the diagnosis of some disorders.

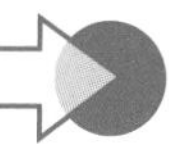

**Practical points**

- Diagnosis is not by exclusion.
- A thorough history, physical examination and stool examination will suggest the diagnosis in most disorders.
- Simple well-directed investigations usually confirm the clinical diagnosis.
- There is no such thing as a 'malabsorption workup'.

# 20.4 Gastro-oesophageal reflux and *Helicobacter pylori* infection

Paul Hammond, Geoffrey Davidson

This chapter discusses gastro-oesophageal reflux (GOR), a very common clinical problem in infants and children, and *Helicobacter pylori*, an infectious agent that colonizes the stomach in more than 50% of the world's population. *H. pylori* infection is acquired in early childhood but its disease manifestations usually do not occur until adulthood. It is possible there may be a relationship between the two, and this will be discussed.

## Gastro-oesophageal reflux

GOR can be defined as the spontaneous or involuntary passage of gastric content into the oesophagus. The origin of the gastric content can vary and includes saliva, ingested food and fluid, gastric secretions, and pancreatic or biliary secretions that have first been refluxed into the stomach (duodenogastric reflux). Gastro-oesophageal reflux disease (GORD) can be defined as significant symptoms or damage arising as a result of GOR. The difference between physiological reflux and GORD is often blurred by the anxiety engendered in parents, particularly first-time parents, by symptoms such as vomiting and irritability. Physiological reflux manifested by spilling, regurgitation and occasional vomiting is seen in more than 60% of healthy infants by 4 months of age, resolves in the majority by 12 months and rarely leads to GORD. Conservative management is important, particularly in an otherwise healthy infant, so as not to label the condition as a disease state when in fact it is not.

The symptoms of GORD in children aged 3–18 years range in frequency from 1.8% to 22%, and are more refractory and associated with complications such as pain, vomiting, haematemesis, oesophagitis, stricture, growth failure, swallowing difficulties, respiratory symptoms and apnoea.

### Pathophysiology (Box 20.4.1)

The main barrier to GOR is the pressure gradient across the lower oesophageal sphincter (LOS) which is formed by the intrinsic LOS (thickened smooth muscle of the lower oesophagus) and the extrinsic striated muscle of the crural diaphragm. Both components work together to generate LOS pressure. The current understanding of LOS function suggests that a pressure of 5–10 mmHg above intragastric pressure is sufficient to maintain an antireflux barrier. Transient lower oesophageal sphincter relaxation (TLOSR) is the major mechanism responsible for GOR in infants, children and adults. A TLOSR is defined as an abrupt decrease in LOS pressure unrelated to swallowing or oesophageal body peristalsis.

Abdominal straining, which occurs frequently in infants, probably exacerbates GOR only when there is simultaneous TLOSR, because both LOS tone and the crural diaphragm are inhibited. The neuroregulation of TLOSR is controlled via a vagovagal reflex. Feeding is a potent stimulus for TLOSR, evidenced by the fact that, in children with GORD, TLOSRs increase from four per hour in the fasting state to eight per hour in the fed state.

Normal oesophageal body peristalsis facilitates clearance of refluxed material including acid. Disordered peristalsis can lead to prolonged acid exposure and oesophageal damage.

The role of gastric emptying in the pathophysiology of GORD is not clear. Delayed gastric emptying could exacerbate GOR by prolonging gastric distension and increasing the frequency of TLOSRs. There are some children at the severe end of the GORD spectrum in whom delayed gastric emptying may be an issue, especially those with neurological or respiratory disease.

### Clinical manifestations

There are many causes of regurgitation and vomiting in infants and children, both within the gastrointestinal tract and external to it. The more common causes are outlined in Box 20.4.2.

Regurgitation can be defined as effortless spilling of gastric content that is usually benign. Vomiting, on the other hand, is a forceful emptying of gastric content that should always be explained. The content of the vomitus is important because of the likely cause, as is the age at onset. Bile staining implies small bowel obstruction and should be examined immediately. Blood staining implies ulceration or gastritis.

**Box 20.4.1 Pathophysiological mechanisms of gastro-oesophageal reflux in infants, children and adolescents**

- Delayed volume clearance
  - Impaired primary or secondary peristalsis
  - Reduced pressure wave amplitude
- Increased occurrence of GOR
  - Transient LOS relaxation
  - Straining
  - LOS sphincter hypotonia
  - LOS pressure drift
- Delayed gastric emptying

LOS, lower oesophageal sphincter.
Modified from Davidson GP, Omari TI 2001 Pathophysiological mechanisms of gastroesophageal reflux disease in children. Curr Gastroenterol Rep 3:257–262.

Table 20.4.1 highlights the symptoms suggestive of GORD in infants and children. Symptoms do vary according to age. Infants more frequently regurgitate but have also been shown to have reflux-related neurobehavioural symptoms including irritability, crying, fussiness and back-arching but not gagging.

**Box 20.4.2 Causes of regurgitation and vomiting in infants and children**

**Gastrointestinal tract**
- Oesophagus
  - Achalasia
  - GOR
  - Foreign body
  - Congenital defects
- Stomach
  - Pyloric stenosis
  - Peptic ulcer disease/gastritis
- Duodenum
  - Malrotation
  - Duodenal ulcer
  - Superior mesenteric artery syndrome
- Small intestine/colon
  - Infectious diarrhoea
  - Intussusception
  - Soy or cow's milk protein intolerance
  - Meconium ileus
  - Inflammatory bowel disease
  - Appendicitis
- Other organs
  - Hepatitis
  - Gallbladder disease
  - Pancreatitis

**Extra-intestinal disorders**
- Generalized sepsis
- Rumination
- Intoxications
- Intracranial lesions (e.g. tumour, hydrocephalus)
- Adrenal insufficiency
- Metabolic disorders

More serious complications include apnoea, acute life-threatening events and recurrent chest disease secondary to aspiration. Chronic cough without associated lung disease is unlikely to be reflux-related.

Older children, usually over the age of 8 years, can describe common symptoms such as heartburn, chest pain, and a sick or sour taste in the mouth, implying refluxate. Some younger children may complain of a hot feeling in the chest, abdomen or throat.

GORD is a common problem in neurologically impaired children and, although regurgitation is the most likely symptom, problems such as recurrent chest disease, feeding difficulties and food refusal, anaemia, weight loss and behavioural changes can all be manifestations of GORD.

There are many potential extra-oesophageal manifestations of GORD; these are highlighted in Table 20.4.2 and need to be considered as they may be the only presenting symptom or sign. Ear nose and throat manifestations such as otitis media, sinusitis and dental erosions are now being recognized. Although a link between many extra-oesophageal manifestations and GORD has been identified, causality has not been proven, and data supporting improvement in symptoms with GORD treatment are sparse.

### Eosinophilic oesophagitis

This condition has been widely recognized only in the past decade. Eosinophilic oesophagitis is distinguished from GORD by the presence of abundant eosinophils in the oesophageal mucosa. Their presence had previously been thought to be due to acid reflux. The density of eosinophils in the mucosa ($<5$ per high-power microscopy field in GORD and $>20$ per high-power field in eosinophilic oesophagitis) defines the difference between these two conditions, although there can be a large overlap in symptoms.

Symptoms include dysphagia with solid food, food impaction, epigastric pain and vomiting. Food allergy is present in more than 60% and at present the only proven effective therapy is strict avoidance of the offending allergen(s). Topical steroids seem capable of inducing remission if a food allergy is not identified.

## Diagnostic tests

Physiological GOR should be diagnosed on clinical grounds; diagnostic tests are not required. There is no single test for the diagnosis of GORD. If there are symptoms or signs of pathological reflux, such as pain, growth failure or respiratory symptoms, then further testing is required (Fig. 20.4.1). The test used will depend on the age of the child, the types of test available, and the type and severity of symptoms. The most commonly used tests are outlined in Box 20.4.3.

**Table 20.4.1 Symptoms suggestive of gastro-oesophageal reflux disease in infants and children**

| | Infants | Children |
|---|---|---|
| **Vomiting** | | |
| Gastrointestinal | Feeding difficulties<br>Failure to thrive<br>Malnutrition<br>Cow's milk protein intolerance | Waterbrash<br>Nausea<br>Dysphagia |
| Respiratory | Cough, stridor<br>Cyanotic episodes<br>Apnoea<br>Acute life-threatening events | Chronic cough |
| **Acid reflux** | | |
| Gastrointestinal | Apnoea, cyanotic episodes<br>Colic, irritability<br>Sleep disturbance<br>Flexion patterns after feeds<br>Hiccoughs<br>Iron deficiency | Heartburn<br>Oesophageal obstruction<br>Dysphagia, odynophagia<br>Night waking<br>Haematemesis |
| Respiratory | Apnoea, cyanotic episodes<br>Stridor | |
| Neurobehavioural | Sandifer syndrome<br>Seizure-like events (similar to infantile spasms) | |

**Table 20.4.2 Potential extra-intestinal manifestations of gastro-oesophageal reflux disease**

| Pulmonary | Ear, nose and throat | Other |
|---|---|---|
| Asthma<br>Chronic bronchitis<br>Bronchiectasis<br>Pulmonary fibrosis<br>Pneumonia | Chronic cough<br>Laryngitis<br>Hoarseness<br>Pharyngitis<br>Sinusitis<br>Vocal cord granuloma<br>Recurrent granuloma | Dental erosions<br>Non-cardiac chest pain<br>Sleep apnoea |

Adapted from Richter JE 2000 Extraesophageal manifestations of gastroesophageal reflux disease. An overview. Am J Gastroenterol 95:51–53.

## Barium oesophagraphy ('barium swallow')

This is the most commonly used but least sensitive test for the diagnosis of GOR. It is useful for detecting structural abnormalities such as pyloric stenosis, malrotation and strictures, and may be useful in the assessment of swallowing function or aspiration. Children with persistent vomiting are most likely to require this test.

## Radionuclide scintigraphy

Radioactive $^{99}$Tc–sulphur colloid is added to an age-appropriate liquid meal and can be used as a direct measure of reflux. It has the benefit of measuring all refluxate. It can also be used to evaluate gastric emptying and to document aspiration due to reflux.

## Upper gastrointestinal endoscopy and biopsies

Endoscopic examination of the upper gastrointestinal tract is indicated in GORD with complications such as chest or epigastric pain, heartburn, haematemesis or persistent unexplained iron deficiency.

Unlike in adult medicine, oesophageal biopsies form an important part of the diagnostic strategy in GORD in children. They can support a reflux aetiology and exclude other less common causes of oesophagitis, such as infection (cytomegalovirus, herpes simplex virus, candidiasis), Crohn's disease or eosinophilic oesophagitis.

## 24-hour intra-oesophageal pH monitoring

This provides an assessment of oesophageal acid exposure. In the majority of infants with GOR, this test is not required and it should be carried out only if it will alter diagnosis, treatment or outcome. Current indications for its use are outlined in Box 20.4.4.

This is not a simple test and should be carried out only in a specialist centre, as many factors need to be considered, including pretest preparation, insertion and positioning of the catheter, symptom assessment and analysis of results.

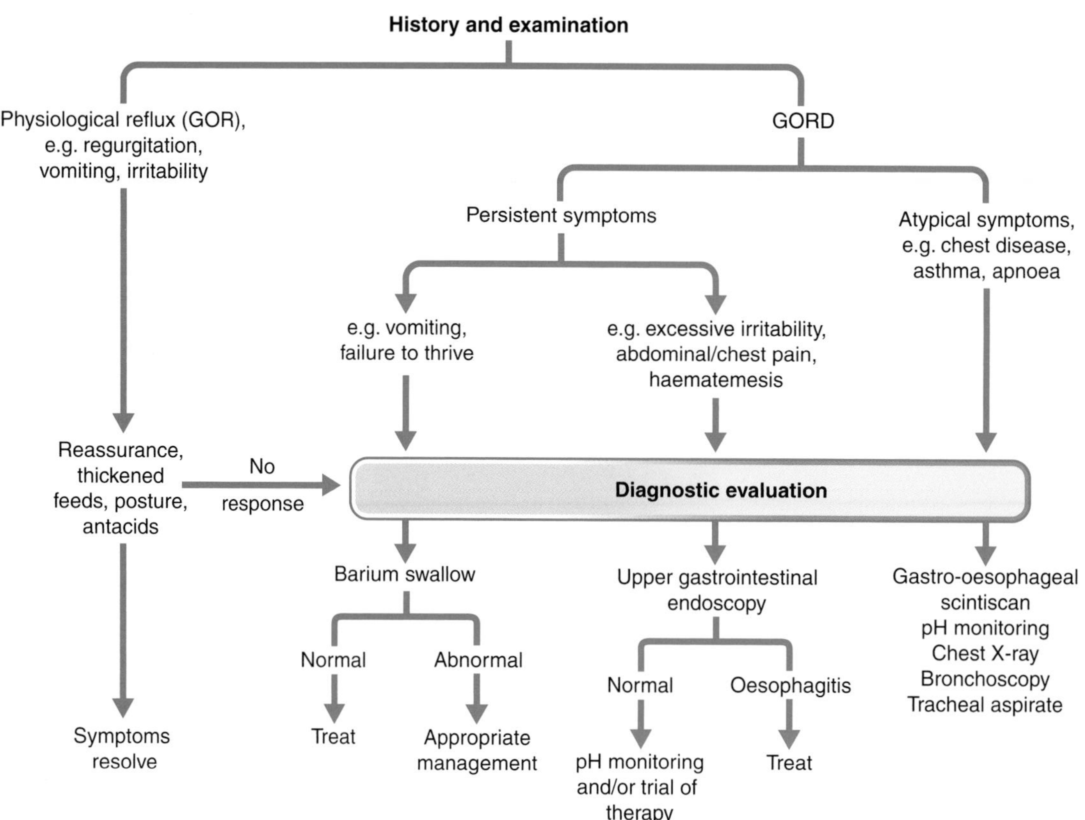


Fig. 20.4.1 Algorithm for diagnostic approach to gastro-oesophageal reflux disease (GORD). (Modified from Youssef NN, Orenstein SR 2001 Clinical Perspectives in Gastroenterology Jan/Feb: 11–17.)

**Box 20.4.3 Commonly used diagnostic tests for gastro-oesophageal reflux disease**

- Barium oesophagraphy
- Upper gastrointestinal endoscopy and biopsies
- Radionuclide scintigraphy (milk scan)
- 24-hour intra-oesophageal pH monitoring
- Oesophageal manometry and multi-channel intraluminal impedance

**Box 20.4.4 Current indications for 24-hour intra-oesophageal pH monitoring**

- Diagnose occult reflux in:
  - unexplained recurrent pneumonia
  - patients with bradycardia, apnoea
  - non-gastrointestinal symptoms caused by reflux, such as stridor, laryngeal symptoms, atypical chest pain, severe irritability
- Assessment of adequacy of medical therapy in cases of severe intractable GORD

## Oesophageal manometry and multi-channel intraluminal impedance

Oesophageal manometry is rarely needed clinically in the diagnosis of GORD in children but may be useful prior to fundoplication in children with a suspected motility disorder. It also has a place in children with swallowing difficulties and in the diagnosis of achalasia.

Multi-channel intraluminal impedance measures the flow of liquid (acid and non-acid) or gas in the oesophagus and thus has an advantage over pH monitoring, which recognizes fluid flow only with a pH <4. It is a relatively new technique and its role in clinical practice is still being evaluated. In young infants and children it is likely to become the 'gold standard' for delineating an association between reflux and a particular symptom such as apnoea, cough or irritability.

Recently both the North American and European Societies for Paediatric Gastroenterology, Hepatology and Nutrition have advocated the use of combined pH/multi-channel intraluminal impedance in investigating symptoms such as excessive crying, distressed behaviour, apnoea and apparent life-threatening events.

### Diagnostic approach to gastro-oesophageal reflux disease

The diagnostic approach depends largely on the nature and severity of symptoms and the presence or absence of complications. In the otherwise healthy infant whose main symptoms are vomiting or regurgitation, parental reassurance is all that is required.

If symptoms persist despite simple therapies such as posture and formula thickening, barium oesophagraphy should be carried out to exclude an anatomical abnormality such as stricture, gastric outlet obstruction or malrotation.

Infants presenting with acid reflux-related symptoms suggestive of oesophagitis require endoscopy and biopsies. In infants with atypical symptoms, the approach is more difficult, but initially aspiration needs to be considered. Barium oesophagraphy, chest X-ray and a gastro-oesophageal scintiscan may provide support for this diagnosis. Referral to a respiratory physician may also be indicated for bronchoscopy and computed tomography (CT). Combined 24-hour pH/impedance monitoring is now more widely available and will detect evidence of GOR and also possible symptom association.

**Clinical example**

Sophie, the 7-month-old daughter of Greek parents, presented with a history of recurrent haematemesis, with bright and altered blood noted in regurgitated fluid and also dark stains on bibs and pillow. She was generally quite happy and thriving, although clinically a little pale. She did not have any evidence of abdominal tenderness.

In view of the recurrent bleeding and the possibility of oesophagitis or gastritis, an upper gastrointestinal endoscopy was carried out. This showed macroscopically ulcerative oesophagitis but normal stomach and duodenum. Sophie was treated with omeprazole 10 mg 12-hourly, and after 4 weeks the bleeding had stopped clinically and the spilling had also decreased. A repeat endoscopy 8 weeks later showed macroscopic healing but still histological evidence of moderate oesophagitis. Sophie remained on omeprazole for a further 4 months but following a trial off therapy her symptoms recurred and she underwent a Nissen fundoplication. When reviewed at the age of 2 years she was well and asymptomatic.

### Treatment approach (Box 20.4.5)

The ideal therapy would include the use of a drug that specifically reduces the frequency of TLOSRs, but this is currently not available. Baclofen is a γ-aminobutyric acid (GABA) agonist frequently used to reduce muscle spasms, particularly in children with neurological handicap. It has been shown to reduce TLOSRs as well as both acid and non-acid reflux in adults and children, but its side-effects preclude it from routine use in clinical practice.

**Box 20.4.5 Treatment approach to gastro-oesophageal reflux disease**

General
- Reassurance
- Positioning
- Thickened feeds

Drug therapy
- Antacids
- $H_2$-receptor antagonists
- Proton pump inhibitors

Continuous nasogastric feeds

Surgery

#### General measures

These include reassurance, positioning and thickening feeds. The importance of reassurance in relation to the otherwise healthy infant cannot be overstated. It is important to avoid numerous dietary changes, unnecessary investigations and multiple drug therapies, which are often recommended by others or tried by parents.

Previously the only posture proven scientifically to be effective was the prone position, but this is no longer recommended because of the increased risk of sudden infant death syndrome (see Chapter 3.10). New evidence suggests that laying children on their left side following a meal significantly reduces regurgitation and the frequency of TLOSRs. Feed thickening has also been shown to reduce symptoms of regurgitation and vomiting by reducing the height by which the refluxate comes up the oesophagus. There are now commercially available infant formulas that contain thickening compounds. The risk is that the attenuation of overt symptoms may mask complications of GORD.

#### Prokinetic drugs

No prokinetic agents have been shown to be beneficial and thus none can be recommended at present.

#### Acid suppression

This is effective in reduction of symptoms due to acid irritation of the oesophagus. Acid suppressing agents are:

- *Antacids.* In infants with mild symptoms suggestive of heartburn such as irritability between feeds, a trial of 0.5–1 mL per kg per dose 3–6 times a day may be worthwhile. Antacids have only a brief duration of action and a response can be noted within several days; if not then do not persist.
- *$H_2$-receptor antagonists.* Ranitidine has proved the most effective, in doses often higher than used in adults. It does have rare serious adverse effects such as fulminant hepatic failure. The dose recommended is 2–3 mg per kg per dose 2–3 times a day.

- *Proton pump inhibitors.* These are the most potent acid-suppressing agents and are used when acid-related symptoms fail to respond to other therapies. They are superior to $H_2$-receptor antagonists in efficacy because of their ability to maintain intragastric pH >4 for longer periods of time and to inhibit meal-stimulated acid secretion. They are often used as first-line treatment where more complete acid suppression is required, for example in chronic respiratory disease, neurologically disabled children and repaired tracheo-oesophageal fistula. In the older child with typical symptoms such as regurgitation and heartburn, response to a short course of a proton pump inhibitor supports GORD as the underlying aetiology.
  - Omeprazole has been most extensively studied in adults and children. It is used in doses ranging from 0.7 to 3.5 mg/kg once daily, just before the first meal of the day. Twice-daily dosing may be indicated in certain situations such as severe oesophagitis, peptic stricture, persistent nocturnal reflux symptoms and extra-oesophageal GORD. There may be a role for 'as required' therapy for symptom control where there are infrequent symptoms and damage is not an issue. Although widely used for infantile irritability, recent studies do not support clinical benefit.

### Continuous feeding

Children with intractable vomiting and growth failure may respond to continuous nasogastric tube or gastrostomy feeding, with catch-up growth, and surgery may be avoided. Transpyloric feeding using a nasojejunal or gastrojejunal tube may rarely have a role, particularly in small infants.

### Surgery

The Nissen fundoplication is the most common surgical procedure; the indications are shown in Box 20.4.6. It is now typically carried out laparoscopically in children. This may work, not by acting as a valve or increasing LOS pressure, but by decreasing TLOSRs due to reduction in the fundal surface area. Fundal distension is an important trigger for TLOSRs.

**Box 20.4.6 Indications for anti-reflux surgery in children**

**Absolute**
- Acute life-threatening event or chronic lung disease due to aspiration
- Continuing severe oesophagitis or oesophageal ulceration despite adequate therapy
- Intractable vomiting with growth failure secondary to GOR

**Relative**
- Oesophageal stricture secondary to GOR
- Severe asthma or respiratory disease unresponsive to therapy
- Family choice to avoid long-term regular acid suppression
- Persistent symptoms with oesophagitis or growth failure

## Summary

It is important to realize that only a small proportion of children with GOR go on to develop GORD. For most infants, symptoms resolve completely before 12 months of age. Unfortunately, many of these children are overdiagnosed and overtreated. It is equally important that those with continuing symptoms are recognized and treated effectively.

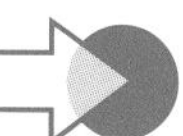

**Practical points**

**Gastro-oesophageal reflux (disease)**
- GOR in infants is usually a benign, self-limiting condition.
- Reassurance and minor interventions such as posture and feed thickening often suffice.
- GORD always requires further assessment and possibly investigation.
- GORD has a number of extra-oesophageal manifestations that need to be considered.
- Proton pump inhibitor therapy should be first-line therapy for treatment of GORD.

# *Helicobacter pylori* infection in children

*Helicobacter pylori* is the commonest bacterial pathogen in humans, infecting more than 50% of the world's population. This infection (initially called *Campylobacter pylori*), discovered in 1982 by Warren and Marshall in Australia, ranks as one of the most important medical discoveries of the last century. They cultured the organism from the gastric antrum of adults with peptic ulcer disease. It meets Koch's postulates as a human pathogen causing chronic active gastritis. *H. pylori* is usually acquired in the first 2 years of life, but the disease consequences rarely arise in childhood.

## Epidemiology

Socioeconomic differences are the most important predictor of *H. pylori* infection prevalence in any population group. In developed countries the prevalence in children seems to be declining, but there is variability in the burden of infection with higher levels in immigrants and Indigenous populations. This is particularly the case in Aboriginal children, where at least

80% are infected. This is similar to developing countries, where up to 80% of children are infected by the age of 2 years, with a lower prevalence in breastfed infants. In developed countries, only 10% of all children are infected by the age of 10 years.

The route of transmission is probably similar to that of other enteric pathogens, being faecal–oral, oral–oral or gastric–oral. *H. pylori* has been detected in vomitus, saliva, faeces, on children's dummies, and also in contaminated water, and food prepared with contaminated water. The housefly has been implicated as a vector. The spread of infection within families is high, most probably from infected mother to child, although there is also evidence of father to child and sibling to sibling spread, especially in households with high infection rates in all family groups. Risk factors for *H. pylori* infection in children are shown in Box 20.4.7.

The natural history of *H. pylori* infection in childhood remains obscure. A significant finding has been spontaneous clearing and reacquisition of gastric infections in preschool children, as spontaneous eradication does not appear to occur in adults. Although *H. pylori* infection rates are decreasing, particularly in developed countries, atopy is increasing. Within populations, the frequency of atopy is less in *H. pylori*-infected individuals, a finding that warrants further research.

## *Helicobacter pylori*-associated disease

### General

In the past, gastric and duodenal ulcers in children have been described as primary or secondary. Secondary ulcers, which are more common in younger children (less than 10 years of age), are caused by systemic stresses such as trauma, burns, septic shock, corticosteroids or non-steroidal anti-inflammatory drugs. Primary ulcers, which usually occur in older children, give rise to symptoms similar to those in adults, with epigastric nocturnal abdominal pain and vomiting, and often a positive family history of peptic ulceration. It is now clear in this latter group that the disease is due to *H. pylori* infection of gastric mucosa.

All *H. pylori* strains produce urease, which is thought to be important in the inflammatory reaction in the stomach and also in maintaining the ideal submucous environment for the organism. The urease reaction is also exploited in a number of diagnostic tests.

**Box 20.4.7 Risk factors for *Helicobacter pylori* infection**

- Poor socioeconomic status
- Household crowding
- Ethnicity
- Migration from high prevalence areas
- Infected parent, particularly mother
- Contaminated water

Genetic analysis of *H. pylori* has demonstrated strains with certain virulence factors, such as vacuolating cytotoxin (Vac A), and cytotoxin-associated genes (*cagA, cagE*). In adult ulcer disease there is a correlation between *cagA* positivity and peptic ulcer, but this is less clear in children. A study has shown a strong correlation between disease severity and the *cagE* genotype in children.

### Gastrointestinal infection (Box 20.4.8)

*Gastritis*
*H. pylori* colonization of gastric mucosa in children is almost always associated with gastritis, which resolves with eradication of the organism. Endoscopy can be negative and biopsy is essential for diagnosis, although on occasions nodular antral hyperplasia can be seen and is diagnostic of infection.

*Duodenal ulcer*
*H. pylori* gastritis is found in 90% of children with duodenal ulcers. Ulcers heal faster if anti-*H. pylori* therapy is given, compared with acid suppression alone. Importantly, ulcers tend not to recur if the infection is successfully eradicated.

*Gastric ulcers*
*H. pylori* infection as a cause of gastric ulcers is much less common in children than adults, probably reflecting the fact that the majority are secondary to systemic causes.

*Gastric adenocarcinoma*
The epidemiological association between *H. pylori* infection and gastric cancer has been judged by the World Health Organization to be sufficiently strong for it to classify *H. pylori* as the first bacterium to be a human carcinogen. *H. pylori*-induced gastric cancer has not been reported in children, but this association may influence a decision regarding whether to treat or not.

**Box 20.4.8 Consequences of *Helicobacter pylori* infection**

**Gastrointestinal**
- Gastritis
- Duodenal ulcer
- Gastric ulcer
- Gastric adenocarcinoma
- Gastric lymphoma and MALT lymphoma

**Extragastric**
- Gastro-oesophageal reflux
- Iron deficiency anaemia
- Short stature

MALT, mucosa-associated lymphoid type.

*Gastric lymphoma and MALT lymphoma*

Sero-epidemiological studies support an association between longstanding *H. pylori* infection and lymphoma and mucosa-associated lymphoid type (MALT) lymphomas. Eradication of *H. pylori* has resulted in regression of MALT lymphoma in some cases. Both of these tumours are rare in children.

*Recurrent abdominal pain*

In adults, a link between non-ulcer dyspepsia (possibly the equivalent of recurrent abdominal pain in childhood) and *H. pylori* has been suggested by a recent meta-analysis of a large number of controlled studies. A comparable study in children with recurrent abdominal pain does not support an association. The major problem with studies in children is the lack of a standardized, validated, reproducible symptom assessment instrument. It is possible that there is a subset of children in whom *H. pylori*-induced gastritis is responsible for recurrent abdominal pain, but more information is required. The current consensus is that recurrent abdominal pain of childhood is not an indication to test for *H. pylori* infection.

### Extra-gastric disease

*Gastro-oesophageal reflux*

It is postulated that certain *H. pylori* strains cause decreased acid production and atrophic gastritis and that, with eradication of *H. pylori*, acid rebound occurs, causing GORD. This is a controversial area in adults, whereas there is contrasting evidence in children supporting a potential link between the presence of *H. pylori* and increased acid production and GORD.

*Iron deficiency/growth stunting*

Iron deficiency has been described in growth-retarded adolescents with *H. pylori* infection. Eradication of *H. pylori* infection corrected the deficiency and led to growth improvement. The current consensus is that testing for *H. pylori* infection should be considered in children with refractory iron deficiency anaemia where no other cause is found.

A large Australian study has shown a relationship between small-for-gestational-age infants and maternal *H. pylori* infection. Growth delay in height and weight has also been shown in *H. pylori*-infected children, but this may be biased by socioeconomic status.

## Diagnostic tests (Box 20.4.9)

Endoscopy and biopsy is the only method that can provide evidence of disease activity such as gastritis or an ulcer. Urease testing of biopsy material gives indirect identification of infection but has only a 50% positive predictive value in children.

**Box 20.4.9 Diagnostic tests for *Helicobacter pylori***

**Endoscopic**
- Biopsy and histology
- Rapid urease test
- Bacterial culture

**Indirect tests**
- Serum antibody (IgA, IgG)
- Stool culture/stool antigen
- $^{13}C$-urea breath test

The $^{13}C$-urea breath test is currently the best non-invasive diagnostic test for *H. pylori* infection in children. It has a greater than 95% positive and negative predictive value. The principle of the test is outlined in Figure 20.4.2. Urea can be labelled with either radioactive $^{14}C$ or stable isotope $^{13}C$. In children and women of childbearing age, the $^{13}C$-urea breath test is recommended. Serology, although commercially available, is frequently unreliable and cannot distinguish between past and present infection. Of the other non-invasive tests under trial the most promising is the use of a monoclonal antibody to detect *H. pylori* antigen in faeces.

The aim of testing is not to detect the presence of infection but to find the cause of clinical symptoms, and therefore the important question is who should be tested (Box 20.4.10).

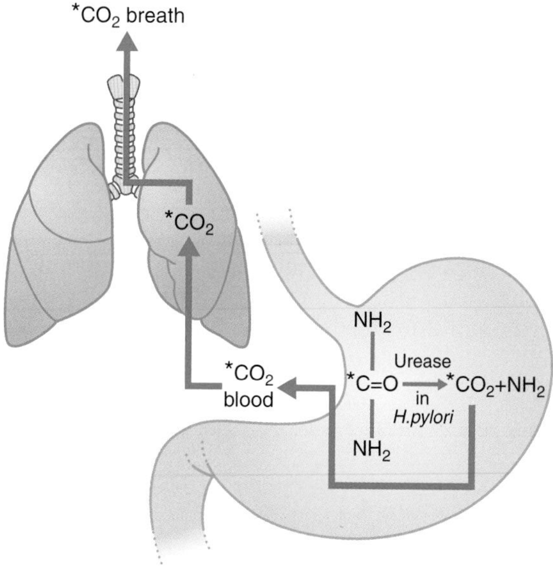


Fig. 20.4.2 The principle of the $^{13/14}C$-urea breath test.

**Box 20.4.10 Who should be tested for *Helicobacter pylori* infection?**

**Yes**

- Endoscopic/radiologically proven gastric or duodenal ulcers
- Confirmation of eradication of *H. pylori* infection

**No**

- Recurrent abdominal pain without ulcer disease
- Asymptomatic children
- Children in families with history of gastric cancer or ulcer disease

**Box 20.4.11 Who should be treated for *Helicobacter pylori* infection?**

- Children with duodenal and gastric ulcers and proven *H. pylori* infection
- Children with histologically proven infection with gastrointestinal symptoms
- Children with gastric lymphoma and proven *H. pylori* infection
- Children with atrophic gastritis with intestinal metaplasia and proven *H. pylori* infection
- Children with refractory iron deficiency and proven *H. pylori* infection

## Treatment

The discovery of *H. pylori* as the cause of primary peptic ulceration and gastric ulcers has dramatically changed their management, because eradication of the organism cures the disease and prevents recurrence. This has meant that peptic ulcer disease is now a curable condition, virtually eliminating the need for long-term or destructive surgery.

If endoscopy is indicated to investigate organic disease and *H. pylori* is found, the child should receive treatment (Box 20.4.11); however, if no ulcer is found the patient/parents should be informed that *H. pylori* eradication may not relieve the symptoms.

The traditional treatments of peptic ulcer do not eradicate *H. pylori* infection, and current treatment in children advocates a combined regimen using two antibiotics and a proton pump inhibitor, based on adult treatment regimens. Bismuth subsalicylate-based treatment is possibly more effective, but access to this treatment in Australia and other countries can be difficult.

The currently recommended first-line treatment is a combination of a proton pump inhibitor, clarithromycin and amoxicillin twice daily for 7 days. Metronidazole can be substituted for either amoxicillin or clarithromycin, but there is a high resistance to this drug and its use may lead to treatment failure. Failure of eradication leads to the use of second-line options, which may include bismuth subsalicylate in a triple or quadruple therapy regimen.

Addition of probiotics to *H. pylori* eradication regimes has led to decreased complication rates and a modest increase in eradication rates.

The burden of illness and socioeconomic costs of *H. pylori*-related illness is considerable, making the development of a prophylactic vaccine to prevent infection or a therapeutic vaccine to eliminate existing infection desirable, but to date no vaccine is available.

**Clinical example**

A 10-year-old Vietnamese child, Than, who had lived in Australia since birth, presented with a long history of recurrent epigastric pain that woke him from his sleep at night. His appetite was described as poor. There was a family history of peptic ulcer disease. Examination revealed a thin child on the 3rd percentile for weight and 25th centile for height. Epigastric tenderness was present. The signs and symptoms suggested peptic ulcer disease, and at endoscopy antral nodular hyperplastic gastritis was noted, as well as an ulcer in the first part of the duodenum. Histological examination showed evidence of *H. pylori* infection. Treatment with triple therapy (clarithromycin, amoxicillin and omeprazole) for 1 week led to resolution of symptoms within 4 weeks. Six weeks after stopping therapy a $^{13}C$-urea breath test was carried out and was negative, confirming eradication. At review 12 months later, Than was well and his height and weight were on the 25th percentile.

# 20.5 Liver diseases

Wolfram Haller, Winita Hardikar

## Introduction

Liver disease is relatively infrequent in childhood. Early recognition is, however, crucial, as the timing of diagnosis has a significant impact on the outcome of many liver disorders. Chronic liver conditions result in a high burden of care for children and their families.

This chapter aims to promote an understanding of the basic concepts of normal liver function, to introduce the concept of biochemical pattern recognition of liver disease, and to enable appropriate differential diagnosis and investigations in the child with suspected liver injury.

## Normal liver anatomy and function

In evaluating liver disease, it is useful to think of the liver as being composed of two morphological and functional subunits. Injury to either compartment gives rise to a specific pattern of symptoms and liver test abnormalities. The first subunit is the parenchymal compartment consisting of hepatocytes, the carriers of anabolic and catabolic enzymes, and non-hepatocytic parenchymal cells. The latter include stellate cells, important for production of fibrous tissue under disease conditions, and the Kupffer cells, resident mononuclear leukocytes fulfilling a crucial role in processing antigens that enter the liver through the portal vein. The second subunit is the biliary compartment consisting of the canalicular and biliary system. This system carries bile produced by the hepatocytes into the bowel, but is also actively involved in resorption of various solutes. Bile acids, comprising 12% of bile, are required for the normal absorption of fat and fat-soluble vitamins in the intestinal lumen.

Blood supply to the liver is predominantly via the portal vein (70%), channelling intestinal nutrients towards the liver. The remaining 30% is provided by the hepatic artery, which supplies oxygen-rich blood to the parenchymal and biliary compartments. The bile ducts are sensitive to reduced arterial flow and may become damaged if hepatic arterial flow is interrupted. Blood flows out of the liver via the hepatic veins, which connect to the inferior vena cava.

The liver plays an indispensable role in whole-body energy homeostasis and provides the necessary enzymatic repertoire for numerous catabolic and anabolic pathways. The main functions of the liver are:

- synthesis of a large number of proteins (e.g. clotting factors and albumin)
- production and excretion of bile
- detoxification and metabolism of endogenous toxins and exogenous drugs
- processing of nutrients – the liver is the central regulator of intermediary metabolism
- immune function
- fluid balance
- regulation of growth and other endocrine functions.

## Pattern recognition in acute and chronic liver dysfunction

Assessment of liver dysfunction in the child is part of a diagnostic process involving a thorough clinical history, clinical symptoms and signs, and a complete panel of 'liver function tests' (see below). The integration of these results will allow further categorization of the disease process. Depending on which morphological and functional compartment is affected, liver disease can be primarily hepatocellular (parenchymal), biliary (cholestatic) or mixed hepatocellular–biliary, and can finally lead to failure of synthetic and detoxification function. Allocation of laboratory tests to a disease pattern results in more targeted investigations (Fig. 20.5.1).

### Laboratory patterns of liver dysfunction

The actual term 'liver function tests' is a misnomer: not all measurements (e.g. alanine aminotransferase (ALT), aspartate aminotransferase (AST)) actually assess the function of the liver, whereas others (e.g. international normalized ratio (INR)) will not be obtained on request of 'liver function tests' on a biochemistry form. For practical purposes, the liver function tests can be divided into four categories, as described below.

**Infectious**

| Disease | Diagnostic test |
|---|---|
| Hepatitis A | HAV-IgG/IgM |
| Hepatitis B | HBsAG<br>Ant-HBc |
| Hepatitis C | Anti-HCV |
| EBV | Serology<br>PCR |
| UTI<br>Sepsis | Serology<br>PCR |

**Immunologic**

| Disease | Diagnostic test |
|---|---|
| Autoimmune hepatitis | Total IGG<br>ANA<br>SMA (type 1)<br>LKM (type 2) |

**Drug toxic**

| Disease | Diagnostic test |
|---|---|
| Paracetamol | Serum level |
| Antiepileptics | Stop medication<br>± liver biopsy |
| Antibiotics | |
| Contraceptives | |



**Immunologic**

| Disease | Diagnostic test |
|---|---|
| Sclerosing cholangitis | pANCA<br>US abdomen<br>MRCP |

**Vascular**

| Disease | Diagnostic test |
|---|---|
| Right heart failure | Echocardiography |
| Budd Chiari syndrome | CT angiography |
| Hepatic artery thrombosis | US abdomen<br>CT angiography |

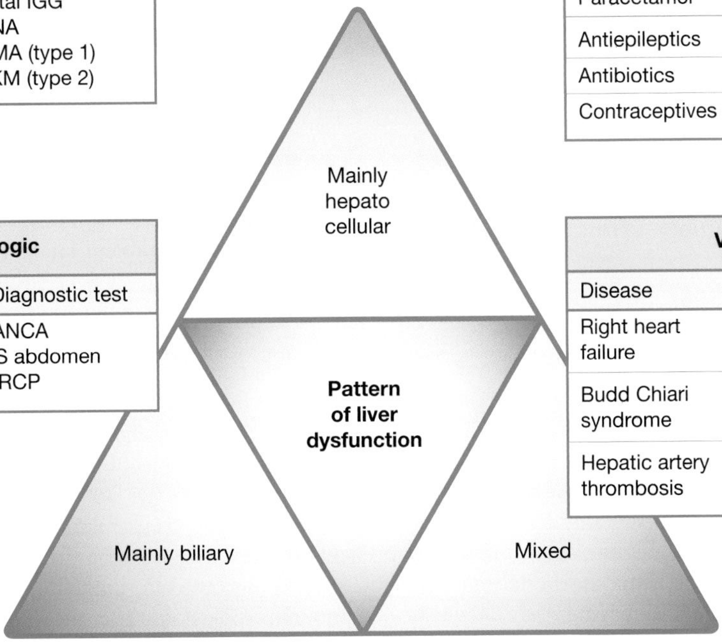

**Obstructive**

| Disease | Diagnostic test |
|---|---|
| Cholelithiasis<br>Sludge | US abdomen |
| Coledochal cyst | US abdomen<br>MRCP |
| Biliary atresia | US abdomen<br>Liver biopsy |
| Alagille syndrome | X-ray spine<br>Ophthalmology<br>Liver biopsy |

**Metabolic**

| | Diagnostic test |
|---|---|
| alpha1 AT deficiency | FeA1AT level<br>Pi type |
| Haemo-chromatosis | Ferritin<br>Transferrin saturation |
| Wilson's disease | Coeruloplasmin<br>Opthalmology |
| Cystic fibrosis | Immunoreactive trypsin<br>Sweat test |

Fig. 20.5.1 Diagnoses and investigations according to the predominant pattern of liver dysfunction. ANA, anti-nuclear antibody; AT, antitrypsin; CT, computed tomography; EBV, Epstein–Barr virus; HAV, hepatitis A virus; HBc, hepatitis B core antigen; HBsAg, hepatitis B surface antigen; HCV, hepatitis C virus; Ig, immunoglobulin; LKM, liver/kidney microsomal antibody; MCS; microscopy, culture, sensitivity; MRCP, magnetic resonance cholangiopancreatography; pANCA, perinuclear anti-neutrophil cytoplasmic antibody; PCR, polymerase chain reaction; Pi, protease inhibitor; SMA, anti-smooth muscle antibody; US, ultrasonography; UTI, urinary tract infection.

### Markers of hepatocellular dysfunction: ALT, AST

ALT is a cytosolic enzyme; AST can be found in both cytosolic and mitochondrial compartments. Both catalyse a chemical reaction called 'transamination' – hence the term transaminases. Hepatocyte damage resulting from infections, drugs, toxins, immunological or ischaemic insults can result in leakage of these enzymes into the circulation. The levels of ALT and AST do not correlate well with the severity of liver damage; for example, low levels of transaminases can be seen in advanced parenchymal necrosis in acute liver failure. ALT is more specific for hepatocellular injury than AST, as the level of AST is also increased in cardiac or skeletal muscle damage as well as in haemolysis. If there is an isolated rise in ALT or AST, consider extrahepatic causes, such as muscle disease or coeliac disease.

### Markers of biliary dysfunction/cholestasis: ALP, GGT, conjugated bilirubin, serum bile acids

Alkaline phosphatase (ALP) is an enzyme of uncertain physiological function. Blockage of bile flow leads to *de novo* production within the bile duct epithelium and to a rise in serum levels, which takes a few days. ALP levels may therefore be normal in acute biliary obstruction. The specificity of ALP is limited, as it is also found in other tissues including bone, intestine and kidney. ALP concentration is therefore often increased in growing children, particularly rapidly growing adolescents. If there is confusion, the origin of the ALP (i.e. liver or bone) can be tested in the laboratory by determining the so-called isoenzymes.

γ-Glutamyltransferase (GGT) is a more sensitive and specific test for biliary disease, and its level increases with biliary obstruction or inflammation. GGT is also induced by certain medications; therefore, if there is an isolated rise in GGT levels, take a full drug history. Bilirubin is the end-product of enzymatic haem breakdown, a component of haemoglobin. This unconjugated bilirubin is lipid-soluble, can cross membranes such as the blood–brain barrier and is therefore toxic, particularly in small infants. Conjugation of the bilirubin to glucuronide in the liver makes it water-soluble and allows excretion (via a transport protein in the cell membrane) into the small bile ducts, called canaliculi. The conjugated bilirubin then drains through the common bile duct into the duodenum. Damage to the transmembranous transport of conjugated bilirubin (e.g. hepatocellular insult) or blockage of the biliary drainage system (e.g. due to gallstones or biliary atresia) impairs bile flow, leading to a clinical phenotype called cholestasis. The water-soluble conjugated bilirubin flushes back into the bloodstream (conjugated hyperbilirubinaemia), is deposited in the skin (jaundice) and filtered in the kidneys (dark urine). The lack of bilirubin in the intestine results in pale (acholic) stools. Determination of conjugated bilirubin is the most important test in any jaundiced patient. A conjugated bilirubin fraction of more than 20% of total bilirubin is called conjugated hyperbilirubinaemia and indicates liver disease and impaired bile flow (cholestasis). Lack of bile flow also leads to retention and blood accumulation of bile acids and other components of bile. It is not known which of these components is the main mediator of the intense pruritus seen in chronic cholestasis.

### Markers of synthetic dysfunction: albumin, INR

Albumin is the most abundant protein produced by the liver with a half-life of 3 weeks. Serum concentrations therefore change slowly in response to acute alterations of synthesis (e.g. in acute liver failure), although albumin is a good marker of chronic synthetic failure. The specificity of a low albumin level is, however, limited as a marker of liver dysfunction. Albumin synthesis is also low in situations of longstanding low protein intake (malnutrition), inflammatory conditions (as a negative acute-phase protein), and can also be lost in the urine (renal disease) or through the intestine (protein-losing enteropathy). The liver synthesizes the majority of coagulation proteins, some of them with the help of vitamin K as a co-factor (factor II, VII, IX, X). Liver synthetic function can therefore be assessed through measurement of the INR. Because most clotting factors have a shorter half-life than albumin (factor VII, 6 hours), the INR is useful in assessing short-term changes in synthetic liver function. In general, an abnormal INR can be attributed to synthetic liver dysfunction if it does not improve 6 hours after a dose of vitamin K.

### Markers of impaired hepatic detoxification: ammonia, lactate

Ammonia is a product of protein catabolism. The liver plays a crucial role in metabolizing this neurotoxic solute. In situations of acute or chronic liver failure, increased concentrations of ammonia may play an important role in the development of hepatic encephalopathy. Lactate is an important carrier of energy in the fasting state and is either oxidized in the citric acid cycle or used as a substrate for gluconeogenesis in the liver. Consequently, liver dysfunction leads to a slowing of these metabolic pathways and to accumulation of lactate within the bloodstream. Lactate is therefore a useful marker of pronounced acute and chronic liver dysfunction.

## Clinical signs of liver dysfunction

A thorough history and clinical examination are essential to guide the diagnostic approach in a child with suspected liver disease. When trying to identify the cause of liver disease, it is useful broadly to categorize children into infants versus older children, acute versus chronic liver disease, and biliary (cholestatic) versus hepatocellular injury. Of course, there will be significant overlap, but the categories are described in detail below and in Table 20.5.1 and Fig. 20.5.1.

The major clinical symptoms and signs of acute and chronic liver dysfunction are (Fig. 20.5.2):

- *Jaundice* due to impaired bile flow is associated with pale stools, steatorrhoea, dark urine and pruritus as described above.
- *Hepatomegaly* can be a consequence of congestion with blood (obstruction of venous outflow), expansion of the parenchymal compartment by storage (fat, glycogen or other storage disease), malignancy (hepatoblastoma, leukaemia), infection (abscess), inflammatory infiltration (infectious and autoimmune hepatitis, drug toxicity) or blockage of biliary outflow. The liver can feel soft and often tender in the acute setting as a consequence of capsular stretching, or hard, firm and irregular in situations of chronic liver insult. Acute biliary obstruction can result in referred right shoulder pain.
- *Splenomegaly* is typically seen acutely with infectious hepatitis, acutely and chronically with metabolic storage diseases, but can also reflect chronic portal and splenic vein congestion in the setting of portal hypertension (see below).

**Table 20.5.1 Clinical and aetiological categories of liver disease in childhood**

| Mode of presentation | Time of presentation: Infancy | Time of presentation: Older child |
|---|---|---|
| **Acute** | Infectious<br>• urinary tract infection<br>• bacterial sepsis<br>• congenital (TORCH)<br>Biliary/obstructive<br>• inspissated bile (sludge)<br>• cholelithiasis<br>Metabolic<br>• galactosaemia<br>• hereditary fructose intolerance<br>• Niemann–Pick C disease<br>• fatty acid oxidation defect<br>• mitochondrial disease<br>Ischaemic<br>• neonatal asphyxia<br>Immunological<br>• neonatal haemochromatosis | Infectious<br>• viral hepatitis (A, B, E, rarely C)<br>• non A–E hepatitis<br>Biliary/obstructive<br>• cholelithiasis<br>Metabolic<br>• Wilson's disease (acute-on-chronic)<br>• mitochondrial disease<br>Drug-induced<br>• paracetamol<br>• antibiotics<br>• antiepileptics (e.g. valproate)<br>• contraceptives |
| **Chronic** | Biliary/obstructive<br>• extrahepatic biliary atresia<br>• Alagille syndrome<br>• choledochal cyst<br>Metabolic<br>• $\alpha_1$-antitrypsin deficiency<br>• cystic fibrosis<br>• tyrosinaemia type 1<br>• glycogen storage disease<br>• Niemann–Pick C disease<br>• mitochondrial disease | Infectious<br>• hepatitis B/C<br>• non-A–E hepatitis<br>Biliary/obstructive<br>• sclerosing cholangitis<br>• choledochal cyst<br>Drug-induced<br>• methotrexate (e.g. chemotherapy)<br>Metabolic<br>• $\alpha_1$-antitrypsin deficiency<br>• cystic fibrosis<br>• Wilson's disease<br>• non-alcoholic fatty liver disease<br>• tyrosinaemia type 1<br>Immunological<br>• coeliac disease<br>• autoimmune hepatitis<br>• sclerosing cholangitis<br>Cardiac<br>• congenital heart disease (+ right ventricular failure) |

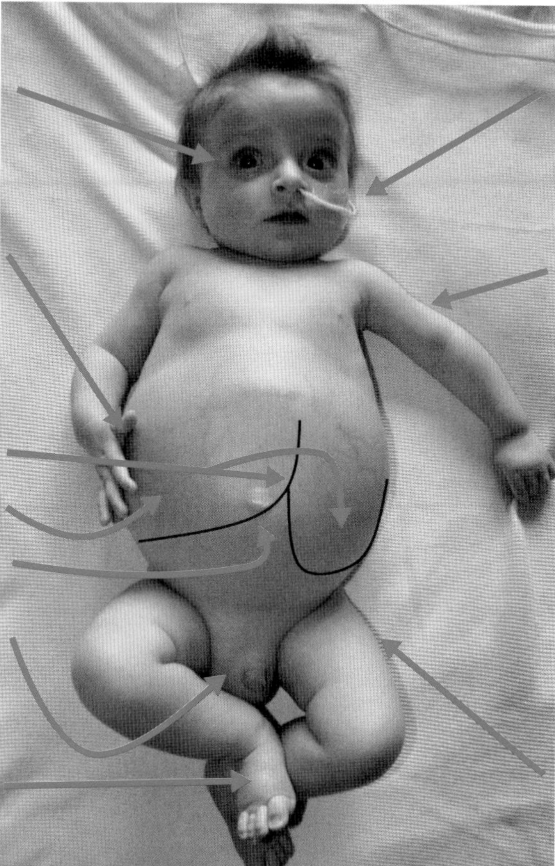


Fig. 20.5.2 Clinical signs of the child with liver disease: an 8-month-old infant with end-stage liver disease due to extrahepatic biliary atresia and failed Kasai portoenterostomy.

- *Encephalopathy* – mental alteration in the setting of acute/chronic liver dysfunction is thought to result from an accumulation of toxins not processed by the failing liver. Encephalopathy is graded according to severity. This is, however, not so straightforward in children, where irritability can reflect many other factors such as hunger or lack of sleep. Early symptoms are reversal of the day/night and awake/asleep pattern in addition to irritability, inconsolability or unusually aggressive behaviour. Lethargy and sleepiness are late signs of hepatic encephalopathy in the child.
- *Skin changes* include palmar erythema, facial telangiectasia, spider naevi, dilated abdominal veins and clubbing, mostly reflecting chronic and severe liver damage with portal hypertension.
- *Portal hypertension* is a result of increased resistance to blood flow into the liver and can be due to blockage of the inflow branch itself (extrahepatic: portal vein thrombosis), parenchymal scarring of the liver in chronic liver disease (intrahepatic: cirrhosis) or as a consequence of obstruction of the vascular outflow branch of the liver (posthepatic: Budd–Chiari syndrome, veno-occlusive disease). The high pressure within the portal vein transmits to the rest of the splanchnic vasculature and results in distension of small venules within the oesophageal, gastric and anal capillary bed, leading to varices. Haematemesis following rupture of oesophageal varices can be the life-threatening first manifestation of portal hypertension, whereas recurrent episodes of melaena or iron deficiency anaemia can be a more insidious sign. Splenic enlargement leads to hypersplenism; a low platelet count can thus be a useful indirect sign of advanced chronic liver disease.

## Liver disease in the neonate and infant

Jaundice is extremely common in the healthy term neonate, affecting more than 50% of newborns. About 5–10% of infants are still jaundiced beyond 3 weeks of age, a condition called prolonged jaundice. It is crucial to distinguish those children with unconjugated hyperbilirubinaemia due to benign breast milk jaundice, haemolysis, blood group incompatibility or inherited conjugation disorders from those with conjugated hyperbilirubinaemia. The latter is commonly associated with liver disease, and hence conjugated and unconjugated bilirubin levels should be determined in any child with severe or prolonged jaundice beyond 2 weeks of age. Common causes of neonatal and infant liver disease are summarized in Table 20.5.1. Manifestation of neonatal liver disease can be acute, chronic or acute-on-chronic.

Taking a detailed history is crucial. Important details and relevance of parental and infant history are summarized in Table 20.5.2.

## The acutely unwell neonate and infant with liver disease

The neonate and infant have a limited array of clinical responses to severe illness, irrespective of aetiology. Significant liver disease should therefore be considered in the setting of any acutely unwell infant. A full set of liver function tests should be performed. Mixed patterns of hepatocellular and biliary dysfunction (with or without synthetic dysfunction) are common; however, there will usually be a predominant category.

Bacterial sepsis and congenital infection are certainly one of the more common causes of liver dysfunction in the young neonate, a septic and TORCH (toxoplasmosis, rubella, cytomegalovirus, herpes simplex and HIV) screen should therefore be part of the workup. Splenomegaly and skin rashes can be additional clinical cues in congenital infections. Congenital infections can also, however, present with prolonged jaundice (see below) later in the neonatal period.

Metabolic liver disease is another important disease complex to consider. Clinical deterioration typically occurs after a honeymoon period of a few days during which toxic metabolites reach a critical blood level. Episodes of hypoglycaemia can further support the diagnosis of a liver-based metabolic disease.

Galactosaemia is a typical example of an autosomal recessively inherited inborn error of metabolism. It is rare, with an incidence of about 1 in 40 000. The lack of an enzyme, galactose-1-phosphate uridyltransferase (Gal-1-PUT), leads to blockage of galactose breakdown and to accumulation of the toxic metabolite, galactose-1-phosphate (Gal-1-P) after a few days of breastfeeding. Towards day 7 of life the newborns display increasing feeding difficulties, vomiting, jaundice, lethargy and/or irritability. Laboratory investigations will show a mixed laboratory pattern of liver dysfunction. There may be associated Gram-negative sepsis (e.g. *Escherichia coli*). Withdrawal of lactose-containing feed (including breast milk) will

**Table 20.5.2 Clinical history in the infant with liver disease**

| Parents | | Infant | |
|---|---|---|---|
| History | Consider | History | Consider |
| Consanguinity | Metabolic | Low birth weight | TORCH, metabolic |
| Miscarriages, early deaths | Metabolic | Vitamin K prophylaxis | Vitamin K deficiency in cholestatic child |
| Pruritus/jaundice during pregnancy | Metabolic | Pale stool colour | Biliary obstruction (e.g. in biliary atresia) |
| Maternal illness during pregnancy | TORCH | Irritability | Early encephalopathy |
| Maternal intravenous drug use | Hepatitis B, C | Lethargy | Late encephalopathy, hypoglycaemia, hyperammonemia |
| Maternal hepatitis | Hepatitis B, C | Slow weight gain | Malabsorption secondary to cholestasis |
| Family history of autoimmune disease | Autoimmune | | |
| Dysmorphic features in parents | Alagille syndrome | | |

improve symptoms rapidly. Cataract, female infertility and developmental delay are common long-term issues. Untreated, galactosaemia leads to liver failure and death. However, a more chronic cholestatic course of disease is also seen.

A significant number of inherited conditions affecting lipid, fatty acid, amino acid and ammonia metabolism, as well as oxidative phosphorylation (mitochondriopathies), share the clinical phenotype of galactosaemia. Further workup should therefore include the determination of urine organic acids, amino acids and succinylacetone as well as plasma amino acids in the acutely unwell neonate.

### Chronic liver disease in the infant

The infants falling into this category typically present with prolonged or new-onset jaundice beyond 2–3 weeks of age, displaying predominantly clinical signs of cholestasis with pale stools and dark urine, but otherwise being clinically well. Baseline laboratory investigations typically show a predominant biliary pattern (conjugated hyperbilirubinaemia) with only mild to moderate hepatocellular dysfunction. Abnormal clotting studies are often related to vitamin K deficiency on the background of longer-standing fat-soluble vitamin malabsorption, and are correctable with vitamin K supplementation. Early diagnostic workup is crucial. Therefore, in any child with jaundice beyond 2 weeks of age, stool colour has to be assessed and conjugated bilirubin should be determined. The approach to the infant with conjugated jaundice is summarized in Fig. 20.5.3.

Chronic infant liver diseases affecting the biliary compartment include extrahepatic biliary atresia and Alagille syndrome. Extrahepatic biliary atresia is characterized by progressive inflammation and obliteration of the extrahepatic and intrahepatic biliary tree, leading to impaired bile flow and secondary damage to the parenchymal compartment. The cause is unknown. Affected babies are typically born at term, appropriate for gestational age with no significant failure to thrive in the early stages of disease. Pale stool colour and prolonged jaundice can be seen early in the course of disease, but are often overlooked. Firm hepatosplenomegaly and failure to thrive will evolve later in the disease. Left untreated, biliary atresia will lead to cirrhosis and death within the first 2 years of life.

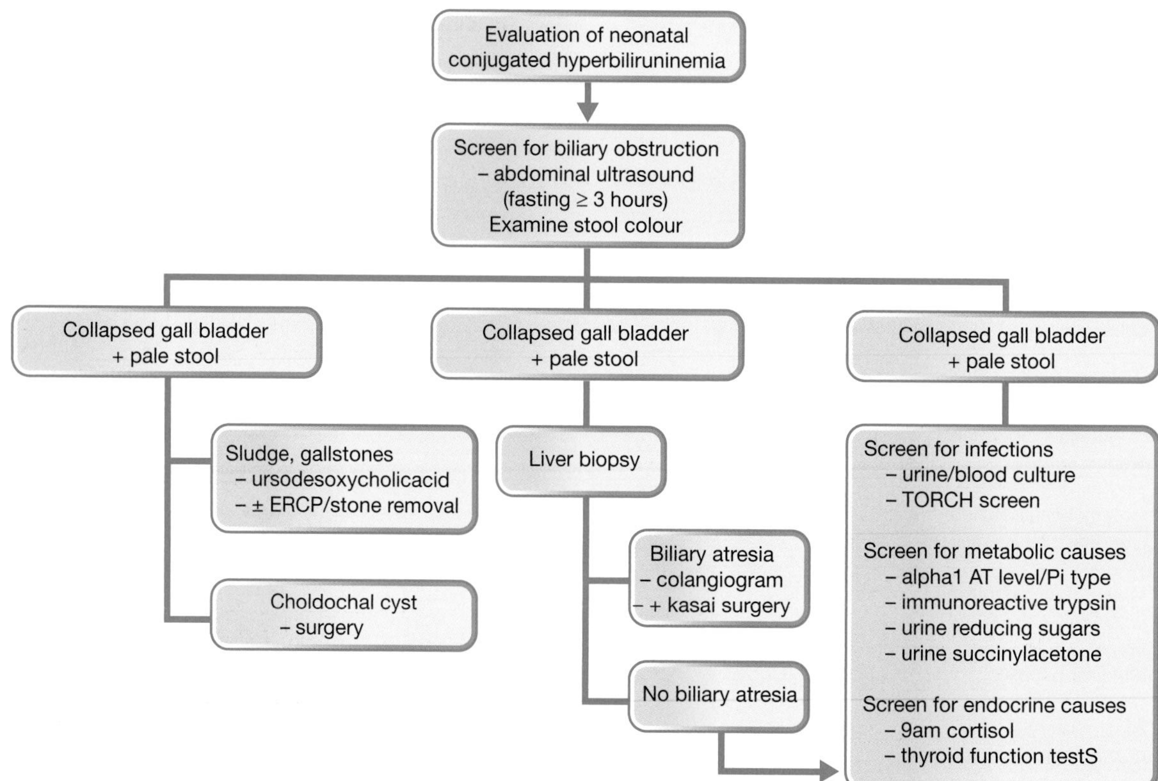


Fig. 20.5.3 The approach to the child with conjugated hyperbilirubinaemia. AT, antitrypsin; ERCP, endoscopic retrograde cholangiopancreatography; Pi, protease inhibitor, TORCH, toxoplasma, others, rubella, cytomegaly, herpes.

Early diagnosis and treatment is crucial, and hence biliary atresia needs to be excluded on an urgent basis in any newborn with conjugated hyperbilirubinaemia. There is no single laboratory test to confirm biliary atresia. Fasting liver ultrasonography often shows a small, collapsed gallbladder, whereas liver biopsy has some characteristic features. The final diagnosis is made with an intraoperative injection of contrast medium into the gallbladder (cholangiography). At the same time, the first-line treatment, the Kasai hepatoportoenterostomy, is performed. This operation restores bile drainage through attachment of a bowel loop to the cut surface of the liver, slows the progression of cirrhosis and development of end-stage liver failure, and thereby delays the need for liver transplantation.

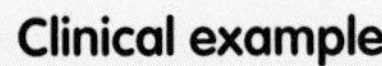

**Clinical example**

Lilah, a 6-week-old breastfed infant, presented with ongoing jaundice from infancy and pale stools but was feeding well. Liver function tests showed a predominantly cholestatic picture with raised conjugated bilirubin and GGT levels. Ultrasonography showed a small contracted gallbladder despite 4 hours of fasting. The $\alpha_1$-antitrypsin level was normal, and liver biopsy showed features consistent with biliary atresia. Operative cholangiography did not identify any extrahepatic biliary tree. Lilah underwent a Kasai operation, which resulted in some biliary drainage. She was able to continue to grow with the help of fortified feeds and fat-soluble vitamin supplementation. By the age of 7 years, Lilah developed end-stage liver disease and underwent liver transplantation.

Alagille syndrome is a rare autosomal dominant condition also presenting with prolonged jaundice. Associated clinical features include a triangular facies, butterfly vertebrae on spinal X-ray (Fig. 20.5.4), posterior embryotoxon on eye examination and pulmonary valve stenosis. Refractory failure to thrive and severe pruritus are frequent late complications. Ultrasound images of the liver and biliary tree can be normal or indistinguishable from biliary atresia. Liver biopsy confirms the diagnosis, displaying a paucity of bile ducts. A subset of patients develop chronic liver failure needing liver transplantation.

Chronic infant liver disease affecting predominantly the parenchymal compartment includes a number of metabolic diseases, of which $\alpha_1$-antitrypsin deficiency is the most common . This is an autosomal recessive genetic disorder in which the defective synthesis of $\alpha_1$-antitrypsin leads to its retention within the liver cell, causing chronic hepatocellular damage. The clinical presentation in the infant can again be indistinguishable from that of biliary atresia with prolonged

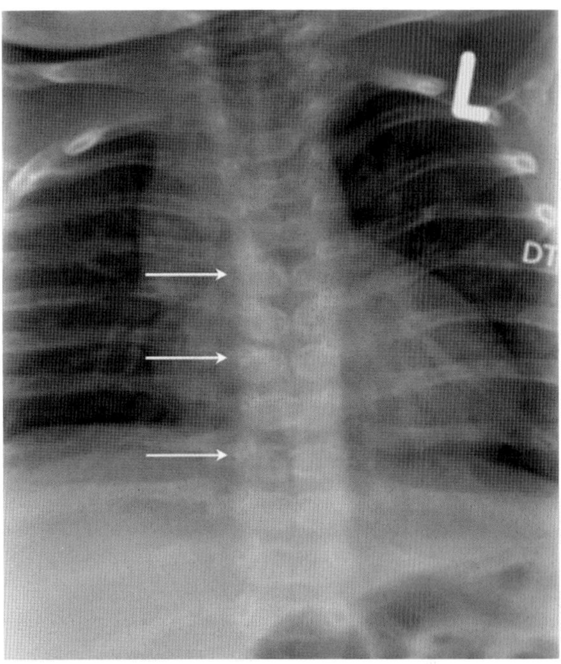


Fig. 20.5.4 X-ray of the thoracic spine with 'butterfly vertebrae' on multiple levels (arrows).

jaundice and the complications of longstanding cholestasis. Liver function tests often show a mixed hepatocellular and biliary picture. Serum levels of $\alpha_1$-antitrypsin are low. A diagnosis can be established by serum protein electrophoresis confirming the abnormal protein – protease inhibitor ZZ (PiZZ) phenotype. The majority of infants clear jaundice spontaneously early during infancy, whilst the hepatitic laboratory pattern persists. A significant number of patients are therefore diagnosed later in life following the incidental finding of hepatomegaly or raised transaminase levels. A minority of patients develops liver failure requiring liver transplantation within the first 2 years of life.

## Liver disease in the older child

The diagnosis of liver disease in the older child is often incidental following detection of hepatomegaly or abnormal transaminases on routine examination and blood testing, unless the child presents already clinically jaundiced. Similar to the infant, clinical history (Table 20.5.3), symptoms, physical examination and liver function tests help to categorize the disease into a predominantly hepatocellular or biliary pattern with an acute, chronic or acute-on-chronic presentation. A range of possible diagnoses with acute and chronic presentation is summarized in Table 20.5.1.

**Table 20.5.3 Clinical history in the older child with liver disease**

| Parents | | Child | |
|---|---|---|---|
| History | Consider | History | Consider |
| Consanguinity | Metabolic | Travel in endemic areas | Hepatitis A, E |
| Miscarriages, early deaths | Metabolic | Surgery, piercing, transfusion | Hepatitis B, C |
| Pruritus/jaundice during pregnancy | Metabolic | Medication (recent new) | Drug-induced |
| Maternal intravenous drug use | Hepatitis B, C | Rash, arthralgia | Drug-induced or autoimmune |
| Family history of coeliac disease, inflammatory bowel disease, rheumatoid arthritis | Autoimmune | New-onset behavioural changes<br>Developmental delay | Metabolic, e.g.<br>Wilson's disease<br>Niemann-Pick C disease<br>Mitochondriopathy |

## The older child with acute liver dysfunction

Older children falling in this category often present with a phenotype of new-onset jaundice and abdominal pain.

In the setting of acute-onset abdominal and right shoulder pain, vomiting and pale stools, biliary obstruction is likely. Abdominal examination is often inconclusive; sometimes a distended and tender gallbladder can be felt. Laboratory investigations display a predominantly biliary pattern of liver function test results. Pancreatic lipase concentration is commonly increased due to ongoing blockage of the distal bile ducts. Diagnosis is confirmed with abdominal ultrasonography, which may demonstrate a dilated biliary tree, an incarcerated stone in the common bile duct, sludge or stones within the gallbladder, or a choledochal cyst. Treatment may consist of endoscopic stone removal (endoscopic retrograde cholangiopancreatography, ERCP) or surgery.

Infectious hepatitis is an important differential diagnosis. Abdominal pain, vomiting, general malaise and, sometimes, fever are present. The degree of symptoms in addition to cholestasis is variable and dependent on the age of the child, with younger children being less symptomatic. Laboratory investigations display a mixed pattern of hepatocellular and biliary features. Ultrasonography may reveal an enlarged or echogenic liver, a normal biliary tree, often a thickened gallbladder wall, portal lymph nodes and a variable degree of splenomegaly. Diagnosis is confirmed with serological testing (see Fig. 20.5.1).

The clinical spectrum of drug toxicity/drug-induced liver disease is very variable. A good clinical history is crucial. Paracetamol overdose is an example of acute and dose-dependent drug toxicity causing profound hepatocellular damage and synthetic dysfunction. Determination of serum paracetamol levels should be part of the diagnostic workup in every child with acute hepatocellular and synthetic injury – even if intake of paracetamol is denied. Nausea, vomiting and abdominal pain are common. Laboratory investigations reveal a predominantly hepatitic picture together with often pronounced synthetic dysfunction. *N*-Acetylcysteine therapy should be started as early as possible, particularly when the amount and timing of paracetamol intake is unclear.

Sodium valproate, an antiepileptic drug, can cause a similar pattern of acute synthetic liver failure, particularly in the child with pre-existing mitochondrial disease. Drug reactions involving liver dysfunction following other drugs, such as antibiotics, are typically less acute and can be accompanied by blood eosinophilia, arthralgia and skin rash.

## The older child with chronic liver dysfunction

Autoimmune hepatitis should be considered in any child with abnormal liver function test results. It is a chronic disease of the parenchymal compartment of the liver. The liver is enlarged and inflamed following infiltration with inflammatory cells. The affected child can be asymptomatic at presentation, display symptoms of acute liver disease with laboratory signs of synthetic failure, or take a more insidious course with intermittent jaundice, loss of energy, abdominal pain and arthralgia. An important laboratory feature is the discrepancy between a high total serum protein and a low–normal albumin concentration, reflecting the polyclonal production of immunoglobulins. Serum autoantibodies allow further classification of the disease into type 1: antinuclear antibody/anti-smooth muscle antibody-positive (ANA/SMA+) and liver/kidney microsomal antibody type 2-positive (LKM-2+). The diagnosis is confirmed by liver biopsy. Treatment involves immunosuppressive medications such as corticosteroids and azathioprine.

**Clinical example**

Troy was a 2-year-old boy, previously well, who developed vomiting and diarrhoea, and was noticed to be jaundiced. Liver function test results showed a predominantly hepatocellular picture with ALT and AST >1000 units/L and raised serum proteins. Serology for hepatitis A, B and C was negative, $\alpha_1$-antitrypsin level was normal, but the LKM autoantibody level was significantly raised. A presumptive diagnosis of autoimmune hepatitis type 2 was made and liver biopsy confirmed evidence of piecemeal necrosis. Troy was treated with corticosteroids, with a significant improvement in his transaminase levels. Because of the severity of the initial presentation, he was commenced and maintained on azathioprine while the steroids were weaned. He remains well 11 years after presentation.

Wilson's disease is an important differential diagnosis to autoimmune hepatitis. It is a rare autosomal recessive disorder presenting beyond 4 years of age. A defective copper-transporting protein leads to retention of copper within the hepatocyte. Intracellular copper overload leads to hepatocellular damage. Once the liver is saturated with copper, copper accumulates in other organs such as the brain, heart, kidneys and bone marrow. As in autoimmune hepatitis, the affected child can be asymptomatic, or present with symptoms of acute liver dysfunction or chronic liver disease. Behavioural changes at school or at home as a consequence of cerebral copper deposition may be reported. An additional clinical feature is the Kayser–Fleisher ring, a circular area of copper deposition in the periphery of the cornea seen on slit-lamp examination. No single diagnostic test is available for Wilson's disease, but, in addition to the clinical features above, diagnosis can be supported by a low serum caeruloplasmin level, increased urine copper excretion or a high concentration of copper within a liver biopsy. Treatment aims to remove copper from the body, for instance with chelating agents (D-penicillamine) or by interfering with copper absorption through the enterocytes (zinc). Patients with an acute presentation often need liver transplantation.

Non-alcoholic steatohepatitis (NASH) is becoming an increasing issue in Western countries. It is associated with the metabolic syndrome (obesity and hyperinsulinism, hyperlipidaemias and hypertension). Mild liver function abnormalities usually improve following lifestyle changes and weight loss. Untreated, NASH can lead to cirrhosis and liver failure. Obesity-related liver disease is best treated by a multidisciplinary team which includes an endocrinologist, dietitian, physiotherapist and psychologist. As childhood obesity is so common, abnormal transaminase levels should not automatically be attributed to 'fatty liver disease'. Other causes of chronic liver disease have to be considered if there are any other clinical warning signs or if raised transaminases do not normalize after a period of lifestyle changes (e.g. 6 months).

**Clinical example**

Sarah was a well adolescent who had liver function tests prior to commencing therapy for acne. The test results showed a mildly abnormal hepatocellular picture. On further questioning, it was discovered that Sarah had been adopted from Bosnia and that her biological mother was thought to have used intravenous drugs. Sarah underwent testing and was found to have hepatitis C infection. She was counselled regarding transmission of blood-borne viruses and was considered for pegylated interferon and ribavirin therapy to eradicate the virus. Depending on the genotype of the virus, successful eradication can occur in 40–80% of patients.

## Liver failure

The described mechanisms of acute or longstanding damage to the hepatocellular and biliary compartment can all lead to temporary or irreversible liver failure. The paediatric definition of liver failure relies on laboratory features, including hepatocellular injury with raised levels of transaminases and synthetic failure with coagulopathy (INR ≥2.0), uncorrectable by intravenous vitamin K administration. Jaundice and hepatic encephalopathy are not prerequisites to establish the diagnosis. Liver failure may be acute (i.e. in someone with no underlying liver disease) or acute on chronic (i.e. decompensation of liver dysfunction in someone with an underlying liver disease). Unfortunately, the underlying chronic liver disease may have been previously unrecognized until the presentation with liver failure. Every effort should be made to establish a diagnosis in order to tailor treatment appropriately and allow recovery of liver function when possible.

In contrast to other end-stage disease states where replacement and supportive therapies exist (dialysis in renal failure, cardiac assist devices in heart failure, ventilatory support in respiratory failure), there is no comparable device for liver failure in routine clinical use. Treatment is mostly supportive: providing adequate nutrition, preventing fat-soluble vitamin deficiency and treating complications such as sepsis, encephalopathy, ascites or variceal bleeding. The only life-saving treatment for refractory acute or chronic liver failure is liver transplantation. Outcome is excellent with 5- and 10-year survival rates beyond 80%. Lifelong immunosuppressive treatment is generally required.

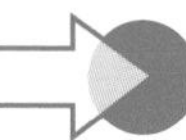

### Practical points

- 'Liver function tests' do not include markers of key liver functions such as synthesis (i.e. INR) and detoxification (i.e. lactate, ammonia). These are important and need to be requested separately.
- Abnormal liver function test results including INR must be repeated to determine the rate of progress of disease. In the setting of the child with abnormal INR and raised transaminases: give vitamin K and check INR 6 hours afterwards. This helps to distinguish vitamin K deficiency from liver failure.
- Any newborn with jaundice persisting beyond the first 2 weeks of age must have the conjugated bilirubin fraction measured and the stool colour examined.
- Pale stools are difficult to detect. Examine infant stool colour yourself.
- Acutely ill infants who are jaundiced are likely to have serious infections or metabolic disorders. Apart from a septic screen, urgent investigations should include a full panel of liver function tests plus creatine kinase.
- In children, encephalopathy is a late sign in the setting of liver dysfunction. Carefully note drowsiness and irritability in the infant, and aggression or unusual behaviour in the older child.

PART 21

# SKIN DISORDERS

# 21.1 Skin disorders

Maureen Rogers, Rod Phillips, Li-Chuen Wong

## Neonatal skin conditions

Many of these conditions will be described below, but the manner of their presentation in the neonatal period will be emphasized in this initial section.

### Pustular lesions in the neonate

There are many conditions that present in the neonatal period with pustules or pustule-like lesions. Some of these are benign and transient and of no systemic significance; however, many potentially serious infections can present with similar pustular lesions and it is vital to exclude infection rapidly in any pustular eruption in a neonate.

#### Sterile benign transient pustular disorders

- *Toxic erythema of the newborn* – widespread red macules each surmounted by a papule or pustule; onset in the first 2 days of life and disappearance by the end of the first week.
- *Transient neonatal pustular dermatosis* – onset at birth of flaccid pustules that dry out in 48 hours, leaving post-inflammatory hyperpigmentation in dark-skinned infants.
- *Infantile acropustulosis* – crops of spontaneously resolving pustules on the hands and feet that occur during the first few months of life.
- *Eosinophilic pustular folliculitis of the scalp* – recurrent groups of pustules on a red base on the scalp in early infancy; later they may occur elsewhere.
- *Pustular miliaria or sweat duct occlusion rash* – short-lived pustules in amongst more typical red papules of miliaria (heat rash), occurring particularly on the face, scalp and upper trunk.

#### Benign transient lesions simulating pustules

- *Milia* – firm, white papules especially on the face, which extrude in early weeks of life; these are sebaceous retention cysts.
- *Sebaceous hyperplasia* – yellow papules on the nose, which resolve in early weeks.

#### Infective disorders presenting with pustules

- *Staphylococcal infection* – particularly impetigo (which more often presents with vesicles); a common site is near an infected umbilical stump.
- *Candida* – multiple widespread small pustules which soon rupture producing a circular lesion with peripheral scale.
- *Herpes simplex* – grouped, often coalescing, pustules; often evolve from initial vesicular lesions. Particularly on presenting part (so usually the head). This may be associated with severe neurological disease (see below and also Chapter 11.4).
- *Varicella* – usually initially vesicles, which may become pustular. Unlike chickenpox in older children, the lesions are often seen in the same stage of development.
- Many other organisms including *Listeria monocytogenes, Pseudomonas aeruginosa* and *Haemophilus influenzae* can cause sepsis and pustules.

### Blistering lesions in the neonate

As indicated there is overlap between pustular and blistering disorders in the neonatal period. Several conditions may present with blisters and then become pustular. The term vesicle refers to a small blistering lesion.

#### Infections

- *Herpes simplex* – grouped coalescing vesicles, particularly on presenting part (so usually the head); rupture to produce deep, punched out, erosions.
- *Varicella* – usually initial vesicles which soon evolve into pustules.
- *Bullous impetigo* – flaccid blisters which soon rupture to produce large superficial spreading erosions (Fig. 21.1.1).
- *Staphylococcal scalded skin syndrome* – widespread erythema followed by superficial erosions, commencing in flexural areas and around the mouth; may be transient blistering.
- *Congenital syphilis* – blisters mainly in buttock area.

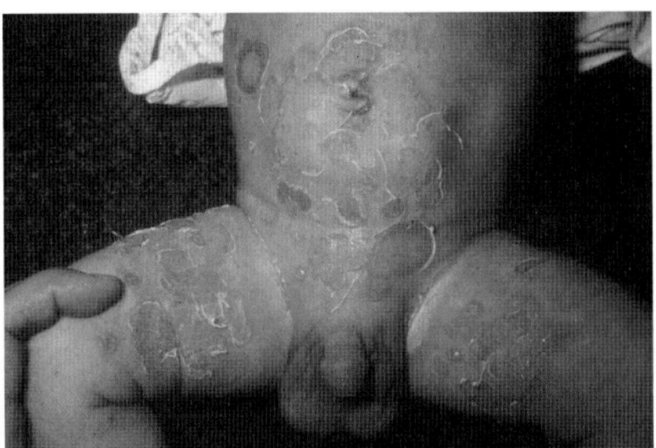

Fig. 21.1.1 Bullous impetigo with flaccid blisters and spreading erosions.

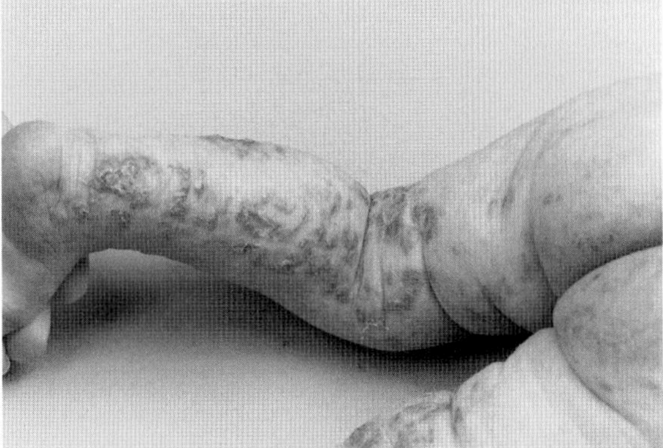

Fig. 21.1.3 Incontinentia pigmenti with a linear array of blisters and pustules.

## Conditions with possible systemic implications

- *Zinc deficiency* – blistered and crusted lesions around mouth, nose and in napkin area.
- *Epidermolysis bullosa* – blistering in areas of trauma; may be mucosal blistering and breathing problems.
- *Bullous ichthyosis* – blisters and erosions on the base of a bright red skin; skin thickens in early days.
- *Mastocytosis* – blisters on the background of localized brownish lesions or a diffuse leathery skin with a *peau d'orange* appearance.
- *Langerhans cell histiocytosis* – vesicles, erosions and purpuric crusted lesions (Fig. 21.1.2); may be self-limiting or can progress to, or reappear as, a serious malignant disease. May be associated lytic bone lesions and hepatomegaly.
- *Incontinentia pigmenti* – a linear arrangement of blisters, particularly on the limbs (Fig. 21.1.3), following the lines of Blaschko (see below). An X-linked recessive disease, so presents predominantly in girls. The mother may have late stigmata of disease, including brown Blaschko-distributed lesions, patchy alopecia and partial anodontia. Infant may have early seizures.

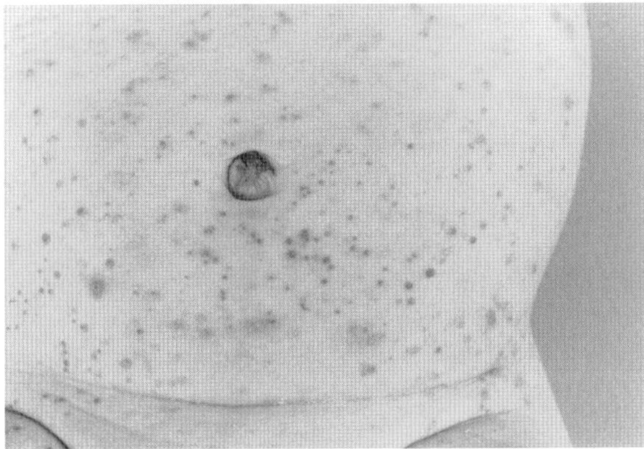

Fig. 21.1.2 Langerhans cell histiocytosis with crusted purpuric papules.

### Purpura in the neonate

This may be due to the early presentation of any cause of childhood purpura (see below), but particular causes in the neonate are mentioned here.

- *Systemic congenital infections* – including rubella, cytomegalovirus, toxoplasmosis, herpes simplex.
- *Haemolytic disease of the newborn* – for example with Rhesus incompatibility.
- *Malignancy* – including neuroblastoma, Langerhans cell histiocytosis, leukaemia.
- *Iatrogenic injury* – including birth trauma, extravasation of drugs, arterial injury during catheterization.

### Red, scaly rashes in the neonate or young infant

A number of important conditions can present with diffuse redness and variable scaliness in the neonate; affected infants often have major problems with temperature regulation and fluid balance, and may seriously fail to thrive.

- *Seborrhoeic dermatitis* – dull red erythema with a greasy, yellow scale involving particularly the scalp, centrofacial area and all flexures, major and minor. The scale may be absent in the flexures, and secondary monilia is common. Usually asymptomatic and self-limiting after the early months of life. Responds to weak steroids and anti-monilial agents. In cases in which there is a failure to respond to appropriate treatment, or the presence of any brownish scale or purpura, the possibility of Langherhans cell histiocytosis, which also occurs in the 'seborrhoeic areas', must be considered.

- *Atopic dermatitis* – rarely this condition presents in very early infancy with a widespread red, scaly and itchy rash. These patients often have food allergies and will go on to develop difficult long-term disease.
- *Ichthyoses* – some of these conditions present with the child covered in a shiny, red membrane that peels off in the early weeks of life to leave a red scaly skin. Some commence with a dramatic degree of redness and scale without the membrane. An early possible complication is hypernatraemic dehydration. The high metabolic state may lead to failure to thrive. Some are associated with neurological abnormalities.
- *Metabolic disorders* – a red, scaly rash can occur in neonates with inherited carboxylase deficiencies and essential fatty acid deficiency secondary to any severe malabsorption. The former may be associated with severe acidosis and coma.
- *Immunodeficiencies* – patients with severe combined immune deficiency (SCID) and other immunodeficiencies may present with a widespread, red, scaly rash in the neonatal period or early infancy. In some cases this represents a congenital graft-versus-host disease.
- *Staphylococcal scalded skin syndrome* – after the blistering and erosive phase there may be a striking scaly and crusted rash, still on a residual erythematous background.
- *Congenital candidiasis* – usually presents with small pustules, but as they resolve a widespread scaly red rash can ensue.

## Birthmarks and other naevoid conditions

Some naevoid conditions are not present till some time after birth, despite being 'programmed' from birth. These will be included in this section.

### Pigmented birthmarks

*Mongolian spot*
These are flat, blue or slate-grey lesions with poorly defined margins. They may be single or multiple and occur particularly on the lumbosacral area, although the shoulders, upper back and other areas may be involved. They are found in over 80% of Oriental and black infants and in up to 10% of white infants, particularly those of Mediterranean origin. They usually fade considerably by puberty, but may remain unaltered throughout life.

*Naevus of Ota*
This is a patchy blue–grey discoloration of the skin of the face, particularly on the cheek, periorbital area and brow. It is usually unilateral and often there is a similar pigmentation of the sclera of the ipsilateral eye. It is most common in Oriental individuals and is present at birth in over 50% of cases. It is a permanent lesion. Associated sensorineural deafness is reported, and very rarely these lesions may be complicated in adult life by development of malignant melanoma.

*Congenital melanocytic naevi (CMN)*
These occur at birth as raised verrucous or lobulated lesions of varying shades of brown to black, sometimes with blue or pink components, with an irregular margin and often growing long dark hairs. They may become increasingly hairy with time. Giant-sized lesions may produce considerable redundancy of skin and often occur in a 'garment' distribution on the trunk and adjacent limbs. In patients with large naevi an eruption of smaller, but essentially similar, lesions may occur during the first few years of life. Malignancy in giant naevi can occur in childhood and the incidence over a lifetime is possibly of the order of 2%. In medium and small lesions the risk is much lower and any development of malignancy is always post-pubertal. When large lesions occur over the axial spine, and in particular when multiple satellite lesions are present, there is a risk of intracranial lesions, both melanocytic involving the meninges and structural in the posterior cranial fossa, which may be further complicated by obstructive hydrocephalus. CMN over the lower spine may be associated with a tethered cord (Fig. 21.1.4). Neuroimaging is required in all these patients.

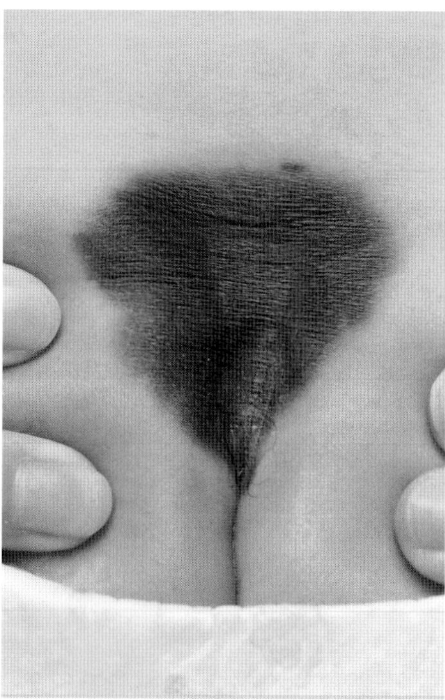

**Fig. 21.1.4** Congenital melanocytic naevus over the lumbosacral area.

*Naevoid pigmentary disorders*

These are flat areas of hyperpigmented or hypopigmented skin, obvious at or very soon after birth. They occur in characteristic patterns – either segmental, or whorled and streaky following the lines of Blaschko (Fig. 21.1.5). These lines represent the tracks taken by genetically identical cells in the embryo and are a marker for genetic mosaic patterns. The lesions usually have rather irregular edges. Sometimes the condition is extensive, resembling a marble cake, and both hypopigmented and hyperpigmented lesions are present in the one individual. These lesions usually occur as isolated phenomena but may be associated, as part of certain mosaic phenotypes, with neurological, skeletal and other abnormalities. One syndrome with hyperpigmented lesions and skeletal abnormalities is McCune–Albright syndrome.

Important in the differential diagnosis of brown lesions are the *café-au-lait* spots of neurofibromatosis, which are rarely present at birth, are more rounded in shape, and which continue to increase in number. In the differential of hypopigmented lesions are the ash leaf-shaped white spots of tuberous sclerosis. These also often appear after birth. Vitiligo, which can occur at any age, is totally depigmented rather than hypopigmented; it usually occurs in otherwise healthy children but can be associated with endocrine diseases. Leprosy is another important cause of acquired hypopigmented lesions.

## Epidermal naevi

Epidermal naevi arise from the basal layer of the embryonic epidermis, which gives rise to skin appendages as well as keratinocytes. These naevi have been classified, according to the tissue of origin, into keratinocytic, sebaceous and follicular types. They can involve any area of skin. They may be present at birth or appear in the first few years of life; subsequently they may simply grow with the patient or new areas of involvement may become evident. On the scalp and face the naevi have a yellowish colour, due to prominent sebaceous glands, and present as a hairless, often linear, plaque, usually flat in infancy and childhood and becoming verrucous at puberty. Lesions elsewhere are usually dark brown but are occasionally paler than the normal skin. They occur as single or multiple warty plaques or lines, often arranged in a linear or swirled pattern (Fig. 21.1.6).

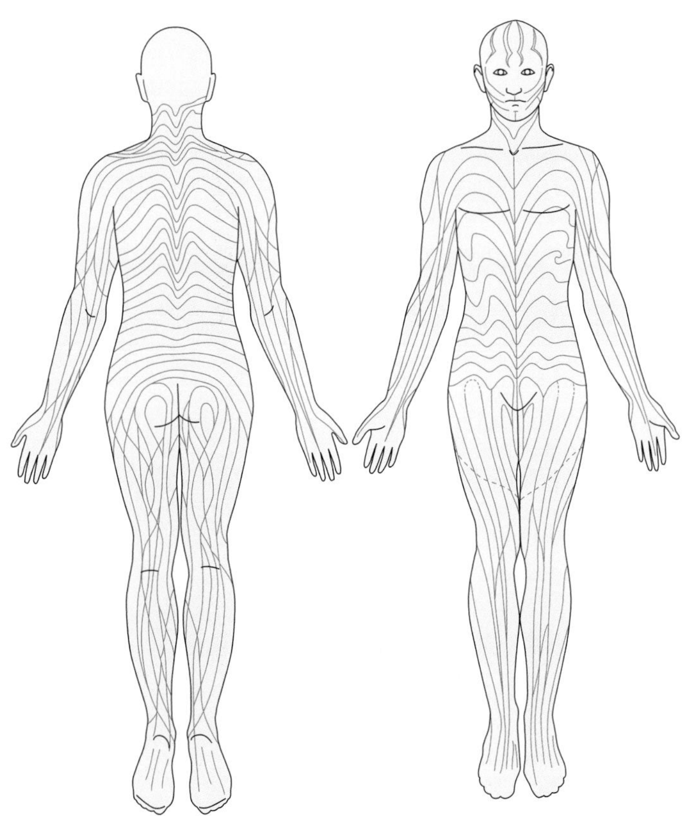

**Fig. 21.1.5** Lines of Blaschko.

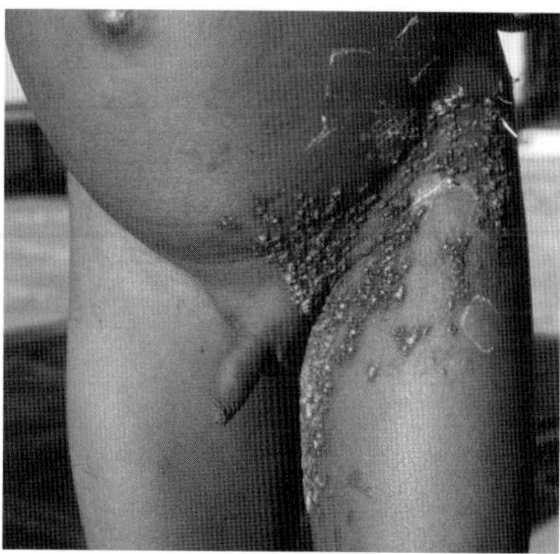

Fig. 21.1.6 Epidermal naevus with brown, warty lesions following the lines of Blaschko.

It is now clear that the linear and swirled patterns taken by epidermal naevi follow the lines of Blaschko and that all epidermal naevi can be explained on the basis of genetic mosaicism, with each type of naevus representing the cutaneous manifestation of a different mosaic phenotype. In most patients the naevus is the only detectable manifestation, but in some patients there are associated abnormalities in other organ systems, particularly skeletal, neurological and ocular. Skeletal abnormalities occur particularly with large naevi of keratinocytic type on the limbs, and neurological and ocular abnormalities with large or centrally located naevi of sebaceous type on the head.

## Vascular birthmarks

These can be divided into haemangiomas, which are proliferative vascular tumours, and vascular malformations, representing fixed collections of dilated abnormal vessels.

*Haemangiomas*

*Presentation and terminology.* Haemangiomas usually appear just after birth, undergo a fast growth phase and then, over a long period, tend to resolve spontaneously. All infantile haemangiomas, whether superficially or deeply located in the skin, have the same structure, being composed in the early stage of proliferating masses of endothelial cells with occasional lumina and later, as they resolve, of large endothelium-lined spaces. The terms capillary, cavernous and capillary–cavernous are misleading and should be abandoned in favour of the simple term haemangioma. However, the terms superficial and deep remain useful.

- Superficial haemangiomas usually appear in the first weeks of life as an area of pallor, followed by a telangiectatic patch. They then grow rapidly into a lobulated, well demarcated, bright red tumour. Rapid growth continues over the first 6 months of life; the growth rate then slows and further growth after 10 months is unusual. After a stationary phase, signs of involution begin, with the appearance of grey areas that enlarge and coalesce. The tumour becomes softer and less bulky and then disappears in 90% of cases by 9 years of age. Residual skin changes at the site may persist.
- Deeper haemangiomas may occur alone or beneath a superficial lesion (Fig. 21.1.7). The overlying skin is normal or bluish in colour. As they resolve, they soften and shrink, and most disappear completely.

*Complications of haemangiomas.* Although many haemangiomas resolve without sequelae, significant complications can occur.

- Incomplete resolution – redundant tissue, residual telangiectasia, scarring following ulceration.
- Ulceration – inevitable scarring, full-thickness tissue loss on 'edge structures' (lip, lid, ala), cicatricial ectropion from scarring of eyelids, cicatricial alopecia.
- Obstruction of vital structures:
  - Large eyelid lesions can obstruct vision producing amblyopia. Lesions that press on the globe, even without obstructing vision, can cause astigmatism and a degree of amblyopia.
  - Lesions around the nares can lead to difficulty in breathing during feeding.
  - Large, or painfully ulcerated, lesions of the lip can lead to problems with sucking.
  - Haemangiomas of the larynx can cause stridor followed by complete obstruction and represent a medical emergency. A 'beard' distribution haemangioma is a marker for possible laryngeal involvement and these patients should be investigated with a lateral airways X-ray even when stridor is not present.

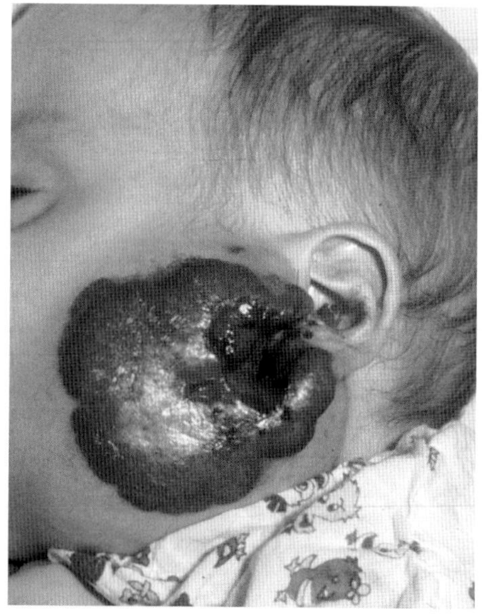

Fig. 21.1.7 Combined deep and superficial haemangioma with ulceration.

**Clinical example**

Harriet was born with a blanched area of skin bilaterally on the lower face, extending under the chin. A week later there was a tracery of telangiectases and over the subsequent 3 weeks bright red, raised dots appeared in the area, gradually coalescing into an extensive red haemangioma. When the baby was 4 weeks old her mother noticed that Harriet's breathing had become noisy when feeding. Urgent referral to investigate the stridor was followed by a lateral airways X-ray, which demonstrated narrowing in the subglottic area. Endoscopy confirmed subglottic haemangioma. The infant was admitted to hospital and observed carefully. Oral propranolol was commenced. After 1 day the stridor had gone and the birthmark was less angry-looking. A tracheostomy was not needed. The propranolol treatment was continued over an 8-month period during which there was considerable fading and shrinking of the haemangiomata. Harriet remained free of respiratory symptoms.

*Possible associations of haemangiomas*

- Lumbosacral lesions – tethered spinal cord.
- Perineal segmental lesions – abnormalities of the genitalia and lower urogenital and gastrointestinal tracts.
- Large segmental facial lesions – posterior cranial fossa malformations, abnormalities of heart, aorta and other major arteries, and ocular abnormalities.
- Multiple small cutaneous haemangiomas – haemangiomas in the liver, brain and other internal organs; high-output cardiac failure.

Appropriate imaging studies should be performed in all patients with these presentations.

*Management of haemangiomas.* Simple observation and reassurance while awaiting natural resolution is the ideal approach for most haemangiomas.

Ulceration should be managed with a combination of topical anaesthetic, topical antibiotic, dressings and/or oral antibiotics as appropriate.

Systemic treatments should be considered for lesions with anticipated long-term appearance problems, an alarming growth rate, ulceration in areas where serious complications could ensue (e.g. lips), interference with vital structures and severe bleeding. The first-line systemic treatment has been high-dose oral prednisolone to try to slow or stop growth. This is associated with predictable steroid side-effects, limiting its use to more serious cases. More recently, oral propranolol has been used as initial treatment. This change has occurred because propranolol appears to be more effective at stopping growth and hastening involution in many haemangiomas and has a better side-effect profile. Unlike the situation with oral steroids, propranolol may shrink lesions that have ceased growing. Some haemangiomas do not respond to propranolol, and propranolol does not help heal ulcerated lesions and might worsen ulceration. This is a new treatment and needs continuing evaluation.

*Vascular malformations*

These are collections of dilated abnormal vessels, classified according to the vessels of origin. All vascular malformations are present at birth (although occasionally not evident) and grow only in proportion to the growth of the child. They show no tendency to involution. The most appropriate terminology refers to the component vessels and many outdated terms (in brackets below) can be abandoned:

*Capillary malformation (port wine stain).* This presents as a flat purple stain, most commonly on the face, but it may occur anywhere. When it involves the upper lid and central forehead it may be a part of Sturge–Weber syndrome, associated with glaucoma, cerebral calcification and seizures. Careful ophthalmological assessment and follow-up, and neuroimaging are indicated in patients with this presentation.

*Venous malformation (varix).* This presents as a bluish tumour that empties with pressure and when elevated, and fills when dependent; phleboliths may develop within it and be seen on ultrasonography or X-ray.

*Lymphatic malformation (lymphangioma, cystic hygroma).* This may be macrocystic, microcystic, or a combination of both. Macrocystic lesions are deep and present as skin-coloured tumours, often with bruising; rarely these lesions become clinically apparent only when bleeding into them occurs. Microcystic lesions are deep or superficial and present on the skin as groups of haemorrhagic vesicles or warty lesions.

*Arteriovenous malformation.* This presents as a pulsatile skin-coloured or erythematous lump. These always need experienced assessment and management because of the significant risk of expansion and problems such as pain and bleeding, particularly at puberty.

*Other mixed malformations.* Some are very complex and associated with limb hypertrophy. Klippel–Trenaunay syndrome is a capillary–venous–lymphatic malformation with limb hypertrophy; Parkes–Weber syndrome is a capillary–arteriovenous malformation with limb hypertrophy and risk of ulceration from the shunting.

## Moles (acquired melanocytic naevi)

These usually first appear after the age of 1 year and increase in number throughout childhood. They commence as brown or black macules, some of which become raised and enlarge laterally as they develop. They are usually of uniform colour and well circumscribed. The risk of melanoma arising from acquired melanocytic naevi is very low (less than 0.1%); melanoma almost never occurs in childhood so their prophylactic removal in young patients is not justified.

*Halo naevi*

A depigmented halo may occur around a melanocytic naevus; the lesion may appear inflamed and often disappears, leaving a white spot, which may eventually repigment. This is a completely benign change. Although often apparently isolated, the condition can occur in the setting of vitiligo (Fig. 21.1.8) and may in some patients indicate a predisposition to this condition.

*Dysplastic or atypical naevi*

A subtype of acquired melanocytic naevi with characteristic clinicopathological features is a marker for an increased risk of developing malignant melanoma. Atypical naevi differ from more typical moles by being larger (more than 5 mm in diameter), having irregular and indistinct margins and irregular tan-brown colouration, often with an erythematous component. They are predominantly macular, sometimes with a central elevated portion. They may appear in childhood as small, typical-appearing naevi, which after puberty develop the atypical features. Characteristic dysplastic naevi may appear on the scalp in childhood. The final confirmation is based on the finding of some or all of a constellation of histopathological features. Patients with multiple dysplastic naevi should be observed frequently and monitored with serial photography. Any such naevus showing significant alteration should be removed immediately.

### Lumbosacral birthmarks

Congenital lesions over the lumbosacral area may be associated with occult spinal abnormalities such as a tethered cord. These spinal anomalies may not cause problems until later in childhood, when they can present insidiously with irreversible bladder, bowel or limb dysfunction. These problems can be prevented by early magnetic resonance imaging (MRI) and surgical correction. Congenital lesions that have been associated with underlying spinal problems include haemangiomas, capillary malformations, lipomas, dimples, sinuses, congenital melanocytic naevi and hairy patches.

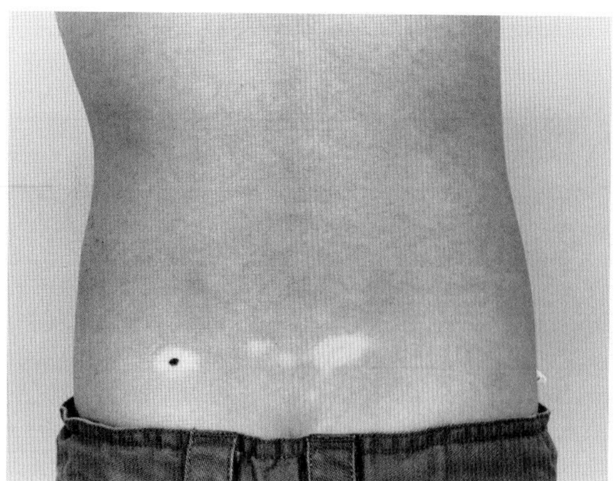

Fig. 21.1.8 Halo naevus in a patient with vitiligo.

## Cutaneous infections and infestations

### Viral exanthems

This term refers to the cutaneous manifestation of a viral illness (enanthem is the manifestation in the mouth).

The patterns may be:

- specific – where the appearance of the exanthem enables a clinical diagnosis of the causative virus.
- non-specific – where the same pattern of exanthem may be caused by many different viruses.

### Specific patterns

The aetiological virus can usually be identified clinically from the pattern of rash in the following situations:

- Chickenpox – scattered vesicles, pustules and dark crusts; lesions occur in crops (see Chapter 12.1).
- Herpes zoster – vesicles and pustules following the distribution of sensory nerves (see Chapter 12.1).
- Herpes simplex – see below.
- Erythema infectiosum – caused by a parvovirus B19, presenting with a slapped cheek appearance followed by a lacy erythematous rash mainly on the limbs (Fig. 21.1.9) (see Chapter 12.1).
- Mollusca – caused by a pox virus (see below).
- Hand, foot and mouth disease – due to one of the Coxsackie group of enteroviruses; presents with pustules and purpuric lesions limited to hands and feet with oral blistering.

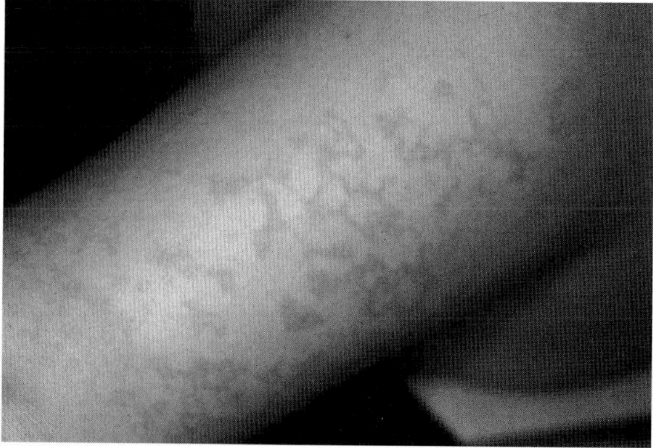

Fig 21.1.9 Lacy erythematous lesions of erythema infectiosum.

### Non-specific patterns

Each of these patterns may be produced by a wide variety of viruses, and the same virus may produce many different patterns of exanthem.

The viruses usually involved are:

- Enteroviruses
- Adenoviruses
- Hepatitis A and B viruses
- Epstein–Barr virus
- Cytomegalovirus
- Human herpesvirus (HHV) 6 and HHV7
- Parvovirus (can produce non-specific as well as specific rashes).

The patterns include:

- *Urticarial exanthems* – raised erythematous lesions that may be annular or figurate; itch is variable and the pattern changes from hour to hour. In young children there may be a central non-palpable purpuric element that resolves over several days rather than hours, leading to misdiagnosis as erythema multiforme. In children under 6 years old, more than 90% of cases of urticaria are caused by a viral illness.
- *Macular exanthems* – these are composed of flat red spots of variable size, sometimes becoming confluent. These are usually widespread and are characteristically difficult to differentiate from allergic reactions to drugs. In general the occurrence of lesions in a linear distribution along scratch marks, exaggeration in areas of sunburn or previous skin disease, and the presence of lymphadenopathy favour a viral over a drug aetiology.
- *Papular exanthems* – papules, which are raised erythematous lesions, may be few or multiple and vary in size from tiny pinpoint lesions to 0.5–1.0 cm in diameter. A linear distribution of groups of lesions is commonly seen and the limbs are usually affected more than the trunk.
- *Purpuric exanthems* – enteroviruses are the commonest causes of purpuric exanthems. Clearly the most important condition to be differentiated is meningococcal septicaemia. The purpuric lesions caused by enteroviruses tend to be small petechial macules but larger, angulated lesions sometimes occur.
- *Vesicular and/or pustular exanthems* – these lesions start as vesicles but often, as in varicella, become pustular and an admixture of lesions is seen. The lesions are often concentrated mainly on the limbs. The buttocks are another common site of involvement.
- *Erythrodermic exanthems* – these are rare, with widespread erythema and variable scaling. They are particularly difficult to differentiate from bacterial toxic reactions and drug reactions.

Conditions that may mimic viral exanthems, or which viral exanthems may mimic, include:

- *Drug reactions* – urticarial, macular, papular or erythrodermic exanthems. History of exposure and timing are helpful in differentiation. An allergic reaction to ampicillin is more common in patients with Epstein–Barr virus infection.
- *Kawasaki disease* – macular, urticarial, erythrodermic exanthems. An erythematous rash accompanied by oedema of the palms and soles is often prominent in Kawasaki disease. Other early features include prolonged high fever, conjunctivitis, redness, swelling or ulceration of mucosal surfaces, and enlargement of lymph nodes. Desquamation of the hands and feet, especially of the digit tips, is a later finding.
- *Meningococcal septicaemia* – purpuric exanthem (see Chapter 12.3). Small purpuric spots and larger stellate areas of purpura developing central necrosis. Associated with high fever and shock.
- *Scarlet fever* – papular exanthem, erythrodermic exanthem. There is significant fever, strawberry tongue, a rough consistency to the rash, and later peeling of palms and soles.
- *Staphylococcal and streptococcal toxic shock* – erythrodermic exanthems. Accompanied by a high fever and significant manifestations of shock.
- *Rickettsial infections* – macular, papular or purpuric exanthems.
- *Miliaria or heat rash* – micropapular exanthem or purpuric exanthem in a thrombocytopenic child with miliaria.
- *Systemic juvenile chronic arthritis* – macular, papular and urticarial exanthems. An erythematous maculopapular rash is often seen in this condition. This rash usually has a salmon-pink colour and tends to come and go, being particularly evident at the time when the fever is at its height. It may also be urticarial.
- *Food-induced urticaria* – urticarial exanthems.
- *Guttate (small spot) psoriasis* – micropapular exanthem.

## Molluscum

This is a poxvirus infection that is uncommon under 1 year of age and occurs particularly in the 2–8-years age group. The spread of lesions is enhanced in warm water and outbreaks occur among children who swim together or share baths or spas. Further spread of mollusca in the individual is also encouraged by being in warm water.

### Clinical features

Typical lesions are spherical and pearly white with a central umbilication, but they may vary from tiny 1-mm papules to large nodules over 1 cm in diameter.

They occur on any part of the skin surface, with common sites being the axillae and sides of the trunk, the lower abdomen and the anogenital area. Rarely they occur on the eyelids, where they may cause conjunctivitis and punctate keratitis. Mollusca on the face in school-aged children are visually unsightly and should be treated.

A secondary eczema often occurs around lesions, particularly in atopic children.

Secondary bacterial infection may occur, producing crusting, redness and pus formation. However, these same changes may be seen during spontaneous resolution, which occurs in most children within several months, leaving normal skin or tiny, varicella-like scars.

#### Management

Each lesion lasts for only weeks and, if the child is kept out of heated pools and spas and has showers rather than baths at home, the proliferation is curbed and the number of lesions usually decreases quickly. If these measures are adhered to rigidly, treatment is rarely required:

- Mollusca are often resistant to chemical therapies but cantharidin and potassium hydroxide may sometimes be effective when applied under strict guidelines.
- The most definitive treatment is deroofing of the lesion with a 21-gauge cutting-edged needle and wiping out the contents.
- With multiple small lesions in a young child, spontaneous resolution should be awaited but, if the lesions are troublesome because of their site, surrounding eczema or frequent secondary infection, removal under nitrous oxide sedation may be considered.
- Treat any secondary eczema.

### Warts

These are benign tumours caused by infection with a variety of papilloma viruses of the papova group:

- The common wart (verruca vulgaris) occurs particularly on hands, knees and elbows.
- Plane or flat warts, 1–3-mm, pink or brown, barely raised papules, occur on the face and often spread along scratch marks or cuts.
- Plantar warts occur particularly over pressure points on the soles and can be differentiated from calluses by a loss of skin markings over the skin surface.
- Warts at mucocutaneous junctions often have a filiform or fronded appearance.
- Anogenital warts may be acquired from maternal infection during delivery but their presence in older children raises the suspicion of sexual abuse.

#### Management

Various forms of treatment are available; they depend on the area, the type of wart and the age of the patient. Because spontaneous disappearance is common, aggressive treatment is often inappropriate. Treatments include:

- Keratolytic wart paints (e.g. salicylic acid, lactic acid and collodion) – for common warts and plantar warts.
- Retinoic acid preparations – for facial plane warts.
- Podophyllotoxin and imiquimod – for anogenital warts, used under strict supervision.
- A 20% formalin solution – for plantar warts, combined with serial paring.
- Cautery or diathermy – useful for lesions on the lips or anogenital area but elsewhere recurrence is fairly frequent following their use and there is also a risk of producing a painful scar, particularly over the joints of digits or on the palms or soles.
- Liquid nitrogen cryotherapy – a successful method of dealing with common warts that is useful for older children.
- Oral cimetidine has recently been demonstrated to be a useful treatment in some cases of multiple refractory warts in young children.
- Topical immunotherapy – creating sensitization with 2% diphencyprone (DCP) followed by application to the warts of a diluted DCP solution or cream will cause an inflammatory reaction, which may hasten resolution of the lesions.

### Dermatological presentations of herpes simplex

Herpes simplex virus (HSV) infections are extremely common in children, and serological studies confirm that more than 90% of the population have been infected by the time of reaching adulthood. The commonest type is HSV1, although HSV2 is more important in adulthood, being the major cause of genital herpes. Several distinct presentations are recognized in childhood.

#### Intrauterine herpes simplex

- Cutaneous lesions include blisters and erosions, sometimes in a dermatomal distribution, and irregular, often linear scars.
- Other features are microcephaly, short digits, cardiac abnormalities and a variety of ocular abnormalities.

#### Neonatal herpes simplex

- The skin lesions are grouped blisters, localized initially on the presenting part, usually the head, with the onset usually between the fourth and eighth days of life. The eruption may become widespread, with individual lesions a few millimetres across coalescing to produce large erosions.

- A rapid immunofluorescence test on material from the blister base enables a diagnosis within a few hours.
- Assess immediately for other organ involvement, of which the most potentially devastating is neurological.
- Immediate treatment with intravenous aciclovir is indicated.

### Primary herpetic gingivostomatitis

The child is systemically unwell with a high fever and there is severe swelling, erosion and bleeding of the gums and the anterior part of the buccal mucosa. Spread to the lips and the facial skin often occurs. There may be considerable soft tissue swelling and prominent lymphadenopathy. If swallowing is impossible, the child will require admission for hydration.

### Primary cutaneous herpes simplex

- Can occur anywhere on the body, depending on the source of infection, as painful grouped blisters or pustules (Fig. 21.1.10) on an erythematous base that soon break to produce erosions or crusted lesions.
- Often there is local swelling and regional lymphadenopathy, and the child may be febrile.
- When a primary lesion occurs on the thick skin of a finger, the blisters do not break easily and intact, grouped pustules last for several days, often misdiagnosed as a bacterial abscess (Fig. 21.1.11).
- When primary herpes simplex occurs in the napkin area it presents as a severe erosive napkin rash. This is usually contracted from a herpes lesion on the lip of a carer, directly or via the hands, but occasionally occurs as a result of sexual abuse.

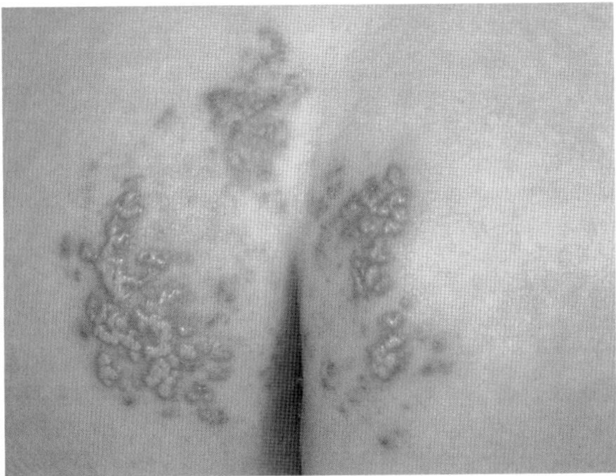

**Fig. 21.1.10** Primary herpes simplex with coalescing, grouped pustules.

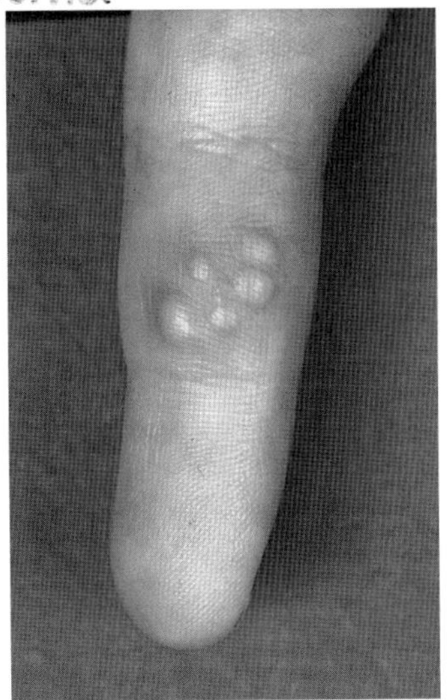

**Fig 21.1.11** Herpes simplex on a finger with grouped, intact pustules.

### Recurrent cutaneous herpes simplex

Recurrent herpes simplex of the face, particularly around the lips (herpes labialis), is common in childhood. As in adults, various factors, including fever and sun exposure, may reactivate the virus. Recurrent herpes can occur at any site.

### Disseminated herpes simplex (eczema herpeticum)

This occurs as a complication of atopic eczema and in immunosuppressed patients. It may originate from a primary or recurrent infection or from external reinfection. Spread is both on the surface of the skin and also by haematogenous dissemination. The lesions are vesicles or pustules 2–4 mm across, which may spread with alarming rapidity and have a tendency to coalescence to produce geographically shaped erosions with scalloped edges (Fig. 21.1.12). If there are more than a very few lesions, the patient should be hospitalized. Secondary bacterial infection should be treated with oral antibiotics, and saline or tap-water packs used to relieve discomfort and dry out the lesions. In severe cases, systemic aciclovir is indicated.

### Indolent ulceration in the immunosuppressed patient

An unusual presentation of herpes simplex in immunosuppressed patients is as a chronic, slowly growing ulcer, often with rather overhanging edges. The outline is usually irregular, reminiscent of the geographical shapes produced by coalescing lesions in the more typical forms of herpes simplex. It requires systemic antiviral therapy.

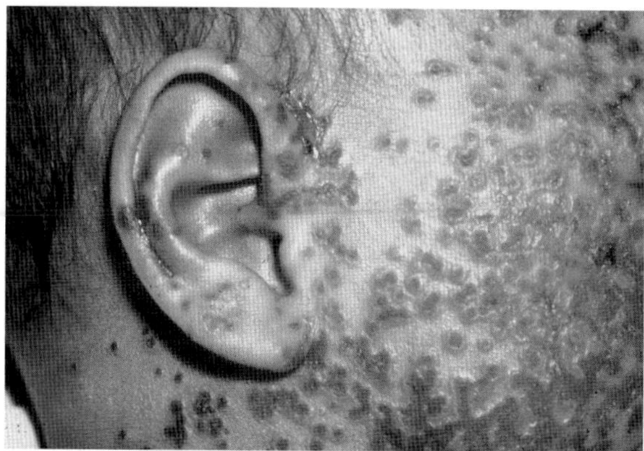

Fig. 21.1.12 Disseminated herpes simplex in an atopic child, with coalescing lesions.

## Impetigo

Impetigo is a bacterial infection caused by *Staphylococcus aureus*, group A streptococcus or a combination of these organisms; it occurs in two forms, bullous and non-bullous (or crusted).

### Clinical features

- Bullous impetigo is always due to staphylococci. Painless blisters arise on previously normal skin and increase rapidly in size and number, soon rupturing to produce superficial erosions with a peripheral brown crust. The erosions continue to expand, sometimes clearing centrally to produce annular lesions. As they dry they may assume a shiny brown-lacquer-like surface.
- Non-bullous impetigo may be due to either organism or to a combination. The lesions begin with a small, transient vesicle on an erythematous base. The serum exuding from the ruptured vesicle produces a thick soft yellow crust, below which there is a moist superficial erosion (Fig. 21.1.13). The deeper the erosion, the more likely the lesion is to be of streptococcal origin.

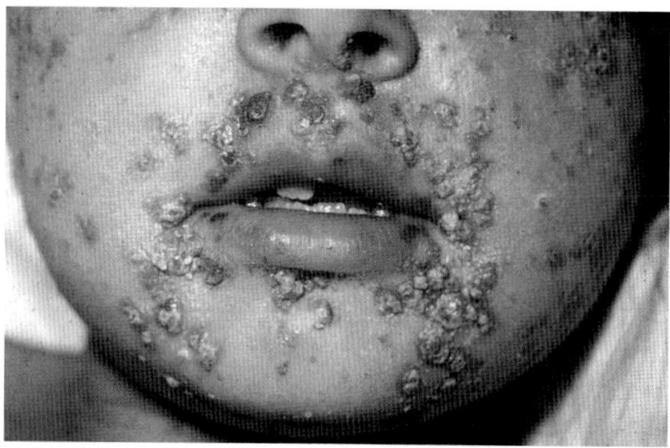

Fig. 21.1.13 Crusted lesions of non-bullous impetigo.

- Impetigo is often superimposed on other skin diseases such as insect bites, scabies, pediculosis and atopic eczema.
- Staphylococcal impetigo does not scar, but deep streptococcal lesions may do so.
- Post-inflammatory pigmentation can occur, particularly in dark-skinned patients.

### Management

- Saline bathing may be used to dry out the lesions.
- Avoid direct contact of the lesions with the skin of other children.
- A swab for culture and sensitivity testing should always be taken.
- Topical mupirocin may be successful for localized early disease. In general, oral antibiotics should be used.
- For bullous impetigo, flucloxacillin or cefalexin is the treatment of choice.
- If the lesions are strongly suggestive of a streptococcal origin or when a group A streptococcus is isolated, the patient should be treated with penicillin or a first-generation cephalosporin and be watched for 8 weeks for signs of glomerulonephritis.

## Staphylococcal scalded skin syndrome

**Clinical example**

At the age of 13 months Oscar developed conjunctivitis. Oral amoxicillin was prescribed by his general practitioner. Four days after starting this treatment Oscar developed a red, macular rash on his face and in the groin and axillary areas. He was febrile and irritable, and screamed when his mother tried to pick him up. The rash was diagnosed as a drug reaction and the antibiotic was ceased. The red rash continued to spread and flaccid blisters appeared in the groin, with the skin lifting off easily. A Gram stain from the blistered groin skin demonstrated no organisms. By this time the result from the conjunctival swab had returned, demonstrating *Staphylococcus aureus* insensitive to penicillin but sensitive to flucloxacillin, which was commenced immediately. The rash worsened over the next 12 hours, with sheeting off of skin all over the body, most marked around mouth and in axilla, groin and neck-fold. The child was brought to a paediatric emergency department, where a diagnosis of staphylococcal scalded skin syndrome was made and intravenous flucloxacillin was started. Over the next 4 days the redness settled, the blisters dried out, and Oscar became comfortable and cheerful. He was discharged on oral flucloxacillin for a further 4 days.

Staphylococcal scalded skin syndrome is a widespread blistering disease caused by the epidermolytic toxin produced by certain strains of *Staphylococcus aureus*, most often of phage group 2, types 70/71 or 51 but occasionally of phage group 1. This toxin produces a superficial splitting of the skin, with the level of split being high in the epidermis. Clinical disease occurs when a sufficient toxin load is produced from infection with these organisms.

### Clinical features

The commonest sites of infection are the umbilicus (in neonates), the nose, nasopharynx or throat, the conjunctiva and deep wounds.

The condition commences with a macular erythema, initially on the face and in the major flexures, and then becoming generalized. The skin is exquisitely tender and the child draws back from contact. After 2 days flaccid bullae develop and the skin wrinkles and shears off. The exfoliation is most marked in the groin, neck-fold (Fig. 21.1.14) and around the mouth, and may involve the entire body surface, but mucosae remain uninvolved.

The child is usually febrile but, because of the superficial level of the split, fluid loss is rarely significant. The erosions crust and dry and heal with desquamation over the next 4–8 days, leaving no sequelae.

Cultures from skin and blister fluid are usually negative. Cultures should be obtained from any area of obvious infection but, if none is apparent, from the nasopharynx and throat.

### Management

- Nurse the child naked on a non-stick material and handle as little as possible.
- Avoid topical agents in the early stages.
- Flucloxacillin is the treatment of choice and is usually given intravenously.
- Analgesia is often necessary in the early stages.
- Emollients are useful once the skin dries and desquamation commences.

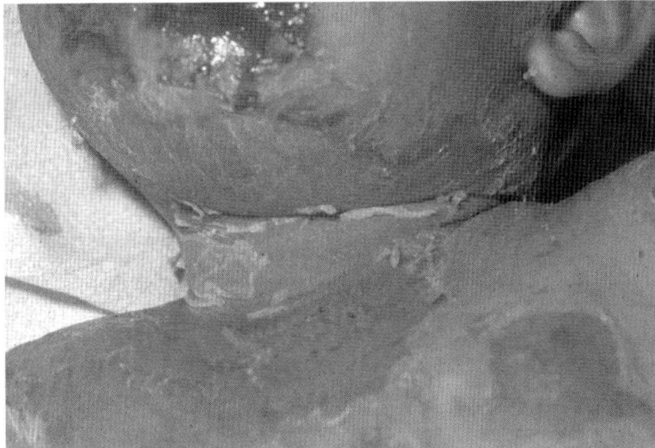

**Fig. 21.1.14** Staphylococcal scalded skin disease with extensive erythema and exfoliation.

## Boils (furuncles)

Boils are cutaneous abscesses, centred on hair follicles, caused by certain species of coagulase-positive *S. aureus*.

### Clinical features

- Local predisposing factors are cutaneous injury, friction and sweating.
- Episodes are often recurrent and many patients with recurrences are found to carry furuncle-producing strains of *S. aureus* in nostrils, axilla or groin, or to have had close contact with someone who does.

### Management

- Early lesions should be treated with warm compresses and oral flucloxacillin or cefalexin.
- For older lesions that have matured and pointed, incision and drainage may occasionally be indicated in conjunction with the use of antibiotics.
- Chronic and recurrent furunculosis should be treated with a course of antibiotics of several weeks' duration. While the patient is on antibiotics, all clothing, towels and bed-linen that have contacted the affected areas should be washed in hot water. Attempts should be made to deal with the carrier state in the patient and/or close contacts. Washing of the groin, axilla and hands with an antiseptic soap can help, as can topical nasal antibiotics such as mupirocin. An oral rifampicin and fusidic acid combination has also been successful in reducing carriage.

## Streptococcal perianal disease

This is a distinctive perianal eruption due to group A β-haemolytic streptococcus (GABHS):

- Peak incidence is in children aged 3–4 years, but it may occur in infants.
- The child complains of pain on defecation and often refuses to open the bowels.
- Bright blood is frequently seen on the stool. A bright pink erythema extends from the anal rim, which is often fissured and macerated, 2–3 cm out from the anus; the skin is tender but not indurated.
- Lymphangitis and lymphadenopathy are absent.
- There may be an associated GABHS balanitis or vulvovaginitis.
- Diagnosis is established by culture, on blood agar, of GABHS from a swab of the perianal skin.
- The treatment of choice is oral penicillin V 50 mg per kg per day in four divided doses, combined with the use of topical mupirocin twice daily. Recurrences are very frequent without this combined therapy, which should be continued for 10 days. Erythromycin is appropriate in penicillin-allergic patients.

## Tinea

This is an infection due to dermatophyte fungi; the source of the fungus is an animal (e.g. dog, cat, guinea-pig, cattle), the soil or another human. Tinea occurs on any part of the skin surface and can involve hair and nails.

### Clinical features and diagnosis

- Classical features of tinea on the general body skin are itchy, annular or geographical erythematous lesions studded with papules or pustules, with a tendency to central clearing and a superficial scale (Figs 21.1.15 & 21.1.16).
- Tinea is often unilateral and always asymmetrical, whereas eczema and psoriasis, which it may resemble, are often symmetrical in distribution.
- Between the toes, maceration with a thick white scale is the main finding, and an annular lesion may extend on to the dorsum of the foot.
- Nail tinea produces a white discoloration and crumbling of the nail plate with an accumulation of subungual debris.
- On the soles there are deep-seated blisters or pustules that dry to produce brown crusts.
- On the scalp there is a characteristic combination of alopecia and inflammation with the hair loss being due to breaking of the hair shafts. Depending on the pattern of hair invasion by the fungus, the hairs are either broken off flush with the scalp or at lengths of up to 2–3 mm, but in an individual case all the hairs break at the same length. The inflammation varies from mild erythema and a fine, dandruff-like scale to a pustular carbuncle-like lesion (kerion).
- A Wood's light (an ultraviolet lamp) is useful in the diagnosis of some varieties of scalp tinea, with the infected hairs fluorescing bright green. Other varieties of scalp tinea produce no typical fluorescence and the Wood's light has no place in the diagnosis of tinea on the skin surface.
- The diagnosis of tinea is confirmed by scraping hairs or scales on to a slide, adding 20% potassium hydroxide and examining the specimen microscopically. Septate branching hyphae are seen in skin scales, and spores are found in hair. The fungus can be cultured on appropriate media.

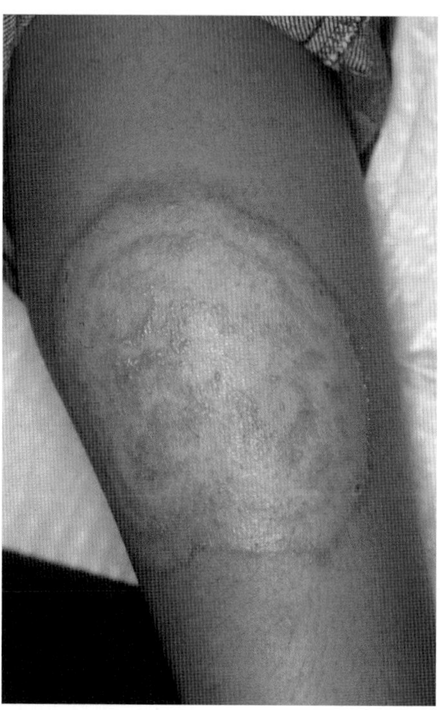

Fig. 21.1.15 Annular lesion of tinea.

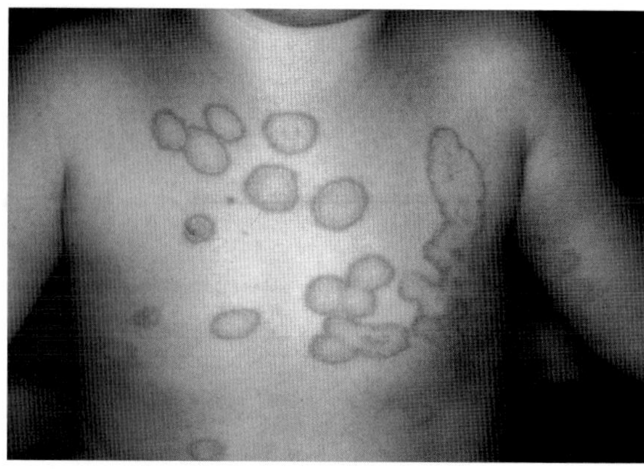

Fig. 21.1.16 Multiple annular lesions of tinea.

### Management

- Topical antifungals may be satisfactory for small, localized patches of tinea on the skin.
- Oral griseofulvin is the treatment of choice for longstanding or severe cutaneous tinea and hair tinea. This fat-soluble drug is best taken after meals, preferably with a glass of milk. For hair tinea, a 3-month course is optimal but shorter treatments of 4–8 weeks may be adequate for cutaneous tinea.
- Nail tinea is not responsive to topical treatment and is treated with oral terbinafine.

## Tinea versicolor

This is an infection with *Pityrosporum* species, which are part of the normal skin flora. It occurs mainly in tropical and temperate zones, and usually affects adolescents and young adults.

### Clinical features and diagnosis

- Presents as well-demarcated, asymptomatic or slightly itchy macules with a fine, branny scale that is often obvious only on light scratching of the lesions. Primary macules 1–10 mm in diameter coalesce into larger patches.
- Lesions occur in two colours – red–brown, especially in the fair-skinned, and hypopigmented in darker-skinned children (Fig. 21.1.17).
- The hypopigmented form must be differentiated from vitiligo, where the depigmentation is total and scale is absent, and pityriasis alba, where lesions are less well demarcated and some erythema may be seen.
- In young children it often presents with only facial lesions, and almost invariably a parent or older relative will have tinea versicolor in the typical distribution.
- Diagnosis is confirmed by microscopic examination of skin scrapings to which 20% potassium hydroxide has been added. Grape-like clusters of spores and short fragments of thick mycelia are seen.

### Management

- Untreated, the condition is persistent, although some improvement may occur in winter.
- The treatment of choice is with topical imidazole creams.
- With the depigmented form, therapy deals with the scale but sun exposure is required for full repigmentation.
- In widespread disease in adolescents, oral ketoconazole once weekly for 6 weeks is effective.

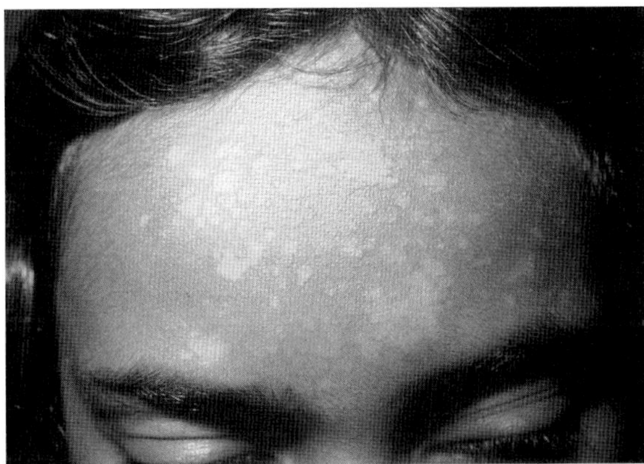

Fig. 21.1.17 Pale lesions of tinea versicolor in a dark-skinned child.

## Scabies

Scabies is due to *Sarcoptes scabei*, an eight-legged, oval-shaped mite less than 0.5 mm in length. The disease is transmitted by close physical contact, with transmission by fomites being exceptional. A small number of mites burrow into the skin in certain sites, particularly between the fingers, the ulnar border of the hand, around the wrists and elbows, the anterior axillary fold, nipples and penis and, in infants, the palms and soles.

### Clinical features and diagnosis

The pathognomonic primary lesion, a typical burrow, may not be seen with the naked eye, but is more easily identified with a dermatoscope. It is a 2–3-mm long, curved grey line with a vesicle at the deeper end.

Other lesions that mark the sites of burrows are small blisters or papules, larger blisters on the palms and soles of infants (Fig. 21.1.18), scratch marks, secondary eczema and secondary bacterial infection.

Eczema or impetigo in the target areas for scabies should always raise suspicion of this disease, as should blisters on the palms and soles of infants.

Often more prominent than the evidence of burrows is the so-called secondary eruption of scabies. This presents as multiple, very pruritic, urticarial papules, which are soon excoriated. They occur particularly on the abdomen, thighs and buttocks.

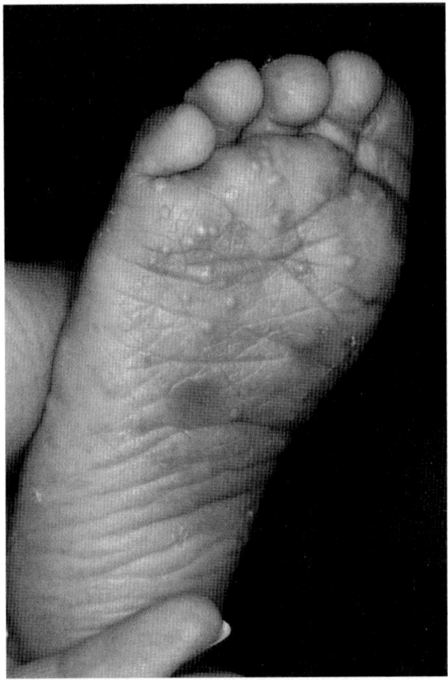

Fig. 21.1.18 Scabies in an infant with pustules on the sole of the foot.

Large inflammatory nodules may form part of the secondary eruption, occurring particularly on covered areas, especially on axillae, scrotum, penis and buttocks. They may, however, be very widespread, producing diagnostic difficulties. They may persist for months after effective scabies treatment.

The diagnosis of scabies is usually a clinical one but can be confirmed by demonstration of the mite. A burrow, which may be softened by the application of 20% potassium hydroxide, is scraped and the material is smeared on a slide for microscopic examination. Burrows may be more easily identified by rubbing a thick, black marking pen over suspicious areas and wiping with an alcohol swab, leaving a burrow outlined with ink.

### Management

- All close contacts should be treated simultaneously with the patient, whether or not they have symptoms.
- 5% permethrin cream is the treatment of choice and should be applied to all body surfaces from the neck down, and left on overnight on two consecutive nights. This treatment should be repeated a week later. The application duration should be reduced to 6 hours in extremely young infants.
- Bedclothes and clothing should be washed in the normal way with no disinfection required.
- An irritant dermatitis may follow scabies treatment, particularly in atopic children, and may require emollients and topical steroids once the miticide therapy is fully completed.
- Persistent nodules may respond to topical corticosteroids but painting with a coal tar solution is preferable for the very resistant ones.

## Pediculosis

Human lice are six-legged arthropods without wings, grey in colour or brown–red when engorged with blood. The body louse and the head louse have a thin body, 2–4 mm long and three similar pairs of legs; the pubic louse is wider and shorter, and the second and third pair of legs are larger than the first, producing a crab-like appearance. The ova (nits) appear as oval, grey–white, 0.5-mm specks, attached by a firm chitin ring to hairs or clothes.

### Pediculosis capitis (head lice)

This is a common infestation, often occurring in epidemics in schools. The occipital area of the scalp is involved preferentially and may be the only site affected. The condition is itchy, leading to scratching with excoriations and also eczematization and secondary infection, which may mask the underlying infestation. Permethrin shampoos are effective pediculicides but may not destroy ova, and a repeat application after a few days is recommended to kill further hatched lice. Removal of nit cases with a fine comb is easier if the chitin is softened by a prior application of vinegar.

### Pediculosis corporis (body lice)

This is rare in children except in severely overcrowded conditions with poor hygiene. The organism infests bedding and clothing, and the nits are not found on the human host. The lice hatch with body warmth and puncture the skin, producing very itchy, small, red papules with haemorrhagic puncta. Spots of dried blood may be found on the clothing and bedlinen. Treatment is directed towards removal of the organisms from materials with hot water laundering and hot ironing or the use of a hot electric dryer.

### Pediculosis pubis (pubic lice, crab lice)

This is mainly an adult disease. The pubic louse has as its normal habitat the anogenital area, but in children it is particularly seen on the eyelashes. Eyelash infestation in children may occur from innocent close contact with an affected adult. Pediculosis of the eyelashes is best treated with petroleum jelly applied thickly twice a day for a week.

## Arthropod bites

Patients with arthropod bites present to a dermatologist in two situations: the severe local allergic reaction and the more chronic hypersensitivity condition called 'papular urticaria'. The arthropods most encountered are mosquitoes, sandflies, fleas and grass mites. The distribution of the bites helps to suggest the causative agent.

### Severe local reactions

- Include blisters, purpura, and cellulitis and lymphangitis even in the absence of secondary infection.
- As the lesions are extremely itchy, scratching occurs, leading to secondary eczematization and secondary infection.

### Papular urticaria

- A very common condition in children, particularly between 10 months and 4 years.
- In a child who has been sensitized by previous exposure, the bite produces an itchy urticarial (hive-like)

weal, which is succeeded by a firm itchy papule that lasts for many days.

- The weal and papule usually show a central punctum and the papule may be surmounted by a tiny blister.
- The persistence and severity of the condition are explained by the fact that new bites by the same species will often cause a recrudescence of activity in resolving lesions.
- Secondary infection and eczematization from scratching also contribute to the chronicity of the condition, which may plague the child through an entire summer.

Management involves avoidance of insect attack, with the use of insect repellents, insecticides, protective clothing and changes in activities, which clearly are difficult in an active child. Wrapping the affected areas in wet dressings overnight as soon as new bites occur is helpful in reducing the itch and preventing scratching, which leads to the secondary eczema and infection. Topical corticosteroids will improve the secondary eczema and have some effect in dampening the severity of the actual bite reaction, but must not be used for prolonged periods. Oral antibiotics are required if there is significant secondary infection.

## Dermatitis

### Atopic dermatitis (atopic eczema)

Note: the terms dermatitis and eczema are often used synonymously.

Atopy is a genetically determined disorder with an increased tendency to form immunoglobulin (Ig) E antibody to inhalants and foods, and increased susceptibility to asthma, allergic rhinitis and atopic eczema. This eczema may begin at any age, but 75% of patients show the first signs by 6 months.

#### Clinical features

The characteristic clinical features are a generalized dryness and a tendency to lichenification or thickening of the skin, pruritus, and excoriations and patches of acute, subacute or chronic eczema. Involvement of the whole cutaneous surface may occur but the predominant areas are the face in infants, extensor aspects of the limbs as the child begins to crawl, and the limb flexures in older children (Fig. 21.1.19). In severe cases the whole skin may be erythematous, and in these patients white dermographism is often a prominent feature; this indicates that the condition is likely to be unstable and difficult.

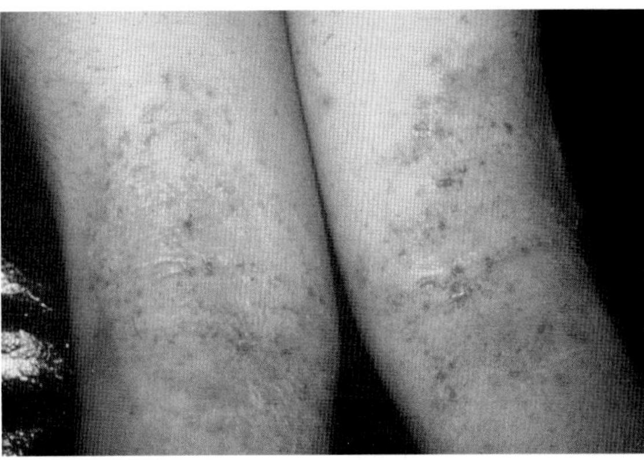

Fig. 21.1.19 Flexural lesions of atopic dermatitis.

#### Complications

Patients with atopic eczema may develop secondary bacterial infection that presents either as yellow crusting impetigo or folliculitis, or simply as worsening eczema. Mollusca are common and atopic patients are at risk of developing severe widespread herpes simplex infections. The usual childhood immunizations are quite safe. Severe eczema can lead to failure to thrive. Psychosocial and behavioural problems may occur in severe cases as a result of the continual discomfort, onerous treatment and restrictions on the child's life. The whole family suffers as a result.

#### Differential diagnosis

- Genetic ichthyoses of various types can lead to a very dry, scaly, and sometimes red skin. In many of these patients only the skin is abnormal but associated abnormalities in some types include cryptorchidism, neurological abnormalities, developmental delay, deafness and cataracts.
- Immunodeficiency syndromes of various types can be associated with dermatitis, and may resemble atopic dermatitis. The condition is usually refractory to treatment and there may be other features such as recalcitrant infections, diarrhoea or haematological abnormalities to suggest an alternative diagnosis.
- Phenylketonuria may present with an eczematous rash.
- Boys with hypohidrotic ectodermal dysplasia, an X-linked disorder, may be more prone to dry skin and eczema; associated abnormalities include deficient hair growth, dentition and sweating, and a tendency to develop respiratory tract infections.

#### Management

*Explanation and education*

The most important aspect of the management of atopic eczema is explanation of the condition to the patient or parents. The family should understand that the child has been born with an inherently dry, irritable skin and that this will be a lifelong tendency. Although the skin does become more stable with time, it will always require extra care. It is essential to talk in terms of control rather than cure, otherwise the family search for an endpoint after which care will no longer be required and this is an unrealistic expectation. The condition should be explained as a multifactorial disorder as it must be appreciated that, just as there is no 'cure', there is no single 'cause'.

*Avoidance of irritants*
Factors that will often irritate the atopic skin should be discussed. Woollen material in direct contact with the skin is a major irritant; apart from the child's own clothing it is important to remember the parent's clothing, carpets, blankets, stroller and car seat covers, furniture and toys. Shiny nylon materials and some acrylics irritate but cotton–polyester mixtures are usually well tolerated. Sand contact is often troublesome, especially with prolonged close contact as in playing in a sandpit. Chlorinated water may aggravate but this is variable. Soap in excess and bubble baths over-dry the skin, and many perfumed and 'medicated' products, disinfectants and strong cleansers cause irritation.

*Dealing with dryness*
Bath oils and oatmeal-containing products are useful and prevent the defatting of the skin that bathing can induce. It is essential to find a suitable moisturizer that can be applied all over twice a day, whether or not there is active eczema. Glycerine 10% in Sorbolene cream is useful in many cases, but more or less greasy preparations are available to suit individual patients and climatic conditions. Urea-containing products sting broken skin and are unsuitable.

*Topical corticosteroids*
These are an essential part of treatment. In general, ointment bases are preferred because they are more emollient than cream bases. Nothing stronger than 1% hydrocortisone should be used on the face or in the axillae or groin. Medium-strength fluorinated corticosteroids are usually adequate for lesions on the trunk and limbs; the stronger preparations are rarely required. These preparations are best used three times a day and ceased as soon as the eczema is clear.

*Wet dressings*
These are useful in severe widespread eczema. A water-based emollient is applied all over; a corticosteroid cream (rather than ointment in this case, because cream is more water-miscible) is applied to the areas of active eczema; sheeting soaked in tap water is applied and bandaged on with a crepe bandage, and a net material is used to hold the dressings in place. The procedure is repeated three times a day. These dressings cool the skin down, reduce itching, physically prevent scratching, increase the hydration of the skin and enhance the penetration of topical steroids. This treatment is usually effective in clearing the eczema in 3–4 days. If dressings are required for longer periods, the corticosteroid should be used only once a day. Particular care should be taken with infants.

*Systemic therapy*
If significant bacterial infection occurs, a swab should be taken and oral antibiotics used. Nocturnal sedation is often valuable during severe episodes but daytime sedation should be avoided; antihistamines are the preferred sedatives. Although they may be essential for associated diseases, oral corticosteroids should never be instituted for the eczema itself; a severe rebound can occur on their withdrawal and after several courses the eczema can become very unstable. Eczema that continues to be widespread and difficult to manage despite all these measures may require oral immunosuppression with azathioprine or ciclosporin, or narrow-band ultraviolet B therapy.

*Dietary manipulation*
No alteration should be made to the patient's diet unless the atopic eczema has failed to respond to conventional therapy properly carried out. There is only a small group of patients with unstable eczema with an associated urticarial element in whom dietary factors are of major significance; skin-prick tests are useful in this group to give a guide for dietary manipulation, which should be instituted only by those with a full understanding of the nutritional requirements of young children.

*Dust mite allergy*
This is important in a selected group of patients. In these children the eczema is usually particularly troublesome on the face and neck. The family should be given details of dust mite reduction strategies, which may be of limited value.

### Discoid eczema

- In children this is often a manifestation of a combined atopic and psoriatic diathesis.
- Well-defined patches of acute eczema occur in a strikingly symmetrical distribution. In infants the commonest sites are the upper back and the tops of the shoulders; in older patients the extensor aspects of the limbs are particularly involved. The lesions may be very thick and exudative and they are very itchy.

- Discoid eczema should be distinguished from tinea and impetigo, which are less symmetrical, and classical psoriasis, which is rarely moist.
- Management involves emollients and topical steroids as for atopic dermatitis, with the continued use of emollient helping to prevent recurrences.

### Pityriasis alba

This condition probably represents a very mild eczema, which, however, produces a striking post-inflammatory depigmentation. The condition is more common in atopics, and occasionally some areas will show erythema and more definite eczematous changes. It is rarely troublesome unless the child has darker skin, making the patches more visible.

- Appears as poorly defined, slightly scaly, hypopigmented patches occurring particularly on the face and the upper arms.
- The mild irritation and signs of mild eczema respond to emollients and weak topical corticosteroids, but the hypopigmentation may be very persistent and require sun exposure over a prolonged period before repigmentation is complete.
- The condition should be differentiated from vitiligo, where there is total depigmentation and no scale, and from tinea versicolor, which is rare on the face, has very well demarcated lesions and has a very fine branny scale.

### Allergic contact dermatitis

- The commonest causative agents in Australia are *Rhus* and a variety of grevilleas, including Robyn Gordon, Ned Kelly and Hookerana.
- The dermatitis is usually severe and blistering often occurs.
- It often occurs in a streaky pattern where the plant has brushed against the skin.
- Initially there may be much oedema, especially on the face (Fig. 21.1.20), and cellulitis is often suspected; however, the child is afebrile and the area is itchy rather than painful.
- The condition may be spread beyond areas of initial contact as a result of retention of allergen on clothing and under the nails.
- A strong topical steroid may be adequate for localized areas but a short course of oral steroids is usually indicated.

> **Clinical example**
>
> Harry, aged 4 years, presented with a swelling and redness around one eye. It was diagnosed by the ophthalmology registrar as preseptal orbital cellulitis, the child was admitted to hospital and intravenous antibiotics were started. It was remarked that a lack of fever and pain was unusual in a child with cellulitis. The next day the area was more swollen and some blistering had occurred. Harry was noted also to have multiple linear blistered red lesions on his arm. Harry's mother told the registrar that Harry's best friend from the preschool had similar lesions on the arms and face, which had been diagnosed by a dermatologist as a plant contact dermatitis. The history obtained was that the preschool garden had been landscaped by parents over the previous weekend and the two children carried Robyn Gordon grevilleas in the car for planting. Harry's antibiotics were ceased and he was discharged from hospital on a 5-day course of oral steroids. The swelling resolved in 2 days, and in 6 days all the rash had disappeared. The following weekend the Robyn Gordon grevilleas were removed from the preschool.

Other occasional causes of allergic contact dermatitis in children include iodine (e.g. wound care, antisepsis for operative field) (Fig. 21.1.21) , nickel (e.g. press-studs on clothing, belt buckles), and topical

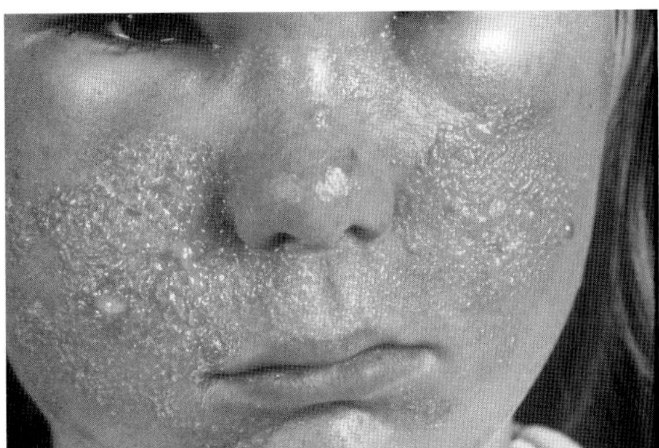

Fig. 21.1.20 Allergic contact dermatitis due to contact with grevillea.

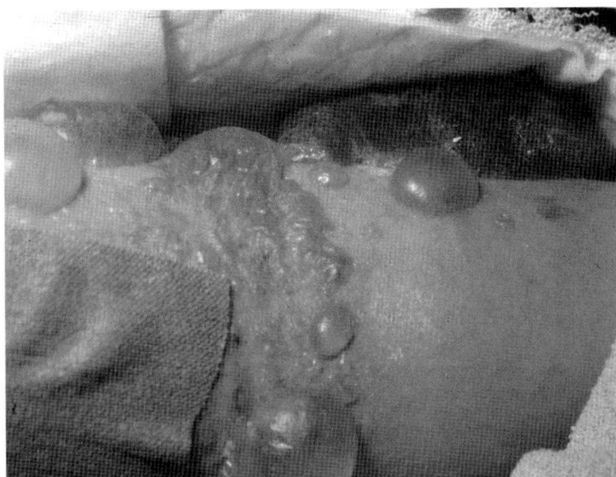

Fig. 21.1.21 Allergic contact dermatitis from iodine used for preoperative skin preparation.

medications (e.g. antihistamine cream), and lime juice (where sun exposure is also required; see photosensitivity, below).

## Napkin rashes

These various causes often occur in combination, and the management of most napkin rashes involves a weak topical steroid, an anti-monilial agent and frequent napkin changes.

### Common causes

- *Seborrhoeic dermatitis* – presents as a dull red rash covering most of the napkin area, sometimes with a greasy yellow scale, although this is characteristically absent in this moist area.
- *Monilia* – manifested as a thick, white material deep in the folds and as small annular lesions with an overhanging white macerated scale at their margin.
- *Irritant dermatitis from urine and faeces* – irritant dermatitis due to urine affects mainly the convex surfaces, with relative sparing of the flexures; irritation due to faeces particularly affects the natal cleft. Napkin dermatitis is rarely caused by irritant or allergic reactions to laundering products.
- *Miliaria* – sweat duct occlusion may occur alone or in combination with other elements. This presents as small red papules, which are very transient, so the pattern varies considerably from hour to hour.

### Variants of common types

- *Gluteal granulomas* – occur on top of a pre-existing napkin rash as purplish nodules that tend to be oval in shape, following the lines of the skin folds.
- *Erosive napkin rash* – occurs in the perianal and natal cleft area, and usually follows a period of diarrhoea. It is seen in infants with lactose intolerance or other causes of malabsorption (Fig. 21.1.22).
- *Ulcerated nodules* – occur most often in the vulval area in a situation of a constant urinary leak in the presence of major congenital anomalies.
- *'Frog plaster' napkin rash* – due to the accumulation of faeces and, to a lesser extent, of urine under the plaster used in cases of developmental dysplasia of the hip; usually of a mixed erosive and ulcerated nodule type.

### Other causes

- *Psoriasis* – produces a bright red, glazed, clearly marginated, napkin rash (Fig. 21.1.23). This may develop into the condition called 'napkin psoriasis'. A few small scaly spots occur on the trunk above the psoriatic napkin rash, followed by a sudden explosion of typical psoriatic lesions on scalp, face and all over the trunk. The infant is well and the condition is usually asymptomatic. The eruption is self-limiting in a few weeks.
- *Impetigo* – presents as small, pus-filled blisters that quickly rupture and expand into large superficial erosions, usually asymptomatic.
- *Herpes simplex* – punched-out 3–8-mm individual erosions that coalesce to form geographical-shaped lesions; considerable swelling is usually seen and there is associated lymphadenopathy and fever.
- *Staphylococcal scalded skin syndrome* – may present in the napkin area with a very painful bright red rash with superficial blistering.
- *Congenital syphilis* – perianal erosions and moist warty lesions may be seen in early infancy, with erythema on the palms and soles, fever, failure to thrive and hepatosplenomegaly.
- *Kawasaki disease* – often presents in the napkin area with a tender red scaly rash in a febrile, irritable child.
- *Langerhans cell histiocytosis* – produces a severe napkin rash with a brownish scale, erosions and purpuric spots, unresponsive to standard napkin

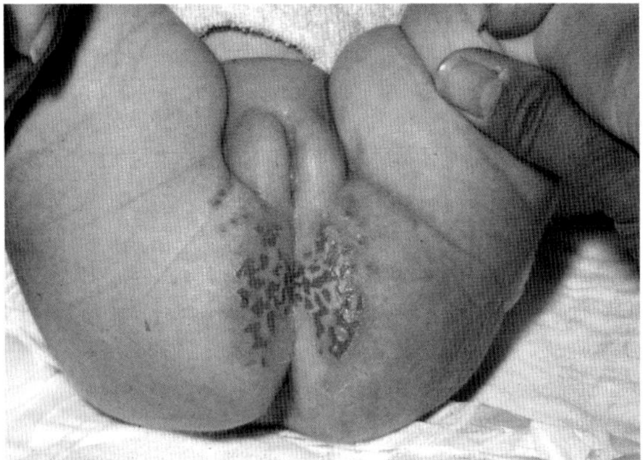

Fig. 21.1.22 Erosive napkin dermatitis.

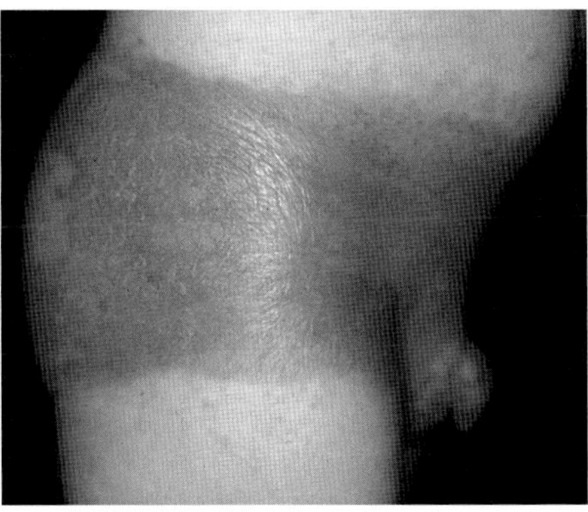

Fig. 21.1.23 Psoriasis in the napkin area with glazed erythema.

rash treatment. A scaly, papular eruption on the scalp or trunk may also appear. Fever, diarrhoea, polyuria and hepatosplenomegaly may be present.

- *Zinc deficiency* – produces a well-marginated shiny rash rather similar to psoriasis, but with a characteristic dark peripheral scale. Similar lesions are present around the mouth and nose. These patients are usually irritable and alopecia may be present.
- *Biotin and essential fatty acid deficiencies* – can cause a rash similar to that of zinc deficiency.
- *HIV infection* – can present as severe, erosive napkin dermatitis, which may be secondarily infected.

## Psoriasis

Psoriasis is an hereditary disease; it is probably an autosomal dominant condition with variable penetrance. It commences during childhood in 30% of patients. It may present in the typical adult form of large erythematous plaques, with a thick, silvery-white scale, predominantly on the knees, elbows, buttocks and scalp, but certain differences are seen in childhood disease:

- Plaques are usually smaller and with a finer scale (Fig. 21.1.24).
- A particularly common presentation is acute guttate psoriasis with the eruption of tiny papules in a widespread distribution. The eruption is often preceded by an intercurrent illness, particularly a streptococcal throat infection.
- The face and intertriginous sites are commonly affected in children.
- Children presenting with vulvitis, balanitis and perianal itching may be found to have psoriasis. In these areas the typical scale is absent and the condition presents as a glazed erythema, often with fissuring.
- Nail involvement is usually absent or minimal with minor pitting.

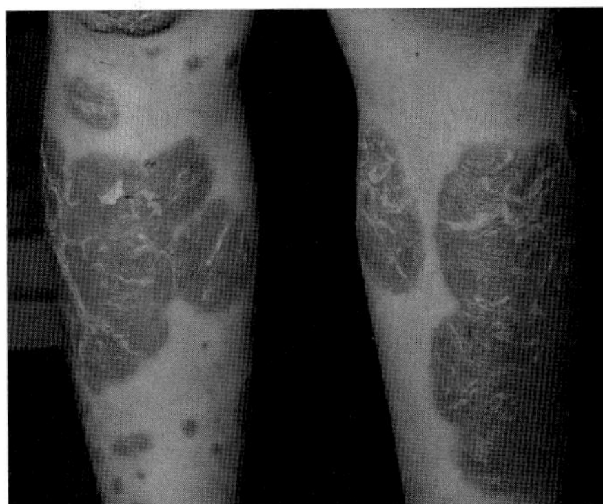

Fig. 21.1.24 Psoriatic plaques with fine scale.

- Pustular psoriasis and psoriatic arthropathy are extremely rare in children.
- There is a particular type of well-marginated, bright red napkin rash, described above, that is a marker for psoriasis.
- Many therapies used in adults are inappropriate in children. In general, psoriasis in children is better treated with tars than topical corticosteroids. No treatment can alter the course of the condition.

## Photosensitivity in children

Photosensitivity may be manifested by exaggerated sunburn, sometimes with blistering, or another rash appearing in a light-exposed area. There are many causes and some are briefly reviewed here.

- *Phytophotodermatitis* – contact with a phototoxic agent (e.g. lime juice, perfumes) followed by sun exposure causes an exaggerated sunburn reaction.
- *Drug reactions* – rare in children.
- *Polymorphous light reaction* – may produce recurring erythematous, itchy vesicles and papules mainly located on the cheeks, ears, upper anterior chest and exposed limbs. The onset of the eruption may be delayed for 1–2 days after sun exposure, but the distribution of the lesions and history of exacerbation in the summer are typical.
- *Solar urticaria* – a transient urticarial rash appearing immediately after sun exposure on exposed areas.
- *Connective tissue diseases*
  - Lupus erythematosus – the skin lesions of systemic lupus erythematosus (SLE) include a characteristic butterfly distribution over both cheeks and the base of the nose. Patchy lesions may also present over the light-exposed areas of ears, neck and limbs. In acute SLE, erythematous macules are also seen about the nail-beds, on the tips of the fingers, the toes, and on the palms of the hands and soles of the feet.
  - Dermatomyositis – an erythematous rash that is distributed over the extensor surfaces of the joints, particularly over the knuckles, elbows and knees, is characteristic of dermatomyositis. In addition, most children with this disorder show a violaceous facial rash and periorbital oedema. Worsening of the condition after sun exposure is typical and some patients show a more widespread scaly red rash in light-exposed areas.
- *Genetic photosensitive disorders* – most very rare, but commoner ones include:
  - Erythropoietic protoporphyria – pain in feet sometimes without much to see, sometimes associated with swelling, redness and blistering; later scarring. May lead to hepatic damage.

- Albinism – dilution or absence of pigmentation; poor vision, photophobia and nystagmus.

## Purpura

The differential diagnosis of purpura in children includes the following:

- *Trauma* – accidental or as part of child abuse; in the latter, bruises of different ages and at unusual sites may be seen.
- *Thrombocytopenia* – purpura in association with a low platelet count is often associated with bruising and signs of bleeding elsewhere. Idiopathic thrombocytopenic purpura is the most common cause (see Chapter 16.2). Children need to be examined and investigated for leukaemia, pancytopenia, splenomegaly, and drug-induced thrombocytopenia or aplastic anaemia (chloramphenicol, anti-thyroid medications).
- *Coagulation disorders* – such as haemophilia; there may be a history of joint pain or swelling, or bleeding from other sites.
- *Infections* – cause vascular damage
  - Purpuric viral exanthems especially due to enteroviruses (see above)
  - Bacterial infections: an unwell febrile child with purpura should be treated for meningococcal septicaemia without waiting for the results of investigations. Septicaemia from *Haemophilus influenzae*, streptococci, staphylococci and some Gram-negative organisms may also cause purpura. Less extensive, but diagnostically useful, are the purpuric lesions of subacute bacterial endocarditis, typhus and typhoid fever.
  - Rickettsial infections such as typhus and, in Australia, Ross River virus.
- *Vasculitis* – in children mainly Henoch–Schönlein purpura (see Chapters 16.2, 18.2). This is quite common in childhood. Purpuric lesions on the legs and buttocks may be the only finding in Henoch–Schönlein purpura, or there may be associated abdominal pain, arthritis or renal involvement. These patients must be followed for months for the development of nephritis.
- *Langerhans cell histiocytosis* – the various rashes that occur in this condition characteristically have a purpuric element.
- *Glucocorticoid excess* – causes skin fragility, which leads to easy bruising and bleeding.
- *Scurvy* – irritability, bone pain, gum sponginess and bleeding may also be present. Wrist X-rays are diagnostic.

## Blistering disorders

The differential diagnosis of blistering in children includes the following (most of these have been described elsewhere in this chapter). Other causes are covered in the neonatal section.

- *Infections*
  - HSV
  - Varicella and other viral exanthems
  - Bullous impetigo
  - Staphylococcal scalded skin syndrome
- *Trauma* – for example, burn; chemical or thermal (accidental or abusive)
- *Contact dermatitis* – for example, plants, iodine
- *Blistering with photosensitivity*
  - Phytophotodermatitis
  - SLE, dermatomyositis
  - Porphyrias
- *The erythema multiforme (EM), Stevens–Johnson syndrome (SJS), toxic epidermal necrolysis (TEN) spectrum* – hypersensitivity reactions
  - EM – target lesions, with peripheral erythema and central blistering and necrosis; occasional moderate mucosal involvement. Main cause is a recent herpes simplex infection.
  - SJS – severe mucosal blistering and erosions. Usually minor skin involvement. Main cause is a *Mycoplasma* infection.
  - TEN – severe widespread sheeting off of skin, severe mucosal involvement. Main cause is drugs.
- *Chronic bullous disease of childhood* – an immunological bullous disease with widespread blisters occurring in rosette patterns.

### Erythema nodosum

Erythema nodosum can occur at any age and presents initially as subcutaneous erythematous lesions, mainly on the anterior lower legs, that may progress to extensive bruise-like lesions. Erythema nodosum may be idiopathic or associated with chronic streptococcal disease, pulmonary or other tuberculosis, Crohn's disease, chronic gastrointestinal infections, sarcoidosis and *Mycoplasma* infection. It may also be secondary to a number of drugs.

## Hair loss in children

There are two major types of hair loss (alopecia): diffuse and patchy. The commonest cause of diffuse alopecia is telogen effluvium, and the main causes of patchy alopecia are tinea, alopecia areata and trichotillomania.

### Diffuse alopecia

- *Telogen effluvium* – high fever causes a large number of hairs to enter the resting or telogen stage of the hair cycle prematurely; 2–3 months later these are inevitably shed. The hairs have a club-shaped end, visible as a white dot with the naked eye. New hairs appear immediately in the empty follicles. The condition may continue for several months but is fully reversible.
- *Some other causes*:
  - drugs
  - malnutrition
  - iron deficiency
  - various aminoacidurias
  - hereditary hair shaft abnormality syndromes
  - congenital atrichia
  - alopecia as a part of other genetic syndromes.

### Patchy alopecia

- *Tinea* – combination of inflammation of varying degree and broken hairs.
- *Alopecia areata* – autoimmune disease with areas of total hair loss and no obvious inflammation; there may be some short, so-called 'exclamation mark', hairs at the edges.
- *Trichotillomania* – hair twisting or plucking; hairs broken at different lengths, usually no inflammation.
- *Some other causes*:
  - hair cutting as a form of artefactual skin disease
  - traction from tight hair styles
  - infections – boils, erysipelas, herpes simplex, herpes zoster, tick bites
  - localized scleroderma (morphoea).

## Excessive hair in children

Hypertrichosis is increased hair that is not in an androgen-dependent distribution. Hirsutism is excessive hair as a result of hyperandrogenism and occurs in a male-pattern distribution.

### Hypertrichosis

Generalized hypertrichosis (increased hair in all areas) may be an isolated finding or may be related to:

- inherited syndromes, including Hurler and De Lange syndromes
- medications, especially minoxidil, phenytoin and ciclosporin
- gastrointestinal disease, including coeliac disease
- hypothyroidism
- anorexia nervosa
- porphyria; look for photosensitivity and blisters.

### Hirsutism

Increased pubic or axillary hair in young children may be due to adrenal, gonadal or central nervous system disease, and requires investigation. Hirsutism in adolescent females may be an isolated finding or may be seen with obesity and amenorrhoea in polycystic ovary syndrome. Cushing syndrome, mild congenital adrenal hyperplasia, virilizing adrenal and ovarian tumours, and thyroid dysfunction may cause hirsutism.

## Acne and acneiform rashes

Some degree of acne is common on the face and upper trunk during puberty and may be the first sign of puberty. Acne, particularly if severe, can lead to significant depression in adolescents and is a risk factor for suicide. Both the depression and the acne need to be recognized and treated.

### Clinical features

Acne affects mainly the forehead and face, but can involve neck, shoulders and upper trunk. Early lesions include blackheads, whiteheads and papules. In more severe cases there may be pustules or inflammatory cysts that can lead to permanent scarring.

### Management

If acne begins before puberty, look for androgen excess, glucocorticoid excess or precocious puberty. If the morphology or distribution is atypical, consider drug-induced acne or tuberous sclerosus (in which facial angiofibromas may mimic acne).

Acne is treatable. No person with acne should just be told it is an inevitable part of adolescence. Effective acne therapies are now available and should be used to control the disease.

For mild disease, the treatment is topical benzoyl peroxide 2.5–5%, a topical keratolytic such as adapalene, and topical antibiotics, either erythromycin or clindamycin. These can be used singly or in combination. Improvement occurs over 1–2 months, not within days.

Treatment of moderate acne often involves the addition of oral antibiotic therapy (e.g. doxycycline) for 3–6 months. Oral hormone therapy can help female patients.

If antibiotics and topical treatment have not resulted in satisfactory clearing within 3–6 months, oral isotretinoin is indicated. Provided pregnancy is avoided, this is safe and highly effective. Isotretinoin is also indicated if there is scarring or cyst formation.

## Recurrent mouth ulcers

These are generally due to aphthous stomatitis. Such ulcers are usually small and resolve in a few days. Recurrent mouth ulcers can also be seen in:

- Iron, folate or vitamin $B_{12}$ deficiency.
- Gastrointestinal disorders – coeliac disease, Crohn's disease and ulcerative colitis are all associated with mouth ulceration. Recurrent abdominal pain, intermittent diarrhoea and failure to thrive may be present.
- Connective tissue disorders – patients with Behçet's disease usually present in late childhood with ulcers at one site (mouth or genitals) and it may be many years before a second site is involved. SLE and juvenile rheumatoid arthritis may cause recurrent mouth ulcers.
- Immunodeficiency states, human immunodeficiency virus (HIV) infection.
- Malignancy – lymphoma and histiocytosis can present with non-healing mouth ulcers.

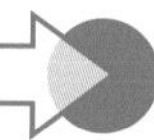

### Practical points

- Purpuric rashes require immediate assessment to exclude life-threatening conditions such as meningococcal disease.
- Apparent cellulitis that is itchy, occurs in a well, afebrile child and begins to blister on the second day suggests allergic contact dermatitis to a plant.
- A bright red, well marginated napkin rash suggests psoriasis.
- Widespread chronic eczema is usually associated with systemic complications including psychosocial and growth problems.
- Painful defaecation, bright blood on the stool and a bright red rash in the immediate perianal area point to streptococcal perianal infection.
- Herpes simplex lesions are grouped and coalesce forming geographical-shaped erosions with a scalloped edge.

PART 22

# ENT, EYE AND DENTAL DISORDERS

# 22.1 Ear, nose and throat disorders

Elizabeth Rose

Paediatric otolaryngologists see children with mucosal diseases of the upper aerodigestive tract (ears, nose, oral cavity, pharynx and larynx), airway obstruction, and pathologies of communication.

The common problems include:

- foreign bodies, in any of these areas
- otitis media, both acute and chronic
- hearing loss, both conductive and sensorineural, and congenital and acquired
- rhinosinusitis and its complications
- tonsillitis and suppuration in the neck
- obstructive sleep apnoea
- noisy and obstructed breathing, especially in infants.

## Growth and development

In infants the face is relatively small compared with the cranium, and elongation occurs with mandibular and maxillary growth as the permanent teeth erupt, from about 6 years of age. This coincides with development of the eustachian tube, as it becomes more vertical and functions more efficiently. During this time there is also growth and maturation of the immune system, with enlargement of the tonsils and adenoids; these increase in size until the age of about 7 years, and then start to involute (Fig. 22.1.1).

Infants are obligate nose-breathers until approximately 5 months, when they are able to mouth-breathe. The nose is small with considerable airway resistance and this explains why infants have difficulty breathing and feeding with a cold.

If there is obstruction at the back of the nose with choanal atresia, intervention is needed in the newborn period, especially if the obstruction is bilateral.

The paranasal sinuses also develop with facial growth. The ethmoid and maxillary sinuses are present at birth; the sphenoid sinus is aerated at 5 years and the frontal sinus at 10 years of age. This has important implications for the complications of acute sinusitis: ethmoid sinusitis can develop intraorbital complications from infancy, but intracranial extension from frontal and sphenoid sinusitis is rare under the age of 10 years.

The temporal bone contains the outer, middle and inner ears. The inner ear is adult size at birth. In the newborn the tympanic membrane (TM) is more horizontal and so difficult to see, and it becomes vertical with growth. At birth there is only one mastoid air cell (the antrum), but there is rapid pneumatization after this.

The paediatric larynx is higher in young children than in adults, and the epiglottis may be seen on tongue protrusion. The larynx is cone-shaped, so the subglottis is the narrowest part and therefore prone to damage and stenosis in prolonged intubation. The laryngeal cartilages are soft and tend to collapse in.

The larynx grows rapidly until the age of 3 years, and then slows before another rapid growth at puberty; the vocal cords lengthen and the angle of the cartilages change, and this accounts for the voice changes that occur.

## Trauma and foreign bodies

Young children can place, inhale or ingest a variety of foreign bodies into each orifice. Small batteries become moist and erode mucosa and cartilage, so need to be removed urgently.

### The ear

A foreign body may be wedged in the canal; if this is vegetable matter, it can expand and cause pain. If not removed easily with a head-light and wax curette, it is best to remove under anaesthesia or sedation to avoid further trauma, especially to the TM.

Trauma from a long or sharp foreign body can perforate a TM, and perforation may also result from a direct hit on the ear. If kept dry, these usually heal spontaneously.

Bleeding from the ear occurs with skull-base fractures, and may contain cerebrospinal fluid (CSF). These should be allowed to heal with minimal intervention, to avoid contaminating the CSF. The child should be examined for nystagmus, hearing loss and facial nerve injury.

An audiogram is performed to identify ossicular and inner ear damage in all cases of trauma and perforation.

### The nose

A foreign body in the nose may present as unilateral rhinorrhoea with an offensive odour; this resolves once the foreign body is removed. This may be accomplished

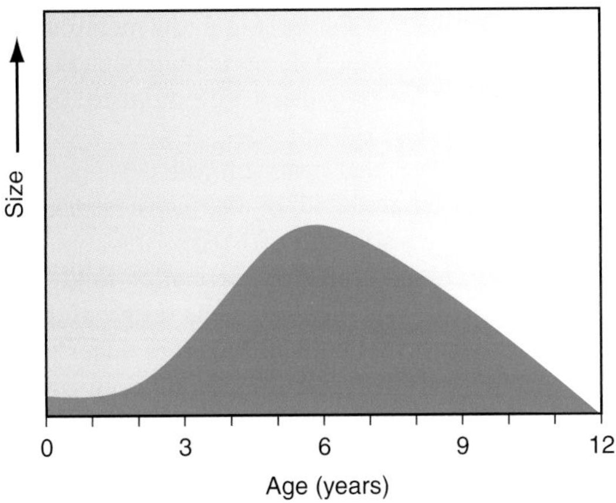


Fig. 22.1.1 Adenoidal size in relation to age. Redrawn with permission from Dhillon RS, East CA, 2006 Ear, Nose and Throat and Head and Neck Surgery: An Illustrated Colour Text, 3e. With permission from Elsevier.

with the child sitting upright and supported against a parent's chest. The nose is sprayed with anaesthetic/decongestant and the foreign body is removed by placing a wax curette behind it and pulling it forwards.

Trauma to the nose is common from falling on to a table or step, or sports injury. There is often swelling and bruising initially, and an assessment for deformity may be needed after this has settled. An assessment of the airway and possible septal haematoma should be performed immediately, as it quickly becomes an abscess and pressure on the cartilage causes necrosis and saddle-nose deformity.

### Pharynx and oesophagus

A child with a pharyngeal foreign body such as a fish bone may present with drooling and can point to the site; a bone is often lodged in the tonsil and can be readily seen and removed.

If a foreign body is further down or in the oesophagus the child will have dysphagia and regurgitation of saliva, and will need general anaesthesia for removal.

Trauma from running with a stick, pencil or other toy in the mouth is common. If it involves the soft palate, flexible nasopharyngeal examination is performed to ensure there is no injury in the retropharynx, as there is the possibility of air and infection tracking down to the mediastinum. Small punctures of the soft palate will heal well, but if there is a large flap, or the injury is on the free edge of the soft palate, it is sutured under general anaesthesia.

### Larynx and bronchi

A child with an inhaled foreign body in the airway may present in the immediate period with choking, gasping and cyanosis, or may have problems later with wheeze, cough and persistent or recurrent pneumonia. A chest X-ray may show ipsilateral hyperinflation from entrapment of air behind the foreign body, but there is a low threshold for performing bronchoscopy if there is a history of choking and no radiological signs. The bronchoscopy is performed under general anaesthesia using a rigid, ventilating bronchoscope and telescopic forceps.

## The ear

### Congenital abnormalities

Differences in the shape and size of the pinna are common. Corrective surgery is performed after the age of 5 years, when the pinna is near adult size.

There is an association of pinna deformity and middle ear abnormalities; the hearing is tested and appropriate intervention with hearing aids may be needed. Often the loss is conductive and the child can be fitted with a bone-conduction hearing aid.

Major deformities of microtia (small ear) and anotia (absent ear) are managed in interdisciplinary clinics with plastic surgeons to determine timing for surgery, both to correct deformities and to improve hearing, by either a tympanoplasty or bone-anchored hearing aid.

### Otitis media

Otitis media is inflammation or infection of the mucoperiosteal lining of the middle ear, and includes the mastoid ear cells and the eustachian tube (ET). There is a spectrum of disease from mild and reversible to chronic and destructive.

- A child with acute otitis media (AOM) usually presents following a cold with severe pain and fever, and may have otorrhoea. Infants and young children may not localize well and present with fever, irritability and sometimes vomiting.
- Otitis media is common in the first year of life, and 75% of children have had at least one episode by the age of 3 years. Recurrent otitis media is defined as at least three episodes in 6 months or four in 12 months. It is most common in autumn and winter as viral infections cause obstruction of the nose and ET.
- The three common causative organisms are *Streptococcus pneumoniae*, *Haemophilus influenzae* (non-typeable) and *Moraxella catarrhalis*.
- The complications of AOM include TM perforation, facial paralysis, mastoiditis, intracranial spread including meningitis and abscess formation, and sigmoid sinus thrombosis.
- A child with mastoiditis has often had symptoms for days before the ear starts to protrude, with erythema and swelling over the mastoid process. The treatment is surgical drainage and antibiotic therapy.

- With unresolved inflammation and eustachian tube obstruction there may be damage and retraction of the TM, with erosion of the ossicles. Retraction pockets form and accumulate keratinizing stratified squamous epithelium, known as a cholesteatoma. This causes bone erosion and usually presents with intermittent otorrhoea with hearing loss. Cholesteatoma may also be congenital and present as a white mass ('pearl') behind an intact TM. This may be an incidental finding.

There are some recognized risk factors for otitis media:

- Race – Australian aboriginal children and some Native Americans (Inuit, Apache and Navajo). There are differences in the eustachian tube and immunological response, but socioeconomic factors are also important.
- Craniofacial abnormalities – including cleft palate and Down syndrome.
- Genetic – both anatomical and immunological.

There are recognized environmental factors, and families can help control these:

- Reduce contact with people with upper respiratory infections, especially large-group childcare centres.
- Avoid tobacco smoke both during and after pregnancy.
- Breastfeed for at least 6 months, preferably 12 months. If bottle-fed, prop the baby up as milk can reflux into the ear if lying flat, causing inflammation.
- Avoid pacifiers/dummies; this is possible from inadvertent sharing in childcare centres.
- Vaccination with the polyvalent pneumococcal vaccine reduces the incidence of AOM by 8%.

**Clinical example**

Maisie is 15 months old; she has a fever and is crying. She has purulent rhinorrhoea, a bulging left ear drum and fluid in the right ear. Her management includes pain relief and, as she is less than 2 years old, an antibiotic – usually amoxicillin. If not clinically improved in 2 days she should be reviewed to determine whether the acute infection has resolved; if not, she should be changed to a β-lactamase-stable antibiotic such as amoxicillin–clavulanate. After this acute infection Maisie might have fluid in her middle ears for some weeks, without having infection.

## Chronic otitis media with effusion (COME)

This is commonly known as 'glue ear'. 'Chronic' implies duration of at least 3 months. There is persistent fluid in the middle ear, usually after AOM, which is asymptomatic apart from hearing loss. The term middle ear effusion (MEE) designates fluid in the ear, without reference to the aetiology or duration.

- COME can be present for 3 months and still resolve spontaneously.
- Biofilms (blankets of bacteria in a low metabolic state and enclosed by a polymeric matrix) may contribute, and the organisms are similar to those that cause AOM.
- There is no evidence that treatment with decongestants, antihistamines, nasal steroids or alternative medications will improve the resolution of MEE.
- The hearing changes in COME are often mild (10–15 dB worse) but there is a wide range, and the criteria for what is a significant loss are uncertain.
- Long-term studies indicate that for children with normal development there are no sequelae for language development from COME.

**Clinical example**

Thien Phuoc is 4 years old and this winter he has had a lot of colds and two episodes of AOM. He often ignores his mother or asks her to repeat what she has said, but she says he speaks clearly in Vietnamese. On examination, he has fluid in both ears. As there is concern about his hearing Thien Phuoc should have an audiogram, but if it is near the end of winter this can be delayed until summer as his mother is not concerned about his speech, and the fluid may resolve spontaneously. If he has persistent middle ear effusions in summer with a conductive hearing loss, then discussions about whether to insert tubes should start. It may be difficult for health workers to determine whether there is a speech delay in a child who does not speak English.

## Diagnosis and management of otitis media

- The diagnosis is often difficult to make as the child may be uncooperative, the ear canals are small, and wax may block the view. In infants it may not be possible to make an accurate diagnosis owing to the slope of the TM.
- The difference between AOM and COME is based on clinical grounds of irritability, fever and pain in acute infection, compared with no symptoms apart from hearing loss if there is chronic fluid.
- In AOM the TM is bulging with loss of the prominence of the handle of the malleus.
- In COME the TM is drawn in and the handle of the malleus is much more prominent.
- The use of pneumatic otoscopy to evaluate mobility of the TM is very useful in determining the presence of middle ear fluid (Fig. 22.1.2).
- All children with pain should be given adequate analgesia.
- Many older children with AOM will not need antibiotic therapy and their pain will be better within 2 days with symptomatic therapy.
- There are groups of children who should be considered for antibiotic treatment:

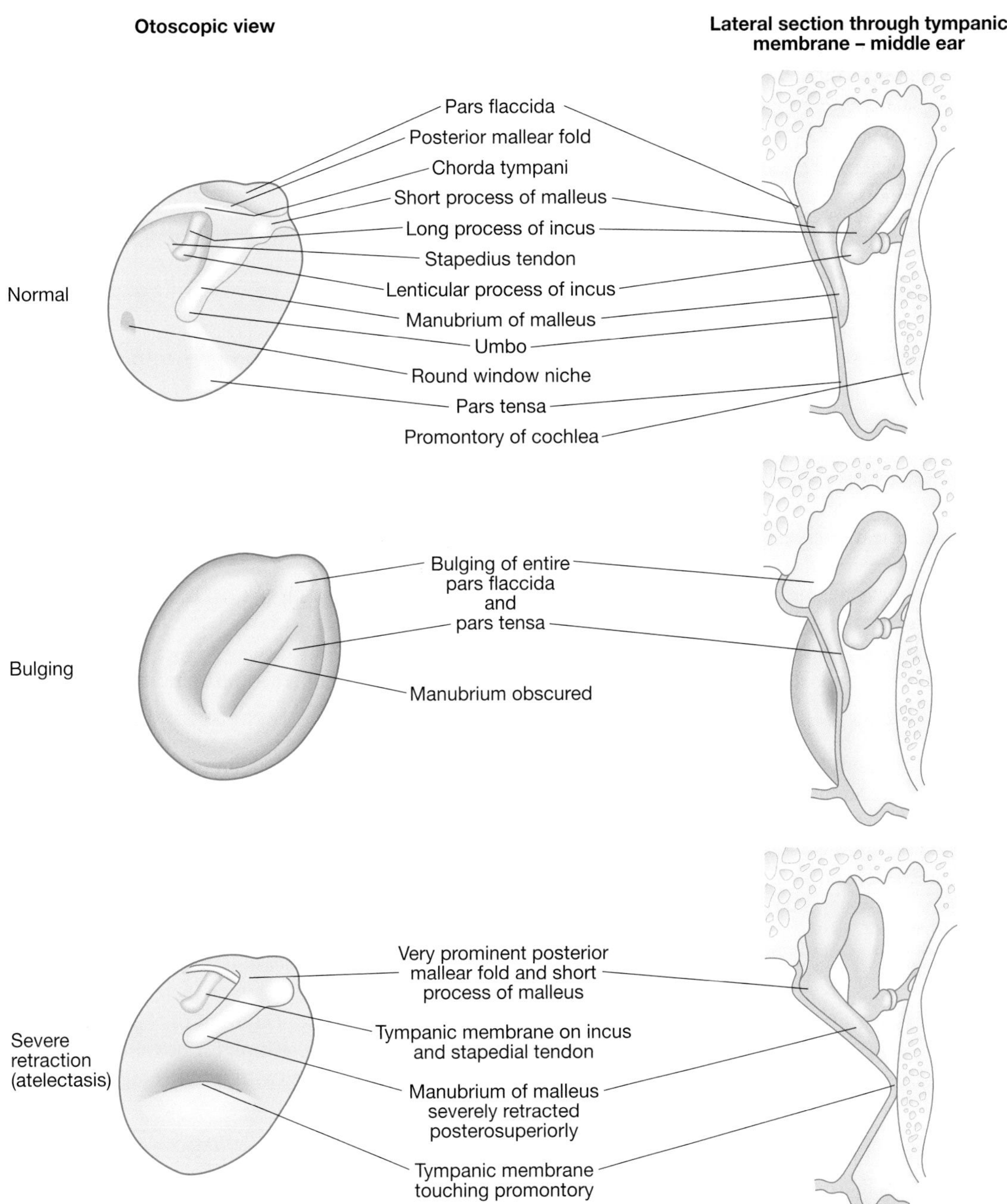


Fig. 22.1.2 Otoscopic view. (Redrawn with permission from Bluestone CD, Stool SE, Alper CM et al (eds) 2003 Pediatric otolaryngology, 4th edn. WB Saunders, Philadelphia, Ch. 10. © Elsevier.) In the normal ear anatomical features such as the manubrium (handle) of the malleus and sometimes the long process of the incus are readily seen. In AOM the TM bulges out with loss of the prominence of the handle of the malleus. With severe retraction of the TM the manubrium is very prominent and is more horizontal. The TM may drape onto the incus and stapes.

- children aged 2 years and under as they are more likely to develop suppurative complications and are not able to describe their symptoms
- severe disease with possible complications, including perforation
- children with known immunosuppression
- Indigenous children
- children with cochlear implants.

- The standard antibiotic therapy for AOM is oral amoxicillin for 5 days. Cefuroxime is an alternative if there is a penicillin allergy.

- If there is no improvement in pain within 2 days the child should be reviewed, and if the infection is not resolving consider changing to a β-lactamase-stable antibiotic such as amoxicillin–clavulanate.
- Otorrhoea in children with chronic TM perforations or who have ventilation tubes in place can often be managed with local therapy. The mucus and pus is mopped out with tissue spears and topical quinolone antibiotic drops are instilled, as they are not ototoxic.
- For children with recurrent AOM, antibiotic prophylaxis gives some benefit, but there may be gastrointestinal side-effects as well as a risk of accelerated bacterial resistance, especially in the childcare setting.
- In children with COME who do not have other problems, start with observation, and request a hearing test if there is no improvement after 3 months. Surgical intervention with middle-ear ventilation tubes should be considered if there is:
  - known language delay
  - learning/intellectual problems
  - significant hearing loss
  - visual impairment in addition to hearing loss from COME
  - damage to the TM with retraction pockets, to prevent permanent ossicular erosion.
- Children with a conductive hearing loss who are not able to have surgery may be referred to Australian Hearing for assessment for a bone-conduction hearing aid.

## Hearing loss

Newborn hearing screening is now universal in Australia, and the aim is to have completed the hearing evaluation by 3 months of age and to have hearing aids fitted by 6 months, to maximize speech and language acquisition.

There are many agencies offering early intervention, and integrated kindergartens and schools for hearing-impaired children. Families are given a folder and information outlining the choices available to them.

### Aetiology

It is not always possible to determine the cause, but the possibilities include: genetic and acquired factors.

*Genetic*

These may be syndromic:

- Autosomal dominant, e.g. Waardenburg syndrome with pigment alterations in the hair and eyes.
- Autosomal recessive, e.g. Usher syndrome (with retinitis pigmentosa), Pendred syndrome (with goitre), Jervell and Lange-Nielsen syndrome (with arrhythmias).

A genetic cause may also be non-syndromic, the most common being abnormalities of the connexin proteins.

*Acquired*

- Prenatal, e.g. intrauterine cytomegalovirus (CMV) infection.
- Perinatal, e.g. hypoxia, prematurity, high bilirubin (kernicterus).
- Postnatal, e.g. meningitis, head injury.

### Management

- Referral to Australian Hearing for hearing aids and early intervention.
- If the hearing loss is greater than 45 dB in the better ear, apply for the Carer Allowance payment from Centrelink.

The investigations performed depend on the wishes of the parents. Some are not ready for genetic testing and counselling at the time of diagnosis, but request referral at a later time.

- Electrocardiography (ECG) to check for prolonged QT interval, seen in Jervell and Lange-Nielson syndrome.
- Imaging of the inner ear at some stage. If the child has profound or total hearing loss, imaging is performed to determine whether there are inner ears and nerves; both computed tomography (CT) and magnetic resonance imaging (MRI) are needed for cochlear implant surgery.
  - If there is mild or moderate loss, the imaging is performed when the child is about 5 years old and able to lie still, unless there is deterioration before this.
  - The main abnormality looked for is widening of the vestibular aqueducts, as this is associated with progressive hearing loss if there is head injury.
- Ophthalmology consultation to check for vision problems but also to look for possible causes such as Usher syndrome (with retinitis pigmentosa).

**Clinical example**

Halil is a 6-month-old baby who was born at 27 weeks' gestation; he had a prolonged stay in the neonatal intensive care unit with ventilation for lung disease, and sepsis requiring intravenous antibiotics. His parents are non-consanguineous and there is no known family history of hearing loss. He was referred from the infant hearing screening programme and objective audiology confirmed that he has severe sensorineural hearing loss in both ears. It is probable that the hearing loss is related to the perinatal problems of prematurity, hypoxia and sepsis. Halil should be referred for hearing aids, and it is likely that he will have sufficient hearing with these to develop speech and language. He should also be referred to ophthalmology to check his eyesight, and to the genetics clinic when his parents are ready.

- There may be a progressive hearing loss, with normal hearing at birth. If parents or teachers are concerned about the hearing, or there is a delay in speech and language, the child should be referred for an audiogram.

## The nose

### Respiratory infection

During the course of an acute respiratory infection there is nasal obstruction/congestion and rhinorrhoea, which starts as thin, becomes mucoid, then purulent, then mucoid again and returns to thin secretions.

Colds last for 10 days, and most preschool children have about 10 colds per year.

Inflammation of the nose (rhinitis) and the sinuses (sinusitis) usually coexist and are difficult to differentiate clinically, so the term used is rhinosinusitis.

- Acute rhinosinusitis (ARS) lasts for between 10 days and 4 weeks.
- Chronic rhinosinusitis (CRS) lasts for more than 12 weeks.
- CRS is common, and the predisposing factors are:
  - exposure to viruses, especially in the childcare setting
  - mucociliary dysfunction and immunoglobulin deficiencies, although there are usually other infections as well
  - allergic rhinitis, including inhaled and ingested allergens.
- Tumours in the nose, such as rhabdomyosarcoma, may also present with chronic rhinorrhoea.

#### Management

- In ARS, symptomatic therapy is all that is required. Nasal saline drops and sprays are effective for eliminating oedema and secretions, and for children older than 3 years topical nasal steroid sprays are safe and effective for reducing rhinorrhoea.
- Cultures from the nose do not correlate well with pathogens within the sinuses, so are not recommended.
- Plain X-rays of the sinuses are usually not useful.
- CT of the sinuses may be requested if there is a poor response to therapy, or if suppurative complications are suspected. This should be with contrast to demonstrate abscess formation in the orbit, extradural space or brain.
- Antibiotics are considered if:
  - the illness is severe
  - suppurative complications are suspected
  - there is also bronchitis or otitis media
  - there are prolonged symptoms.
- In CRS, topical saline sprays or lavage and nose-blowing is usually all that is needed, but in severe cases consider investigations for allergies, immune deficiencies and adenoid hypertrophy.
- Sinus surgery is rarely indicated except for management of suppurative complications; however, in CRS adenoidectomy may be effective, especially if there is associated nasal obstruction and chronic snoring.

See Figures 22.1.3 and 22.1.4.

### Epistaxis

This is common and often results from a combination of infection and trauma (nose-picking). It is more likely if there is a haematological disorder with low platelets or a bleeding diathesis.

Most bleeding comes from the anterior septum, and in the short term can be controlled by pressure on the nasal septum for 10 minutes.

If there is crusting, the main treatment is application of an antibiotic ointment and avoidance of trauma.

If there is recurrent bleeding, this is managed with application of silver nitrate using topical local anaesthesia, although in younger children a general anaesthetic may be needed.

Nasopharyngeal angiofibroma is a rare tumour that occurs in adolescent males and presents with severe epistaxis and nasal obstruction; the diagnosis is made by nasendoscopy, or by CT with contrast.

## The oropharynx

### Acute sore throat

This is a common problem and may be caused by:

- viruses including rhinovirus, influenza and parainfluenza, and Epstein–Barr virus
- bacteria, especially *Streptococcus pyogenes*
- fungi, including *Candida albicans*, especially if immunosuppressed.

Tonsillitis is a clinical diagnosis based on:

- the child presents with sore throat, fever and dysphagia
- inflammation is confined to the tonsils and there may be exudate on them
- enlarged tender cervical lymphadenopathy
- the absence of coryza and cough, which would indicate a viral upper respiratory illness.

The throat should also be examined for possible suppurative complications:

- peritonsillar (quinsy) abscess
  - associated trismus (difficulty opening the mouth)
  - displacement of the tonsil medially

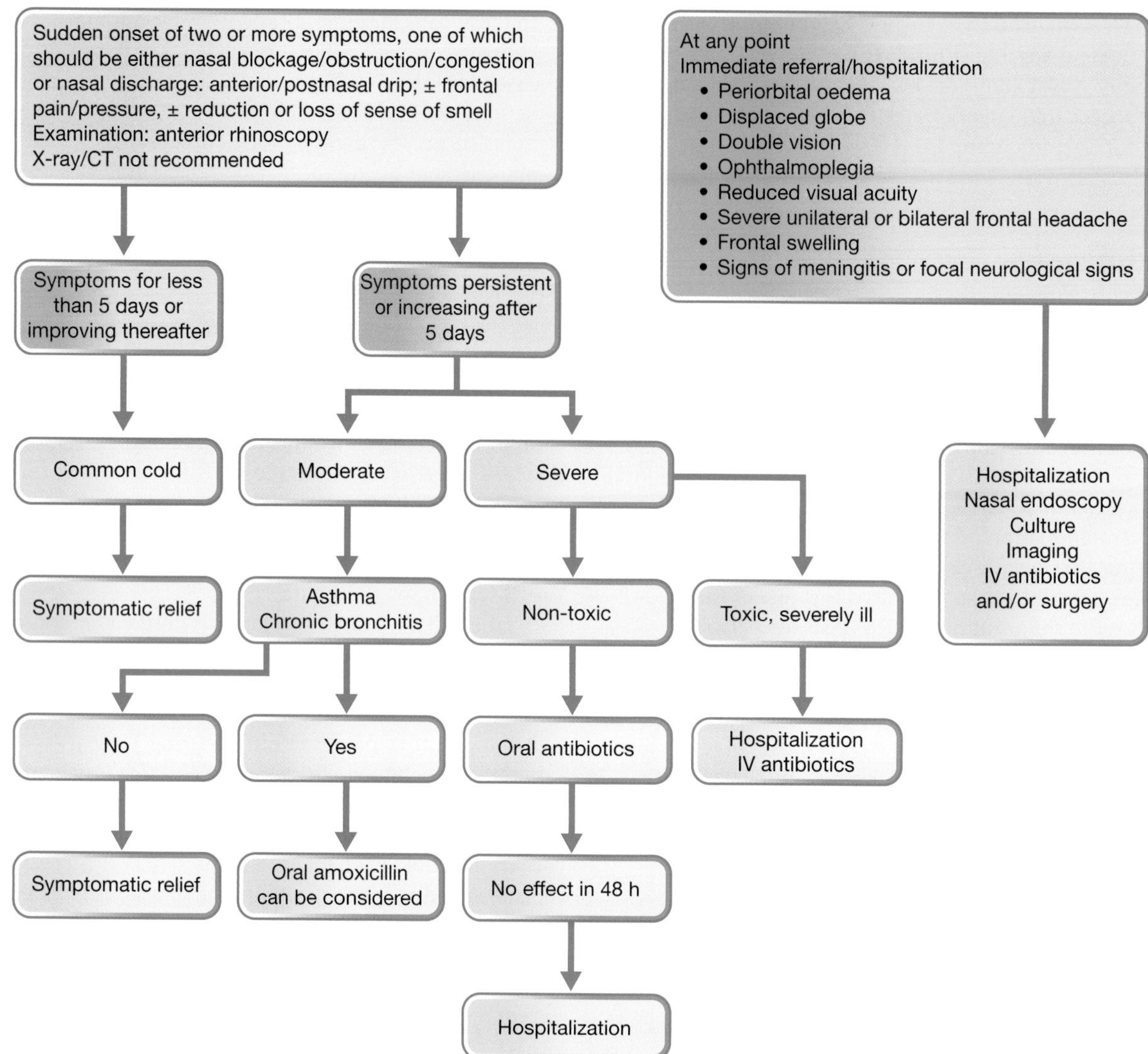


Fig. 22.1.3 Evidence-based scheme for children with acute rhinosinusitis. CT, computed tomography; IV, intravenous. (Reproduced with permission from Fokkens W, Lund V, Mullol J 2007 Rhinol Suppl 20:103.)

- parapharyngeal abscess, often with swelling in the pharynx and neck
- retropharyngeal abscess
- suppurative lymph nodes in the neck.

Throat cultures are usually not needed and may be inaccurate, as it is possible to be a carrier of *Streptococcus pyogenes* and not have infection.

Antibiotic therapy is usually not necessary unless:

- there is a suspected suppurative complication
- the child is immunosuppressed
- the child is Indigenous or a Pacific Islander, as these children are more likely to develop rheumatic fever
- at present, strains of *Streptococcus pyogenes* that cause rheumatic fever are rare, but the recommendation to avoid antibiotic therapy may change in the future.

When indicated, the recommended antibiotic therapy is penicillin V for 10 days.

Suppurative complications in the pharynx usually require:

- evaluation with CT or MRI
- intravenous antibiotics
- surgical drainage as there is a risk of:
  - spontaneous rupture and aspiration into the lungs
  - spread into the mediastinum
  - thrombosis or erosion of major vessels in the neck.

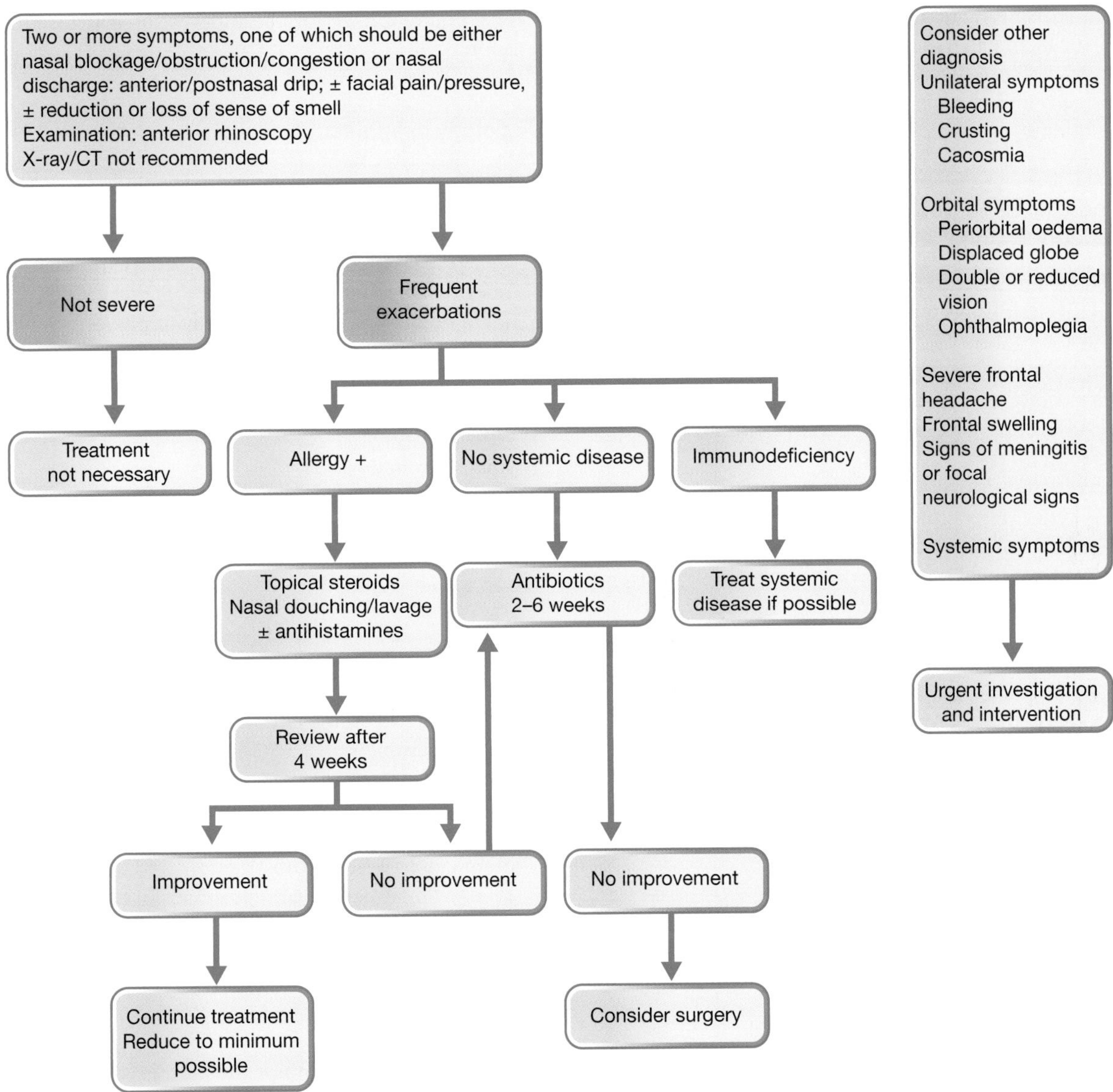


Fig. 22.1.4 Evidence-based scheme for children with chronic rhinosinusitis. CT, computed tomography. (Redrawn with permission from Fokkens W, Lund V, Mullol J 2007 Rhinol Suppl 20:104.)

### Clinical example

Vasuki is 10 years old and in grade 4 at school. She has had recurrent tonsillitis every 6–8 weeks since she was in kindergarten. With each illness she has a sore throat with exudate on the tonsils and cervical lymphadenopathy, and misses 3–4 days from school. It is not likely that Vasuki will improve as she has had recurrent tonsillitis for 6 years, and she misses several days from school each time. She would probably benefit from tonsillectomy.

## Obstructive sleep apnoea

This is airway obstruction resulting in temporary apnoea while sleeping with pauses greater than 6 seconds, respiratory effort, restless sleep and awakenings.

The child is often hard to wake in the mornings and has daytime somnolence. There may be poor school performance, or a younger child may be thought to have a developmental delay. In severe cases there is failure to thrive and even cor pulmonale.

Predisposing features are:
- tonsil and adenoid hypertrophy
- craniofacial disorders
- neurological impairment/hypotonia
- obesity.

### Indications for tonsillectomy and adenoidectomy

There are several reasons why a child might benefit from tonsillectomy and adenoidectomy. Caution must be taken when removing adenoids to examine for structural or functional problems with the palate, as removal of the adenoids may cause velopharyngeal insufficiency with nasal escape of air and indistinct speech.
- recurrent tonsillitis – at least seven episodes in 1 year. Many children starting in kindergarten and school have a year of tonsillitis and the next year will be improved, so observation over 2 years or more is warranted. A good guide is the severity of each episode and whether the child has missed more than 2 weeks from school in a year.
- obstructive sleep apnoea
- recurrent quinsy
- biopsy for possible malignancy, especially lymphoma.

*Indications for adenoidectomy only*
- Chronic mouth breathing and discomfort
- Chronic rhinorrhoea and recurrent sinusitis
- Chronic otitis media with effusion.

## Noisy and obstructed breathing

- Stridor is noisy breathing from narrowing of the airway at or below the larynx.
- A child may also have noisy or obstructed breathing from problems in the:
  - pharynx (especially tonsils and adenoids)
  - chest (e.g. diaphragmatic hernia)
  - abdomen (e.g. a large abdominal mass).
- Inspiratory stridor is usually from extrathoracic pathology.
- Expiratory stridor is from intrathoracic pathology.

Features of upper *airway obstruction* include:
- stridor
- tachypnoea, tachycardia, chest retraction
- cyanosis.

There may also be:
- a weak cry
- recurrent aspiration
- recurrent or prolonged croup.

See Figure 22.1.5 for the differential diagnosis of stridor.

### Aetiology in infants

*Congenital*
- Laryngomalacia – also called 'floppy larynx'. The baby has high-pitched inspiratory stridor and on awake flexible nasendoscopy there is an omega-shaped larynx and the aryepiglottic folds fall in on inspiration. This usually improves by 12–18 months, but rarely the obstruction is severe with failure to thrive, and the child needs surgery with a supraglottoplasty to remove redundant mucosa.
- Webs and cysts
- Subglottic stenosis
- Bilateral vocal cord paralysis, associated with abnormalities such as the Arnold–Chiari malformation in the central nervous system, but may also be idiopathic.

*Acquired*
- Subglottic stenosis – with good neonatal care acquired stenosis is uncommon. Severe cases require tracheostomy and later laryngotracheal reconstruction.
- Subglottic haemangioma – this usually becomes symptomatic in the first few months of life and then, like other haemangiomas, involutes. The infant can have severe obstruction, and the current standard treatment is with propranolol to avoid the need for a tracheostomy.
- Subglottic cysts occur in premature babies who had prolonged intubation; these are opened in the operating theatre under general anaesthesia.
- Recurrent juvenile papillomatosis; this is caused by human papilloma virus (HPV) and the child presents as a toddler with hoarseness and stridor. The mainstay of treatment is laser therapy. With the new HPV vaccine it is hoped that this distressing disease will become a disorder of the past.
- Unilateral vocal cord paralysis may occur after surgery in the neck and chest (congenital heart disease, tracheo-oesophageal fistula and thyroid surgery) and causes a hoarse voice, but rarely airway obstruction.

### Aetiology in older children

- Acute laryngotracheobronchitis (croup)
- Epiglottitis (which is uncommon now with the *H. influenzae* type B vaccine)
- Foreign body
- Retropharyngeal abscess.

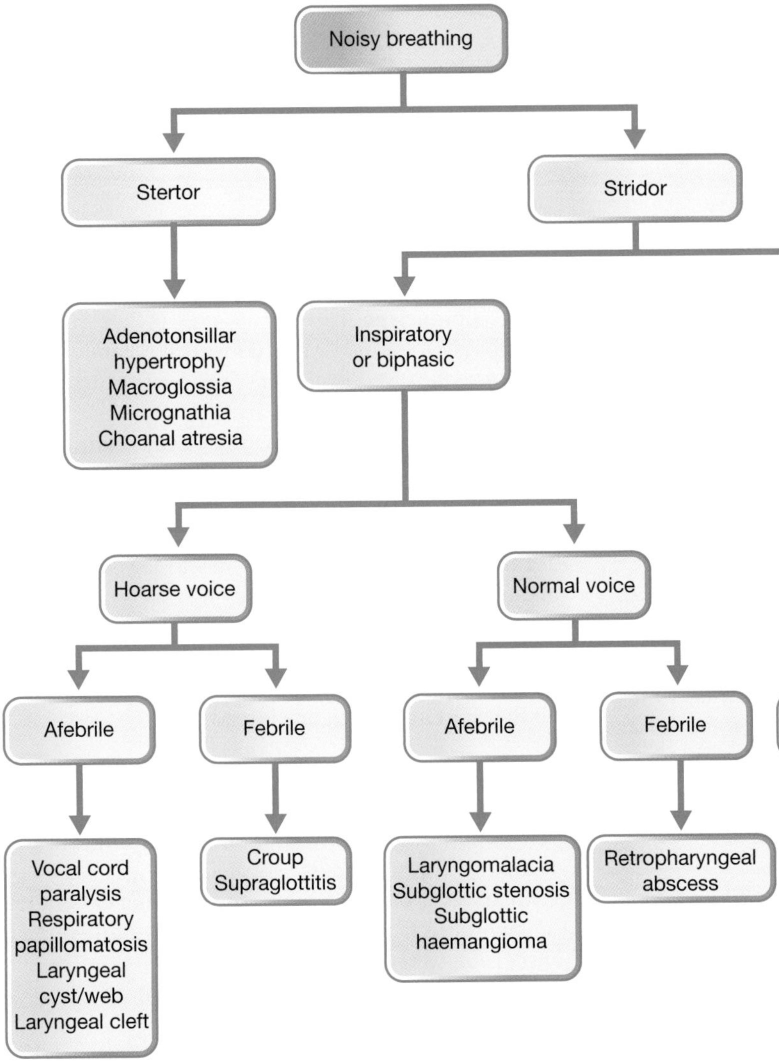

- Noisy breathing
  - Stertor
    - Adenotonsillar hypertrophy<br>Macroglossia<br>Micrognathia<br>Choanal atresia
  - Stridor
    - Inspiratory or biphasic
      - Hoarse voice
        - Afebrile
          - Vocal cord paralysis<br>Respiratory papillomatosis<br>Laryngeal cyst/web<br>Laryngeal cleft
        - Febrile
          - Croup<br>Supraglottitis
      - Normal voice
        - Afebrile
          - Laryngomalacia<br>Subglottic stenosis<br>Subglottic haemangioma
        - Febrile
          - Retropharyngeal abscess
    - Expiratory
      - Afebrile
        - Foreign body<br>Bronchial asthma
      - Febrile
        - Bronchiolitis

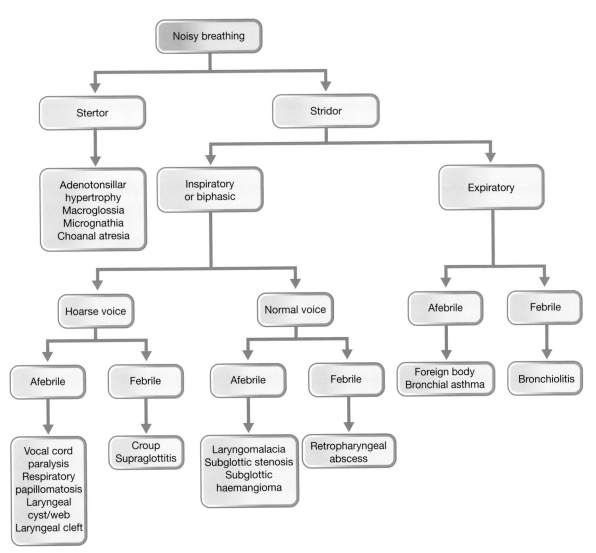

Fig. 22.1.5 Differential diagnosis of stridor in children. (Redrawn with permission from Ludman H, Bradley PJ (eds) 2007 ABC of Ear, Nose and Throat, 5th edn. John Wiley, Chichester, p56.)

## Assessment

Assessment of the child requires careful history and examination. Investigations may include:

- flexible awake endoscopy, to assess vocal cord mobility, and look for other cysts, oedema, webs
- radiology, which may include:
  - chest X-ray
  - barium swallow, to assess for a vascular ring
  - MRI/magnetic resonance angiography (MRA) of the chest for possible vascular anomalies
  - ultrasonography or MRI of the brain for Arnold–Chiari malformation
  - echocardiography
- bronchoscopy under general anaesthesia, if no other cause is found.

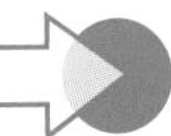

**Practice points**

- A child with an inhaled foreign body may present with unilateral wheeze or unresolved pneumonia.
- If there is concern about a child's hearing or speech and language development, an audiogram should be performed, even if the child passed the newborn screening hearing test.
- In many children with epistaxis there are crusts and infection in the nose and antibiotic ointment can treat both the infection and the bleeding.
- Tonsillitis is a clinical diagnosis in a child with sore throat, fever, dysphagia, exudate on the tonsils, cervical lymphadenopathy and the absence of coryza and cough.
- The most common cause of stridor in newborn babies is laryngomalacia.

# 22.2 Eye disorders

Susan Carden, James Elder

Examination of the eyes should be included in all general medical paediatric checks because it is only through timeliness of diagnosis of ophthalmic pathology that the best vision can be achieved.

## Development of vision

At birth, an infant has a visual acuity of approximately 6/120 and by 12 months this has improved to about 6/12. This rapid development is the result of retinal maturation, myelination of the visual pathways, the ability to accommodate (change the focal length of the eye) and maturation within the visual cortex. The maturation of vision occurs probably until 14 years of age, with the most rapid phase being in the first 2 years, and subtle changes occurring after 8 years of age.

## Measurement of vision in children

Asking a parent 'Does your child see well?' or 'How well do you think your child sees?' often gives useful information about an infant's visual function. If a parent expresses concern about an infant's vision, take note, as this concern is often well founded.

An understanding of normal visual behaviour is vital to estimating visual function in infancy. At birth, when alert, an infant should be able to fix on a face briefly. By 6 weeks of age most infants smile in a visually responsive fashion to a face. At this age the infant will also be able to follow a face or light. By 6 months of age an infant can actively follow objects in the visual environment. Comments on an infant's ability to 'fix' and/or 'follow' are very useful qualitative measures of vision. Forced preferential looking tests are used to measure vision quantitatively.

Picture-naming tests can be done by children between 2 and 3 years of age, and single letter-matching tests are within the abilities of most 3–4-year-olds. The standard Snellen chart test is generally not performed well until the child is between 5 and 6 years of age.

Children with specific language delay or intellectual delay will have difficulty with some tests of visual acuity, and forced preferential looking tests may be more appropriate.

The vision should be tested for each eye individually.

Repeat the test on another occasion if the test results seem inaccurate.

The notation for documenting visual acuity is often based on the Snellen fraction (e.g. 6/6). Most visual acuity tests use standard distances of 3 or 6 m between subject and chart. The numerator of the Snellen fraction is the distance from the chart, whereas the denominator indicates which line on the chart was the smallest to be seen. If the vision is poor, the subject should be brought closer to the chart. The vision then may be recorded as 2/18 or 1/60, etc., depending on how close the subject is to the chart and which line is read.

### What level of vision is abnormal?

An infant who is not fixing and following must be examined further and investigated.

In an older child, a vision of worse than 6/9 is a reasonable cut-off for referral. In addition, a difference in visual acuity between the two eyes of two or more lines indicates the need for further assessment.

## Assessment of a child with a possible eye problem

### History

Prematurity, perinatal difficulties (e.g. birth asphyxia), significant syndromes (e.g. Down syndrome) and other sensory impairment (e.g. deafness) are all associated with an increased risk of eye disease. Common childhood eye problems such as strabismus and refractive errors have a familial tendency, although the precise genetics are not well understood. Finally, the parents' perception of a child's visual function is important, particularly if there is concern that the vision is poor.

### Examination

As with any paediatric medical examination, observation of the child in the environment of the waiting room, walking towards your clinical room and in the

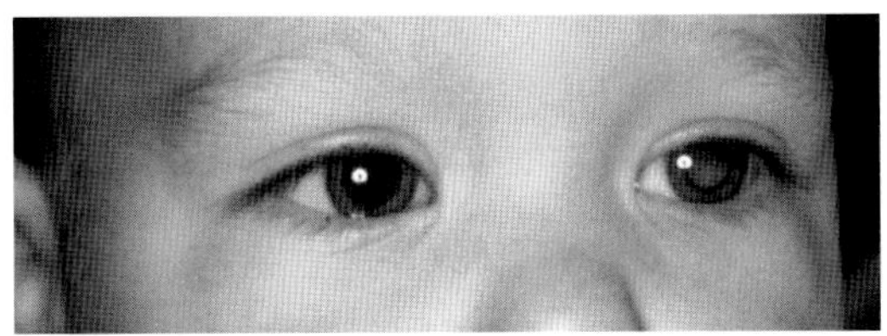

Fig. 22.2.1 Retinoblastoma. 'White' light reflex in left pupil.

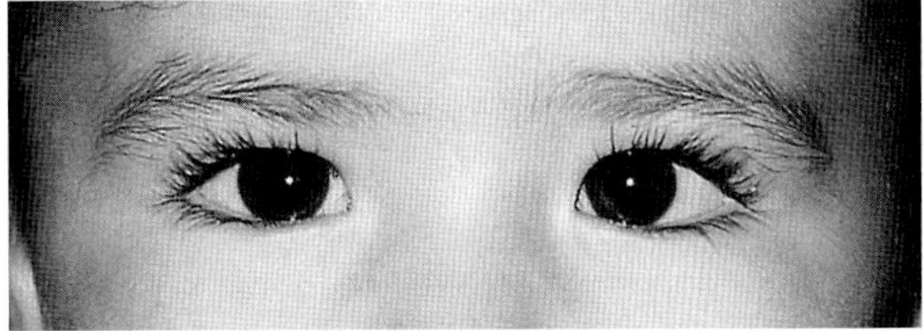

Fig. 22.2.2 This infant has prominent epicanthic folds, giving rise to the appearance of misaligned eyes. This is pseudostrabismus. Note that the corneal light reflections are symmetrical. Cover testing failed to reveal misalignment of either eye.

clinical room is generally the key to diagnosis. Observe whether the child smiles at a face, looks around the room or follows moving objects.

Systematic examination of the eye involves dividing the areas into three: external (eyelids, eyelashes and periorbital region), anterior segment (cornea, pupil, iris and lens) and posterior segment (vitreous cavity, optic nerve and retina).

Most eyelid, eyelash and ocular surface abnormalities can be detected by observation. Many intraocular abnormalities can be detected by examination of the 'red reflex'. This is the red to orange colour seen within the pupil when the line of illumination and observation are approximately coaxial (that is, the same). This situation is most easily obtained by observing the child's eye with a direct ophthalmoscope from a distance of about 1 m. The light reflex for each eye can be compared. A dull or absent red reflex indicates an opacity, such as a cataract, in the normally clear media of the eye. A white reflex results from an abnormally pale reflecting surface within the eye, such as a white retinal tumour (retinoblastoma; Fig. 22.2.1) Although these intraocular disorders are rare, they are important in terms of the severe effect on vision or threat to life.

## Misalignment of the eyes

Strabismus or squint occurs in 3–4% of children. Observation will confirm the presence of a large-angle strabismus. However, a broad nasal bridge or prominent epicanthic folds will mimic milder degrees of strabismus, especially in younger infants. This condition is known as pseudostrabismus (Fig. 22.2.2). The epicanthic folds cover the sclera on the medial aspect of the globe, while the lateral sclera is easily visible. This creates the appearance of misalignment, particularly when the child looks laterally. Examination of the symmetry of corneal light reflections will aid in determining whether there is an esotropia (in-turning of the eyes) or only pseudostrabismus.

A cover test is a reliable method of detecting strabismus. The cover test is done by first getting the child to fix on an object while the observer determines which eye appears to be misaligned. The eye that appears to be fixing on the object (and not misaligned) is then covered while the apparently misaligned eye is observed. If strabismus is present, a corrective movement of the misaligned eye will be seen as this eye takes up fixation on the object of regard (Fig. 22.2.3). If no movement is seen, the eye is uncovered.

The cover test is then repeated, covering the other eye this time; the eye that is not covered is again observed for a corrective movement and, if present, strabismus is confirmed. The test can be repeated as many times as necessary. If no movement is seen following repeated covering of either eye, then strabismus is not present. Care must be taken to allow the child to fix with both eyes open before covering either eye, otherwise normal binocular control may be prevented and a small latent squint (phoria) may be detected. Latent squints are normal variants and are of no significance.

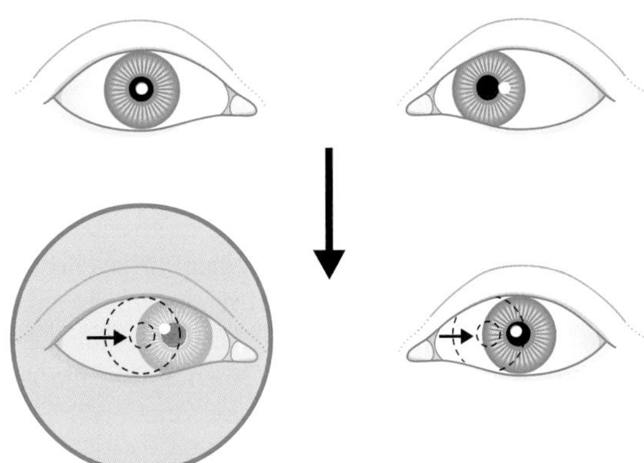

Fig. 22.2.3 Cover test. First the child's attention is attracted with a toy (top). Then the eye that appears to be looking directly at the toy is covered and the other eye is observed for a refixation movement (bottom). In convergent squint there will be an outward movement of the uncovered eye (pictured), and in divergent squint there will be an inward movement of the eye. If no movement is detected, the test should be repeated but covering the other eye first.

# Common eye problems in childhood

## Amblyopia

Amblyopia, the cortical response to abnormal input from the eyes and manifest as reduced visual acuity in one or both eyes, results from refractive (spectacle) error (in one or both eyes), strabismus or from deprivation (e.g. cataracts). Amblyopia usually responds to treatment if detected in a timely fashion. Detection of amblyopia is one of the major reasons for routine visual screening in childhood as the earlier it is detected the more chance there is that treatment will be successful.

Refractive errors cause a poorly focused image to be transmitted from the retina to the cortex. Such input does not stimulate normal cortical development and amblyopia results.

Strabismic (misaligned) eyes each send a different view of the world to the cortex. If the brain 'paid attention' to the image from each eye, diplopia would ensue. However, the immature visual cortex is capable of ignoring the image from one eye. Eventually the cortex may suppress the input from a deviating eye, with resulting amblyopia.

Treatment of amblyopia involves the correction of any focusing errors with appropriate spectacles and forcing the brain to use the amblyopic eye by depriving the brain of clear input from the better-seeing eye. This is commonly done with a patch. Unfortunately, realigning strabismic eyes is not enough to overcome amblyopia secondary to strabismus.

## Strabismus

A squint or misaligned eye is frequently associated with amblyopia. Childhood strabismus is often the result of failure of binocular control at a cortical level. Less commonly it is the result of cranial nerve lesions or extraocular muscle disease. In most children, strabismus is not associated with neurological or intellectual problems. However, children with widespread central nervous system abnormalities have an increased risk of developing strabismus. Down syndrome is a good example of this, with an approximately 10-fold increased risk of developing strabismus.

The following is a brief description of frequent patterns of strabismus seen in childhood and an outline of their management.

### Infantile esotropia

This is a large-angle convergent squint seen before 6 months of age. Strabismic amblyopia is common in infantile esotropia, but refractive errors are rare. Occlusion therapy and surgery are the most common treatments. Children with infantile esotropia need to be followed up throughout childhood: approximately one-third require further surgery, and amblyopia can occur despite adequate eye alignment.

### Intermittent divergent strabismus (exotropia)

While exotropia can occur in infancy, it is more common from 18 months of age. It is often more noticeable on distance fixation and may be associated with monocular closure in bright light. Amblyopia is less commonly associated with exotropia than with esotropia because the deviation is intermittent and, presumably, when the eyes are straight normal visual development proceeds. In some cases the divergence becomes more constant and surgery may be undertaken to improve alignment.

### Accommodative esotropia

This occurs in children who are excessively 'long-sighted' (hypermetropic). To overcome hypermetropia and focus a clear image on the retina, accommodative effort is used. Accommodation consists of the combination of changing focal length of the lens together with convergence of the eyes (so that both are directed at the near object of regard). Thus, in children with excessive hypermetropia there is increased focusing and at times excessive convergence; a convergent squint (esotropia) appears as a result of the increased accommodative effort used by these children. Accommodative esotropia can be completely or partially corrected by prescribing glasses that compensate for the appropriate amount of hypermetropia. Amblyopia, sometimes in both eyes, is often seen in association with an accommodative esotropia. Occlusion therapy may be required. If glasses only partly correct the esotropia, surgery may be indicated to obtain optimal alignment.

**Clinical example**

A 3-year-old girl presented with a history of a worsening inward turn of her left eye over 4 months. The cover test confirmed a left convergent squint and the red reflex was normal in each eye. Subsequent assessment by an ophthalmologist confirmed the findings and the girl's visual acuities were 3/3 in the right eye and 3/9 in the left, with refraction showing that she was hypermetropic. When seen 4 months later she was wearing glasses and had been patching her right eye for 2 hours a day. Her eyes were straight to cover test, her left eye vision was improving and strabismus surgery was less likely to be appropriate.

## Refractive errors

Common refractive errors include hypermetropia, myopia and astigmatism. These are the result of defects in the focusing components of the eye (the optics of the eye). Hence, any defect in the shape of a surface of the eye can cause a refractive error: an abnormality of corneal curvature (a frequent cause of astigmatism), abnormalities of lens power and axial length of the eye that is too long (causing myopia) or too short (causing hypermetropia). Children rarely complain of poor vision related to refractive error. Children with poor vision, due to any significant refractive error, often hold objects of regard very closely.

Significant refractive errors can be equal in both eyes or they can be different in each eye (anisometropia). Bilateral equal refractive errors can cause amblyopia in both eyes, whereas anisometropia can lead to unilateral amblyopia.

Vision screening in preschool children aims to detect silent, significant, refractive errors that are amenable to treatment. Amblyopia becomes less amenable to treatment the older a child becomes.

If a refractive error is suspected in a young child because of strabismus or poor visual acuity, objective testing with cycloplegic retinoscopy is required. If a child is prescribed glasses, these should be worn the majority of the time. Occlusion therapy with a patch is a frequent mainstay of treatment and needs to be monitored very carefully to avoid under-patching or over-patching (reverse amblyopia).

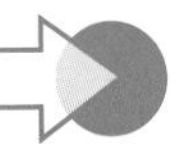

### Practical points

**Vision assessment and strabismus**

- Parental assessment of their infant child's vision is often very accurate; if they are concerned their child is not seeing, you should be concerned also.
- Carefully observe the child's visual behaviour before actively examining the child. Red reflexes can be observed from a distance. Urgent referral is required if an abnormal red reflex is found.
- Vision screening programmes aim to detect silent, significant refractive errors in children. Children under 7 years of age rarely complain of poor vision relating to a refractive error (reduced visual acuity).
- Strabismus is a common cause of amblyopia. Suspected cases of strabismus should be referred to an ophthalmologist for further assessment and management.
- Cover testing is a helpful method to diagnose strabismus.
- Amblyopia can often be treated effectively with glasses and/or occlusion therapy if it is detected in a timely manner. An optimal time is at about 3 years of age (or earlier).

## Nasolacrimal duct obstruction

Obstruction of one or both nasolacrimal ducts is a common problem during infancy. It can present as a watery and sticky eye in the first few weeks of life. Despite the persistent discharge, the eye is 'white' and not red or inflamed. An inflamed eye suggests an alternative diagnosis such as conjunctivitis. If the obstruction persists, the lower lid may become red and sometimes slightly scaly as a result of prolonged skin irritation.

The differential diagnosis includes trauma, conjunctivitis and infantile glaucoma. These conditions are described below.

Most congenital nasolacrimal duct obstructions resolve spontaneously during the first year of life. Persistence after 1 year of age is generally an indication for probing of the duct under general anaesthesia.

## Trauma

Trauma to the eye may be physical (blunt or sharp) thermal, electromagnetic or chemical.

Direct blunt trauma to the eye may cause disruption of iris blood vessels (leading to a hyphaema, i.e. blood in the anterior chamber of the eye), iris tears (iridodialysis), dislocation of the lens, rupture of the choroid, retinal haemorrhages and, rarely, rupture of the sclera. Gross inspection of the eye will reveal most injuries. Choroidal and global rupture may be suspected on the basis of the nature of the injury and associated poor vision. Referral to an ophthalmologist is necessary for confirmation of the injury and further management.

Surface trauma can be diagnosed with the help of fluorescein staining and a cobalt blue light. It is helpful to instil local anaesthetic drops at the beginning of the examination. Areas of epithelial abrasion will fluoresce green. If a round ulcer and/or vertical linear abrasions are seen, suspect a subtarsal foreign body. The upper lid should be everted and any subtarsal foreign bodies can be removed with a moistened cotton-bud. Superficial trauma is treated with antibiotic ointment and daily review until any epithelial defect (ulcer or abrasion) has healed.

If the cornea or sclera has been penetrated, intraocular contents can prolapse out through the wound. In such cases, the iris and pupil may appear distorted or the anterior chamber may be shallower than normal. Any patient with a suspected penetrating eye injury must be referred to an ophthalmologist. During transport of the patient, the eye should be protected with a cone that does not exert any pressure on the eye. If vomiting is likely, an antiemetic should be given to prevent further prolapse of intraocular tissue.

Thermal injuries to the eyes are uncommon because closure of the eyelids tends to protect the eyes. With time, facial burns may cause cicatricial scarring that interferes with lid function, leading to exposure and drying of the eye's surface. If a primary thermal injury to the eye is suspected, fluorescein dye should be used to detect any ulceration. If ulceration is found, treatment with antibiotic ointment and regular review is important.

Radiation injuries to the eye are generally the result of medical radiation therapy for facial or ocular neoplasia. Typical complications can be cataract, dry eye syndrome, radiation retinopathy and optic neuropathy. These changes are seen some considerable time after the irradiation.

Chemical burns to the eye in childhood are potentially very serious, especially if the chemical is alkaline. Burns may occur with accidental access to a domestic cleaning agent, many of which are alkaline in nature. Strong alkali will denature and dissolve protein and penetrate deeply into the cornea. Acids tend to coagulate the corneal structures and this often prevents deeper penetration of the acidic chemical into the eye. Immediate first aid should consist of copious irrigation with water at the site of the accident and this should be continued for at least 10 minutes. Following adequate irrigation, all patients with chemical burns of the eye should be referred to an ophthalmologist.

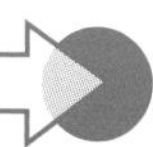

**Practical points**

**Blocked tear ducts and eye injury**

- Most congenital blocked tear ducts resolve spontaneously by 1 year of age.
- Inspection with the addition of local anaesthetic drops and fluorescein staining will enable the diagnosis of most physical trauma to the eye.
- All chemical injuries to the eye should be regarded as serious and require copious irrigation.

## Conjunctivitis

Conjunctivitis may be infective, allergic or due to chemical irritation. The main symptoms are itch, pain, irritation or a gritty sensation. The main signs are epiphora (watering), discharge, and erythema of conjunctiva and lids. The relative prominence of different symptoms and signs varies with the cause of the conjunctivitis (Table 22.2.1).

Ophthalmia neonatorum is bacterial conjunctivitis contracted during delivery from the maternal birth canal. It can be due to *Neisseria gonorrhoeae* or *Chlamydia trachomatis*. These are serious diseases that both cause conjunctivitis with copious discharge and marked erythema. Gonococcal conjunctivitis can cause perforation of the cornea, resultant loss of vision and generalized sepsis. Chlamydial conjunctivitis can also lead to a generalized sepsis and pneumonia. Microbiological diagnosis is required urgently, and conjunctival swabs and scrapings need to be done. Antibiotic treatment often requires topical and systemic measures for the infant, and systemic treatment of the mother and her partner(s).

Bacterial conjunctivitis occurring outside the first few weeks of life in children is usually the result of relatively innocuous organisms (e.g. *Staphylococcus* spp. and *Haemophilus* spp.) Microbiological investigation is not usually indicated and a broad-spectrum topical antibiotic should be prescribed (e.g. chloramphenicol, framycetin sulphate, neomycin).

Viral conjunctivitis is common at all ages. The discharge from viral conjunctivitis is often less than with bacterial conjunctivitis. Viral conjunctivitis is frequently associated with upper respiratory tract

**Table 22.2.1 Signs and symptoms of conjunctivitis**

| Cause of conjunctivitis | Symptoms | Signs |
|---|---|---|
| Viral | Moderate discomfort | Moderate epiphora<br>Mild discharge<br>Mild to moderate erythema |
| Bacterial | Moderate to severe discomfort | Moderate epiphora<br>Copious discharge<br>Moderate to severe erythema |
| Allergic | Excessive blinking and eye rubbing | Mild to moderate epiphora<br>Stringy discharge<br>Mild erythema |
| Chemical | Pain intense | Severe epiphora<br>Mild discharge<br>Moderate to severe erythema |

The descriptions in this table are intended to be a guide; there may be considerable variation and overlap in the signs and symptoms of conjunctivitis from different causes.

infection symptoms. Treatment usually involves eye toilets and prevention of the sharing of towels in the family.

Allergic conjunctivitis is common in children of all age groups and empirically seems to be worsening as the climate changes. Children tend to complain of itch much less than adults but will often be noted to rub their eyes vigorously. Many children may present only with excessive blinking and may have been thought to have a tic. House-dust mite, grass and other plant pollens are common allergens that precipitate allergic conjunctivitis. Therapy depends on the severity of the symptoms. If mild, cold compresses may be all that is needed. For more severe symptoms, topical eye-drop mast cell stabilizers are helpful. In more persistent and severe cases, topical steroid preparations may be indicated. Topical steroids should be used only under the supervision of an ophthalmologist because of the risk of side-effects, including cataract, glaucoma and keratitis.

**Clinical example**

A 4-year-old boy presented with a 12-hour history of a red and watery eye. He complained of pain and his parents had not observed any discharge. Examination revealed a red eye with no obvious trauma or foreign body on the surface of the eye. After topical local anaesthetic drops had been instilled, fluorescein staining demonstrated a round ulcer on the upper part of the cornea. Eversion of the upper eyelid revealed a small foreign body. It was removed with a moistened cotton-bud. The ulcer was treated with antibiotic ointment and healed in 1 day.

## Lid infections and inflammation

These are common in children and most arise in the skin appendages of the eyelids (lash follicles and meibomian glands). Infection of a lash follicle is called a stye. Unless there is significant secondary erythema of the surrounding lid, topical and systemic antibiotics are not indicated. Occasionally, severe preseptal cellulitis will follow a focal lid infection and systemic (often intravenous) antibiotics will then be needed for treatment.

Inflammation of a meibomian gland is known as a chalazion. This is the result of inflammation due to blockage of the duct of the gland, rather than infection. A chalazion will appear as a lump in the substance of the lid. It can be inflamed in appearance. Warm compresses may give symptomatic relief and help drainage. Chalazia may persist for many months. Some will discharge their contents through either the conjunctiva or the skin. Occasionally, surgical drainage is indicated for a persistently inflamed and large chalazion.

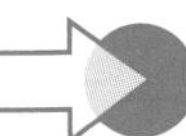

**Practical points**

**Conjunctivitis and chalazia**

- Neonatal conjunctivitis may be sight-threatening and a threat to the newborn infant's health. Immediate investigation with appropriate treatment is needed.
- Children do not always complain of itchiness with allergic conjunctivitis. Excessive blinking may be the key to the diagnosis.
- Most chalazia are not infected, and redness and swelling is the result of sterile inflammation. Consequently topical and oral antibiotics are of little use in treatment. Most chalazia resolve spontaneously.

## Ptosis

Ptosis, also called blepharoptosis, is a droopy upper eyelid and results from innervational or muscular defects of the levator superioris or Müller muscles. Innervational defects include third cranial nerve palsy, Horner syndrome (sympathetic nervous system) and myasthenia gravis. Congenital ptosis is the commonest type of ptosis in children, and is caused by a defect in the levator superioris muscle. Ptosis can cause amblyopia in young children. This is usually the result of occlusion of the visual axis. On occasion, ptosis is a cosmetic concern; surgical correction can be offered in many cases.

## Learning difficulties

Learning difficulties are common in school-aged children. Affected children are often sent for an ophthalmic examination to rule out a disorder of vision. It is uncommon to find a cause, although allergic eye disease (in particular vernal allergic eye disease) is an increasing cause of poor concentration. It is commonly assumed that there may be a visual abnormality that contributes to, or even causes, the learning difficulty. This assumption is ill-founded and arises because vision is obviously involved with activities such as reading and writing. Children with learning difficulties are no more or less likely to have visual problems than children without evidence of learning problems. Rather than expending effort on therapies for perceived ocular abnormalities, parents should be encouraged to take an educational approach to their child's learning difficulties.

## Visual handicap

Visual handicap in childhood may be the result of ocular and/or cortical visual abnormalities, and may be associated with other abnormalities, such as deafness, motor defects and intellectual deficits. Intervention and support for a particular child needs to be planned after a thorough assessment of the child's visual and associated handicaps. From a purely visual point of view, interventions may include mobility training, low vision aids, such as magnifiers and closed-circuit television, and training in alternative means of communication, such as Braille and the use of a computer to write.

The presence of an additional handicap, such as deafness or an intellectual deficit, compounds the situation and necessitates skilled intervention over many years.

## Other important eye problems in childhood

These are mentioned briefly because prompt recognition enables early treatment and optimal outcomes.

### Poor vision in infancy

This first comes to attention when a child fails to achieve normal milestones of visual development (see Measurement of vision in children, above). If the cause of severe visual impairment is within the eye, sensory nystagmus will develop by 3–4 months of age. This nystagmus is often slow and somewhat pendular rather than jerky in appearance, due to its immaturity. Severe visual loss due to cortical visual impairment tends not to cause nystagmus.

Causes of poor vision in infancy include:

- cataracts
- albinism
- retinal colobomas
- infantile glaucoma
- congenital retinal dystrophy
- retinoblastoma
- delayed visual maturation
- cortical visual impairment.

Prompt recognition is vital as there may be a treatable cause (e.g. cataracts) and, even if no treatment is possible, early and appropriate intervention minimizes the negative effects of severe visual impairment on general development.

### Cataract

A cataract is any opacity within the lens. Bilateral congenital cataracts will often cause poor vision in infancy, whereas unilateral congenital cataract may go unrecognized as one eye has normal vision. Both bilateral and unilateral congenital cataracts are treatable if diagnosed early. Cataracts are detected readily by inspection of the red reflex with the direct ophthalmoscope.

There are numerous causes of congenital cataract, including: hereditary (dominant, recessive and X-linked); metabolic (e.g. galactosaemia); association with systemic syndromes (e.g. Down syndrome); and congenital infection (e.g. rubella embryopathy). Many, especially unilateral cataracts, are idiopathic.

### Retinoblastoma

This is a rare childhood cancer arising within the retina. Sporadic and hereditary forms are recognized. The sporadic form is the result of two separate mutations that negate the action of the retinoblastoma (Rb) gene within a single retinoblast cell, and thus is always unilateral (see Fig. 22.2.1). The hereditary form arises when the first of these two mutations occurs in one Rb gene within a germ cell (most often a sperm). The second mutation occurs within the retinoblast. As all retinoblasts descended from an affected germ cell have the first mutation, by chance more than one retinoblastoma will usually develop and hence the hereditary form is often, but not always, bilateral.

Retinoblastoma often presents with leukocoria (white pupillary reflection – the white tumour is seen immediately behind the lens), strabismus, poor vision, or a known family history of retinoblastoma. Prompt recognition is vital as early treatment will increase the possibility of preserving vision and life. With current treatments the 5-year survival rate for this childhood cancer is about 98%.

### Glaucoma

Glaucoma in infancy presents with a cloudy and enlarged cornea (buphthalmos) with associated epiphora (watery eye) and photophobia (see Fig. 22.2.4). It may be unilateral or bilateral, and is usually an isolated ocular abnormality. If unrecognized it will result in severe and untreatable visual loss over weeks

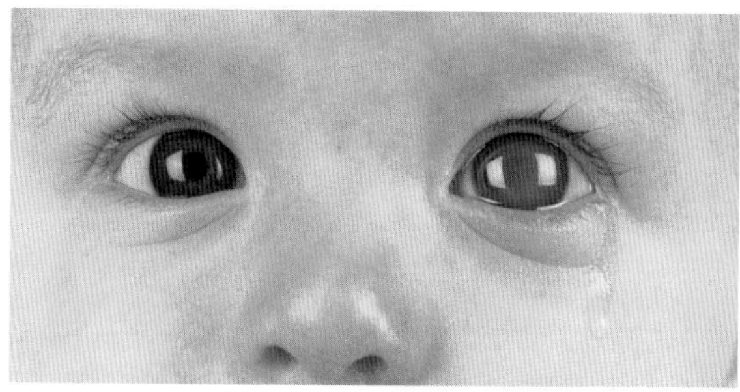

Fig. 22.2.4 Congenital glaucoma. The left eye has a corneal diameter larger than that on the right eye, a hazy cornea, and is watery.

to months. Surgical treatment, aimed at increasing the drainage of aqueous fluid out of the eye, is indicated as in most instances, medical therapy with anti-glaucoma medication is usually a temporizing or adjunctive measure.

### Colobomas

A coloboma is a defect resulting from failure of complete fusion of the embryonic fissure of the developing eye between the fourth and sixth week of gestation. If the optic nerve or macular area of the retina is involved, vision will be affected significantly. An iris coloboma may or may not be present in association with a visually more important posterior pole coloboma.

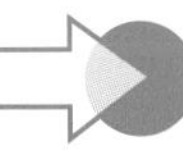

**Practical points**

**Further important considerations**

- Learning difficulties are seldom the result of eye problems.
- Examine the red reflexes of all infants suspected of having poor vision and all infants with strabismus. An abnormal red reflex may be due to retinoblastoma and urgent referral is mandatory.
- Think of congenital glaucoma if a child has one eye that is bigger than the other. Then look for coexisting clouding of the cornea and seek a history of a watery eye and photophobia.

## The eye in paediatric systemic disease

The following is a brief account of the common ocular features of some paediatric systemic diseases.

### Extreme prematurity

Marked prematurity gives rise to eye problems by interfering with the orderly development of retinal blood vessels. This disorder is known as retinopathy of prematurity (ROP). Mild ROP is seen in 30–50% of infants weighing less than 1250 g at birth and then regresses without ill effect on vision. In some infants the ROP progresses and a fibrovascular proliferation develops within the eye that detaches the retina, with resultant loss of vision.

Excess oxygen administration to premature infants has been known since the 1950s to be a cause of severe ROP. Curtailment of oxygen use to amounts sufficient to limit respiratory and neurological sequelae has greatly reduced the incidence of blinding ROP, but has not completely prevented it, particularly as infants of even lower gestation survive.

Regular screening of at-risk infants (birth weight <1500 g or gestation <32 weeks) by an ophthalmologist enables timely detection of significant ROP before retinal detachment ensues. Retinal ablation with laser surgery greatly reduces the risk of the development of retinal detachment and subsequent blindness.

### Juvenile chronic arthritis

Childhood chronic arthritis is associated with inflammation of the iris (iritis or anterior uveitis). Those at particular risk are young girls with oligoarticular juvenile chronic arthritis who are antinuclear antibody positive, although it also occurs in other presentations of juvenile arthritis. The iritis that occurs in these children is painless and chronic, and may, if untreated, cause cataract and glaucoma. Periodic assessment by an ophthalmologist will detect early uveitis. The mainstay of uveitis treatment is topical steroid drops. Glaucoma can be associated with the disease and also with steroid treatment. Regular review by an ophthalmologist is important.

### Down syndrome

Down syndrome is associated with an approximately 10-fold increased risk of developing eye problems during childhood when compared with the average incidence. Blocked tear ducts and blepharitis are significant problems. Squint, nystagmus, poor vision, refractive error, keratoconus, cataract and anomalous optic nerve heads can frequently be found. An increased index of suspicion for eye problems should be maintained for children with Down syndrome.

### Physical child abuse

Non-accidental injury may involve the eye. Direct trauma to the eye or eyelids will be obvious on inspection. Violent shaking of a small child is often associated with the development of retinal haemorrhages and a severe closed brain injury. Although not pathognomonic of child abuse, the presence of retinal haemorrhages is highly suggestive of abuse in cases of unexplained severe brain injury in a young child.

### Diabetes mellitus

Insulin-dependent diabetes mellitus (type 1) is increasing in frequency in childhood. Screening for eye complications occurs regularly in adults. Severe diabetic eye disease is uncommon in childhood because the diabetes is usually kept under strict control. In cases where the control is poor, regular eye checks can be commenced early (e.g. at 6 years of age). In developing countries, where medical treatment may be erratic and blood sugar level control is poor, severe diabetic eye disease (cataracts, retinal haemorrhages and neovascularization) can occur before the age of 10 years. Significant retinal abnormalities are seen in a small number of diabetic children in mid to late adolescence, particularly if the disease was of early onset and control is poor.

## Summary

It is important for the paediatrician to become familiar with examination of children's eyes and to incorporate this into their general medical examination technique. Timely diagnosis of ophthalmic problems is essential so that a referral to an ophthalmologist can rapidly initiate sight-saving treatment.

# Teeth and oral cavity disorders 22.3

Nicky Kilpatrick, Kerrod Hallett

The oral cavity can be considered the gateway to the body. It is the start of the alimentary tract and is integrally involved in the initial phases of digestion. The oral cavity consists of teeth sitting in sockets in the alveolar processes of the maxillary and mandibular bones supported by a fibrous sling known as the periodontal ligament. The oral cavity is lined by a combination of attached gingival tissue (gums) and more generalized mucous membranes. As with the rest of the body, the oral cavity is susceptible to both developmental and acquired disorders that can occur in isolation or as part of more general medical conditions or genetic syndromes.

It is becoming increasingly well recognized that oral health plays a significant role in maintaining good general health and wellbeing. This chapter will, therefore, summarize the key features of normal oral development and highlight the common disorders that affect both the teeth and their supporting structures. It will also identify the oral manifestations of some of the more common paediatric diseases.

## Development

Teeth start to form from the fifth week *in utero* and may continue until the late teens or early twenties with the eruption of the third permanent molars (or wisdom teeth) (Table 22.3.1). The first tooth to erupt is usually a lower central incisor at around 7 months of age. By the age of 2.5 years most children will have a complete primary dentition consisting of 20 teeth: 8 incisors, 4 canines, 8 molars. At around the age of 6 years, the primary incisors become mobile and fall out. Most people have 32 permanent teeth, the first of which to erupt is usually the lower first permanent molars at around 6 years of age. The period that follows, referred to as the mixed dentition phase, is highly variable.

Permanent upper incisors are usually more prominent than their predecessors; this allows the mandible to grow forward and encourages the development of what is described as a normal occlusion – a class I occlusion. Variations of the norm are common particularly in the anteroposterior dimension, and cause changes to the relationship between the upper and lower incisors. When the maxilla is forward relative to the mandible and the upper incisors protrude, creating an increase in 'overjet', this is known as a class II malocclusion. Conversely, in those cases where the mandible is relatively prognathic and the upper front teeth develop behind the lower ones, the result is a class III malocclusion, or reverse overjet.

These malocclusions may result from growth anomalies in either or both jaws and may be complicated further by the pattern of eruption of the dentition, size of the teeth and other external influences such as thumb-sucking. Recognizing malocclusions is important not only in determining the need for and nature of treatment, but also in diagnosing growth disorders and in syndrome identification, as jaw discrepancies are common in such conditions.

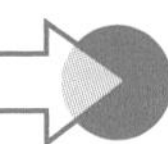

**Practical points**

- Eruption times vary widely.
- Provided the sequence of eruption of the teeth is in order (central incisors before lateral incisors, etc.), delays *per se* are not a cause for concern.
- Asymmetrical eruption, particularly of the permanent incisors, should be reviewed by a dentist in order to check that there is no obstruction (such as an extra tooth) to the eruption of the appropriate tooth.
- The simultaneous presence of primary and permanent teeth during the mixed dentition phase is generally not a problem.
- Premature loss of primary teeth can be a sign of underlying systemic disease and should be reviewed by a paediatric dentist.

### Teething

Teething is a normal process by which an infant begins to cut their first teeth (primary dentition). A variety of symptoms can accompany teething, including sensitive and painful gums, mouth ulceration, drooling, feeding difficulties, lack of sleep, fevers, diarrhoea and crying. There is no scientific evidence that any of these symptoms is directly related to tooth eruption; nevertheless, they are commonly reported and can cause significant distress to the child and anxious parent. Similarly there is no evidence base to support any particular management strategy. The use of chilled teething rings, hard sugar-free rusk biscuits and finger

**Table 22.3.1 Summary of the eruption times for primary and permanent teeth**

| Primary dentition (months after birth) | | | | | | | |
|---|---|---|---|---|---|---|---|
| Central incisors | Lateral incisors | | Canines | | First molars | | Second molars |
| 6–12 | 9–16 | | 16–23 | | 13–19 | | 23–33 |
| **Permanent dentition (years of age)** | | | | | | | |
| Central incisors | Lateral incisors | Canines | First premolars | Second premolars | First molars | Second molars | Third molars |
| 6–8 | 6.5–8.5 | 9–13 | 9.5–11.5 | 10–13 | 5.5–7.0 | 11–13 | 17+ |

pressure appears to help. Over-the-counter teething preparations are of limited use. Not only do many contain choline salicylate and significant amounts of ethanol, which are contraindicated in very young infants, but also repeated use can cause ulceration of the gums. Some lidocaine-based gels are thought to be slightly more effective and may be mildly antiseptic. Mildly increased temperature can be managed with systemic oral medication, but temperatures of 38°C and above, or other serious symptoms (e.g. convulsions), should not be ascribed to teething and should be assessed independently.

## Developmental anomalies

A few developmental anomalies occur in the newborn or very young child. As it is unusual for infants to be seen by a dental health professional, it is important that the medical practitioner examine the oral cavity periodically and refer to a paediatric dentist as appropriate. Amongst the more common are Epstein pearls, Bohn nodules, eruption cysts and natal teeth.

### Oral alveolar developmental cysts

#### Epstein pearls

- Whitish-yellow nodules appear on the roof of the mouth in a neonate.
- Composed of trapped epithelial remnants during palatal fusion.
- The cysts usually burst and disappear by 90 days.

#### Bohn nodules

- Multiple 1–5-mm creamy nodules on the outer surface of the alveolar ridges (normally shed *in utero*).
- Composed of epithelial remnants.
- Sometimes mistaken for prematurely erupting teeth.
- No treatment indicated as the contents discharge spontaneously by the third month.

#### Eruption cysts

- A blue or clear swelling overlying the crown of an erupting tooth, most frequently in the incisor region of the maxilla.
- Eruption is slightly delayed and discomfort or pain may occur.
- Management is symptomatic only. Surgical intervention is contraindicated.

#### Natal and neonatal teeth

- Present in 1 in 3000 births, or erupt in the neonatal period – usually in the lower incisor region.
- Most are prematurely erupted normal primary teeth, but some may be 'supernumerary' or extra teeth.
- Can interfere with breastfeeding (nipple trauma).
- Can cause an ulceration under the tongue in breastfed infants, called Riga–Fede disease, that often necessitates tooth removal.
- Removal is commonly indicated to alleviate parental anxiety and is simple (using topical local anaesthesia and a haemostat). Suggest checking vitamin K-dependent coagulation factors before removing teeth.

### Developmental defects of enamel

Teeth start forming from the fifth week *in utero*. Any disturbance in metabolism can cause damage to, or even the death of, the sensitive enamel-forming cells (the ameloblasts). Such a disturbance will leave a permanent developmental defect on the tooth surface which will be apparent as a loss of tooth substance (hypoplasia) or a deficiency in the quality of the enamel (hypomineralization) once the tooth erupts. Such defects in enamel have in the past been related to:

- prenatal events such as maternal rubella virus or cytomegalovirus (CMV) infection, maternal syphilis and pregnancy toxaemia
- natal events such as prematurity, hypoxia and hyperbilirubinaemia
- postnatal events – measles virus infection, gastrointestinal disease and hypoparathyroidism.

The first permanent molars (the so-called 6-year-old molars) and incisors are particularly susceptible to enamel defects as they are developing at the time of birth. Children with other health issues such as congenital heart disease or cerebral palsy are more likely to have developmental defects of their teeth, possibly as a result of systemic illness, fevers and periods of hypoxia in infancy and early childhood. Early identification of these defects is important as the quality of the tooth enamel is compromised; the teeth may be sensitive, particularly to oral hygiene measures, and more likely to develop decay.

### Clinical example

Miranda, now aged 2 years, was born normally at term with a normal birth weight. Since then she has demonstrated slow developmental milestones and mild hemiplegia with no obvious cause. Dental examination revealed a caries-free primary dentition, which, however, had chronologically distributed enamel hypoplastic (developmental) defects, affecting the teeth at 4–7 months *in utero*. On questioning, the grandmother had recorded in her diary the dates when her daughter had a severe viral infection and was in bed for several days.

Antibodies to CMV were detected on testing. CMV was the presumptive cause of the enamel defects and possibly also of the mild neurological defect and hemiplegia. This diagnosis helped early planning for future care. These enamel defects can increase the risk of developing dental caries as the surface of the teeth are often more porous and retain plaque, and they can be quite sensitive. Such teeth can be protected with a tooth-coloured adhesive material and the parents should be encouraged to assist Miranda with her oral hygiene and to maintain regular dental visits.

## Acquired disorders of the teeth

### Dental caries

Dental caries (decay) remains one of the most common chronic diseases in childhood, and recent epidemiological data show that disease prevalence and severity in childhood is increasing. As with many diseases, there are considerable inequalities in terms of caries experience with around 80% of all decay being experienced by just 20% of children. It is therefore important to identify children at high risk of developing decay and target them for proactive prevention. Given the fact that very few preschool-aged children are seen by a dental health professional, responsibility lies with medical and nursing professionals to identify infants at risk of developing decay and to refer to a paediatric dentist for appropriate anticipatory preventive advice.

Dental caries (or decay) is an infectious disease caused by the presence of certain bacteria, predominantly mutans streptococci (MS), in the oral cavity. The MS metabolize sugars and starches to produce acids; this lowers the pH of the oral cavity and promotes loss of minerals from the tooth surface. Minerals in the saliva, including calcium, phosphate and fluoride, are re-deposited on the tooth surface once neutral pH is restored (normally after about 20 minutes). This process is dynamic and as long as minerals are replaced the tooth surface remains sound and intact. If, however, the drop in pH is prolonged and/or frequent, there will be a net loss of minerals leading to a weakening and eventual breakdown (cavitation) of the tooth surface. The early sign of mineral loss is characterized by pre-cavitated or 'white spot' lesions (Fig. 22.3.1A), usually around the necks of the teeth where the MS tend to colonize the oral biofilm

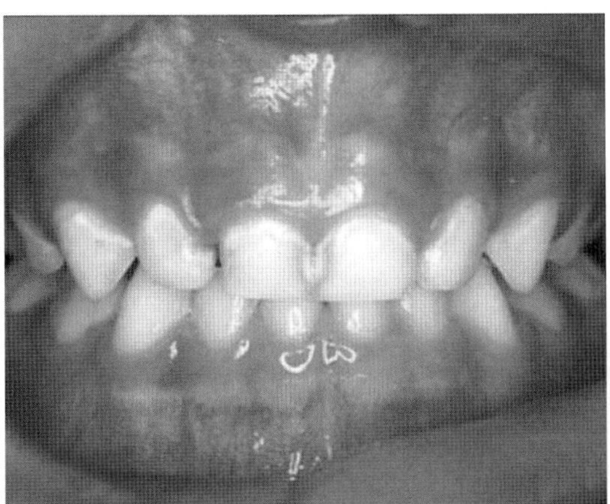

A

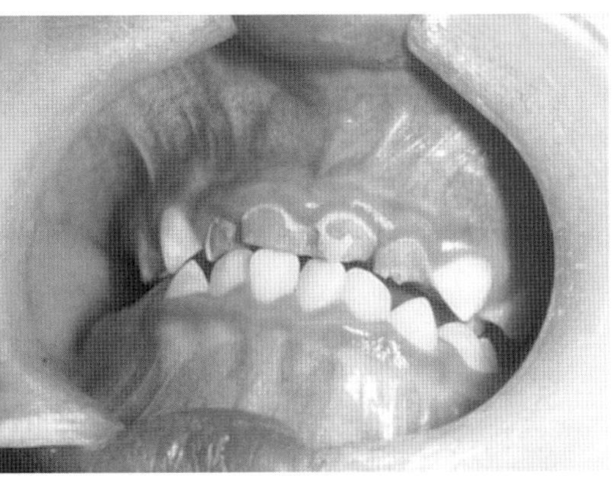

B

Fig. 22.3.1 **(A)** Typical appearance of an early carious lesion. The white spot lesion represents demineralization of the enamel caused by the presence of bacterial plaque creating an acidic environment. If left unmanaged, the white area will continue to demineralize until cavitation occurs **(B)** If identified early enough, remineralization of the enamel is possible through exposure to topical fluoride (particularly toothpaste) and other calcium-based products such as casein phosphopeptide–amorphous calcium phosphate (CPP-ACP).

(known clinically as dental plaque) on the teeth. Early identification of these pre-cavitated lesions is important because they signal the need for proactive preventive measures to encourage remineralization. If the disease does progress to cavitation, restorations (fillings and crowns) are necessary to rehabilitate function and aesthetics.

Early childhood caries (ECC – historically also referred to as nursing-bottle caries, baby-bottle decay, and many other terms) is a distinct form of dental caries affecting preschool-aged children. ECC is particularly virulent, causing massive destruction to the primary dentition in children as young as 14 months of age (Fig. 23.3.1B). At birth, MS do not inhabit the oral cavity; however, the earlier colonization occurs, the greater the risk of ECC. The most common source for transmission of MS has been shown to be the primary caregiver, usually the mother. Poor maternal oral health coupled with inappropriate feeding behaviours such as prolonged on-demand breastfeeding, particularly through the night after 18 months of age, and putting a child to sleep with a bottle, places an infant at high risk of developing ECC. Medical practitioners, paediatricians and maternal child health nurses are all in a strategically good position to identify individuals at risk of developing ECC (Table 22.3.2).

## Prevention of dental caries

Strategies to prevent dental caries should start as soon as the first primary teeth erupt (Table 22.3.3).

*Fluoride*

Fluoride is the single most effective way to protect teeth from decay. It acts in two ways: it can enhance the ability of teeth to resist demineralization caused by intraoral acids, and it can also inhibit oral bacterial enzymes to reduce the conversion of sugars to acids. However, the latter effect is relatively small in comparison to its biochemical modification of the structure of tooth enamel.

Fluoride can be delivered both systemically and topically. Fluoridation of the water supplies allows for both effects. Water ingested during development of the teeth allows fluoride to be incorporated into the developing dental enamel. However, it is as a topical agent that water has its most beneficial effect as low-dose fluoride comes into frequent contact with the teeth before being ingested. As such, water fluoridation is considered a very cost-effective public health intervention. However, many homes in rural and remote areas do not enjoy 'town water' and so miss out on the advantages of water fluoridation. The other common source of fluoride comes in the form of toothpaste. In Australia and New Zealand (and most parts of Europe) there are two common strengths of fluoride toothpaste; most adult toothpastes contain around 1000 parts per million (ppm) fluoride, whereas child toothpastes contain lower concentrations of fluoride, around 400 ppm. Early exposure to fluoridated toothpaste is very effective in preventing caries as the newly erupted immature tooth surface is highly susceptible to the beneficial maturation effect of fluoride. The use of additional fluoride supplements (tablets or drops)

**Table 22.3.2 Common risk factors for dental caries**

| Risk factor | Influence |
|---|---|
| Fluoride exposure | Exposure to fluoridated water source and the regular use of fluoridated toothpaste are two key factors that reduce caries risk |
| Sugar exposure | Infant feeding habits are very important, with frequency of exposure being most relevant. High risk associated with prolonged bottle-feeding and on-demand night-time breast feeds (>18 months of age) |
| Family oral health history | Poor parental oral health places child at risk of decay as cariogenic bacteria can be transmitted to infants from their primary caregiver (usually the mother) |
| Social and family practices | Poor, Indigenous, ethnic and migrant groups have higher levels of dental disease |
| Medical history | Medically compromised children are at greater risk of dental decay, the impact of which on their general health can be considerable. They are also less likely to receive appropriate treatment |
| Saliva flow | Children with reduced salivary flow are at significant risk of developing caries as the acids in the oral cavity cannot be diluted, buffered and cleared effectively. Examples of such children are those taking specific medications for management of asthma, those with ADHD, childhood cancer, or with certain head and neck tumours managed by radiotherapy |

ADHD, attention-deficit/hyperactivity disorder.

**Table 22.3.3 Summary of caries preventive strategies**

| Factor | Strategy |
|---|---|
| Fluoride | A smear of child's fluoridated toothpaste should be applied regularly to an infant's teeth within 6 months of their eruption<br>Teeth should be brushed twice a day with nothing to eat or drink after the night-time brushing<br>Parents should supervise tooth-brushing until around 8 years of age<br>The use of additional fluoride supplements (tablets or drops) is no longer recommended due to the risk of unsupervised ingestion |
| Diet | Reduce the frequency of intake of sweetened foods and drinks, particularly between mealtimes<br>Avoid on-demand feeding through the night-time<br>Limit sugary snacks to meal times when salivary flow is optimal<br>Avoid sugary snacks close to bedtime<br>Increase water intake for hydration |
| Dental attendance | Parents should be encouraged to take their infant to a dental professional within 6 months of the eruption of their first teeth<br>Regular monitoring by a dental professional should continue into adulthood |
| Remineralizing products | Products containing fluoride concentrates and calcium phosphopeptides are available through dental practitioners. These promote remineralization of early carious lesions (e.g. Tooth Mousse®; GC Corporation, Itabashi-ku, Tokyo, Japan) |

is no longer recommended in Australia and New Zealand, but varies around the world. Advice regarding the appropriate use of fluoride prescription should be sought from the local paediatric dentists and/or professional bodies.

*Oral hygiene measures*

In comparison to early and effective tooth-brushing with fluoridated toothpaste, other oral hygiene measures are relatively less important for children. Flossing, although useful for adults in the prevention and control of both caries and periodontal disease, is difficult for children as it requires a high level of manual dexterity. In those at high risk of caries, parents can be shown how to floss between the primary molars after tooth-brushing with a fluoridated toothpaste, which will optimize the topical effects of fluoride. Mouth rinses may be a useful adjunct to routine care and are starting to gain a foothold in preventive dentistry. However, at this stage they are best prescribed by a dental professional and should not be viewed as an alternative to effective tooth-brushing.

*Diet*

In addition to encouraging optimal exposure to fluoride, providing advice on healthy dietary practices that reduce the length of time that the saliva pH is below the threshold 5.5 for enamel demineralization will also reduce the risk of caries development and progression. At all ages, diet modification to reduce the frequency of intake of both sugary foods and drinks is important. In particular, children put to bed and allowed to sleep with a nursing bottle are likely to develop decay. As children get older, encouraging water drinking and limiting sugary snacks/drinks to meal times, when salivary flow is optimal, will optimize the buffering capacity of the saliva.

*Remineralization products*

Recently new products have been developed that contain casein phosphopeptide–amorphous calcium phosphate (CPP-ACP). These products, as either a chewing gum (Recaldent®; Cadbury Japan Limited, Adams Division) or a topical cream (Tooth Mousse®; GC Corporation, Itabashi-ku, Tokyo, Japan), act as a reservoir for calcium phosphate, maintaining a state of supersaturation around the tooth with respect to calcium and phosphate, thereby depressing the demineralization of tooth tissue and promoting its remineralization. These products can be used in conjunction with fluoride products such as toothpaste, as they act synergistically to promote remineralization in the oral cavity. With the exception of individuals with milk protein allergy, they are safe and effective. These products are currently available only through dental surgery outlets, but are being used increasingly, particularly in individuals who continue to develop caries despite optimal fluoride exposure.

## Fluorosis

High serum levels of fluoride can produce a developmental abnormality of enamel maturation known as fluorosis. Mild cases appear clinically as a white flecking or linear opacity of the enamel; more severe cases can have quite marked brown mottling. When recommending fluoride strategies, the risks of developing fluorosis (which potentially can create minor aesthetic challenges in the permanent dentition) need to be weighed against the risk of developing dental caries and all its potential sequelae. Discussion between a paediatric dentist and the family is important in order to optimize prevention but reduce unwanted side-effects.

### Dental abscesses

If dental caries is undiagnosed, untreated or treated inappropriately, it can cause pain, systemic infection and abscesses. In the primary dentition an abscess can be superficial, pointing beneath the gum usually on the cheek side of the tooth, and often relatively unpainful. Alternatively and more seriously, an infection from a necrosed tooth can spread into the deeper soft tissue planes and lymph nodes (Fig. 22.3.2). Cellulitis is accompanied by systemic illness, high fever, facial swelling and often limited mouth opening. In the upper jaw this can cause closure of the eye, whereas in the lower jaw it can compromise the airway as the submandibular and sublingual spaces become involved. In most cases a simple clinical examination will identify the affected tooth; however, an orthopantomogram is useful to confirm the diagnosis. Once the infection has reached this stage, extraction as soon as possible (often under general anaesthesia) is usually the best course of action.

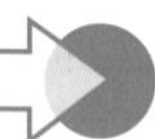

**Practical point**

- When presented with any facial swelling, consider a dental cause as part of the differential diagnosis.

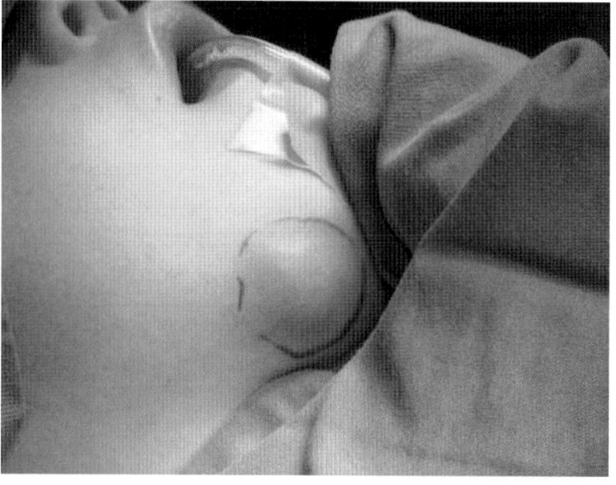

Fig. 22.3.2 An example of the potential sequelae following the failure to treat a carious lower primary molar in a 4-year-old boy. The necrotic tooth has become infected and resulted in cellulitis, pus tracking extraorally, and systemic illness. Treatment includes intravenous antibiotics, extraction of the tooth and drainage of the abscess.

**Clinical example**

Jimmy, aged 3 years and 6 months, presented with his mother because he had been crying when he ate or drank at the daycare centre. Recently his mother had noticed that he sometimes woke up at night crying because of the pain in his mouth. On being asked about his health, his mother reported that he had seen a heart doctor at the children's hospital because he had a 'hole in the heart'. She also acknowledged that Jimmy still took a bottle of milk to bed at night and that she sometimes put a little of his favourite chocolate powder in the milk to help him sleep.

Oral examination confirmed the presence of early childhood dental caries with extensive decay involving the incisor teeth in both upper and lower jaws as well as the upper first primary molars, with some white areas of early enamel demineralization on the recently erupted second molars. In addition, his gums were slightly inflamed and there were widespread deposits of white furry plaque over his teeth and gums.

From the history of spontaneous pain, particularly at night, it was apparent that the decay was well advanced and involved the nerve (pulp) of at least some of the teeth. The presence of generalized plaque deposits around the teeth and gums suggested that tooth-brushing did not happen regularly, if at all. In addition to posing a risk of bacteraemia (and hence for endocarditis in Jimmy who had a pre-existing cardiac history), the presence of gingivitis also suggested that he was not receiving the optimal benefits to be gained from regular topical fluoride exposure.

Management was in two stages. First, the immediate relief of pain and elimination of infection was performed by the removal of all pulpally involved teeth and the restoration of non-pulpally involved teeth; this was completed under general anaesthesia. Prophylactic antibiotic cover is no longer recommended for this child, but proactive preventive advice was required and provided at ongoing outpatient appointments. This advice included recommending (and demonstrating) tooth-brushing using an adult fluoridated toothpaste (1000 ppm). This should be done by Jimmy's parents twice a day, and at the same time to stop immediately the night-time use of the infant feeding bottle. Finally, information was provided to Jimmy's mother on the particular importance of good oral health for people with congenital heart disease.

Oral health for children who have other health-care needs is often not high on the list of parental priorities. Close cooperation is necessary between doctors, paediatricians and paediatric dentists to assist parents of such children in appreciating the importance of oral health for their child and to provide advice on how to minimize potential future problems. It is never too early to start to talk about teeth.

## Trauma

Almost a third of children will experience dental injury to either their primary or permanent teeth. The peak ages are between 18 months and 3 years when infants are learning to walk and prone to falling, and again in early teens when they (boys in particular) are participating in more adventurous games and sports. Most injuries in children are accidental in nature as opposed to adults, where fights and traffic accidents are not uncommon.

Dental injuries can affect the teeth, bone and soft tissues, or any combination of the three, with injuries to the teeth and lacerations of the tongue and lips being the most common. Jaw fractures are relatively uncommon in children and not covered further here.

## Primary dentition

Injuries to the primary dentition most commonly involve displacement of the upper primary incisors from their sockets with or without some soft tissue lacerations (Fig. 22.3.3). In general, infants are very resilient and parents are often more stressed than the affected child.

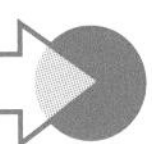

### Practical points

- Check that there are no other signs of injury such as limb fractures or head injury.
- Refer to an appropriate dental professional.
- If the displacement is mild and not affecting function (i.e. the child can bring their teeth together), regular monitoring may be appropriate.
- If the tooth is more severely displaced, it should be removed, under either local or general anaesthesia depending on the age of the child and nature of the injury.
- An avulsed primary tooth is never repositioned.

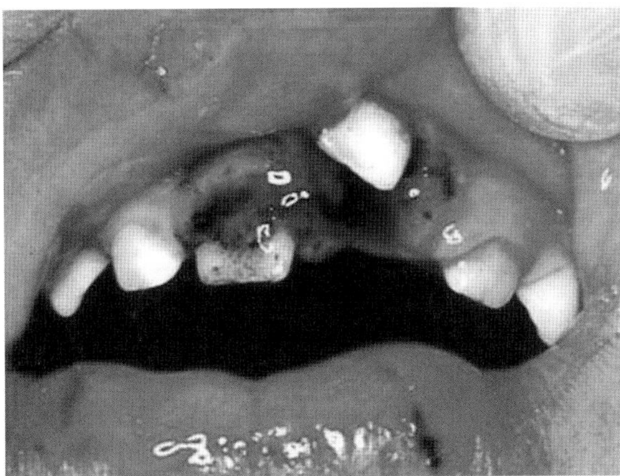

Fig. 22.3.3 Tooth displacement injuries such as this occur commonly in the primary dentition. These teeth create interference when this child tries to close his teeth together. In the primary dentition one does not try to reposition the teeth as this may cause further damage to the permanent successor, the crowns of which are located close to the apices of the primary tooth roots. Removal of these teeth is the best treatment.

Injury to the primary teeth can, in some instances, affect the development of the underlying permanent successor. Primary teeth are never re-implanted as this too can have a detrimental effect on the permanent successor; however, parents can be reassured that early loss of primary incisors has no lasting effect on speech, function or appearance.

## Permanent dentition

Injuries to the permanent dentition range from a small tooth fracture to complete loss (avulsion) of multiple teeth and significant soft tissue lacerations. Injuries to the permanent dentition are often missed or incorrectly diagnosed. Appropriate emergency management of traumatized teeth impacts significantly on the ultimate outcome of the injury.

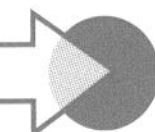

### Practical points

- All injuries should be carefully examined intraorally.
- Ideally an avulsed permanent tooth should be replanted immediately, if possible.
- Irrespective of the degree of seriousness of the injury, trauma to the permanent dentition should be referred promptly (by telephone) to a dental professional.

Unless replaced immediately, the long-term prognosis for an avulsed permanent tooth is guarded. Given that this rarely occurs, the avulsed tooth should be handled as little as possible and stored in milk. The child should be referred by telephone immediately to an emergency dental provider. Direct contact with the dentist will ensure that they are prepared to accept the child for treatment, hence avoiding further delays. Often this will be a paediatric dentist or hospital-based dental unit.

Dental management of displaced teeth usually involves repositioning accompanied by placement of a thin wire splint bonded to the affected and some unaffected teeth to stabilize the injury for several days. In some cases further endodontic (root canal) therapy may be required and treatment can continue for many years after the initial injury. In many cases the prognosis for retaining traumatized teeth in the long term is very good. However, avulsion and severe intrusion injuries, particularly those with additional bony fractures, do not have a good prognosis in the long term. The aim of treatment in these cases is often to retain a child's natural teeth through adolescence so that once growth is complete the permanent prosthetic replacement of the compromised teeth can be considered.

### Non-accidental injury (child abuse)

Orofacial trauma is commonly reported in cases of child abuse. Bruising and laceration of lips and alveolar mucosa, damage to teeth, alveolar bone fractures, finger and bite marks on face and neck are all frequent signs of child abuse. These result from slapping, punching, hand over mouth, forcible feeding with spoon or fork, and forcible intrusion or removal of a feeding bottle, dummy or toy from the mouth. Tears to the upper midline fraenum in pre-ambulatory infants is highly suspicious, and oral bruising and palatal contusion can be seen in cases of sexual abuse. Oral signs should not be neglected when considering the possibility of child abuse, and an intraoral examination should form part of routine surveillance.

## Dental erosion

Dental erosion is defined as a chronic localized loss of dental hard tissue, chemically etched away from the tooth surface without bacterial involvement (which differentiates it from caries, which is bacterial in aetiology). Many young children show wear of their primary incisors but more worrying is the fact that almost one-third of adolescents have significant wear of their permanent teeth as well. The appearance of erosive tooth wear is quite characteristic, but challenging for most non-dental professionals to diagnose. There is a general loss of lustre from the surface enamel, thinning and chipping of the upper incisors, and there may be smooth exposed dentine, pulpal exposure and sensitivity.

As with dental caries, the aetiology is multifactorial but is associated with an increased exposure of the teeth to acid (Table 22.3.4). These non-bacterial acids may be extrinsic (essentially dietary) or intrinsic (from the gastric tract). Children with dysphagia and other conditions associated with abnormal muscle tone tend to have more gastric reflux and are more likely to have dental erosion. In addition, children with muscle spasticity tend to grind their teeth which, superimposed upon the softening caused by acidic erosion, can lead to rapid tooth tissue loss.

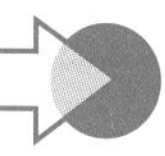

**Practical point**

- Any child with a history of gastric reflux should be counselled as to the potential for erosive tooth tissue loss, and advised to seek dental review.



**Table 22.3.4 Potential sources of acid responsible for dental erosion**

| Extrinsic | Intrinsic |
|---|---|
| Dietary<br>• citrus fruits and juice<br>• carbonated drinks (including 'diet' products)<br>• sports drinks<br>• wine<br>Environmental/occupational<br>• swimming (poorly regulated pool water)<br>• nutrition regimes for elite athletes<br>Lifestyle<br>• recreational drugs<br>Medications<br>• topical effect – aspirin, vitamin C, phenylketonuria supplements, nebulized asthma medications without spacer<br>• systemic effect on saliva – asthma, ADHD, antidepressants, anticholinergic medications<br>• ethanol-containing mouthwashes | Gastro-oesophageal reflux<br>• infancy<br>• early childhood<br>Cyclical vomiting<br>Eating disorders<br>• bulimia nervosa<br>Rumination |

ADHD, attention-deficit/hyperactivity disorder.

The role of the medical practitioner in managing dental erosion is to be aware of the risk factors, to provide generic preventive advice (Table 22.3.5) and to refer the child to a dentist for ongoing monitoring. If caught early enough, little active dental treatment will be required; however, if significant tooth tissue loss occurs in the young permanent dentition, pain and aesthetic considerations may mean that restorative treatment is required.

## Acquired disorders of the soft tissues

### Bleeding gums

Gingivitis is the most common cause of bleeding gums. Gingivitis is a non-specific inflammation of the gingival tissues (gums) that reflects the bacterial challenge to the host when dental plaque accumulates. Dental plaque is a complex biofilm that starts to accumulate around the teeth immediately after toothbrushing. It consists of 70% microorganisms and 30% food debris, and if brushing is ineffective the gums

**Table 22.3.5 Strategies to prevent dental erosion**

| Factor | Strategy |
|---|---|
| Reducing acid exposure | Inform patients of types of food and drink that have greatest erosive potential<br>Consumption of still/non-carbonated drinks as an alternative<br>Limiting the intake of acidic foods/drinks to mealtimes<br>Advocate consumption of a neutral food immediately after a meal (e.g. cheese)<br>Rinsing mouth out after acid exposure (i.e. after episode of vomiting), but delay brushing teeth immediately after the exposure as this increases wear of tooth tissue |
| Optimizing salivary function | Increased water intake<br>Use of water bottles in schoolbags<br>Advise use of sugar-free chewing gum to enhance salivary flow |
| Enhancing resistance to erosion | Suitable products include: neutral fluoride mouthwashes, Recaldent® chewing gum and Tooth Mousse® |

organize a subclinical inflammatory response within 2 days that will become clinically apparent by 10 days. The characteristic signs of chronic gingivitis include red inflamed gums that bleed when brushed and that can deteriorate to a point where there is bleeding on eating and, in some cases, even spontaneous bleeding (Fig. 22.3.4). Gingivitis is easily reversed with appropriate oral hygiene practices to remove the plaque.

If certain anaerobic organisms predominate in the subgingival biofilm, gingivitis may progress to periodontitis in which the inflammatory mediators and cytokines destroy the underlying supporting tissues. This can lead to significant bone loss around the teeth, which become mobile and may ultimately be lost. There is a high degree of individual susceptibility to periodontal disease, with certain subgroups with a compromised immune response being particularly prone to destructive periodontal disease (e.g. individuals with Down syndrome). Fortunately, with the exception of some rare connective tissue disorders (e.g. Ehlers–Danlos syndrome) and immunocompromised individuals (e.g. those with cyclic neutropenia), children and adolescents do not experience periodontal disease.

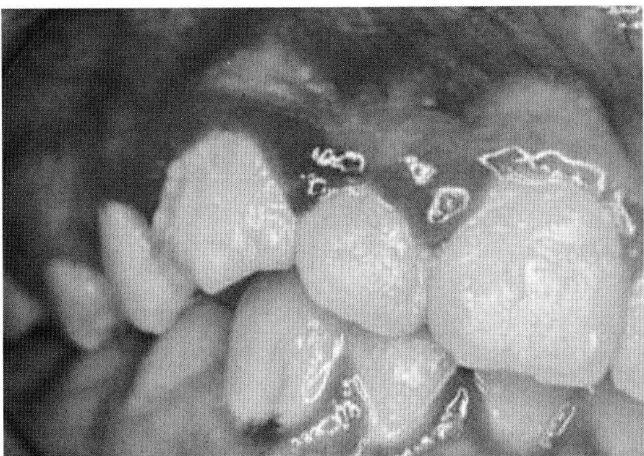

Fig. 22.3.4 The appearance of plaque-induced gingivitis. Note the build-up of soft white bacterial plaque associated particularly with the gingival margins. Good oral hygiene not only reduces the bacterial load but, if using fluoridated toothpaste, increases exposure of the underlying enamel to the protective benefits of fluoride.

## Oral ulceration

Ulceration of the oral cavity is often a sign of underlying systemic disease and, if present, treatment of the oral lesions will be essentially symptomatic whilst the underlying disorder is attended to appropriately. A careful history and examination should be completed in order to assist with the diagnosis.

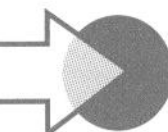

**Practical points**

- Take a good history of:
  - general health status including appetite, weight loss, fever
  - the ulcers, including frequency, position, duration, stimuli.
- Complete a thorough examination of:
  - general health, including appearance, weight, psychological state, signs of inflammatory bowel disease
  - oral cavity, including location, size, appearance, obvious traumatic aetiology.
- Useful special tests – full blood screen, full blood count (FBC), erythrocyte sedimentation rate (ESR), iron, serum $B_{12}$, folate, as well as markers for inflammatory bowel disease.

### Infections

The most common oral infection seen in children is primary herpetic gingivostomatitis (Fig. 22.3.5). The signs are of a systemic viral infection with fever, lassitude, lack of appetite and very sore oral cavity with characteristic painful ulcerated gingival tissues as well as occasionally on the tongue and buccal mucosa. Other viral infections can involve the oral cavity including hand, foot and mouth disease, and chickenpox.

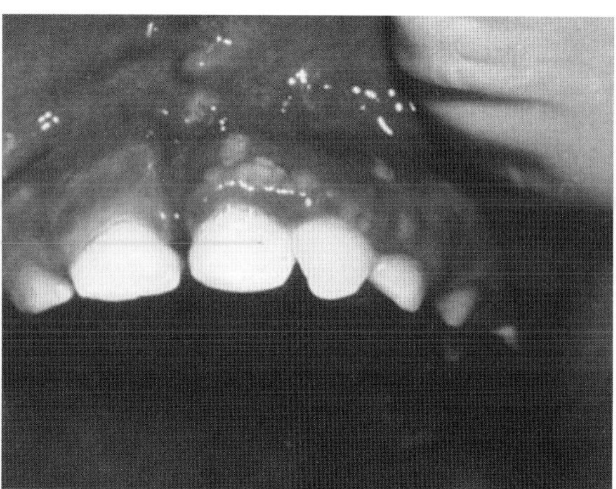

Fig. 22.3.5 The early appearance of primary herpetic gingivostomatitis. The gums become fiery-red, covered with fluid-filled blisters that later burst and ulcerate. Typically the child presents with fever and dehydration requiring supportive medical care.

*Treatment*

Treatment is symptomatic, involving fluids and analgesia and encouraging the parents to maintain oral hygiene to prevent secondary bacterial infection of the ulcers.

## Trauma

Single ulcers located in specific sites around the oral cavity can be caused by both physical and chemical trauma. Use of a toothpick to relieve food packing between teeth can cause ulceration interdentally, and the placement of an aspirin tablet directly on to the buccal gum in order to relieve toothache has been known to produce a nasty chemical ulcer. In most cases of traumatic ulcer, the aetiology will be relatively clear; however, it is important to bear in mind the potential for self-inflicted injury. Particularly in instances of apparently random and repeated episodes of traumatic ulceration, there may be an associated condition involving insensitivity to pain such as Riley–Day syndrome.

*Treatment*

Treatment involves the elimination of the irritant, such as a fractured filling or poorly contoured orthodontic appliance, or cessation of the injurious behaviour.

## Aphthous ulcers

In many situations an obvious aetiology is not forthcoming. These are referred to as aphthous ulcers. Fortunately they are relatively uncommon in children, as they are difficult to treat. They are non-infective, extremely painful ulcers, occurring most commonly on the labial and buccal mucosa and tongue borders. A prodromal burning sensation precedes breakdown of an initially white papule to form an ulcer with a crater-form base that heals slowly over 8–10 days. Aphthous ulcers may be of minor or major type and may be associated with stress; however, they may also be associated with an underlying iron or folate deficiency.

*Treatment*

Aphthous ulcers are difficult to manage and rarely is treatment totally successful. Chlorhexidine gluconate or a tetracycline–nystatin combination mouth rinse along with diligent tooth-brushing help relieve pain and control secondary infection. Other strategies for aphthae include topical anaesthetics, systemic analgesics, and topical anti-inflammatories including steroids. However, these medications, at best, will reduce the duration of the ulcer experience rather than cure it.

## Haematological causes

Children suffering from an underlying haematological disorder, including neutropenia and leukaemia, can experience oral ulceration. Children with leukaemia may present initially with bleeding gums in the *absence* of poor oral hygiene. Those with cyclic neutropenia, in particular, experience cyclical bouts of severe gingivitis accompanied by significant periodontal bone loss, resulting in premature loss of both primary and later permanent teeth. Children with this condition need regular review and management by a paediatric dentist or periodontist in order to try to slow the process.

## Gastrointestinal causes

As the oral cavity is the start of the gastrointestinal tract, it is common that disorders affecting the rest of the tract can present in the mouth. Individuals with inflammatory bowel conditions such as Crohn's disease, coeliac disease and ulcerative colitis may experience oral ulceration. In addition, those with Crohn's disease can have other significant oral manifestations, often described as orofacial granulomatosis, including:

- marked lip enlargement, together with enlargement of the buccal mucosa
- alveolar mucosal erythematous granulomatosis in the anterior regions of the maxilla
- large, linear ulceration in the buccal mucosa posteriorly.

These oral findings can occur on their own, or together with anal fissuring, genital swelling and gastrointestinal changes.

*Treatment*

If there are any concerns about gastric symptoms (e.g. weight loss, blood in the stools), the child should be referred to a paediatrician (or paediatric gastroenterologist) and paediatric dentist for a combined evaluation.

### Dermatological causes

Oral ulcers occur in many of the rarer dermatological conditions such as epidermolysis bullosa, pemphigus and pemphigoid. However, these conditions are usually diagnosed from their more general manifestations rather than their oral symptoms.

### Malignancy

Oral malignancy is rare in children; however, single, persistent, large ulcers that have no obvious traumatic aetiology and are not associated with acute systemic illness should be viewed with suspicion and referred for investigation to a paediatric dentist/maxillofacial surgeon.

### Gingival swellings

Swelling of the gingival tissues can be congenital or acquired, although the former are relatively rare. Individuals with any of the mucopolysaccharidosis disorders may have very enlarged gums, often to the extent that teeth fail to erupt or are ectopically displaced. Similar disruption to the developing dentition can occur in individuals with vascular anomalies, such as a lymphangioma, that may affect both soft and hard tissues of the jaws.

Of the acquired causes of gum enlargement, drugs are most commonly implicated – most specifically the anti-seizure medication, phenytoin, and the immunosuppressant cyclosporin A. The latter has been widely used in organ transplant protocols, and in children has caused significant aesthetic and psychological problems as the gums enlarge in an unsightly fashion and teeth are covered in excess gum tissue. The advent of tacrolimus as an alternative to cyclosporin A has improved significantly the quality of life of these children by reducing not only the gum overgrowth but also the hirsutism. Most of the enlargement resolves once the causative drug is stopped. Other more localized swelling of the gingival tissues includes giant cell granuloma, histiocytosis and lymphoma, and, although rare, such swellings are of obvious clinical significance and should be reviewed by a paediatric dentist.

## Children with special health-care needs

Children with significant medical conditions, developmental disabilities and craniofacial disorders face multiple health issues, amongst which is often an increased risk of dental disease, coupled with barriers in accessing appropriate dental services. Given that many dental problems are relatively simple to prevent and manage if diagnosed early, close collaboration between the general health-care providers (medical practitioner, paediatrician or nurse) and the dental care provider is essential. Identifying an appropriate 'dental home' for children with special health-care needs is important so that these complex children have access to timely and appropriate oral health care. Many general dentists are not comfortable managing children with special health-care needs, whereas paediatric dentists are trained specifically in this area.

### Medications

Many children with special health-care needs are on multiple medications for prolonged periods of time. There is an increased risk of developing caries associated with the long-term use of sugar-based liquid medications. As many of the common liquid medications are 'over-the-counter' formulations, parents should be warned to check that, where possible, they purchase a sugar-free brand of medications such as cough linctus or analgesic.

Given the high prevalence of asthma, particularly in Australia and New Zealand, a suggested association between asthma medication (particularly $\beta_2$-agonist inhalers) and dental erosion/caries is relevant. This association appears to be more of a problem in adults than in children, and one large study in children showed no such association. There are theoretical reasons why this might occur, for example: chronic mouth-breathing from associated allergic rhinitis leading to mouth dryness; a higher incidence of gastro-oesophageal reflux, which may result in more acid in the oral cavity; an acidic base to some nebulizer solutions. The use of both spacers and oral rinsing with water afterwards will minimize the potential oral health risks, which should not be viewed as a contraindication to positive asthma prevention.

### Congenital heart disease

Children with congenital heart defects (CHD) are predisposed to infective endocarditis (IE), which is associated with high morbidity and mortality. Traditionally attention has focused on the risk of developing IE following bacteraemia associated with dental treatment, with the resultant implementation of aggressive prophylactic antibiotic regimens. However, the lack of substantive evidence that preoperative antibiotics are effective in preventing IE, coupled with the realization that bacteraemia originating in the oral cavity occurs daily (resulting from chewing, tooth-brushing, etc.), has led to a dramatic rethinking of the guidelines for prophylactic antibiotic usage in individuals with CHD; see the UK National Institute for Health and

Clinical Excellence (NICE) guidelines (http://guidance.nice.org.uk/CG64).

Recommendations regarding antibiotic cover vary widely around the world, and it is important that clear, concise and consistent information is provided to families regarding this issue. When taking their child to a dental professional, parents should be provided with written confirmation of the child's cardiac status together with a clear indication of the risk of IE and the need for prophylaxis endorsed by their cardiologist. This will facilitate the smooth provision of appropriate dental care and minimize the unnecessary prescription of antibiotics. Educational resources exist for parents in most paediatric cardiology units; these should be reviewed regularly and informed by contemporary evidence (http://www.rch.org.au/emplibrary/cardiology/dentalheart.pdf). Finally, irrespective of antibiotic regimen, emphasis should be placed on optimizing the oral health of children with CHD and thus reducing the need for dental intervention and minimizing the risk of additional exposure to infection.

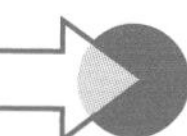

**Practical points**

- Every child with a special health-care need should have a regular dentist familiar with the implications of their medical history.
- Good communication between paediatricians and paediatric dentists will optimize health outcomes for individuals and their families.
- The specific prescription of sugar-free alternatives should be part of routine clinical practice.
- Parents of children with a congenital heart defect should be provided with written confirmation of their child's cardiac status with respect to endocarditis.
- Standard protocols for prophylactic antibiotic cover should be followed when a child with a significant congenital heart defect requires any invasive dental procedure (protocols can be accessed at: http://www.rch.org.au/cardiology/health-info.cfm?doc_id=3482).

# Index

Note: Page numbers in *italics* refer to boxes, figures and tables.

## B

## C

## D

## E

## F

## G



## H

## I

## N

## O

## P

## Q



## R

## S